Specific Nursing Care Plans

General Nursing Care Plans

Danger Signs

Emergency Procedures

ESSENTIALS OF
MATERNITY NURSING

ESSENTIALS OF MATERNITY NURSING

IRENE M. BOBAK, RN, MS, PhD
Professor,
San Francisco State University,
San Francisco, California

MARGARET DUNCAN JENSEN, RN, MS
Professor Emeritus,
San Jose State University,
San Jose, California

THIRD EDITION

with 622 illustrations

Mosby Year Book
St. Louis Baltimore Boston Chicago London Philadelphia Sydney Toronto

Mosby Year Book

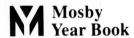

Dedicated to Publishing Excellence

Editor: Nancy L. Coon
Sr. Developmental Editor: Susan R. Epstein
Project Manager: Patricia Gayle May
Production Editor: Deborah Vogel

Great care has been used in compiling and checking the information in this book to ensure its accuracy. However, because of changing technology, recent discoveries, and research and individualization of prescriptions according to patient needs, the uses, effects, and dosages of drugs may vary from those given here. Neither the publisher nor the authors shall be responsible for such variations or other inaccuracies. We urge that before you administer any drug you check the manufacturer's dosage recommendations as given in the package insert provided with each product.

THIRD EDITION

Printed in the United States of America

Mosby–Year Book, Inc.
11830 Westline Industrial Drive, St. Louis, MO 63146

Library of Congress Cataloging-in-Publication Data

Bobak, Irene M.
Essentials of maternity nursing / Irene M. Bobak, Margaret Duncan Jensen.
p. cm.
Includes bibliographical references.
Includes index.
ISBN 0-8016-0233-5
1. Obstetrical nursing. I. Jensen, Margaret Duncan. II. Title.
[DNLM: 1. Obstetrical Nursing. 2. Perinatology—nurses' instruction. WY 157 B663e]
RG951.B66 1991
610.73'678—dc20
DNLM/DLC
for Library of Congress 90-13311
CIP

CL/VH 9 8 7 6 5 4 3 2

Contributors

VICKI AKIN, RN, MSN
Associate Professor
University of San Francisco
San Francisco, California

JOEA E. BIERCHEN, RSN, MSN, EdD
Professor of Nursing
St. Petersburg Junior Community College
St. Petersburg, Florida

DEBRA I. CRAIG, RN, MSN
Assistant Professor of Nursing
Point Loma Nazarene College
San Diego, California

BARBARA DERWINSKI-ROBINSON, RNC, MSN
Associate Professor
Montana State University
Billings, Montana

LINDA A. DRAPP, RN, BSN
Program Assistant
Young Parents Young People
University of Missouri-St. Louis
St. Louis, Missouri

DOROTHY K. FISCHER, RN, PhD
Assistant Professor
University of Delaware
Newark, Delaware

CHERYL HARRIS, RN, BS
Staff Nurse, Neonatal Intensive Care Unit
Children's Mercy Hospital
Kansas City, Missouri

DEITRA LEONARD LOWDERMILK, RNC, PhD
Clinical Associate Professor
University of North Carolina
Chapel Hill, North Carolina

MARY COURTNEY MOORE, RN, RD, MSN, CNSN
Graduate Student
Vanderbilt University
Nashville, Tennessee

SHANNON E. PERRY, RN, PhD, FAAN
Professor
San Francisco State University
San Francisco, California

EDNA QUINN, RN, CNM, PhD
Associate Professor
Salisbury State University,
Salisbury, Maryland

FANNIE M. RANKIN-HIRSCHHAUT, RN, BS, MBA
Certified Diabetes Educator
Clinical Education Coordinator
Mills-Peninsula Hospitals

JANICE M. SPIKES, RN, PhD
Project Director, Young Parents Young People
University of Missouri-St. Louis
St. Louis, Missouri

M. COLLEEN STAINTON, RN, DNS
Professor
Assistant Dean, Research and Scholarly Development
University of Calgary
Calgary, Alberta, Canada

SUSAN M. TUCKER, RN, BSN, PhN
Assistant Director of Nursing
Kaiser-Permanente Medical Center
Panorama City, California

MARY L. TURGEON, EdD, MT(ASCP)
Dr. Mary L. Turgeon & Associates
Waverly, New York

VIVIAN WAHLBERG, RN, CM
Dr. Med Sc
Stockholm, Sweden

DIANE TRACE WARLICK, RN, JD
Attorney at Law
St. Croix, U.S. Virgin Islands

RHEA WILLIAMS, RN, PhD
Associate Professor
California State University, Los Angeles
Los Angeles, California

Consultant Panel

STUART BARGER, RN, MSN
Instructor
Department of Nursing
Everett Community College
Everett, Washington

CLAUDIA ANDERSON BECKMAN, RN, PhD
Associate Professor
Department of Maternal Child Nursing
University of Tennessee
Memphis, Tennessee

JOEA E. BIERCHEN, MSN, EdD
Professor of Nursing
St. Petersburg Junior College
St. Petersburg, Florida

CONSTANCE BOBIK, RN, BSN, MSN
Assistant Professor
Department of Nursing
Brevard Community College
Cocoa, Florida

KAREN JOHNSON-BRENNAN, BSN, MS, EdD
Associate Professor
Department of Nursing
San Francisco State University
San Francisco, California

ELEANOR F. BROWN, RNC, MSN
Assistant Professor
Macon College
Macon, Georgia

IRIS CAMPBELL, RN, SCM, MTD, MN
Assistant Professor
Department of Nursing
University of Alberta
Edmonton, Alberta, Canada

MARY LOU DRAKE, EdD
Associate Professor
Department of Nursing
University of Windsor
Windsor, Ontario, Canada

GLORIA ESSOKA, RN, BSN, MSN, PhD
Associate Professor
Director, Undergraduate Program
Department of Nursing
Hunter College
New York, New York

MARY KAY FALLON, RNC, MS, MA
Perinatal Clinical Nurse Specialist
Barnes Hospital
St. Louis, Missouri

KATHY HANNOLD, RN, MS
Director of Women and Infant Services
Barnes Hospital
Faculty
University of Missouri-St. Louis
St. Louis, Missouri

JANET KENNEY, RN, PhD
Associate Professor
Arizona State University College of Nursing
Tempe, Arizona

DIANE NELSON, RN, CNM, MSN
Instructor
Department of Nursing
Southern Connecticut State University
New Haven, Connecticut

RICHARD PFLANZER, PhD
Indiana University
School of Medicine
Indianapolis, Indiana

KAREN PROTROWSKI, RN, MSN
Assistant Professor
Department of Nursing
D'Youville College
Buffalo, New York

DONNA RIOS, RN, MSEd
Assistant Director
School of Nursing
St. Elizabeth Hospital Medical Center
Youngstown, Ohio

RACHEL SPECTOR, RN, PhD
Associate Professor
Boston College School of Nursing
Chestnut Hill, Massachusetts

JANE STARN, RN, PhD
Associate Professor
University of Hawaii School of Nursing
Honolulu, Hawaii

MARY VEACH, RN, PhD
Adjunct Professor
Kansas-Newman College
Associate Director of New Life Center
St. Francis Regional Medical Center
Wichita, Kansas

MARGUERITE WILCOX, RNC, BSN, MN
Associate Professor
Department of Nursing
Boise State University
Boise, Idaho

SUE WILLIAMS, PhD, MPH, RD
President, SRW Production, Inc. and Director, The Berkeley Nutrition Group, Berkeley, California;
Metabolic Nutritionist, Kaiser-Permanente Northern California Regional Newborn Screening and Metabolic Program, Kaiser-Permanente Medical Center, Oakland, California;
Field Faculty, M.P.H.-Dietetic Internship Program and Coordinated Undergraduate Program in Dietetics, University of California, Berkeley, California

To the following members of our families who, by virtue of their belief in us, prompted the courage and motivation to complete this book:

Marianne K. Zalar
Albert B. Bobak
Irene L. Bobak
Stephen J. Bobak
Veronica Bobak
Sister Mary Eleanor, VSC
IRENE M. BOBAK

John and Russ Duncan
Carlo and Marjory Jensen
James Duncan
Erin Duncan
Bruce and Kathleen Duncan
Rita Jensen
Bill, Robert, and Stephen Danner
and to the memory of our daughter
Jeanne Jensen Danner
MARGARET DUNCAN JENSEN

Preface

Maternity nursing offers a unique combination of challenge and opportunity. Nurses are challenged to assimilate a tremendous, ever-growing body of scientific knowledge and to develop the technical and analytic skills necessary to apply that knowledge to practice. Each client presents a new challenge, for individual needs must be identified and met. The opportunities, however, are sufficiently extraordinary to make maternity nursing one of the most fulfilling specialities in nursing practice; nothing is more wondrous than the creation of a new human life. Assisting the woman and her family through the childbearing process—teaching, counseling, supporting, providing expert care—makes the nurse an integral part of this incredible experience.

The goal of nursing education is to prepare today's student to meet tomorrow's challenge, and to recognize and seize the opportunity inherent in that challenge. This preparation must extend beyond mastery of facts and skills. Nursing students must be able to combine competence with caring. They must address both physiologic and psychosocial needs. Above all, they must look beyond the condition and see the client as an individual with specialized needs.

Essentials of Maternity Nursing was developed to provide students with the knowlege they need to become ***competent*** nurses and the sensitivity they need to become ***caring*** nurses. This third edition has been revised and refined in response to comments and suggestions from both students and educators. It includes the most accurate, current, and clinically relevant information available, and it presents that information in a concise, logical format.

❑ APPROACH

Professional nursing practice continues to evolve and adapt to society's changing health priorities. Nursing education must also reflect these changes, as well as the needs of nursing students. This third edition of *Essentials of Maternity Nursing* was designed to meet the unique needs of maternity clients and students in the nineties.

Today's students are challenged to learn more than ever before and often in less time than their predecessors. We therefore carefully selected the content ***essential*** to the practice of safe and thoughtful maternity nursing. We presented this material in language that is ***easily understandable*** to students in all types of nursing programs to enable them to readily master this essential content. Students will find that the ***attractive two-color design*** highlights important content. Hundreds of ***photographs and drawings*** illustrate important concepts and techniques to further enhance comprehension.

Health care today emphasizes a focus on ***wellness.*** This focus is an integral part of our philosophy that pregnancy and childbirth are part of the natural developmental process. We therefore present the entire normal childbearing cycle before discussing potential complications. We believe that students need to thoroughly understand and recognize the ***normal*** processes and conditions before they can identify complications and comprehend their implications for care.

In order to implement ***preventive*** care, maternity nurses must be able to recognize signs and symptoms of emergent problems. Throughout the discussions of assessment and care we alert the nurse to deviations from normal and provide references to the pertinent content in the complications unit.

Today's clients include representatives from virtually every ethnic group. ***Cultural differences*** are highlighted throughout the text to emphasize the wide range of ethnic diversity that may be encountered, as well as its impact on maternity care. We stress the importance of determining each client's cultural preferences rather than relying on information based on broad stereotypes.

To truly meet the specific needs of each client the nurse must include family members and significant others in the plan of care. ***Family dynamics*** are rarely more prominent than in relation to pregnancy and childbirth, and the nurse is often the family's primary advocate. We therefore continually remind the student to consider the needs of family members, including grandparents and siblings, as well as the support they can provide for the client.

❑ FEATURES

Each chapter begins with ***learning objectives*** to focus students' attention on important content to be mastered. A list of ***key terms*** alerts students to new vocabulary; these terms are then boldfaced and defined within the chapter.

The ***five-step nursing process*** is used consistently and conspicuously as the organizing framework for discussing nursing care. Two different kinds of care plans help students learn to apply the nursing process in the clinical setting. ***General nursing care plans*** detail the overall care for a particular condition or situation. ***Specific nursing care plans*** guide students in tailoring care to meet the needs of a particular client. Both types of care plans follow the five-step nursing process, use only NANDA-approved nursing diagnoses, include client-centered goals, and provide rationales for each nursing action.

Maternity nursing has traditionally emphasized involving clients in their own care. Shorter hospital stays mandate an increased focus on teaching self-care measures. ***Guidelines for client teaching*** identify content that clients need to know and provide strategies for effective teaching.

The practice of maternity nursing requires expert performance of a wide array of diagnostic and therapeutic interventions. To assist students in mastering these skills, we have provided detailed, ***step-by-step procedures.*** Rationales for each step promote learning and understanding. Students in maternity settings must be alert to potentially dangerous situations and they must be prepared to quickly and effectively intervene. ***Danger boxes*** highlight signs and symptoms to watch for, and ***emergency procedures*** are tabbed for easy access.

At the end of each chapter we have provided several tools to help students assess their comprehension and broaden their understanding. Brief ***chapter summaries*** and ***key concepts boxes*** highlight essential chapter content and provide students with a basis for evaluating mastery of important material. ***Learning activities*** offer students opportunities to implement their knowledge and practice new skills. Current, relevant ***references*** and ***bibliographies*** provide a springboard for additional study and research in related topics.

NEW to this edition is the ***Quick Reference for Maternity Nursing*** that accompanies each copy of this text. This unique, handy reference features essential information and nursing implications for sixteen drugs commonly used in the maternity setting and provides checklists for critical assessments and teaching topics. This portable, accessible booklet will be invaluable to students in the clinical setting.

❑ ORGANIZATION

Essentials of Maternity Nursing is composed of six units organized to enhance learning and understanding. The first five units present the entire normal childbearing cycle; Unit VI discusses complications and their potential impact on the woman, fetus, newborn, and family.

Unit I, "Introduction to Maternity Nursing," begins with an overview of maternity nursing practice, then addresses the family as a unit of care. A chapter on legal and ethical issues prepares students to deal with these important areas in the context of maternity nursing. The biologic and psychologic aspects of human sexuality provide the foundation for care before, during, and after pregnancy. ***A new chapter on immunology*** emphasizes the importance of this body system in relation to pregnancy and fetal development. The unit ends with a chapter detailing the nurse's role in fertility management, stressing the importance of teaching, counseling, and supporting clients.

Unit II, "Normal Pregnancy," describes nursing care of the woman and her family from conception through preparation for childbirth. A separate chapter on maternal and fetal nutrition emphasizes this important aspect of care, highlighting the impact of cultural variations on diet and the importance of early recognition of nutritional problems.

Unit III, "Normal Childbirth," focuses on the collaboration between the physician, nurse, woman, and family during the process of labor and delivery. Separate chapters deal with the nurse's role in the pharmacologic relief of discomfort and fetal monitoring. Both of these chapters familiarize students with the modalities currently in use and focus on interventions to support and educate the woman and her family.

Unit IV, "Normal Newborn," addresses the immediate assessment and care of the neonate during the critical period of adjustment to extrauterine existence. Information on the nutritional needs of the newborn and nursing care associated with breastfeeding or formula-feeding is highlighted in a separate chapter.

Unit V, "Normal Postpartum Period," deals with a time of significant change for the entire family. The mother requires both physical and emotional support, and family members have new roles to assume as the newborn becomes established as part of the family unit.

Unit VI, "Complications of Childbearing," discusses the conditions that place the mother, fetus, newborn, and family at risk. Nursing interventions focus on achieving the best possible outcome, as well as supporting the woman and family when their expectations are not met. The chapter on loss and grief helps the nurse understand the grieving process and provide compassionate care to the entire family.

The text concludes with a glossary of all important terms, appendices that provide resource information, and a detailed, cross-referenced index.

❏ TEACHING AND LEARNING PACKAGE

To assist faculty and promote student learning we have developed the following supplements to the text:

- The Instructor's Manual with Test Bank is keyed chapter by chapter to the text to help coordinate course objectives to chapter content. Each chapter in the manual includes a student worksheet that can be copied and used as a hand-out to reinforce learning and evaluate comprehension. Unique to this manual are guidelines for prioritizing reading assignments so students in briefer courses can use the text to its fullest potential. The test bank includes more than 500 new questions formulated to prepare students for the NCLEX. The answer key provides page references and coding of questions according to the NCLEX test plan categories of nursing process and client needs.
- A *computerized test bank* is available for use on the IBM PC or Apple IIe and IIc microcomputers. These questions, taken from the test bank in the instructor's manual, are designed to be used as the basis for individual test construction. Directions for rearranging, adding, and deleting questions are included.
- A set of *more than 50 two-color overhead transparencies* completes this ancillary package. These illustrations were selected for their instructional value during lectures and classroom discussions.

▪ ▪ ▪

We are fully aware of the increasingly important contribution men are making to the nursing profession, as well as the growing number of women entering the medical profession. We hope this trend will continue. The construction of the English language, however, sometimes makes it awkward to eliminate totally the feminine and masculine pronouns. Therefore to present material clearly and smoothly, we have occasionally used the feminine pronoun to refer to the nurse and the masculine pronoun to refer to the physician.

Over the years we have received many comments and suggestions regarding our maternity nursing texts. We have incorporated many of these suggestions in the organization and development of this text. We welcome comments from instructors, students, and practitioners who use this text so that we may continue to be responsive to the needs of the profession.

❏ ACKNOWLEDGMENTS

We wish to thank everyone whose comments and suggestions prompted this collaborative effort and reviewers who provided valuable criticism of the manuscript.

We offer thanks for shared expertise and photographs to the staffs of Stanford University Medical Center, Stanford, California; Kaiser-Permanente Hospital and Santa Clara Valley Medical Center, Santa Clara, California; St. Luke's Hospital, Kansas City, Missouri; Jewish Hospital and Barnes Hospital, St. Louis, Missouri; Mills Memorial Hospital, San Mateo, California; Fountain Valley Community Hospital, Fountain Valley, California; and The Woman's Hospital of Texas, Houston, Texas.

We would like to thank the following photographers: Judith Bamber, San Jose, California; Joan Edelstein, San Jose, California; and M. Colleen Stainton, Calgary, Alberta, Canada. A special thank you goes to Marjorie Pyle, RNC, Lifecircle, Costa Mesa, California.

Several families in addition to our own have made unique contributions to the original photographs in this text, especially David and Carolyn Carlton and their son, Mathew, and Paul and Janet Ho and their children Shubert and Candice.

We are indebted to these families, who embody the philosophical basis for our text—family-centered nursing care.

This edition contains artwork by George Wassilchenko, Oral Roberts University, Tulsa, Oklahoma, whose precise, detailed anatomic drawings have made a substantial contribution to facilitating the study of complex theory. We look forward to a continuing association with this outstanding medical illustrator.

Special words of gratitude are extended to Nancy Coon, Suzi Epstein, and Debbie Vogel of Mosby–Year Book, Inc. for their encouragement, inspiration, and assistance in the preparation and production of this text. We acknowledge the assistance of our families, both concrete and supportive, and we thank each other for the stimulation, support, and mutual respect generated by this collaboration.

Irene M. Bobak

Margaret Duncan Jensen

Contents in Brief

Contents

UNIT I Introduction to Maternity Nursing

UNIT V Normal Postpartum Period

UNIT VI Complications of Childbearing

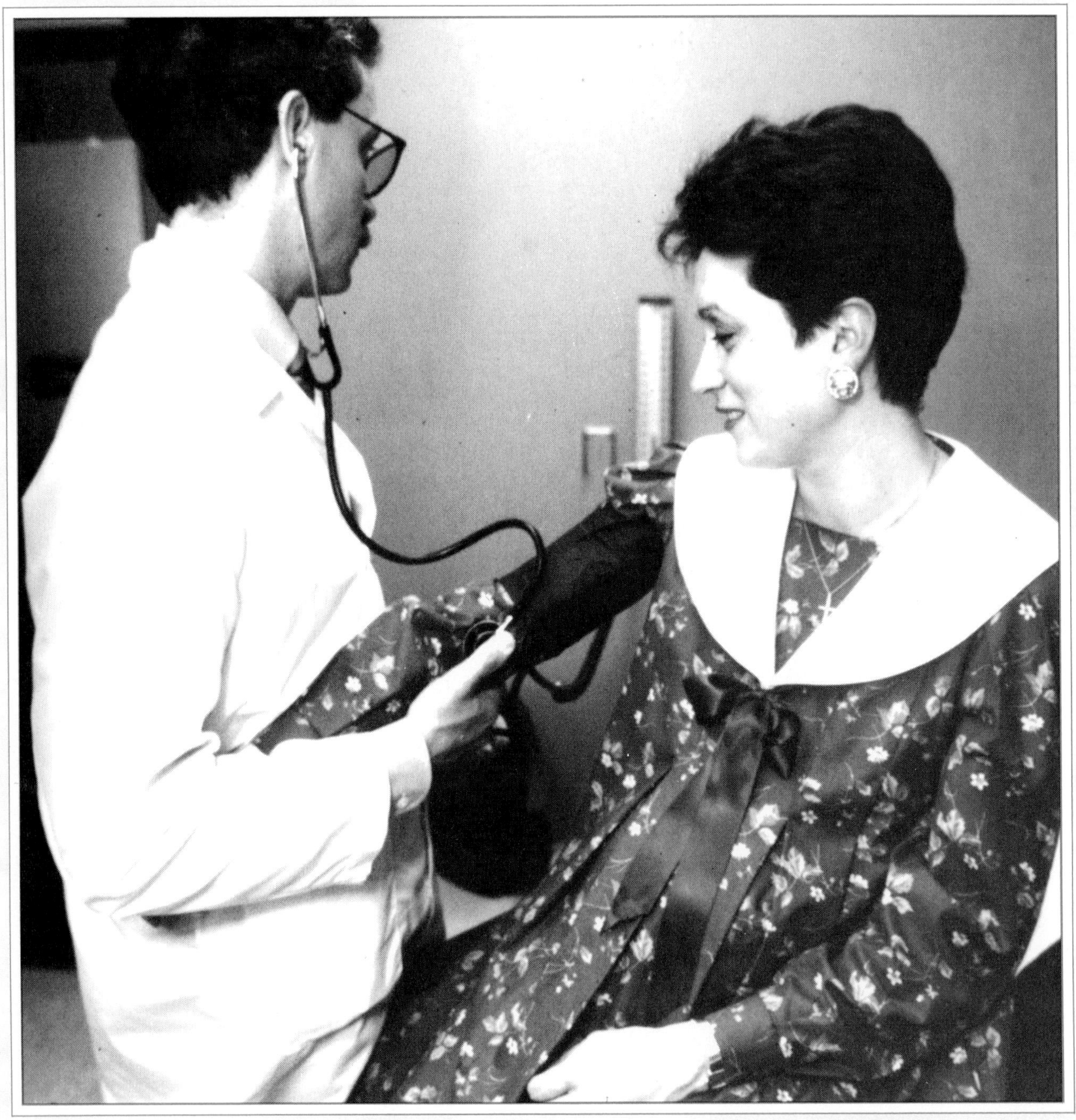

UNIT

I

INTRODUCTION TO MATERNITY NURSING

CHAPTER I

The Client, the Nurse, and the Nursing Process

Irene M. Bobak and Joea E. Bierchen

Learning Objectives

Correctly define the key terms listed.

Examine the nature and scope of contemporary maternity nursing.

Describe the roles of the nurse in contemporary maternity care.

Differentiate between preventive, curative, and rehabilitative nursing functions.

Discuss the role of the nurse as health advocate.

Summarize nursing actions associated with each phase of the helping relationship.

Outline the teaching/learning process.

Key Terms

advocacy
contemporary maternity care
curative aspects
helping relationship
nursing process
  assessment
  nursing diagnosis
  planning
  implementation
  evaluation
preventive aspects
rehabilitative aspects
teaching/learning process

Since recorded time, birth has evoked strong emotions. Birth is one of the most dramatic episodes in life—a moment in time when the past merges with the present, and the present holds all the potential for a new future. Wonder and excitement, as well as awe and reverence are stirred by the creation of another human; a creation that began with conception, progressed through an orderly process of biologic development, and culminated in birth. Yet, the beginnings of this new human cycle, and many of the factors that determine each baby's potential life pattern, lie hidden in the days before birth. The newborn is the expression of multiple genetic and environmental events that occurred during the generations of family reproductive cycles that preceded this birth. Genetic and environmental factors have influenced the growth, development, and health of the parents—and of their new child. Cultural values and beliefs have influenced parental behavioral adaptations to the pregnancy and birth.

Contemporary maternity care involves the client and her family in a collaborative relationship with physicians, nurses, registered dieticians, and other health professionals. Clients and their families are encouraged to be active participants in the management of their childbearing experiences. Health team efforts are directed toward the goals of a healthy pregnancy and an optimum outcome. The general objectives of maternity care are to minimize potential risks and maximize the client's potential for successful childbearing. Maternity nurses are active members of the health care team; effective application of the nursing process enables nurses to help clients achieve their childbearing goals.

This chapter discusses the nature and scope of maternity nursing, the nursing process, the client, and the nurse. Emphasis is placed on application of the nursing process in developing a collaborative, goal-oriented nurse-client relationship. Brief discussions of the nursing process and selected psychosocial concepts are included to review, reinforce, and facilitate integration of previous learning, as well as to assist beginning nursing students in developing a cognitive organizational framework for maternity nursing.

❑ NATURE AND SCOPE OF MATERNITY NURSING

Over the past several decades, the nature and scope of maternity nursing have broadened. Contemporary maternity nursing is concerned with all aspects of maternity care; nurses are influencing the quality and cost of care, the environment in which care is given, and social issues that affect the health and welfare of clients and their families.

Maternity nursing focuses on helping clients and families meet health needs associated with the childbearing experience. Client needs are those associated with (1) avoiding or achieving pregnancy, (2) maintaining and monitoring or interrupting pregnancy, (3) the normal anatomic, physiologic, and psychologic adaptations to pregnancy and childbirth, (4) preexisting and coexisting medical disorders, and (5) pregnancy-related health problems. Nursing actions encompass the health-illness continuum and include prevention, cure, and rehabilitation. Interventions are directed toward promoting and maintaining health, early diagnosis and effective management of emerging health problems, and minimizing maternal and infant disability. Nursing interventions are designed also to encourage and enable the client and family to make informed decisions and take an active part in pregnancy-related care. Maternity nurses provide counseling and referral, client teaching, and direct care from preconceptional family planning through pregnancy, birth, and the early adjustment of the family to a newborn child. Nursing activities may be carried out in such settings as clinics, physician's offices, hospitals, and alternative birthing centers. In addition, maternity nurses serve as maternal-infant health advocates on the local, state, and national level.

Table 1-1 **Maternal-Infant Biostatistic Terminology**

Term	Definition
Rate	Relates to total population at risk; includes affected and unaffected
Fertility rate	Number of births per 1000 women between the ages of 15 and 44 (inclusive) calculated on a yearly basis
Birthrate	Number of live births per 1000 population
Maternal mortality rate	Number of deaths from deliveries and complications of pregnancy, childbirth, and the puerperium (the first 42 days after termination of the pregnancy) per 100,000 live births
Infant mortality rate	Number of deaths of infants under 1 year of age per 1000 live births
Neonatal mortality rate	Number of deaths of infants under 28 days of age per 1000 live births
Fetal mortality rate	Number of fetal deaths before 20 weeks gestation to number of live births and fetal deaths
Ratio	Relates affected to unaffected population.
Fetal mortality ratio	Number of deaths in utero before 20 weeks gestation per 1000 live births
Induced abortion ratio	Number of induced abortions to 1000 live births

Biostatistical Picture

Biostatistics is the application of statistical analyses to biologic data. Rates and ratios describe the incidence of specific events (e.g., birth, death, disease) among a given population. Population data can be separated by specific demographic variables (descriptive characteristics), such as age, sex, and marital status, thereby enabling health professionals to compare the incidence of specific events among subgroups. Knowledge and understanding of basic maternal-infant biostatistics enables nurses to identify clients who are at increased risk for pregnancy-related health problems. Identifying potential risk factors is important in planning and providing goal-directed care to maximize client potential for an uneventful and successful pregnancy. Relevant maternal-infant biostatistics include fertility, birth, and death rates, as well as the ratio of induced abortions to live births. Data may be grouped or combined by demographic characteristics of age, race, marital status, level of education, occupation, income, and other variables. Table 1-1 defines selected maternal-infant biostatistic terminology.

Nursing Implications. Over the past few years, statistical findings have shown small increases in fertility and birthrates and changes in the demographic characteristics of the childbearing population. Changes in infant and maternal mortality are not statistically significant. Societal health indices reveal a continuing natural increase in total population; that is, more births than deaths. This finding has implications for our society, the economy, and for health care services.

The young and poor are vulnerable to maternity complications and maternal/infant death. Many women still do not receive adequate prenatal care, and many women categorized as being at "high-risk" are still without specialized treatment (U.S. Institute of Medicine, 1988). Efforts should be increased to: (1) educate members of high-risk populations about health promotion, health maintenance, and self-care; (2) encourage early entry into the health care system when pregnancy is suspected; (3) emphasize the value of consistent prenatal visits in reducing the risk of pregnancy-related problems to both the woman and her fetus; and (4) support programs that accomplish these objectives. Several government programs provide services to promote and protect maternal-child health.

❑ NURSING PROCESS AND MATERNITY CARE

Contemporary maternity nursing is based on application of the **nursing process,** which provides an organizational framework for effective nursing care. The nurse assesses the client's general physical and emotional health; pregnancy status; response to the anatomic, physiologic, and psychologic changes associated with pregnancy; and the influence of life experiences, values, and beliefs on pregnancy-related behaviors. The nurse identifies the client's level of relevant knowledge and her individual needs for nursing, and establishes nursing diagnoses. She then collaborates with the client to set client-centered goals. The nurse implements goal-directed nursing care and coordinates the efforts of the health care team, as well as evaluates the effects of nursing actions and client progress toward established goals. Integrating the process into a written nursing care plan enables consistency and continuity of individualized, goal-directed client care.

Each stage of the nursing process contains several phases (Fig. 1-1). The rate of progression through the phases depends on the stage of development of the nurse-client relationship, the nature of the health problem, the setting, the available resources, and the nurse's level of knowledge and skill.

Assessment

The **assessment** stage involves at least two phases: data collection and formulation of inferences, or hypotheses, from the data. Assessment begins when the nurse is alerted to a client's need. The stimulus itself forms part of the data base. The stimulus may be the client's posture or gait as she walks into the clinic, her facial expression while waiting or during the initial contact, her opening comments, a change in color, increased activity, elevated vital signs, or data on written health record forms.

Once alerted, the nurse begins the essential first phase in the assessment stage—the collection of accurate data to formulate nursing diagnoses. Data is collected from interviews, physical examination, and laboratory tests. Sources of data include the client, her family and friends (if this is acceptable to the client, or when the client is unable to provide essential information), and health care records.

Inferences are subjective conclusions; that is, the nurse's interpretation of the data collected. The nurse's knowledge, skill, experience, personal and professional values, and beliefs influence the formulation of inferences. Often, during data collection, assessment findings suggest a pattern.

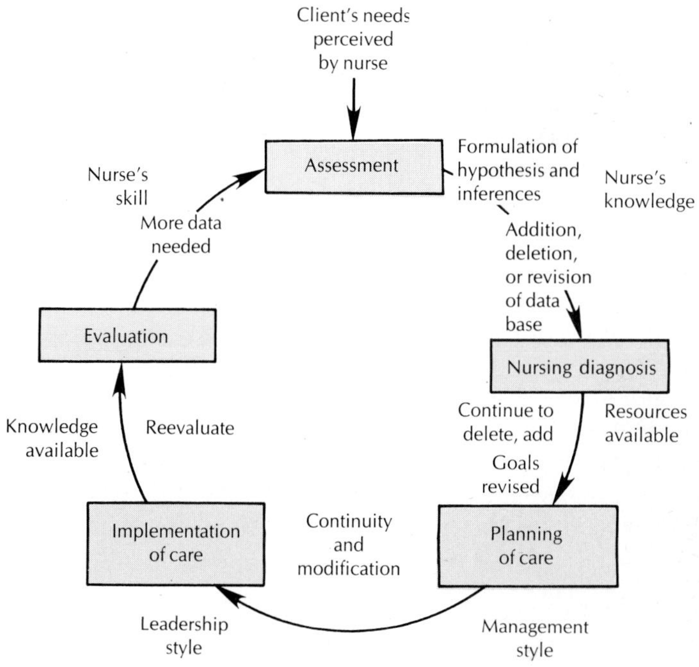

Fig. 1-1 Stages of the nursing process.

Nursing Diagnosis

During the **nursing diagnosis** stage of the nursing process, the collected data is organized, interpreted, analyzed, and validated. Knowledge and understanding of the implications of normal anatomic, physiologic, and psychosocial adaptations to pregnancy is essential to making accurate nursing diagnoses. Assessment findings are compared with established normal physical and psychosocial parameters. Integrating and grouping information from the total current data base enables the nurse to identify relationships between history and physical findings with client behaviors and suggests specific provisional nursing diagnoses.

The accuracy of the diagnoses depends on the comprehensiveness of the data base. Analysis, synthesis, and validation are required to achieve accurate, meaningful nursing diagnoses. *Analysis* identifies categories of client concerns or needs. *Synthesis* is concerned with looking for relationships and patterns (Benner and Tanner, 1987). *Validation* is concerned with determining both the accuracy of the data collected and its interpretation (i.e., nursing diagnosis). This may be done in three ways: (1) with the client for relevance and completeness, (2) with others on the nursing team concurring that the diagnoses fit the data available, and (3) with a member or members of the client's interpersonal system.

Nursing diagnoses are statements summarizing the

analyzed data. The nursing diagnosis is a two-part statement (Christensen and Kenney, 1990). The first part consists of the diagnostic title, usually drawn from the current North American Nursing Diagnosis Association (NANDA) list of nationally accepted nursing diagnoses, and ". . . describes a human response, health state, or altered interaction pattern" (Christensen and Kenney, 1990). The second part of the diagnosis specifies the related etiologic or contributing factors. Each nursing diagnosis indicates the nature and extent of a client's specific health problem. The second part of the statement provides direction for nursing interventions, which are aimed at prevention. This falls within the boundaries of nursing practice as stated in various nurse practice acts. The following are examples of nursing diagnoses formulated from analysis of common assessment findings associated with pregnancy.

Knowledge deficit related to
- Contraceptive options available for effective family planning

Potential self-concept disturbance related to
- Developmental tasks of pregnancy

Potential altered parenting related to
- Lack of experience with newborn care

Ineffective individual coping related to
- Physical discomfort of afterpains and episiotomy

Once the nursing diagnoses have been established, the nurse explores any personal value judgments about the family that may affect or impede effective nursing interventions. Nursing diagnoses therefore are crucial because they guide selection and implementation of effective nursing interventions.

Planning

Planning is the formulation of nursing interventions designed to meet client needs and manage or resolve health-related problems. Essential phases in planning are prioritizing the nursing diagnoses, establishing client-centered, diagnosis-related goals, prioritizing the goals, selecting nursing interventions that will help the client achieve the goals, and identifying methods of evaluating client progress toward goals.

Usually several nursing diagnoses are identified during the stage of analysis; priorities for care are established on the basis of the immediacy (threat to the client's survival) and importance of the actual and potential client problems. For example, for the postpartum client, the diagnosis of "Potential fluid volume deficit related to immediate postpartum hemorrhage caused by uterine atony" takes precedence over the diagnosis of "Pain related to cesarean delivery incision."

Setting Goals

Goal-setting should be a collaborative process between the nurse and client. Clients whose life-styles and other responsibilities are considered in developing the plan of care will be more likely to participate actively in their own health care plan. On occasion, this may not be possible (e.g., if the client is unconscious, too ill, or a newborn infant). In some cases, the nurse assumes responsibility for clarifying the objectives of care with family members; in other situations, the nurse may seek peer review of client goals by health care conferences.

Goals should be related to the specific nursing diagnosis. They should be explicit (i.e., stated in terms of observable/measurable changes in client status or behavior), and they should be realistic or achievable by the client within the allotted time. Short-term goals should be accomplished by the client within a limited amount of time, and they should contribute to the achievement of long-term goals. The method of evaluating client progress toward each goal should be identified and specific outcome criteria that demonstrate client progress should be described. The following is an example of one diagnosis-related goal.

Nursing diagnosis: Sleep pattern disturbance related to increased nocturnal urination

Goal: Alters daily pattern of fluid intake to minimize need for nocturnal urination

Outcome (evaluative) criteria: Client reports—(1) drinks 800 to 1000 ml of fluids between 8 AM and 4 PM daily; (2) limits fluid intake after 8 PM; (3) sleeps uninterrupted for 6 to 8 hours

The goal in this example considers the client's waking time and provides for less intake of fluids after 4 PM to minimize interference with sleep. Outcome (evaluative) criteria identify client compliance with plan and effectiveness of the intervention.

As with nursing diagnoses, goals are prioritized on the basis of the immediacy of the problem or on the client's and nurse's preference. The nurse's preference is determined by the resources available, commitments to other clients, and the need for further data or plans of other health team members.

Selecting Nursing Interventions

Nursing interventions are selected on the basis of the goals and outcome criteria desired by the client and nurse; anticipated effectiveness in helping the client achieve the goals; the amount of risk to the client; the availability of resources, facilities, and personnel; and the client's ability to comply with the proposed care (Glass, 1983). Representative nursing interventions include providing direct care, counseling and referral, role-modeling, and client teaching (e.g., discussion, demonstration, and "hands-on" learning activities).

The nurse may select goal-directed nursing actions from a repertoire of known, effective nursing interventions; from the literature; and by consulting with other nurses, as well as the client. Information from the client and family regarding ways in which the client has coped with similar health problems or situations in the past is helpful in planning an individualized approach to care. Wherever possible, the client's self-care patterns should be incorporated into the nursing plan of care. As personal knowledge increases, an expanding repertoire of nursing skills enables the nurse to develop a plan of care that correlates nursing actions with the client's needs and goals and accommodates the client's individual preferences and cultural proscriptions. The written nursing care plan facilitates consistency and continuity of care and enables other members of the health care team to effectively help the client achieve the established goals and evaluate the outcomes of nursing interventions.

To illustrate the development of nursing care plans, two different types are included in this text. To administer individualized care, the nurse must first be knowledgeable about the general care for a particular condition or situation. *General nursing care plans* provide this information. *Specific nursing care plans* guide the student in tailoring care to meet the individual needs of a specific client.

Implementation

Implementation is the stage of the nursing process in which the plan is put into action; the nurse initiates and completes the interventions designed to help the client achieve the goals and demonstrate the specified outcome criteria. Many *procedures* for nursing care are described in the text to help in the implementation phase of the nursing process. Implementation also may include referral to, and interaction with, other team members. Coordinating nursing care with that provided by other members of the health care team is important in maximizing the effectiveness of the total approach toward goal achievement. During the implementation stage of the nursing process, the nurse continues to gather and validate data and to modify the plan of care as necessary (Potter and Perry, 1989).

The overall management of the health care setting is an essential, indeed critical, aspect of implementation. *Each nurse contributes to the setting by supporting colleagues through review of nursing care plans, willing consultation and assistance in client care, and appropriate praise.*

Evaluation

Evaluation is a joint process between the nurse, the client, and the family. This stage involves reassessing client status and behavior to determine progress toward, or attainment of, the goals. To evaluate client progress, the nurse compares the client's current status, abilities, and knowledge with those of previous assessments and with the specified outcome criteria.

Commonly, evaluation is concurrent with implementation. While implementing the plan of care, the nurse reassesses the client and her response to the planned interventions. The nurse may modify the plan as indicated by client reactions, or redefine the expected outcomes (Potter and Perry, 1989). The outcome of the evaluation stage determines the need for additional assessment data, for revising current goals, for adding new goals, for continuing the planned interventions, or for implementing alternative nursing actions. For example, the nurse reviews a maternity client's written record of her daily diet to evaluate the effectiveness of previous client teaching/nutrition counseling. The nurse discovers that, because of cultural beliefs, the woman has failed to comply with the recommended diet. This finding suggests a need to collaboratively develop a list of client-acceptable foods that will effectively meet her antepartal nutrition needs.

❑ CLIENT

Usually a woman's childbearing years are identified as between the ages of 15 and 44 (Monthly Vital Statistics Report, 1989). However, maternity clients include the fetus, neonate, adolescent, young adult, and the woman entering her middle years. Most commonly, clients are under 35 years of age and are in good health; some, however, will be designated at *high-risk* because of maternal, familial, or fetal factors (Chapter 22). Many will enter the health care system early, whereas others may not seek care until health problems arise. Some will have strong family support systems; others will be alone. Motivation and psychologic adaptation to pregnancy vary among women. Most will be delighted by their pregnancies; some will be angry, defensive, or apathetic. Knowledge and understanding of the psychosocial, physiologic, and cultural factors that influence a woman's response to pregnancy enables the nurse to make accurate, holistic, comprehensive, nursing assessments of client status; formulate appropriate nursing diagnoses; plan and implement effective, client-centered, goal-directed interventions; and evaluate client progress.

Accurately identifying current and projected client

problems and needs is vital to planning and implementing effective maternity nursing care. Williams (1989) suggests that awareness of the psychologic significance (i.e., personal meaning) of pregnancy, childbearing, and parenting enables the nurse to provide competent, individualized client care. Thus holistic nursing assessments of maternity clients require a basic knowledge and understanding of biologic and psychosocial factors that influence pregnancy-related behaviors (e.g., client motives and adaptations).

Childbearing is an intensely personal experience. A variety of motives may lead to pregnancy. Some women seek pregnancy to meet their own needs for someone to love—and to love them; others may want to punish a significant other, such as a parent. For most, the pregnancy is perceived as an outcome of their love and desire for a family.

Individual perceptions of the personal meaning of pregnancy and childbirth are influenced greatly by the person's previous life experiences, cultural values and beliefs, and needs and desires. Usually childbirth is a family-centered event, with every family member being affected by the birth. The birth of a child often unifies a family. Many partners insist on sharing this important event with the mother by actively participating in the pregnancy and labor. For some people, this sharing extends beyond the immediate participants to siblings, extended family members, friends, and community members.

Parenthood, beginning as it does with the excitement of pregnancy and birth, can serve many purposes. To some it is a life-fulfilling state, a chance to help their children become the adults of the future. Children born to such parents are wanted children whose dependency is recognized and accepted.

Other pregnancies are neither planned nor desired. Children born under these conditions may suffer parental and material deprivation. One of the greatest needs such children have is for parents who have learned the art of "gentle socialization of children," and who create a nurturing environment peopled with interested, concerned, and loving adults (Edwards, 1973). Giving the child up for adoption may present a viable solution to the client experiencing an unplanned or undesired pregnancy.

❑ MATERNITY NURSE

Maternity nurses are in a unique position to effect change in the care women receive. Nurses have early, frequent, and continuing contact with the woman and her family. The nurse acts in a variety of roles and settings to bring comprehensive health care to people during the childbearing years. Nurses act as caregivers, teachers, counselors, technicians, advocates, managers, and researchers. They provide services to maternity clients in hospital maternity units and birthing centers, physician's offices and clinics, family planning agencies, and homes. The services nurses provide and the degree to which they function autonomously depend on their educational preparation, amount of experience, level of competence, and practice setting.

The high-technology environment for contemporary maternity nursing practice requires competence in applying, operating, monitoring, and interpreting data from biomedical systems. Orientation, inservice, guided practice, and continuing education programs enable beginning maternity nurses to develop and maintain skills needed to maximize the value of biomedical adjuncts.

Benner's work (1983, 1984) describes how a body of practical knowledge is developed as the nurse acquires expertise. The nursing process may be implemented with varying degrees of effectiveness depending on the nurse's competence. Nurses progress from novice to expert, acquiring further knowledge, skill, and confidence through experience and continued learning; excellence in nursing requires commitment and involvement (Benner, 1984).

Nursing Roles

Caregiver. The holistic concept of the nurse as caregiver includes creating a climate for the helping/healing relationship (Benner, 1984). Caring is the essence of nursing. Caring is expressed through the skillful combination of interpersonal and technical skills. In high-technology settings, the warmth, hope, and shared concern of the nurse balance the often dehumanizing aspects of the situation and help mobilize the client's energy for coping. The care given by maternity nurses includes basic physical care and comfort measures, emotional support, and assistance in decision-making. Nursing interventions are directed toward the **preventive aspects, curative aspects,** and **rehabilitative aspects** of pregnancy-related care for childbearing families and their infants.

Teacher and Counselor. Maternity nursing emphasizes the preventive aspects of health care. Much of this is accomplished through teaching and counseling clients. As a teacher or counselor, the nurse tries to help women learn how to make the best possible health care decisions for themselves and their children. The nurse provides a nonjudgmental environment in which this learning can take place and helps clients realistically evaluate their efforts. The nurse acts as a role model for clients, demonstrating self-care, infant care, and parenting skills and attitudes.

The nurse also intervenes to minimize the emotional impact of the high-technology environment on clients and families by explaining and teaching the functions and value of biomedical adjuncts to therapy (e.g., fetal monitors). With supportive teaching, the nurse can help even the most anxious or uninformed client learn to accept and adjust to needed therapeutic procedures and to provide effective self-care.

Advocate. As health care becomes more complex, nurses are assuming liaison, or **advocacy,** roles between the client and other personnel or health care agencies. The maternity nurse encourages the client to become aware of her health care rights and responsibilities. Because the nurse is committed to a holistic view of health care, she often knows more about the client than do other health workers. Furthermore, the nurse is in a position to explain, interpret, defend, and protect client rights. As an advocate, the nurse also attempts to modify health services on a local or national level so they reflect a humanitarian approach to health care. Participation in professional organizations and politics (such as health-related legislation) is an important feature of the nursing commitment to ensuring health care for all persons (Archer and Goehner, 1982; Wilson, 1981).

Manager. All nurses participate in the management of nursing care by prioritizing client needs, providing client-centered, goal-directed care, and organizing the delivery of care for maximum benefit and minimum expense in time and materials. Nurse managers coordinate and facilitate the many services required in the health care of clients (Etheredge, 1985). Team leaders or charge nurses are examples of nurse managers, since they direct the care of groups of clients and nursing personnel. Additional dimensions of the management role include cost containment and quality assurance. Managerial efforts are directed toward maximizing the benefits of care, minimizing expense to client and health agency, and evaluating the quality of care provided for compliance with established nursing standards (Chapter 3). Nurse managers need to be knowledgeable about client care and able to communicate and collaborate effectively with workers at all levels of the health care system.

Researcher. Research has had an invaluable effect on shaping nursing practice and developing ideas for further inquiry that will keep our future practice alive. The purpose of nursing research is to improve client care. The idea of scientific research in nursing dates back to Florence Nightingale, who encouraged nurses to develop the habit of systematically making and recording accurate observations and then contemplating their meaning. Observations should focus on discovering and verifying knowledge useful for saving lives, expediting recovery, and reducing disability. Nurses need to evaluate the effectiveness of established clinical nursing methods and protocols by measuring the outcomes in client health status. Nursing research (e.g., documenting the benefits of alternative models of treatment and care) can improve the quality of care with resulting savings in costs to clients. Nurses should evaluate findings of current research for relevance to their own practice and client care.

Expanded Roles

Credentialed Specialist. Specialists are those who have consciously and formally increased their knowledge and skill in a specific area of nursing; formal education and experiential career ladders prepare nurses for advanced levels of practice. Credentialed nursing specialists include clinicians, nurse practitioners, and nurse-midwives. Many state nurse practice acts provide for additional licensure for advanced practice; eligibility is determined on approval of the program completed and preceptor certification of proficiency in practice.

Whereas licensure is mandatory and granted by the state, certification is voluntary and provided by national professional nursing specialty practice organizations. Licensure signifies the nurse has met the minimum requirements for general nursing practice (i.e., is a registered nurse [RN]) or for advanced nursing practice in that state (i.e., is an advanced registered nurse practitioner [ARNP]). Certification signifies the nurse has met minimum standards established by professional peers in a specific nursing specialty (i.e., certified nurses have met national standards of practice limited to one special area in nursing).

The Organization for Obstetrical, Gynecologic, and Neonatal Nurses (formerly the Nurses' Association of the American College of Obstetrics and Gynecology [NAACOG]), the American Nurses' Association (ANA), and the American College of Nurse-Midwives certify performance at advanced levels of maternity nursing practice by examination. Certified nurses are entitled to use the designation Registered Nurse Certified (RNC). Nurses who meet the requirements of the American College of Nurse-Midwives are entitled to use the designation Certified Nurse-Midwife (CNM). The ANA House of Delegates (1985) passed a resolution requiring a master's degree in nursing as the minimum requirement for nurse practitioner certification by 1995.

Nurse-Midwives. The American College of Nurse-Midwives was founded in 1969. It is the official accrediting agency for educational programs in midwifery. It defines qualifications, delineates professional roles and functions, and establishes standards of practice. Since 1971, the college has administered the National Certification Examination to graduates of accredited programs. In January of 1987, the college listed nine approved certificate programs, 15 university programs granting master's degrees, and one doctoral program in midwifery (American College of Nurse-Midwives, 1987).

In affiliation with physicians for consultation and referral, the nurse-midwife functions independently to provide safe, effective, reproductive health care to healthy women; provide family-centered care to healthy mothers and newborns; and perform emergency procedures in the absence of a physician. High-risk clients and clients who experience unexpected complications are referred promptly to physicians. More than 2500 certified nurse-midwives provide services in health maintenance organizations, private practice settings, alternative birthing centers, clinics, and hospitals throughout the 50 states (American College of Nurse-Midwives, 1987).

❑ NURSE-CLIENT RELATIONSHIPS

Establishing an open, interactive, therapeutic nurse-client relationship is essential to (1) assessing client health status accurately and determining the woman's perceptions and present level of adaptation to pregnancy, childbearing, and parenthood; (2) identifying actual and potential client needs and problems and setting mutual goals; (3) planning and (4) implementing client-centered, goal-directed care; and (5) evaluating effects of nursing interventions. Intrapersonal and interpersonal factors influence the development and growth of the nurse-client relationship. Interactions and relationships with others are affected by the way we perceive ourselves, others, the situation and setting, and others' responses to us. The expectations, perceptions, and behaviors of nurses and clients are influenced by self-awareness, self-concept, perception of social and professional roles, and personal, professional, and cultural values and beliefs.

Pregnancy, childbearing, and parenting have been identified as life crisis events (Williams, 1989). The client's health needs are influenced by the personal meaning of these events. Her responses to the altered physiology, psychologic adaptations, and developmental tasks of pregnancy and parenting influence how she feels about herself. Commonly, maternity clients seek understanding, acceptance, and help with decision-making and coping with pregnancy-related changes. They expect the nurse to provide information, encouragement, and support (i.e., they seek a helping relationship).

Helping Relationship

The **helping relationship** is purposeful and goal-directed (Rodgers, 1961). Characteristics of an effective helping relationship include trust, empathy, caring, autonomy, and mutuality (Sundeen et al, 1989). Inherent in the relationship is the expectation that nurse and client work collaboratively toward the expected outcomes, which are that the client will make informed decisions, meet her health needs, and gain new coping and adaptation skills (Brady, 1989).

The maternity nurse uses the nursing process to help the client adapt to her changing body and self-concept and to prepare her for entry into her new role as parent. Supportive maternity nurse-client relationships and open communication encourage clients to verbalize anxieties and concerns, seek or gain assistance in problem-solving, establish and achieve appropriate goals, and develop effective coping abilities.

Both client and nurse are influenced by the interplay of intrapersonal and interpersonal perceptions. Knowledge of one's own dynamic concept of "self," and the intrapersonal and interpersonal factors that influence each individual's perceptions, actions, and interactions enables the nurse to interpret and understand client behavior, relate effectively with clients, establish therapeutic rapport, and initiate and maintain the helping relationship.

Knowledge of the factors that generate or reduce stress, as well as support or interfere with the development of productive human relationships enables nurses to create an environment that provides psychologic security, facilitates an open, interactive nurse-client relationship, and promotes shared responsibility for the achievement of the desired outcomes. The nurse's interpersonal skills and ability to communicate acceptance, empathy, concern, and desire to help are essential to developing and maintaining the helping relationship.

Implementing the Helping Relationship

The helping relationship is a dynamic process that evolves sequentially. Each phase builds on a previous phase and accomplishes certain tasks. The process of developing a relationship is the same regardless of the time frame (short- or long-term) in which it occurs. Table 1-2 summarizes nursing actions associated with each phase of the nursing relationship.

Effective, situation-appropriate communication encourages positive interpersonal perceptions; the effective interchange of information; a shared understanding of roles, goals, and objectives; and collaborative decision-making. With practice, nurses can develop a repertoire of techniques that enhances their skill and accuracy in eliciting and validating assessment data,

Table 1-2 Phases of the Helping Relationship

Phase	Nursing Action
Preparation	Preliminary assessment; review health form, laboratory tests, prenatal record, report sheet, chart
Initiation	Ensure privacy, confidentiality; open communication, establish rapport, assure mutual understanding of expectations; assessment—history, physical; planning—establish nursing diagnoses, set mutual goals, identify outcome criteria; implementation—client teaching and care; evaluation—client acceptance of goals and understanding of teaching
Consolidation and growth	Continue developing relationship; reassess status, evaluate for outcome criteria; planning—clarify, continue, expand, or delete goals as needed; identify alternative interventions as needed; implementation—support client problem-solving, decision-making; reinforce, expand client teaching
Termination	Evaluation—review goals that have been accomplished; end relationship with invitation to make contact or return if needed

analyzing the personal meaning of the experience to the client, and identifying primary and ancillary concerns.

Nonverbal factors also influence effective, open communication. The nurse's nonjudgmental attitude; relaxed, unhurried approach; and appropriate use of space, vocal tone, touch, and eye contact to convey understanding, acceptance, trust, and empathy are important in establishing a productive interpersonal relationship.

The setting in which nurse-client interactions take place is an important factor in developing rapport and facilitating open communication. Maternity nursing interviews often explore sensitive, personal aspects of the client's health and life. The interview setting should assure client privacy. Furthermore, when possible, diagnostic and treatment equipment, as well as supplies and teaching materials should not be visible. Commonly, such equipment and materials distract the client's attention and may engender anxiety.

Sending and receiving clear messages is critical to any helping relationship. Language used in nurse-client interactions must promote and ensure mutual understanding. The social or lay language of any culture contains elements that are known and recognized by all who speak it. However, within any culture, each subgroup develops a language of its own. Subgroups may be determined by ethnic origin, age, or profession. When nurses are involved in caring for clients from a specific cultural group, fluency in their language minimizes the potential for misunderstandings, frustration, and anxiety, and increases the potential for active client participation in effective, goal-directed activities.

The nurse learns a professional language as part of being initiated into the nursing profession. For transactions between colleagues, a professional language facilitates precise, meaningful exchange of information. However, many clients are not familiar with medical terminology (Bentz, 1980). Language that is not clear to both the sender and the receiver of information will result in unmet goals. Nurses may have to translate or define terms that are unfamiliar to the client. Information must be given in familiar language, with feedback for mutual understanding. Otherwise much of what is said is either unclear or lost.

Another element in nonverbal communication is time—its meaning and use. The use of time may be either a barrier or an aid to meaningful communication. Clients who are kept waiting, or who feel rushed, may interpret this as a comment on their level of importance to the nurse. This can cause irritability and block effective communication. However, the nurse who appears relaxed and allows adequate time for interactions has a positive effect on the client's response to assessment interviews, client teaching, and direct care.

Knowledge of sociocultural variations is vital to developing therapeutic nurse-client relationships with members of ethnic groups. The traditional American value for directness and expression of feelings is not shared by members of many other cultures. Nursing assessments must be individualized to identify and accommodate the client's cultural preferences for space, time, and patterns of social interactions (e.g., eye contact, touch, pace) (Le Veck, 1987). Nursing interventions must be appropriate to behaviors accepted and valued by the client's cultural group.

Nurses who are observant and sensitive to the client's behaviors and responses are able to modify interpersonal techniques appropriately to accommodate individual personal and cultural preferences. A personalized approach to interactions enhances the development and maintenance of a productive, collaborative, nurse-client relationship.

Both client and nurse actively establish a shared understanding of expectations for the helping relationship. Through discussion of assessment findings and the sharing of perceptions and information, roles are clarified, expectations are described, and goals are set by mutual collaboration and agreement (Potter and Perry, 1989).

Determining appropriate nursing care for a particular client is largely the responsibility of the nurse, who analyzes the assessment findings, establishes nursing diagnoses, and outlines the goals. Many clients expect to share in planning their care and to make informed choices concerning their health management. The extent to which the client understands, accepts, and complies with the nursing recommendations is an essential element in the success of the process. The nurse and the client review the goals for care; then they discuss the client behaviors needed to achieve these goals.

Often, nurse-client discussions elicit innovative solutions to client difficulties. Involving clients in the nursing care process increases their awareness of their responsibility for health maintenance. During the process of care, the nurse and client mutually make periodic evaluations. Although the nurse has a leadership role, a conscious effort is made to maintain a partnership.

Compliance with Care. Once mutual goals have been established, the nurse may use various techniques to prompt client compliance with the plan of care. A relaxed atmosphere encourages voicing of client needs and exchanging of ideas. Ensuring client understanding about the relationship between the behaviors recommended and the goals to be achieved facilitates compliance with the therapy. Barriers to understanding arise in various ways. Cultural differences can preclude understanding. Language differences may necessitate an interpreter. High anxiety levels may make it impossible for the client to "take in" the meaning of prescribed treatments. Evaluating client understanding and repeating teaching and counseling as needed increase the potential for successful compliance with the plan of care.

Noncompliance with the plan of care may have serious consequences to both mother and fetus. Much of maternity care is preventive in nature. The effectiveness of preventive care depends on maintaining the health of mother and fetus, prompt detection of disease, and institution of remedial measures. Collaboration between client and nurse is essential for success. Since the client and nurse share accountability for successful health care, each needs to participate in a responsible way in the decision-making process.

❑ THE TEACHING-LEARNING PROCESS

Holistic health care is part of a broad effort to create humane, democratic alternatives to large, impersonal, unresponsive health care services and institutions (Redman, 1988). Given impetus by consumerism and self-care movements, the emphasis in holistic health care is on education and self-care (**teaching-learning process**), rather than on treatment or dependence. Holistic nursing incorporates the view that adequate client knowledge is essential to competent self-care, and any setting where health care is provided is a place for education. Client teaching is an essential nursing intervention in implementing the preventive, curative, and rehabilitative aspects of maternity nursing. Health teaching helps clients minimize their potential for pregnancy-related problems. Furthermore, anticipatory teaching can help clients cope more effectively with many situations that arise throughout the childbearing experience.

Both the client and the nurse bring a highly personal definition of health to the nurse-client interaction. The free exchange of information that characterizes the helping relationship enables collaborative identification of client assets, deficits, and learning needs. General goals for client teaching are that clients will (1) make informed decisions on the basis of adequate, accurate, current knowledge, and (2) maintain or, if necessary, alter their life-styles and behavior to achieve optimum health. Through client teaching, nurses can help clients prevent, promote, maintain, or modify a number of health-related behaviors (Redman, 1988).

Learning has been separated into three classifications: cognitive (understanding), psychomotor (motor skills), and affective (attitudes) (Redman, 1988). Each of these areas of learning is activated most effectively by a particular method of learning. *Cognitive:* facts and concepts are taught by written materials, audiovisual aids, and lecture/discussion. *Psychomotor:* motor skills are best learned through skills demonstration, guided practice, and return-demonstration. *Affective:* attitudes can be examined and (perhaps) altered by discussions that encourage insight into affective behavior (Redman, 1988). Attitudes also may be affected by guided values clarification and role modeling. The teaching process uses the same steps as those of the nursing process (Fig. 1-2).

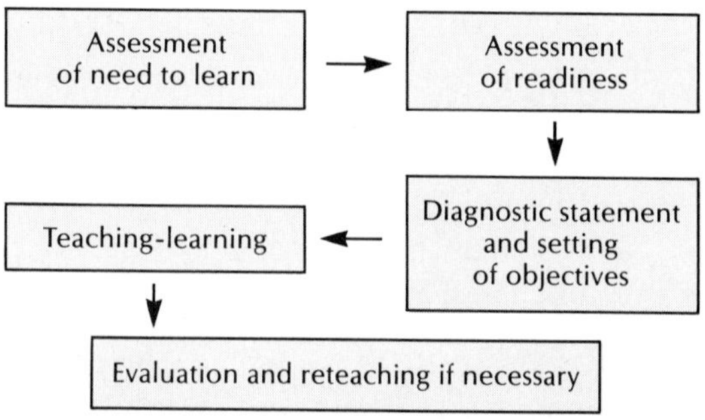

Fig. 1-2 Integration of the teaching, learning, and nursing processes. (From Redman BK: The process of patient education, ed 6, St Louis, 1988, The CV Mosby Co.)

Assessment

The first step is to identify the client's *need for teaching.* An individual may request information or express a desire to learn a task. The information requested may be about promoting health or preventing or treating a problem, or it may be about a health facility and its services.

Learning requires motivation. People who are not convinced they need to learn will resist efforts to be taught. Several conditions affect motivation (e.g., cultural values and socioeconomic class) (Redman, 1988). People vary in their *readiness for health learning* because of their intellectual capabilities, general educational backgrounds, and attitudes toward responsibility (Redman, 1988; Loughrey, 1983; Taylor, 1984). According to Redman (1988), two factors decide readiness to learn: (1) motivation, which determines the individual's willingness to expend the effort required; and (2) individual background (experiences, skills, and attitudes) and the ability to learn that which is perceived as needed or desired. The *theory of learned helplessness* (Redman, 1988) suggests that if the expected outcome is associated with independence, some persons experience fear and are unable to cope with the anticipated outcome. Other people feel that nothing they do can affect their environment or what happens to them. These people are described as having no internalized locus of control or internal motivation.

Timing is another factor that affects a person's ability to learn. The person must recognize an unmet need and yet be comfortable (physically, and in that environment) to be able to learn (McHatton, 1985; Miller, 1985; Redman, 1988).

Analysis and Setting of Objectives

The nursing diagnosis can identify an existing knowledge deficit. Teaching objectives and provisional learning goals are established to meet the client's need for learning. The following illustrates one nursing diagnosis derived from assessment of needs verbalized by couples in a prenatal class.

Nursing diagnosis: Potential altered parenting related to knowledge deficit regarding physical care of the newborn

Teaching objective: To develop client competence and confidence in ability to perform basic newborn care procedures

Planning and Implementation

Once the nursing diagnoses and teaching objectives are established and validated, the nurse establishes goals in collaboration with the client. Taking the client's cultural or ethnic values and beliefs into consideration, the nurse plans goal-directed teaching/learning activities and selects the teaching method and tools.

The nurse plans teaching methods to activate all three learning classifications. For the diagnosis listed, the nurse may select the following methods: audiovisual aids, discussion, demonstration, and guided practice. To promote cognitive learning, a film is used to present a visual overview of the procedure and identify essential concepts and principles. Discussion and demonstration at the client's intellectual and educational levels reinforce concepts and principles and enable understanding. Affective learning is encouraged through discussion of giving the baby a shampoo. This helps the mother work through her attitudes about the activity. Psychomotor skills are learned through guided practice in shampooing an infant model. This helps develop needed motor skills and increases confidence in ability to perform this task.

Teaching tools also can be developed to help nurses present information. An example of a teaching tool used in this text is the guidelines for client teaching format found in the clinical chapters. The nurse changes the teaching tool as knowledge increases from client interactions. The long-term goal for the above client is that she will develop competence and confidence in her ability to provide basic infant care. The client's short-term goal will be to perform an infant shampoo safely and accurately using a life-size infant model. Once the client has accomplished this short-term goal, she should: demonstrate increasing comfort in handling infant model (body language, eye contact); perform procedure safely and accurately with minimum guidance and assistance; and verbalize confidence in ability to perform procedure safely.

Timing is based on the client's verbalized unmet need for assistance in gaining skills needed for newborn care, and on the client's collaboration in goal-setting. For hospitalized clients who demonstrate the same unmet need, teaching is offered when the mother is rested, comfortable, and has asked to learn the activity. When the same teaching methods are used, visual aids, discussion, and demonstration can be provided while the mother rests in bed or a chair. Most women tire easily in the early postpartum period, so the session should be limited by the woman's tolerance.

Readiness to learn is an important consideration in deciding the timing for client teaching. Rubin's research (1984) reveals that new mothers progress through time-related stages of adjustment to the childbearing experience, and suggests that client teaching should be postponed until the mother has entered the stage of "taking-hold" (Chapter 21). However, as a result of the current short (48 hours or less) postpartum inhospital stay, nurses must expedite identifying and meeting the client's learning needs. New mothers often express the need and desire for anticipatory guidance and teaching in self-care, infant care, and problems that may occur after discharge (Davis et al, 1986). Effective anticipatory client teaching minimizes potential postdischarge feelings of insecurity, incompetence, and anxiety that effect the new mother's self-concept, and it enables new mothers to cope more effectively with the demands of caregiving and the changes in role and lifestyle (Pridham, 1986). Recent nursing research indicates that effective client teaching can be implemented early in the postpartum period (Gay, Edgil, and Douglas, 1988; Martel and Mitchell, 1984).

Evaluation

During each nurse-client interaction, the nurse will focus on reassessment, evaluate client progress toward goals, and consequently restructure plans. Ongoing evaluation allows the nurse and client to examine the effects of current health behaviors and modify plans to meet emerging needs.

Evaluation activities also characterize the termination phase of the helping relationship. The nurse and client review the goals they have accomplished and plan for future health care. This final phase of the helping relationship leaves the client with a positive impression of the health care system. A positive impression can affect the client's future health maintenance. Satisfied clients are more likely to return for preventive health care, rather than seeking only curative care.

SUMMARY

Nursing is a combination of interwoven processes, knowledge, skills, roles, and functions. Achieving excellence in the art of becoming alert to meaningful cues and responding effectively requires a comprehensive knowledge base and skillful use of the nursing process. Nurse-client responsibility is at the heart of providing effective, client-centered, goal-directed nursing care. Although all human relationships have characteristics in common, the nurse-client relationship is initiated by the nurse for the benefit of the client. The nurse utilizes professional communication and decision-making skills to facilitate the nursing process. The nurse's responsive dimensions, trust, and empathic understanding are essential to the nurse's role in establishing and maintaining the helping relationship. Awareness of the influence of intrapersonal and interpersonal perceptions on client and nurse facilitates acceptance of and progress toward mutually defined goals. Teaching is a vital component of effective nursing care, enabling clients to make informed decisions and to set and achieve realistic goals. Contemporary maternity nurses assume both traditional and new roles and responsibilities as they meet the challenges of the present and the future.

KEY CONCEPTS

- Caring is the essence of nursing.
- Maternity nursing involves actions that can be identified as preventive, curative, and rehabilitative.
- Through advocacy, nurses can influence the health and well-being of present and future generations.
- The nursing process involves both client and nurse in all five stages: assessment, nursing diagnosis, planning, implementation, and evaluation.
- Health and illness behaviors are influenced by cultural values and beliefs, personal definition of health, and personal preferences.
- Individuals have the capability to make decisions about their health and affect their health by the choices they make.
- Client teaching is directed toward enabling individuals to make informed choices regarding health-related behaviors.

References

American College of Nurse-Midwives, Today's certified nurse-midwives, Washington, DC, May, 1987, The College.

American Nurses' Association, Summary of proceedings, house of delegates, Kansas City, Mo, 1985, The Association.

Archer S and Goehner P: Nurses, a political force, Belmont, Calif, 1982, Wadsworth Publishing Co.

Benner P and Tanner C: Clinical judgment: how expert nurses use intuition, Am J Nurs 87 1:23, 1987.

Benner P: From novice to expert, excellence and power in clinical nursing practice, Menlo Park, Ca, 1984, Addison-Wesley Publishing Co, Inc.

Benner, P: Uncovering the knowledge embedded in clinical practice, Image 15(2):36, 1983.

Bentz, J: Missed meanings in nurse/patient communication, MCN 5:55, 1980.

Brady, P: Therapeutic relationships. In Johnson B: Adaptation and growth, psychiatric-mental health nursing, ed 2, Philadelphia, 1989, JB Lippincott Co.

Christensen PJ and Kenney JW: Nursing process: Application of theories, frameworks, and models, ed 3, St Louis, 1990, The CV Mosby Co.

Davis J et al: A study of mother's postpartum teaching priorities, Matern Child Nurs J 15:41, 1986.

Edwards M: Communications: dimensions in childbirth education, Pacific Grove, Ca, 1973, M Edwards.

Etheredge ML: Nurse-manager . . . try that title on for size, Nurs '85 15(8):26, 1985.

Gay JT, Edgil AE, and Douglas AB: Reva Rubin revisited, JOGN Nurs 11:394, Nov/Dec, 1988.

Glass H: Interventions in nursing: goal or task-oriented? Int Nurs Rev 30(2):53, 1983.

LeVeck P: The role of culture in mental health and illness. In Cook S and Fontaine K: Essentials of mental health nursing, Menlo Park, Calif, 1987, Addison-Wesley Publishing Co.

Loughrey L: Dealing with an illiterate patient . . . you can't read him like a book, Nurs '83 13(1):64, 1983.

Martel LK and Mitchell SK: Rubin's puerperal change reconsidered, JOGN Nurs 13:145, May/June, 1984.

McHatton M: A theory of timely teaching, Am J Nurs 85 (7):798, 1985.

Miller A: When is the time ripe for teaching? Am J Nurs 85 (7):801, 1985.

Monthly Vital Statistics Reports, 37:12, Births, marriages, divorces, and deaths for 1988. National Center for Health Statistics, US Department of Health and Human Services Public Health Service, Centers for Disease Control, March 28, 1989.

Potter P and Perry A: Fundamentals of nursing: concepts, process and practice, ed 2, St Louis, 1989, The CV Mosby Co.

Pridham K: The meaning for mothers of a new infant: relationship to maternal experience, Matern Child Nurs J 16(2):103, 1986.

Redman B: The process of patient education, ed 6, St Louis, 1988, The CV Mosby Co.

Rodgers C: On becoming a person, Boston, 1961, Houghton Mifflin Co.

Rubin R: Maternal identity and the maternal experience, New York, 1984, Springer Publishing Co, Inc.

Sundeen S et al: Nurse-client interaction: implementing the nursing process, ed 4, St Louis, 1989, The CV Mosby Co.

Taylor J: Are you missing what your patients can teach you? RN 47(6):63, 1984.

US Institute of Medicine: Prenatal care: reaching mothers, reaching infants, Washington, DC, 1988, National Academy Press.

Williams R: Issues in women's health care. In Johnson B: Psychiatric-mental health nursing, ed 2, Philadelphia, 1989, JB Lippincott Co, 1989.

Wilson J: Nurses and politics, Can Nurse 77:40, 1981.

Bibliography

Kim M, McFarland G, and McLane A: Pocket guide to nursing diagnoses, ed 3, St Louis, 1989, The CV Mosby Co.

McFarland G and McFarlane E: Nursing diagnosis and intervention: planning for patient care, St Louis, 1989, The CV Mosby Co.

Rew I: Nursing intuition: too powerful—and too valuable—to ignore, Nurs '87 17(7):43, 1987.

Smith C: Patient teaching: it's the law, Nurs '87 17(7):67, 1987.

Taptich B et al: Nursing diagnosis and care planning, Philadelphia, 1989, WB Saunders Co.

Tucker S et al: Patient care standards: nursing process, diagnosis, and outcome, ed 4, St Louis, 1988, The CV Mosby Co.

CHAPTER

2 The Family, a Unit of Care

Rhea Williams

Learning Objectives

Correctly define the key terms listed.

Identify key factors in determining the quality of family health.

Explain the functions carried out by a family for the well-being of its members.

Distinguish the properties of family dynamics and the criteria for family decision making.

List three major family theories. Evaluate the components and implications for nursing of each theory.

Define and give examples of maturational and situational crises.

Identify factors that can alter one's perceptions of an event.

Differentiate between constructive and destructive coping mechanisms.

Relate the role of culture in the nursing care of individuals and families during the childbearing and child-rearing periods.

Outline important components of a family care plan.

Key Terms

blended family
communal family
coping mechanisms
cultural context
developmental theory
extended family
family dynamics
family functions
family theories
homosexual family
interactional theory
maturational crises
nuclear family
single-parent family
situational crises
structural-functional theory
support systems

Every newborn comes into this world surrounded by a family, be it a single-parent family or a large extended family. Regardless of the family structure, the maternity nurse is in a unique position to influence the care and well-being of these childbearing families. In so doing, the nurse acknowledges the family unit as the focus of care.

As one of society's most important institutions, the family represents a primary social group that influences and is influenced by other people and institutions. It is recognized as the fundamental social unit because most people have more continuous contact with this social group than with any other. The family assumes major responsibility for the introduction and socialization of persons. It serves to transmit to members the fundamental cultural background of a given family. Despite the stresses and strains to which it now is subject, the family forms a social network that acts as a potent support system for its members.

To deliver safe, comprehensive, and holistic care within the context of the nursing process, nurses working with childbearing families need a clear understanding of the family as an institution in our society.

❑ DEFINING THE FAMILY

Families are defined in many ways. Definitions of the family involve delineation of family *structure, functions, composition,* and *affectional ties.* A household is composed of the person or persons who occupy a housing unit. Although a majority of households consist of a family-type of living arrangement, many do not. Two major categories of households are identified by the U.S. Bureau of the Census as family and nonfamily. A *family* or *family household* requires the presence of at least two persons: the householder and one or more additional family members related to the householder through birth, adoption, or marriage. A *nonfamily household* is composed of a householder who either lives alone or with persons who are not related to the householder.

The concept of household encompasses not only traditional forms of family structure but also other designated groups: (1) the never-married, (2) one parent and children living together as a one-parent family, (3) two homosexuals living together in a stable union, and (4) stable consensual unions, with or without children (WHO, 1978).

Friedman (1986) offers a broad definition of family, emphasizing the importance of emotional involvement as a necessary characteristic. She says, "the family is composed of people (two or more) who are emotionally involved with each other and live in close geographic proximity."

Various family forms have been defined. Descriptions of these forms follows.

Nuclear Family. The **nuclear family** is a family group consisting of parents and their dependent children. The family lives apart from either the husband's or wife's family of origin, and is usually economically independent.

The nuclear family has long represented the traditional American family. In this family group, parents are expected to play complementary roles of husband-wife and father-mother in giving emotional and physical support to each other and their children. Recent trends in contemporary society, however, have caused many variations in this often considered ideal family structure. The "idealized" two-parent, two-child nuclear family where the father is the sole provider and the mother is the homemaker may be a myth of the past (Fig. 2-1). In fact, reporting on a recent family conference, Libman (1988), states that today, couples in an intact first marriage, with two children and the mother at home represent only 8% of the nation's families.

Extended Family. By definition the **extended family** includes three generations. The family is a central focus for all members who live together as a group. Through its kinship network it provides supportive functions to all members. This family structure serves to prescribe the responsibilities and actions of family members.

Variations of the traditional nuclear and extended families have always existed. Until recently, most of these *alternative family forms* have been considered deviations from the norm. Parents outside of matrimony were pressured to conform by either marrying or releasing the newborn for adoption (Evans et al, 1989). Today, single parenthood, unintentional or planned, is becoming an acceptable option in many communities within the United States. Single parenthood can be a voluntary choice that does not result in rejection by family, ostracism by society, or loss of job. In addition, biologic and adoptive parenthood is becoming a socially acceptable option for women and men who do not choose to marry; lesbian and gay parenthood by artificial insemination is another alternative (Evans et

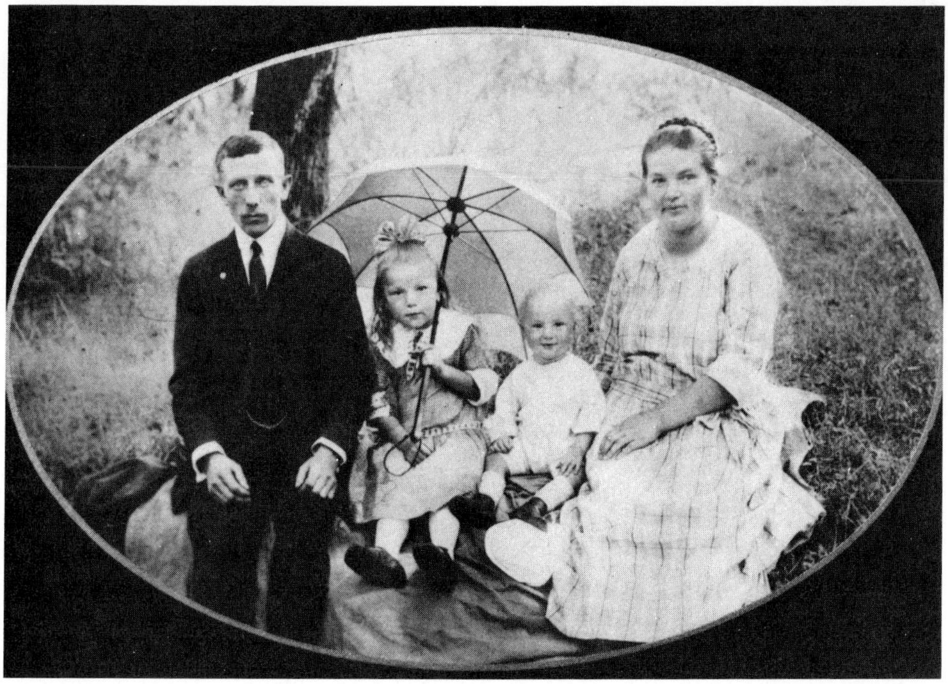

Fig. 2-1 Nuclear family in the 1920s.

al, 1989). The emergence of single parenthood as a planned choice reflects a belief that one has the "right" to choose to be a parent.

Single-parent Family. The **single-parent family** is becoming an increasingly recognized structure in our society. The single-parent family may result from loss of a spouse by death, divorce, separation, or desertion; from the out-of-wedlock birth of a child; or from the adoption of a child. The 1986 U.S. Bureau of the Census reveals that there were 8.9 million one-parent family groups in 1986 compared with 3.8 million in 1970. Of all children 17 years old or younger, 26% live in a family with a single parent, another relative, or a nonrelative. It is estimated that of all children born in the 1980s, 35% will have experienced living in single-parent families twice by 1990 (Libman, 1988).

The single-parent family tends to be vulnerable economically and socially. Unless buttressed by a concerned society, it may create an unstable and deprived environment for the growth potential of children (Norton and Glick, 1986).

For other adults the single-parent family is a chosen life-style that provides a free and open system for development of parents and children. In these families, decision making and communication are seen as joint commitments between parent and child, and the parent-child relationship is considered a major source of life fulfillment.

Blended Family. The **blended family** includes stepparents and stepchildren. Separation, divorce, and remarriage are common phenomena in our society, in which approximately 50% of marriages end in divorce. Divorce and remarriage may occur at any time in the family life cycle and therefore will have different impacts on family function. Whatever the timing, effort is required to restabilize old family groups and constitute and stabilize new family groups. This emotional work must be accomplished before family and individual development can proceed.

Homosexual Family. **Homosexual families** are being recognized increasingly in Western society. Children in such families may be the offspring of previous heterosexual unions of the homosexual parent or be conceived by one member of a lesbian couple through artificial insemination. Homosexual couples have the same biologic and psychologic needs as do heterosexual couples. They too seek quality care for themselves and their children.

Communal Family. **Communal family** groupings vary from the highly formalized structure of the Amish community in Lancaster County, Pennsylvania, to the loosely knit groups found in the Santa Cruz Mountains near Boulder Creek, California. These latter communities are formed for specific ideologic or societal purposes. They are considered an alternative life-style for people who feel alienated from a predominantly economically oriented society. Some communes consist of nuclear groups living in an extended or expanded family community and are envisioned as persisting over time. Others may provide temporary shelter. In some communes all parents participate in caregiving activities for all children. In many of these groups the combination is fluid; individuals and families are free to come and go as their needs dictate.

Family Unit. Despite the difficulty of defining the family precisely, members of a family can readily describe its composition, who is kin and who is not, how the family has affected their lives, and what family style they believe in.

However the family is defined, the *family unit* is incomplete without an adult. From an adult's perspective the family can be composed of persons of any age or sex bound by a blood or love relationship. From the child's perspective, the family is a set of relationships between the child's dependent self and one or more protective adults.

Regardless of the form it assumes or the society in which it is found, the family possesses enduring characteristics that have far-reaching personal and societal effects. According to Blehar (1979):

> Despite disagreement about the state of the family and its definition, a consensus might be reached on three points: (1) the family is currently in a state of flux precipitated by economic and social pressures; (2) imperfect though it may be, it is difficult to imagine substituting an alternative that could perform all its functions as well; and (3) it is more desirable to bolster families than to attempt to supplant them with untried structures.

What then are the functions that families must perform, and how can nurses best bolster families facing economic and social pressures?

❑ FAMILY FUNCTIONS

As the family progresses through its life cycle (see Table 2-1) from young adulthood to the commitment of two people to share a life and ending with the dissolution of the family through death or other separations, it carries out certain functions for the well-being of its members. The **family functions** extend over five basic areas: biologic, economic, educational, psychologic, and sociocultural (WHO, 1978). The interdependent functions depend on the physical and mental health of family members. As a supportive structure for these functions, each family develops certain common *beliefs, values,* and *sentiments* that are used as criteria in the choice of alternative actions.

Biologic functions include reproduction, care and rearing of children, nutrition, maintenance of health, and recreation. The ability to carry out such functions implies certain prerequisites: a healthy genetic inheritance, fertility management, care during the maternity cycle, good dietary behavior, intelligent use of health services, companionship, and nurturing of its members.

Economic functions include earning enough money to carry out the other functions, determining the allocation of resources, and ensuring the financial security of family members. To accomplish these tasks, the family must have the necessary skills, opportunities, and knowledge.

Educational functions include the teaching of skills, attitudes, and knowledge relating to the other functions. To be able to do this, family members must have knowledge, skills, and experience.

The family is expected to provide an environment that promotes the natural development of personality, offers optimum psychologic protection, and promotes the ability to form relationships with people outside the family circle. These tasks require stable emotional health, common bonds of affection between individuals, and the ability to be mutually supportive, to tolerate stress, and to cope with crises.

Sociocultural functions are associated with the socialization of children. The socialization of children includes the transfer of values relating to behavior, tradition, language, religion, and prevailing or previous social mores. It results in the conditioning of family members to a variety of behavior norms appropriate to all stages of adult life. To be able to do this, the family must possess accepted standards and be sensitive to the varying social needs of children according to their ages. It must also accept and exemplify behavioral norms and be willing to explain, defend, and promote them. Although certain functions are relegated to or emphasized more in one phase of the family's life cycle than another (e.g., the care and socialization of children are part of the childbearing and child-rearing phase of the cycle), many of the functions are continuous for the survival and progress of the family.

❑ FAMILY DYNAMICS

Families work cooperatively to accomplish family functions. Through **family dynamics,** family members assume appropriate social roles. Social roles are learned in the family, the first social group, and are learned in pairs (e.g., mother-father, parent-child, and brother-sister). A social role does not exist by itself but is designed to mesh with that of a role partner. Pairing of roles enables social interactions to take place in an orderly, predictable manner—the roles are said to be complementary. Some families maintain a traditional pairing of roles, whereas other families have changed the behavior patterns to suit a change in family lifestyle. The process by which paired roles are brought into a new alignment is known as *negotiation.* Negotiation is essential if family equilibrium is to be maintained. Negotiation occurs among family members, as well as among outsiders.

From the time it is formed, the family sets up *boundaries* between itself and the outside. People are extremely conscious of those considered members of their family and those who rank as outsiders—those who do not have kinship status. Some families isolate themselves from the outside community. Others have a wide community network to help in times of stress. Although boundaries exist for every family, family members set up *channels* through which they mediate external forces and attempt to protect the family from disturbances. The channels also ensure that the family receives its share of social resources.

Ideally the family uses its resources to provide a safe, intimate environment for the biopsychosocial development of children and its adult members. The family provides for the *nurturing* of the newborn and the gradual *socialization* of the growing child. It is the source of first relationships with others. The relationships children form with parents (or parenting persons) are the earliest and closest and persist throughout a lifetime. For better or worse, parent-child relationships influence a person's concepts of self-worth and ability to form later relationships. The family also interprets and mediates the child's perceptions of the complex outside world. The family provides the growing child with an identity that possesses both a past and a sense of the future. The family transmits cultural values and rituals from one generation to the next (Friedman, 1986).

Through everyday interactions the family develops and uses its own patterns of verbal and nonverbal *communication.* These patterns give insight into the feeling exchange within a family and act as reliable indicators of interpersonal functioning. Family members not only react to the communication or actions of other family members but also interpret and define them.

Over time the family develops protocols for *problem solving,* particularly regarding decisions deemed important to the family, such as having a baby, buying a house, or sending children to college. The criteria used in making decisions are based on *family values* and *attitudes* concerning the appropriateness of the behavior of its various members and the moral, social, political, and economic events of the wider social system. The *power* to make critical decisions is conferred on a family member through tradition or negotiation. This power may be overt or covert and reflects the family's concepts of male or female dominance and cultural practices, social customs, and community norms. As a result family members are positioned into certain *statuses* or *hierarchies* and play out these statuses by assuming various *roles*. Most families have a member who "takes charge" or "is supportive" or "can't be expected to do anything."

❑ FAMILY THEORIES

Many academic disciplines have studied the family and have developed theories that provide differing perspectives for assessing it. Knowledge of these theories provides the nurse with guides to understanding family functioning and dynamics. They provide a basis for planning the day-to-day care of families and help predict certain future events that may necessitate a modification of care. A brief discussion of three **family theories** (structural-functional, developmental, and interactional) is presented here.

Structural-functional Theory

The **structural-functional theory** originated with the work of social anthropologists Malinowski (1945) and Radcliffe-Brown (1952), who documented the interrelatedness and interdependence of the national social system and all subsocial systems. According to this theory the family is a social system with components (family members) with specific roles and role behaviors, such as the father role or the mother role. Family dynamics are directed toward maintaining *equilibrium* between complementary roles to permit family functioning within the family unit and in relation to society. Family structure is culturally determined. The United States represents a pluralistic culture in which varying family forms are recognized and accepted in differing degrees. Classification of families according to their structure provides insight into stresses that families may experience as they differ from the normative structures supported by the society.

Implications for Maternity Nursing. The structural-functional approach allows the nurse to examine relationships between the family and other social systems. According to Friedman (1986):

> The structural-functional perspective is a very useful framework for assessing family life because it enables the family system to be examined holistically (as a unit), in parts (as subsystems or dimensions), and interactionally (as a system interacting with other institutions, such as the educational and health system, the family's reference group[s], and the wider society).

Insights gained from the structural-functional approach can help the nurse become aware of family relationships. First the nurse can recognize the family's *relationship to the larger social system*. Some families establish rigid boundaries, outsiders are kept at a distance, and input from the community is curtailed. Other families are isolated, and when crisis strikes, they often find their inner resources inadequate as coping mechanisms. A third group of families maintains open boundaries through work, school, or community involvement. Energy can flow in both directions, and assistance often is given and accepted.

Second, noting the *internal relationships* of the family may reveal sources of strength or weakness. Commonly the socially conceptualized roles, such as husband and wife, may not fit reality. Hence people establishing or attempting to maintain the so-called normal family roles often face frustration. The interplay of traditionally designed complementary roles may be a source of role conflict. In many families today the husband's and wife's roles are interchangeable; that is, the wife assumes some instrumental functions (earning an income) and the husband assumes some expressive functions (caring for an infant). The ability to negotiate such exchanges is necessary to maintain equilibrium.

Third, the nurse needs to be aware of the development of *reciprocal relationships* within a family that can stunt a person's growth. Some families mold a family member to act as scapegoat; others designate a member to be forever dependent. As an example of the latter, the child born prematurely may always be treated as a sick child.

The major drawback of the structural-functional theory is that its rigid adherence to roles and associated tasks requires a constant updating of the tasks assigned. In addition, this approach tends to "freeze the family in time," minimizing the importance of growth, change, and disequilibrium.

Developmental Theory

The **developmental theory** approach to the study of the family incorporates ideas from a number of theoretical and conceptual approaches to the study of society and the individual (social systems approach, structural-functional approach, life cycle concepts of developmental needs and tasks, and concepts of interacting personalities). Familiar proponents of the life cycle concept are Duvall (1977), Wright and Leahey (1984), and Carter and McGoldrick (1988). The central theme in the developmental theory is noting "the changes in the process of internal development with the dimensions of time as central" (Bower and Jacobson, 1978). The family is described as a *small group, semiclosed* system that engages in interactive behavior within the larger cultural social system. The significant unit in this theory is the *person* rather than the role. The family process is one of *interaction* over the *life cycle* of the family.

Family members pass through phases of growth, from dependence through active independence to interdependence. The family also demonstrates variations in structure and function over time. Together these constitute the *family life cycle*. Stages and tasks of the family life cycle as outlined by Carter and McGoldrick are found in Table 2-1.

Mercer (1989) summarizes the essence of the developmental approach in family nursing:

> Developmental concepts include movement to a higher level of functioning. This implies continuous, unidirectional progression. However, during transitional periods from one stage or phase to the next, disequilibrium occurs, during which time the individual may revert to an earlier level of developmental responses. Families face normative and unexpected transitions that also create a period of disorganization, during which the family functions at a lower level than usual. Resolution of the disequilibrium or crisis has potential to lead to a higher level of family functioning.

Implications for Maternity Nursing. The developmental theory has provided many useful insights into family functioning. Knowledge of types of problems, identified during certain phases of the life cycle, can assist nurses in providing anticipatory guidance for families. For example, helping childbearing families prepare for the birth of a newborn may minimize the development of crisis situations.

Because the family as a group and the family as individuals are simultaneously engaged in developmental tasks (Duvall, 1977; Erikson, 1968), disharmony (dissonance) is possible if the developmental task of the family is not synchronous with the developmental task of the person. There are many examples of such dissonance. The adolescent father grappling with his need to break from his family ties is expected to establish monetary and other support for the new family he has created. A toddler learning socially acceptable behaviors who is introduced to a new sibling may revert to more infantile behavior. Awareness of the implications of situations such as these can be useful in helping the family develop appropriate coping mechanisms.

The developmental approach presents a concept of

Table 2-1 Stages of the Family Life Cycle

Family Life Cycle Stage	Emotional Process of Transition: Key Principles	Second-Order Changes in Family Status Required to Proceed Developmentally
Leaving home: single young adults	Accepting emotional and financial responsibility for self	Differentiation of self in relation to family of origin Development of intimate peer relationships Establishment of self re work and financial independence
The joining of families through marriage: the new couple	Commitment to new system	Formation of marital system Realignment of relationships with extended families and friends to include spouse
Families with young children	Accepting new members into the system	Adjusting marital system to make space for child(ren) Joining in child-rearing, financial, and household tasks Realignment of relationships with extended family to include parenting and grandparenting roles
Families with adolescents	Increasing flexibility of family boundaries to include children's independence and grandparents' frailties	Shifting of parent child relationships to permit adolescent to move in and out of system Refocus on midlife marital and career issues Beginning shift toward joint caring for older generation
Launching children and moving on	Accepting a multitude of exits from and entries into the family system	Renegotiation of marital system as a dyad Development of adult-to-adult relationships between grown children and their parents Realignment of relationships to include in-laws and grandchildren Dealing with disabilities and death of parents (grandparents)
Families in later life	Accepting the shifting of generational roles	Maintaining own and/or couple functioning and interests in face of physiologic decline; exploration of new familial and social role options Support for a more central role of middle generation Making room in the system for the wisdom and experience of the elderly, supporting the older generation without overfunctioning for them Dealing with loss of spouse, siblings, and other peers and preparation for own death; life review and integration

From Carter B and McGoldrick M: The changing family life cycle: a framework for family therapy, ed 2, New York, 1988, Gardner Press, Inc.

family that is fluid and changing and thus more in tune with reality. It is less difficult to plot the phases of the life cycle in the nuclear family than in an extended family. The extended family may involve many generations. Sometimes it is difficult to document the life cycle of a family; often we can only catch glimpses of it. It changes or disintegrates before we can grasp its significance.

Interactional Theory

Burgess (1926) first postulated the idea that the family could be perceived within an interactional framework. Mead (1934) presented the first concepts; Hills and Hansen (1960), Rose (1962), and Stryker (1959) made later additions.

The major theme of the **interactional theory,** also known as action theory or role theory, conceives of the family as a *unit of interacting personalities,* not bound necessarily by legal or contractural agreements, that exists as long as the interaction is taking place. The significant unit is *the individual.* The family process is one of *role taking.* This process is dynamic: family members are constantly testing the concept they have of the role of another and adjusting their own self-concept. The process is accomplished through *symbolic communication,* and all family behaviors stem from family members playing their many roles.

Implications for Maternity Nursing. The interactional theory is particularly useful as a basis for nurse-family interactions. It is broad enough and inclusive enough to encompass various insights into human nature. It transcends family configuration and cultural, ethnic, or social class boundaries of families, such as nuclear family or extended family, and emphasizes *communication* as a central process (Schvaneveldt, 1966). It helps the nurse understand how family members relate to one another. For example, the communication or interaction between mother and child on issues of discipline can give the nurse insight about the family's functioning. The interactional approach to working with families does have some limitations, however. For example, it does not consider the consequences of family-environment influence and interaction. Friedman (1986) asserts "Since the family actively and constantly interacts with its environment, that family-environmental interface must be included in an assessment if comprehensive family nursing care is to be provided."

All three of the theories presented here provide the nurse with a useful view of the family. Nurses use the knowledge from family theories to assist in establishing working relationships with families. When nurses question "who is doing what work," they are using knowledge from the structural-functional theory. When they ask about the significance of events such as birth, children leaving home, or death, they are using family developmental approach. When they assess the effect the birth of a child may have on a husband-wife relationship, they are using interactional family theory.

All three theories offer the maternity nurse a basis for understanding the family unit and an approach for using the nursing process to promote family health among childbearing families.

❑ KEY FACTORS IN FAMILY HEALTH

Certain factors have proved important in determining the quality of family health. For example, family dynamics (previously discussed on p. 19) encompasses coordination of intrafamilial roles, distribution of power in the family, and the process of decision making. It also affects the use of health services.

Family socioeconomic characteristics are important. Social class affects expectations, obligations, and rewards, all of which affect use of health services. In addition, the family acts as the primary economic unit in which incomes may be pooled, expenditure decisions made jointly, and services rendered internally.

Friedman (1986) considers a family's social class as a prime molder of family life-style. Social class, she says, along with cultural background:

> . . . Exerts the greatest overall influence on family life, influencing our early socialization, the role expectations we hold, the values we stress, the types of behavior we consider acceptable or deviant, or the world experiences we have.

❑ CULTURAL CONTEXT OF THE FAMILY

The family process in its **cultural context** is a central concern in nursing. The reproductive beliefs and practices of a culture are embedded in its economic, religious, kinship, and political structures. Concepts focus on four components of a cultural system: (1) the moral and value system, (2) the kinship system, (3) the knowledge and belief system, and (4) the ceremonial and ritual system. Because of cultural pluralism in North America and the rapid expansion of international nursing, nurses are becoming increasingly aware of the need to focus on cultural variations in perceptions of life events and use of health care systems. Clients have a right to expect that their cultural needs relative to health care will be met, as well as their physiologic and psychologic needs. Newton (1972) suggested that health professionals distinguish between health practices based on necessity and those based on social custom. Those social customs need to be maintained and supported that help comfort or make more meaningful the reproductive events that occur to women and their families.

Culture has many definitions. Spradley (1981) defines culture as the "acquired knowledge people use to interpret experience and generate behavior." Each cultural group passes this knowledge to its members from generation to generation. Cultural knowledge includes beliefs and values about each facet of life from birth to death. A person's worldview results from one's cultural knowledge and provides rules for interaction with others, with nature, and with the supernatural (Powers, 1982). These rules have been tested over time and relate to food, language, religion, art, health and healing practices, kinship relationships, and all other systems of behavior. Within each culture may be found many subcultures.

Subculture refers to a group existing within a larger cultural system that retains its own characteristics; individuals identify themselves as members of the group. A subculture may be an ethnic group or a group organized in other ways. For example, there is a subculture of nursing and a subculture of medicine.

Each subculture has rich and complex traditions, including health practices that have proven effective over time. These traditions vary from group to group. In a pluralistic society, these traditions and practices are subject to the influences from many groups. As cultural groups become associated with each other, the processes of acculturation and assimilation may occur.

Acculturation refers to changes that take place in one or both groups when people from different cultures come in contact with one another. People may retain some of their own culture and also reformulate cultural elements. This familiarization among cultural groups results in much overt behavioral similarity. Individuals exchange and adopt mannerisms, styles, and practices of the other group. Changes are evident when one observes such things as dress, language patterns, food choices, and health practices among cultural groups within the society. An example of acculturation would be the adoption of food practices of ethnic groups in the United States. For example, the original recipe for pizza, which is of Italian origin, has been accepted and adopted by many other groups.

Assimilation, on the other hand, occurs when a cultural group loses its identity and becomes a part of the dominant culture. According to Friedman (1986), "Assimilation denotes the more complete and one-way process of one culture being absorbed into the other." Assimilation is the process by which groups "melt" into the mainstream, thus accounting for the notion of a "melting pot," a phenomenon that has been said to occur in the United States. Spector (1979), however, asserts that in the United States, the "melting pot," with its dream of a common culture "has proved to be a myth and faded; it is now time to identify and both accept and appreciate the differences among people."

Nurses must recognize that a wide range of cultural diversity may exist within a society. Assessment of the beliefs and practices of a group and those within the group is essential for the health care provider striving to provide culturally sensitive health care. The nurse must also be aware of factors that may prevent some individuals from providing this optimum care. Understanding the concepts of ethnocentrism and cultural relativism may be helpful to nurses caring for families in a pluralistic society.

Ethnocentrism is "being centered in one's own ethnic or cultural system, judging the world in general by the standards established in that particular system" (Downs, 1971). Essentially it supports the notion that "my group is the best." Socialization into the profession of nursing occurs within the framework of the Western health care system. This system emphasizes the biomedical model, which in the United States is based primarily on the white, middle-class value system. The biomedical model presents pregnancy and childbirth as phenomena with inherent risks, most appropriately managed through specific knowledge and technology. The nurse encountering behavior in women incongruent with this model may become perplexed and label the women's behavior inappropriate and in conflict with good health practices. If the Western health care system provides the only standards for judging, the behavior of the nurse is termed *ethnocentric.*

Cultural relativism, the opposite of ethnocentrism, involves learning about and applying the standards of another person's culture to activities within that culture. To be culturally relativistic means the nurse recognizes that people from different cultural backgrounds actually see the same objects and situations differently. There are reasons why people behave the way they do, and these reasons are for the most part culturally determined.

Cultural relativism does not require nurses to accept the beliefs and values of another culture; rather, nurses recognize that the behavior of others may be based on a system of logic different from their own. Cultural relativism is an affirmation of the uniqueness and value of every culture. Spector (1979) sees this as mandatory for health professionals. Spector states that ". . . because health care providers learn from their culture the way and the how of being healthy or ill, it behooves them to treat each client with deference to his own cultural background."

Table 2-2 Cultural Beliefs and Practices: Childbearing and Parenting

Pregnancy	Childbirth	Parenting
MEXICAN-AMERICAN (Kay, 1978) Pregnancy desired soon after marriage Expectant mother influenced strongly by mother or mother-in-law Cool air in motion considered dangerous during pregnancy Unsatisfied food cravings thought to cause a birthmark Some pica observed in the eating of ashes or dirt (not common) Milk avoided because it causes large babies and difficult deliveries Many predictions about the sex of the baby May be unacceptable and frightening to have pelvic examination by male doctor Use of herbs to treat common complaints of pregnancy Drinking chamomile tea thought to assure effective labor	**Labor** Use of "partera" or lay midwife preferred in some places After delivery of baby, mother's legs brought together to prevent air from entering uterus **Postpartum** Diet may be restricted after delivery, for first 2 days only boiled milk and toasted tortillas permitted Bed rest for 3 days after delivery Mother's head and feet protected from cold air—bathing permitted after 14 days Mother often cared for by her own mother Forty-day restriction on sexual intercourse	**Newborn** Breastfeeding begun after the 3rd day; colostrum may be considered "filthy" Olive oil or castor oil given to stimulate the passage of meconium Male infant not circumcised Female infant's ears pierced Belly band used to prevent umbilical hernia Religious medal worn by mother during pregnancy; placed around infant's neck Infant protected from the "evil eye" Various remedies used to treat "Mal ojo" and fallen fontanel (depressed fontanel)
BLACK (Carrington, 1978) Acceptance of pregnancy depends on economic status Pregnancy thought to be state of "wellness," which is often the reason for delay in seeking prenatal care, especially by lower income blacks Old wives tales include having your picture taken during pregnancy will cause stillbirth; reaching up will cause the cord to strangle the baby Craving of certain foods including chicken, greens, clay, starch, dirt	**Labor** Use of "Granny midwife" in certain parts of the country Stoic behavior exhibited to avoid calling attention to selves Mother may arrive at hospital in far-advanced labor Emotional support often provided by other women, especially own mother **Postpartum** Vaginal bleeding seen as sign of sickness; tub baths and shampooing of hair prohibited Sassafras tea thought to have healing power Liver thought to cause heavier vaginal bleeding because of its high "blood" content Pregnancy may be viewed by black men as a sign of their virility Self-treatment for various discomforts of pregnancy including constipation, nausea, vomiting, headache, and heartburn	**Newborn** Feeding very important: "Good" baby thought to eat well Early introduction of solid foods May breastfeed or bottle feed; breast-feeding may be considered embarrassing Parents fearful of spoiling baby Commonly call baby by nicknames May use excessive clothing to keep baby warm Belly band used to prevent umbilical hernia Abundant use of oil on baby's scalp and skin Strong feeling of family, community, and religion

Table 2-2 Cultural Beliefs and Practices: Childbearing and Parenting—cont'd

Pregnancy	Childbirth	Parenting
ASIAN (Chung, 1977) Pregnancy considered time when mother "has happiness in her body" Pregnancy seen as natural process Strong preference for female physician Belief in theory of hot and cold May omit soy sauce in diet to prevent dark-skinned baby Prefer soup made with ginseng root as general strength tonic Milk is usually excluded from diet because it causes stomach distress	**Labor** Mother attended by other women Father does not actively participate **Postpartum** Must protect self from Yin (cold forces) for 30 days Ambulation limited Shower prohibited Chinese mother avoids fruits and vegetables Diet Some clients are vegetarians Korean mother is served seaweed soup with rice Chinese diet high in hot foods	Concept of the family is important and valued Father is head of the household; wife plays a subordinate role The birth of a boy is preferred

Modified from Williams RP: Issues in women's health care. In Johnson BS, editor: Psychiatric mental health nursing: adaptation and growth, Philadelphia, 1989, JB Lippincott Co.

Childbearing in Various Cultures

Childbearing is one facet of health that is related to all aspects of a woman's life. Although most cultures do not regard pregnancy or childbirth as an illness, both conditions are considered times of heightened susceptibility to dangerous elements. Stern et al (1980) noted that "pregnant women seek security measures and court benevolent gods with ritualized behavior, whether anointing their abdomens with herbal oils in an African village or practicing daily yoga in California." Perception of the time of greatest vulnerability varies among cultures, with some groups placing greatest emphasis on the prenatal stage and others on labor and delivery or the puerperium. Western health care culture places the greatest emphasis on the prenatal and labor and delivery stages and least on the postpartum stage.

Childbearing in all cultures is complete with norms and behavioral expectations for each stage of the perinatal cycle. All relate to each culture's view of how a person maintains health and prevents illness. Health practices reflect theories of balance and harmony among opposing forces. The intrinsic factors influencing balance and harmony include heat and cold. The extrinsic factors include air and water, food and drink, sleep and wakefulness, movement, exercise and rest, evacuation and retention, and passions of the spirits, or emotions. Thus for pregnant women of many cultures, maintenance of health during childbearing implies a balance and harmony in each woman's relationship to her physical, social, and spiritual environment.

Beliefs and Practices. Nurses working with childbearing families in the United States and Canada care for families from various cultures and ethnic groups. To provide a high level of care to all families, the nurse should be aware of the cultural beliefs and practices that are important to these families. There are countless beliefs and practices that are of either a religious or ethnic derivation and may or may not still be followed by families from diverse cultural backgrounds.

Table 2-2 provides examples of some cultural beliefs and practices surrounding childbearing that may be important to Mexican-Americans, Asians, and blacks. Most of these cultural beliefs and customs are reflective of the traditional culture and are not universally practiced by all members of the cultural group in all parts of the country. Variables such as degree of acculturation, educational and income levels, and amount of contact with the older generations influence the extent to which these customs are practiced. Women from these cultural-ethnic groups may adhere to some, all, or none of the practices listed.

It is important that the nurse become familiar with the woman as an individual and validate which, if any, cultural beliefs are meaningful to her. Equipped with this knowledge, the nurse supports and nurtures those beliefs that promote physical or emotional adaptation. However, if certain beliefs are identified that might be harmful, the nurse should carefully explore those beliefs with the client and use them in the reeducation and modification process.

FAMILY AND CRISIS

We live in a stressful society. For the family system, stress can arise internally or externally. Although many families cope with stress, the situation may become acute and take on the characteristics of a crisis. Crisis may be defined as a disturbance of habit: a disruption in a family's or an individual's usual means of maintaining control over a situation. If faced with a crisis, the family or person attempts to resolve it using customary values and behaviors. If the family's usual behaviors are inadequate to resolve the crisis, new behavior patterns must be developed through crisis intervention.

One of the goals of crisis intervention is to help the client learn new ways of dealing with conflicts or problems. Although the client may seek help for a specific problem, the strategies learned may be applied to future difficulties. Crises can be centered around maturational or situational events.

The experience of childbearing is accompanied by both maturational and situational events that make it a significant turning point in the life of a family. Indeed, childbearing is often considered a time of crisis. Maternity nurses who understand crisis theory can readily assist those families who are unable to cope with the stress of these events.

Maturational Crisis

Maturational crises develop as a result of normal growth and development. They characteristically evolve over time and involve *role* and *status* changes. They include events such as birth, infancy, childhood, adolescence, adulthood, and old age. Each phase of the family life cycle produces characteristic crises or events capable of creating stress of such severity that it can affect the health of one or more family members.

The birth of a child represents one of the most important events in the life of a family. Births and the subsequent care of the children require parental, intellectual, and psychologic maturity, and this may account for periods of crisis in a family.

Nurses assist with the birth of children and can provide support as the adults undertake active parenting roles. Nurses can provide knowledge of human psychosocial development, which will help parents both see their children realistically and establish appropriate criteria for children's behavior. Nurses may use this unique relationship with a family to promote birth as a family-centered happening with great potential for growth for all participants.

Situational Crisis

Situational crises include such events as preterm birth, mental or physical illness, loss of financial or social support, changed body image, experience of violence or serious illness, divorce, death, and grief. These crises involve a threat to a person's sense of integrity, or an actual or potential loss or deprivation of some kind. Anxiety and depression are characteristic responses. If the situational crisis causes severe strain, it can result in impairment of health.

Response to Crisis

In both maturational and situational crises, the family plays a critical role in the alleviation of distress, successful adaptation, and healthy rehabilitation. The nurse's knowledge of a family's reactions to crisis prompts a more rational assessment of the family's ability to withstand the stress. The nurse can help the family mobilize its problem-solving abilities to deal with the problem (Chapter 1).

Aguilera and Messick (1990) have devised a stratagem for assessing a family's or an individual's potential or actual response to a crisis. They maintain that three key areas or components act as balancing factors affecting equilibrium: (1) the client's perception of the crisis event, (2) the client's coping mechanisms, and (3) the client's support system. The interplay between these three areas is critical for the outcome or resolution of a problem. A brief discussion of each of the three areas follows.

Perception of Event. What one person considers a crisis may or may not be perceived as a crisis by someone else. Factors such as *age* and *prior experience* can alter perception. For example, an event viewed as a crisis by an adolescent may not be seen as a crisis by a 30-year-old adult. *Emotional states, anxiety,* or *hostility* may color a person's perception. The highly anxious young mother of a firstborn child may become disorganized by her infant's crying, whereas a mother of four may accept the crying as normal.

Nursing intervention relative to a client's perception of a crisis-provoking event may be limited to helping the client state "what the problem is." However, if the event can have a negative effect on the client, the infant, or the family, more intervention is required as indicated in the following example.

In some cultures pregnancy is seen as such a natural event that no medical or nursing supervision is considered necessary. Since complications of pregnancy can arise with detrimental effects for mother and child, the nurse should encourage the family to participate in ongoing health care.

Coping Mechanisms. Coping mechanisms can be defined as patterns of behavior that people or families have developed for dealing with threats to their sense of well-being (Stuart and Sundeen, 1987). Coping mechanisms may be constructive or destructive. *Con-*

structive coping mechanisms lead to a resolution of a problem. They vary with the level of anxiety being experienced. For mild anxiety the individual may resort to crying, sleeping, eating, exercise, or smoking and drinking. In interpersonal situations, avoiding eye contact or limiting close relationships to those who cause no anxiety may be successful.

If the threat and consequent level of anxiety become severe, people will resort to the use of task-oriented reactions or ego-oriented reactions. Task-oriented behaviors are aimed at relieving the stress situations. They are consciously directed and have been objectively appraised by the person using them. Ego-oriented reactions are also known as ego-defense mechanisms. They include repression, projection, and displacement. These reactions protect the person from feelings of inadequacy and worthlessness. However, such responses can be used to the person's detriment. They can distort reality, interfere with interpersonal relationships, and limit working ability. If misused they become *destructive coping mechanisms.*

Nurses use knowledge of human coping mechanisms to assess the type of defense mechanism the person or family uses and the success of the mechanism in ameliorating problems. Attempts are made to substitute more beneficial behaviors, while supporting and reinforcing constructive coping, if the defense is recognized as destructive. However, coping mechanisms, whether constructive or destructive, appear to be essential for all individuals and groups if they are to maintain emotional stability.

Support Systems. **Support systems** refer to the support that people may expect from others in their environment during a time of crisis. Caplan (1959), one of the developers of crisis intervention, maintains that the successful resolution of a crisis often depends on the client's support system. If a client's support system is strong, only minimum intervention may be necessary to resolve a crisis and help the client recover. If the client's support system is not strong, disorganization may occur and the client may not recover without considerable intervention from health care professionals.

A client's support system may include family, friends, and significant others in the environment. Other people who function as part of support systems are health personnel, or "community caretakers" (Caplan, 1959). Community caretakers are people in the various agencies that represent the organized health resources of a community. These individuals are knowledgeable and experienced. They may be able to assist those who are unable to handle crises on their own or with the help of family and friends. Maternity nurses are in an ideal position to offer help throughout the maternity cycle. The assistance may take the form of teaching or counseling, or it may involve helping the client learn the procedures for enlisting the aid of other community agencies. For example, nurses have developed *parent education programs* to provide women and men with mechanisms for coping with the stress of labor. These programs also help parents learn about their infants' needs and about child-care activities, so that the parents are better able to cope with the changing needs of a growing child and to understand the impact of a newborn on the family.

These key factors, family dynamics, socioeconomic status, cultural patterns, and coping responses viewed from a theoretical perspective should all be considered as nurses formulate nursing care plans for the childbearing family.

❑ FAMILY CARE PLAN

Assessment

To plan for the care of a family or particular family member, the nurse must remember that a family operates as a system. That is, no one family member has a problem, if a problem exists, the whole family has a problem. Solutions to problems can evolve best through family participation.

Data Collection Process. The *process* of an assessment in planning family care is often more difficult and complicated than that involved in assessing the physical health of individual clients. It requires adept skill in communication and the ability to establish a trusting relationship with each member of the family simultaneously. In every family group, areas of openness and privacy exist, and all groups resent interrogation by an outsider. The reasons for obtaining information must be explained to family members in a clear manner.

Information such as the address, marital status, and family members' ages can be obtained readily because it is generally given freely. Other information is attained by (1) *observing* and noting relationships, attitudes, and stress responses (who is doing what), (2) *listening* to conversation about community and family involvements or hopes and aspirations, and (3) *being aware* of cultural and socioeconomic factors that might affect the family's behaviors.

As previously discussed, cross-cultural variations in reproductive practices can greatly influence the family's response to childbearing. It is therefore important that the nurse include cultural considerations when assessing families.

The model developed by Stern (1980) for improving communication between individuals and families from a variety of ethnic and cultural backgrounds and Western health care providers can be useful for nurses when doing family assessment. This model identifies barriers in communication that exist on three levels: approach, custom, and language.

Approach includes numerous factors one considers in interpersonal relationships. The American approach to most issues in health care is to address the problem directly. With many cultures (Stern, 1980) engaging in small talk is vital before a serious discussion. Commenting on flowers or pictures and having tea or a cold drink are equated with showing respect. To begin talking to an expectant mother about the need for prenatal care before commenting on the other children, the pretty chair, or the weather might set up an atmosphere of distrust. In some cultures, women prefer a caregiver of the same sex. Therefore it may be critical that the initial encounter be with a woman. Showing respect and patience is essential in building trust.

Custom includes practices and behaviors characteristic of a culture. Understanding that a cultural reason exists for all behaviors and making a sincere effort to ascertain the person's rationale for behavior are important steps in establishing trust. The clients themselves may be the most helpful in helping the nurse understand their cultural logic and individual differences. Assessment of health beliefs and practices is essential for the health care professional who is striving to achieve a holistic approach to care. For the client, adherence to a particular cultural custom provides a sense of constancy with one's cultural heritage.

Language is an important factor. Stern (1980) emphasizes the use of clear, jargon-free English. When the family does not speak English, a bilingual nurse is ideal for assessing the family. If such a nurse is not available, an interpreter, either a family member or a member of the same cultural group, may be used. When an interpreter is being used, it is important to address questions and responses to the client and not to the interpreter.

The following questions illustrate ways to elicit cultural explanations regarding childbearing.

1. What do you and your family think you should do to keep healthy during pregnancy?
2. What are the things you can do or not do to affect your health and the health of your baby?
3. Who do you want with you during your labor?
4. What things or actions are important to you and your family to do after the baby is born?
5. What do you and your family expect from the nurse or nurses caring for you?
6. How will family members participate in your pregnancy, childbirth, and parenting?

A nurse cannot be expected to know all there is to know about every culture and subculture, as well as their many life-styles. Understanding one's own culture is necessary to come to a better realization of why we believe as we do. Understanding clients' cultures, through interview, study, contact, and a demonstrated sincere interest, is invaluable. This understanding enables nurses to render culturally sensitive and relevant nursing care.

Analysis, Synthesis, Validation. Following the data-gathering phase the nurse analyzes and synthesizes the findings. Inferences about the data are formulated. The nurse formulates inferences about the data by asking herself questions, such as, what aspects of family theories are represented by this family: structural-functional, developmental, or interactional? What are the significant stressors influencing this family? Do the family's beliefs reflect myth or old wives' tales? Do these beliefs promote physical or emotional well-being or might they be harmful to the family? Is this family's immediate support system adequate for their coping with potential crises during childbearing? Does family communication respect all family members in light of individual's developmental stage?

Because inferences are subjective and based not only on the nurse's competence level but also on individual values and beliefs, the nurse needs to validate the interpretation of the data with the client. Validation of inferences is followed by the development of nursing diagnoses.

Nursing Diagnoses

Nursing diagnoses are formulated to reflect the family's perception of its needs, as well as the nurse's perception. *It is important to determine the family's perception of its nursing care needs rather than the perception of any one family member.*

Examples of nursing diagnoses (Christensen and Kenney, 1990) commonly encountered with childbearing families include:

Altered parenting related to
- Impaired parent-infant attachment

Altered family processes related to
- Birth of a child with a defect

Anxiety related to
- Expectations of parenting experience

Knowledge deficit related to
- Infant care activities

Social isolation related to
- Lack of interaction with peers

Spiritual distress related to
- Conflict between ideal and personal religious practices associated with childbearing

Once the nursing diagnoses are established, the nurse takes time to explore personal value judgments about the family that may affect and impede nursing interventions. It is also essential for the nurse to validate the diagnoses. In addition to direct validation with the family, a review of the literature, an analysis of norms within a cultural context, and discussion with other persons involved in the family are means of validation.

Planning

The next step is to set goals and outcome criteria related to each diagnosis. These are established as a joint enterprise between nurse and family. They are evaluated for realism and acceptance by family members. Goals for care are both short- and long-term. Once agreed on, the goals are assessed to determine priority. Certain health needs require immediate attention (e.g., unexplained vaginal bleeding). Other health needs require more time to resolve (e.g., anger over birth of a child of undesired sex).

Working with the available data, the nursing diagnoses, and the health goals, the nurse proceeds to organize a plan for implementing the most appropriate interventions. The nurse identifies the nursing role, that is, whether the role is teacher, direct care provider, or referrer.

Teaching must be at a level that is understandable and supportive to individual family members. Different strategies may be necessary for different family members. As a direct care provider, the nurse promotes activities that will lead to the family's own self-care and independence. The nurse plans for the best use of resources available to the family, both internal and community support systems. The nurse must determine whether the resources are appropriate and whether the family is able or willing to use them.

Implementation

The selected nursing actions are implemented; they are preventive, curative, or rehabilitative, and are tailored to the individual needs of the family and its members. Nurses may also use their knowledge and skills in guiding family members who will actually implement the interventions.

Evaluation

Evaluation is a joint process between nurse and family. Mutually determined goals and outcome criteria need to be stated precisely and behaviorally so that the degree to which goals are met can be determined. The criteria need to be realistic and flexible enough to permit modification as circumstances change.

Friedman (1986) suggests six questions that should be asked when evaluating the family nursing process.

1. Were family expectations set in relative and accurate terms?
2. Is there a consensus between the family and other health team members on the evaluation?
3. What additional data need to be collected to evaluate progress?
4. Were the nursing diagnoses, goals, and approaches realistic and accurate?
5. If the family's behavior and perception indicate that the problem has not been satisfactorily resolved, what are the reasons?
6. Were there any unforeseen outcomes that need to be considered?

SUMMARY

The family is the fundamental social unit of every society. It has many functions. One function is to serve as a crucial support system for the individual. Family dynamics are complex. Family theories provide guides to understanding family functioning and its developmental stages and tasks. The family faces and must cope with maturational and situational crises. Families function within a cultural context. All of the components of the nurse and individual client relationship and of the nursing process are utilized when the client-family unit is the focus of care.

LEARNING ACTIVITIES

1. Develop a family care plan for a childbearing family.
2. Select a family whose cultural origins are different from your own. Interview an adult member of the family regarding cultural variations related to childbearing and child-rearing. Pay particular attention to taboos.
3. Select one of the family theories and analyze a childbearing family using the major concepts identified in the theory.

KEY CONCEPTS

- The family forms a social network that acts as a potent support system for its members.
- Ideally, the family provides a safe, intimate environment for the biopsychosocial development of children and its adult members.
- Family theories provide the nurse with useful guides from which to understand family function.
- Sometimes it is difficult to document the life cycle of a family; often we can only catch glimpses of it.
- The reproductive beliefs and practices of a culture are embedded in its economic, religious, kinship, and political structures.
- Differences between the dominant culture of North America and other cultures in general are reflected in how the roles of parents are expressed and how children are viewed.
- North American culture is a pluralistic one in which varying family forms are recognized and accepted in differing degrees.
- In both maturational and situational crises the family plays a critical role in the alleviation of distress, successful adaptation, and healthy rehabilitation.
- Balancing factors affecting equilibrium in a family include the client's perception of the crisis event, the client's coping mechanisms, and the client's support system.

References

Aguilera DC and Messick JM: Crisis intervention: theory and methodology, ed 5, St Louis, 1990, The CV Mosby Co.
Blehar MC: Families and public policy. In Corfman E, editor: Families today, vol 2, National Institute of Mental Health, Division of Scientific and Public Information, Science Monograph No 1, Washington, DC, 1979, US Government Printing Office.
Bower F and Jacobson M: Family theories: frameworks for nursing practice. In Archer S and Fleshman R, editors: Community health nursing: patterns and practice, N Scituate, Mass, 1978, Duxbury Press.
Burgess EW: The family as a unit of interacting personalities, Family 7:3, March, 1926.
Caplan G: Concepts of mental health and consultation, Children's Bureau, US Department of Health, Education and Welfare, Washington, DC, 1959, US Government Printing Office.
Carrington BW: The Afro-American. In Clark AL, editor: Culture/child-bearing/health professionals, Philadelphia, 1978, FA Davis Co.
Carter B and McGoldrick M: The changing family life cycle: a framework for family therapy, ed 2, New York, 1988, Gardner Press, Inc.
Christensen P and Kenney S: Nursing process: application of theories, frameworks, and models, ed 3, St Louis, 1990, The CV Mosby Co.
Chung HQ: Understanding the oriental maternity patient, Nurs Clin North Am 12:67, March, 1977.
Downs JF: Cultures in crisis, Beverly Hills, Calif, 1971, Glencoe Publishing Co.
Duvall ER: Marriage and family development, ed 5, Philadelphia, 1977, JB Lippincott Co.
Erikson EH: Identity: youth and crisis, New York, 1968, WW Norton & Co, Inc.
Evans MI et al: Fetal diagnosis and therapy: science, ethics, and the law, Philadelphia, 1989, JB Lippincott Co.
Friedman MM: Family nursing theory and assessment, New York, 1986, Appleton-Century-Crofts.
Hills R and Hansen D: The identification of conceptual frameworks used in family study, Marriage Fam Living 22:311, 1960.
Kay MA: The Mexican-American. In Clark AL, editor: Culture child-bearing health professionals, Philadelphia, 1978, FA Davis Co.
Libman J: The American ideal is kin through thick and thin, Los Angeles Times, November 20, 1988.
Malinowski B: The dynamics of cultural change, New Haven, Conn, 1945, Yale University Press.
Mead GH: Mind, self and society, Chicago, 1934, University of Chicago Press.
Mercer RT: Theoretical perspective on the family. In Gillis CL et al, editors: Toward a science of family nursing, Menlo Park, Cal, 1989, Addison-Wesley Publishing Co, Inc.
Newton N: Childbearing in broad perspective: pregnancy, birth and the newborn baby, Boston, 1972, Delacorte Press.
Norton A and Glick P: One parent families: a social and economic profile, Fam Relations 35(1):9, 1986.
Powers BA: The use of orthodox and Black-American folk medicine, Adv Nurs Sci 4:35, 1982.
Radcliffe-Brown A: Structure and function in a primitive society, New York, 1952, Free Press.
Rose A: Human behaviors and social processes: an interactional approach, Boston, 1962, Houghton Mifflin Co.
Schvaneveldt J: The international framework in the study of the family. In Nye FA and Bernardo FM, editors: Emerging conceptual frameworks in family analysis, New York, 1966, Macmillan Publishing Co.
Spector RE: Cultural diversity in health and illness, New York, 1979, Appleton-Century-Crofts.
Spradley BW: Community health nursing, Boston, 1981, Little, Brown & Co, Inc.
Stern PN et al: Culturally-induced stress during childbearing: the Filipino-American experience, Issues Health Care Women 2(3-4):67, 1980.
Stryker S: Symbolic interaction as an approach to family research, Marriage Fam Living 21:111, May, 1959.
Stuart GW and Sundeen SJ: Principles and practice of psychiatric nursing, ed 3, St Louis, 1987, The CV Mosby Co.
Williams RP: Issues in Women's Health Care. In Johnson BS, editor: Psychiatric mental health nursing: adaptation and growth, Philadelphia, 1989, JB Lippincott Co.

Wright LM and Leahey M: Nurses and families: a guide to family assessment and intervention, Philadelphia, 1984, FA Davis Co.

World Health Organization: Health and the family: studies in the demography of family life cycles and their health implication, Geneva, 1978, The Organization.

Bibliography

Affonso D: A cognitive framework for cultural diversity: implications for health professionals, International Childbirth Education Association International Symposia, Honolulu, 1988.

Alvarez RR: Familia, Berkeley, Cal, 1987, University of California Press.

Bampton B et al: Initial mothering patterns of low income black primiparas, JOGN Nurs, May, 1981.

Boyle JS: The practice of transcultural nursing, Transcultural Nursing Society Newsletter 7(2):9, 1987.

Doherty W: Family interventions in health care, Fam Relations 34(1):129, 1985.

Griffith S: Childbearing and the concept of culture, JOGN Nurs 11:181, 1982.

Gross C et al: The Vietnamese American family—and grandma makes three, MCN 6:177, May/June, 1981.

Hollingsworth AO et al: The refugees and childbearing: what to expect, RN 43:45, 1980.

Kaptchuk T and Croucher M: The healing arts, New York, 1987, Summit Books.

Kulin J: Childbearing Cambodian refugee women, Can Nurse, p 46, June, 1988.

Lee PA: Health beliefs of pregnant and postpartum Hmong women, Nurs Res 8(1):83, 1986.

Lee RV: Understanding Southeast Asian mothers-to-be, Childbirth Educ 8(3):32, 1989.

Lee RV et al: Southeast Asian folklore about pregnancy and parturition, Obstet Gynecol 71:243, 1988.

Leininger MM, editor: Transcultural nursing care—teaching, practice, research, Salt Lake City, 1980, University of Utah Press.

McGoldrick M: Normal families: an ethnic perspective. In Walsh F, editor: Normal family processes, New York, 1982, The Guilford Press.

McLemore SD: Racial and ethnic relations in America, Boston, 1980, Allyn & Bacon, Inc.

Meleis AI and Sorrell L: Bridging cultures: Arab American women and their birth experiences, MCN 6:171, 1981.

Monroe P, Garand J, and Price S: Family health plan choices: the health maintenance organization option, Fam Relations 34(1):71, 1985.

Muecke M: Caring for the southeast Asian refugee patients in the USA, Am J Public Health 73:431, 1983.

NPA Bulletin: Increasing culturally relevant practice with Hispanic clients 3(4):23, 1988.

Painter MT: With good heart, Vaqui beliefs and ceremonies in Pascua village, Tucson, 1986, The University of Arizona Press.

Perry DS: The umbilical cord: transcultural care and customs, J Nurse Midwife 27(4):25, 1982.

Sklare M: Understanding American Jewry, New Brunswick, Conn, 1982, Center for Modern Jewish Studies, Brandeis University.

Spector RE: Cultural diversity in health and illness, ed 2, New York, 1985, Appleton-Century-Crofts.

Stern PN, Tilden VP, and Maxwell EK: Culturally induced stress during childbearing: the Philipino-American experience, 1985, Hemisphere Publishing Corp.

The Single Parent Family, Special issue of Family Relations, Fam Relations 35:1, Jan, 1982.

Thernstrom S, editor: The Harvard encyclopedia of American ethnic groups, Cambridge, Mass, 1980, Harvard University Press.

Tien JL: Do Asians need less medication? Issues in clinical assessment and psychopharmacology—a nursing perspective, J Psychosoc Nurs Ment Health Serv 22:19, 1984.

Tien JL and Johnson H: Black mental health client's preference for therapists: a new look at an old issue, Int J Soc Psychiatry 31(4):258, 1985.

Torres E: Green medicine, Kingsville, Tex, 1983, Nieves Press.

Unschuld PU: Medicine in China, a history of pharmaceuticsm, Berkeley, 1986, University of California Press.

Zepeda M: Selected maternal infant care practices of Spanish-speaking women, JOGN Nurs 11:371, 1982.

CHAPTER

3 Legal and Ethical Issues

Cheryl Harris and Diane Trace Warlick

Learning Objectives

- Correctly define the key terms listed.
- Identify examples of duty: the standard of care.
- List three ways in which a nurse may commit professional malpractice.
- Describe examples of liability and causation.
- Summarize the independent practice of nursing.
- Assess risk management through practices of prevention and appropriate reporting, and discovery procedures.
- Discuss two purposes for maintaining accurate client records.
- List 10 steps in a bioethical decision-making model.
- Explore ethical dilemmas in relation to in vitro fertilization and embryo transplantation, elective abortion, neonatal intensive care, and AIDS.
- Assess mother surrogates and genetic counseling in relation to legal-ethical issues.

Key Terms

Legal Terms

battery
breach
civil law
discovery and privileged communication
expert witness
incident report
informed consent
liability and causation
malpractice
nurse practice act
professional competency and currency
professional liability insurance
quality assurance
reasonably prudent person
risk management
standard of care
tort

Ethical Terms

beneficence
cost-containment
ethical dilemmas
ethical perspective
ethics committee
nonmalfeasance

Legal Issues

Diane Trace Warlick

The law affects nursing practice in many ways through statutes, regulations, and judicial opinions. The nurse is required by public health laws to administer eye prophylaxis for newborns and to report venereal disease and child abuse cases. Governments apply criminal laws to nurses who violate narcotic and drug statutes or who are accused of being instrumental in a client's death. Regulations are mandatory rules that are developed by boards or agencies established under laws that authorize rulemaking. Boards of nursing are generally established by such laws, which authorize their adoption of regulations to govern the licensure and practice of nursing. The violation of these regulations may subject the nurse to charges by the board of practicing without a license, practicing outside the scope of nursing, or aiding and abetting an unlicensed person to practice nursing. The discussion that follows is concerned with **civil law** that seeks to compensate parties who have been injured or damaged by the negligence of a professional nurse. This body of civil law has been termed the law of torts. A **tort** is a noncriminal offense in which a person seeks monetary compensation from another person for injuries suffered as a result of that person's actions.

❑ MALPRACTICE

Malpractice is a form of negligence that is a part of tort law. When the standard of care is breached and that **breach** is a cause of injury to the client, the nurse may be guilty of professional malpractice. The legal definition of malpractice is "professional misconduct, improper discharge of professional duties, or failure to meet the standard of care of a professional which resulted in harm to another" (Black, 1979). Professional malpractice is a form of negligence. The legal definition of negligence is "carelessness, failure to act as an ordinary, prudent person, or action contrary to what a reasonable person would have done" (Black, 1979). These definitions state the three ways in which a nurse might commit professional malpractice: (1) by performing a duty carelessly or improperly, (2) by failing to perform a duty when it is indicated, or (3) by performing an unauthorized act.

The sequence of events preceding a legal claim for damages caused by negligence is as follows:

1. The state licenses a professional nurse to practice nursing according to the guidelines established by the state nurse practice act.
2. A member of the general public enters into a relationship with a professional nurse in which the nurse offers and delivers health care services.
3. By virtue of the license to practice, the nurse has certain duties and obligations. These duties and obligations are called the standards of care.
4. The nurse fails to fulfill these duties and obligations and breaches a standard of care. The nurse need not *intend* to do harm. Harm may be inflicted unintentionally through negligence.
5. As a direct or indirect but foreseeable result of that breach, an actual injury is sustained. The injury must be actual rather than potential or "at risk for" injury. Actual injury includes both physical and emotional distress. However, in most cases, emotional distress by itself is not enough for a successful lawsuit.
6. The client or client's family may be compensated for the injury by monetary damages assessed against the nurse. "General damages" include monetary compensation for pain and suffering experienced by the injured party. "Special damages" include income lost by absence from work or inability to work and the cost of health care and rehabilitation.

Standard of Care

The **standard of care,** or external code of behavior or expected performance for a professional nurse is defined as the average degree of skill, care, and diligence exercised under similar circumstances by a **reasonably prudent person** with similar background, training, and experience (Black, 1979). Standards are developed by professional organizations and through the recognition by courts of standards based on the opinion of expert witnesses in the same profession.

Major points of the American Nurses' Association, Standards of Maternal-Child Health Nursing are presented in Appendix B.

The Organization for Obstetric, Gynecologic, and Neonatal Nurses (formerly the Nurses' Association of the American College of Obstetrics and Gynecology [NAACOG]) has published standards that are presented as recommendations and general guidelines (NAACOG, 1986). Examples of standards for electronic fetal monitoring appear in Chapter 14.

Standards of care reflect minimum acceptable requirements for performance. To be successful in a lawsuit against a nurse, the plaintiff must first establish the nurse's "duty" or the standard of care that the nurse is expected to follow. The plaintiff must then prove that the nurse's action or inaction in the particular case failed to conform to that standard of care. The standard of care is generally established through expert testimony in malpractice lawsuits. It is enforced by the court system in the form of verdicts in lawsuits or settlements.

To determine the standard of care for professional nursing, the appropriate starting point is the state's **nurse practice act** and the state regulations pertaining to nursing practice. These laws and regulations define the scope of nursing practice, standards for nursing education, and the point of articulation between the profession of nursing and the profession of medicine. To exceed the legal base of nursing practice is, by definition, to violate the standard of care and to be negligent. For instance, if a particular state declares it illegal for the nurse to dispense medications without a physician's order and the professional nurse hands a woman a month's supply of birth control pills, that action is a violation of the standard of care. If there are no written policies or procedures to permit such nursing interventions, the nurse's actions are negligent.

Standards of care are determined by the nursing profession in its definition of nursing practice, policies and protocols for nursing practice, standards of nursing education, and proscription of activities considered outside of nursing. Standards of care are further delineated by nursing specialist organizations and joint boards of medicine and nursing who define appropriate behavior in special and specific circumstances.

Other standards of care established by the profession are the policies and protocols governing nursing practice in a particular agency or unit of an institution. These policies and protocols define behavior expected of all professionals within their domain. They may act to expand behavior expected in a particular situation beyond the customary practice of nursing and into the practice of medicine. For instance, special or standardized procedures may permit a nurse in an intensive care unit to initiate drug therapy if a client displays a particular symptom. They may also permit a nurse to dispense birth control pills under special circumstances where otherwise that behavior would be illegal (Calif. Bus. and Prof. Code).

Professional nurses have a legal obligation to know

and understand the standard of care or duty imposed on them. *Ignorance of a policy or protocol will not be accepted as an excuse for failure to follow it.*

The failure of the agency or institution in which the nurse is employed to update its policies in keeping with recent scientific developments will not protect the individual nurse from liability if client harm results. This is one of the reasons it is critical for nurses to keep current in their specialities.

Some recent cases have established the duty of the nurse to oversee the behavior of other professionals and to report situations in which other professionals' behavior fails to conform with the established standard of care (Cushing, 1985). For instance, when a physician writes an erroneous drug order, the nurse has a duty to report the error and obtain a corrected order (Annas, Glantz, and Katz, 1981). When the client is exposed to danger as a result of action by other professionals, the nurse has a duty to protect that client. That duty extends beyond mere reporting of the incident and requires the nurse to follow up on reporting until the client is returned to safety (Darling, 1965). Labor and delivery room nurses occasionally deal with this situation when they call for physician assistance and fail to get it. They must continue to ask for physician assistance until they do get it. Nurses' responsibilities extend beyond the care of clients directly assigned to them and encompasses the behavior of other professionals functioning in the same area.

Breach: Failure to Conform to Standard of Care

In a court of law, a breach of the standard of care, as with the standard itself, is established by the testimony of expert witnesses, who are commonly leaders in their fields. To qualify as an **expert witness** in a trial, the expert must convince the court that he possesses special knowledge of the subject. Credentials that help establish this "special knowledge" include administrative responsibility, teaching, and research in addition to clinical competence. Based on the testimony about the actual situation or a "hypothetical" situation that is an exact duplicate of the case under consideration, expert witnesses are asked to state whether the behavior of the nurse met or failed to meet the standard of care required under the circumstances. Experts are expected to give the reasons for their opinions and to cite recent professional literature that supports the opinion. Both sides in the case generally have their own expert witnesses in a malpractice case. The judge or jury makes the final determination regarding whether the defendant-nurse in the actual situation had breached the standard of care.

Liability and Causation

Professional nurses are liable for the consequences of their actions. This is called **liability and causation.** The best synonym for *liable* is *responsible.* Nurses are responsible for both the direct and indirect results caused by their actions. If a client falls out of bed as a consequence of the nurse's failure to put up the side rails, the nurse is responsible for the harm to the client directly caused by that failure to act. If the nurse fails to report the improper behavior of another health care professional and a client is injured by that other person, the nurse is responsible for that injury indirectly caused by the failure to act.

Until the last 20 years, courts rarely found nurses to be independently liable for their actions (Fiesta, 1983). Most courts found that nurses acted on the basis of orders given and were not autonomous or independent providers of services. The nurse functioned either as an agent of the physician, in which case the physician assumed all liability, or as an employee of the hospital, in which case the hospital assumed all liability. The legal doctrine that assigns liability for the entity controlling the nurse is *respondeat superior* (Black, 1979). It literally means "let the master answer" and assigns liability for nursing action to the employer of the nurse. This sort of liability of the hospital and physician is called vicarious liability.

Over the past several years, however, a change in the legal perspective of nursing practice has occurred. Increasingly, nurses are viewed as autonomous health care providers who practice independently in certain clearly defined situations. Recent cases have found nurses to be independently liable and did not assign the liability to physicians and hospitals where nurses were acting outside of the direction of physicians and hospitals (Black, 1979).

It is important for the professional nurse to understand the distinction between the dependent practice of nursing, which is the implementation of the physician-directed management of care, and the independent practice of nursing. Based on the California Nurse Practice Act, the California Nurses' Association's definition of the independent practice of nursing is:

1. Direct and indirect client care services that ensure the safety, comfort, personal hygiene, and protection of clients and the performance of disease prevention and restorative measures.
2. The performance of skin tests and immunization techniques and the withdrawal of human blood from veins and arteries.
3. The observation of signs and symptoms, reactions to treatment, and general behavior or physical condition and the determination of whether such observations exhibit abnormal findings and

the appropriate reporting and referral of such abnormalities (Calif. Bus. and Prof. Code).

The independent practice of nursing encompasses those decisions and actions taken by the nurse based on nursing judgment and a nursing management plan rather than on a management plan directed by the physician.

The independent practice of nursing has become the basis for expanding liability for the professional nurse. Whereas cases against professional nurses are still a small percentage of the malpractice lawsuits brought to court, nurses are increasingly being held personally accountable for client injuries resulting from the performance of their duties.

❑ RISK MANAGEMENT AND QUALITY ASSURANCE

In the early 1980s, the American Hospital Association established a task force to define the relationship between hospital risk management and quality assurance. It recognized that there are areas of overlapping function, but also significant differences. The differences and similarities are shown in Table 3-1. The task force concluded that the functions of quality assurance and risk management should be integrated, but that a role remains for both programs in a hospital. The distinctions are discussed in the following sections.

Risk management is a concept adapted from the general insurance industry in response to escalating losses sustained by hospitals, physicians, nurses, and professional liability insurance carriers as a result of malpractice lawsuits. The increased number of malpractice lawsuits and the dramatic rise in the cost of professional liability insurance has been the impetus for the development of hospital programs to control losses. These hospital risk management programs were developed as a means for the prevention of malpractice lawsuits and reduction of associated financial losses. The risk management process seeks to minimize losses by identifying risks, establishing preventive practices, developing reporting mechanisms, identifying potential malpractice claims, and delineating procedures for managing a lawsuit once it has been filed.

The nurse should be familiar with the concepts of risk management and their implications for nursing practice. An effective risk management program requires the active involvement of the nursing staff in a system of checks and balances that ensures a high quality of client care. Risk management procedures minimize the risk of loss by improving the quality of nursing care, thereby reducing the likelihood of client injury. Effective risk management thus minimizes the risk of a lawsuit against the nurse and other health care providers.

Quality assurance is an umbrella term used to encompass those activities that review and evaluate actual client care and institute remedial actions to bring client care into conformity with the standard of care. Quality assurance involves a retrospective search for trends in client care, using tools such as chart review, chart audit, peer review, and performance evaluation. The goal of quality assurance is to establish that all professional conduct meets the applicable standard of care.

Occurrence Criteria

A major tool developed for hospital risk management programs is known as ***occurrence criteria.*** These are criteria designed to detect potential malpractice

Table 3-1 **Comparison of Quality Assurance and Risk Management**

	Quality Assurance	Traditional Risk Management
Purpose	Assure that quality of care provided is optimum—evaluate practitioner performance and protect clients	Minimize the hospital's losses—protect the hospital
Character	Educational/remedial	Crisis intervention
Function	Measure actual care against standards, and where care does not meet standards, take remedial action	Detect risks to the hospital, then prevent their recurrence or minimize their effect when they occur
Clients involved	Single client or group of clients, discharged or still hospitalized—patterns	Single client discharged or still hospitalized—isolated events
Time frame	Retrospective or concurrent with client stay	Concurrent with notice of potential loss
"Standard"	Written explicit clinically-based criteria	Unwritten implicit criteria (what people think is an "incident")

claims on the basis of unexpected outcomes for the particular diagnosis. For example, a postoperative client requiring second surgery; the readmission of a client for the same illness within 3 days of discharge; or an emergency room client's return within 24 hours necessitating admission to the hospital. These occurrences, which would not generally trigger the filing of an incident report, are nevertheless significant occurrences with potential legal implications.

The nursing staff should be actively involved in risk management through the detection and reporting of significant occurrences. The risk management office should promptly undertake chart review to evaluate the individual case and take the necessary follow-up steps. The goal is to identify potential malpractice claims before a lawsuit is filed, carry out a thorough investigation, initiate appropriate remedial measures, and ideally resolve the situation without litigation. The Joint Commission on Accreditation of Health Care Organizations developed risk management standards that became effective in 1989 and included outcome criteria beginning in January 1990.

Informed Consent

The doctrine of **informed consent** invokes elements of both risk management and quality assurance. It developed from the common law recognition of the right of persons to be free from all forms of unconsented touching. Violation of that right is called **battery.** In some states, the informed consent doctrine is established by specific legislation, while in others it is the result of judicial decisions.

There are two distinct legal viewpoints in regard to the requirements for legally valid informed consent. Nurses should be aware of which standard applies in the state in which they practice. In the majority of states, informed consent requires that the client be provided with all information regarding the procedure, its risks, its anticipated results, and any alternative treatments that would be important to the average person in making a decision about whether to undergo the procedure. In the remaining states, the law only requires that the client be given the information about a procedure that is normally given by other practitioners in the same locality. It is the responsibility of the person who will perform the procedure to obtain the informed consent. Informed consent may also be required for the withdrawal or withholding of life-sustaining treatments.

Many health care providers have experienced legal difficulties with respect to the obligation to obtain informed consent (Cushing, 1984). A major problem for providers arises from the need to rely on a client's assertion that she understands the information provided and consents to the procedure to establish informed consent. If at a later date the client denies that she understood, the provider may have to prove that the consent process was adequate. If the only documentation of the informed consent is a short statement on the chart that "informed consent was obtained," the provider may experience great difficulty in establishing that the requisite information was provided.

To reduce the problem concerning informed consent issues, the nurse should be aware of and apply the following rules regarding informed consent.

1. *Responsibility for obtaining informed consent rests with the person performing the procedure and should not be delegated to the nurse.* The nurse may contribute to the education process by providing background information about the procedure or by witnessing the client's signature.

2. *Informed consent should be obtained for all invasive procedures;* including those routinely performed by nurses, such as starting intravenous fluids, and inserting Foley catheters. In these circumstances, it is the nurse's obligation to obtain the informed consent. Although consent is generally presumed from the fact that the client allows the procedure to be performed, and is conscious during the procedure, the nurse should document in the nurses' notes the fact that the procedure, its purpose and potential risks have been explained to the client.

3. *The information provided must be geared to the client's level of understanding.* It must be done in the language and with the words that the client is capable of understanding.

4. *Consent must be obtained from an individual with the capacity to consent.* Minors generally do not have the capacity to consent to medical treatment without parent approval. Clients whose minds are impaired by drugs or injury do not have capacity to consent, since they are incapable of understanding the information and making an informed decision. Special considerations apply if the client is a minor or is mentally incompetent, or if an emergency is in progress.

5. *Blanket consents* ("I consent to everything") *and blanket releases* ("I release everyone from liability") *are traditionally disregarded by the courts.* They are not based on a full disclosure of the information and may be viewed as a means to deceive the client or avoid the disclosure required by the informed consent doctrine.

6. *The consent is only as good as its documentation.* Oral consents are legal and binding, however, they are extremely difficult to prove several years later in the process of a lawsuit. Prudent practitioners now provide complete written information on the intended procedure, its purpose, its risks, and its alternatives to the client and ask the client to acknowledge its receipt by

signing the document. Ideally, clients would also write on the written informed consent document that they understand the information, have had an opportunity to ask questions, and have had the questions answered. A copy of this document should be given to the client, and the original put in the medical record.

7. *Client's refusal of treatment should also be an informed decision.* The nurse should carefully document the potential consequences of refusal of which the client has been informed, and these wishes should thereafter be respected.

Consent to Sterilization or Abortion. Informed consent is obviously required for voluntary sterilization and abortion, as with any invasive procedure. Since the ability to produce children and the decision to terminate a pregnancy are emotionally charged issues that affect both partners in a relationship, many institutions require the consent of both partners before performing either procedure (Rhodes and Miller, 1984). Under certain circumstances, some state laws may also require the consent of both biologic parents before performing an abortion.

Professional Liability Insurance

Professional liability insurance is a risk management tool that allows nurses to protect their assets from potential losses as a result of malpractice claims filed against them. It helps nurses avoid financial losses as a result of a settlement of a lawsuit or a judgment against them based on a finding that their conduct failed to meet accepted standards of care. Liability insurance can also protect nurses against unfounded malpractice claims by paying for the costs and attorneys' fees incurred in being defended against the lawsuit.

Liability insurance is a contract between the nurse and the insurance company in which the nurse agrees to pay a periodic premium and the company agrees to cover the nurse against claims of malpractice. Coverage is limited to a predetermined amount ("ceiling") per claim, whether the case is settled or goes to judgment; and by an aggregate amount per year. The insurance policy should be investigated carefully for the type of coverage, limits of coverage, and exceptions to coverage. For example, some policies do not cover nurses in expanded roles. Others may not cover nurses working in independent practice settings.

Nurses must decide whether to carry their own liability insurance or to rely solely on the protection offered by their employers. There are many factors that should be taken into consideration before making this decision. A commonly used argument against personal coverage is that it adds to the cost of litigation because it involves an additional insurance company who will hire separate legal counsel, which may delay the proceedings. The major argument in favor of separate coverage is to supplement coverage carried by the employer. Personal insurance coverage allows the nurse to obtain independent legal representation. It should also cover the nurse for activities outside the scope of the nurse's employment. It will ensure that the nurse's interests, as well as the interests of the hospital and the physician, are represented. The nurse must be aware that the insurance policy will impose responsibilities on the nurse as a condition of coverage. Conditions of coverage usually include a requirement that any claim be reported to the insurance company promptly. These conditions of coverage must be complied with.

Professional Competency and Currency

Maintaining **professional competency and currency** by keeping up to date on practices and standards of care is a critical factor in risk management and the reduction of potential liability. The standard of care applied by the courts in a malpractice lawsuit presumes that the average health care provider stays informed of, and practices according to, the most current information. The plaintiff's expert witness will rely on recent professional literature that supports a finding of liability and will testify that it establishes the standard of care under the circumstances. The nurse's ignorance about recent developments in the field will not be an acceptable defense. The American Nurses' Association (ANA) Code of Ethics requires that nurses maintain their competence in nursing; and nurses should expect to be held to that standard by a court of law.

As a result of the present nationwide nursing shortage, nurses commonly find themselves in situations in which their professional competency is impeded by external factors. "Short staffing" and "floating" are two common occurrences that impair the nurse's ability to perform in accordance with recognized standards of practice. It is ultimately the hospital's duty to assure that it has sufficient staff to provide acceptable care to all clients in accordance with their needs. It is the nurse's duty, however, to bring staffing problems to the hospital's attention (Horsley, 1981). The professional nurse has a duty to report situations in which the standard of care is compromised by an inadequate number of staff or by a staff that is insufficiently trained to provide the care required by the circumstances. The duty requires nurses to clearly communicate their concerns to a person who has the power to remedy the situation—generally beginning with their immediate supervisors.

A nurse who is "floated" to a specialty unit without orientation or experience in the area has a duty to ask for assistance, supervision, and orientation. If not provided, the nurse may have an obligation to reject the assignment. Nurses' duty not to abandon clients may, however, ultimately conflict with the duty to reject an assignment they do not feel competent to fulfill. In that situation, reporting their concerns to the appropriate person is the nurses' only means of protecting themselves from liability in the event an injury occurs. The following steps should be taken, and documented by the nurse in handling this situation.

1. The nurse must report the potential breach of the standard of care to her supervisor.
2. If the nurse's immediate supervisor is unwilling or unable to remedy the situation, the nurse should request the supervisor to report the problem to the next higher supervisor, or the nurse should do so.
3. If the nurse's rejection of the assignment would place the clients in greater danger from abandonment, the assignment should be completed to the best of the nurse's ability.
4. The nurse should prepare a written report for submission to the risk management office. The report should contain the nurse's concerns and the steps taken to remedy the situation.

Quality of Nurse-Client Relationship

The quality of the nurse-client relationship is the most significant factor in the prevention of financial loss to the nurse or hospital for nursing acts or omissions. It has been clearly documented that clients who feel angry, frustrated, or depersonalized by their health care workers are more likely to sue when an injury occurs (Wecht, 1982). Anger and frustration are common accompaniments to illness and adjustment to the post-illness state, but these feelings can be deflected away from the provider and channeled into a more positive outlet by a supportive nurse-client relationship.

The nurse cannot make clients happy about serious illnesses or less than optimum outcomes. However, the competent, caring nurse possesses the judgment and skill necessary to support a client through illness to recovery, or to enable a client to cope with chronic conditions. The early identification of situations that have upset the client, especially where those feelings are directed toward the staff, will allow intervention designed to redirect or resolve the negative feelings. Involvement of the client in the management plan, special attention to comfort measures, and changes in nursing assignments where indicated may help the client feel less victimized and more in control of the situation.

❑ REPORTING PRACTICES

A major aspect of any risk management program is the appropriate documentation of client care and effective communication of those incidents that may give rise to a malpractice lawsuit. The documentation of client care is accomplished by the complete and accurate charting of occurrences and observations on the client record. The communication of problem situations from the caregiver to the administration is generally handled by filing incident reports. In addition, occurrence reports may be utilized to report unexpected outcomes that may forecast potential liability. It is critical for the nurse to be aware of the differences between the client record, and incident and occurrence reports, as well as to distinguish between their functions.

Incident Reports

The **incident report** documents situations that could result in injury to the client, thereby resulting in liability of the institution or the health care professional. They may be used to report errors or omissions in care, irresponsible professional behavior, accidents, or unexpected outcomes that lead to client injury, disability, or death. The nurse is generally required to submit the report to the supervisor, who in turn forwards it to the hospital or agency administrator and the risk manager. Incident reports are considered confidential communications between the institution's staff and administration. They are generally not considered part of the medical record, but rather an internal tool for the purpose of investigation of the particular situation and ultimately the improvement of the quality of care.

Incident reports were long considered to be immune from mandatory disclosure in malpractice lawsuits as "privileged communications" between the institution's attorney and the institution. The courts have increasingly found that incident reports are not confidential attorney-client communications. They are reviewed by other individuals or committees within the institution's hierarchy. In addition their use is not limited to communication with the institution's legal counsel. For these reasons, recommendations as to the use and content of incident reports are changing.

Risk management principles mandate that incident reports be utilized solely for the reporting of an incident. Incident reports are not for follow-up investigation, evaluation, or determination of the actual cause of or responsibility for the incident. It is preferable to include only the basic objective facts about what occurred, who witnessed the incident, and the results of the follow-up medical examination. The risk management office should conduct the follow-up investigation to determine exactly what occurred and why. The risk manager should promptly interview the client and all witnesses to the incident. If the investigation and subsequent reports by the risk manager are made in contemplation of a potential lawsuit and/or in consultation with the institution's lawyer, they are much more likely to be protected from disclosure in litigation.

Some guidelines for the use of incident reports follow:

1. The report should be written accurately and clearly, and it should include all of the essential facts. Accusations, admissions, and conclusions should be avoided.
2. Nurses should never include opinions as to fault for the incident or speculate about what occurred. For example, the nurse should chart, "client found on floor beside bed; bedrails down; client alert, vital signs. . ." The nurse should not write, "client fell out of bed" unless the fall was actually observed.
3. The nurse should not write "incident report filed" on the client's chart. Lawyers who are unfamiliar with hospital records and procedures may not know to ask to see an incident report unless the client's chart makes reference to one.
4. The report should be submitted to the individual designated by the institution's policy/procedure manual, and no one else. The more copies of the incident report that are distributed, the weaker the assertion that the report is confidential and privileged, and the more likely a court will require its production in discovery.

Charting

The main purposes for keeping client records are (1) to produce a clear and accurate history of the client's illness or medical problem; (2) to document the management plan and its effectiveness, or lack thereof; and (3) to serve as a means of communication between the many health care providers who render services in the specific situation. Charting must therefore be accurate, legible, objective, and comprehensive.

Nurses must be careful to chart only actual observations, rather than subjective opinions or unsupported conclusions. The charting of conclusions that may have a negative impact on the client's character or reputation—such as alcoholism, substance abuse, a violent nature, or mental impairment—may precipitate a legal action if the statements are conveyed to third parties. The charting of such conclusions unsupported by actual observations serves no purpose in a medical record. Conclusions should only be included if they represent a confirmed diagnosis or are properly considered in a differential diagnosis. Instead, the nurse should chart actual behavior observed, which can be relied on to support a subsequent diagnosis. For example, instead of charting that the client "was drunk," the nurse should chart, "the client was unsteady, unable to walk, and had an odor of alcohol on his or her breath." The nurse should also chart supporting laboratory values.

Comprehensiveness

The realities of nursing practice in most facilities rarely afford nurses the opportunity to record their activities and observations immediately on completion of each specific assignment. Whereas immediate charting is desired, delays invariably occur. These delays may contribute to gaps and omissions in charting, resulting in a medical record that is not comprehensive. The following guidelines will assist the nurse in charting more accurately and comprehensively.

1. Nurses can carry notepads to make brief notes that will refresh their memories when charting at a later time.
2. Significant observations or changes in a client's condition should be charted immediately, with the date and exact time being recorded.
3. The nurse must never chart an action, such as the giving of medications, before it is done.
4. Care is taken not to record nursing observations out of sequence. If an omission does occur, however, the nurse should not try to squeeze the note between two other notes in order to put it in the proper sequence. Instead, the note is placed after the last entry and includes a statement of the circumstances accounting for the delay in the charting.
5. When the nurse is too involved with client care to chart each action simultaneously, as in emergency situations, a specific member of the health care team should be designated to record actions and observations as they occur. The charting should include an accurate reporting of times and actions, as well as the identity of the person taking each action.
6. Nurses should always sign their full names and professional titles at the end of each entry on the record.

Errors. A critical issue in the documentation of nursing care is how to handle errors when charting. Some helpful guidelines follow.

To correct an error in charting, the nurse should clearly draw one line through the error, write "error" above it and initial the entry. It is acceptable practice to also include a brief explanation of the error, such as "wrong chart," but only if the individual correcting the error is the individual who made it. An error should never be completely obliterated. The correct entry should be legibly written, dated, and signed following the last entry on the nurses' notes.

The nurse must never change or correct another person's charting. If a note is clearly inaccurate, the nurse should bring it to the attention of the individual who wrote it so that person can make the necessary correction. If the nurse who detects a charting error by another professional has an entry to make on the chart, the nurse should chart only her own observations.

The nurse should never make accusations of error directly in the client chart, such as "Mrs. X charted in error." If the person who made a charting error refuses to correct it, or if the error is a treatment error rather than charting error, the appropriate place to report it would be in an incident report.

Omissions. The omission of essential information from the medical record may result in the information not being communicated to other members of the health care team, thereby compromising the quality of care. In the event of a malpractice lawsuit, the omission may be interpreted to mean that the care was not provided or the observations not made. The client record is the only official written piece of evidence, created at the time of the occurrences in question, that documents the actual facts and circumstances surrounding the client's health care and condition. Because the chart is compiled by health care providers who have a duty to make a complete and accurate record, a lack of comprehensiveness or objectivity in the record implies a failure to meet the standard of care. It is therefore critical for risk management purposes to chart all pertinent observations.

Since malpractice lawsuits are usually not filed until months, or even years, after the events in question, nurses may not be able to recall the details necessary to accurately present a case in court if such details are not recorded in the client chart. In the absence of a well-documented record, health care providers must rely on their recollection of events to support their position. With the passage of time, it is difficult, if not impossible, to remember the details of care provided in any given case. For example, if vital signs are not charted and the client claims that they were not taken, will the nurse remember several years later specifically whether they were taken, and if so, whether they were normal? Furthermore, providers' unsupported statements from the witness stand that the care complied with recognized standards of care tend to sound self-serving and insincere when contested by the word of an injured client. There is simply no substitute for a careful, accurate, and objective medical record.

❑ DISCOVERY AND PRIVILEGED COMMUNICATION

Discovery is a formal part of every civil lawsuit. It was developed by the judicial system to end the former practice of "litigation by surprise." Until the adoption of the discovery process, trial lawyers attempted to keep the opposition from learning its legal position and facts within the knowledge of its witnesses, which resulted in frequent surprises and unfair results at trials.

Discovery is the legally required exchange of information between the plaintiff and the defendant so that each side has a reasonable opportunity to learn the facts about the case before a trial. There are specific rules that must be followed in discovery. Each side is allowed to direct written questions (interrogatories) to the other side and to ask questions of witnesses face-to-face (deposition). The questions must be answered truthfully and under oath, but it is not necessary to volunteer information about which a question has not been asked.

Privileged communications are exempt from the discovery process and need not be disclosed. The attorney-client privilege protects communications between the attorney and his/her client from mandatory disclosure. Communications, investigations, and reports made in contemplation of litigation or at the direction of one's attorney are also privileged. These privileges have been the basis for nondiscovery of incident reports in the past, but as discussed previously, this protection has been lost in many states. The physician-client relationship (and some nurse-client communications) is ordinarily privileged, except when the client puts the relationship at issue in a malpractice lawsuit. In that situation, the client is not allowed to raise a claim of privilege to protect his/her medical records, and all aspects of the relationship are discoverable by the other side. Some helpful guidelines on the discovery process follow.

All unprivileged documents are discoverable, including private journals. If the nurse has kept a private record of the event, she is required to produce it for the other side to review, if requested.

Whereas nurses are generally cautioned not to keep private records of occurrences on the job, it may be the best means for their protection from personal liability in the event of a dispute with the institution, such as short-staffing situations or mandatory floating over the nurse's objection. It is important, however, that these situations be reported to the administration via incident reports to allow the institution to correct policies that may be harmful to the clients' well-being.

Communication with the client, the client's attorney, and the client's investigators should take place in the presence of the institution's lawyer or the nurse's legal counsel, and with their prior knowledge and consent.

Conversations are discoverable in the same manner as written documents. The opposing side is entitled to ask witnesses about the content of conversations about the event in question. No outside discussion of the event should occur except in the presence of the attorney for the nurse or institution. This prohibition includes discussions with nursing colleagues, the nurse's family members, and particularly the client, the client's family, or attorney.

Discussions of the event within the context of quality assurance, risk management, or peer review proceedings may be privileged from discovery under certain circumstances in some states. Before participating in these proceedings, however, the nurse should check with her attorney to determine whether and under what circumstances the privilege may apply.

Nurses should be aware of their rights to hire their own attorneys to protect their interests in the event of a malpractice suit against them personally or as an employee of the institution that has been sued. When nurses carry their own liability insurance coverage, the insurance company should provide separate legal counsel to protect their interests. Although the hospital has an obligation to defend an employee from claims of malpractice arising in the course of employment, there are situations in which the institution's interests are in conflict with the nurse's interests. A conflict occurs when the institution's defense and the nurse's defense are incompatible. In conflict or potential conflict situations, the nurse should always have separate legal representation.

If a nurse who has not been sued directly in a malpractice case against the employer has received an official request (subpoena) for information from the plaintiff-client, the nurse is required to cooperate fully and comply with the request in good faith. Before responding, however, the nurse should have her attorney (and/or the institution's) review the request and any proposed response. There are legal grounds that may be applicable for objecting to subpoenas. A determination whether a basis for not responding exists in a particular case must obviously be made before the response is given.

Ethical Issues

Cheryl Harris

Ethical dilemmas occur in every field of nursing practice; perinatal nursing is not immune. Technical advances in the medical field have proceeded at a breakneck pace, often outstripping society's ability to consider the ethical implications of these new techniques. Fetal experimentation, neonatal intensive care, amniocentesis resulting in a recommendation for abortion, genetic engineering, and the humane treatment of persons with AIDS are just a few areas in which nurses must determine an ethical stance. For this reason, it is important for nurses to develop a rational, systematic, well-considered **ethical perspective** with which to analyze these ethical questions.

Flanagin (1988) describes the case of a 27-year-old woman from Washington, D.C. who was 26 weeks into pregnancy and terminally ill with cancer. A court ordered that a cesarean delivery be done to save the baby. The infant girl was delivered alive, but died after a few hours. The mother died 2 days later. Flanagin is disturbed to note that although attorneys and physicians were involved in the decision-making process, nurses were not. She asserts that nurses must become more involved in ethical decision making in order to inject the nurse's unique perspective into resolving these difficult questions. Approximately 60% of hospitals now have an **ethics committee.** Weeks (1987) agrees that it is crucial for nurses to become involved as representatives to such committees to help resolve these profound issues. This section will not address all of the ethical decisions a nurse must make, but it should help nursing students develop this aspect of their practice.

❑ ETHICAL DECISION MAKING

During their early years, nurses begin to form their ethical and moral values within their own family structure and through religious affiliations. Nurses have responsibilities and commitments to use ethical conduct in relationships with clients, other nurses, physicians, and their employing institution (Curtin, 1982). Inherent in the values of most nurses are **beneficence** (the practice of doing good) and **nonmalfeasance** (to do no harm). In some circumstances, it is difficult to prevent these two principles from conflicting. For example, in newborn intensive care, some treatment is painful. Decisions must be made about whether future quality of life justifies the pain inflicted on the infant and his/her parents during treatment.

Several different professional associations, including the ANA, have developed codes of ethics for nurses to follow (see box, p. 42). These frameworks for ethical conduct are helpful when applied to a given client circumstance in which ethical questions have arisen.

According to a study by Berseth, Kenny, and Durand (1984), newborn intensive care nurses are often reluctant to assist in making ethical decisions about various critical issues in neonatal intensive care. These nurses believe that the physician and parents of the child should make such decisions. However, nurses who serve as primary caregivers have unique insights about the entire family unit and therefore could be helpful if they joined in the dialogue of decision making.

Thompson and Thompson (1985) have presented a bioethical model for a logical reasoning process that nurses may use to make ethical decisions (see box, p. 42). Through use of the 10 steps described in this

CODE FOR NURSES

1. The nurse provides services with respect for human dignity and the uniqueness of the client unrestricted by considerations of social or economic status, personal attributes, or the nature of health problems.
2. The nurse safeguards the client's right to privacy by judiciously protecting information of a confidential nature.
3. The nurse acts to safeguard the client and the public when health care and safety are affected by the incompetent, unethical, or illegal practice of any person.
4. The nurse assumes responsibility and accountability for individual nursing judgments and actions.
5. The nurse maintains competence in nursing.
6. The nurse exercises informed judgment and uses individual competence and qualifications as criteria in seeking consultation, accepting responsibilities, and delegating nursing activities to others.
7. The nurse participates in activities that contribute to the ongoing development of the profession's body of knowledge.
8. The nurse participates in the profession's efforts to implement and improve standards of nursing.
9. The nurse participates in the profession's efforts to establish and maintain conditions of employment conducive to high quality nursing care.
10. The nurse participates in the profession's effort to protect the public from misinformation and misrepresentation and to maintain the integrity of nursing.
11. The nurse collaborates with members of the health professions.

A BIOETHICAL DECISION MODEL

Step One	Review the situation to determine health problems, decision needed, ethical components, and key individuals
Step Two	Gather additional information to clarify situation
Step Three	Identify the ethical issues in the situation
Step Four	Define personal and professional moral positions
Step Five	Identify moral positions of key individuals involved
Step Six	Identify value conflicts, if any
Step Seven	Determine who should make the decision
Step Eight	Identify range of actions with anticipated outcomes
Step Nine	Decide on a course of action and carry it out
Step Ten	Evaluate/review results of decision/action

From Thompson JE and Thompson HO: Ethics in nursing, New York, 1981, Macmillan Publishing Co, Inc, with permission.

bioethical model, the nurse will be able to analyze critically ethical situations as they arise. Thompson and Thompson suggest that nurses and other professionals form small discussion groups to address ongoing ethical problems within their areas of practice.

❑ ETHICAL ISSUES IN MATERNITY NURSING

Within the scope of maternity and newborn intensive care are numerous subjects with ethical questions.

In Vitro Fertilization and Embryo Transplantation

A recent ethical dilemma brought to focus by modern obstetrics is the technique of in vitro fertilization with subsequent embryo transplantation, the results of which are known as test-tube babies. Since the first live birth with this technique in 1978, numerous infants have been born as a result of this procedure.

The issue of in vitro fertilization is legally, ethically, and morally significant. As the use of this technique proliferates, questions will probably increase. Nurses may wish to apply the Thompson bioethical decision model to this complex question.

Elective Abortion

The abortion issue has dramatically polarized American society. The legal aspects continue to rage in the courts and legislative bodies across the United States.

"Pro-life" and "pro-choice" public groups have dramatically focused ethical and legal attention on the issue of abortion. Fromer (1982) reminds us that, like it or not, nurses are very much involved in abortion issues. Nurses may assist as an abortion is performed or may refuse to do so. Nurses are asked to give advice about abortions and to provide information about where a client may obtain one. To provide service to a client seeking an abortion, nurses must understand their personal ethical position on abortion (Thompson and Thompson, 1981).

From an ethical perspective, abortion is essentially the removal of the woman's support from the fetus. This leads to fetal death, since the fetus cannot sustain its life without the mother. Bok (1978) suggests that if an abortion is performed after the diagnosis of a fetal defect, the parents have consented to remove support from that particular fetus.

Wertz and Fletcher (1989) voice concern over a new trend as parents base choices of sex selection on information gained through the use of prenatal diagnostic techniques. These authors suggest that an increasing number of physicians regard "sex choice as a logical extension of parents' rights to control the number, timing, spacing, and quality of their offspring." Wertz and Fletcher conclude that physicians should stop being neutral on the abortion issue, and instead offer "moral guidance" to couples involved in such decision-making situations. These authors suggest this as an alternative to waiting until either the courts or governmental agencies begin to intervene.

Summarizing the abortion controversy is difficult, but basically the pro-choice proponents believe that the mother's rights take precedence and that she should have freedom of choice and privacy. Many pro-choice advocates believe that abortions should be used only as a last resort, with contraception and adoption being other alternatives. Most pro-life proponents believe that the fetus is human from the moment of conception and as such should be protected from abortion, which ends life.

Neonatal Intensive Care

Hundreds of neonatal intensive care units (NICUs) are available throughout the United States. They are confronted with difficult ethical questions and legal problems of all types.

Some of the ethical dilemmas in decision making are ironically caused by the dramatic advances in neonatal-perinatal care. The medical and nursing knowledge base has increased rapidly in a relatively short time. Infants who would have automatically died 10 years ago now have a good chance to survive with few undesirable consequences. In essence, the joint disciplines of perinatology and neonatology have pushed back the point of viability to unimagined degrees. A preterm infant of less than 1500 g (3 lb, 5 oz) had a slim chance of survival in 1965. Whereas an infant of 1000 g (2 lb, 3 oz) has a good chance today. The advances in neonatal surgery have significantly improved the outcome for many infants born with heart defects or other congenital anomalies. This section will explore some of the issues faced by nurses who work in an NICU.

Costs of Treatment. One ethical problem that arises not only in the NICU but in all areas of perinatal care involves societal pressures about money. Newborn intensive care and fetal surgery are costly. Considering the dwindling public funds available for health care, many persons question the appropriateness of diverting monies from preventive programs (such as immunization programs for the poor) to the care of one critically ill infant. The hospitalization cost for one NICU baby can easily exceed $100,000. Federal, state, and local funds used for this type of care will not be available for other health care programs. Morreim (1988) notes that formerly shortages in resources were described in either ***access*** to health care, as some clients did not live close to health care, or ***commodity scarcities*** of such items as organs for transplantation or equipment such as dialysis units. Now to those scarcities, he adds ***fiscal scarcity*** caused by decreased financial resources.

Veatch (1986) describes the ethical dilemmas of **cost-containment** caused by diagnosis related groups (DRGs). For example, if a hospital discovers that DRG 386 (extreme prematurity, neonates) is "losing money" for the hospital, they might decide to close their NICU, transfer out severely affected neonates, or change their guidelines for resuscitation based on a higher birth weight. Veatch believes the ethics of cost-containment decisions deserve examination.

Unpredictable Prognoses. Many infants who receive care in the NICU have an unpredictable prognosis, which presents ethical dilemmas for all personnel. For example, neonatal asphyxia has a variable outcome depending on the severity of the original episode. If the infant suffers a subsequent cardiac arrest, the appropriate care might be in question. Is resuscitation of the infant ethically correct? How long should resuscitation efforts be continued? Is there an ethical imperative to save all infants?

The NICU is designed to facilitate diagnosis and treatment of infants with immediate and acute but essentially life-threatening problems, such as aspiration pneumonia or respiratory distress syndrome. Proper care can result in a dramatic reduction in morbidity and mortality in these infants. However, an ethical question arises as to whether it is appropriate to use equipment and intensive care skills to keep an infant with a poor prognosis alive while "neglecting" an infant with a better prognosis.

Cohen (1977) discusses violation of the ethical principle of aiding one client while harming another. He suggests that if one assumes the obligation to provide intensive care to a client, terminating this care later because another client has a higher potential for survival violates the original obligation. However, he recognizes the difficult dilemma that intensive care personnel face when they do not want to sustain infants who are beyond salvage (e.g., an infant who has suffered a massive intracranial hemorrhage). Persons who care for these infants have difficulty deciding which infant would be better served if allowed to die.

Steinfels (1978) poses the question of whether the emphasis on neonatal intensive care for smaller and smaller preterm infants has resulted in decreased efforts in the prevention of prematurity. Although a birth weight of 1000 g was formerly the lower limit of saving preterm infants, many NICUs now use heroic efforts to save infants weighing as little as 600 to 700 g. Steinfels also suggests that more attention be paid to the impact on the family of the preterm infant who is saved but severely impaired.

Silverman (1981) suggests that many parents may believe that producing an infant with severe handicapping conditions is worse than having an infant who dies. Furthermore, he deplores the "rescuer" role of many health professionals. In this role providers make unrestrained heroic efforts to prolong even the most fragile life with no concern for the parents' wishes. Silverman asserts that because parents will have the day-to-day responsibilities for consequences of neonatal intensive care, they should be among the primary decision makers regarding the care of their infant.

Since outcome for neonates is often difficult to predict, Rhoden (1986) suggests the adoption of guidelines to help make decisions in life and death situations. She describes guidelines adopted by other countries as they make decisions about neonatal care. Every case must be decided on an individual basis, but Rhoden suggests that such guidelines can help in the decision-making process for many of the infants who receive care in NICUs.

Many authorities have suggested that an ethics committee composed of clergy, ethicists, lawyers, physicians, nurses, and lay persons could review each case. Watchko (1983) recommends a model in which the physician and parent would make the original decision and then review their decision with an ethics committee. If disputes resulted about what was correct, the courts would be asked to intervene. In this solution, the parents represent a noninstitutional perspective and are subject to review by other family members, social agencies, such as churches, and close friends. The physician, who represents an institutional viewpoint, is subject to peer review. The hospital-based committee serves as a consultant. If the courts are involved, they assume the primary authority.

The ethical issues surrounding provision of newborn intensive care has produced a great amount of discussion and debate for the past 20 years. Experts from many different perspectives met 15 times between 1984 and 1987 to discuss these important issues. Although this group was unable to reach a consensus, their published opinions provide fascinating additional reading for the interested student (Caplan, 1987).

AIDS

Acquired immunodeficiency syndrome (AIDS) was first identified and brought to public attention in 1981. The epidemic of this lethal syndrome poses physical, emotional, legal, and ethical challenges to nurses regardless of their area of practice. Maternity nurses who manage health issues for pregnant women and their newborns with AIDS must examine their own values. Chow (1989) challenges nurses to examine their own fears and prejudices against AIDS clients and to assume a leadership role in setting a national nursing agenda to promote excellent and compassionate nursing care for people who face the anguish of this disease.

Brown (1987) states that the AIDS epidemic has an impact on nurses at all levels of practice from staff nurses, to administrators, to educators. Nurses are confronted with many ethical issues involved in AIDS, such as the client's right to human dignity, privacy, and confidentiality. Often nurses may have intrapersonal conflicts about the client who lives an alternative lifestyle, or who is a drug abuser. Nurse administrators must confront issues of resource allocation and personnel management for those under their supervision. Nurses must be educated about the physical nature of this disease process to assist their clients, as well as to protect themselves from contracting this incurable disease.

Steele (1986) notes that AIDS is a "catastrophic health problem." She recommends that nurses must examine their own reactions and engage in values clarification to help society cope with this crisis. Finally, Steele reminds all nurses that they may be in a position to help AIDS victims develop a high quality of life for whatever time they have remaining, since they know that their disease is always fatal.

SUMMARY

A wide variety of ethical and legal issues arise in maternity and newborn nursing. This chapter presents a review of current ethical and legal positions involved in the care of clients. Many of the ethical dilemmas are a result of the rapid advances taking place in all specialties. The new medical technology and expanded roles for nurses have increased the chances of survival for normal infants and improved the care for all newborns. Because family-centered maternity health care raises ethical and legal questions of monumental proportions, it is essential for all nurses who care for women, new mothers, and their infants to understand these issues.

LEARNING ACTIVITIES

1. Determine from the nursing service at your hospital if a "conscience clause" for nurses is written into the policies. If so, read and discuss it with your student group.
2. Determine what policy is written or unwritten concerning "no-code" and withholding of treatment in the neonatal intensive care unit at your hospital.
3. Research recent medical malpractice suits to determine the type and frequency of obstetric-related suits. Report on such questions as: How often was the nurse named as defendant? and Are there any areas of obstetric practice that seem particularly hazardous in relation to lawsuits?

4. Interview several registered nurses on the subject of "floating." Obtain answers to these questions for discussion with the group:
   a. Does their facility make a practice of floating nurses?
   b. How do they personally feel about floating?
   c. What do they do if they feel unqualified to float to a certain area?
   d. What pressures have they felt relative to floating?
   e. Have any of them floated to an area and had a serious problem develop while there?

KEY CONCEPTS

- The conduct of all legally competent individuals is held to a standard of care—that degree of care exercised by a reasonably prudent person under similar circumstances.
- Professional nurses are liable for the consequences of their actions.
- The independent practice of nursing encompasses those decisions and actions taken by nurses based on *nursing judgment* and *nursing management* plan.
- The concept of risk management seeks to minimize losses by establishing preventive practices, appropriate reporting practices, and discovery procedures.
- In the event of a lawsuit, the client record is the only piece of evidence created at the time of the event.
- Ethical dilemmas occur in every field of nursing practice.
- Nurses have responsibilities and commitments to use ethical conduct in relationships with clients, other nurses, physicians, and their employers.
- Inherent in the values of most nurses are beneficence and nonmalfeasance.

References

Annas G, Glantz L, and Katz B: The rights of doctors, nurses and allied health professionals, Cambridge, Mass, 1981, Ballinger Publishing Co.

Berseth CL, Kenny JD, and Durand R: Newborn ethical dilemmas: intensive care and intermediate care nursing attitudes, Crit Care Med 12(6): June, 1984.

Black HC: Black's law dictionary, St Paul, 1979, West Publishing Co.

Bok S: Ethical problems of abortion. Hastings Center Rep 19(4):19, 1978.

Brown ML: AIDS and ethics: concerns and considerations, Oncol Nurs Forum 14(1):69, 1987.

California Business and Professions Code, section 2725. California Administrative Code, section 1470 et seq.

Caplan A, editor: Special report re: imperiled newborns, Hastings Center Rep 17(6): Dec, 1987.

Chow M: Nursing's response to the challenge of AIDS, Nurs Outlook 37(2): Mar/April, 1989.

Cohen CV: Ethical problems of intensive care, Anesthesiology 47:217, 1977.

Curtin L and Flaherty MJ: Nursing ethics: theories and pragmatics, Bowie, Md, 1982, Robert Brady Co.

Cushing M: Informed consent—an MD responsibility? Am J Nurs 84:437, April, 1984.

Cushing M: Lessons from history: the picket-guard nurse, Am J Nurs 85:1073, Oct, 1985.

Darling v. Charleston Community Memorial Hospital, 211 NE 2nd 253 (IL 1965).

Fiesta J: The law and liability: a guide for nurses, New York, 1983, John Wiley & Sons, Inc.

Flanagin A: The ethical voice of nursing—I can't hear it, can you?" JOGN Nurs May/June, 1988.

Fromer MJ: Abortion ethics, Nurs Outlook 30(4):234, 1982.

Horsley JE: Short-staffing means increased liability for you, RN 44(2):73, 1981.

Morreim EH: Cost containment: challenging fidelity and justice, Hastings Center Rep 16(6): Dec, 1988.

NAACOG: Standards for obstetric, gynecologic and neonatal nursing, ed 3, Washington, DC, 1986.

Rhoden NK: Treating baby Doe: the ethics of uncertainty, Hastings Center Rep 16(4): Aug, 1986.

Rhodes A and Miller R: Nursing and the law, ed 4, Rockville, Md, 1984, Aspen Publishers, Inc.

Silverman WA: Mismatched attitudes about neonatal death, Hastings Center Rep 11(6):12, 1981.

Steele SM: AIDS: clarifying values to close in on ethical questions, Nursing and Health Care 7:5, May, 1986.

Steinfels M: New childbirth technology: a clash of values, Hastings Center Rep 8(9): Feb, 1978.

Thompson JE and Thompson HO: Ethics in nursing, New York, 1981, Macmillan Publishing Co, Inc.

Thompson JE and Thompson HO: Ethical decision making for nurses, Norwalk, CT, 1985, Appleton-Century-Crofts.

Veatch RM: DRGs and the ethical reallocation of resources, Hastings Center Rep 16(3): June, 1986.

Watchko JF: Decision making on critically ill infants by parents, Am J Dis Child 137:795, 1983.

Wecht C, editor: Legal medicine 1982, Philadelphia, 1982, WB Saunders Co.

Weeks LC: Consider this column re: ethics committees, J Nurs Adm 17(10): Oct, 1987.

Wertz DC and Fletcher JC: Fatal knowledge? Prenatal diagnosis and sex selection, Hastings Center Rep 19(3): May/June, 1989.

Wilson D: An overview of sexually transmissable diseases in the perinatal period, J Nurse Midwife 33(3):115, 1988.

Bibliography

American Nurses Association: Nursing: a social policy statement, Kansas City, Mo, 1980, American Nurses Association.

Annas GJ: Baby M: babies (and justice) for sale, Hastings Center Rep 17(3):13, 1987.

Buley DD: When the burden of proof falls on you, Nurs '86 16:41, Feb, 1986.

Cushing M: Legal side: how a suit starts, Am J Nurs 85:655, June, 1985.

Driscoll ME: AIDS: legal aspects of occupational exposure, Calif Nurs Review 10(3):10, 1988.

Erlen JA and Holzman IR: Anencephalic infants: should they be organ donors? Pediatr Nurs 14(1):60, 1988.

Ethics Grand Rounds: When refusing treatment jeopardizes another life, Nurs '88 18(5):145, 1988.

Kim M, McFarland G, and McLane A: Pocket guide to nursing diagnoses, ed 3, St Louis, 1989, The CV Mosby Co.

Lagerloff J: Ethics: maternal-fetal conflict, Calif Nurs Rev 10(1):34, 1988.

LaRocco SA: Dilemmas in practice: a case of patient abuse, Am J Nurs 85:1233, Nov, 1985.

Larson DR: Ethics: should anencephalic neonates be organ donors? AORN J 47(3):778, 1988.

Northrop CE and Kelly ME: Legal issues in nursing, St Louis, 1987, The CV Mosby Co.

Penticuff JH: Ethics in obstetric and gynecologic nursing, NAA-COG update series, lesson 26, vol 1, 1984.

Rabinow J: Where you stand in the eyes of the law, Nurs '89 19(2): Feb, 1989.

Roland R: Technology and motherhood: reproductive choice reconsidered, SIGNS 12(3):512, 1987.

Shaffer MK and Pfeiffer IL: Dilemmas in practice: nursing research and patients' rights, Am J Nurs 86:23, Jan, 1986.

Van Lier DJ and Roberts JE: Promoting informed consent of women in labor, JOGN Nurs 15(5):419, 1986.

CHAPTER

4 Human Sexuality

Irene M. Bobak

Learning Objectives

Correctly define the key terms listed.

Identify the internal, external, and accessory structures of both the female and male reproductive systems.

Explain the functions of the structures of both the female and male reproductive systems.

Summarize the menstrual cycle in relation to hormonal response, ovarian response, and endometrial response.

Discuss the clinical significance of human sexual response.

Explain two theories of human development.

Relate the nurse's role in parental counseling regarding sex education.

Delineate the six developmental tasks of adolescence.

Differentiate expected behaviors in the three phases of adolescence.

List the developmental tasks of the three phases of adolescence.

List the developmental tasks of the three phases of adulthood.

Assess personal belief system regarding sexuality and the impact such beliefs have on one's ability to counsel and teach sexually related material.

Key Terms

autonomy
climacterium
cognitive development
concrete operations stage
core gender identity
developmental tasks
ego integrity
endometrial cycle
gender preference
generativity
heterosexuality
homosexuality
hypothalamic-pituitary cycle
identity
industry
initiative
intimacy
living ligature
masturbation
menarche
menopause
menstruation
mittelschmerz
myotonia
orgasm
ovarian cycle
ovulation
personality development
premenstrual syndrome (PMS)
preoperational stage
primary dysmenorrhea
promiscuous
prostaglandins
pubarche
secondary dysmenorrhea
sensorimotor stage
sex role standards
sexuality
spinnbarkheit
squamocolumnar junction
taboo
trust
vasocongestion
withdrawal bleeding

The purposes of this chapter are twofold: (1) to review sexual and reproductive anatomy and physiology, and (2) to trace the psychosocial development of sexuality from birth through adulthood.

Nurses providing maternity health care to women require a greater depth and breadth of knowledge of female anatomy and physiology than is usually taught in general courses. Often, the reproductive system, including the breasts, is the last system taught, if there is time. Knowledge of the anatomy and physiology of the structures, both female and male, involved in reproduction is basic to planning for, implementing, and evaluating nursing care of the maternity client and her family.

Although the female and male reproductive systems differ markedly in appearance, their structures are homologous (having the same embryonic origin) (Figs. 4-1 and 4-2). Each structure performs a vital role in the continuation of the human species and the generation and maintenance of secondary sexual characteristics. Through hormonal influences the genitals, pelvis, and breasts acquire the unique adaptations necessary to childbearing. Both female and male reproductive systems consist of the following four principal components:

1. External genitals
2. A pair of primary sex glands (gonads)
3. Ducts leading from the gonads to the body's exterior
4. Secondary (accessory) sex glands

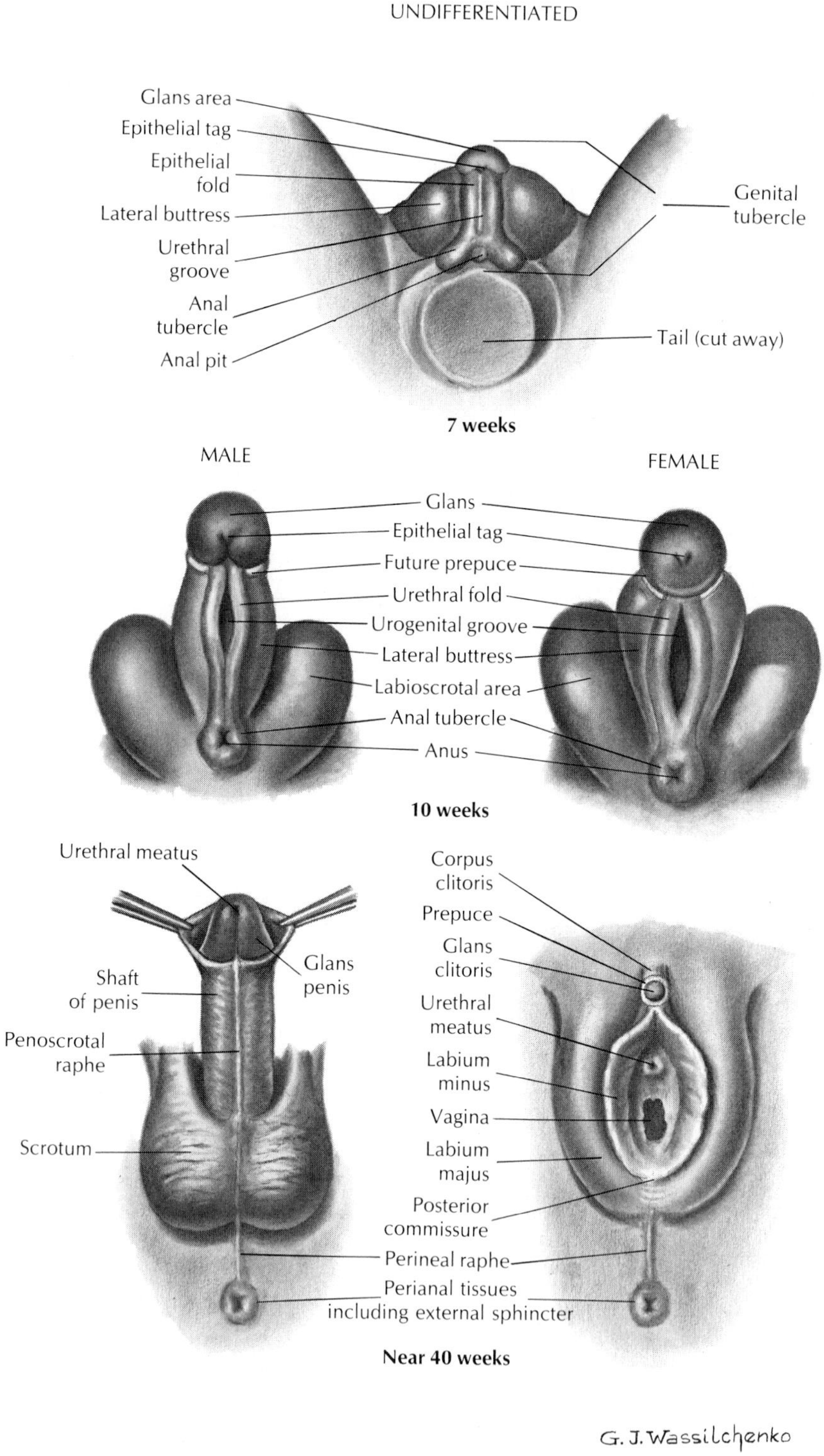

Fig. 4-1 Homologues of external genitals.

❑ FEMALE REPRODUCTIVE SYSTEM

The female reproductive system consists of internal organs, located in the pelvic cavity and supported by the pelvic floor, and external genitals, located in the perineum. The female's internal and external reproductive structures develop and mature in response to estrogens and progesterones, starting in fetal life and continuing through puberty and the childbearing years. The reproductive structures atrophy (decrease in size) with age or a drop in ovarian hormone production. An extensive and complex innervation and a generous blood supply support the functions of these structures. The appearance of the external genitals varies greatly from woman to woman, since the size, shape, and color are determined by heredity, age, and race and the number of children a woman has borne.

External Structures

The external female genitals (vulva, pudenda) are located in the perineum. The external structures are presented in the following order (from anterior to posterior).

1. Mons pubis (mons veneris)
2. Labia majora (sing., labium majus) and minora (sing., labium minus)
3. Clitoris
4. Prepuce of clitoris

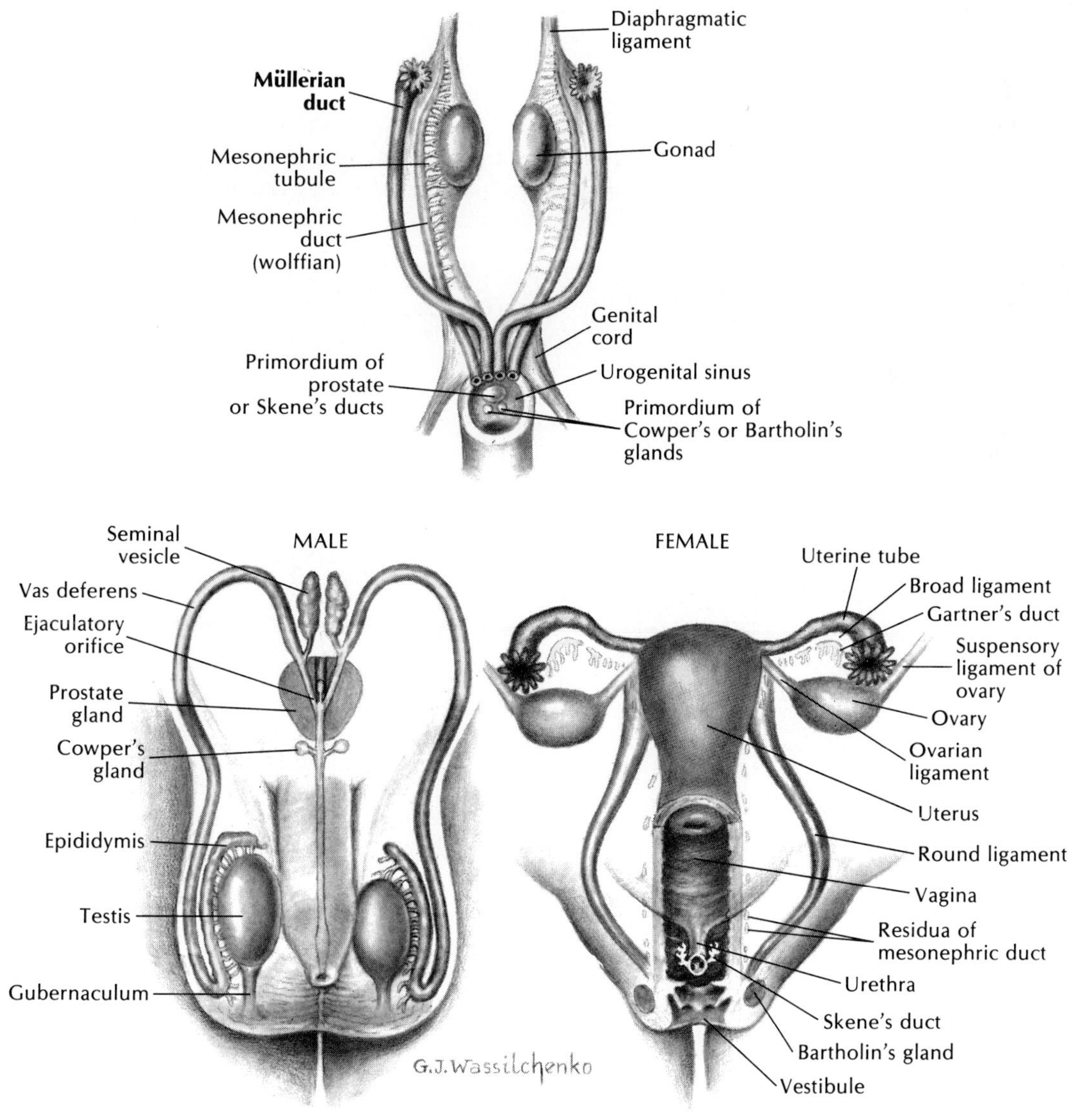

Fig. 4-2 Homologues of internal genitals.

5. Vestibule
   a. Urethral or urinary orifice (meatus)
   b. Lesser vestibular, paraurethral, or Skene's glands
   c. Hymen and vaginal introitus, or orifice
   d. Greater vestibular, vulvovaginal, or Bartholin's glands
6. Fourchette
7. Perineum

The external genitals are illustrated in Fig. 4-3.

Mons Pubis. The mons pubis, or mons veneris, is the rounded, soft fullness of subcutaneous fatty tissue and loose connective tissue over the symphysis pubis. It contains many sebaceous (oil) glands and develops coarse, dark, curly hair at **pubarche,** about 1 to 2 years before the onset of the menses. Menarche (the onset of menses) occurs on the average at 13 years of age. Characteristics of pubic hair vary from sparse and fine among Oriental women to thick, coarse, and curly among black women. The functions of the mons are to play a role in sensuality and to protect the symphysis pubis during coitus.

Labia Majora. The labia majora are two rounded lengthwise folds of skin-covered fat and connective tissue that merge with the mons. They extend from the mons downward around the labia minora, ending in the perineum in the midline. The labia majora function as protection for the labia minora, urinary meatus, and vaginal introitus. In the woman who has never experienced vaginal childbirth, the labia majora come together in the midline, obscuring the vaginal introitus. Some labial separation and even gaping of the vaginal introitus follow childbirth and perineal or vaginal injury.

On their lateral surfaces the labial skin is thick, usually pigmented darker than the surrounding tissues, and covered with coarse hair (similar to that of the mons) that thins out toward the perineum. The medial (inner) surfaces of the labia majora are smooth, thick, and without hair. They contain an abundant supply of sebaceous glands and sweat glands and are highly vascular. The extreme sensitivity of the labia majora to touch, pain, and temperature is caused by the extensive network of nerves; thus they function during sensual arousal.

Labia Minora. The labia minora, located between the labia majora, are narrow, lengthwise folds of hairless skin extending downward from beneath the clitoris

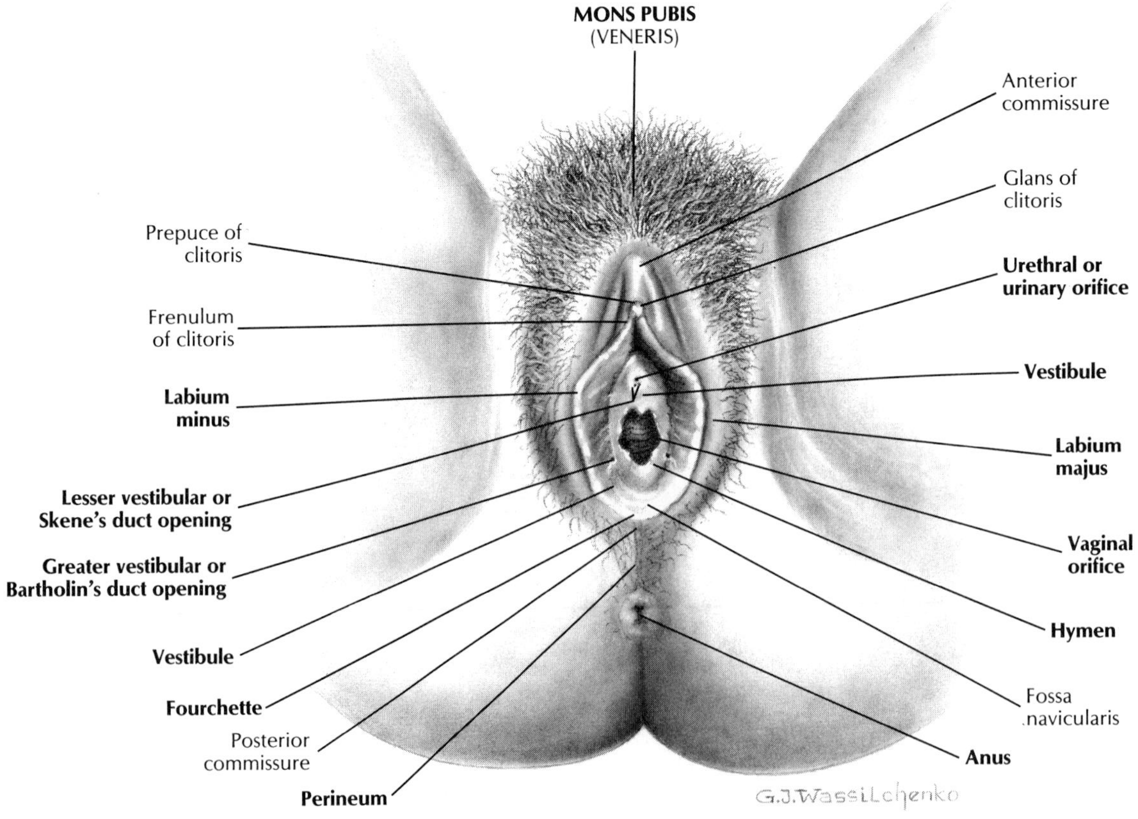

Fig. 4-3 External female genitals.

and merging with the fourchette. Whereas the lateral and anterior aspects of the labia are usually pigmented, their medial surfaces are similar to vaginal mucosa: pink and moist. Their rich vascularity gives them a reddish color and permits marked turgescence (swelling) of the labia minora with emotional or physical stimulation. The glands in the labia minora also lubricate the vulva. A rich nerve supply makes them sensitive, enhancing their erotic function. The space between the labia minora is called the vestibule.

Clitoris. The clitoris is a short, cylindric, erectile organ fixed just beneath the arch of the pubis; the visible portion is about 6 × 6 mm or less in the unaroused state. The tip of the clitoral body is called the glans and is more sensitive than its shaft. In healthy women the length of the clitoral body varies from 2 mm to 1 cm, and the width is usually estimated at 4 to 5 mm. When sexually aroused, the glans and shaft increase in size.

Sebaceous glands of the clitoris secrete smegma, a fatty substance with a distinctive odor, which serves as a pheromone (an organic compound that provides communication with other members of the same species to elicit a certain response, which in this case is erotic stimulation of the human male). The term *clitoris* comes from a Greek word meaning "key," because the clitoris was seen as the key to female sexuality. Its rich vascularity and innervation make the clitoris highly sensitive to temperature, touch, and pressure sensation. The clitoris contains many nerve endings, as does its male homologue, the glans penis. Its main function is to stimulate and elevate levels of sexual tension.

Prepuce of Clitoris. Near the anterior junction the right and left labia minora separate into medial and lateral portions. The lateral portions unite above the clitoris to form its prepuce, a hoodlike covering; the medial portions unite below the clitoris to form its frenulum. Sometimes the prepuce covers the clitoris. As a result this area has the appearance of an opening that can be mistaken for the urethral meatus if the nurse does not identify vulvar structures carefully. Attempts to insert a catheter into this sensitive area can cause considerable discomfort.

Vestibule. The vestibule is an ovoid or boat-shaped area formed between the labia minora, clitoris, and fourchette. The vestibule contains the openings to the urethra, paraurethral (lesser vestibular, Skene's) glands, the vagina, and the paravaginal (greater vestibular, vulvovaginal, or Bartholin's) glands. The thin, almost mucosal, surface of the vestibule is easily irritated by chemicals (feminine deodorant sprays, bubble bath salts), heat, discharges, and friction (tight jeans).

Although not a true part of the reproductive system, the *urinary* (urethral) *meatus* is considered here because of its closeness and relationship to the vulva. The meatus is a pink or reddened opening of varying shapes, often with slightly puckered margins. The meatus marks the terminal, or distal, part of the urethra. It is usually about 2.5 cm (1 in) below the clitoris.

The *lesser vestibular* (paraurethral, Skene's) *glands* are short tubular structures situated posterolaterally just inside the urethral meatus, at about the 5 and 7 o'clock positions around the meatus. They produce a small amount of mucus, which functions as lubrication.

The *hymen* (see Fig. 4-3) is a partial, rarely complete, elastic but tough mucosa-covered fold around the *vaginal introitus.* In virginal females the hymen may be an impediment to vaginal examination, insertion of menstrual tampons, or coitus. The hymen may be elastic and allow distension, or it may be torn easily. Occasionally the hymen covers the orifice completely, resulting in an imperforate hymen that prevents passage of menstrual flow, instrumentation (e.g., with a speculum), or coitus. A hymenotomy may be necessary in some cases. After instrumentation, use of tampons, coitus, or vaginal delivery, residual tags of the torn hymen (hymenal caruncles or carunculae myrtiformes) may be seen.

One common myth is that one can tell by the condition of the hymen whether a female is a virgin. Sexually active and even parous females may have intact hymens. For other women the hymen may be torn during strenuous physical work or exercise, masturbation, or use of tampons. Some cultural groups cleanse the female infant so vigorously that the hymen is torn, leaving only hymenal tags in its place. Therefore the "test for virginity"—evidence of bleeding following sexual intercourse—is an unreliable criterion.

The *greater vestibular* (vulvovaginal, Bartholin's) *glands* are two compound glands at the base of the labia majora, one on either side of the vaginal orifice. Each gland is drained by several ducts, about 1.5 cm long. Each opens into the groove between the hymen and the labia minora. Usually the gland openings are not visible or palpable. The glands secrete a small amount of clear, viscid mucus, especially during coitus. The alkaline pH of the mucus is supportive of sperm.

Fourchette. The fourchette is a thin, flat, transverse fold of tissue formed where the tapering labia majora and minora merge in the midline below the vaginal orifice. A small depression, the fossa navicularis, lies between the fourchette and the hymen.

Perineum. The perineum is the skin-covered muscular area between the vaginal introitus and the anus. The perineum forms the base of the perineal body (see Fig. 4-15, p. 61). The terms *vulva* and *perineum* occasionally but inaccurately are used interchangeably.

Internal Structures

The internal reproductive organs are discussed in the order that reflects the path of the ovum. Supportive tissues are discussed along with the internal reproductive organs they support. Internal organs include the ovaries, uterine (fallopian) tubes, uterus, and vagina. A brief description of the bony pelvis follows.

Ovaries: Female Gonads. One ovary is located on each side of the uterus, below and behind the uterine tubes. The ovaries are held in place by two ligaments, the mesovarian portions of the uterine *broad ligament,* which suspend them from the lateral pelvic side walls at about the level of the anterosuperior iliac crest, and the *ovarian* ligaments (see Figs. 4-5 and 4-9), which anchor them to the uterus. The ovaries are movable with palpation.

The ovaries are similar in origin (homologous) to the testes in the male. Each ovary resembles a large almond in size and shape (Fig. 4-4). Each is whitish and rounded but flattened, weighs about 3 g, and measures approximately 3 × 2 × 1 cm. At the time of ovulation, ovarian size may double temporarily. The oval-shaped ovaries are firm in consistency and slightly tender. The surface of the ovary is smooth before menarche. After sexual maturity, scarring from repeated ruptures of follicles and ovulation roughens the nodular surface.

The two functions of the ovaries are **ovulation** and hormone production. At birth the normal female's ovaries contain countless thousands of primordial (primitive) ova. At intervals during the reproductive life (generally monthly), one or more ova mature and undergo ovulation. The ovary is also the major site of production of steroid sex hormones (estrogens, progesterone, and androgens) in amounts required for normal female growth, development, and function.

Uterine Tubes (Oviducts). The paired uterine (fallopian) tubes are attached to the uterine fundus (Figs. 4-5, 4-6, and 4-9). The tubes extend laterally, enter the free ends of the broad ligament, and curl around each ovary.

The tubes are approximately 10 cm (4 in) long and 0.6 cm (¼ in) in diameter. Each tube has an outer coat of peritoneum, a middle, thin muscular coat, and an inner mucosa. The mucosal lining consists of columnar cells, some of which are ciliated and others of which are secretory. The mucosa is at its thinnest during the time of menstruation. Each tube, along with its mucosa, is continuous with the mucosa of the uterus and of the vagina.

The structure of the uterine tube changes along its length. Four distinctive segments can be identified (Figs. 4-5 and 4-6): (1) the infundibulum, (2) the ampulla, (3) the isthmus, and (4) the interstitial part. The *infundibulum* is the most distal portion. Its funnel, or trumpet-shaped opening, is encircled with fimbriae. The fimbriae become swollen, almost erectile, at ovulation. The *ampulla* makes up the distal and middle segment of the tube. It is in the ampulla that the sperm and the ovum unite and fertilization occurs.

The *isthmus* is proximal to the ampulla. It is small and firm, much like the round ligament. The *insterstitial* (or intramural) portion passes through the myo-

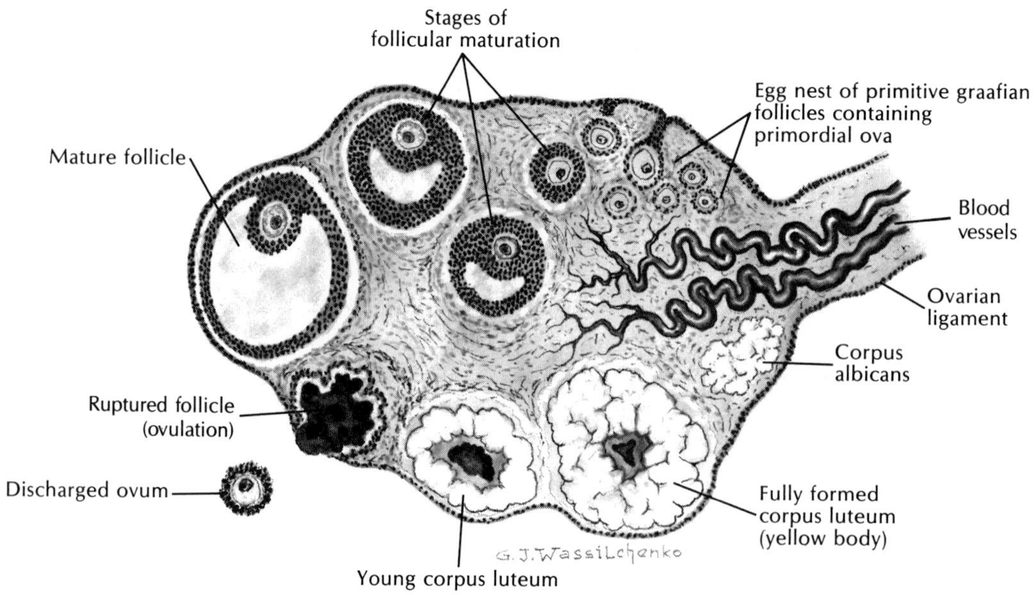

Fig. 4-4 Cross section of ovary showing sequence of events leading to maturation of follicle, ovulation, and luteinization and involution of corpus luteum (corpus albicans).

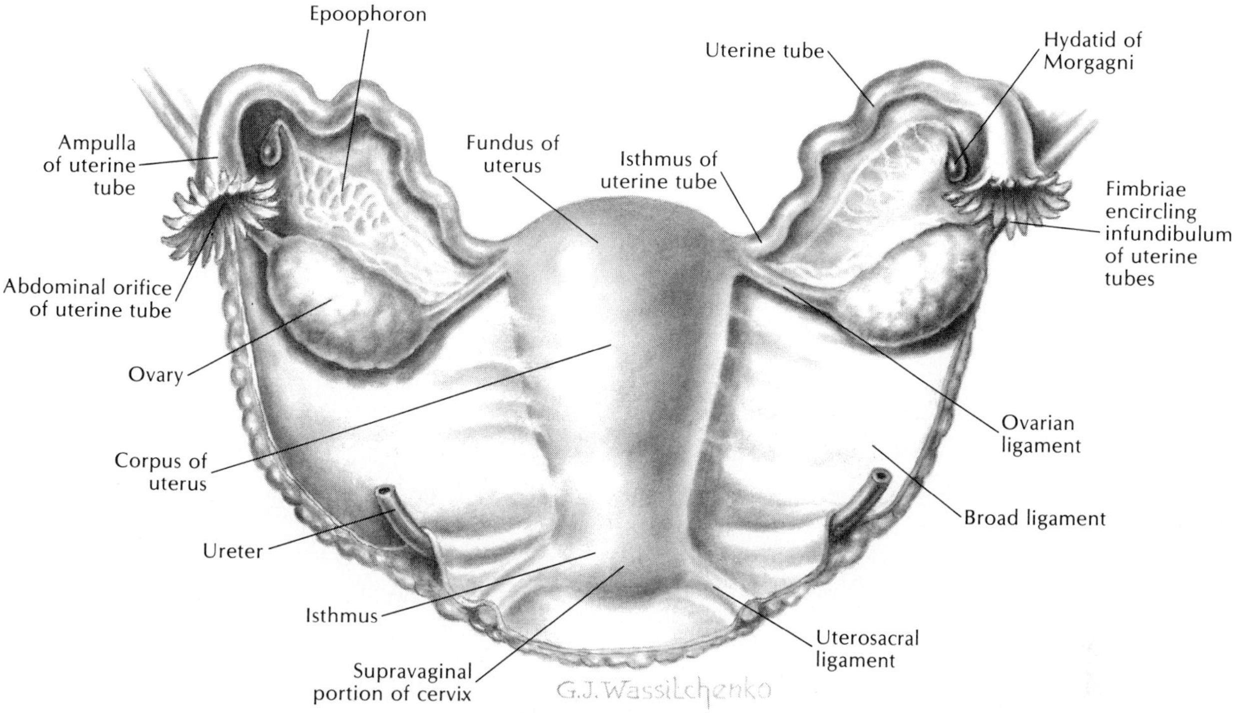

Fig. 4-5 Uterus and adnexa, posterior view.

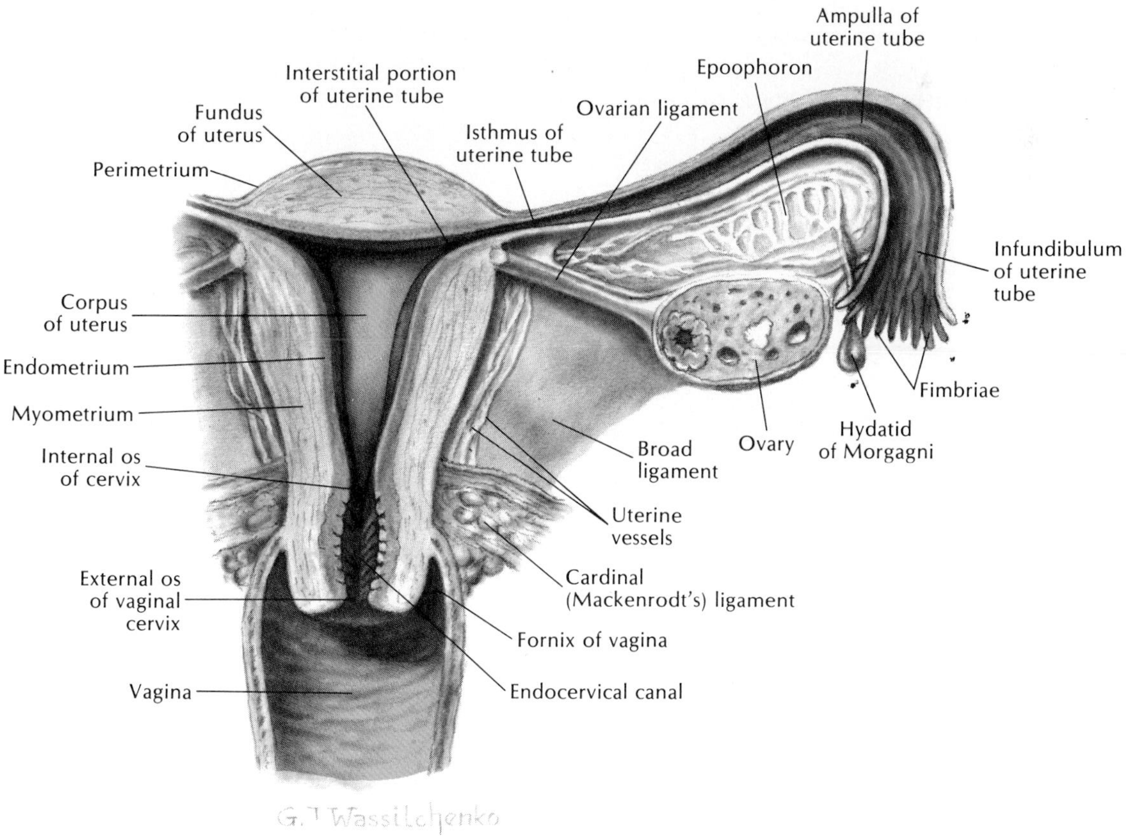

Fig. 4-6 Cross section of uterus, adnexa, and upper vagina.

metrium between the fundus and the body of the uterus and has the smallest lumen. Before the fertilized ovum can pass through this lumen, or tunnel, measuring less than 1 mm in diameter, it has to discard its crown of granulosa cells.

The uterine tubes provide a passageway for the ovum. The fingerlike projections (fimbriae) of the infundibulum pull the ovum into the tube with wavelike motions. The ovum is propelled along the tube, partially by the cilia but primarily by the peristaltic movements of the muscular coat, toward the uterine cavity. Peristaltic motion is influenced by estrogen and prostaglandins. Peristaltic activity of the uterine tubes and the secretory function of their mucosal lining are greatest at the time of ovulation. The columnar cells secrete a nutrient to sustain the ovum while it is in the tube.

Uterus. Between birth and puberty the uterus descends gradually into the true pelvis from the lower abdomen. After puberty the uterus is usually located in the midline in the true pelvis posterior to the symphysis pubis and urinary bladder and anterior to the rectum.

For most women, with the urinary bladder empty, the uterus is anteverted (tipped forward) and slightly anteflexed (bent forward), with the corpus lying over the top of the posterior wall of the bladder. The cervix is directed downward and backward toward the tip of the sacrum so that it is usually at approximately a right angle to the plane of the vagina. For other women the uterus may be in the midposition or tipped backward (retroverted). The uterus that is bent more than usual so that the fundus is closer to the cervix is said to be anteflexed, or retroflexed (Fig. 4-7).

A full bladder pushes the uterus back toward the rectum. A full rectum moves the uterus forward against the bladder. Uterine position also changes depending on the woman's position (e.g., lying supine, prone, on her side, or standing), her age, and pregnancy. The free mobility permits the uterus to rise slightly during the sexual response cycle so that the cervix is placed in a position to increase the likelihood of fertilization.

The uterus is supported by ligaments and by muscles of the pelvic floor, including the perineal body. A total of 10 ligaments stabilize the uterus within the pelvic cavity (see Figs. 4-5, 4-6, and 4-9): four paired ligaments—broad, round, uterosacral, and cardinal (transverse, Mackenrodt's); and two single ligaments—anterior (pubocervical) and posterior (rectovaginal). The posterior ligament forms the deep rectouterine pouch known as the *cul-de-sac of Douglas* (Figs. 4-8 and 4-15).

The uterus is a flattened, hollow, muscular, thick-walled organ that looks somewhat like an upside-down

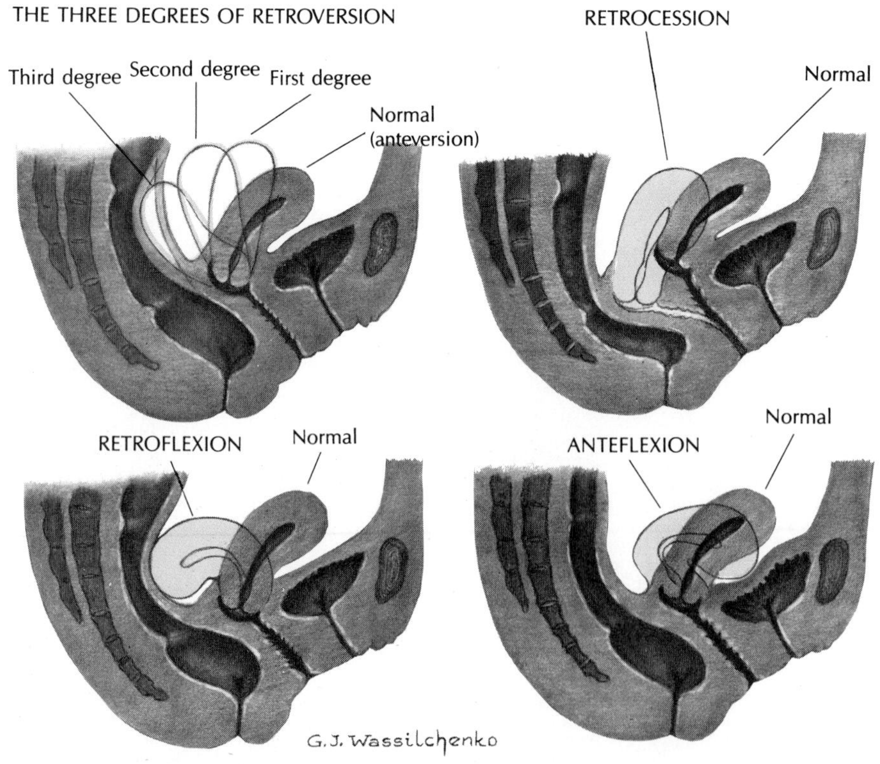

Fig. 4-7 Uterine positions.

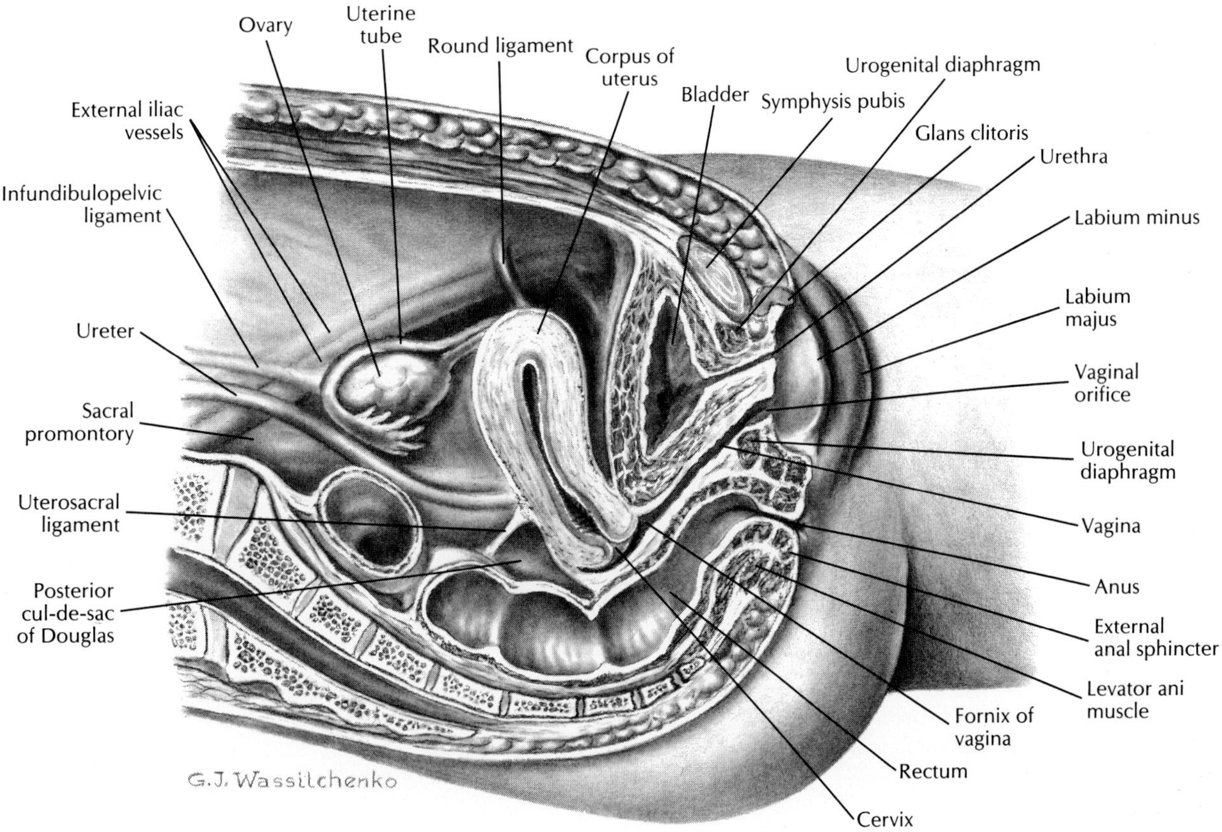

Fig. 4-8 Midsagittal view of female pelvic organs, with woman lying supine.

pear (Fig. 4-8). Its length, width, and thickness vary, averaging about 7.5 × 3.5 × 2 cm (3 × 1½ × ¾ in). In the adult woman who has never been pregnant the uterus weighs 60 g (2 oz). The uterus normally is symmetric in shape and nontender, smooth, and firm to the touch. The degree of firmness varies with several factors; for example, it is spongier during the secretory phase of the menstrual cycle, softer during pregnancy, and firmer after menopause.

The uterus has three parts (see Figs. 4-5 and 4-6): the *fundus,* the upper, rounded prominence above the insertion of the uterine tubes; the *corpus,* or main portion, encircling the intrauterine cavity; and the *isthmus,* the slightly constricted portion that joins the corpus to the cervix and is known as the lower uterine segment during pregnancy.

Uterine Wall. The uterine wall is made up of three layers: the endometrium, the myometrium, and a partial outer layer of parietal peritoneum (see Fig. 4-6).

The highly vascular *endometrium* is a lining of mucous membrane composed of three layers: a compact surface layer, a spongy middle layer of loose connective tissue, and a dense inner layer that attaches the endometrium to the myometrium. (The upper two layers are also referred to as the functional layer; and the inner layer, as the basal layer.) During menstruation and following delivery, the compact surface and middle spongy layers slough off. Just after menstrual flow ends, the endometrium is 0.5 mm thick; near the end of the endometrial cycle, just before menstruation begins again, it is about 5 mm (less than ¼ in) thick.

Layers of smooth muscle fibers that extend in three directions (longitudinal, transverse, and oblique) make up the thick *myometrium* (Fig. 4-9). The smooth muscle fibers interlace with elastic and connective tissues and blood vessels throughout the uterine wall and blend with the dense inner layer of the endometrium. The myometrium is particularly thick in the fundus, thins out as it nears the isthmus, and is thinnest in the cervix.

The *outer* myometrial layer, found mostly in the fundus, is made up of longitudinal fibers and is therefore well suited for expelling the fetus during the birth process. In the thick *middle* myometrial layer the interlaced muscle fibers form a figure-eight pattern encircling large blood vessels. Contraction of the middle layer produces a hemostatic action (Fig. 4-10). Only a few circular fibers of the *inner* myometrial layer are

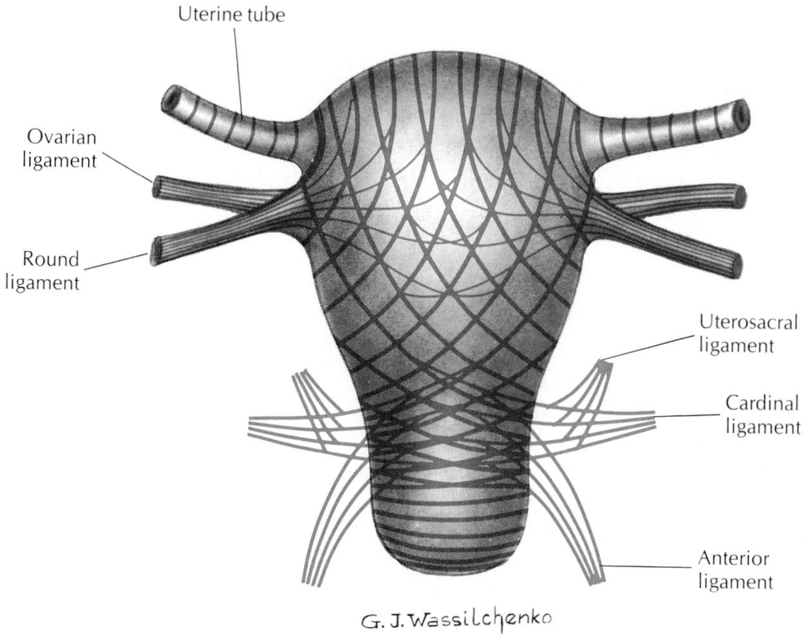

Fig. 4-9 Schematic arrangement of directions of muscle fibers. Note that uterine muscle fibers are continuous with supportive ligaments of uterus.

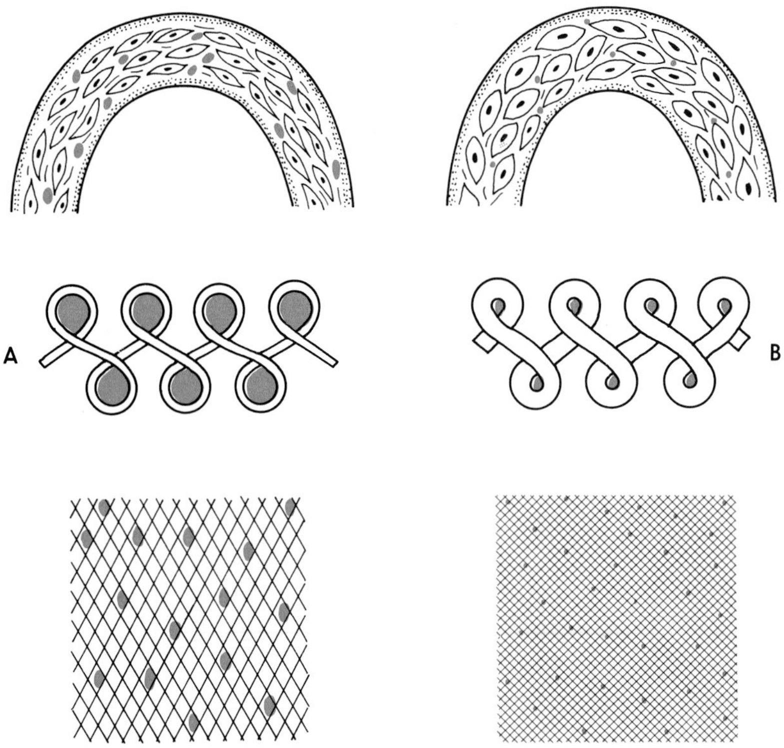

Fig. 4-10 The living ligature: interlacing smooth muscle fibers of the thick middle myometrium. Color denotes blood vessels. **A**, Relaxed muscle fibers. **B**, Contracted muscle fibers ligating the blood vessels.

found in the fundus. Most of the circular fibers are concentrated in the cornua (the place where the uterine tubes join the uterine body) and around the internal os. The sphincter action of this layer prevents the regurgitation of menstrual blood out of the uterine tubes during menstruation. Their sphincter action around the internal cervical os helps retain the uterine contents during pregnancy. Injury to this sphincter can weaken the internal os and result in an incompetent internal cervical os (see Chapter 23).

For clarity and interest, each muscle layer and its function were described individually. It must be remembered that the myometrium works as a whole. The structure of the myometrium, which gives strength and elasticity, presents an example of adaptation to function:

1. To thin out, pull up, and open the cervix and to push the fetus out of the uterus, the fundus must contract with the most force.
2. Contraction of interlacing smooth muscle fibers that surround the blood vessels controls blood loss after abortion and childbirth. Because of their ability to close off (ligate) blood vessels between them, the smooth muscle fibers of the uterus are referred to as the **living ligature** (Fig. 4-10).

The *parietal peritoneum,* a serous membrane, coats all the uterine corpus except for the lower one fourth of the anterior surface, where the bladder is attached, and the cervix. Because parietal peritoneum does not completely cover this organ, it is possible for diagnostic tests and surgery involving the uterus to be performed without entering the abdominal cavity.

Cervix. The lowermost portion of the uterus is the cervix, or neck. The attachment site of the uterine cervix to the vaginal vault divides the cervix into the longer supravaginal (above the vagina) portion (see Fig. 4-5) and the shorter vaginal portion (see Fig. 4-6). The length of the cervix is about 2.5 to 3 cm, of which about 1 cm protrudes into the vagina in the nongravid woman.

The cervix is composed primarily of fibrous connective tissue with some muscle fibers and elastic tissue. The cervix of the nulliparous woman is a rounded, almost conical, rather firm, spindle-shaped body approximately 2 to 2.5 cm in external diameter. The narrowed opening between the uterine cavity and the endocervical canal (canal inside the cervix that connects the uterine cavity with the vagina) is the internal os. The narrowed opening between the endocervix and the vagina is the external os. The external os is a small circular opening in women who have not borne children. Childbirth changes the circular os to a small transverse opening dividing the cervix into an anterior and a posterior lip (Fig. 4-11).

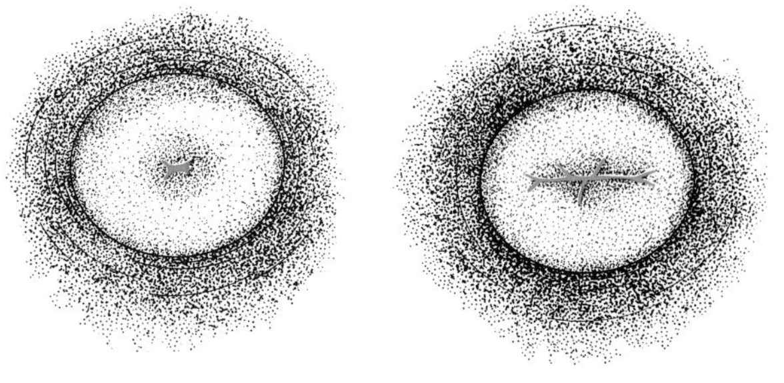

Fig. 4-11 External cervical os as seen through speculum. **A,** Nonparous cervix. **B,** Parous cervix.

When the woman is not ovulating or pregnant, the tip of the cervix feels firm, much like the end of one's nose, with a dimple in the center. The dimple marks the site of the external os.

The most significant characteristic of the cervix is its ability to stretch during vaginal childbirth. Several factors contribute to cervical elasticity: high connective tissue and elastic fiber content, numerous infoldings in the endocervical lining, and a muscle fiber content of about 10%.

Canals. There are two cavities within the uterus, which are known as the uterine and cervical canals (see Fig. 4-6). The uterine canal in the nonpregnant state is compressed by thick muscular walls so that it is only a potential space, flat and triangular in shape. The base of the triangle is formed by the fundus. The uterine tubes open into either end of the base. The apex of the triangle points downward and forms the internal os (opening) of the cervical canal.

The endocervical canal with its many infoldings has a surface layer of tall, columnar, mucus-producing cells. *Columnar epithelium* is beefy red, deeper, and rougher looking than the epithelial outer covering of the cervix. After **menarche** (the start of menstruation) *squamous epithelium* covers the outside of the cervix (ectocervix). This external covering of flat cells gives a glistening pink color to the cervix. A deeper bluish red color is seen when the woman is ovulating or pregnant. A reddened (hyperemic) cervix may indicate inflammation.

The two types of epithelium meet at the **squamocolumnar junction.** This junction line is usually just inside the external cervical os but may be found on the ectocervix in some women. The squamocolumnar junction is the most common site of neoplastic cellular changes. Therefore cells for cytologic study, the Papanicolaou smear, are scraped from this junction.

The columnar epithelial cells produce odorless and nonirritating mucus in response to ovarian endocrine hormones—estrogen and progesterone.

Blood Vessels. The abdominal aorta divides at about the level of the umbilicus and forms the two iliac arteries. Each iliac artery divides to form two arteries, the major one of which is the hypogastric artery. The uterine arteries branch off from the *hypogastric arteries*. The closeness of the uterus to the aorta ensures an ample blood supply to meet the needs of the growing uterus and conceptus.

In addition the ovarian artery, a direct subdivision of the aorta, first supplies the ovary with the blood and then proceeds to join the uterine artery, thus further adding to the blood supply (Fig. 4-12).

In the nonpregnant state the uterine blood vessels are coiled and tortuous. With advancing pregnancy and an enlarging uterus, these blood vessels straighten out. The uterine veins follow along the arteries and empty into the internal iliac veins.

Innervation. The internal genitals have a rich supply of afferent and efferent autonomic nerves, both motor and sensory.

Parasympathetic fibers from the sacral nerves are probably responsible for producing vasodilatation and inhibiting muscular contraction. Efferent sympathetic motor nerves arise from the ganglia of T-5 (thoracic 5) to T-10, come together over the sacrum, and reach the uterus through ganglia that lie near the base of the uterosacral ligaments. These efferent sympathetic motor nerves are believed to cause vasoconstriction and muscular contraction. The autonomic nerves just described (parasympathetic and efferent sympathetic motor) regulate the action of the uterus, but the uterus has an intrinsic motility (i.e., it can contract and relax even if the nerves to it are cut). This means that even if a woman suffers an accident that injures the spinal cord

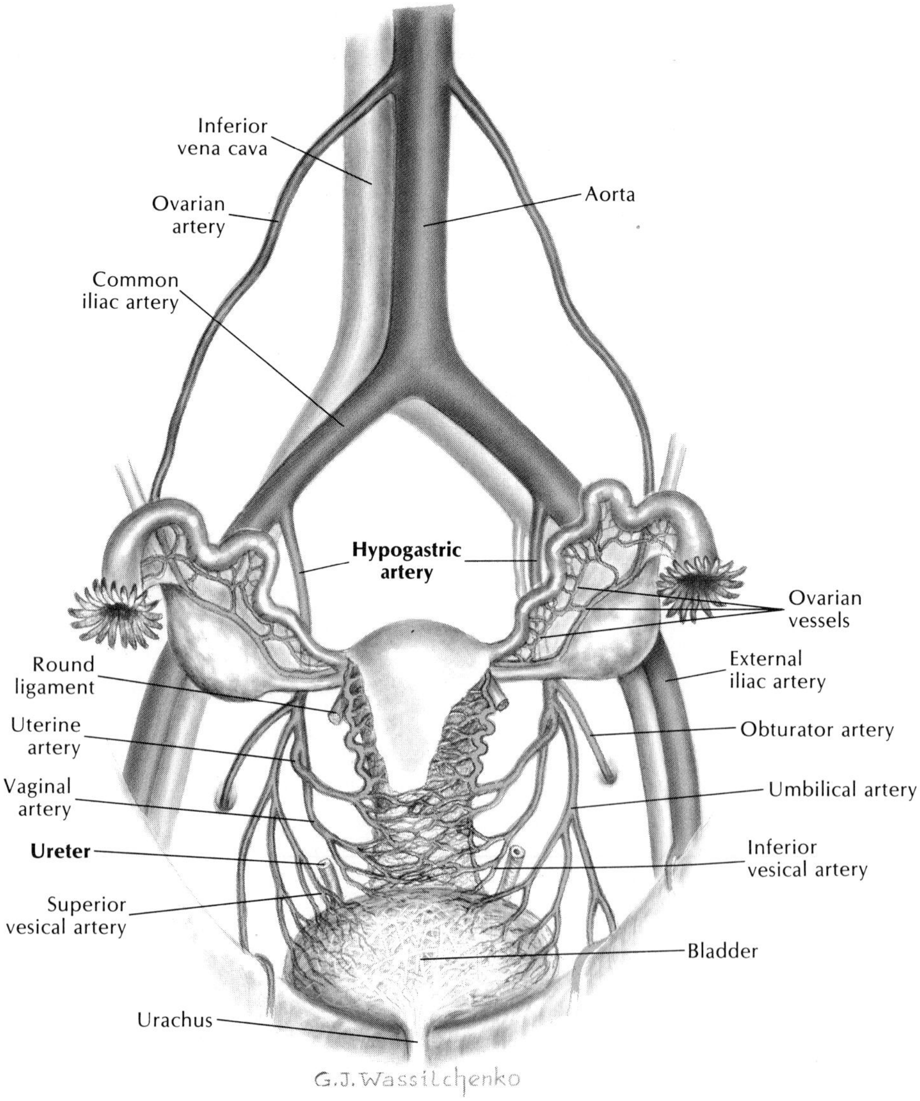

Fig. 4-12 Pelvic blood supply.

at or above T-5, she may still be able to have uterine contractions sufficient to deliver an infant vaginally (see spinal cord injury, p. 721).

Sensory fibers carrying pain sensation from the uterus come together in the paracervical areas and proceed upward to pass just below the division (bifurcation) of the aorta, and then travel to the spinal cord at the level of T-11 and T-12. Because of this arrangement, pain that originates in the ovary or in the ureters may mimic pain that originates in the uterus, any of which may be felt in the flank and down to the inguinal and vulvar areas.

Functions. The three functions of the uterus are essential for the survival of the species but not for the physiologic survival of the individual. These functions include cyclic menstruation with rejuvenation of the endometrium, pregnancy, and labor.

Vagina. The vagina is a tubular structure located in front of the rectum and behind the bladder and urethra (see Fig. 4-8). The vagina extends from the introitus, the external opening in the vestibule between the labia minora of the vulva, to the cervix. When the woman is standing, the vagina slants backward and upward. It is supported mainly by its attachments to the pelvic floor musculature and fascia.

The vagina is a thin-walled, collapsible tube capable of great distension. Because of the way the cervix protrudes into the uppermost portion of the vagina, the length of the anterior wall of the vagina is only about 7.5 cm, while that of the posterior wall is about 9 cm. The recesses formed all around the protruding cervix are called fornices: right, left, anterior, and posterior. The posterior fornix is deeper than the other three (see Figs. 4-6 and 4-15).

The smooth muscle walls are lined with glandular mucous membrane. During the reproductive years this mucosa is arranged in transverse folds called *rugae.*

The vaginal mucosa responds promptly to estrogen and progesterone stimulation. Cells are lost from the mucosa, especially during the menstrual cycle and pregnancy. Cells scraped from the vaginal mucosa can be used to estimate steroid sex hormone levels.

Vaginal fluid is derived from the lower or upper genital tract. The continuous flow of fluid from the vagina maintains relative cleanliness of the vagina. *Therefore vaginal douching in normal circumstances is not necessary.* A spread of vaginal mucus from the posterior vaginal fornix and a scraping from the squamocolumnar junction of the cervix, fixed in ethyl ether and alcohol and then treated with trichrome nucleocytoplasmic stain, constitute the *Papanicolaou (Pap) smear* used throughout the world for cancer detection by cell examination (cytology).

The copious blood supply to the vagina is derived from the descending branches of the uterine artery, the vaginal artery, and the internal pudendal arteries (see Fig. 4-12).

The vagina is relatively insensitive. There is some innervation from the pudendal and hemorrhoidal nerves to the lowest one third. Because of this minimal innervation and lack of special nerve endings, the vagina is the source of little sensation during sexual excitement and coitus and causes less pain during the second stage of labor than if this tissue were well supplied with nerve endings.

The *G-spot* is an area on the anterior vaginal wall beneath the urethra defined by Graefenberg as analogous to the male prostate gland. During sexual arousal it may be stimulated to the point of orgasm with ejaculation into the urethra of fluid similar in nature to prostatic fluid (Droegemueller et al, 1987).

The vagina functions as the organ for copulation (coitus) and as the birth canal.

Pelvic Floor and Perineum. The pelvic floor and perineum are composed of the pelvic diaphragm, the urogenital diaphragm or triangle, and the muscles of the external genitals and anus. The perineum is sometimes defined as including all the muscles, fascia, and ligaments of the upper (pelvic) and lower (urogenital) diaphragms. The perineal body adds strength to these structures.

The *upper pelvic diaphragm,* composed of muscles and their fascia and ligaments, extends across the lowest part of the pelvic cavity like a hammock (Fig. 4-13). The largest and most significant portion of the diaphragm is formed by the pair of broad, thin *levator ani muscles* that extend sheetlike between the ischial spines and coccyx, and the sacrum. The levator ani group of muscles is made up of three muscle pairs: puborectalis, iliococcygeus, and pubococcygeus muscles. The pubococcygeus muscle is particularly significant for women. It plays a role in sexual sensory function, in bladder control, in controlling perineal relaxation during labor, and in expulsion of the fetus during birth.

The second paired muscles of the upper pelvic diaphragm are the closely joined *coccygeus muscles.* These muscles extend from the ischial spines to the coccyx and lower sacrum. The several parts of the pelvic diaphragm provide a slinglike support to abdominal and pelvic viscera.

The strength and resilience of this sling are derived from the way in which the layered parts of this sling are interwoven and interlaced. *The layers are not fixed; that is, they slide over each other.* This unique arrangement strengthens the supportive capacity of the pelvic diaphragm, allows for dilatation of the vagina during the birth process and for its closure after delivery, and assists with constriction of the urethra, vagina, and anal canal, which pass through the diaphragm.

The *lower pelvic diaphragm* is located in the hollow

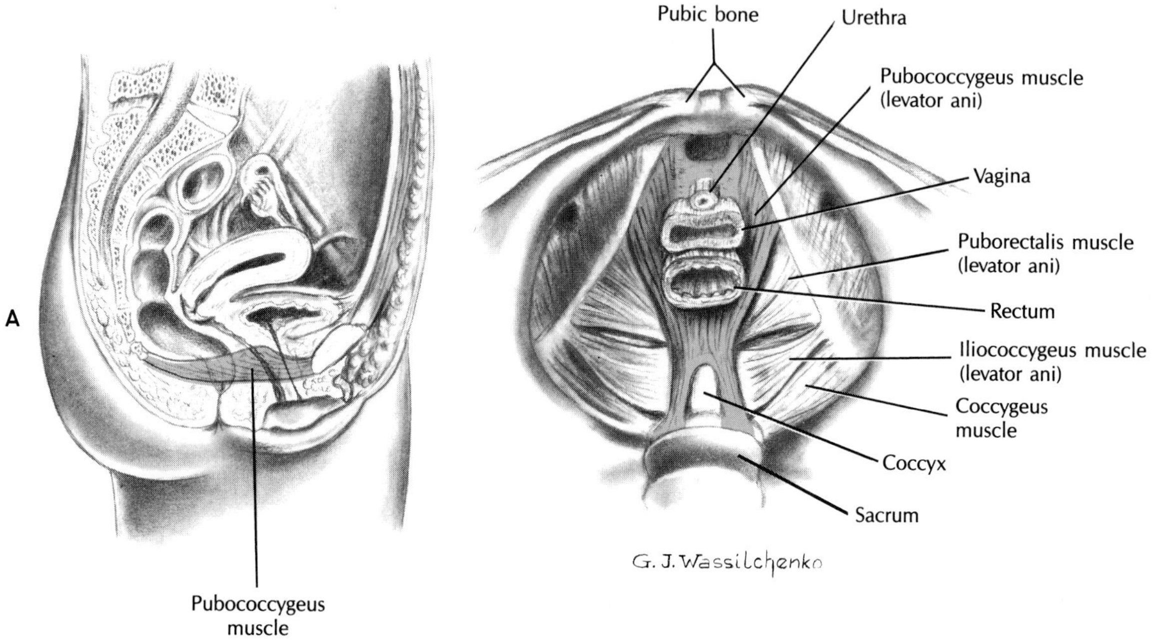

Fig. 4-13 Upper pelvic diaphragm. **A,** Pubococcygeus portion of the levator muscles, midsagittal view. **B,** View from above.

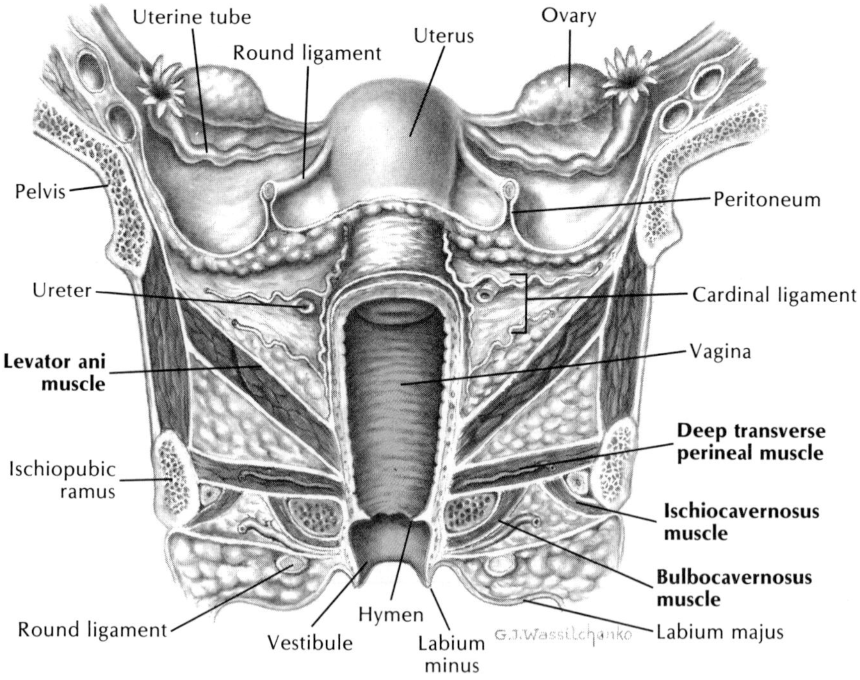

Fig. 4-14 Levator ani muscles of upper pelvic diaphragm and urogenital (lower pelvic) diaphragm, anterior view.

of the pubic arch and consists of the transverse perineal muscles, which originate at the ischial tuberosities and insert into the perineal body. The strong muscle fibers provide support to the anal canal during defecation and to the lower vagina during delivery. The deep transverse perineal muscles join to form a central seam, or raphe. Some of their fibers encircle the urinary meatus and vaginal sphincters.

The *perineum* is located below the upper and lower pelvic diaphragm. Its muscles and fascia reinforce the strength of the pelvic diaphragm and aid in constricting the urinary, vaginal, and anal openings. The *bulbocavernosus muscle* (Fig. 4-14) fibers originate in the perineal body and surround the vaginal opening as the muscle fibers pass forward to insert into the pubis.

The *ischiocavernosus muscles* originate in the tuberosities of the ischium and continue at an angle to insert next to the bulbocavernosus muscles (see Fig. 4-14). These muscle fibers contract to cause erection of the clitoris.

Anal sphincter muscle fibers originate at the coccyx, separate to pass on either side of the anus, fuse, and then insert into the transverse perineal muscles.

The bulbocavernosus, transverse perineal, and anal sphincter muscle fibers can be strengthened through Kegel's exercises (see Chapter 10).

The *perineal body,* the wedge-shaped mass between the vaginal and anal openings, serves as an anchor point for the muscles, fascia, and ligaments of the upper and lower pelvic diaphragms (Fig. 4-15). The skin-covered base of the body is known as the perineum. The perineal body, about 4 cm wide by 4 cm deep, is continuous with the septum between the rectum and vagina. This tissue is flattened and stretched as the fetus moves through the birth canal.

Bony Pelvis. The nurse needs to be thoroughly familiar with the bony pelvis to understand the female reproductive tract and perineum. The pelvis serves three primary purposes: (1) Its bony cavity produces a protective cradle for pelvic structures. (2) Its architecture is of special importance in accommodating a growing fetus throughout pregnancy and during the birth process. (3) Its strength provides stable anchorage for the attachment of supportive muscles, fascia, and ligaments.

In a study of the bony pelvis, the following structures and *landmarks* are especially important (Fig. 4-16): iliac crest and superior, anterior iliac spine; sacral promontory; sacrum; coccyx; symphysis pubis; subpubic arch; ischial spines; and ischial tuberosities.

The pelvis (Fig. 4-16, *A*) is made up of four bones: (1) and (2) the right and left innominate bones, each of which is made up of the right or left pubic bone, ilium, and ischium, which fuse after puberty; (3) the sacrum; and (4) the coccyx. The two *innominate bones* (hip bones) form the sides and front of the bony passage, and the *sacrum* and *coccyx* form the back.

Below the *ilium* is the *ischium,* a heavy bone terminating posteriorly in the rounded protuberances known as the *ischial tuberosities* (see Fig. 4-16, *B*). The tuberosities bear the body's weight in the sitting position. The *ischial spines,* the sharp projections from the posterior border of the ischium into the pelvic cavity, may be blunt or prominent.

The *pubis,* forming the front portion of the pelvic cavity, is located beneath the mons. In the midline the

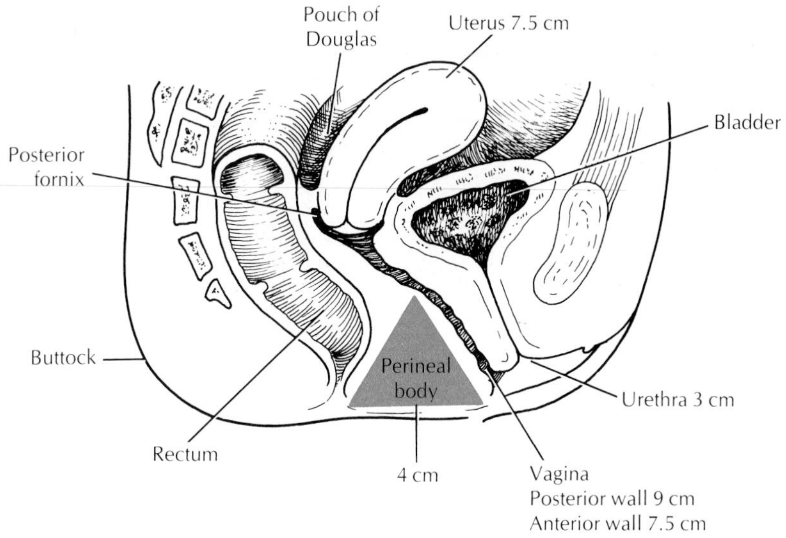

Fig. 4-15 Perineal body. Location and size relative to surrounding tissues, with woman sitting.

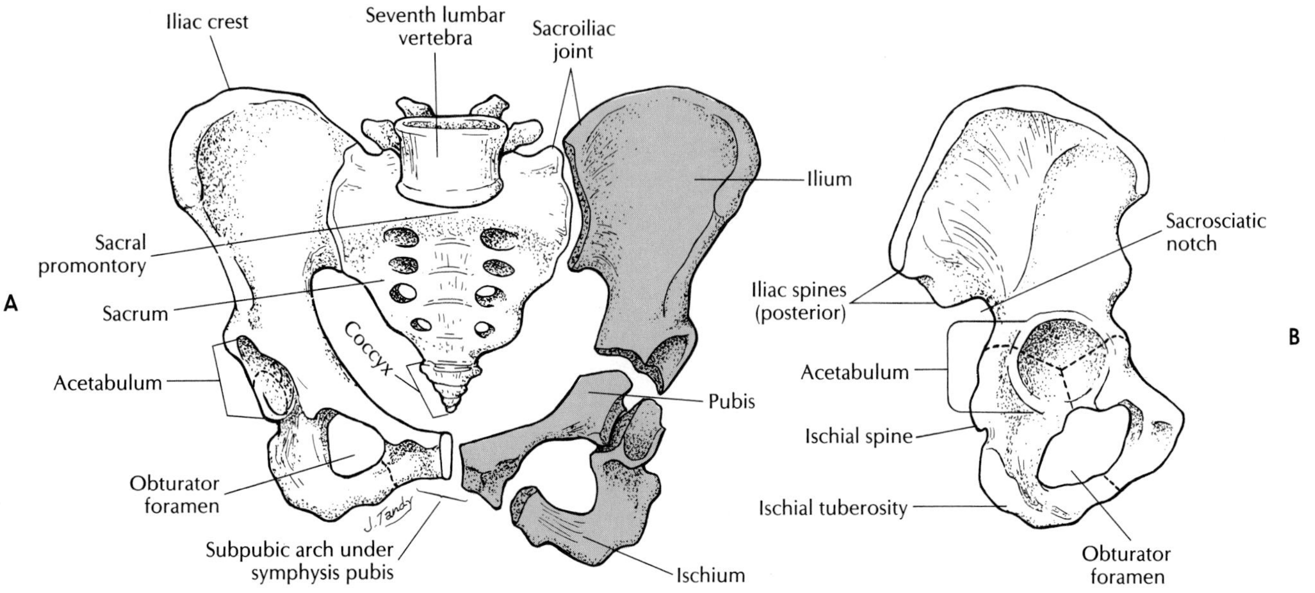

Fig. 4-16 Adult female pelvis. **A,** Anterior view. The three embryonic parts of the left innominate bone are lightly shaded. **B,** External view of right innominate bone (fused).

two pubic bones are joined by strong ligaments and a thick cartilage to form the joint called the symphysis pubis. In the female the angle formed by the subpubic arch optimally measures slightly more than 90 degrees.

The *sacrum* is formed by five fused vertebrae. The upper anterior portion of the body of the first sacral vertebra, the promontory, forms the posterior margin of the pelvic brim.

The *coccyx* (tailbone), composed of three to five fused vertebrae, articulates with the sacrum. The coccyx projects downward and forward from the lower border of the sacrum.

The pelvis is divided into two sections, the shallow upper basin, or false pelvis, and the deeper lower, or true, pelvis (Fig. 4-17, *A*). The *false pelvis* lies above the linea terminalis (brim, inlet) and varies considerably in size in different women. The *true pelvis* consists of the brim, or inlet, and the area below.

Pelvic planes include those of the *inlet,* the *midpelvis,* and the *outlet.* The cavity of the mid true pelvis resembles an irregularly curved canal (Fig. 4-17, *B*) with unequal anterior and posterior surfaces. The anterior surface is formed by the length of the symphysis (4.5 cm). The posterior surface is formed by the length of the sacrum (12 cm).

Age, sex, and race are responsible for the greatest variations in pelvic shape and size. There is considerable change in the pelvis during growth and development. Pelvic ossification is complete at about 20 years of age or slightly later. Smaller people have smaller, lighter bones than larger people.

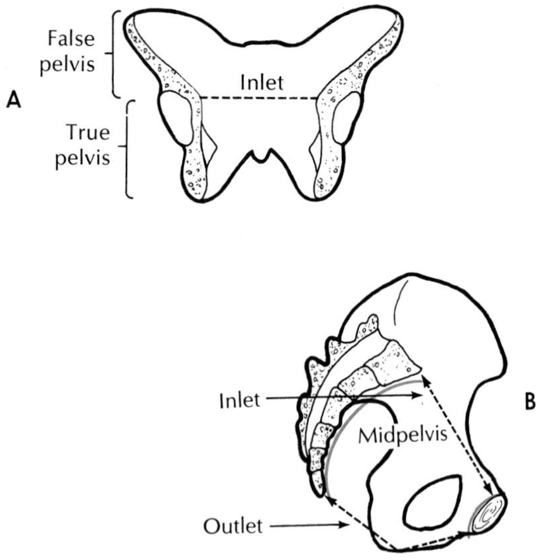

Fig. 4-17 Female pelvis. **A,** Cavity of false pelvis is shallow basin above inlet; true pelvis is deeper cavity below inlet. **B,** Cavity of true pelvis is an irregularly curved canal.

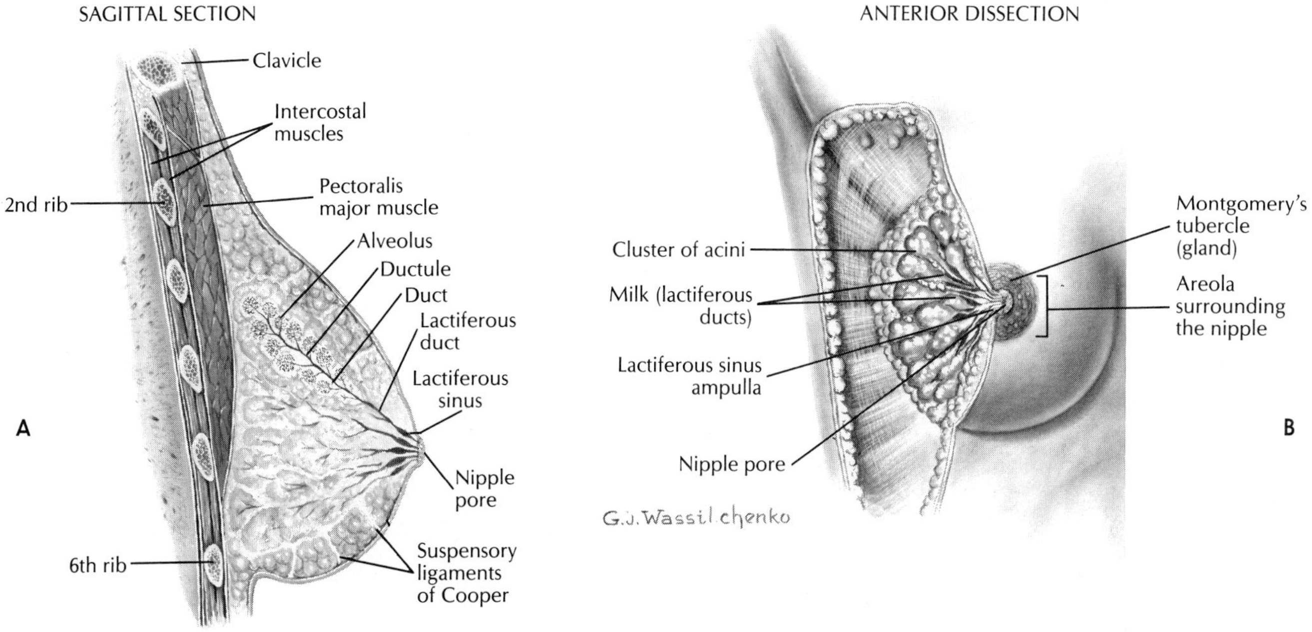

Fig. 4-18 Position and structure of mammary gland. **A,** Sagittal section. **B,** Anterior dissection. (**A,** From Seidel HM et al: Mosby's guide to physical examination, St Louis, 1987, The CV Mosby Co.)

Breasts

The breasts are paired mammary glands located between the second and sixth ribs (Fig. 4-18). About two thirds of the breast overlies the pectoralis major muscle, between the sternum and mid axillary line, with an extension to the axilla referred to as the tail of Spence. The lower one third of the breast overlies the serratus anterior muscle. The breasts are attached to the muscles by connective tissue or fascia.

The breasts of healthy mature women are approximately equal in size and shape but are often not absolutely symmetric. The size and shape vary depending on the woman's age, heredity, and nutrition. However, the contour should be smooth with no retractions, dimpling, or masses.

True glandular tissue is called *parenchyma;* supporting tissues, the fat, and fibrous connective tissue are called *stroma.* It is the relative amount of stroma that determines the size and consistency of the breast.

Estrogen stimulates growth of the breast by inducing fat deposition in the breasts, development of stromal tissue (i.e., increase in its amount and elasticity), and growth of the extensive ductile system. Estrogen also increases the vascularity of breast tissue.

Once ovulation begins in puberty, progesterone levels increase. The increase in progesterone causes maturation of mammary gland tissue, specifically the lobules and acinar structures. During adolescence fat deposition and growth of fibrous tissue contribute to the increase in the size of the gland. Full development of the breast is not achieved until after the end of the first pregnancy or in the early period of lactation.

Each mammary gland is made up of 15 to 20 lobes, which are divided into lobules. Lobules are clusters of acini. An acinus is a saclike terminal part of a compound gland emptying through a narrow lumen or duct. In discussions of mammary glands the correct anatomic term *(acinus)* is often used interchangeably with *alveolus.* The acini are lined with epithelial cells that secrete colostrum and milk. Just below the epithelium is the myoepithelium (*myo,* muscle), which contracts to expel milk from the acini (Fig. 4-19).

The ducts from the clusters of acini that form the lobules merge to form larger ducts draining the lobes. Ducts from the lobes converge in a single nipple (papilla) surrounded by an areola. Just as the ducts converge, they dilate to form common lactiferous sinuses,

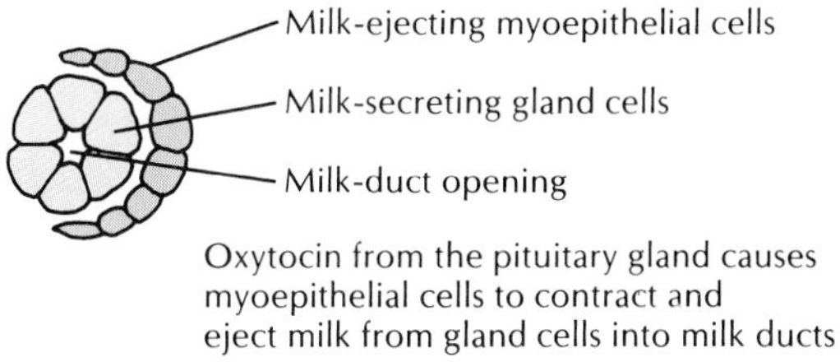

Fig. 4-19 Acinus in cross section.

which are also called ampullae. The lactiferous sinuses serve as milk reservoirs. Many tiny lactiferous ducts drain the ampullae and exit in the nipple.

The glandular structures and ducts are surrounded by protective fatty tissue and are separated and supported by fibrous suspensory *Cooper's ligaments*. Cooper's ligaments provide support to the mammary glands while permitting their mobility on the chest wall.

The round nipple is usually slightly elevated above the breast. On each breast the nipple projects slightly upward and laterally. It contains 15 to 20 openings from lactiferous ducts. The nipple (mammary papilla) is surrounded by fibromuscular tissue and covered by wrinkled skin. Except during pregnancy and lactation, there is no discharge from the nipple.

The nipple and surrounding areola are usually more deeply pigmented than the skin of the breast. The rough appearance of the areola is caused by sebaceous glands, *Montgomery tubercles* (see Fig. 4-18), directly beneath the skin. These glands secrete a fatty substance that is thought to lubricate the nipple. Smooth muscle fibers in the areola contract to stiffen the nipple to make it easier for the breastfeeding child to grasp.

Blood Vessels and Lymphatics. The vascular supply to the mammary gland is abundant. In the nonpregnant state the skin does not have an obvious vascular pattern. The normal skin is smooth without tightness or shininess.

The skin covering the breasts contains an extensive superficial lymphatic network that serves the entire chest wall and is continuous with the superficial lymphatics of the neck and abdomen. In the deeper portions of the breasts the lymphatics form a rich network as well. The primary deep lymphatic pathway drains laterally toward the axillae.

Besides their function of lactation, breasts function as organs for sexual arousal in the mature adult.

Changes in Response to the Menstrual Cycle. The breasts change in size and nodularity in response to cyclic ovarian changes throughout reproductive life. Increasing levels of both estrogen and progesterone in the 3 to 4 days before menstruation increase vascularity of the breasts, induce growth of the ducts and acini, and promote water retention. The epithelial cells lining the ducts proliferate in number, the ducts dilate, and the lobules distend. The acini become enlarged and secretory, and lipid (fat) is deposited within their epithelial cell lining. As a result, breast swelling, tenderness, and discomfort are common symptoms just before the onset of menstruation. After menstruation, cellular proliferation begins to regress, acini begin to decrease in size, and retained water is lost.

After breasts have undergone changes numerous times in response to the ovarian cycle, the proliferation and involution (regression) are not uniform throughout the breast. In time, after repeated hormonal stimulation, small persistent areas of nodulations may develop. This normal physiologic change must be remembered when breast tissue is examined. Nodules may develop just before and during menstruation, when the breast is most active. The physiologic alterations in breast size and activity reach their minimum level about 5 to 7 days after menstruation stops. Therefore breast self-examination is best carried out during this phase of the menstrual cycle (Fig. 4-20).

Menstrual Cycle

Menstrual Myths. Many myths have their origin in the mystery that surrounded the woman, her hidden reproductive organs, and her uniqueness in adding new members to society. As a consequence a vast store of folklore, fancies, and superstitions have evolved. Because of their recurring nature and similar sequence, menstrual cycles were thought to be under the control

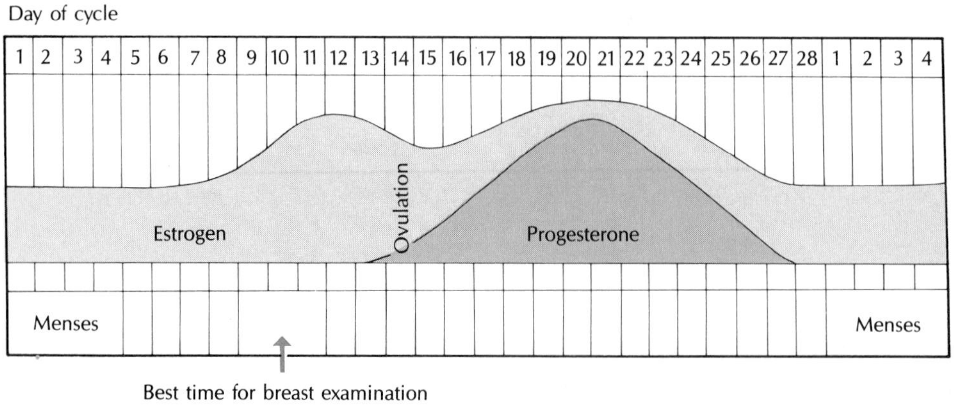

Fig. 4-20 Changes in breast tissue in response to menstrual cycle.

of the moon. Before the discovery of ovulation in humans, it was thought that an egg was produced during menstruation only when fruitful intercourse had occurred. Not until the nineteenth century was knowledge available about the existence of the human egg, ovulation, and ovarian functioning.

An awareness of some myths about menstruation is necessary to use the nursing process effectively with both female and male clients. The menstruating woman is seen as being vulnerable to physical and psychologic stress. Recall some of the myths you may have heard: "Don't wash your hair," "Don't take a bath," "Watch out, you'll catch cold," "That's too heavy for you to carry now."

As late as the second half of this century the many behavioral changes falsely attributed to women during their menstrual cycles have been used to argue, for example, why it would be unwise to have a woman for president of the United States. Historical literature contains many references to dangers attributed to menstruating women. Should a menstruating woman walk through a farmer's fields, the crops would not grow and the flowers would wilt; if she tried to bake bread, the dough would not rise. The danger also exists for her husband so that physical contact, especially sexual intercourse, was and in some places still is prohibited. In many cultures the menstruating woman is kept in a separate menstrual hut or in separate quarters. Following a ritualized "cleansing" the woman returns to her place in her family.

Menarche. Although young girls secrete small, rather constant amounts of estrogen, a marked increase occurs between 8 and 11 years of age. Moreover, increasing amounts and variations in gonadotropin and estrogen secretion develop into a cyclic pattern at least a year before menarche or the first menstrual period. This occurs in most girls in North America at about 13 years of age.

Initially periods are irregular, unpredictable, painless, and anovulatory in the majority of young girls. After one or more years a hypothalamic-pituitary rhythm develops, and adequate cyclic estrogen is produced by the ovary to mature a number of graafian follicles. Approximately 14 days *before* the beginning of the next menstrual period, pituitary follicle-stimulating hormone (FSH) rises, a surge of luteinizing hormone (LH) is released by the anterior pituitary, and ovulation (extrusion of the ovum) occurs.

Ovulatory periods tend to be regular, monitored by progesterone. In some women ovulatory periods are associated with *dysmenorrhea* (painful uterine cramping), which may be an effect of progesterone or prostaglandins or both. This discomfort is rarely serious and is readily relieved by a hot water bottle, exercise, or simple analgesics. When viewed in its proper perspective, slight cramping may be reassuring to the girl and her parents as an indication of normal ovulatory function.

Although pregnancy may occur in exceptional cases of true (constitutional) precocious puberty, most pregnancies in young girls occur well after the normally timed menarche. *However, all girls would benefit from knowing that pregnancy can occur at any time after the onset of menses.*

Endometrial Cycle. **Menstruation** is periodic uterine bleeding that begins with the shedding of secretory endometrium approximately 14 days after ovulation. The first day of the menstrual discharge has been designated as *day 1* of the **endometrial cycle.** The average duration of menstrual flow is 5 days (range of 3 to 6 days), and the average blood loss is approximately 50 ml (range of 20 to 80 ml), but there is great variation. During menstruation the average daily loss of iron is 0.5 to 1 mg. If the woman's usual blood loss is over 80 ml, she will most likely need iron supplementation to prevent secondary anemia.

For about 50% of women, menstrual blood does not appear to clot. The menstrual blood clots within the uterus, but the clot is liquefied before it is discharged from the uterus. If the discharge leaves the uterus too rapidly, liquefaction may not be complete so that clots will appear in the vagina. Uterine discharge includes mucus and epithelial cells in addition to blood.

It is generally assumed that the purpose of the menstrual cycle is to prepare the uterus for pregnancy. When pregnancy does not occur, menstruation follows. The individual's age, physical and emotional status, and environment influence the regularity of her periods.

The four phases of the menstrual cycle are (1) the menstrual phase, (2) the proliferative phase, (3) the secretory phase, and (4) the ischemic phase. During the *menstrual phase,* shedding of the functional two thirds of the endometrium (the compact and spongy layers) is initiated by periodic vasoconstriction of the spiral arterioles most marked in the upper layers of the endometrium. The basal layer is always retained, and regeneration begins near the end of the cycle from cells derived from the remaining glandular remnants or stromal cells in the basalis.

The *proliferative phase* is a period of rapid growth that extends from about the fifth day to the time of ovulation, which would be, for example, day 10 of a 24-day cycle, day 14 of a 28-day cycle, or day 18 of a 32-day cycle. The endometrial surface is completely restored in approximately 4 days or slightly before bleeding ceases. From this point on an eightfold to tenfold thickening occurs, with a leveling off of growth at ovulation. Early in the proliferative phase the functional layer is moderately dense and only slightly vascular. Three or four days before ovulation the glands develop and vascularity is increased. The proliferative phase depends on estrogen stimulation derived from ovarian (graafian) follicles.

The *secretory phase* extends from the day of ovulation to about 3 days before the next menstrual period. After ovulation, larger amounts of progesterone are produced. This hormone causes the glands to become tortuous, serrated, and widened. An edematous, vascular, functional endometrium is now apparent. The cells lining the glands secrete a thin, glycogen-containing fluid.

At the end of the secretory phase the fully matured secretory endometrium reaches the thickness of heavy, soft velvet. It becomes luxuriant with blood and glandular secretions, a suitable protective and nutritive bed for a fertilized ovum, should one be available.

Implantation (nidation) of the fertilized ovum generally occurs about 7 to 10 days after ovulation. If fertilization and implantation do not occur, the corpus luteum (yellow body) regresses. With the rapid fall in progesterone and estrogen levels the spiral arteries go into a spasm. During the *ischemic phase* the blood supply to the functional endometrium is blocked and necrosis develops. The functional layer separates from the basal layer, and menstrual bleeding begins, marking day 1 of the next cycle.

Hypothalamic-Pituitary Cycle. Toward the end of the normal menstrual cycle, blood levels of estrogen and progesterone fall. Low blood levels of these ovarian hormones stimulate the hypothalamus to secrete gonadotropin-releasing hormone (Gn-RH). Gn-RH in turn stimulates anterior pituitary secretion of FSH. FSH stimulates development of ovarian graafian follicles and their production of estrogen. Estrogen levels begin to fall, and hypothalamic Gn-RH triggers the anterior pituitary release of LH. A marked surge of LH and a smaller peak of estrogen precede the expulsion of the ovum from the graafian follicle by about 24 to 36 hours. LH peaks about the thirteenth or fourteenth day of a 28-day cycle. If fertilization and implantation (nidation) of the ovum have not occurred by this time, regression of the corpus luteum follows. Therefore the levels of progesterone and estrogen decline, menstruation occurs, and the hypothalamus is once again stimu-

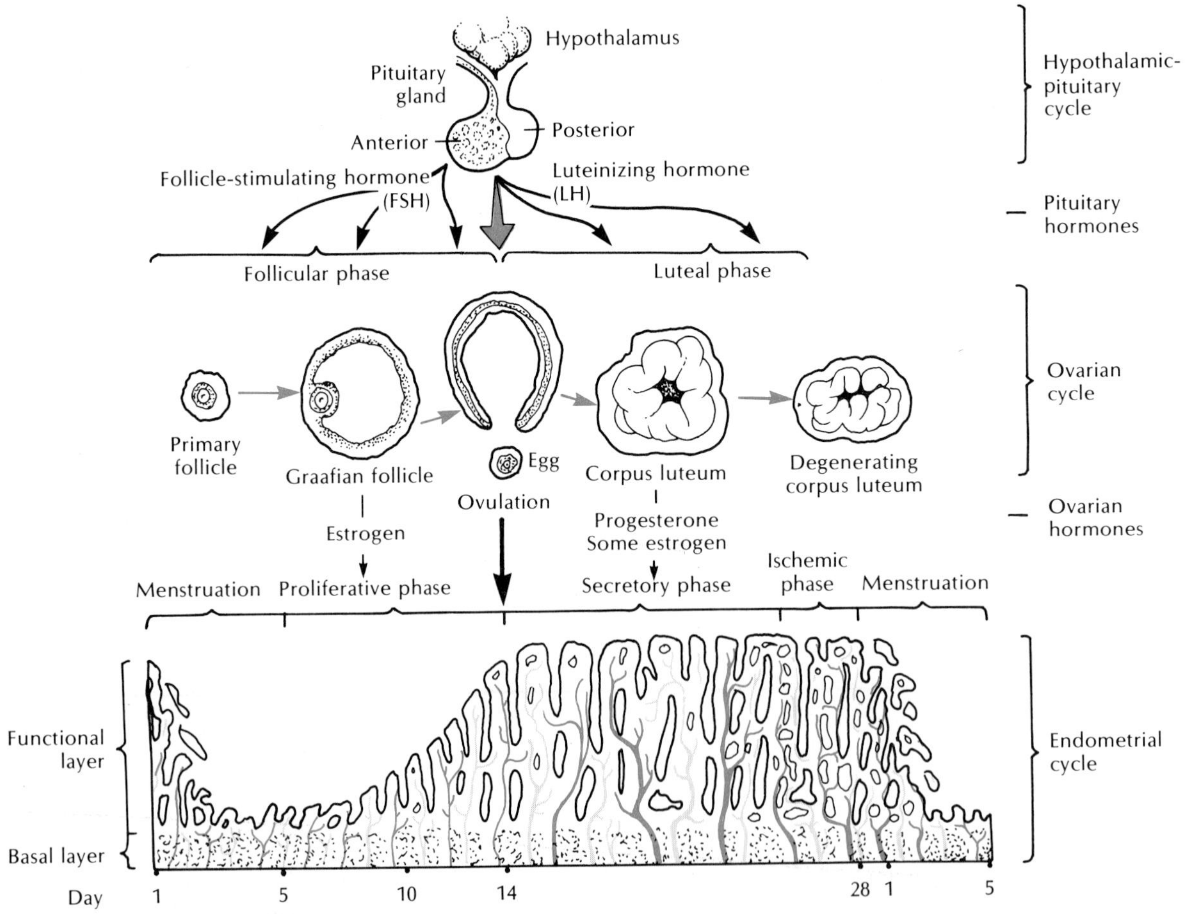

Fig. 4-21 Menstrual cycle.

lated to secrete Gn-RH. This is called the **hypothalamic-pituitary cycle.**

Ovarian Cycle. The primitive graafian follicles contain immature oocytes (primordial ova; see Fig. 4-4). Before ovulation, from 1 to 30 follicles begin to mature in each ovary under the influence of FSH and estrogen. The preovulatory surge of LH affects a selected follicle. Within the chosen follicle the oocyte matures, ovulation occurs, and the empty follicle begins its transformation into the corpus luteum. This *follicular phase* (preovulatory phase; Fig. 4-21) of the ovarian menstrual cycle varies in length from woman to woman. *Almost all variations in* ***ovarian cycle*** *length are the result of variations in the length of the follicular phase.* On rare occasions (1 in 100 menstrual cycles), more than one follicle is chosen and more than one oocyte matures and undergoes ovulation (see discussion of twins, Chapter 7).

After ovulation, estrogen levels drop. For 90% of women, only a small amount of **withdrawal bleeding** occurs so that it goes unnoticed. In 10% of women there is sufficient bleeding for it to be visible, resulting in what is known as *midcycle bleeding.*

The *luteal phase* begins immediately after ovulation and ends with the start of menstruation. This postovulatory phase of the ovarian cycle usually requires *14 days* (range of 13 to 15 days). The corpus luteum reaches its peak of functional activity 8 days after ovulation, secreting both of the steroids, estrogen and progesterone. Coincident with this time of peak luteal functioning the fertilized egg is implanted in the endometrium. If no implantation occurs, the corpus luteum regresses, and steroid levels drop. Two weeks after ovulation, if fertilization and implantation do not occur, the functional layer of the uterine endometrium is shed through menstruation.

Other Cyclic Changes. When the hypothalamic-pituitary-ovarian axis is functioning properly, other tissues undergo predictable responses. Before ovulation the woman's basal body temperature (BBT) is lower, often below 37° C (98.6° F); after ovulation, with rising progesterone levels, her BBT rises (see also Chapter 6). Changes in the cervix and cervical mucus follow a generally predictable pattern (Figs. 4-22 and 4-23). Preovulatory and postovulatory mucus is viscous (sticky) so that sperm penetration is discouraged. At

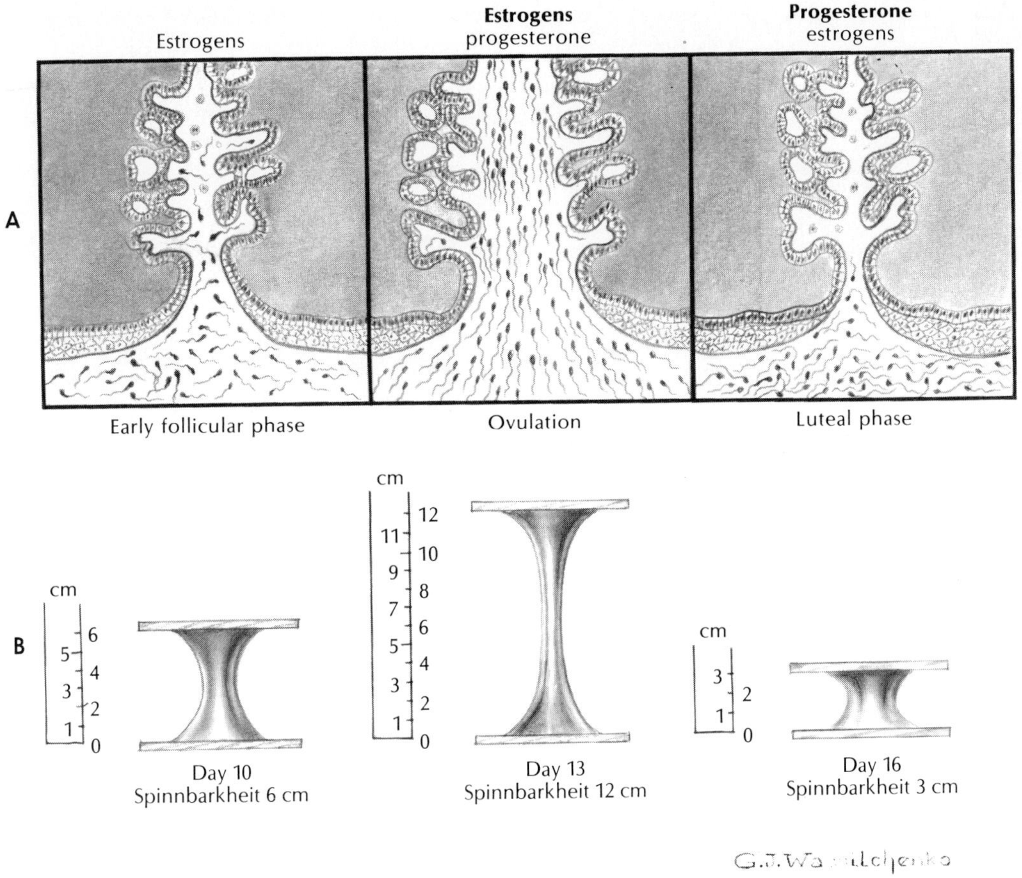

Fig. 4-22 Changes in cervix and in cervical mucus during menstrual cycle. **A,** Changes in opening of the cervix that facilitate sperm migration. **B,** Characteristic stretchable quality of cervical mucus demonstrated between two glass slides.

the time of ovulation, cervical mucus is thin and clear. It looks, feels, and stretches like egg white. This stretchable quality is termed **spinnbarkheit** (Fig. 4-22). Some women experience localized lower abdominal pain called **mittelschmerz** that coincides with ovulation.

These and other cyclic changes enhance fertility awareness and form the basis for the symptothermal method used for conception and contraception. The subjective and objective signs are biologic markers of the phases of the menstrual cycle (Table 4-1). Examination of women with impaired fertility includes a thorough documentation of the presence or absence of these biologic markers (Chapter 6).

Climacterium. The **climacterium** (perimenopause) is a transitional phase during which ovarian function and hormone production are declining. This phase spans the years from the onset of premenopausal ovarian decline to the postmenopausal time when symptoms stop. **Menopause** (from the French *meno,* menstruation, and *pause,* stop) refers only to the last menstrual period. However, unlike menarche, menopause can be dated with certainty only at 1 year after menstruation ceases. The average age at natural menopause is 51.4 years, with a range of 35 to 60 years. Menopause is an unmistakable biologic marker for the end of reproductive function.

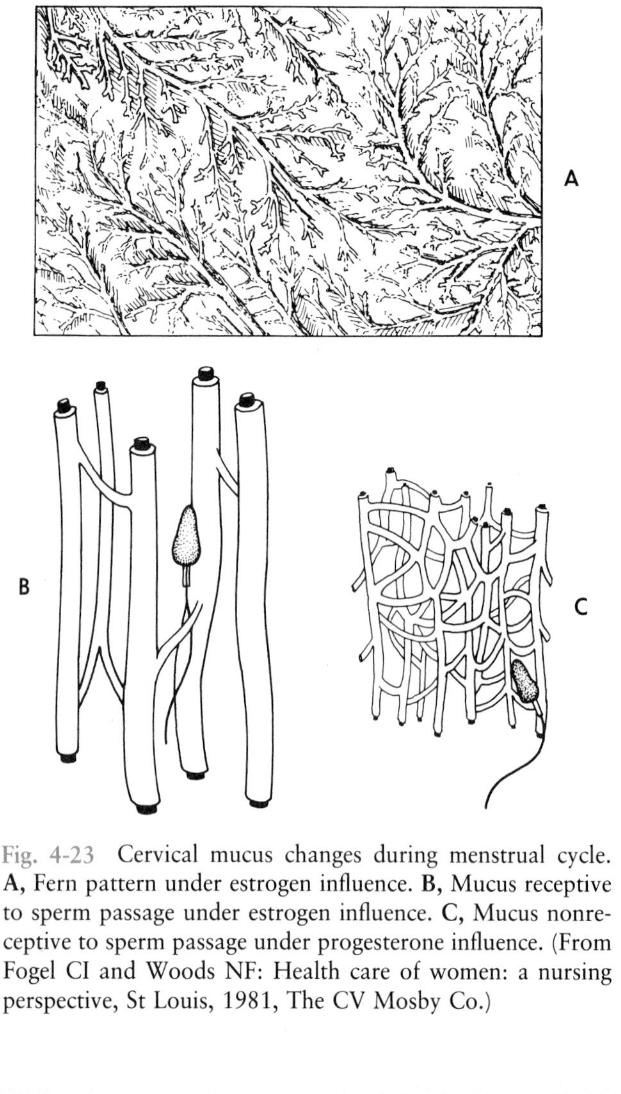

Fig. 4-23 Cervical mucus changes during menstrual cycle. **A,** Fern pattern under estrogen influence. **B,** Mucus receptive to sperm passage under estrogen influence. **C,** Mucus nonreceptive to sperm passage under progesterone influence. (From Fogel CI and Woods NF: Health care of women: a nursing perspective, St Louis, 1981, The CV Mosby Co.)

Changes in reproductive organs and hormones occurring during the climacterium may be viewed as cessation of endocrine events that began at puberty (Fig. 4-24). One of the initiating events of the climacterium may be the diminishing number of primordial follicles in the ovary. During the reproductive period, 400 to 500 follicles mature and several thousand more atrophy. Eventually fewer and fewer follicles exist, producing less and less estrogen, and fewer and fewer corpus lutea are present, producing less and less progesterone. The level of gonadal hormone production decreases gradually, until there is no longer enough to stimulate endometrial growth and initiate endometrial sloughing. Circulating pituitary gonadotropin levels rise as ovarian hormone concentrations decrease. Levels of FSH and LH remain high after menopause has occurred.

Diminishing levels of ovarian estrogen gradually affect target organs. The cells of reproductive organs and surrounding tissues shrink in size or atrophy slowly. The *uterus* becomes smaller in size or involutional. The endometrium becomes thinner. *Menstrual cycles* become irregular or cease abruptly. Several patterns of irregular menstrual cycles may occur. Some women state that their menses come regularly but are lighter and last fewer days. Other women note that they may skip one cycle every few months. A few women describe irregular cycles that are also heavier in flow.

As estrogen stimulation is withdrawn from the muscles that support the uterus, the *levator ani* (see Figs. 4-13 and 4-14), which already may have been stretched or torn during childbirth, undergoes further relaxation and loss of tone. The *vaginal walls* grow thinner, smoother, and shorter. The *vestibular glands* (see Fig. 4-3) produce less mucus. Lubrication during coitus takes longer, since the vagina produces less fluid. The *labia* lose subcutaneous fat.

Urethral atrophy is related to withdrawal of ovarian hormones. The terminal portion of the *urethra* has the same embryonic origin as the vagina. Consequently the cells of the distal urethra shrink in size, shortening the urethra after menopause. *Bladder walls* become thin, and bladder support weakens.

Estrogen and calcitonin are needed to maintain equilibrium between the breaking down or resorption of bone and continuous bone formation. Estrogen inhibits bone resorption by raising calcitonin levels, which control the rate of bone formation. Decreasing estrogen levels lower calcitonin concentration. Concurrently lev-

Table 4-1 Signs and Symptoms of the Phases of the Menstrual Cycle

Sign	Preovulation	Ovulation	At Least 2 Days After Ovulation up to Menses
SUBJECTIVE SIGNS			
Physical discomfort			
Breasts	Unreported	Unreported	Heaviness, fullness; enlarged, tender*
Abdomen	Dysmenorrhea: uterine cramping; nausea, vomiting, and diarrhea; dizziness	Intermenstrual pain (mittelschmerz) occurs 1.7 days after peak of cervical mucus and 2.5 days before increase in BBT	Premenstrual syndrome: backaches; feeling of increasing pelvic fullness
General	Increased weight; feeling of heaviness	Unreported	Headache†; acne
Affective changes‡			
Moods	Some depression may persist from premenses	Sense of well-being	Premenstrual syndrome (PMS): increased irritability, passivity, depression
Libido	Unreported	Increases sexual desire	Unreported
Energy levels	Unreported	Unreported	Spurt of energy, followed by fatigue
OBJECTIVE SIGNS			
BBT	Individualized, often below 37° C (98.6° F)	Slight drop in BBT	Rise of about 0.2-0.4° C (0.4°-0.8° F)
Respiration	Unreported	Unreported	Hyperventilation with decrease in alveolar P_{CO_2}
Heart rate	Unreported	Unreported	Increased slightly
Breasts	Time of least hormonal effect and smallest breast size	Increased nipple erectility; increased areolar pigmentation	Increased nodularity; enlarged
Cervix (see Figs. 4-22 and 4-23) Mucus characteristics	"Dry" (no mucus) progressing to viscous, opaque; no ferning	Abundant, thin, clear (egg white) mucus with spinnbarkheit (4 cm often up to 10 cm) that dries in a fern pattern (arborization); facilitates sperm transport	Cloudy, sticky, impenetrable to sperm; dries in granular pattern (no ferning)
Mucus pH	About 7.0	7.5	Unreported
Os	Gradual, progressive widening	Open, with mucus seen spilling out	Gradual closing of os
Color of exocervix	Pink	Hyperemic (red)	Gradual return to pink
Body	Firm to touch (like tip of nose)	Soft (like earlobe)	Gradual return to firm

*Sociocultural influences may affect symptoms reported by women. Breast tenderness is rarely reported by Japanese women.

†Headaches reported with greater frequency by Nigerian women.

‡NOTE: Literature usually attributes negative premenstrual symptoms to biology, while good moods and rational behavior are not. When men and women are compared in activity patterns, mood changes, and symptoms, similar variability has been found in *both* men and women even though the changes in women are given more attention by society.

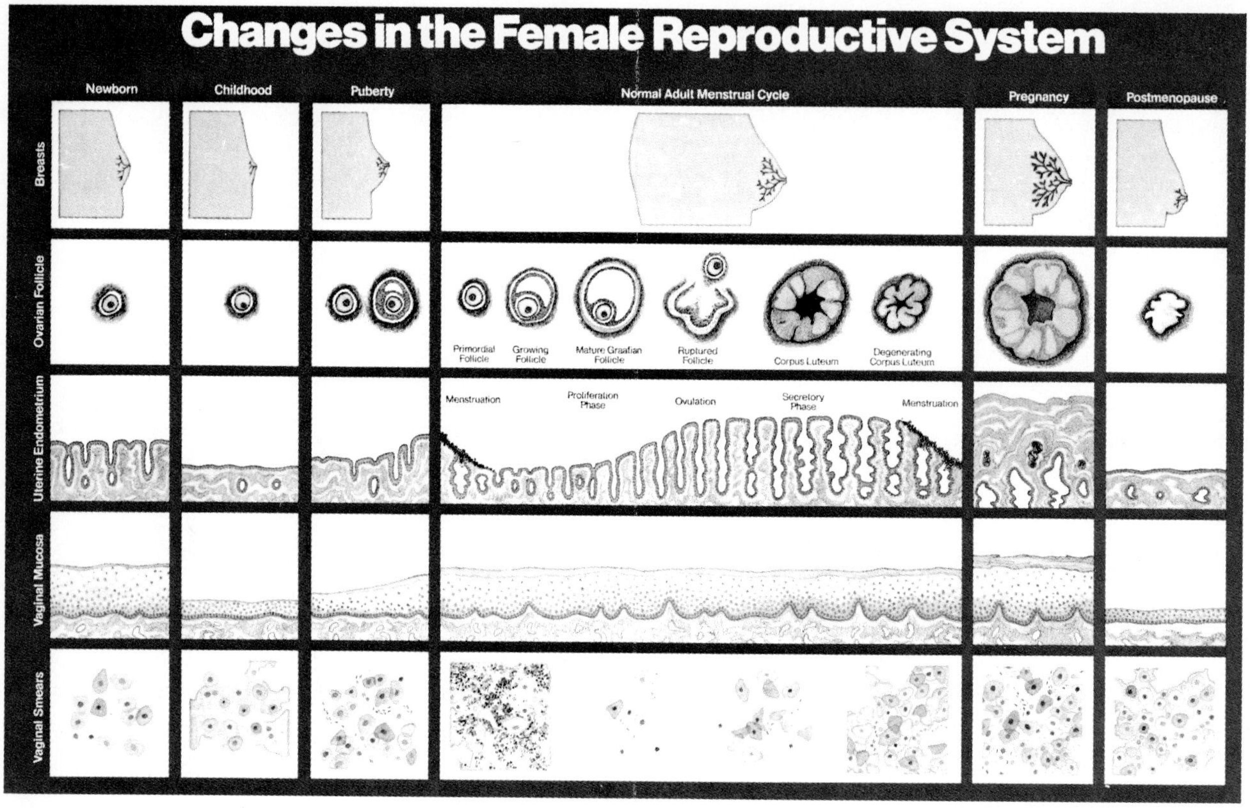

Fig. 4-24 Summary of changes in female reproductive system over life span. (Courtesy Merrill-National Laboratories, Division of Richardson-Merrill, Inc, Cincinnati.)

els of parathyroid hormone rise, enhancing bone breakdown. Estrogen also increases the metabolism of vitamin D, which is essential for absorption of calcium from the intestine; as estrogen levels decline, calcium uptake declines. As a result, *bone density* decreases.

Vasomotor instability, evidenced by hot flushes ("hot flashes"), can be annoying. The dilatation of blood vessels may be caused by surges of anterior pituitary hormones (FSH or LH), which would connect hot flushes with hormonal disturbances in the hypothalamus, the heat regulatory center of the brain. An accompanying release of prostaglandins may contribute to dilatation of the blood vessels.

Later in the postmenopausal period the outer portion of the ovary ceases production of hormones. The ovarian core produces a male hormone, testosterone. Following menopause the female hormone influence declines, while the male hormone influence remains static or increases in response to high levels of FSH and LH. At this time some women may note a growth of dark, coarse facial hairs on the chin, as well as increased amounts of fuzzy facial hair. After the ovarian core ceases to function, the adrenal gland is the sole producer of steroid hormones.

Menstrual Disorders

Dysmenorrhea. Dysmenorrhea, painful menstruation, is one of the most common gynecologic problems in women of all ages. **Primary dysmenorrhea** occurs in the absence of organic disease; the initial episode occurs when ovulation begins, about 6 to 12 months after menarche. **Secondary dysmenorrhea** is associated with organic pelvic disease.

Primary dysmenorrhea begins when the ovary is fully developed, ova mature, and progestin is secreted; it often improves by age 25 or following pregnancy with vaginal delivery. Although psychogenic factors may be significant in the perception of and reaction to dysmenorrhea, a physiologic basis exists. Discomfort depends on ovulation; it does not occur when ovulation is suppressed.

If ovulation occurs, during the progesterone-induced luteal phase and subsequent menstrual flow, prostaglandin F_2 alpha ($PGF_{2\alpha}$) is found. Excessive secretion and subsequent excessive release of $PGF_{2\alpha}$ during menstrual shedding of the endometrium increase the amplitude and frequency of uterine contractions. Pain is described as a low abdominal pain. Cramplike cyclic aching of dysmenorrhea results from ischemia after strong muscle contractions. Increased production of $PGF_{2\alpha}$ may be responsible for systemic responses such as aching (back, lower abdomen, thighs), gastrointestinal symptoms (anorexia, nausea, vomiting, diarrhea) (Heitkemper, Shauer, and Mitchell, 1988), central nervous system (CNS) symptoms (dizziness, syncope, headache, poor concentration), weakness, and sweats. The initial event that causes prostaglandin release to precipitate symptoms remains unknown (Lublanezki and Fischer, 1987).

Secondary dysmenorrhea occurs in association with pathologic changes such as endometriosis (Chapter 6), pelvic inflammatory disease, cervical stenosis, uterine or ovarian neoplasms or uterine polyps. The presence of an intrauterine device (IUD) is also a factor. Pregnancy must be ruled out to avoid confusion with complications of early pregnancy.

For some women heat (heating pad, hot bath), massage, distraction, exercise, and sleep are sufficient to achieve relief for primary dysmenorrhea. Heat is especially effective because it reduces muscle tone and increases circulation; both effects relieve ischemia. For some women **orgasm** brings relief. Uterine contractions of orgasm facilitate menstrual flow and relieve pelvic vasocongestion. The pleasurable experience of orgasm can reduce tension and increase the woman's sense of well-being. The addition of natural diuretics to the diet helps some women reduce edema and related discomforts. Asparagus, parsley, and caffeine have a diuretic effect.

Several over-the-counter (OTC) menstrual pain preparations are available (Lublanezki and Fischer, 1987). Aspirin, a mild inhibitor of prostaglandin synthesis, may provide sufficient relief. Acetaminophen is useful for relief of noninflammatory pain associated with primary dysmenorrhea (Sohn, Korberly, and Tannenbaum, 1986). Relief is usually obtained with the recommended dosage, 650 mg every 4 hours not to exceed 4000 mg in a 24-hour period. Ibuprofen (Motrin, Advil, Nuprin) also inhibits prostaglandin synthesis. In doses of 200 to 400 mg every 4 to 6 hours, ibuprofen is rated as superior to aspirin and acetaminophen as an analgesic by most women (Lublanezki and Fischer, 1987). These prostaglandin-synthesis* inhibitors are most effective if started several days before the onset of the menstrual flow. However, this could expose an early pregnancy to the drugs. Other commonly used prostaglandin-synthesis inhibitors include naproxen (Naprosyn and Anaprox) and mefenamic acid (Ponstel) (Droegemueller et al, 1987).

Some products, such as Cope and Midol, contain both aspirin and caffeine; Midol also contains cinnamedrine, a mild uterine relaxant. Many products contain pamabrom, which is similar to caffeine in its diuretic effect. Pyrilamine maleate, an antihistamine, is also in many OTC products. Its mechanism of action is unknown and has some sedative and analgesic effect. Pyrilamine is marketed only in combination with a diuretic or with a diuretic and analgesic.

Surgical intervention may be indicated as a last resort for women with intractable dysmenorrhea. Presacral neurectomy or sympathectomy brings relief to 70% of women who undergo the surgery.

Premenstrual Syndrome (PMS). **Premenstrual syndrome** (PMS) refers to a diffuse, loosely defined set of both physical and behavioral symptoms that begins approximately 7 to 10 days before menses and ends with the onset of menses (Table 4-2). Commonly there

*Prostaglandin-synthesis inhibitors block the effect of prostaglandins on tissue.

Table 4-2 **Dysmenorrhea and Premenstrual Syndrome (PMS): Comparison of Onset and Duration, Range of Response, and Incidence**

	Dysmenorrhea	PMS
Onset and duration	Acute 24-48 hr before or coincident with onset of menses, with pelvic pain that decreases or ends with end of menses	Diffuse 7-10 days before menses, resolves with onset of menses
Range of response	From mild to severe and disabling for 24-48 hr	From awareness of physiologic changes to incapacitation or disruption of life-style
Incidence	Some discomfort; 80% of all women Severe enough to interfere with normal activities for 1-2 days: 35% of older adolescents; 25% of college women; 60%-70% of single women in their 30s and 40s Incapacitation: 10% of all women	5%-95% of all women

is a positive family history for PMS, although the relative influence of heredity versus environment is unclear.

PMS may be expressed positively in heightened creativity and ability to concentrate and in increased mental and physical activity. However, these reactions receive little notice in the media or literature.

For most people PMS refers to the variety of negative symptoms, among which are those related to edema or emotional instability: abdominal distension or bloating, pelvic fullness, swelling of extremities, breast tenderness, weight gain, irritability, depression, crying spells, insomnia, fatigue, feelings of unreality and panic, headache, and backache (Droegemueller et al, 1987). Some women feel more sexually arousable, whereas others react with indifference to even the thought of sex. For a small percentage of women PMS is so incapacitating that their normal activities are totally disrupted for 1 to 2 or more days during each cycle.

In part because of the elusiveness of the cause of PMS, there is little agreement and great variety in methods of management. Data from a careful, detailed history and a daily log of somatic symptoms and mood fluctuations spanning several cycles give direction to a plan for management. Cultural affective influences must be separated from physiologic influences (Fogel and Woods, 1981).

Psychosocial aspects may be the first priority for care. Support groups may affect the self-esteem of women with PMS (Walton and Youngkin, 1987). Lack of understanding of PMS may stress relationships to the breaking point. Couple counseling is scheduled before the anticipated onset of PMS.

Medications may be required for relief from some distress, for example, diuretics for edema. A well-balanced diet low in sodium or with addition of naturally diuretic foods may ease some symptoms.

Table 4-2 presents a comparison of onset and duration, range of response, and incidence of dysmenorrhea and PMS.

❑ MALE REPRODUCTIVE SYSTEM

The male reproductive system consists of external genitals and internal organs, located in the pelvic cavity. The male's reproductive system begins to develop

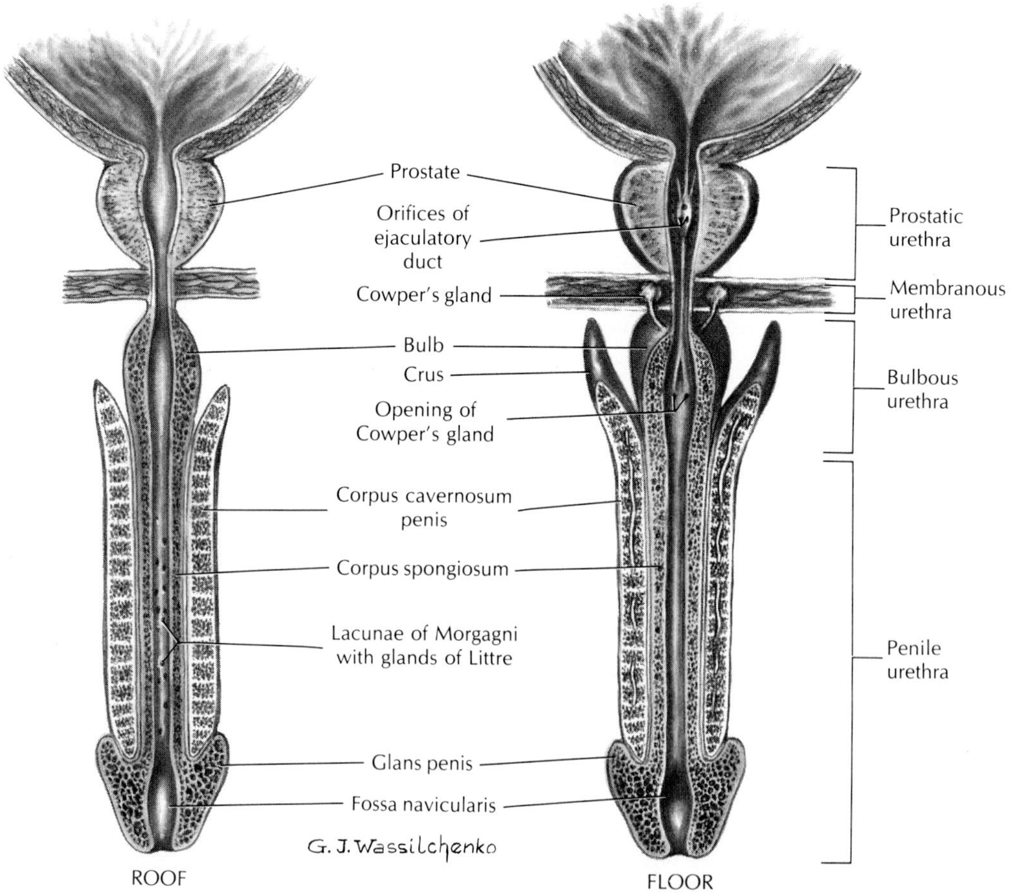

Fig. 4-25 Anatomy of urethra and penis.

in response to testosterone during early fetal life. Essentially no testosterone is produced during childhood. Resumption of testosterone production at the onset of puberty stimulates growth and maturation of reproductive structures and secondary sex characteristics.

External Structures

The structures that make up the external genitals are presented in the following order:

1. Mons pubis
2. Penis
3. Scrotum

At maturity, pubic hair is long, dense, coarse, and curly over the symphysis pubis. It is referred to as the *mons pubis.*

The *penis,* an organ of urination and copulation, consists of the shaft or body and the glans (Fig. 4-25). The shaft of this external male reproductive organ, which enters the vagina during coitus, is composed of three cylindric layers and erectile tissue, two lateral *corpora cavernosa* and a *corpus spongiosum,* which contains the urethra. These corpora terminate distally in the smooth, sensitive *glans penis,* which is the counterpart of the female glans clitoris.

Skin and fascia loosely envelop the penis to permit enlargement during erection. The glans is the enlarged end of the penis that contains many sensitive nerve endings and a urethral meatus at the tip (usually). The *prepuce* (foreskin), an extended fold of skin, covers the glans in uncircumcised males (Fig. 4-26). In the newborn the foreskin is generally not retractable and may not be retractable for 4 to 6 months or even as long as 13 years. It is easily retractable in the adolescent and the adult. With sexual arousal, neurocirculatory factors cause considerable increase in blood flow to the erectile tissue of the corpora, and enlargement and erection of the penis occur.

The *urethra* is a common passageway for both urine and semen (see Figs. 4-25 and 4-26).

The *scrotum,* a wrinkled pouch of skin, muscles, and fascia (see Fig. 4-26), is divided internally by a sep-

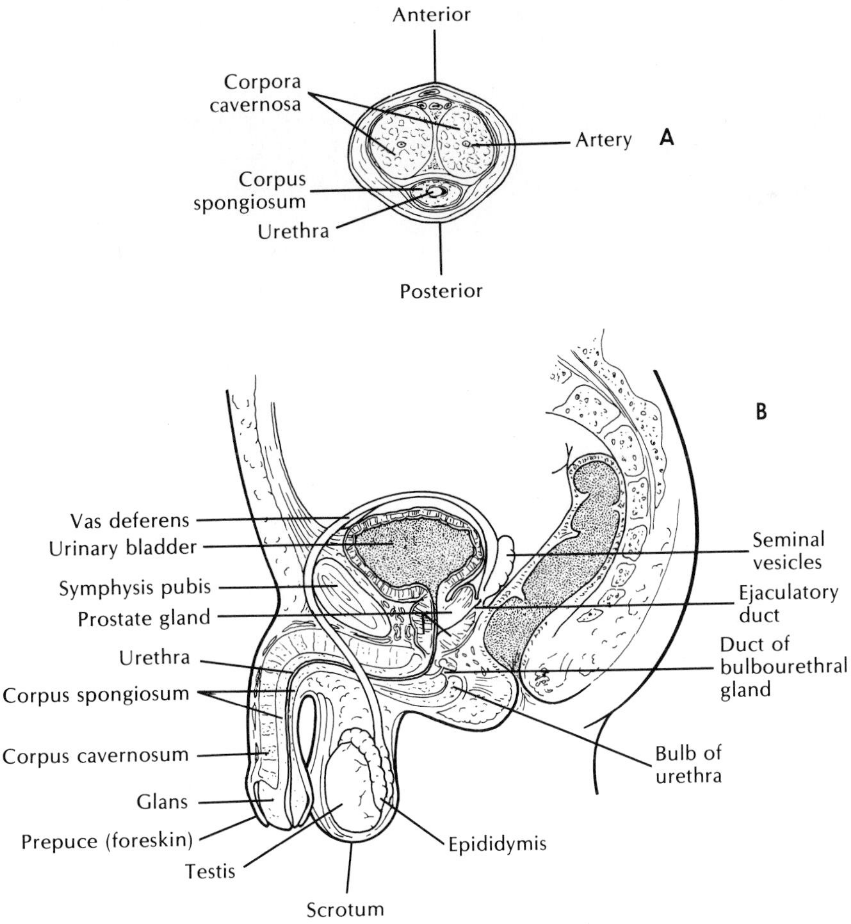

Fig. 4-26 Fascial planes of male lower genitourinary tract. **A,** Transverse section of penis. **B,** Relationship of bladder, prostate, seminal vesicles, penis, urethra, and scrotal contents.

tum, and each compartment normally contains one *testis, epididymis,* and *vas deferens* (seminal duct). The left side of the scrotum hangs somewhat lower (about 1 cm) than the right. The skin is abundantly supplied with sebaceous and sweat glands and is sparsely covered with hair. Under the skin are found the *cremaster* fascia and thin smooth muscle layer. Contraction and relaxation of this smooth muscle result in retraction of the testes to protect them from external trauma and cold. During hot external (environmental) or internal (fever) temperature the cremaster muscle relaxes, lowering the testes away from the body. Conversely, cold external temperature stimulates contraction of the cremaster muscle to bring the testes close to the body.

The purpose of this mobility is to maintain the testes within an optimum temperature range for the production and viability of sperm. Hot tubbing, tight underwear (jockey shorts) and pants, and long-term sitting (long-distance truck drivers) present too hot an external environment or prevent testicular mobility so that spermatogenesis and sperm are jeopardized.

Internal Structures

Internal structures include the following (see Figs. 4-25 and 4-26):

1. Testes: male gonads
2. Ducts of the testes
3. Accessory reproductive tract glands
   a. Seminal vesicles
   b. Prostate glands
   c. Bulbourethral glands

Testes: Male Gonads. The testes are two small ovoid glands located within the scrotal sac. Both are suspended by attachment to scrotal tissue and the spermatic cord. Originally located in the abdomen, the testes descend through the inguinal canal by the end of the seventh lunar month of fetal life. At term birth one or both of the testes may still be within the inguinal canals with final descent into the scrotal sac occurring in the early postnatal period. The testes must be within the scrotum for spermatogenesis to occur.

The testes are similar in origin (homologous) to the ovaries in the female. Each testis is whitish, somewhat flattened from side to side, measures about 4 or 5 cm in length, and weighs 10 to 15 g. White fibrous tissue encases each testis and divides it into several lobules. Within each lobule are one to three long (about 75 cm), narrow, coiled *seminiferous tubules* and clusters of *interstitial cells* (Leydig's cells). Spermatids attach to the germinal epithelium (Sertoli cells) within the seminiferous tubules and develop into sperm. The interstitial cells are large connective and supportive tissue (stromal) cells responsible for the production of the androgen hormone testosterone.

The two principal functions of the testes are spermatogenesis and hormone production. Primitive sex cells (spermatogonia) are present in the seminiferous tubules of the male newborn. Spermatogenesis, the maturation process that results in sperm, begins during puberty and normally continues throughout a man's lifetime. The testes secrete the steroid sex hormone testosterone in the amounts that are required for normal male growth, development, and function.

Ducts (Canals) of the Testes. For sperm to exit the body they must travel the full length of the duct system in succession: seminiferous tubules, epididymides (pl.), vasa deferentia (pl.), ejaculatory ducts, and the urethra. The seminiferous tubules are mentioned earlier. Each testis has one tightly coiled tube, about 6 m (20 ft) in length. The tube, the *epididymis* (see Fig. 4-26) lies along the top and side of each testis. The epididymides are storage sites for maturing sperm and produce a small part of the seminal fluid (semen). Seminiferous tubules are continuous with the epididymides, which in turn connect to the vasa deferentia.

Accessory Reproductive System Glands. Accessory reproductive glands secrete fluids that support the life and function of sperm. These glands include the paired *seminal vesicles,* located along the lower posterior surface of the bladder; the *prostate gland,* which surrounds the prostatic urethra; and the *bulbourethral* (or Cowper's) *glands,* located below the prostate, one at either side of the membranous urethra (see Figs. 4-25 and 4-26).

Semen. Semen is the fluid ejaculated at the time of orgasm. It contains sperm and secretions from the seminal vesicles, prostate gland, and bulbourethral glands. An average volume per ejaculate is 2.5 to 3.5 ml (range: 1 to 10 ml) after several days of continence (no ejaculations). The volume of semen and sperm count decrease rapidly with repeated ejaculations. Semen contains constituents that provide nourishment, support and enhance sperm motility, and buffer the acidic environment of the cervical and vaginal fluids.

Semen is white to opalescent in color with a specific gravity of 1.028. The pH is alkaline, ranging from 7.35 to 7.5. Sperm count averages 100 million/ml with fewer than 20% abnormal forms. About 60% of the total fluid is derived from the seminal vesicles; about 20% from the prostatic glands. Some fluid is secreted by the bulbourethral glands and probably the urethral glands.

Less than 5% of the ejaculate consists of sperm and fluid from the testes and epididymides. Since vasectomy affects only the production of this portion of the ejaculate, there is no noticeable change in volume, even after sperm are no longer available for transport through the remaining canal system.

A high concentration of prostaglandin is produced

by the seminal vesicles. However, their function in semen production is not fully understood (Ganong, 1987). Prostaglandins are discussed on p. 77.

❑ FEMALE AND MALE DEVELOPMENT AND RESPONSE PATTERNS

The hypothalamus and anterior pituitary gland in females and males regulate the production of FSH and LH. The target tissue for these hormones is the gonad. In the female the ovary produces ova and secretes estrogen and progesterone; in the male the testis produces sperm and secretes testosterone. A *feedback mechanism* between hormone secretion from the gonads, hypothalamus, and anterior pituitary aids in the control of the production of sex cells and steroid sex hormone secretion (Figs. 4-21 and 4-27).

Physiologic Response to Sexual Stimulation

Although the first outward appearance of maturing sexual development occurs at an earlier age in females, both females and males achieve physical maturity at about the age of 17. However, great variation is possible between individuals' rates of development. Anatomic and reproductive differences notwithstanding, women and men are more alike than different in their physiologic response to sexual excitement and orgasm. For example, the glans clitoris and the glans penis are homologues with the same number of nerve endings (see Fig. 4-1). This explains why the clitoris is so sensitive to sexual stimulation. Not only is there little difference between female and male sexual response, but it is now accepted that the physical response is essentially the same whether the source of stimulation is coitus, fantasy, or mechanical or manual masturbation.

Currently there are two theories to explain the physiologic response to sexual stimulation. The first and most widely used theory is the four-phase response cycle described by Masters and Johnson. The second is Helen Kaplan's biphasic sexual response cycle.

Physiologically, sexual response, according to Masters and Johnson (1966), can be analyzed in terms of two processes: vasocongestion and myotonia.

1. **Vasocongestion.** Sexual stimulation results in reflex dilatation of penile blood vessels (erection) and circumvaginal blood vessels (lubrication), causing engorgement and distension of the genitals. Venous congestion is localized primarily in the genitals, but it also occurs to a lesser degree in the breasts and other parts of the body.
2. **Myotonia.** Arousal is characterized by increased muscular tension, resulting in voluntary and involuntary rhythmic contractions. Examples of sexually stimulated myotonia are pelvic thrusting, facial grimacing, and spasms of the hands and feet (carpopedal spasms).

The response cycle is arbitrarily divided into four phases: excitement phase, plateau phase, orgasmic phase, and resolution phase. One moves through the four phases progressively, and there is no sharp dividing line between any two phases. However, there are specific body changes that take place in sequence. The time, intensity, and duration for cyclic completion also vary for individuals and situations.

Excitement Phase. The woman's first observable

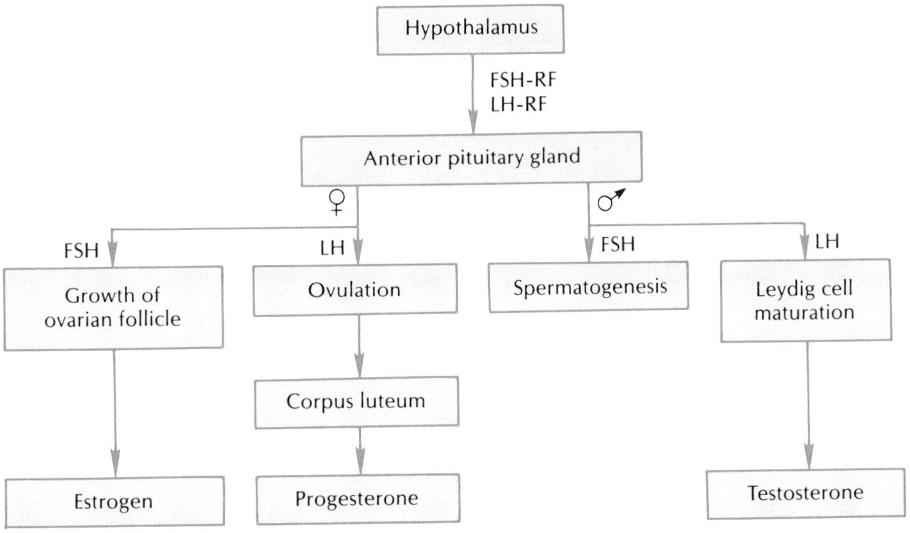

Fig. 4-27 Hypothalamic-pituitary-gonadal axis; comparison of female and male (RF = releasing factors).

reaction to sexual stimulation is vaginal lubrication, which has the biologic function of preparing the vagina for penile penetration. The inner two thirds of the vaginal barrel lengthen and distend. The cervix and fundus are pulled upward. The external genitals become congested and darker in color. The clitoris increases in diameter and in tumescence (vascular congestion and swelling).

The man's first observable reaction to sexual stimulation is erection of the penis (increase in length and diameter). The scrotal skin becomes congested and thick. The testes elevate because of contraction of the cremasteric musculature.

Plateau Phase. In the woman, the wall of the outer one third of the vagina becomes greatly engorged, along with the labia minora, forming the "orgasmic platform." The clitoris retracts under the clitoral hood to protect the clitoris from intense, direct stimulation.

In the man, preorgasmic emission of two or three drops of mucoid substance is released from the Cowper's glands. The testes continue to elevate until they are situated close to the body to facilitate ejaculatory pressure.

Orgasmic Phase. Strong, rhythmic (every 0.8 second), muscular contractions occur in the woman's orgasmic platform. The number of contractions ranges from 3 to 15. The uterus also contracts rhythmically.

This phase may be subjectively described as follows:

Stage 1: sensation of "suspension," followed by "intense sensual awareness, clitorally oriented and radiating upward into the pelvis"

Stage 2: "suffusion of warmth" especially in the pelvic area

Stage 3: "pelvic throbbing" located in the vagina and lower pelvis

In men, the testes are held at maximum elevation. Rhythmic contractions of the penis and rectal sphincter occur at 0.8-second intervals for the first three to four major responses.

This phase may be subjectively described as follows:

Stage 1: point of "inevitability," which occurs just before ejaculation and lasts 2 or 3 seconds; awareness of presence of fluid in the urethra

Stage 2: ejaculation with rhythmic contractions capable of expelling semen up to 60 cm (24 in)

Resolution Phase. Blood returns from the engorged walls of the woman's vagina, and the labia majora and minora rapidly return to their unexcited state. The clitoris rapidly returns from under the hood; however, return to normal size may take longer. Uterus descends, and cervix dips into seminal pool.

In the first stage of the man's resolution phase 50% of erection is lost rather rapidly. The second stage can last much longer, depending on the maintenance of physical condition.

Refractory Period. The *refractory* period is the time necessary to complete the cycle again. The time varies from a few minutes to a few days, depending on the age and state of physical and emotional health.

Biphasic Response. Kaplan (1974) has presented an alternative to the four-phase sexual response cycle of Masters and Johnson. She believes clinical and physiologic evidence suggests that sexual response is biphasic, with the following two distinct and relatively independent components:

1. Genital vasocongestive reaction—produces vaginal lubrication and swelling in the female and penile erection in the male
2. Reflex clonic muscular contractions—constitute orgasm in both sexes

Phase 1: Vasocongestive Reaction. Erection in the male is a local vasocongestive response. During erection the corpora cavernosa become engorged with blood. Special valves in the penile veins are closed by reflex action, preventing loss of blood. This mechanism is regulated by the parasympathetic division of the autonomic nervous system. This system controls the diameter and valves of the penile blood vessels, thus causing erection or loss of erection. Once erection has occurred, excitement can be maintained for some time. Men are physically capable of losing and regaining several erections during love play.

Kaplan calls the vasocongestive reaction in females the "lubrication-swelling" phase. During this phase, dilatation of the circumvaginal venous plexus causes a transudate on the walls of the vagina, which results in lubrication. The tissues become the "orgasmic platform" (analogous to erection in the male). In addition the uterus becomes engorged and begins to rise slightly out of the pelvic cavity so that the cervix is placed in a position to increase the likelihood of fertilization.

Phase 2: Reflex Clonic Muscular Contractions. The visceral aspects of the ejaculatory reflex are under control of the sympathetic division of the autonomic nervous system, as opposed to the parasympathetic division that is involved with erection. Male orgasm has two phases: *emission* and *ejaculation*. Emission comprises contractions of the vasa deferentia, the prostate, the seminal vesicles, and the internal part of the urethra. Masters and Johnson (1966) have called the subjective response to emission "ejaculatory inevitability." Ejaculation is the external mechanism that causes spurts of semen to be forced outward from the penis.

The biphasic nature of the response cycle is dramatically explained by the impact of aging on the refractory period. For example, a man's frequency of ejaculation may be reduced, but his ability to have erections may remain relatively the same.

The woman, like the man, has orgasms consisting of a series of reflex, involuntary rhythmic contractions of the orgasmic platform.

Clinical Significance. There are four important findings from the research of Masters and Johnson that have significance for nurses working with pregnant women and their families. These findings concern (1) multiple orgasm, (2) simultaneous orgasm, (3) clitoral versus vaginal orgasm, and (4) variations in orgasmic patterns.

Since women never physically have a refractory period, they are capable of having one orgasm after another until exhausted. *Multiple orgasms* are most commonly reported by women in their late thirties and early forties. Some women have reported being multiply orgasmic for the first time during the second trimester of pregnancy. The reason is that because of the increased vasocongestion of pregnancy, total completion of the resolution phase never occurs.

Many couples have considered *simultaneous orgasm* the ultimate goal of sexual bliss. The findings of Masters and Johnson and of others show the illogic of such goals, because many couples progress through the response cycle at different rates. The myth of the desirability of simultaneous orgasm has harmed many relationships because of the difficulty of achieving this goal. Although possible, simultaneous orgasm is the exception rather than the rule and is achieved when the woman reaches orgasm easily.

Freud taught that women transfer sexual sensation from the clitoris to the vagina when they reach psychosexual maturity. A clitoral orgasm was considered therefore to be an immature orgasm. This belief existed until Masters and Johnson demonstrated that an orgasm is a total body response to sexual stimulation, with the most intense response located in the pelvic area. The response is essentially the same regardless of whether it is experienced through coitus, masturbation, or mechanical stimulation. The clitoris is defined as the "transmitter and conductor" of erotic sensation. Hite (1976) reported that 30% of the women in her sample of 300 were orgasmic during intercourse without additional clitoral stimulation.

There are many response patterns for both women and men. These patterns vary in both intensity and duration.

Prostaglandins

Prostaglandins (PGs) are oxygenated fatty acids now classified as hormones. The different kinds of PGs are distinguished by letters (PGE, PGF), numbers (PGE_2), and letters of the Greek alphabet ($PGF_{2\alpha}$).

PGs are produced in most organs of the body but most notably by the prostate and the endometrium. Therefore semen and menstrual blood are potent prostaglandin sources. PGs are metabolized quickly by most tissues. They are biologically active in minute amounts in the cardiovascular, gastrointestinal, respiratory, urogenital, and nervous systems. They also exert a marked effect on metabolism, particularly on glycolysis. Prostaglandins play an important role in many physiologic, pathologic, and pharmacologic reactions. $PGF_{2\alpha}$, PGE_1, and PGE_2 are most commonly used in reproductive medicine.

Prostaglandins affect smooth muscle contractility and modulation of hormonal activity. Indirect evidence supports PGs' effects on the following events:

1. Ovulation
2. Fertility
3. Changes in the cervix and cervical mucus that affect receptivity to sperm
4. Tubal and uterine motility
5. Sloughing of endometrium (menstruation)
6. Onset of abortion, spontaneous and induced
7. Onset of labor, term and preterm

After exerting their biologic actions, newly synthesized PGs are rapidly metabolized by tissues in such organs as the lungs, kidneys, and liver.

PGs may play a key role in ovulation. If PG levels do not rise along with the surge of LH, the ovum remains trapped within the graafian follicle. After ovulation, PGs may influence production of estrogen and progesterone by the corpus luteum.

The introduction of PGs into the vagina or into the uterine cavity (from ejaculated semen) increases the motility of uterine musculature, which may assist the transport of sperm through the uterus and into the oviduct. High concentration of PGs in the semen (about 55 μg/ml) may be necessary for normal fertility in males.

PGs produced by the woman cause regression (return to an earlier state) of the corpus luteum, regression of the endometrium, and sloughing of the endometrium, which results in menstruation. PGs increase myometrial response to oxytocic stimulation, enhance uterine contractions, and cause cervical dilatation. They may be one factor in the initiation or maintenance of labor or both. In addition, prostaglandins may be involved in the following pathologic states: male infertility, dysmenorrhea, hypertensive states, preeclampsia-eclampsia, and anaphylactic shock. Further discussion of PGs relevant to abortion may be found in Chapter 23; for a discussion of PGs' role in pregnancy and childbirth, see Chapter 26.

PSYCHOSOCIAL NATURE OF HUMAN SEXUALITY

Nurses providing maternity health care require a foundation in psychosocial aspects of growth and development. The nurse is expected to provide counseling and guidance to sexually maturing and sexually active individuals, as well as to expectant and new parents. New parents often need information about the growth and development of the individuals who comprise their family. The following assists in the development of comprehensive individualized nursing care plans.

A holistic approach to sexual development takes into account the psychosocial nature of human sexuality, as well as the biologic nature. These spheres are interdependent and involve processes that progress in an orderly manner resulting in the ultimate physical and psychologic maturation of an individual. A brief description of cognitive development as proposed by Piaget is included in the presentation. Intellectual response is a critical factor in developing a socially responsible use of sexual potential. As a person's sense of sexual identity is influenced by mastery of psychologic developmental tasks, Erikson's stages of personality development are presented. Social forces that strengthen the concepts of femaleness or maleness are reviewed. The review begins with gender identity in the young child and progresses through the life cycle. Family members are the first significant others in the child's sexual, cognitive, and personality development. As the child matures and ventures into the wider world, peer, educational, and other social groups provide environments that may promote or retard development.

Cognitive Development

Cognition is the process by which people recognize, accumulate, and organize the knowledge of their world and use this knowledge to solve problems and change behavior. A young woman is used for an example. **Cognitive development** begins when she *perceives* or recognizes an event as a problem. She then searches her *memory* to see if the problem is similar to any past experience. Next she *generates ideas* as to a possible solution. Finally she *evaluates* the accuracy of the choice. Obviously the richer the source of ideas, concepts, and past experiences used in successful resolution of problems, the greater the odds for success in resolving current difficulties. Both innate intellectual ability and the quality of the environment are decisive factors in cognitive development.

Piaget (1950), a Swiss scientist, developed theories about how the adult process of thought develops. According to Piaget, cognitive development progresses in an orderly and sequential manner through four stages. The process is one of gradual evolution, with each stage building on the specific attainments of the previous one. Table 4-3 summarizes cognitive and personality development across the life span.

Sensorimotor Stage (Birth to 2 Years). Reflex activity dominates the beginning of the **sensorimotor stage.** It gives way to repetitive and finally to imitative behavior. Any problem solving is the result of trial and error, but a sense of "what causes what" begins to emerge. Discovery can be exciting as a child becomes aware of her or his own body, as well as other familiar objects. Language begins in a limited fashion, mostly single or double words such as "mine" or "me too." By the end of this period an object can exist without being present (object permanence). As a result, hide-and-seek is no longer frightening but has become a pleasurable game.

Preoperational Stage (2 to 7 Years). During the **preoperational stage** children are extremely self-centered or egocentric. As Whaley and Wong (1990) express it, "they are unable to see things from any perspective other than their own; they cannot see another's point of view, nor can they see any reason to do so." They live in a well-defined world made up of what they see, hear, or otherwise experience. Characteristically, children are "centered" in that they see one aspect of a situation but are unable to take any other factors into account. They are unaware of the transition process between one static state (the beginning) and another static state (the end). Gradually their language becomes more complex, and single words progress to phrases and then to sentences. Children grow dramatically through direct experience and an increasing ability to use symbolic communication. Behavior appears to assume *cyclic trends* of equilibrium and disequilibrium.

Concrete Operations Stage (7 to 12 Years). The **concrete operations stage** is characterized by a gradual increase in problem-solving ability. The method of reasoning used is inductive. Solutions to problems are not based on abstractions but are derived from what has been perceived and categorized. The "social self" appears. Children are no longer exclusively egocentric but can relate to the feelings and thoughts of others.

Formal Operations Stage (12 to 18 Years). Progress through the formal operations stage may be erratic and difficult for the adolescent. By the end of this stage, successful people can consider hypotheses and analyze scientifically. They can deduce conclusions from a set of observations, consider alternatives, and assess risks. In short, they are capable of reasoning logically by using abstractions and of assuming responsibility for the actions taken as solutions to their problems. Piaget notes that formal thinking involves two major dimensions: the use of propositional logic (the ability to think about a problem and thus rearrange as-

Table 4-3 Summary of Cognitive and Personality Development

Stage	Significant Others	Cognitive Development (Piaget)	Personality Development (Erikson)
Infancy (birth to toddlerhood)	Maternal person ↓	Sensorimotor: reflex→repetition→imitation	Trust vs. mistrust
Early childhood (2-7 yr)	Parental persons and other family members ↓	Preoperational, direct experience (seeing, hearing, feeling) within a well-defined world	Initiative vs. guilt
Middle childhood (7-12 yr)	Neighborhood and school ↓	Concrete thinking (not abstract), humanized (limited inductive reasoning)	Industry vs. inferiority
Adolescence (12-18 yr)	Peer groups and models of leadership ↓	Formal thinking (deductive and abstract reasoning) may be limited up to 15 yr	Identity vs. identity confusion
Early adulthood	Partners in friendship, sex, competition, and cooperation ↓	Formal thinking includes problem solving and separation of fantasy and fact	Intimacy and solidarity vs. isolation
Young and middle adulthood	Divided labor and shared household ↓	Formal thinking includes problem solving and separation of fantasy and fact	Generativity vs. self-absorption
Later adulthood	Humankind, family, and friends	Formal thinking includes problem solving and separation of fantasy and fact	Ego integrity vs. despair

pects of it until it becomes clear) and the ability to separate fantasy from fact.

Personality Development

Personality is a complex of characteristics that distinguishes a particular individual in her or his relationships with others. It includes emergent tendencies to act and to interact and thereby influence the individual's environment.

Erikson (1959) proposed a theory of **personality development** that defines the process in stages. Each stage focuses on a central conflict and depends on the ones before it. These problems are envisioned as conflicts between opposites; for example, trust versus mistrust. As each conflict is resolved or mastered to a greater or lesser degree, the individual is ready to move on to the next level. Unresolved conflicts can hamper a person's further development and may persist in residual form throughout life. (See Table 4-3.)

Trust versus Mistrust (Birth to 1 Year). Basic **trust** develops as a response to being loved and cared for by a giving and concerned adult. The period from birth to 1 year is a time of "taking in" for the infant, who needs nurturing, security, and a feeling of continuity to develop trust. If such care makes up the bulk of the infant's experiences, trust takes precedence over mistrust. Successful completion of this stage results in a sense of trust in the child's responses to others throughout life.

Autonomy versus Shame and Doubt (1 to 3 Years). A sense of **autonomy** develops with the gradual unfolding of the child's control of body, self, and people in the immediate environment. If those who provide care applaud the child's efforts toward self-control and increasing motor skills, autonomy will result. Conversely, feelings of self-doubt and shame can occur if the child experiences frequent failures and frustrations.

Initiative versus Guilt (3 to 6 Years). The stage of **initiative** versus guilt ushers in an active exploratory phase in children's development. They learn much from their world by playing games and asking endless questions. They show more evidence of being guided by an inner conscience: the "parent" has been increasingly internalized. This is a time for fears and phobias. Children's developmental tasks revolve around directing their efforts toward purposeful activity and achieving a balance between daring and caution.

Industry versus Inferiority (6 to 12 Years). During the period of **industry** versus inferiority, children develop a sense of being a productive worker. They need opportunities to complete activities and be rewarded for their efforts. Introduction to formal schooling takes place now, and success or failure in this respect can set the stage for later career choice.

Identity versus Identity Confusion (12 to 18 Years). The period of adolescence comes after a period of relative calm. During this time of transition between childhood and adulthood, adolescents have certain tasks to perform: they must establish sexual roles, select an occupation, become independent of the family, and develop a social rather than egocentric response to people and the wider society. The adolescent must accept a new body image that includes the ability to reproduce. Successful mastery of these tasks helps adolescents develop a sense of self and **identity** that both they and society can accept. With this sense comes the ability for devotion and fidelity. Without it people know not "who they are" or "where they are going," and identity confusion persists.

Intimacy versus Isolation (Early Adulthood). Once people have sense of identity, they can move toward **intimacy**—intimate relationships with others. This can be expressed on a personal level as friendship, sexual intimacy, or the intimacy of parent-child relationships. On a social level love of fellow humans is expressed in concern for the welfare of others. Without this sense of freedom to love and be loved, people are isolated and may develop a sense of alienation from family, friends, and society.

Generativity versus Self-absorption (Young and Middle Adulthood). During the period of **generativity** versus self-absorption, people are concerned with creating the next generation and providing the necessary nurturing and caregiving. The tasks in this stage include preparation for assuming the role of parent, participating in the birth of children, and adapting to the reality of parenthood. Some people may become substitute parents in myriad ways: adopting children, being friends to adolescents, teaching, or nursing. Self-absorption is minimized when involvement of the self with others takes place. Growth of the personality, as a person seeks balance between commitment to self and commitment to others, leads to a sense of productiveness and fulfillment.

Ego Integrity versus Despair (Late Adulthood). Staying productive and involved in the welfare of others increases the satisfaction, or **ego integrity,** of elderly people. (In the United States old age arbitrarily begins at 65 years.) In most cases an elderly person's physical and mental abilities gradually decline, imposing limitations and curtailing his sphere of activity. As people confront the limitations, they must balance acceptance against despair. Wisdom and a sense of satisfaction in their accomplishments come to those who succeed in the search for personal meaning.

❑ DEVELOPMENT OF SEXUALITY

Sexual identity begins at conception. At that time, through the chance combination of an ovum and a sperm, a person's biologic sex is determined. Thereafter, intrauterine and extrauterine environmental influences both play their part in the realization of each person's sexual potential. Biophysical, psychologic, sociocultural, and ethical factors all contribute to the molding of an individual's **sexuality.**

We are born into a sexually oriented world, and from birth onward we assume socially defined sexual roles that reflect the basic pattern prescribed by the society. These roles are learned informally through being part of a social group. Development of a concept of sexual roles and sexual identity begins at an early age and continues as a series of developmental tasks throughout a person's life span.

Infancy and Childhood

Developmental Tasks. One of the first questions parents ask when their child is born is "Is it a boy or a girl?" The answer sets in motion a series of social influences that will be reflected in the child's concept of "who I am" and "what I can do." The **developmental tasks** relative to forming a sexual identity include developing core gender identity, acquiring prescribed sex role standards, identifying with the parent of the same sex, and establishing gender preference.

Core Gender Identity. **Core gender identity** is the earliest and most stable form of gender identity. By 2 years of age children can differentiate between girls and boys through awareness of dissimilarities in hair and clothing and some awareness of anatomic differences. Core gender identity is developed in normal children by the time they have reached 3 or 4 years of age.

Efforts to determine the importance of biologic versus environmental contributions to a person's gender identity have generated much controversy and research. Some studies indicate certain different biologic responses in female and male newborns and suggest differences in the infants' responses to the environment and readiness for various learning experiences. Other studies reveal the importance of gender labeling on the eventual acceptance of gender identity. Infants whose sex was uncertain at birth accepted the sex role assigned by their parents and identified with that role (Maccoby, 1974).

From the child's perspective, knowing oneself as either a girl or a boy begins before full realization of the implications of sexual identity. The infant establishes her or his gender identity from interactions with the parents. It is largely accomplished by acceptance of parental labeling; for example, "Be a good boy," "That's my girl," and "That is my big boy."

Communication, verbal or nonverbal, provides the child with cues about the sex-appropriateness of her or his behavior. A sense of trust in sexual identity develops through the early reaffirmations of femaleness or maleness.

Sex Role Standards. The term **sex role standards** refers to the various behaviors, attitudes, and attributes that differentiate the roles. Even 2-year-olds are exposed to this conditioning, because parents choose for them the kinds of clothing, toys, and activities that reflect the parents' expectations of sex role standards.

The child learns by observing the behavior of women, men, girls, and boys. The child formulates a concept of who should perform what tasks, who provides the comforting, who provides the active play, and who is nurturing when there is sickness. The feelings children develop about themselves as people in general and as sexual people in particular are directly related to their experiences with their bodies and the attitudes and values they derive from many sources. One of the most important ways children learn about their bodies is through exploratory sexual behavior (sex play). *Sex play* is defined by Kinsey et al (1948, 1953) as "actual genital play." Four categories of sex play are listed as follows:

1. *Self-exploration and self-manipulation:* most common forms of sex play. Fondling of penis and manual stimulation of the clitoris are most common. Infants begin the process of exploring their bodies even by 2 to 3 months of age. As they grow they discover they are able to experience sexual pleasure through self-stimulation. Parents who feel masturbation is harmful will rebuke even young children and forbid them "to play with themselves."
2. *Same-sex comparisons:* comparison of size and shape. Prepubescent homosexual behaviors do not necessarily lead to adult homosexuality. Children need reassurance that their genitals are similar to those of others.
3. *Coital play:* when a boy lies on top of a girl. The activities are largely experimental, imitative, and exploratory. Children become aware of parental sleeping arrangements, bathing, and privacy. They begin differentiating sex role behaviors and will play at being Mommy and Daddy.
4. *Exhibitionism:* showing and handling genitals in public, especially in the presence of companions. Most children engage in sex play activities only sporadically, especially when these activities are ignored by adults. For example, one out of four boys who had engaged in sex play had done so only during 1 year, and some had participated in such play only once before puberty (Kinsey et al, 1948). Kinsey et al (1948, 1953) found that 9 years of age was the peak age for girls, when 14% engaged in some form of sex play. For boys the peak was 12 years of age, when 38% were similarly involved.

During early childhood (2 to 7 years) children are vulnerable to shaming experiences. Caregivers often use the sense of shame or guilt to encourage children to limit acting out sexually to appropriate places. Children need to be encouraged to develop self-control without loss of self-esteem or the feeling that sexual activity is sinful. During middle childhood the child interacts more freely outside the family. Biologic drives are less pronounced as the child strives for body competence and mastery. Sex role mastery centers on competitiveness, such as "being the fastest runner," or "throwing the ball farther than anyone else."

In Western society the adjectives used to describe a female predominantly express a mothering capacity, that is, "gentle, loving, submissive, patient, warm, and concerned." These qualities suit a person whose central reason for being is assumed to be the care and nurturing of the young and, by extension, anyone who needs such care. Those adjectives used to describe the male, namely, "dominant, aggressive, impatient, objective, and ambitious," portray a person capable of independent, decisive action. These are seen as the qualities needed in the marketplace and the basis for career orientation.

In reality, people of both sexes possess these qualities in common. Some personalities lean more toward the socially defined concept of either female or male; others have no clear demarcation of roles. These latter people, termed *androgynous personalities,* use those qualities most needed at the moment without feeling guilty about usurping another's role. A male nursing student made the following comment during a discussion of mothering:

> It is not a case of one or the other, it is what the time calls forth. The most nurturing behavior of "mothering," if you want to call it that, that I've ever seen was in Vietnam when a man was trying to get a wounded friend out of range of fire. He protected him, covering him with his own body, gave him his food and water. No mother could have shown more devotion.

A common way children prepare for a future parenting role is through sibling caregiving. Older children from either the nuclear or extended family care for younger children. Older children are used to provide role flexibility for mothers and for the development of caregiving skills by children. Stereotyped sex roles, so important in many cultures, are maintained when children assume child care responsibilities for younger family members (Weisner and Gallimore, 1977).

Identification with Parent of Same Sex. As a child comes to identify with the parent of the same sex the child internalizes the values, attitudes, and ideals of that parent. The exact method by which the process of identification is accomplished is not yet known. The child does perceive physical and psychologic similarities and is told about similarities by others. Adoption of the same-sex parent's behavior may be motivated by fear of loss of the love of this important person or by awareness of that person's power to control rewards. For a girl to forgo identification with her father, she must love her mother sufficiently to form a positive identification with her. A boy needs to relinquish his early identification with his mother and form a strong commitment to his father.

Gender Preference. **Gender preference** implies not only a knowledge of one's gender and the appropriate sex role but also a liking for it. Development of gender preference involves three elements: (1) success in the role, (2) liking the same-sex parent, and (3) reinforcement from family, ethnic group, and social institutions as to the value of the role (Newman and Newman, 1975). As with other attitudes, fluctuations in preference occur as people face situations in which one sex role either enhances or hinders personal goals. Deep-seated sex preferences on the part of parents can affect initial parent-child relationships if the child is not of the preferred sex. The parenting lag that results can last a day or a lifetime, depending on whether the parent succeeds or fails in resolving conflicting emotions. Certain ethnic groups have welcoming rituals for one sex and not for the other. These seemingly innocuous societal and personal preferences eventually lead a person to make value judgments about the worthiness of her or his sex. As a result the individual's self-esteem is either increased or diminished.

By the time puberty occurs the person has completed most of the developmental tasks of early childhood. Acceptance of childhood sexual identity will have consequences for self-esteem, peer relations, and selection of skills and interest. The concomitant development of moral standards such as honesty and fidelity results in a linkage between sexual identity (role) and moral commitments. Feelings of self-acceptance or guilt can be generated by either upholding or violating standards in these spheres.

Table 4-4 describes the sex-related behaviors of infancy, early childhood, and late childhood. In addition, the function for each behavior is given. As the reader will see from this table and the following two tables, human sexuality is a developmental process throughout the life cycle.

Implications for Nursing. A knowledgeable maternity nurse has many opportunities to help young parents provide a supportive environment for their children's sexual development. *Nurses and parents must be careful not to ascribe adult motives to the sexual behaviors of children.* Katchadourian and Lunde (1972) stated: "It is particularly important not to label the sex play of children as deviant or perverse, no matter what it entails. To do so would be like calling a child who believes in ghosts and fairies delusional or mentally ill." Kolodny et al (1979) caution nurses that contradictory messages about the body (parental encouragement to be aware of the body but to exclude the genitals from awareness) are among the earliest recognizable common determinants of adult sexual problems. For example, parents tell their children to "wash behind their ears" and then remind them to "wash down there." Parents and many health professionals respond to their own insecurities about sex when confronted by the overt but innocent sexuality of children.

Adolescence

Adolescence, the transitional period between childhood and adulthood, begins with puberty. The onset of puberty varies for each person. Biologically the first visible signs of puberty are the development of the secondary sexual characteristics. Menstruation can be a first indication of puberty. Shortly thereafter most teenagers experience a rapid increase in linear growth. Concomitantly, emotional changes such as moodiness, tearfulness, or withdrawal are suddenly noticeable in a previously serene youngster. For example, one mother related, "My daughter (aged 12) asked me where I had put her baby teeth. When I replied that I had thrown them away, she burst into tears and cried that I didn't think much of her to throw away something so precious."

It is not until adolescence that the socially and parentally defined sex role is openly questioned. In recent years changes in the concepts of what constitutes female and male roles have had great impact on teenagers. Conflict can result when the teenager chooses standards consistent with the peer group's attitude rather than with parental expectations.

Developmental Tasks. Erikson (1959) has described the adolescent stage of development as the one in which the major task is achieving identity versus identity confusion. A person's identity has many di-

Table 4-4 Infancy and Childhood Sexual Development

Age	Behavior	Function
Infancy (birth to 18 mo)	Oral exploration, sucking, mouthing; explores own body	Erotic attachments and pleasures achieved from self-stimulation are forerunners of future development
	Quality and quantity of touch by caregiver; color of clothes, blankets, room; style of clothes	Beginning of formation of core gender identity
	Mothers look at and talk to girls more than boys and respond to girl's irritability more quickly; boys are touched, held, rocked, and kissed more as infants	Parental acceptance of general societal roles for females and males
	Boys: erection in first few days of life; girls: vaginal lubrication	Reflex response, not yet eroticized
Early childhood (18 mo to 3 yr)	Act of releasing contents of bowel and bladder is source of enjoyment	Learns to associate genitals with privacy, and cleanliness or dirt
	Phallic exhibitionistic period (discovers genitals and finds they can bring pleasure)	Beginning of lifelong association between sexual feelings and genitals
	Sporadic investigation of playmate's genitals; sex play probably more homosexual than heterosexual	Knowledge seeking; experimental, imitative, exploratory play, precursor to future sociosexual encounters
Middle childhood (3 to 5 yr)	Observes relationship between parents (kiss, hug, talk to each other)	Works through beginning relationships with parent of opposite sex; much of warmth the child experiences from close relationships with parents is later transferred to relationships with persons of opposite sex
	Self-exploration and self-manipulation	Learns erotic potential
Late childhood (5 to 11 yr)	Transition from home environment to school	Develops meaningful relationships with peers of same sex; solidifies sexual identity with homosocial relationships
	Begins to read, watch movies, and television	Latent erotic inquiry develops; moral categories are learned
	Learns "dirty" words	Cognitive and affective meanings of words and symbols are not understood and possibly may be distorted by child
	May be labeled as "tomboy" or "sissy"	Early gender distinction; learns early that male role is more important than female role

Adapted by Marianne Zalar from Sadock BJ, Kaplan HD, and Freedman AM: The sexual experience, Baltimore, 1976, The Williams & Wilkins Co.

mensions, including intellectual, interpersonal, and sexual. It is now recognized that the adolescent developmental process proceeds in sequence through three phases. These phases—early, middle, and late adolescence—put a characteristic stamp on the manner of accomplishing the developmental tasks. The developmental tasks of adolescence may be defined as follows (adapted from Havighurst, 1972):

1. *Achieving awareness and acceptance of body image.* The body image is well established by about 15 years of age. Adolescents must cope with normal but rapid changes in physical appearance and alterations in functional capacity. They must accept their physique and learn to use their bodies effectively. Deviations from the "norm" are a source of stress and may or may not be incorporated into the adolescent's body image.
2. *Achieving emotional independence of parents and other adults.* The movement away from dependence on parents that was begun with the school years is completed in this period of development. Successful accomplishment results in affection and respect for one's parents without a childish dependence on them.
3. *Achieving new and more mature relations with age mates of both sexes.* Adolescents accomplish a satisfactory social adjustment through social activities and experimentation with the peer

group. Here they learn to behave as adults as they create, on a small scale, the society of their elders. The influence of the peer group increasingly takes precedence over that of the family.

4. *Achieving a feminine or masculine social role.* Although sex is biologically determined, the feminine and masculine roles are culturally established behavior sets that must be learned.
5. *Establishing a life-style that is personally and socially satisfying.* This includes the choice of a career, as well as contemplation of sexual relationships, marriage, family interdependence, and parenthood.
6. *Acquiring a set of values and an ethical system as a guide to socially responsible behavior.* This includes assuming responsibility for her or his own behavior and recognizing the effect that behavior may have on another's welfare.

Table 4-5 outlines the sexual behaviors and sexual functions of early, middle, and late adolescence.

Early Adolescence. Early adolescence begins approximately between 11 and 13 years and merges with midadolescence at 14 or 15 years (Johnson, 1983). It is characterized by an increase in height and the appearance of the secondary sexual characteristics.

In terms of cognitive powers early adolescent thought represents a mixture of two stages, the concrete operational stage and the beginning of the formal operational stage (Piaget, 1950). Although there is a greater capacity for logical reasoning, adolescent thought is still based largely on concrete evidence rather than on abstractions. Some adolescents never reach the final level of cognition (the ability to deal with abstractions), whereas others move smoothly through the intervening period.

Young adolescents tend to see the world around them only in relation to the effect it has on *them*. As their capacity for abstract thought increases, they become intensely interested in themselves, their thoughts, ideas, and fantasies, and what effect they have on others. As a result they are introspective, self-conscious, and easily hurt by real or imagined slights. They feel that everyone is looking at them critically so they demand privacy. The slamming of the bedroom door, the NO ADMITTANCE signs put on retreats, and the long periods of self-enforced isolation from the family are typical of this phase.

The major task of early adolescence is acceptance of a new body image. The rapid changes in appearance cause adolescents to spend much time thinking about their bodies and comparing their physiques with those of others. Girls are interested in their developing breasts and often want to wear brassieres before they are needed. They tend to idealize body structure and feel depressed when their skin, hair, and legs do not compare favorably with the "ideal."

Parents are still in control, and the young adolescent is aware of vulnerability and need for dependence. However, parents and brothers and sisters notice a beginning of the critical appraisal to which they will be increasingly subjected. The adolescent becomes aware of the status of the family in the community and is anxious that her or his family measure up to certain standards.

This is the time of intense relationships with members of the same sex, and these relationships are used primarily for support and mutual understanding. Young adolescents have endless face-to-face and telephone conversations about hypothetical activities; for example, "If Peter speaks to me, I will say . . . ." Through these conversations they weigh alternatives, assess risks, evaluate results and in fact practice the problem-solving approach.

Vocational choice is not a source of conflict. The young adolescent's choice is often unrealistic or idealistic. Young adolescents fantasize about what they are able to do, and although their increasing cognitive powers make them accept this as daydreaming, they are defensive about their abilities. They do like to work for money and often take newspaper routes or babysit.

Midadolescence. Midadolescence begins around 14 or 15 years and merges with late adolescence at about age 17. Almost all adolescents have reached their growth peak by midadolescence. Many aspects of the body have attained their adult form. For example, in boys the development of the lower jaw alters the contour of the face from the round, childish one to that of the adult. Both boys and girls generally accept their bodies, although this acceptance is tempered by a desire to look otherwise. As a result the interest in their bodies is expressed through efforts to improve themselves. Grooming, makeup, and the right clothes become all important. Stabilizing the body image is important in developing a sense of identity. Adolescents of this age can remember that they looked much the same a year ago; body structure has begun to assume permanence.

The midadolescent phase is characterized by increasing competence in abstract thought (Johnson, 1983). The adolescent is capable of perceiving future implications of current acts and decisions. The ability to think in this manner fluctuates. In times of stress the adolescent reverts to concrete operations.

The major task during this phase is emancipation from the family. Adolescents vacillate between acting like responsible adults and acting like dependent children. Their ability to step into the adult role, even if

Table 4-5 Adolescent Sexual Development

Behavior	Function
EARLY ADOLESCENCE (12 TO 15 YR)	
Talking; being given greater autonomy and less direct adult supervision	Enlargement of the testing of superego formation
Greater involvement in and importance of peer groups, especially same sex (homosocial peer involvement); social recognition of sexual interest even if premature in terms of biologic development	Reflects commitment to anticipated roles
Masturbation, necking, petting, and especially heterosexual intercourse	Commonly generates feelings of anxiety and guilt
Boys	Directly linked to sexual pleasure
Capacity to ejaculate; first orgasm within 2 years of puberty for all but a few boys	
Pattern of masturbation initiated	Leads to independent commitment to sexuality (i.e., capacity to engage in sexual activity without social or emotional attachments); exploring of biologic capacities
Active fantasy life	Helps reinforce commitments to heterosexual behavior
Girls	
Menstruation	Serves as direct reminder that intercourse can result in pregnancy
Masturbation to orgasm rare at this age	
Homosocial peer involvement	Reflects a commitment to anticipated roles as girlfriend, wife, and mother
MIDDLE ADOLESCENCE (15 TO 18 YR)	
Rating and dating system becomes central aspect of adolescent society	Heterosociality becomes fairly normative in terms of both adult and youth culture expectations
Masturbation, especially for boys, is an important sexual outlet	Represents way station in transition from infantile to adult sexuality and from narcissism to object relatedness
Sociosexual activity colored by homosocial attachments (activity involves sharing stories about scoring, going steady, etc.)	Role confirmation
Petting, genital involvement without coitus; when there is coital involvement, relationships are usually not serious and do not generate numerous repetitions	Associated with involvement in peer social life (i.e., general popularity, frequency of dating, number of partners dated)
LATE ADOLESCENCE (18 TO 20 YR)	
Premarital intercourse virtually normative	Period of maximum interpersonal and intrapsychic sexual self-consciousness
Beginning of superficial problems of sexual competence (i.e., secondary impotence, premature ejaculation, penis size, failure to achieve orgasm)	One's sexual status is a matter of public concern
Unresolved problems of relating erotic to sentimental (residual of good girl vs. bad girl syndrome, masturbation)	
Girl's anxieties about unintended pregnancy and concern for effect on her reputation if relationship does not culminate in marriage	

Adapted by Marianne Zalar from Sadock BJ, Kaplan HD, and Freedman AM: The sexual experience, Baltimore, 1976, The Williams & Wilkins Co.

briefly, increases their resentment of being considered children. Role experimentation becomes a central process in the search for identity. Adolescents "try out" many roles in fantasy. They may select movie stars or sports heroes as role models. Vocational choice is related to the midadolescents' concern about obtaining the life-style they desire. The settled occupations of their parents and their parents' friends may seem too confining. They want to do something new, different, and monetarily rewarding.

There is a definite movement away from the family. Midadolescents are critical of their parents, and the parents' appearance, behavior, dress, and social manners are all subjected to intense scrutiny and disparagement. Brothers and sisters are considered a nuisance, and the adolescent sees herself as being treated unfairly in terms of other members of the family. An adult outside the family group—a nurse, a physician, a coach, or a school counselor, for example—may be taken as a role model. There is increased participation in the adult world. Adolescents become advocates of various ideologies and enjoy debating the merits of current ideas. Many show evidence of leadership potential as they engage in developing their cognitive skills. Rebellion is usually couched in verbal terms rather than physical ones and is more destructive than constructive. Running away is a common phenomenon for adolescents between the ages of 15 and 17 years as an attempt to solve problems and to prove they are not children.

Peer relationships now dominate over family ones. The adolescent looks to the peer group for definitions of the behavioral code. There is a strong need to affirm the newly developed self-image through the affirmation of peers. Most conflicts with parents reflect this change, and communication patterns that were once open may become closed.

There is a change from relationships with members of the same sex to heterosexual relationships (**heterosexuality**). Adolescents test their ability to attract the opposite sex. They continue to define the parameters of femininity and masculinity. They tend to develop plural or rapidly changing serial relationships. As one mother remarked, "I couldn't keep up with the girls' names. I use to just say 'Hello there.' I was afraid I'd call Brenda, Linda or make some other terrible mistake."

Late Adolescence. The late adolescent phase extends from age 17 through 21. The upper limit of the phase depends on cultural, economic, and educational factors (Johnson, 1983). The late adolescent is physically mature. Most late adolescents have achieved a stable body image, and the agonizing over this or that real or fancied disability is largely over.

Cognitive development in late adolescence reflects the decentering of thought and production of a life plan, as described by Elkind (1968) and Piaget (1972). They have established abstract thought processes. They are future oriented and capable of perceiving and acting on long-range options.

One of the major tasks confronting the late adolescent is to become a fully *independent* productive citizen. This occurs as the adolescent moves from being an idealistic reformer to an achiever. Adolescents finally realize that criticism alone will not bring about changes and that ideals must be linked to a commitment and work. They become self-supporting or begin their professional education. They have become socially functioning adults (Handwerker and Hodgman, 1983). The choice of career pattern is reasonably set. Whatever it may be, it will establish the adult life-style. Although young women are now assuming the right to choose careers rather than early marriage, many still suspend the final shaping of a career until after commitments to parenthood are fulfilled.

Late adolescents are more tolerant of their families, in part perhaps because they sense the ending of the intense dependent relationship. If, on the whole, parents have permitted growth through role experimentation and have supported the need for increasing independence, the conflicts of parent and child seem to fade. On the other hand, the now self-supporting person may feel totally alienated and break all family ties.

Late adolescents' relationships are still peer-centered, but they realize that with the changes in locale necessitated by job or education these early friendships may end and be replaced by others. The need for approval by the peer group is still strong.

The late adolescent is capable of forming stable relationships. She or he is ready for mutuality and reciprocity in caring for another, in contrast to the former self-centered orientation. Marriage and family become part of present or future plans.

Adolescent Sexuality. The adolescent's heightened sexual awareness brings to the surface sexual concerns. These include myths about masturbation and concerns about possible homosexuality, sexual activity and the presence, frequency, and content of sexual fantasies and dreams. Although physically sexually mature, they are trying to cope with emerging sensations and social situations while they are still psychologically immature.

Masturbation. Young adolescents may fear that any variation from normal, particularly of the genitals, has resulted from masturbation. The adolescent needs to learn that **masturbation** is a normal, universal behavior that causes neither physical nor mental harm. It is a natural part of learning about human sexuality and can be a useful means of relieving sexual tension (Brookman, 1983).

Masturbation is also a common mode of discharge of tension for adolescents, particularly when alone, unhappy, or frustrated. It serves to fuse psychologic and physical sexuality. It is not always associated with sexual fantasies. The value of masturbation may be lessened by the shame and guilt that accompany it. Male adolescents often fear discovery of evidence of ejaculation and females often fear changes in their genitals as a result of masturbation. Fears are not limited to discovery by others but also are caused by the expansive experience of orgasm, with the resulting feelings of loss of ego boundaries. If masturbation is used as a continual source of comfort or with inappropriate exposure (exhibitionism), it is indicative of disturbance (Stuart and Sundeen, 1987).

Mutual masturbation can also serve the purposes of tension release and fusing of identity. If mutual masturbation is the primary focus of the relationship, without the enrichment of other aspects of a relationship, then it may be maladaptive. Mutual masturbation is often acceptable to adolescents as long as it does not lead to intercourse. It can help dispel anxieties about sexuality by assuring adolescents that they are sexually adequate.

Homosexuality. Homosexual experience to some degree is part of the psychosexual development of many individuals. The adolescent who is overly affectionate with same-sex peers or adults may cause considerable parental concern. This is a result of society's unresolved position on the meaning or acceptance of homosexuality. Fantasies about sexual encounters with members of the same sex can be very disturbing to the adolescent. Memories of early same-sex explorations compound the adolescent's fear of becoming homosexual. The fear is probably a reaction to society's negative valuation of homosexuality.

For many years the medical profession, including psychiatry, has searched for causes of **homosexuality.** The message in looking for the cause of a condition is that it is a maladaptive state that can be treated or cured. Many theories of the cause of homosexuality have been formulated; however, no cause has ever been established. Today emphasis is placed on learning more about homosexuality and viewing it as a sexual preference or mode of sexual expression (Kinsey, 1948).

Marmor (1980) defined the homosexual person as "one who is motivated in adult life by a definite preferential erotic attraction to members of the same sex and who usually (but not necessarily) engages in overt sexual relations with them." Marmor's definition excludes transitory incidental homosexual activity in adolescence and in primarily heterosexual persons.

The incidence of homosexuality in the United States today has been conservatively estimated at 10% to 15% of the population (APA, 1987). If these estimates are accurate, nurses come into contact with homosexuals on a daily basis. Despite this incidence of homosexuality, nurses generally know little about homosexuality and almost always assume that all clients are heterosexual (Stuart and Sundeen, 1987).

Sexual Activity. Adolescents are surrounded by mixed messages. Parents, religious groups, teachers, health professionals, and others tell them to refrain from sexual contact, to control sexual impulses, and to keep away from temptation. Many of these same adults are asking adolescents to refrain from activities they themselves openly practice. At the same time books, movies, music, and advertisements are laden with sexually stimulating messages.

Questions about whether and when to be sexually active and whether one needs to have sex to be popular become a major part of the lives of adolescents. They express confusion about love and how one expresses love, and concern about sexual adequacy. Pajama parties and locker room discussions are often the only outlet the adolescent has to discuss some of these concerns and to obtain information—and a great deal of misinformation—about sex.

Interest in dating stems from the adolescent's need for companionship and emotional and physical closeness. Intimacy includes hand-holding, kissing, embracing, petting, and sexual intercourse. Approximately two thirds of all teenage males and one half of all teenage females have had intercourse at least once (Brookman, 1983). Many younger adolescents may use intercourse as a means of conforming to peer group expectations, as a challenge to parents, as experimentation, or as a means of relieving loneliness or stress. Some adolescents develop sincere commitments to one another that may persist and lead to marriage. Many have "a series of close committed single-partner relationships, each lasting weeks, months, or longer" (Brookman, 1983). Few adolescents are **promiscuous;** that is, they do not have multiple partners with little or no commitment.

Adolescents are hesitant to talk to adults, especially parents, because the adult often discounts or invalidates their feelings. Some parents are threatened by their adolescent's budding sexuality. They (and some nurses) deal with their own uncertainty about sex by ignoring the reality of adolescent sexuality or by becoming hostile and punitive. At times little attention is given to the teenager who is reluctant to engage in dating at all. The young person who fails to show any interest may need careful evaluation.

Implications for Nursing. Health professionals need to be knowledgeable and comfortable with their own sexuality to work effectively with adolescents. Glossing over important issues and making broad generalizations about sexual concerns can be more confusing than helpful. Nurses who counsel young people about specific sexual issues need (1) knowledge of sexual anatomy, physiology, and behavior; (2) recognition of the importance of local peer influences; and (3) understanding of the adolescent's family and ethnocultural background. The approach to adolescents is based on their intellectual and psychosocial maturation. Provision of privacy and reassurance of confidentiality are essential to building trust and confidence between adolescent and nurse. The adolescent usually is willing to express concerns if the discussions are held in a comfortable and nonjudgmental setting.

An increased incidence of adolescent pregnancy and the increased number of adolescents with sexually transmitted diseases, including AIDS, make sex education and sex counseling a major task for nurses working with adolescents (see Chapter 27). Information about their bodies' sexual responses, contraception, pregnancy, and sexually transmitted disease can be made available to them to help them become sexually responsible adults.

It is important for nurses working with adolescents to be aware of adolescents' concern about masturbation and homosexuality. Factual information about masturbation can be given to adolescents, but it is not appropriate for the counselor to advocate masturbation. The decision should be made by each person and includes personal values, such as religious belief.

Brookman (1983) states that reassurance concerning homosexuality may be offered by sharing these points:

1. Strong attraction to same-sex adults is a normal event for most adolescents, representing displacement of such feelings for parents onto others in the separation-individuation process.
2. Strong attraction to same-sex peers is the first step in the shifting of a person's love-object relationship from the parents to age mates. It is also an intermediate early-adolescent stage in the development of the capacity to form intimate interpersonal relationships.
3. Exhibitionism, voyeurism, and mutual masturbation are common experimental experiences, especially among boys age 8 to 13. Group masturbation and ejaculation, often as a contest, are common methods of declaring maturity and superiority in the peer group.
4. In many cultures, the expression of affection between same-sex friends and relatives through embracing and kissing is a normal and accepted practice for males, as well as females.
5. People who have had a homosexual episode in adolescence do not necessarily retain a homosexual preference as adults. There is nothing predictive in such an act alone.
6. Adult sexual identity is not solidified until late adolescence, but as this is most influenced by early childhood factors, ultimate sexual gender preference is well established, albeit nascent, by the advent of adolescence.

It is important to note that some adult homosexuals report awareness of their homosexuality as early as adolescence. The nurse counseling such adolescents needs to be accepting and comfortable in communicating with people who exhibit a sexual preference that may differ from their own. The incidence of sexually transmitted diseases and other infections encountered in sexual relationships makes it essential to secure appropriate medical and counseling sources for all individuals. Nurses who are not comfortable with these clients need to refer them to other professionals or agencies who can help them. "Counseling support from within the gay community can be a valuable adjunct to whatever the health professional can provide" (Brookman, 1983).

Adulthood

Adulthood encompasses the period from adolescence to a person's death. Three phases are discernable: early, middle, and late adulthood. Table 4-6 outlines the sexual behaviors and sexual functions of these three phases.

Early Adulthood. Early adulthood encompasses that portion of the life cycle devoted to parenting, consolidation of relationships, whether marital or nonmarital, and commitment to a life work. The young adult has attained physical and intellectual maturity. Stature and reproductive growth are virtually complete. The process of aging, beginning in the twenties and continuing in the thirties and forties, causes minimum overt change.

Cognitive powers include the ability to think abstractly, to be future oriented, and to act on long-range options (Piaget, 1950). Personality development is related to the task of developing intimacy and solidarity as opposed to existing in isolation (Erikson, 1959). Intimacy involves learning to give and receive love, choosing whether to marry and choosing a sexual partner or partners (Duvall, 1977).

Body image remains a concern for the young adult, particularly in terms of body contour and size (Woods, 1984). Nonacceptance of one's body may inhibit the establishment of sexual relationships.

Family ties are important, but the relationship of parent and child takes on an adult quality. The young adult is expected to be moving toward financial and social independence from the family. She or he is also expected to choose a vocation and obtain the necessary education for it. Establishing a career and advancing in it are major concerns throughout this part of the life cycle.

Social groupings include varying age levels and are

often based on similar interests. The need for strong friendships with peers diminishes as individual friendships assume permanence.

Sexuality. Early adulthood has been described as a period of maximum sexual self-consciousness (Offer and Simon, 1976). There is social acceptance and legitimization of sexual experiences. The tasks of sexual development for the young adult include maintaining a long-term commitment to a sexual relationship, practicing responsible reproductive health care, and making rational decisions about childbearing.

1. *Commitment to a relationship* is strengthened by the need to give and receive pleasure. Commitments vary in length and type. For example, some couples remain monogamous throughout their marriage. Others have open marriages, in which the couple agrees that one or both may participate in other sexual encounters. Some couples remain in relationships without formal marriage. Relationships can be terminated by divorce or death. Finally, serial monogamy is practiced by many people in the United States. Serial monogamy is characterized by repeated marriages and divorces. The person is married to only one person at a time but is married a number of times throughout her or his life.
2. *Responsible reproductive health care* includes such actions as women having a Papanicolaou smear at prescribed intervals and both women and men avoiding sexually transmitted diseases.
3. *Rational decisions about childbearing* are important to ensure that every child is a wanted child. The couple is responsible for using reliable contraceptive means when pregnancy is not desired. Unwanted and unplanned children often become targets of abuse and neglect.

Table 4-6 **Adult Sexual Development**

Behavior	Function
EARLY ADULTHOOD (23 TO 30 YR)	
Formal engagement and marriage	Sexual access legitimized and regularized; as sexual access ceases to be a problem, more attention focused on activity
Sexual dysfunction problems become more meaningfully symptomatic	Problems with gender competence, regularization of sexual access plus sheer density of interaction may result in declining eroticism especially for men
Pregnancy and child rearing	Many pressures (fatigue, economic, time, occupational) contribute to decreased eroticism
Beginning of extramarital affairs	More common among men of low socioeconomic class because of weaker commitment to occupational success and resulting loss of homosocial masculinity
MIDDLE ADULTHOOD (30 TO 46 YR)	
Rates of marital intercourse decline	Maximum involvement in careers, family, and child rearing
Men's interest in marital competence decreases	Much of decline caused by (1) de-eroticization of wife-mother role and (2) husband's alternative attachments
Women's interest in marital competence increases	Commitment to the sensual and away from continuing confirmation of emotional attachment
Period of rising extramarital activity	For men, homosocial validation of masculinity; for women, justification
LATE ADULTHOOD (46 TO 65 YR)	
Imperative to continue sexual activity	Harder for either sex to continue to function because of long sexual abstinence
Loss of sexual partner through death or illness	Commonly have guilt feelings about sexual fantasies
Performance problems (particularly erectile difficulties)	Source of anxiety
Menopause	Can be freedom from pregnancy worries and also source of concern in youth-oriented society
OLD AGE (65 + YR)	
Sexual feelings still experienced although desire and ability have decreased somewhat	Result in guilt feelings because of cultural **taboo** against sexuality among aged persons

Adapted by Marianne Zalar from Sadock BJ, Kaplan HD, and Freedman AM: The sexual experience, Baltimore, 1976, The Williams & Wilkins Co.

Myths. In a culture characterized by a rapid increase in knowledge and technology, many people still are misinformed about human sexuality. Listed below are common myths about reproduction and birth control (Stuart and Sundeen, 1987):

1. A couple must have simultaneous climaxes if conception is to take place
2. A woman can become pregnant only through penile penetration or artificial insemination
3. Urination by the woman after coitus or having sexual intercourse in a standing position will prevent pregnancy
4. The woman determines the sex of the child
5. Excessive masturbation is harmful
6. Sex during menstruation is unclean and harmful
7. Advancing age means the end of sex

Middle and Late Adulthood. These phases of the life cycle represent the greatest maximizing of early potential and then a gradual lessening of biopsychosocial attainment through the normal process of aging. Changes in family structure from events such as children leaving home, death of a spouse or role reversal in dealing with aging parents necessitate major changes in life-style. The critical task for these years is maintaining feelings of self-esteem versus despair. The need to love and be loved, to be successful, and to feel meaningful prompts involvement in community service and in leisure pursuits.

Cognitive powers continue unabated until physical insults such as Alzheimer's disease or cerebral vascular accident cause a decline. Body image remains an important concern. Western society's accent on health and youth make grooming, weight, nutrition, and exercise a continuous part of an adult's daily life.

Sexuality. The sexual developmental tasks of middle and late adulthood focus primarily on adapting to the physical and emotional changes in sexual performance caused by the aging process. The childbearing years are coming to an end. This is a relief for many couples because the threat of pregnancy can be removed from their lovemaking. Others may mourn the loss of the chance for another child.

The fear of growing older in a youth-oriented society can be a source of depression and anxiety. Bodily changes, lower hormone production, and menopause may contribute to anxiety and depression.

The research of Masters and Johnson (1966) has shown that aging does not decrease libido or the capacity to be orgasmic. Men and women are capable of sexual activity well into their old age. Disinterest and abstinence are probably caused by loss of a partner, boredom, ill health, or cultural attitudes about the appropriateness.

Many older people do not understand the impact of aging on their physical response to sexual stimulation. They see these changes as an indication they should terminate sexual activity rather than merely as a need to make minor adaptations. For example, vaginal lubrication in women is slower and decreased in amount; in men, erection is slower and erectile firmness decreased. Love play will probably need to be extended, with more direct genital stimulation to produce lubrication and erection. Woman have a shortened orgasmic phase and men's need to ejaculate decreases, resulting in decreased force and volume of ejaculation. These physiologic changes require adaptations in sexual behavior and not cessation of sexual activity.

Mims and Swenson (1980) have stated:

> Sexual fulfillment throughout adulthood and into old age is not only possible but likely. The feeling that older people are not interested in sex (except if they are abnormal—the "dirty old man" syndrome) is largely caused by our inability to imagine our parents or our grandparents as sexually active people. The greatest danger of such attitudes is that they tend to comprise a "self-fulfilling prophecy": if people believe that sexual interest ceases with advancing age, they will find that it does cease. Or, if sexual interest persists, people may believe themselves to be abnormal, sinful, or psychologically sick.

Implications for Nursing. The nurse is in a unique position to help adults with health maintenance and detection of problems concerning sexuality. Contacts with adults occur at clinics or hospitals when people seek counseling or care for contraception. Giving nursing care during the pregnancy cycle is an important part of the maternity nurse's role.

The role of sex educator is an important one for nurses working with families during the childbearing and child rearing years. Parents often need help with teaching their children about sex because adults commonly are misinformed about many aspects of reproduction and how their bodies function. Parents therefore need accurate sex information to teach their children to be healthy, responsible sexual beings.

Besides helping with childhood and adult sexuality, the nurse can help prepare clients for the sexual problems and changes occurring with age. Many nurses have not been aware of the importance of sex education for older people because of the myth that the elderly are no longer interested in sex.

Sexual dysfunction problems often begin after children are born. The mother especially may become so involved with child rearing that her relationship with her husband suffers. At the same time the husband may be actively involved in career establishment, thereby leaving little energy for home life. The nurse needs to be aware of how the demands of parenting can adversely affect the marital relationship. Simple counseling provided during these early years may prevent serious marital problems in later years.

The older woman, in particular, who has been able to move gracefully into old age and who continues to recognize herself as a sexual being is probably better able to accept the sexuality of the young. The pregnancy of a daughter then may be accepted as a continuation of her own sexuality rather than as a threat or reminder of her lost youth.

A knowledgeable, nonjudgmental nurse who recognizes personal sexual biases can contribute a great deal to the sexual health of young families. The nurse can recognize potential problems within the marriage and either intervene or refer the couple for further counseling.

SUMMARY

Basic knowledge about the female and male reproductive systems is a prerequisite to understanding the process of conception. A systematic investigation of the human reproductive system provides the nurse with a firm foundation for gaining insight into the client's needs and health concerns.

Basic concepts of the psychosocial nature of human sexuality provide guidelines for anticipatory guidance of the childbearing family. Each individual's cognitive and personality development influence his or her mastery of developmental tasks from infancy through adulthood. The atmosphere in which the child is raised will affect future attitudes and behaviors. Sexual identity begins early and is shaped by societal expectations. Mixed messages about sexuality, peer pressures, and confusion about the relationship of love and sex may cause conflicts. During adulthood childhood potential is realized and key social roles are assumed. The importance ascribed to the roles of man-woman, husband-wife, and parent-child reflect society's concern with the biopsychosocial nature of adult sexuality. Nurses need to understand that everyone's feelings and values regarding sexuality are not going to match their own feelings and values.

LEARNING ACTIVITIES

1. Using a teaching model, identify the external and internal structures of both female and male reproductive systems.
2. In group discussion, describe myths and misunderstandings encountered regarding menstruation and menopause.
3. Assess some of the popularized books on sexual response and bring findings to class for a discussion of how this material relates to anatomic and physiologic facts, accepted theories of sexual response, and the challenges of client education for the nurse.

Continued.

KEY CONCEPTS

- The myometrium of the uterus is uniquely designed to expel the fetus and promote hemostasis after birth.
- The uterus has an intrinsic motility allowing uterine contractions even after spinal cord injury.
- Normal feedback regulation of the menstrual cycle depends on an intact hypothalamic-pituitary-gonadal mechanism.
- Ovulation occurs 14 days *before* the first day of menstruation.
- The female's reproductive tract structures and breasts respond predictably to changing levels of sex steroids across the life span.
- Prostaglandins play an important role in reproductive functions by their affect on smooth muscle contractility and modulation of hormones.
- Disorders associated with menstruation have a negative effect on the quality of life for affected women and their families.
- Premenstrual syndrome (PMS) refers to a diffuse, loosely defined set of symptoms that begins approximately 7 to 10 days before menses and ends with the onset of menses.
- Nurses need to know themselves and to be aware of their own feelings and values regarding sexuality before they can adequately and competently help clients meet their needs for information or refer them for further counseling.
- Adolescence can best be understood in three phases, involving six developmental tasks: achieving more mature relations with age mates of both sexes, achieving a feminine or masculine social role, accepting one's physique, achieving emotional independence of parents and other adults, establishing a satisfying life-style, and acquiring a new set of values.
- Responsible sexuality includes commitment to a relationship, responsible reproductive health care, and rational decisions about childbearing.

4. Identify nurse-held attitudes that may make it difficult for nurses to support the sexuality of the following:
   A. Children
      (1) Preschool age group (ages 3 to 5 years)
      (2) School age group (ages 5 to 11 years)
      (3) Adolescents (ages 12 to 15 years)
   B. Older parent group (40 years old or over)
   C. Mentally or physically impaired persons
   D. Drug-dependent persons (alcoholics, heroin addicts)
5. Write down personal belief systems related to sexuality and discuss how these may affect one's ability to counsel and teach sexuality-related material.

References

American Psychiatric Association: Diagnostic and statistical manual of mental disorders, ed 3, revised, (DSM-III-R), Washington, DC, 1987, The American Psychiatric Association.

Brookman R: Adolescent sexuality and related health problems. In Hoffman A, editor: Adolescent medicine, Menlo Park, Calif, 1983, Addison-Wesley Publishing Co, Inc.

Droegemueller W, et al: Comprehensive gynecology, St Louis, 1987, The CV Mosby Co.

Duvall ER: Family development, ed 5, Philadelphia, 1977, JB Lippincott Co.

Elkind D: Cognitive development in adolescence. In Adams JF, editor: Understanding adolescence, Boston, 1968, Allyn & Bacon, Inc.

Erikson E: Identity and the life cycle; selected papers. In Psychological issues, New York, 1959, International Universities Press.

Fogel DI and Woods NF: Health care of women: a nursing perspective, St Louis, 1981, The CV Mosby Co.

Ganong WE: Review of medical physiology, ed 13, Norwalk, Conn, 1987, Appleton & Lange.

Handwerker L and Hodgman C: Approach to adolescence by Perinatal Staff. In McAnarney E, editor: Premature adolescent pregnancy and parenthood, New York, 1983, Grune & Stratton, Inc.

Havighurst RJ: Developmental tasks and education, ed 3, New York, 1972, David McKay Co, Inc.

Heitkemper MN, Shaver JF, and Mitchell ES: Gastrointestinal symptoms and bowel patterns across the menstrual cycle in dysmenorrhea, Nurs Res 37(2):109, 1988.

Hite S: The Hite report: nationwide study of female sexuality, New York, 1976, Dell Publishing Co, Inc.

Johnson R: Adolescent growth and development. In Hoffman A, editor: Adolescent medicine, Menlo Park, Calif, 1983, Addison-Wesley Publishing Co, Inc.

Kaplan HS: The new sex therapy, New York, 1974, Brunner/Mazel, Inc.

Katchadourian HA and Lunde DT: Fundamentals of human sexuality, New York, 1972, Holt, Rinehart and Winston.

Kinsey AC et al: Sexual behavior in human male, Philadelphia, 1948, WB Saunders Co.

Kinsey AC et al: Sexual behavior in human female, Philadelphia, 1953, WB Saunders Co.

Kolodny RC et al: Textbook of human sexuality for nurses, Boston, 1979, Little, Brown & Co, Inc.

Lublanezki N and Fischer RG: Pediatric drug information, Pediatr Nurs 13(6):435, 1987.

Maccoby EE and Jacklin C: The psychology of sex differences, Stanford, Calif, 1974, Stanford University Press.

Marmor J, editor: Homosexual behavior: a modern reappraisal, New York, 1980, Basic Books Inc, Publishers.

Masters WH and Johnson VE: Human sexual response, 1966, Little, Brown & Co, Inc.

Mims FH and Swenson M: Sexuality, a nursing perspective, New York, 1980, McGraw-Hill Book Co.

Newman B and Newman R: Development through life: a psychosocial approach, Homewood, Ill, 1975, The Dorsey Press.

Offer D and Simon W: Sexual development. In Sadock B, Kaplan H, and Freedman A, editors: The sexual experience, Baltimore, 1976, The Williams & Wilkins Co.

Piaget J: The psychology of intelligence, Boston, 1950, Routledge & Kegan Paul.

Piaget J: Intellectual evolution from adolescence to adulthood, Hum Dev 15:1012, 1972.

Sohn C, Korberly B, and Tannenbaum R: Menstrual products, Handbook of Nonprescription Drugs 17:371, 1986.

Stuart GW and Sundeen SJ: Principles and practice of psychiatric nursing, ed 3, St Louis, 1987, The CV Mosby Co.

Walton J and Youngkin E: The effect of a support group on self-esteem of women with premenstrual syndrome, JOGN Nurs 16(3):174, 1987.

Weisner TS and Gallimore R: My brother's keeper: child and sibling caretaking, Curr Anthropol 18:169, 1977.

Whaley LF and Wong DL: Nursing care of infants and children, ed 4, St Louis, 1990, The CV Mosby Co.

Woods NF: Human sexuality in health and illness, ed 3, St Louis, 1984, The CV Mosby Co.

Bibliography

Anthony CP and Thibodeau GA: Textbook of anatomy and physiology, ed 12, St Louis, 1987, The CV Mosby Co.

Forrest JD: American women—a sexual profile, Contemp OB/GYN 29(special issue): 75, April, 1987.

Hacker SS: Students' questions about sexuality: implications for nurse educators, Nurse Educator 10(4):28, 1984.

Havens B and Swenson I: Menstrual perceptions and preparation among female adolescents, JOGN Nurs 15(5):406, 1986.

Krozy R: Becoming comfortable with sexual assessment, Am J Nurs 78(4):1036, 1980.

Malasanos L, Barkauskas V, Moss M, and Stoltenberg-Ollen K: Health assessment, ed 4, St Louis, 1989, The CV Mosby Co.

Marsman JC and Herold ES: Attitudes toward sex education and values in sex education, Fam Relations 35(3):357, 1986.

Nass GD, Libby RW, and Fisher MP: Sexual choices: an introduction to human sexuality, ed 2, Monterey, Calif, 1984, Wadsworth Health Science Division.

Ryan KJ: Interpreting the controls of the menstrual cycle, Contemp OB/GYN 26(3):107, 1985.

Sherwen LN: Psychosocial dimensions of the pregnant family, New York, 1987, Springer Publishing Co, Inc.

Seidel HM et al: Mosby's guide to physical examination, ed 2, St Louis, 1989, The CV Mosby Co.

Storch ML: Taking a sexual history, Contemp OB/GYN, 29 (special issue): 111, April, 1987.

Thornton NG and Dewis M: Multiple sclerosis and female sexuality, Can Nurse, p 16, April, 1989.

Woods NF: Relationship of socialization and stress to perimenstrual symptoms, disability, and menstrual attitudes, Nurs Res 34(3):145, 1985.

CHAPTER

5 Immunology

Mary L. Turgeon

Learning Objectives

Correctly define the key terms listed.

Explain immunologic benefits of colostrum and breast milk to the newborn.

Compare and contrast active and passive immunity using the Rh factor as an example.

Discuss the relationship between allergic and immunologic phenomena.

Explain helper, suppressor, and killer cells using AIDS as an example.

Describe the action of vaccination using rubella as an example.

Discuss the effect on the functioning of the immune system of factors such as age, life-style, environment, and nutrition.

Key Terms

acquired immunodeficiency syndrome (AIDS)
active immunity
adaptive immunity
anaphylaxis
congenital rubella syndrome
helper cells
hemolytic disease of the newborn
immunocompetent
immunoglobulin
immunology
killer cells
natural immunity
passive immunity
supressor cells
vaccination

Immunology is defined as the study of the molecules, cells, organs, and systems responsible for the recognition and disposal of foreign (nonself) material, as well as of how the human body defends itself against this material. A system such as the human immune system is necessary for survival. Nonself substances can be as diverse as life-threatening infectious microorganisms or a life-saving organ transplant. The desirable consequences of immunity include natural resistance, recovery, and acquired resistance to infectious diseases. A deficiency or dysfunction of the immune system can cause many disorders. Undesirable consequences of immunity include allergy, rejection of a transplanted organ, or an autoimmune disorder (a condition in which the body's own tissues are attacked, as if they were foreign material). In medical science, the immune system can be advantageously manipulated to protect against a disorder such as hemolytic disease of the newborn.

❑ BODY DEFENSES

The first barrier to infection is unbroken skin and mucosal membrane surfaces. These surfaces are of utmost importance in forming a physical barrier against many microorganisms. Secretions such as mucus or those produced in the process of eliminating liquid and solid wastes (e.g., the urinary and gastrointestinal processes) are also important as nonspecific mechanisms for removing potential pathogens from the body. The acidity and alkalinity of the fluids of the stomach and intestinal tract, as well as the acidity of the vagina, can destroy many potentially infectious microorganisms. These fluids can also have chemical properties that are of value in defending the body. Lysozyme is an enzyme found in tears and saliva. This enzyme attacks the cell wall of susceptible bacteria, particularly certain gram-positive bacteria, and destroys the organism. Another chemical of importance in tears and saliva is immunoglobulin A (IgA) antibody.

The body has a wide variety of barrier-assisting defenses that initially protect the body against disease. Although these barriers vary between individuals, they do assist in the general resistance to infectious organisms. Problems associated with nonspecific body defenses that are important in the nursing care of maternity and neonatal clients are presented in Table 5-1.

Natural Immunity

Natural (innate or inborn) resistance is one of the two ways that the body resists infection after microorganisms have penetrated the first line of resistance. The

Table 5-1 Examples of Maternity and Neonatal Immunologic Problems

Client	Immunologic Dysfunction	Potential Problem
Obstetric		
Pregnancy	Decrease in stomach acidity as a result of self-medication with excessive sodium bicarbonate for heartburn (pyrosis)	Increased vulnerability to the invasion of pathogenic bacteria in the gastrointestinal tract
Labor and delivery	Disruption of intact skin as a result of third or fourth degree extension of perineal laceration (episiotomy)	Possible contamination of the suture line and infection (with intestinal [enteric] bacteria) of the perineum, vagina, uterus, uterine tubes, and peritoneum
Postpartum	Drying or cracking of nipples and areola area of the breasts may cause the lubricating glands of Montgomery to cease adequate functioning Retention of moisture as a result of plastic liners in breast pads	Drying can produce a change in the secretion of fatty acids and increased susceptibility to bacterial infection and possibly mastitis
Neonatal	Facial palsy (e.g., Bell's palsy) can cause the eye on the affected side to remain open	Drying of the mucous membrane (conjunctiva) can increase susceptibility to infection

second form, adaptive or acquired resistance, specifically recognizes and selectively eliminates exogenous (or endogenous) agents.

Natural immunity is characterized as a nonspecific mechanism. If a microorganism penetrates the skin or mucosal membranes, cellular and humoral defense mechanisms become operational. The elements of natural resistance are phagocytic cells, complement, and the acute inflammatory reaction. Despite their relative lack of specificity, these components are essential, because they are largely responsible for natural immunity to many environmental microorganisms.

Cellular Components

Mast cells (tissue basophils)
Neutrophils
Macrophages

Humoral Components

Complement
Lysozyme
Interferon

Adaptive Immunity

If a microorganism overwhelms the body's natural resistance, another form of defensive resistance, acquired or **adaptive immunity,** allows the body to recognize, remember, and respond to a specific stimulus—an antigen. Adaptive immunity can eliminate microorganisms, and it commonly leaves the host with specific immunologic memory. This condition of memory or recall, *acquired resistance,* allows the host to respond more effectively if reinfection with the same microorganism occurs. Adaptive immunity, like natural immunity, is composed of cellular and humoral components.

Cellular Components

T lymphocytes
B lymphocytes
Plasma cells

Humoral Components

Antibodies
Lymphokines

The major cellular component of this mechanism is the lymphocyte; the major humoral component is the antibody. Lymphocytes selectively respond to nonself materials—antigens—which leads to immune memory and a permanently altered pattern of response or adaptation to the environment. The majority of the actions of the two categories of the adaptive response—humoral-mediated and cell-mediated immunity (Table 5-2)—are exerted by the interaction of antibody with complement and the phagocytic cells of natural immunity, as well as of T cells with macrophages.

Antibody-mediated Immunity

If specific antibodies have been formed to antigenic stimulation, they are available to protect the body against foreign substances. The recognition of foreign substances and subsequent production of antibodies to these substances is the specific meaning of immunity. Antibody-mediated immunity to infection is *acquired* if the antibodies are formed by the host or received from another source. These two types of acquired immunity

Table 5-2 **Characteristics of Humoral-mediated and Cell-mediated Immunity**

	Humoral-mediated Immunity	Cell-mediated Immunity
Mechanism	Antibody-mediated	Cell-mediated
Cell type	B lymphocytes	T lymphocytes
Mode of action	Antibodies in serum	Direct cell-to-cell contact or soluble products secreted by cells
Purpose	Primary defense against bacterial infection	Defense against viral and fungal infections, intracellular organisms, tumor antigens, and graft rejection

(Table 5-3) are called *active* and *passive* immunity, respectively.

Active immunity can be acquired by natural exposure in response to an infection or natural series of infections, or it may be acquired by an injection of an antigen. This intentional injection of antigen, called **vaccination,** is an effective method of stimulating antibody production and memory (acquired resistance) without suffering from the disease. The selected antigenic agent should produce the antibodies without the clinical signs and symptoms of the disease in an **immunocompetent** host (a person whose immune system is able to recognize a foreign antigen and build specific antigen-directed antibodies) and produce permanent antigenic memory. Booster vaccinations may be needed in some cases to expand the pool of memory cells.

Artificial **passive immunity** is achieved by infusion of serum or plasma containing high concentrations of antibody. This form of passive immunity provides immediate antibody protection against microorganisms such as hepatitis A. The antibodies have been produced by another person or animal that has been actively immunized, but the ultimate recipient has not produced them. The recipient will only temporarily benefit from passive immunity for as long as the antibodies persist in his or her circulation. Passive immunity can also be acquired naturally by the fetus through the transfer of antibodies by the maternal circulation in utero. Maternal antibodies are also transferred to the newborn after parturition in the prelactation fluid called colostrum. For the newborn to have lasting protection, active immunity must occur.

Table 5-3 **Types of Acquired Immunity**

Type	Mode of Acquisition	Antibody Produced by Host	Duration of Immune Response
ACTIVE			
Natural	Infection	Yes	Long*
Artificial	Vaccination	Yes	Long*
PASSIVE			
Natural	Transfer in vivo or through colostrum	No	Short
Artificial	Infusion of serum/plasma	No	Short

*In the immunocompetent host.

Hypersensitivity Reactions

Immediate hypersensitivity comprises a subset of the body's antibody-mediated effector mechanisms. This subset consists of the reactions primarily mediated by immunoglobulin E (IgE), a class of immunoglobulins with unique biologic properties. Expression of immediate hypersensitivity results from:

1. Exposure to antigen (allergens)
2. Development of an IgE antibody response to the antigen
3. Binding of the IgE to mast cells
4. Reexposure to the antigen
5. Antigen-interaction with antigen-specific IgE bound to the surface membrane of mast cells
6. Release of potent chemical mediators from sensitized mast cells
7. Action of these mediators on various organs

Atopic diseases are processes mediated by or related to IgE-immediate hypersensitivity. The most dramatic and devastating systemic manifestation of immediate hypersensitivity is **anaphylaxis.** Anaphylaxis is an immediate hypersensitivity reaction characterized by local reactions such as *urticaria* (hives) and *angioedema* (redness and swelling), or by systemic reactions in the respiratory tract, cardiovascular system, gastrointestinal tract, and skin. This type of reaction can be fatal. Other types of atopic diseases include allergic rhinoconjunctivitis, asthma, gastrointestinal allergy, and atopic dermatitis, an eczematous skin eruption.

In addition to IgE-dependent hypersensitivity, two other immunoglobulin-dependent (antibody-dependent) mechanisms and a cell-mediated, delayed hypersensitivity mechanism exist. A system of classification for hypersensitivity was developed over two decades ago. Characteristics of this classification of hypersensitivity are presented in Table 5-4.

Although antihistamines have a role to play in the treatment of mild allergic phenomena, they cannot be effective in situations of severe manifestations of allergy (as anaphylaxis). In these cases epinephrine (Adrenalin) is the drug of choice (by injection) to reverse the pathophysiologic condition by dilating the bronchi; by constricting the blood vessels, causing an increase in blood pressure; and by increasing the rate and strength of the heartbeat (and therefore the circulation of oxygen through the body).

The desensitization process—by which minute amounts of the allergen are gradually introduced into the client's system (increasing the exposure, but in amounts that are too small to produce allergic symptoms)—is technically an immunologic treatment aimed at helping the body become immune to the allergen by developing IgM antibodies specific to the substance.

Some clients have developed a sensitivity to certain foods, soaps, or drugs as allergens. Although it should be standard procedure for the nurse to assess all clients for sensitivity to foods and substances (including adhesive tape), occasionally the nurse is involved in producing an inadvertant allergic reaction in a client. Such an incident may even occur while the nurse is administering a protective immunization to a client (as the rubella vaccine), since the vaccine is derived from duck egg or human (foreign protein) culture.

Cell-mediated Immunity

Cell-mediated immunity consists of immune activities that differ from those of antibody-mediated immunity. Cell-mediated immunity is moderated by the link between T lymphocytes and phagocytic cells (i.e., monocyte-macrophage cells). Lymphocytes (T cells) do not recognize the antigens of microorganisms or other living cells, such as *allografts* (a graft of tissue from a genetically different member of the same species [e.g., a human kidney]), directly, but do so when the antigen is present on the surface of an antigen-presenting cell—the macrophage. Lymphocytes are immunologically active through various types of direct cell-to-cell contact and by the production of soluble factors, such as *lymphokines,* for specific immunologic functions. These include the recruitment of phagocytic cells to the site of inflammation. The term *delayed hypersensitivity* is often used synonymously with the term *cell-mediated immunity. Delayed hypersensitivity,* however, refers to the slow appearance of a secondary response in the skin. The term dates back to the time when antibody responses were detected by immediate hypersensitivity and reflected the subtle difference in the length of time that it took for a delayed response to occur (e.g., tuberculin skin test). The process of cell-mediated immunity can be seen in the sequence of events resulting in poison ivy dermatitis caused by binding of the substance to the skin:

1. Delayed hypersensitivity (contact dermatitis)
2. Immunity to viral and fungal antigens
3. Immunity to intracellular organisms
4. Rejection of foreign-tissue grafts
5. Elimination of tumor cells bearing neoantigens
6. Formation of chronic granulomas (undegradable material such as tubercle bacilli, streptococcal cell walls, asbestos, or talc sequestered in a focus of concentric macrophages that also contain some lymphocytes and eosinophils)

Under some conditions, the activities of cell-mediated immunity may not be beneficial. Suppression of the normal adaptive immune response *(immunosuppression)* by drugs or other means is necessary in conditions such as organ transplantation, hypersensitivity, and autoimmune disorders.

Table 5-4 Classification of Hypersensitivity Reactions

	Type I Anaphylactic	Type II Cytotoxic	Type III Immune Complex	Type IV T Cell–Dependent
Antibody	IgE	IgG, possibly other	IgG, IgM	None
Cells involved	Mast cells, basophils	Red cells, white cells, platelets	Host tissue cells	T cells, macrophages
Examples	Anaphylaxis, hay fever, food allergy	Transfusion reactions, hemolytic disease of the newborn, thrombocytopenia	Arthus reaction, serum sickness, pneumonitis	Allergy of infection, contact dermatitis

Modified from Barrett JT: Textbook of immunology: an introduction to immunochemistry and immunobiology, ed 5, St Louis, 1988, The CV Mosby Co.

Cells and Cellular Activities

The entire leukocytic cell system is designed to defend the body against disease. Each cell type, however, has a unique function and behaves both independently and in many cases in cooperation with other cell types. Leukocytes can be functionally divided into the general categories of granulocyte, monocyte-macrophage, and lymphocyte-plasma cell. The primary phagocytic cells are the polymorphonuclear neutrophilic (PMN) leukocytes and the mononuclear monocyte-macrophage cells. The lymphocytes participate in body defenses primarily through the recognition of foreign antigen and production of antibody. Plasma cells are antibody-synthesizing cells.

In normal circulating blood, the following types of leukocytes can be found in order of frequency: neutrophils, lymphocytes, monocytes, eosinophils, and basophils. The lymphocytes participate in defending the body against disease through recognition of foreign antigens and antibody production. Several major categories of lymphocytes are recognized as functionally active. These categories are the *T cells, B cells,* and the *natural killer (NK)* and *K-type* lymphocytes.

T cells are responsible for cellular immune responses and are involved in the regulation of antibody reactions either by helping or suppressing the activation of B lymphocytes. Sensitized T lymphocytes protect humans against infection by mediating intracellular pathogens that are viral, bacterial, fungal, or protozoan. These cells are responsible for chronic rejection in organ transplantation. T cells are divided into two subsets: the *helper/inducer* (CD_4 [T_4]) and the *suppressor/cytotoxic* (CD_8 [T_8]). Functionally, the helper T cells signal B cells to generate antibodies, control production and switching of types of antibodies formed, and activate suppressor cells. The normal functioning of **helper cells** and **suppressor cells** in the immune response can be reversed under certain conditions, such as autoimmune disorders, and acquired immunodeficiency syndrome (AIDS). The normal ratio of helper cells and suppressor cells (approximately 2:1) can be reversed under certain conditions.

B cells serve as the primary source of cells responsible for humoral (antibody) responses. Participation of B cells in the humoral immune response is accomplished by their maturation into plasma cells with subsequent synthesis and secretion of immune antibodies (immunoglobulins). Stimulation of B cells to produce antibodies is a complex process usually requiring interactions between macrophages (that phagocytize, process, and present antigens to T cells), T cells, and B cells. B lymphocytes aid in the body's defense against encapsulated bacteria, such as streptococci. The condition of hyperacute rejection of transplanted organs is mediated by the B cell.

Lymphocytes that lack the recognizable surface markers of mature T or B lymphocytes include the natural killer (NK) cells and **killer** (K) **cells.** The NK and K cells destroy target cells through an extracellular nonphagocytic mechanism referred to as a *cytotoxic reaction.* NK cells have the ability to nonspecifically attack certain types of tumor cells and cells infected with a number of different viruses. NK cells are stimulated by interferon (an antiviral substance) released by an intracellular virus. NK cells will actively kill the virally infected target cell and if this is completed before the virus has time to replicate, they will combat viral infection. NK cells are classified as a population of effector lymphocytes that produce such mediators as *interferon* and *interleukin-2* (IL-2). K cells exhibit a different kind of cytotoxic mechanism than NK cells; the target cell must be coated with low concentrations of IgG antibody. This is referred to as an antibody dependent cell-mediated cytotoxicity (ADCC) reaction. An ADCC reaction may be exhibited by both K cells and phagocytic and nonphagocytic myelogenous type leukocytes. K cells are capable of lysing tumor cells.

Antibody Classes

Five distinct classes of **immunoglobulin** molecules are recognized in most higher mammals: IgM, IgG, IgA, IgD, and IgE. These immunoglobulin classes differ from each other in such things as molecular weight and carbohydrate content. In addition to the differences between classes, the immunoglobulins vary within each class.

IgG. The major immunoglobulin in normal serum is IgG. This immunoglobulin diffuses more readily into the extravascular spaces than other immunoglobulins and neutralizes toxins or binds to microoganisms in extravascular spaces. It is capable of crossing the placenta. IgG accounts for 70% to 75% of the total immunoglobulin pool.

IgM. IgM accounts for about 10% of the immunoglobulin pool. It is largely confined to the intravascular pool because of its large size. This antibody is produced early in an immune response and is largely confined to the blood. IgM is effective in agglutination and cytolytic reactions. In humans, it is found in smaller concentrations than IgG or IgA.

IgA. IgA represents 15% to 20% of the total circulatory immunoglobulin pool. It is the predominant immunoglobulin in secretions, such as tears, saliva, colostrum, breast milk, nasal fluids, and intestinal secretions. Secretory IgA is of critical importance in protecting body surfaces against invading microorganisms. It provides external surfaces of the body with protection from microorganisms because of its presence in seromucous secretions.

IgD. IgD is found in very low concentrations in plasma. It accounts for less than 1% of the total immunoglobulin pool and is very susceptible to proteolysis. This immunoglobulin is primarily a cell membrane immunoglobulin found on the surface of B lymphocytes in association with IgM.

IgE. IgE is a trace plasma protein in the blood plasma of unparasitized individuals. IgE is of major importance because it mediates some types of hypersensitivity (allergic) reactions, allergies, and anaphylaxis. It is generally responsible for an individual's immunity to invading parasites. The IgE molecule is unique because it mediates the release of histamines and heparin.

Antibody Synthesis. Production of antibodies is induced when the host's immune system comes into contact with a foreign antigenic substance and reacts to this antigenic stimulation. When an antigen is initially encountered, the cells of the immune system recognize the antigen as nonself and either elicit an immune response or become tolerant to it depending on the circumstances. An immune reaction can take the form of cell-mediated immunity (immunity dependent on T cells and macrophages) or involve the production of antibodies directed against the antigen. Whether a cell-mediated response or an antibody response takes place depends on the way in which the antigen is presented to the lymphocytes; many immune reactions display both kinds of responses. The antigenicity of a foreign substance is also related to the route of entry. Intravenous and intraperitoneal routes are stronger stimuli than subcutaneous and intramuscular routes. Subsequent exposure to the same antigen produces a memory response, an *anamnestic response,* and reflects the outcome of the initial challenge. In the case of antibody production, both the quantity and class of immunoglobulins produced varies.

❑ IMMUNOLOGIC CONDITIONS IN MATERNITY NURSING

Immunologic problems have an impact in every area of nursing practice, including maternity nursing. Problems can affect the fetus, neonate, or pregnant woman. The nurse must be knowledgeable about the nature of these problems to provide competent care. Hemolytic disease of the newborn, rubella, and AIDS are of particular concern to the maternity nurse.

Hemolytic Disease of the Newborn

Hemolytic disease of the newborn (HDN), formerly called erythroblastosis fetalis, results from excessive destruction of fetal red cells by maternal antibodies. In HDN, the erythrocytes of the fetus become coated with maternal antibodies that correspond to specific fetal antigens. This hemolytic process reduces the normal life span of fetal erythrocytes. The fetal liver, spleen, and bone marrow respond to hemolysis by increasing production of erythrocytes. Increased erythrocyte production outside of the bone marrow can cause enlargement of the liver and spleen and premature release of nucleated erythrocytes into the fetal circulation. If increased erythropoiesis cannot compensate for erythrocyte destruction, a progressively severe anemia develops. Severe anemia may cause the fetus to develop cardiac failure with generalized edema (hydrops fetalis), resulting in death in utero. In newborn infants, severe anemia can produce heart failure shortly after birth. Less severely affected infants experience erythrocyte destruction after birth, which generates large quantities of unconjugated bilirubin. This produces the threat of accumulation of free bilirubin in lipid-rich tissue of the central nervous system. Total plasma bilirubin levels approaching 20 mg/dl can cause mental retardation or death.

Prenatal and Postpartum Testing. The following procedures are generally employed in prenatal testing under various conditions. These procedures are ABO blood grouping; Rh testing for D and D^u; alloantibody screening (if negative, should be repeated again at 34 weeks of gestation); alloantibody identification, if the antibody screening test is positive; antibody titer, if an alloantibody is present; and amniocentesis. Amniocentesis is an analysis of fluid from the amniotic cavity that is obtained by the transabdominal insertion of a needle into the amniotic cavity (Chapter 22).

Various laboratory procedures are helpful in addition to the procedures listed as prenatal assays. These procedures may be useful in determining the presence and assessment of the severity of HDN, or quantitating the extent of fetal-maternal hemorrhage. Postpartum testing of umbilical cord or infant blood includes hemoglobin and hematocrit determination, serum bilirubin assay, ABO and Rh grouping, direct anti-globulin test (DAT), or Coombs' test, and antibody elution and identification. If the DAT is positive, a peripheral blood smear for quantitation of the number of immature erythrocytes in the infant's blood is performed.

An analysis of bilirubin is valuable in determining the severity of HDN, because a relationship between cord bilirubin concentration and the severity of HDN exists. The normal infant's cord bilirubin level ranges from 0.7 to 3.5 mg/dl. A cord bilirubin of 4 mg/dl or more may be an indication for exchange transfusion. Severe cases of HDN commonly have cord bilirubin values in excess of 6 mg/dl. About 40% of infants born with a positive DAT require no treatment; others need exchange transfusions to prevent kernicterus from developing. An exchange transfusion removes bilirubin and circulating maternal antibodies from the infant's plasma and replaces antibody-coated erythrocytes with compatible Rh negative red blood cells.

Intervention. Severe intrauterine hemolysis in the fetus can be treated by intraperitoneal fetal transfusion (IPT) or intrauterine transfusion. In addition, administration of Rh immune globulin (Rh IgG) to the pregnant woman at 28 weeks gestation (antenatal) has decreased the incidence of primary immunization in Rh_o (D) negative women to 0.07%. The use of Rh IgG after conditions such as abortion, ectopic pregnancy, or hemorrhage during pregnancy has also contributed to the decreased incidence of D antigen immunization.

For prophylactic treatment using Rh IgG to be effective, appropriate amounts must be administered to previously unsensitized Rh (D) negative women within 72 hours after delivery or obstetric intervention. Administration of immune prophylaxis is performed after delivery of an Rh (D) positive infant; following amniocentesis, abortion, or ectopic pregnancy; or before delivery in selected cases (antenatal) (p. 884). Requirements include the following: the mother must be D and D^u negative, the screening (Coombs') test for alloantibodies must be negative for anti-D antibody, the infant must be D or D^u positive (in cases where the Rh cannot be determined, it must be assumed that this criterion has been met), and the DAT on cord cells or infant's cells, if available, must be negative. These criteria must be met *each time* an Rh negative mother delivers. If the conditions are met with each delivery, the mother must receive Rh IgG each time. Rh IgG does not provide permanent prevention of HDN.

Rubella Infection

The **rubella** virus was first isolated in 1962. Acquired rubella, also known as German or 3-day measles, is caused by a ribonucleic acid (RNA) virus. Because the virus is endemic to humans, the disease is highly contagious and is transmitted through respiratory secretions. Before widespread rubella immunization in the United States and Canada, rubella infections occurred in epidemic proportion at 6- to 9-year intervals. In 1964, more than 20,000 cases of **congenital rubella syndrome** and an unknown number of stillbirths occured in the United States as the result of an epidemic that year. In countries where vaccination is uncommon, the incidence of rubella infection continues to be high, and epidemics are frequent. Contracting the infection and receiving a vaccination against rubella are the only routes to developing immunity.

It is critical to continue to determine the rubella immune status of women of childbearing age and to vaccinate those who are not immune. Other individuals requiring rubella immune status determination include preschool and school-age children, all women at or just prior to childbearing age, women who are about to be married, married women, pregnant women, and health care personnel. If a woman is not rubella immune, she should be vaccinated. She is advised not to become pregnant for 3 months, because there is a remote possibility that the vaccination could lead to an infected fetus. In pregnant women, a positive test confirms immunity, but to rule out any possibility of unsuspected current infection, an IgM screening procedure may also be ordered. If the pregnant woman is not rubella immune, she should be cautioned to avoid exposure to rubella infection. Vaccination is contraindicated in a pregnant woman. However, the woman should be vaccinated immediately after termination of the pregnancy (Chapter 21).

Rubella infection is usually a mild self-limiting disease with only rare complications in children and adults. Rubella infections in pregnant women, especially those infected in their first trimester of pregnancy, can have devastating effects on the fetus. In utero infection can result in fetal death or manifestation of rubella syndrome. This syndrome represents a spectrum of congenital anomalies. In addition to stillbirth, fetal abnormalities associated with maternal rubella infection include encephalitis, hepatomegaly, bone defects, mental retardation, cataracts, thrombocytopenic purpura, cardiovascular defects, splenomegaly, and microcephaly. In neonates with cogenital rubella syndrome, low birthweight (Chapter 28) and failure to thrive are common. Of newborns infected in utero, 10% to 20% fail to survive past the first 18 months of life. The point in the gestation cycle at which maternal rubella infection occurs greatly influences the severity of congenital rubella syndrome. In the first month, the risk of anomaly is 50%; during the first trimester the risk is 25%; by the third month the risk drops to less than 10%; by the fourth or fifth month the risk is only 6%; and after the fifth month there is no risk for anomalies (American College of Obstetricians and Gynecologists, 1981).

The extent of congenital anomalies varies from one infant to another. Some infants manifest nearly all of the defects associated with rubella, while others exhibit few if any consequences of infection. Clinical evidence of congenital rubella infection may not be recognized for months or years after birth.

In a person suffering from a primary rubella infection, the appearance of both IgG and IgM antibodies is associated with the appearance of clinical signs and symptoms. IgM antibodies become detectable a few days after the onset of signs and symptoms and reach peak levels at 7 to 10 days. These antibodies persist but rapidly diminish in concentration over the next 4 to 5 weeks until antibody is no longer clinically detectable. The presence of IgM antibody in a single specimen suggests that the person has recently experienced a rubella infection. In most cases, the infection probably occurred within the preceding month. Production of IgG is also associated with the appearance of clinical signs and symptoms. Antibody levels increase rapidly for the next 7 to 21 days, then level off or even decrease in strength. IgG antibodies, however, remain present and protective indefinitely. The detection of IgG antibody is a useful indicator of rubella infection *only* in cases where the first (acute) and second (convalescent) blood specimens are drawn several weeks apart. Optimum timing for paired testing for the diagnosis of a recent infection is 2 or more weeks apart, with the acute specimen taken before or at the time signs and symptoms appear or within 2 weeks of exposure. Demonstration of an unequivocal increase in IgG antibody concentration between the acute and convalescent specimens is suggestive of either a recent primary infection or a secondary (anamnestic) antibody response to rubella in an immune individual. In the case of an anamnestic response, IgM antibodies are not demonstrable, but IgG production begins quickly. No other signs or symptoms of disease are exhibited. If both IgM and IgG test results are negative, the person has never suffered from rubella infection or been vaccinated. These people are susceptible to infection. If no IgM is demonstrable but IgG is present in paired specimens, the person is immune.

Because IgG antibody is capable of crossing the placental barrier, there is no way of distinguishing between IgG antibody of fetal origin and IgG antibody of maternal origin in a neonatal blood specimen. Testing for IgM antibody is invaluable in the diagnosis of congenital rubella syndrome in the neonate. IgM does not cross an intact placental barrier, therefore demonstration of IgM in a single neonatal specimen is diagnostic of congenital rubella syndrome.

Acquired Immunodeficiency Syndrome

In 1983, researchers at the Pasteur Institute in Paris isolated a retrovirus (see glossary) from a homosexual man with lymphadenopathy. The virus was named the lymphadenopathy-associated virus (LAV), but the researchers were unable to prove that this agent caused **acquired immunodeficiency syndrome** (AIDS). The American research team headed by Dr. Robert Gallo also isolated the same class of virus, which it labeled human T-lymphotropic retrovirus (HTLV) type III. In 1984, the American team was able to demonstrate conclusively through virologic and epidemiologic evidence that this virus was the cause of AIDS. When it was demonstrated that LAV and HTLV-III were the same virus, an international commission changed the name of the virus to human immunodeficiency virus (HIV).

The AIDS pandemic is still in its early stages, and its ultimate dimensions are difficult to assess accurately. HIV has been isolated from blood, semen, vaginal secretions, saliva, tears, breast milk, cerebrospinal fluid (CSF), amniotic fluid, and urine. To date, however, only *blood, semen, vaginal secretions,* and possibly *breast milk* have been implicated in transmission of HIV. Pediatric AIDS cases are usually related to the receipt of unscreened blood or blood products, or to the mother being infected with HIV during pregnancy.

HIV has a marked preference for the helper-inducer subset of lymphocytes. It displays an affinity for these cells because the CD_4 (T_4) surface marker protein on these cells serves as a receptor site for the virus. The extensive destruction of T cells leads to the gradual depletion of helper/inducer and suppressor/cytotoxic subsets of T lymphocytes. This abnormality exists in the lymph nodes as well as in circulating T cells. Normally, this ratio is 2:1 in heterosexuals and 1.5:1 in homosexuals. A reversal of these subsets is evident in, but *not* diagnostic of, AIDS. In people with AIDS, the lymphocyte subset ratio is usually less than 0.5:1. A diminished ratio can also be seen in individuals with other disorders, such as cutaneous T cell lymphoma, systemic lupus erythematosus (SLE), and acute viral infections. This disease additionally demonstrates defective NK cell activity.

After initial infection, the body mounts a vigorous immune response against the viremia. Immunologic activities include the production of different types of antibodies against HIV. Some antibodies neutralize it, others prevent it from binding to cells, and others stimulate cytotoxic cells to attack HIV infected cells. A *"window" period* of seronegativity exists from the time of initial infection to 6 or 12 weeks or longer thereafter. Increased production of core antigen is believed to be associated with a burst of viral replication and host cell lysis. A detectable antibody response appears about 6 weeks after the time of infection.

❑ ASSESSING IMMUNE RESPONSIVENESS

Cell-mediated Immune Defects

Deficiencies of cell-mediated immunity are often suspected in individuals with recurrent viral, fungal, parasitic, and protozoan infections. Persons with AIDS exhibit some of the most severe manifestations of cell-mediated immunity.

One avenue of testing involves delayed hypersensitivity skin testing to determine the integrity of an individual's cell-mediated immune response. Over 90% of normal adults will react to one of the following antigens within 48 hours after antigen exposure: *Candida albicans,* trichophyton, tetanus toxoid, mumps, and streptokinase-streptodornase (SKSD). Reactivity to histoplasmin or purifed protein derivative (PPD) is positive in individuals with active infection or previous exposure to histoplasmosis or tuberculosis, respectively; therefore they are not useful in the assessment of anergy.

Hematologic testing can include determination of the absolute number of lymphocytes, which is the total number of lymphocytes compared with the total number of leukocytes.

The number of T lymphocytes, the primary effector cell in cell-mediated reactions, can be determined by a number of different techniques. The "gold standard" has previously been the E (erythrocyte rosette formation) technique. Development of monoclonal antibodies, however, has permitted a quick and specific method for determining the number of T cells. It is by use of immunofluorescent techniques, in which the fluorescent microscope or fluorescence-activated cell sorter (FACS) is used. Additional testing can include functional testing or the measurement of biologic response modifiers, such as IL-2 (T cell growth factor), using bioassay and radioimmunoassay.

Humoral System Defects

The humoral system can be screened for abnormalities by quantitating the concentration of IgM, IgG, and IgA. Serum protein electrophoresis, however, may not be sensitive enough to detect selective immunoglobulin (Ig) class deficiencies. IgD and IgE are not useful in the determination of a suspected humoral deficiency.

The number of B lymphocytes in the peripheral blood and lymphoid organs can be determined by several different techniques. The most common procedure involves the detection of surface Ig. Most B cells bear IgM and/or IgD. Flouresceinated anti-human Ig antibody can be added to isolated cells in suspension and the percent of B cells determined. Normally, 5% to 15% of peripheral blood lymphocytes are B cells, while 40% of splenic and lymph node lymphocytes are surface Ig-bearing. Although surface Ig is the only membrane characteristic unique to B cells, other markers such as Fc receptors, C3 receptors, and gene production of the HLA-DR region are present. B cell function, such as proliferation and antibody production, can be assessed in vitro. These techniques generally use mitogens or antigens to detect polyclonal antigen-specific responses.

Factors Associated with Immunologic Disease

Factors such as general health and the age of an individual are important considerations in the functioning of the immune system in defense against infectious disease. In the case of noninfectious diseases or disorders, however, additional factors may be of importance.

In the maternity setting, the nurse must consider the development of the immune system in the fetus and newborn, environmental factors, nutritional status, and life-style considerations.

Immunity in the Newborn. Although nonspecific and specific body defenses are present in the unborn and newborn infant, many of these defenses are not completely developed in this group. A healthy newborn does not sweat, has no tears, and is not born with "normal" skin or intestinal microbial flora. Young children are at greater risk for diseases, particularly infectious diseases. If the integrity of the skin is broken, the newborn is predisposed to tissue and blood invasion by foreign cells such as bacteria. Infants who are preterm, small-for-gestational age, or postterm have different skin qualities that increase their susceptibility to invasive agents.

Full-term infants usually have passively acquired natural immunity because of the presence of maternal IgG antibodies. These antibodies are transferred from mother to infant through the placental circulation and provide short-term resistance to the specific antigens to which the mother produced antibodies. The preterm infant may be deficient in this type of immunity, especially if born before the thirty-sixth week of gestation. The other antibody type that a newborn can acquire passively is IgA. This class of antibody is present in colostrum and can be acquired in the newborn by breastfeeding.

The fetus is capable of forming IgM antibodies in response to an intrauterine infection. The newborn can also develop IgM antibodies as the initial humoral response to exposure to an antigenic substance (e.g., bacteria or viruses). In addition, a healthy newborn usually demonstrates the presence of IgA in tears and mucous secretions within a few months after birth.

Environment. The environment of each person is significant in determining the challenges posed to one's immune system. The various component factors of one's environment—the quality of air, water, and food, the ventilation, refrigeration, crowding, and cleanliness in the setting—contribute to the risks that a person encounters from microorganisms and substances. With the infectious diseases of tuberculosis and toxoplasmosis, one can readily appreciate the influence of environment in acquisition and transmission. Not every person is exposed to the tubercle bacillus or to the parasite that causes toxoplasmosis (Chapter 23).

However, if one lives in a setting in which tubercle bacillus is endemic (e.g., an urban, overcrowded area with poor ventilation), then the risks of exposure are much greater. The cat owner whose pet harbors the toxoplasmosis parasite is at increased risk of acquiring the disease, especially if the person has contact with the cat's feces (i.e., through emptying the litter pan). It is recognized that the infection can be transmitted from mother to fetus via placental transfer.

The environment of the newborn in a hospital setting is a factor over which a nurse can exert some control to effect fewer challenges to the neonate's immune defense system. Persons who harbor infectious diseases should be barred from the nursery, and the medical aseptic technique employed in the nursery environment should be meticulous (Chapter 17). This is not to suggest that the normal newborn should be provided with a sterile environment but that there is no reason to overtax a relatively meager set of immune defense mechanisms. An overwhelming systemic infection, such as that caused by herpes virus in the neonate, can not only interfere with healthy growth and development of the parent-child relationship because of prolonged separation but can also threaten the newborn's life. For this reason the environment into which a fetus will be born must be assessed for its risk potential in posing harm to the newborn.

Nutritional Status. The importance of good nutrition to good health has always been emphasized. Good nutrition is known to be important to growth and development, and it is now suggested that a healthy diet is of importance in the aging process and in the triad of nutrition, immunity, and infection. The consequences of diet, however, in multiple aspects of the immune response have been documented in many disorders. Every constituent of body defenses, including phagocytosis and humoral and cellular immunity, appears to be influenced by nutritional intake. Deficient or excessive intake of some dietary components, such as vitamins and minerals, can exert negative effects on the immune response. Therefore a healthy diet is important to the maximum functioning of the immune system.

Malnutrition caused by extremely reduced caloric intake or a deficiency, complete or partial, of a specific nutrient can produce abnormal immune function. Protein deficiency is an example of a disorder that compromises the immune system. Individuals with such a deficiency have altered immune defenses, such as decreased levels of IgA in secretions and decreased total levels and abnormal ratios of lymphocytic white cells. Imbalanced intake of minerals can also cause immunologic abnormalities.

Breast milk is supportive of the body's immune defense system because it favors the growth of *Lactobacillus bifidus* in the infant's intestinal system. This microorganism converts lactose into lactic acid. Lactic acid diminishes the growth of pathogenic organisms in the intestinal tract. Breast milk also provides the necessary amounts of nutrients, such proteins and essential minerals, that support the healthy functioning of the immune system.

Life-style. Certain infectious diseases are associated with the patterns of living that people establish for themselves. For instance, the sexually transmitted diseases of syphilis and gonorrhea are more likely to be acquired by people with multiple sex partners. Many other aspects comprise the concept of *life-style* besides sexual preference patterns and sexual behavior. These factors include the numerous health behaviors that people practice—such as their patterns of rest, exercise, food and drug intake, relaxation, work performance, self-care, and use of health care professionals. It is important for the nurse to assess carefully the numerous details about clients' life-styles because these factors affect the clients' susceptibility to invasion by harmful substances. For instance, a pattern of heavy alcohol consumption is associated with certain nutritional deficiencies (notably the B vitamin complex) that decrease the individual's immune responsiveness to vaccines and depress the cell-mediated and humoral lymphocytic activity (Whitney and Cataldo, 1983). Individuals who assume responsibility for their health and who practice health maintenance and preventive strategies (as acquiring artificial active immunity) are more likely to enjoy a competent immune defense system.

Principles of Nursing Care with Compromised Immune Responsiveness

When clients have any degree of compromised immune responsiveness, the nurse must take steps to ensure their protection from sources of infection in the hospital and the home environment. Scrupulous attention must be given to practicing medical asepsis by all caregivers who come in contact with the client to prevent superimposed iatrogenic nosocomial infections. In some cases reverse or protective isolation should be instituted to further protect the client.

To devise an individualized plan the nurse assesses for factors that place a person at risk, such as the client's age, overall health status, environment, and life-style. The client requires supportive therapy to maintain good fluid and nutritional status and to maintain the integrity of this first-line defense mechanism. In some situations the client is further protected with passive immunity support via IgG antibody injections. Those clients who have a poor prognosis (as those with AIDS) and their families also need to have supportive psychosocial care and opportunities to discuss and design their own future. Specific care needs that are induced for clients with problems of immune responsiveness are discussed in Chapter 23.

It is essential that nurses appreciate the complexity of the immune system. It is important to fully understand how to:

1. Support the healthy defense mechanisms of clients
2. Protect those clients whose immune responsiveness is impaired
3. Avoid the unintentional stimulation of potentially dangerous (allergic) defense mechanisms

SUMMARY

Immunologic conditions of importance in maternity nursing include hemolytic disease of the newborn, rubella, and AIDS. Factors such as general health and the age of an individual are important considerations in the functioning of the immune system in defense against infectious disease. In the case of noninfectious diseases or disorders, additional factors may be of importance. These factors can include genetic predisposition to many disorders, nutritional status, environment, and life-style. It is essential that nurses be familiar with the complexity of the immune system in order to support the healthy defense mechanisms of clients, protect immunologically impaired clients, and avoid unintentional stimulation of allergic reactions.

LEARNING ACTIVITIES

1. Have each person in your clinical group examine different prenatal and postnatal client records. Make a list of immunology-related assessments (e.g., interview questions in the history, physical examinations, and laboratory tests). Within a group setting, compare and contrast the findings.
2. Prepare a teaching guide for expectant and new parents about the immunologic advantages of colostrum and breast milk for the newborn.
3. Discuss health practices that help keep an individual immunocompetent.
4. In a postclinical seminar, discuss the immunology of the three examples of immunologic conditions in maternity nursing given in this chapter:
   a. Hemolytic disease of the newborn
   b. Rubella infection
   c. AIDS

KEY CONCEPTS

- The desirable consequences of immunity include natural resistance, recovery, and acquired resistance to infectious diseases.
- With medical science, the immune system can be advantageously manipulated to protect against disorders such as congenital rubella syndrome and hemolytic disease of the newborn, as well as many environmental microorganisms. It can also be manipulated to effect tissue repair after trauma or infection.
- Vaccination is an effective method of stimulating antibody production and memory without having to suffer from the disease.
- IgG, the major immunoglobulin in normal serum, is capable of crossing the placenta.
- IgA, the predominant immunoglobulin in secretions (including colostrum and breast milk), is of critical importance in protecting body surfaces (internal and external) against invading microorganisms.
- Three examples of immunologic conditions of critical importance in maternity nursing are hemolytic disease of the newborn, rubella infection, and AIDS.
- Factors such as fetal/neonatal development, life-style, environment, and nutrition affect the functioning of the immune defense system.

References

American College of Obstetricians and Gynecologists: Rubella-A clinical update, ACOG Technical Bulletin 62:7, 1981.

Whitney EN and Cataldo CB: Understanding normal and clinical nutrition, New York, 1983, West Publishing Co.

Bibliography

Adams MM et al: Cost implications of routine antenatal administration of Rh immune globulin, Am J Obstet Gynecol 149(6):633, 1984.

Bowman JM: Prevention of Rhesus isoimmunization, Am J Obstet Gynecol 148(8):1151, 1984.

Bowman JM, editor: Rh_o (D) immune globulin, Berkeley, Calif, 1984, Cutter Biological.

Caswell AK and Caswell M: Antenatal treatment to prevent Rh immunization, Lab Med 14(10):655, 1983.

Cheng MS and Lukomskyj L: Postpartum D^u-positive women and Rh immune globulin, Lab Med 17(12):748, 1986.

Chernesky MA and Mahoney JB: Rubella virus. In Rose NR, Friedman H, and Fahey HJL, editors: Manual of clinical laboratory immunology, ed 3, Washington, DC, 1986, American Society of Microbiology.

Epstein LB et al: Progressive encephalopathy in children with acquired immune deficiency syndrome, Ann Neurol 17:488, 1985.

Froberg JH: The anemias: causes and courses of action, RN, p 42, May, 1989.

Gallo RC and Montagnier L: AIDS in 1988, Scientific American 259(4):40, 1988.

Ganong WF: Review of medical physiology, ed 14, Norwalk, Conn, 1989, Appleton & Lange.

Haseltine WA and Wong-Stall F: The molecular biology of the AIDS virus, Scientific American 259(4):52, 1988.

Kaiser HB: Allergy and immunology: new discoveries, new treatments, better results, Contemp OB/GYN 21:90 (special issue), May 1983.

Papsidero L et al: Acquired immune deficiency syndrome: detection of viral exposure and infection, Am Clin Prod Rev p 17, Oct, 1986.

Phipps WJ, Long BC, and Woods NF: Medical-surgical nursing: concepts and clinical practice, ed. 4, St Louis, 1991, The CV Mosby Co.

Reckling JB and Neuberger GB. Understanding immune system dysfunction, Nurs '87 17(9):34, 1987.

Redfield RR and Burke DS: HIV infection: the clinical picture, Scientific American 259(4):90, 1988.

Roitt I: Essential immunology, ed 4, Oxford, England, 1983, Blackwell Scientific Publications.

Thompson JM et al: Mosby's manual of clinical nursing, ed 2, St Louis, 1989, The CV Mosby Co.

Turgeon ML: Clinical hematology, Boston, 1988, Little, Brown & Co, Inc.

Turgeon ML: Fundamentals of immunohematology, Philadelphia, 1989, Lea & Febiger.

Ungvarski P: Coping with infections that AIDS patients develop, RN p 53, Nov, 1988.

US Department of Health and Human Services: Human immunodeficiency virus infection in the United States: a review of current knowledge, MMWR 36:1, 1987.

US Department of Health and Human Services: Universal precautions for prevention of transmission of HIV, hepatitis B virus, and other blood borne pathogens in health care settings, MMWR 37:377, 1988.

US Department of Health and Human Services: Update: acquired immunodeficiency syndrome and HIV infection among health care workers, MMWR 37:229, 1988.

Wiley K and Grohar J: Human immunodeficiency virus and precautions for obstetric, gynecologic, and neonatal nurses, JOGN Nurse 17(3):165, 1988.

CHAPTER

6 Fertility Management

Irene M. Bobak and
Barbara Derwinski-robinson

Learning Objectives

Correctly define the key terms listed.

List common causes of impaired fertility.

Describe the different methods of contraception.

State the advantages and disadvantages of commonly used methods of contraception.

Evaluate the alternatives available to a woman experiencing an unplanned pregnancy.

Develop a nursing care plan for techniques for surgical intervention of pregnancy for each trimester.

Key Terms

autoimmunization
basal body temperature (BBT)
calendar method
cervical cap
cervical mucus method
condom
contraception
dilatation and curettage (D&C)
diaphragm
elective abortion
fertile period
GIFT
impaired fertility
intrauterine device (IUD)
in vitro fertilization-embryo transplant
isoimmunization
laminaria
male contraception
oral hormonal contraceptives
periodic abstinence
predictor test
referred shoulder pain
safe period
semen analysis
spermicide
spinnbarkheit
therapeutic intrauterine insemination
thermal shift
vacuum (suction) curettage
vaginal sponge
withdrawal bleeding

This chapter addresses several fertility-related issues, associated tests, and common therapies. The reproductive spectrum is addressed covering everything from impaired fertility, to voluntary control of fertility, to surgical interruption of pregnancy.

❑ IMPAIRED FERTILITY

The inability to conceive and bear a child comes as a surprise to 15% to 20% of otherwise healthy adults (Evans et al, 1989). It is difficult to be denied the experiences of pregnancy and birth, parenthood, and the expression of love through the care and nurturing of another human being. Disturbance in one's sexual self-concept is often experienced. Couples requesting assistance with impaired fertility problems have already decided that they want a child. They seek acceptance and assistance from the nurse and physician in coping with and possibly resolving these problems.

The traditional definition of **impaired fertility** is the inability to conceive after at least 1 year of adequate exposure when no contraceptive measures were used. It is also the inability to deliver a live infant after three consecutive conceptions. A contemporary definition does not consider a time limit. It is the inability to conceive or carry to live birth at a time the couple has chosen to do so.

Impaired fertility is *primary* if the woman has never been pregnant or the man has never impregnated a woman. It is *secondary* if the woman has been pregnant at least once but has not been able to conceive again or sustain a pregnancy.

Sterility implies that conception is not possible and the cause cannot be remedied. The incidence of impaired fertility seems to be increasing. An estimated one out of every six couples in the United States is involuntarily childless (Willson and Carrington, 1987). Probable causes include the trend to delay pregnancy until later in life when fertility decreases naturally, the increase in pelvic inflammatory disease, and the increase in substance abuse. Diagnosis and treatment of impaired fertility require considerable physical, emotional, and financial investment over an extended period. The attitude, sensitivity, and caring nature of those who are involved in the assessment of impaired fertility lay the foundation for the client's ability to cope with the subsequent therapy and management. All members of the health team must respect the clients' rights to privacy and the confidentiality of client records.

Religious Considerations. Civil laws and religious proscriptions about sex must always be kept in mind by the clinician. For example, the Orthodox Jewish husband and wife may face infertility investigation and management problems because of religious laws that govern marital relations. According to Jewish law the couple may not engage in marital relations during menstruation and through the following 7 "preparatory days." The wife then is immersed in a ritual bath (Mikvah) before relations can resume. The 5 menstrual days and 7 preparatory days collectively are called the "nida state." Any vaginal bleeding of physiologic origin marks the beginning of the nida state. Fertility problems can arise when the woman has a short cycle (i.e., a cycle of 24 days or less, when ovulation would occur on day 10 or earlier). Small doses of estrogen may delay ovulation to allow for the time needed to complete the nida state. Other procedures that induce bleeding may delay intercourse for another 12 days to allow for the nida state. Thus Orthodox Jewish clients, as well as observant Catholics, may at times question proposed diagnostic and therapeutic procedures because of religious proscriptions. These clients are encouraged to consult their rabbi or priest for a ruling.

Other religions teach that a marriage can be annulled if a woman is found to be infertile, though the reverse is not true if a man is found to be infertile. Religious influences over fertility and hence impaired fertility account for many of the sociocultural attitudes displayed toward childless couples (Menning, 1977).

Psychosocial Considerations. Within the United States, feelings connected to impaired fertility are many and complex.* The origin of some of these feelings are myths, superstitions, misinformation, or "magical" thinking about the cause of infertility. Other feelings arise from the need to undergo many tests and examinations and from being "different" from others.

Menning (1977) and Speroff et al (1983) have tried to debunk some common myths. These myths include:

1. *Infertility has a psychologic origin.* For 80% to 90% of all cases of impaired fertility, there is a discernible physiologic explanation.
2. *Adopting improves a couple's chance of conceiving.* A classic, often quoted, study by Rock et al (1965) found no significant increase in conception among 113 couples with impaired fertility who had adopted and 249 couples who had not adopted.
3. *Being infertile is a sexual disorder.* For most couples, impaired fertility is not related to their ability to perform sexual intercourse.
4. *It is immoral to wish to bear children and to actively pursue that goal.* For those who wish to have children, their impaired fertility is an involuntary barrier to their choice of parenthood.

Veevers' report (1973) on the social meaning of parenthood and nonparenthood provides further insight into the psychosocial impact of impaired fertility. To the extent to which a society perceives nonparenthood as unnatural, as an avoidance of responsibility, a rejection of gender role, a sign of immaturity, or a hindrance to positive marital adjustment is the extent to which couples with impaired fertility may perceive their society as being nonsupportive. Under such circumstances, an infertile couple might have problems not only accepting their impaired fertility but also in discussing their feelings with health care providers.

Cultural Considerations. Worldwide, cultures continue to employ symbols and rites that celebrate fertility. One fertility rite that persists today is the custom of throwing rice at the bride and groom. Other fertility symbols and rites include the passing out of congratulatory cigars, candy, or pencils by a new father, and baby showers held in anticipation of a child's birth. Last but not least is the American image of motherhood. Mothers and motherhood are paid homage, especially in the communications media of the United States. It is no wonder that Mother's Day is the busiest day for telephone companies and one of the busiest for florists.

The person without children in Samoa is pitied. According to Brownlee (1978), in many cultures a woman's inability to conceive may be due to her sins, to evil spirits, or to the fact that she is an inadequate person. The virility of a man in some cultures remains in question until he demonstrates his ability to reproduce by having at least one child.

Determination of a culturally defined cause for sterility is usually accompanied by a culturally proposed solution for the problem. These proposed solutions may or may not be effective. For example, Vietnamese men thought sterility was caused by loss of sperm during wet dreams or through daytime discharge (Coughlin, 1965). Tonics consisting of licorice, aconite, and

*See Chapter 4 for psychosocial aspects and Chapter 29, Loss and Grief.

ginseng might be used to counteract the effect. Certain foods such as cereal were to be eaten, and substances such as alcohol were to be avoided.

In most cultures, responsibility for impaired fertility is usually attributed to the woman. If infertility is believed to be caused by a misplaced uterus, methods are used to replace it. A Samoan woman may go to a bush doctor who will massage the abdomen over the uterus with oil and attempt to put it back in place (Clark and Howland, 1978).

For Mexican-American women and others who subscribe to heat/cold balance and imbalance theories, barrenness is considered to result from having a "cold womb" (Clark, 1970). The cold womb may be heated through external and internal means. Clark (1970) describes two methods used by Mexican-American women. One method requires a barren woman to sit over a washtub of hot water, to which rosemary is added, so that the vapors warm the womb. The other method attempts to build up body heat over a period of 3 days. This is done by avoiding cold foods and water, using a belladonna plaster over the sacral area, and ingesting cathartic pills and hot chocolate.

Factors Associated with Infertility

The couple is a "biologic unit" of reproduction. Many factors, both male and female, contribute to normal fertility. A normally developed reproductive tract is essential. Normal functioning of an intact hypothalamic-pituitary-gonadal axis supports gametogenesis—the formation of sperm and ova. The life span of the sperm and ovum is short. Although sperm remain viable in the female's reproductive tract for 48 hours or more, probably only a few retain fertilization potential for more than 24 hours. Ova remain viable for about 24 hours, but the optimum time for fertilization may be no more than 1 to 2 hours (Cunningham, MacDonald, and Gant, 1989). It is likely that viable sperm may need to be present in the uterine tube at the time of ovulation for optimum fertilization (Cunningham, MacDonald, and Gant, 1989). Thus timing of intercourse becomes critical.

The male must produce sperm that are normal, adequate in number, and motile. Accessory glands must provide supportive secretions to the sperm to form semen. The tube system to the urethra must be patent. Ejaculation must deposit semen around the cervix at the appropriate time of the female's menstrual cycle. After being deposited, sperm must be able to penetrate and be sustained by receptive and supportive cervical mucus. Sperm must undergo capacitation (Chapter 7) to prepare for fertilization. Then they migrate through the uterus to the ampulla of the uterine tube to fertilize a receptive normal ovum.

In the female, a graafian follicle must mature and release a healthy ovum able to be fertilized. The ovum must be drawn by the fimbria into a healthy, patent uterine tube and fertilized within a few hours. The conceptus must migrate down the tube into a well-developed normal uterus. Implantation of the blastocyst must occur within 7 to 10 days in a hormone-prepared endometrium. The conceptus must develop normally, reach viability, and be delivered in good condition for extrauterine life.

An alteration in one or more of these structures, functions, or processes results in some degree of impairment of fertility. Causes of impaired fertility are sometimes difficult to assign to either the male or the female (Willson and Carrington, 1987). A male factor may be solely responsible in 30% of infertile couples, but it may be contributory in another 10%. Tubal factors are identified in about 25% of infertile couples, an ovulatory disorder in about 20%*, or a cervical factor in approximately 15%. Miscellaneous factors (5%) or unknown (unexplained) factors (5%) account for the remaining causes.

Unexplained infertility and recurrent (habitual) abortion may be the result of aberrations of the immune system (e.g., antisperm antibodies, failure of implantation and growth of a blastocyst) (Evans et al, 1989).

❑ INVESTIGATION OF FEMALE INFERTILITY

The investigation of impaired fertility is conducted systematically, since multiple factors involving both partners are common. Both partners must be interested in the solution to the problem. The medical investigation requires time and considerable financial expense, as well as causes emotional distress and strain on the couple's interpersonal relationship. A thorough investigation usually requires 3 to 4 months of time.

Investigation of impaired fertility begins with a complete history and physical examination (see box, p. 108). The history explores the duration of infertility, past obstetric events, and contains a detailed sexual history. Medical and surgical conditions are evaluated. Exposure to reproductive hazards in the home (e.g., mutagens such as plastic-vinyl chlorides, teratogens such as alcohol, and emotional stresses) and workplace are explored.

A complete general physical examination is followed by a specific assessment of the reproductive tract. Evidence of endocrine system abnormalities is sought. In-

*Other authors (Evans et al, 1989) suggest that ovulation disorders are implicated in 40% to 50% of infertile couples.

ASSESSMENT OF THE WOMAN

HISTORY

1. Duration of impaired fertility: length of contraceptive and noncontraceptive exposure
2. Fertility in other marriages of self or spouse
3. Obstetric
   a. Number of pregnancies and abortions
   b. Length of time required to initiate each pregnancy
   c. Complications of any pregnancy
   d. Duration of lactation
4. Gynecologic: detailed menstrual history and leukorrheal history
5. Previous tests and therapy done for impaired fertility
6. Medical: general medical history including chronic and hereditary disease (e.g., endocrine dysfunction); drug use
7. Surgical: especially abdominal or pelvic surgery
8. Sexual history in detail: libido, orgasm capacity, techniques, frequency of intercourse, and postcoital practices; number of sexual partners
9. Occupational and environmental exposure to chemicals, x-ray equipment, or extreme therapy changes; physical nature of occupation or hobbies; vacations and work habits
10. Personal: motivation for childbearing; attitude toward partner, career aspirations; reason for seeking advice regarding impaired fertility at this time

PHYSICAL EXAMINATION

1. General: careful examination of other organs and parts of body; special attention given to habitus, fat and hair distribution, acne
2. Genital tract: state of hymen (full penetration); clitoris; vaginal infection, including trichomoniasis and candidiasis; cervical tears, polyps, infection, patency of os, accessibility to insemination; uterus, including size and position, mobility; adnexae, tumors, evidence of endometriosis

LABORATORY DATA

1. Routine urine, complete blood count, and serologic test for syphilis; additional laboratory studies as indicated
2. Basic endocrine studies in women with irregular menstrual cycles or in amenorrhea, hirsutism, acne, or excessive weight gain
3. For women with irregular menstrual cycles: protein-bound iodine (PBI) or other thyroid tests, 17-ketosteroid assay test, 17-hydroxycorticosteroid test, glucose tolerance test (GTT), endometrial biopsy, and progesterone levels
4. For women with amenorrhea: tomographic x-ray films of skull, T_4 or other thyroid tests, 17-ketosteroid assay test, 17-hydroxycorticosteroid test, GTT, endometrial biopsy, gonadotropin follicle-stimulating hormone (FSH), luteinizing hormone (LH) determination, and buccal smear and chromsomal studies

Other laboratory tests added as desired for a more complete diagnosis of endocrine problems

5. Rh factor and antibody titer tests—important in abortion and premature delivery problems
6. *Sperm antibody agglutination studies:* special laboratory procedure involves obtaining a fresh semen specimen from man and a blood sample from the woman; sperm are incubated in the blood serum of the woman and checked at intervals for agglutination; the test is negative if no agglutinated sperm are found
7. Chromosome studies, where indicated

adequate development of secondary sex characteristics (e.g., inappropriate distribution of body fat and hair) may point to problems with the hypothalamic-pituitary-ovarian axis or genetic aberrations (e.g., Turner's syndrome). Women with Turner's syndrome are typically short, have underdeveloped breasts, and abnormal gonads. These women are infertile. Other women may have an abnormal uterus and tubes as a result of exposure to diethylstilbestrol (DES) in utero. Evidence of past infection of the genital urinary system is sought. Bimanual examination of the internal organs may reveal lack of mobility of the uterus or abnormal contours of the uterus and adnexa.

Laboratory data is assembled. Data from routine urine and blood tests is obtained along with other tests (see box, above).

Tests and Examinations

There are several examinations and tests for impaired fertility. The basic infertility survey involves evaluation of the cervix, uterus, tubes, and peritoneum; detection of ovulation; assessment of immunologic compatibility; and evaluation of psychogenic factors (Scott et al, 1990). Procedures commonly used include the following:

Detection of ovulation: basal body temperature (BBT), cervical mucus characteristics, endometrial

Table 6-1 **Tests for Impaired Fertility**

Test/Examination	Timing (Menstrual Cycle Days)	Rationale
Hysterosalpingogram	1-4	Late follicular, early proliferative phase will not disrupt a fertilized ovum. May open uterine tubes before time of ovulation.
Postcoital (Huhner test)	Peak cervical mucus flow*	Ovulatory late proliferative phase—look for normal motile sperm in cervical mucus.
Sperm immobilization antigen-antibody reaction		Immunologic test to determine sperm and cervical mucus interaction.
Assessment of cervical mucus		Cervical mucus should have low viscosity, high spinnbarkheit.
Ultrasound observation of follicular collapse	Ovulation	Collapsed follicle is seen after ovulation.
Serum assay of plasma progesterone	20-25	Midluteal midsecretory phase—check adequacy of corpus luteal production of progesterone.
Basal body temperature (BBT)		Elevation occurs in response to progesterone.
Endometrial biopsy	26-27	Late luteal, late secretory phase—check endometrial response to progesterone and adequacy of luteal phase.

*Exogenous estrogen may be given to induce mucus flow if spontaneous and reasonably regular ovulation does not occur.

biopsy, radioimmunoassays of hormones essential for fertility, laparoscopic and sonographic examination

Assessment of tubal patency and peritoneum: hysterosalpingography, laparoscopic examination, culdoscopy

Assessment of the uterus: hysterosalpingography, timed endometrial biopsy, laparoscopic examination, serum progesterone levels

Evaluation of the vagina and cervix: BBT, cervical mucus characteristics, postcoital test of interaction between sperm and cervical mucus, in vitro test of cervical mucus penetration by sperm

Evaluation of immunologic compatibility: sperm agglutination tests, sperm immobilization tests

Nurses can alleviate some of the mystery associated with impaired fertility by explaining to clients the timing and rationale for each test (Table 6-1). Fertility test findings favorable to fertility are summarized on p. 116. A discussion of the most common tests follows.

Detection of Ovulation. Documentation of time of ovulation is important in the investigation of impaired fertility. Direct proof of ovulation is pregnancy or the retrieval of an ovum from the uterine tube. There are several indirect or presumptive methods for detection of ovulation. These include assessment of BBT and cervical mucus characteristics, as well as endometrial biopsy. These clinical tests more or less determine whether progesterone is secreted in significant amounts (Table 6-1; Willson and Carrington, 1987) to accommodate implantation and maintain pregnancy. Occurrence of mittelschmerz and midcycle spotting provides unreliable presumptive evidence of ovulation (Scott et al, 1990).

Hormone Analysis. Hormone analysis is performed to assess endocrine function of the *hypothalamic-pituitary-ovarian axis.* Blood and urine specimens are obtained at varying times during a woman's menstrual cycle. Blood specimens are drawn to determine levels of progesterone, estrogen, FSH, and LH. Urine specimens provide information about the levels of 17-ketosteroids and 17-hydroxycorticosteroids. The venipuncture may cause some discomfort. Collecting urine specimens and bringing them to the laboratory can be inconvenient.

A venipuncture specimen is drawn late in the woman's menstrual cycle to assess the function of the *corpus luteum.* This test can be done in a serial manner to determine if the levels of plasma progesterone correlate well with the client's BBT and cervical mucus characteristics (pp. 129 and 130).

Timed Endometrial Biopsy. Endometrial biopsy is scheduled after ovulation during the luteal phase of the menstrual cycle. Late in the menstrual cycle, 3 to 4 days before expected menses, a sample of the endometrium is removed for histologic study to assess the function of the corpus luteum and the receptivity of the endometrium for implantation. There are two methods of performing a timed endometrial biopsy; neither method requires hospitalization. The first method is implemented 3 to 4 days before expected menses. With the woman draped and in the lithotomy position, a vaginal speculum is inserted into the vagina. Using a small lumen vabra aspirator, a sample of the endometrium is obtained.

The second method includes the following steps:

1. Couple is cautioned to abstain from intercourse during preceding "fertile" period to avoid dislodging a possible embryo during the procedure.
2. The cervix is dilated with laminaria 4 to 24 hours before the procedure, which requires no analgesia. (**Laminaria** are small, thin inserts of packed seaweed which, when inserted into the cervix, absorb moisture, expand in size, and thus dilate the cervix.)
3. The woman assumes the lithotomy position, is draped, and the speculum is inserted.
4. The laminaria are removed (Fig. 6-1).
5. If not previously dilated with laminaria, the cervix is dilated at this time with metal rod dilators. Analgesia or anesthesia is often necessary.
6. A small specimen of endometrium is removed from the side wall in the fundus to avoid dislodging an embryo should conception have occurred. (When implantation occurs, it is usually high in the fundus, either in the anterior or posterior portion.)

Findings favorable to fertility include an endometrium that is negative for tuberculosis, polyps, or inflammatory conditions and that reflects secretory changes normally seen in the presence of adequate luteal (progesterone) phase.

Hysterosalpingography. Radiographic (x-ray) film allows visualization of the uterine cavity and tubes after the instillation of radioopaque contrast material through the cervix (Fig. 6-2). It is possible to see abnormalities of the uterus such as congenital defects (Fig. 6-3) or defects produced by submucous myomas and endometrial polyps. Distortions of the uterine cavity or uterine tubes as a result of current or past pelvic inflammatory disease (PID) are identified. Scar tissue and adhesions from inflammatory processes can immobilize the uterus and tubes, kink the tubes, and surround the ovaries. PID may follow infection from sexually transmitted diseases (STDs) or rupture of an inflamed appendix.

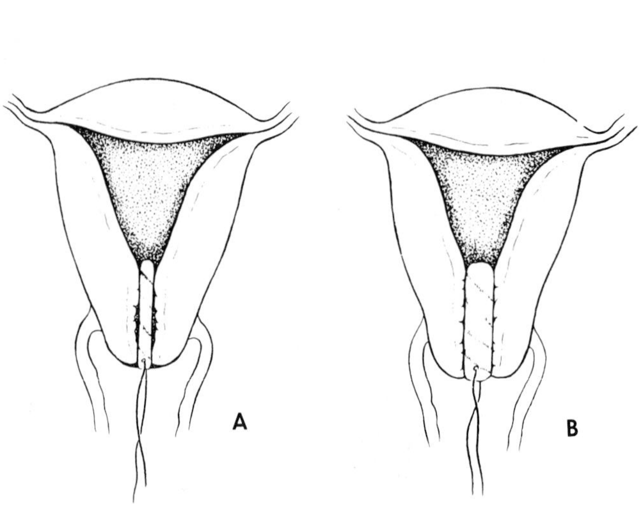

Fig. 6-1 Laminaria tents. **A,** Inserted through narrow cervical canal beyond the internal os. **B,** Cervix dilated 4 to 12 hours later. (From Sandberg EC: Synopsis of obstetrics, ed 10, St Louis, 1978, The CV Mosby Co.)

Hysterosalpingography is scheduled 2 to 5 days after menstruation to avoid flushing a potential fertilized ovum out through a tube into the peritoneal cavity. Also at this time there are no open vessels and menstrual debris has all been discharged. This decreases the risk of embolism or of forcing menstrual debris out through the tubes into the peritoneal cavity. If the woman has PID, she is treated with antimicrobials and the test is rescheduled in 2 to 3 months.

Referred shoulder pain may occur during this procedure. The referred pain is indicative of subphrenic irritation from the contrast material if it is spilled out of the patent uterine tubes or if the tubes are occluded. The discomfort subsides with position change. It usually disappears within 12 to 14 hours and can be controlled with mild analgesics.

This procedure may be therapeutic as well as diagnostic. The passage of contrast medium may clear tubes of mucous plugs, straighten kinked tubes, or break up adhesions within the tubes (secondary to salpingitis). The procedure may stimulate cilia in the lining of the tubes to facilitate transport of the sex cells. It also may aid healing as a result of the bacteriostatic effect of the iodine within the contrast medium.

Laparoscopy. During laparoscopy, a small telescope is inserted through a small incision in the anterior abdominal wall. Cold fiberoptic light sources allow for superior visualization of the internal pelvic structures (Fig. 6-4). The woman is usually admitted shortly before surgery, having taken nothing by mouth (NPO) for 8 hours. She voids before surgery. A general anesthetic is given and the woman is placed in the lithotomy position. Her pubic hair is shaved only if this examination is likely to be followed by laparotomy. A needle is inserted and a pneumoperitoneum with carbon dioxide gas is established to elevate the abdominal wall from the organs, thereby creating an empty space that permits visualization and exploration with the laparoscope. If tubal patency is being assessed, a cannula is used to instill a dye contrast medium through the cervix. Visualization of the peritoneal cavity in infertile women may reveal endometriosis, pelvic adhesions, tubal occlusion, or polycystic ovaries. Fulguration (destruction of tissue by means of electricity) of small endometrial implants, lysis of the adhesions, and taking of ovarian biopsies are some of the procedures possible through the use of a laparoscope. After surgery, deflation of most of the gas is done by direct expression. Trocar (and needle) sites are closed with a single subcuticular absorbable suture or skin clip, and an adhesive bandage is applied. Postoperative recovery requires taking of vital signs, assessing level of consciousness, preventing aspiration, monitoring intravenous fluids, and reassuring the client regarding referred shoulder discomfort. Discharge from the hospital usually occurs in 4 to 6 hours. Referred shoulder pain or subcostal discomfort (from pneumoperitoneum) usually lasts

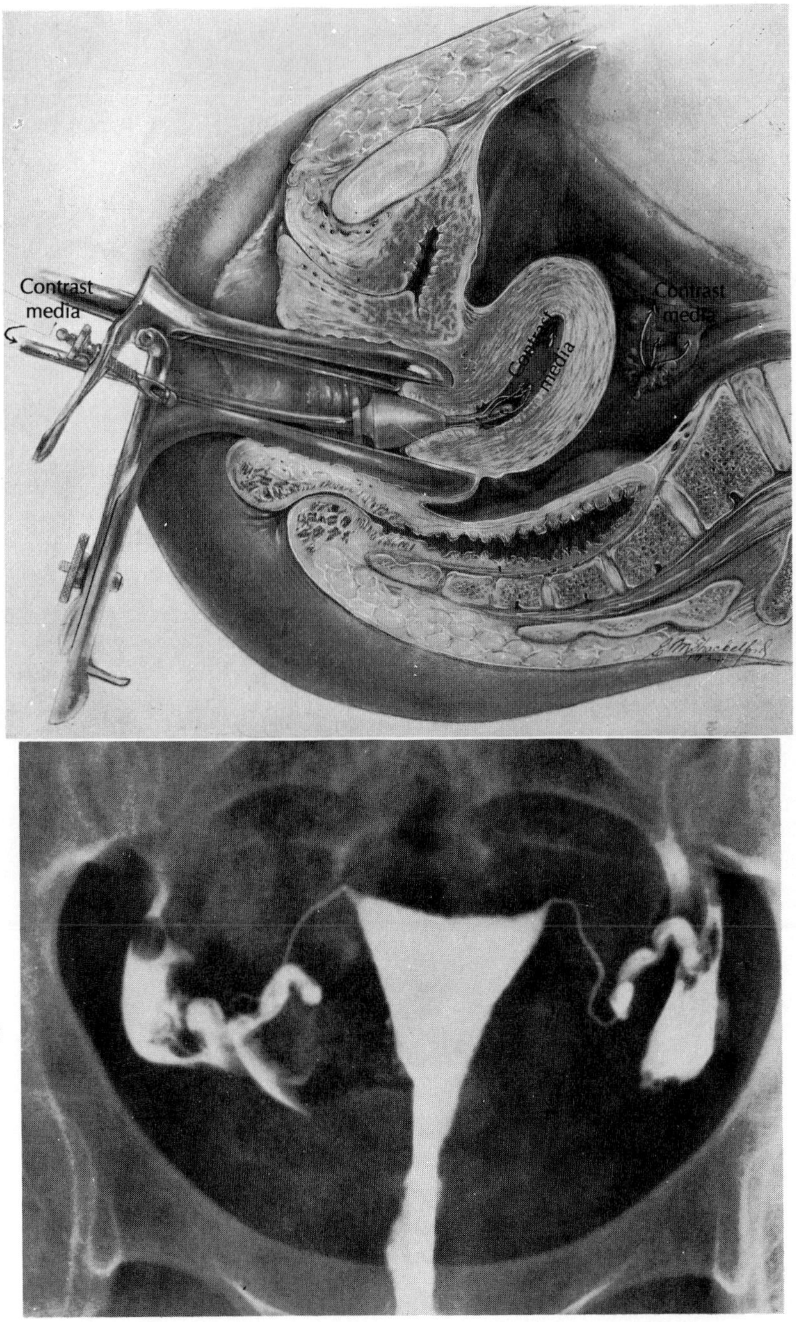

Fig. 6-2 **A,** Hysterosalpingography. Sagittal section showing technique. Contrast media flows through intrauterine cannula and out through tubes, the cervix being closed by a rubber stopper. **B,** Normal hysterosalpingogram showing passage of radiopaque material through fimbriated ends of tubes. (From Willson JR: Management of obstetric difficulties, ed 6, St Louis, 1961, The CV Mosby Co.)

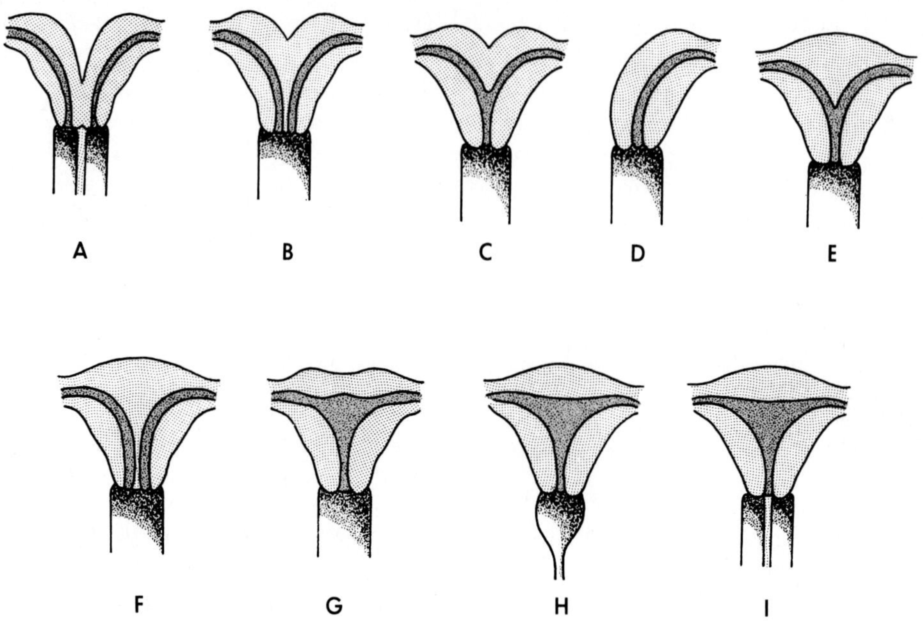

Fig. 6-3 Abnormal uteruses. **A,** Uterus didelphys bicollis (septate vagina). **B,** Uterus bicornis bicollis (vagina simplex). **C,** Uterus bicornis unicollis (vagina simplex). **D,** Uterus unicornis. **E,** Uterus subseptus. **F,** Uterus septus. **G,** Uterus arcuatus. **H,** Congenital stricture of vagina. **I,** Septate vagina. (Modified from Willson JR and Carrington ER: Obstetrics and Gynecology, ed 8, St Louis, 1987, The CV Mosby Co.)

only 24 hours and is relieved with a mild analgesic. The woman must be cautioned against heavy lifting or strenuous activity for 4 to 7 days, at which time she is usually asymptomatic.

Ultrasound Pelvic Examination. Abdominal or transvaginal ultrasound (Chapter 22) is also used to assess pelvic structures (Fig. 6-5). This procedure is used to visualize pelvic tissues for a variety of reasons (e.g., to identify abnormalities, to verify follicular development and maturity, or to confirm intrauterine [vs. ectopic] pregnancy).

❑ REPRODUCTIVE STRUCTURES AND FACTORS IMPLICATED IN INFERTILITY

Congenital or Developmental Factors. If the woman has abnormal external genitals, surgical reconstruction of abnormal tissue and construction of a functional vagina may permit normal intercourse. If internal reproductive tract structures are absent, there is no hope for fertility. Surgical intervention depends entirely on the anatomic development, the surgical feasibility, and the individual's actual gender role.

Vaginal and uterine anomalies and their surgical repair vary from individual to individual. If a functional uterus can be reconstructed, pregnancy may be possible. After surgical repair of the uterus, cesarean delivery is necessary to prevent uterine rupture during labor. Women with ovarian agenesis or dysgenesis are sterile, and no treatment will improve their fertility.

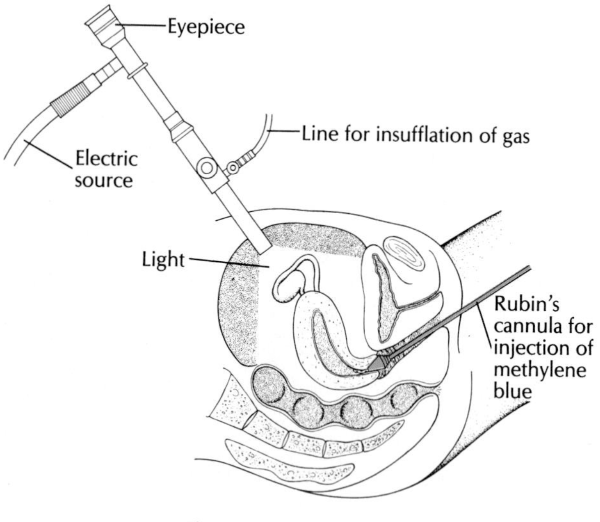

Fig. 6-4 Laparoscopy.

Ovarian Factors

Within healthy ovaries, graafian follicles respond to FSH and LH by the maturation of an ovum and ovulation. The graafian follicle produces estrogen; the empty

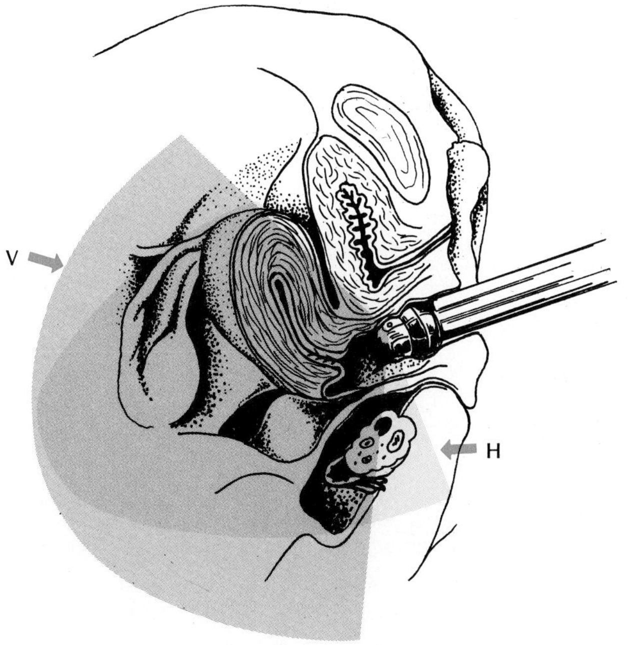

Fig. 6-5 Vaginal ultrasonography. Major scanning planes of transducer: H = horizontal, V = vertical.

graafian follicle becomes the corpus luteum and produces estrogen and progesterone.

Anovulation may be primary. *Primary anovulation* may be caused by a pituitary or hypothalamic hormone disorder or an adrenal gland disorder such as congenital adrenal hyperplasia. *Secondary anovulation* may be caused by ovarian disease. In amenorrheic states and instances of anovulatory cycles, hormone studies usually reveal the problem.

Treatment and Prognosis. Drug therapy is often an important but expensive component of client care. *Ovulatory stimulants* may be warranted. *Clomiphene* (Clomid, Serophene), an oral preparation, is a follicular maturing agent. It is used to treat anovulation caused by hypothalamic suppression when the hypothalamic-pituitary-ovarian axis is intact. *Bromocriptine* (Parlodel), a synthetic ergot alkaloid that inhibits the release of prolactin, is used to treat anovulation caused by elevated levels of prolactin. *Thyroid-stimulating hormone* (TSH) is indicated if the woman has hypothyroidism; *human menopausal gonadotropin* (hMG) (Pergonal), if she has hypogonadotropic amenorrhea. When anovulation is caused by hypothalamic-pituitary dysfunction, hypothalamic failure, or failure to respond to clomiphene, *gonadotropin-releasing hormone* (GnRH) may be prescribed.

Hormone replacement therapy may be indicated. The woman who has low levels of estrogen is a candidate for *conjugated estrogens and medroxy-progesterone.* A hypoestrogenic condition may result from a high-stress level or decreased percentage of body fat as a result of an eating disorder (e.g., anorexia nervosa) or excessive exercise. *Hydroxyprogesterone* supplementation with vaginal suppositories or intramuscular injection is used to treat luteal phase defects.

The nurse may encounter other medication as well. In the presence of adrenal hyperplasia, *prednisone,* a glucocorticoid is taken orally. *Danazol* is the drug of choice in the management of endometriosis. Infections are treated with appropriate antimicrobial formulations.

The nurse's role is that of teacher/counselor. Although the physician is responsible for informing clients fully about the prescribed medications, the nurse must be ready to answer clients' questions. Clients often ask the nurse to confirm their understanding of the drug, its administration, potential side effects, and expected outcomes. Since information varies with each drug, the nurse needs to consult the medication package inserts, pharmacology references, physician, and pharmacist as necessary.

Ovarian tumors must be excised. Whenever possible, functional ovarian tissue is left intact. Scar tissue adhesions caused by chronic infection may cover much or all of the ovary. These adhesions usually necessitate surgery to free and expose the ovary so that ovulation can occur.

Thyroid gland dysfunction may be associated with menstrual abnormalities, impaired fertility, or recurrent fetal wastage. Therapy consists of management of the thyroid condition coupled with careful scrutiny of BBT charts (p. 129) to promote sperm deposition at the same time as ovulation. Continuous monitoring and management of thyroid function during pregnancy are also carried out.

In the presence of severe emotional problems the woman is referred to a mental health therapist. Her condition may require the teamwork of the mental health therapist, the endocrinologist, and an obstetrician-gynecologist.

Diazepam (Valium) ingestion may be responsible for menstrual irregularities or failure to ovulate, changes in libido, and gynecomastia, possibly by raising estrogen levels. These effects can be reversed simply by withdrawing from the drug.

Tubal (Peritoneal) Factors

The fingerlike processes of the fimbriated end of the uterine tube and the tube itself need to be freely movable to approach the ovary to "catch" the ovum. The tube must be open, sufficiently long, and capable of ciliary action and peristalsis to carry the ovum into and down the tube. In most cases fertilization occurs in the ampulla of the tube. Some unknown factor, possibly an enzyme, supplied by the ampulla of the tube seems to be required for the physiologic change or "conditioning" of the sperm called capacitation (Chapter 7).

The motility of the tube and its fimbriated end may be reduced or absent as a result of infections, adhesions, or tumors. In rare instances there may be congenital absence of one tube. It is also possible to find one tube relatively shorter than the other. This condition is often associated with an abnormally developed uterus.

Inflammation within the tube or involving the exterior of the tube or the fimbriated ends represents a major cause of impaired fertility. Tubal adhesions resulting from pelvic infections (e.g., ruptured appendix) may impair fertility. When infection with purulent discharge eventually heals, scar tissue adhesions form. In the process the tube may be blocked anywhere along its length. It can be closed off at the fimbriated end, or it can be distorted and kinked by adhesions. Adhesions may permit the tiny sperm to pass through the tube but may prevent a fertilized egg from completing the journey into the intrauterine cavity. This results in an ectopic pregnancy that may completely destroy the tube (see discussion of ectopic pregnancy, Chapter 23).

In other cases, adhesions of the tubes to the ovary or bowel may follow *endometriosis*. Endometriosis is a disease in which endometrial tissue, ordinarily found only within the uterus, is present outside the uterus attached to other organs or tissue in the woman's body (Fig. 6-6). The ectopic endometrial tissue responds to hormonal stimulation in the way that uterine endometrium does. In endometriosis, periodic monthly bleeding from endometrial implants causes dense adhesions, making pregnancy difficult or impossible.

Treatment and Prognosis. Treatment must include prevention and early adequate management of infection with appropriate antibiotics. Surgery may be necessary when drainage of a serious focus of infection is required. Hysterosalpingography is useful for identification of tubal obstruction and also for the release of blockage. During laparoscopy, delicate adhesions may be divided and removed and endometrial implants may be destroyed by electrocoagulation or Nd:YAG laser. Laparotomy and even microsurgery may be required to do extensive repair of the damaged tube. Prognosis is dependent on the degree to which tube patency and function can be restored.

Uterine Factors

The uterus must be of sufficient size and shape to permit maintenance of a pregnancy to term gestation. The endometrium must be prepared by estrogen and progesterone and must be healthy for implantation to occur.

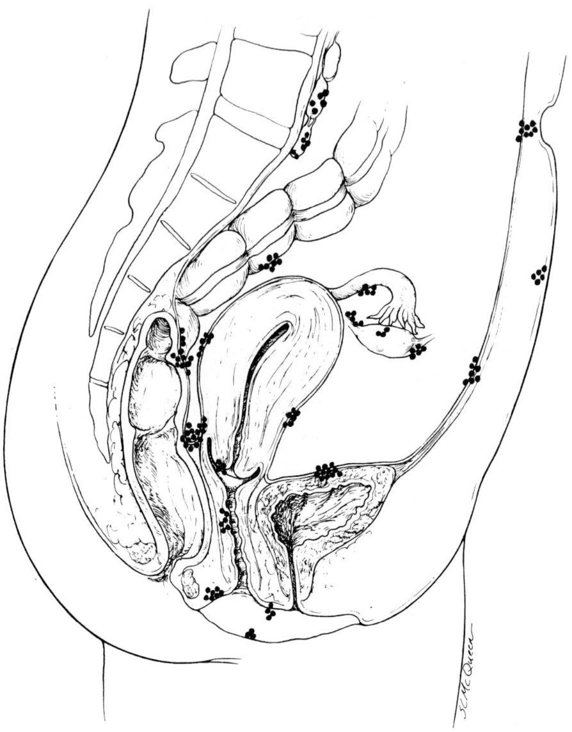

Fig. 6-6 Common sites of endometriosis. (From Droegmueller W et al: Comprehensive gynecology, St Louis, 1987, The CV Mosby Co.)

Congenital abnormalities of the uterus are far more common than might be expected. Minor developmental anomalies of the uterus are fairly common; major anomalies occur rarely (see Fig. 6-3). Hysterosalpingography may reveal a double uterus or other anomalous congenital variations that include a T-shaped uterus and a boxlike uterus. These types of uteruses have been described in daughters of women who took diethylstilbestrol (DES) during the early months of pregnancy. Endometrial and myometrial *tumors* (e.g., polyps or myomas) may also be revealed by x-ray studies of infertile women.

Asherman's syndrome, uterine adhesion or scar tissue, is characterized by hypomenorrhea or amenorrhea. The adhesions, which may partially or totally obliterate the uterine cavity, are sequelae to surgical interventions such as too vigorous curettage (scraping) after an abortion (elective or spontaneous). The hysteroscope is useful in the verification of intrauterine scars as well as for the localization and removal of displaced or broken intrauterine devices (IUDs).

Endometritis (inflammation of the endometrium) may result from any of the causes of infection of the uterine tubes. Women who have numerous sex partners are more susceptible to endometrial infection than are women in monogamous relationships.

Treatment and Prognosis. A woman with a relatively small uterus may become pregnant, but the uterus may be incapable of accommodating the enlarging fetus, and a spontaneous abortion may result. In such cases recurrent or habitual (three or more) spontaneous abortions often occur. No medical therapy has been effective for the enlargement of an abnormally small uterus. Observation suggests that women who do become pregnant but who miscarry, often abort at a later time with each successive pregnancy. Finally, after two or three pregnancy losses, they may deliver a viable infant. Apparently actual "growth" of the uterus occurs with each pregnancy. Plastic surgery—for example, the unification operation for bicornuate uterus—often improves a woman's ability to conceive and carry the fetus to term.

Impaired fertility may result from infections such as endometrial tuberculosis (from an acid-fast bacillus) or schistosomiasis (from a fluke parasite), which are significant health problems in many parts of the world including the Near East, Puerto Rico, and South America. These disorders often involve the tubes and ovaries. Medical cure of the infection may permit pregnancy despite some scarring of the endometrium.

Surgical removal of tumors or fibroids involving the endometrium or uterus often improves the woman's chance of conceiving and maintaining the pregnancy to viability. Surgical treatment of uterine tumors or maldevelopment that results in successful pregnancy requires delivery by cesarean surgery near term gestation. The uterus may rupture as a result of weakness of the area of surgical healing.

Vaginal-Cervical Factors

Vaginal fluid is acidic (pH of 4 or less), whereas cervical mucus is normally alkaline (pH of 7 or more). Ejaculation should place the sperm at or near the cervical os. The alkalinity of cervical mucus helps support sperm and permits the ascending transportation of sperm at the time of ovulation.

In addition, endocervical mucus normally obstructs or plugs the cervix, acting as a barrier against infection. The latter is important because, in the woman, ascending infection to the peritoneum is virtually unimpeded with a normally patent genital tract. Alkaline mucus in the cervix not only controls procreation but also is a specific protection to life and health. The amount of cervical mucus and its characteristics are influenced by the hormones estrogen and progesterone (see Figs. 4-22 and 4-23).

Vaginal-cervical infections (e.g., trichomoniasis vaginitis) increase the acidity of the vaginal fluid and reduce the alkalinity of the cervical mucus. Thus vaginal infection often destroys or drastically reduces the number of viable, motile sperm before they enter the cervical canal. The amount of mucus and its physical changes are influenced by the presence of blood, pathogenic bacteria, and such irritants as an IUD or a tumor. Severe emotional stress, antibiotic therapy, and diseases such as diabetes mellitus alter the acidity of mucus.

About 20% of infertile women have sperm antibodies. The production of antibodies by one member of a species against something that is commonly found within that species is termed **isoimmunization.** Sperm may be immobilized within the cervical mucus, or they become incapable of migration into the uterus (see postcoital test, p. 118). A greater incidence of sperm agglutination occurs in women with otherwise unexplained impaired fertility. However, the true significance and reliability of tests for sperm immobilization or agglutination are uncertain.

Treatment and Prognosis. Therapy for lower genital infection requires the elimination of vaginitis or cervicitis (Chapter 23). Appropriate antibiotic or chemotherapeutic drugs generally resolve this problem. In addition to antibiotics, radial chemocautery (destruction of tissue with chemicals) or thermocautery (destruction of tissue with heat, usually electrical) of the cervix, cryosurgery (destruction of tissue by application of extreme cold, usually liquid nitrogen), or conization (excision of a cone-shaped piece of tissue from the endocervix) is effective in eliminating chronic infection. When the cervix has been deeply cauterized or frozen or when extensive conization has been performed, extreme limitation of mucus production by the cervix may result. Therefore sperm migration may be difficult or impossible because of the absence of a mucous "bridge" from the vagina to the uterus. Therapeutic intrauterine insemination may be necessary to carry the sperm directly through the *internal os* of the cervix.

If the cervical os is unusually small, it is often called a pinhole os. In such cases, gentle dilatation of the cervix or several shallow radial incisions followed by dilatation are often sufficient to open the lower cervix. In contrast, if the cervix is grossly lacerated after delivery and widely gapping, suturing the cervix (trachelorrhaphy) or cryosurgery may be required to reduce the size of the external os. Prevention of recurrent infection helps maintain a column of mucus.

Good general hygiene must be practiced to minimize vaginal infections. The woman benefits from good hand washing before and after elimination of urine and stool. To avoid self-contamination, she must wipe from front to back once with each tissue and never wipe back and forth over the perineal area. Feminine deodorants, soaps that are heavily colored and perfumed, bubble-bath salts that cause chemical irritation, and tight clothing that provide a dark damp milieu favorable to microbial growth are avoided. Good nutrition is practiced with the avoidance of large amounts of unrefined sugars, which raise the pH of vaginal fluids. To maintain a healthy vaginal-cervical pH during antibiotic therapy, the woman may insert one or two applicators full of cultured yogurt (not pasteurized) once or twice daily. As a general rule, douching is avoided unless by prescription from a physician.

Good mental health helps prevent some forms of vaginitis that could become secondarily infected. Stress from anxiety, worry, and emotional discomfort increases the vaginal pH so that vaginal infections are more likely to take hold. Concurrent medical conditions such as diabetes mellitus must be controlled to maintain vaginal-cervical pH within normal range.

Treatment is available for women who have *immunologic reactions to sperm.* Exposure to semen via the orogenital and anal modes is avoided. The use of condoms during genital intercourse for 6 to 12 months will reduce female antibody production in the majority of women who have elevated antisperm antibody titers. After the serum reaction subsides, condoms are used at all times except at the expected time of ovulation. Approximately one third of couples with this problem conceive by following this course of action. A summary of fertility test findings favorable to fertility is outlined in the box below.

The prognosis for the infertile woman is generally good provided a serious genital or inflammatory disorder is not identified. Most women present numerous so-called minor problems that, although compounded, may be relatively easy to correct (e.g., chronic cervicitis, hypothyroidism). If successful treatment has not been achieved after a year, for example, other alternatives may be considered (e.g., adoption, childlessness, therapeutic insemination, or in vitro fertilization).

SUMMARY OF FERTILITY TEST FINDINGS FAVORABLE TO FERTILITY

1. Follicular development, ovulation, and luteal development are supportive to pregnancy:
   a. BBT (presumptive evidence of ovulatory cycles)
      (1) Is biphasic
      (2) Reveals temperature elevation that persists for 12 to 14 days just before menstruation
   b. Cervical mucus characteristics change appropriately during phases of the menstrual cycle
   c. Findings from endometrial biopsies taken at different times during menstrual cycle are consistent with day of cycle
   d. Laparoscopic visualization of pelvic organs verifies follicular and luteal development
2. The luteal phase is supportive to pregnancy:
   a. Levels of plasma progesterone are adequate
   b. Endometrial biopsy findings indicate a secretory endometrium
3. Cervical factors are receptive to sperm during expected time of ovulation:
   a. Cervical os is open
   b. Cervical mucus is clear, watery, abundant, and slippery and demonstrates good spinnbarkheit and arborization (fern pattern)
   c. Cervical examination is negative for lesions and infections
   d. Postcoital test findings are satisfactory (adequate number of live, motile, normal sperm present in cervical mucus)
   e. No immunity to sperm can be demonstrated
4. The uterus and uterine tubes are supportive to pregnancy:
   a. Uterine and tubal patency is documented by
      (1) Passage of carbon dioxide into peritoneal cavity
      (2) Spillage of dye into peritoneal cavity
      (3) Outlines of uterine and tubal cavities of adequate size and shape with no abnormalities
   b. Laparoscopic examination verifies normal development of internal genitals and absence of adhesions, infections, endometriosis, and other lesions
5. The male's reproductive structures are normal:
   a. There is no evidence of developmental anomalies of the penis, testicular atrophy, and varicocele (varicose veins on the spermatic vein in the groin)
   b. There is no evidence of infection in the prostate, seminal vesicles, and urethra
   c. The testes are more than 4 cm in the largest diameter
6. Semen is supportive to pregnancy:
   a. Sperm are adequate in number per milliliter of ejaculate
   b. Majority of sperm show normal morphology
   c. Sperm are motile, forward moving
   d. No autoimmunity* exists
   e. Seminal fluid is normal

*The production of antibodies against one's own tissues or secretions is termed **autoimmunization.**

❑ INVESTIGATION OF MALE INFERTILITY

The systematic investigation of impaired fertility in the male, as it does for the female, begins with a thorough history and physical examination (see box below). Assessment of the male proceeds in a manner similar to that of the female (p. 108), starting with noninvasive tests. Male reproductive failure may be caused by many of the difficulties that also affect women, such as nutritional, endocrine, and psychologic disorders. Exposure to reproductive hazards in the workplace and home is evaluated.

Substance abuse can be a major factor in male infertility. *Alcohol* consumption causes erectile problems (impotence). Cigarette smoking has been associated with abnormal sperm, a decreased number of sperm,

ASSESSMENT OF THE MAN

HISTORY

1. Fertility in other marriages of self or spouse
2. Medical: general medical history, including infections (e.g., sexually transmitted diseases, mononucleosis), mumps orchitis, chronic diseases, recent fever, drug use
3. Surgical: herniorraphy, injuries to genitals, or other surgery in genital area
4. Occupational and environmental exposure to chemicals, x-ray equipment, or extreme therapy changes; physical nature of occupation and hobbies; vacations and work habits
5. Previous tests and therapy done for study of impaired fertility; duration of impaired fertility
6. Sex history in detail, with discussion of actual coital techniques such as frequency and ability to ejaculate, adequacy of erection, number of sex partners
7. Personal: motivation for childbearing; attitude toward partner; career aspirations

PHYSICAL EXAMINATION

1. General examination: careful examination of other organs and parts of body, with special attention given to habitus, fat and hair distribution
2. Genital tract: penis and urethra; scrotal size; position, size, and consistency of testes; epididymides and vasa deferentia; prostate size and consistency
3. Careful search for varicocele, with man in both supine and upright positions

LABORATORY DATA

1. Routine urine, complete blood count, and serologic test for syphilis
2. Complete semen analysis—essential
   a. Liquefaction: usually complete within 10 to 30 minutes
   b. Semen volume — 2-5 ml (range: 1 to 7 ml)
   c. Semen pH — 7.2 to 7.8
   d. Sperm density — 20 to 200 million/ml
   e. Normal morphology (%) — ≥60% normal oval
   f. Motility (important consideration in sperm evaluation); percentage of forward-moving sperm (swim-up test) estimated in relationship to abnormally motile and nonmotile sperm. This requires evaluation by a technician with some degree of experience, but since the test provides a more accurate diagnosis, it is well worth the time involved; ≥50% is normal
   g. Cell count: average normal, 60 million or more per milliliter or a total of 150 to 200 or more million per ejaculate; minimum normal standards: 40 million/ml, with a total count of at least 125 million per ejaculate (average of counts on two or preferably three separate specimens)

   NOTE: These values are not absolute, but only relative to the final evaluation of the couple as a single reproductive unit.

   h. Ovum penetration test
3. Additional laboratory studies as indicated
   a. Basic endocrine studies indicated in men with oligospermia or aspermia:
      (1) Tomographic x-ray films of skull
      (2) T_4 or other thyroid tests
      (3) 17-Ketosteroids
      (4) Gonadotropin FSH, LH determination
      (5) 17-Hydroxycorticoids and pregnanediol
      (6) Buccal smear and chromosome studies (e.g., Klinefelter's syndrome, XXY sex chromosomes)
      (7) Test for sperm antibodies; **autoimmunization.** Autoimmune antibodies (produced by the man against his own sperm) agglutinate or immobilize sperm in less than 5% of men with impaired fertility
   b. Testicular biopsy, where correct interpretation is available (may give a more accurate diagnosis and prognosis in cases of azoospermia and severe oligospermia), vasography if indicated and available

and chromosome damage. The degree of abnormality is related to the number of cigarettes smoked per day (Mattison et al, 1989). *Marijuana (cannabis sativa)* adversely affects spermatogenesis (e.g., it depresses the number and motility of sperm and increases the percentage of abnormally formed sperm.) *Monoamine oxidase* (MAO), an antidepressant, adversely affects spermatogenesis. *Amyl nitrate, butyl nitrate, ethyl chloride,* and *methaqualone* (used to prolong orgasm) cause changes in spermatogenesis. *Heroin, methadone,* and *barbiturates* decrease libido.

Tests and Examinations

The basic infertility survey of the male includes a semen analysis. The postcoital test evaluates characteristics of the sperm within the cervical mucus of the man's sexual partner.

Semen Analysis. Examination of semen is an important part of investigation of impaired fertility, since the male is often at least partially responsible (Willson and Carrington, 1987). A complete **semen analysis,** study of the effects of cervical mucus on sperm forward motility and survival, and evaluation of the sperm's ability to penetrate an ovum provide basic information. Sperm counts vary from day to day and are dependent on emotional and physical status and sexual activity. Therefore a single analysis may be inconclusive (Willson and Carrington, 1987). Usually three specimens taken at monthy intervals are evaluated.

Semen is collected by ejaculation into a clean, widemouthed plastic or glass jar with a screw top (Willson and Carrington, 1987). The specimen is usually collected by masturbation following 2 to 5 days of abstinence from ejaculation. Some couples are unable to collect the semen in the manner described. These couples can collect the semen in a special, non-rubber, unpowdered condom that has been punctured in several places.

For other couples, most but not all of the semen can be aspirated from the vaginal vault immediately after intercourse. These latter two methods allow for the possibility of pregnancy. The collection jar is tightly capped and taken to the laboratory within 1 hour of ejaculation. Exposure to excessive heat or cold is avoided. Normal values for semen characteristics are given in the box on p. 117.

The fertility potential of sperm is difficult to evaluate solely by semen analysis, which gives little insight into sperm survival, cervical penetration, migration to the uterine tubes, or capacity for ovum penetration and fertilization (Cunningham, MacDonald, and Gant, 1989). It addition, there is insufficient knowledge of the method by which male and female antibodies can act to inhibit fertility potential of sperm. An immunologic disorder as yet not identified may be the basis for unexplained infertility (Cunningham, MacDonald, and Gant, 1989).

Seminal deficiency may be attributable to one or more of a variety of factors. The male is assessed for these factors (Scott et al, 1990): hypopituitarism, nutritional deficiency, debilitating or chronic disease, trauma, exposure to environmental hazards such as radiation and toxic substances, gonadotropic inadequacy, and obstructive lesions of the epididymis and vas deferens. A genetic basis such as Klinefelter's syndrome is ruled out. Hormone analyses are done for testosterone, gonadotropin, FSH, and LH. Testicular biopsy may be warranted.

Postcoital Test. The postcoital test is one method used to test for adequacy of coital technique, cervical mucus, sperm, and degree of sperm penetration through cervical mucus. The test is performed within 2 hours after ejaculation of semen into the vagina. A specimen of cervical mucus is obtained. Intercourse is synchronized with the expected time of ovulation (as determined from evaluation of BBT, cervical mucus changes, and usual length of menstrual cycle). It is performed only in the absence of vaginal infection. Couples may experience some difficulty abstaining from intercourse for 2 to 4 days before expected ovulation and then having intercourse with ejaculation "on schedule." Sex "on demand" may strain the couple's interpersonal relationship. A problem may arise if the expected day of ovulation occurs when facilities or physician are unavailable (such as over a weekend or holiday). If no sperm is found, the coital technique used must be evaluated (e.g., extreme obesity may prevent adequate penile penetration).

General Therapies

The difficulty may be caused by timing and frequency of intercourse. The couple is taught about the menstrual cycle, the peak cervical mucus symptom, and appropriate timing of intercourse.

Penile intromission is often difficult because of chordee and obesity. The couple is advised to alter positions used for intercourse. Heavy use of alcohol makes penile erection difficult to achieve and maintain until ejaculation. The man is advised to avoid imbibing alcohol during the time of the woman's ovulation.

Medical therapy for male infertility has been disappointing, especially when pituitary or testicular disease is discovered. Occasionally it is possible to suppress the production of sperm with injections of testosterone and in that way cause a reduction in the number of autoimmune antibodies present in the man. Following the reduction in sperm autoantibodies, sperm quality improves, and a pregnancy sometimes occurs.

Drug therapy may be indicated for male infertility.

Infections are identified and treated promptly with antimicrobials. Problems with the thyroid or adrenal glands are corrected with appropriate medications. Testosterone enanthate (Delatestryl) and testosterone cypionate (Depo-Testerone) by injection are used to stimulate virilization, especially in the adolescent. Human chorionic gonadotropin (hCG) (Pregnyl) given intramuscularly virilizes a hypogonadotropic male to restore Leydig cell function and spermatogenesis. FSH and hMG aid hCG for completion of spermatogenesis. Bromocriptine, an ergot derivative and dopamine agonist, is used to treat hypogonadotropic hypogonadism–associated prolactin-producing hypothalamic or pituitary tumors and may reduce the tumor. Clomiphene may be given for idiopathic subfertility.

Surgical repair of varicocele has been relatively successful. A varicocele on the left side is found in a substantial number of subfertile men. Ligation of the varicocele does lead to improvement of the sperm quality and commonly to pregnancy.

Simple changes in life-style may be effective in the treatment of subfertile men. Poor nutritional state is corrected if it exists. High temperatures in the groin area reduce the number of sperm produced. High temperatures may be caused by the wearing of brief shorts and tight jeans that keep the scrotal sac pressed against the body regardless of environmental temperature changes. The testes are kept at temperatures too high for efficient spermatogenesis. Frequent and prolonged hot tubbing has also been implicated in relative infertility. It must be remembered that these conditions only lead to relative infertility and should not be employed as a means of contraception.

Lubricants used during intercourse should not contain spermicides or have spermicidal properties (i.e., K-Y Jelly). If lubrication is needed, Personal, manufactured by Ortho, is suggested.

Assessment

The nurse assists in obtaining data relevant to fertility through interview and physical examination. The data base needs to include information to identify whether infertility is primary or secondary. Religious, cultural, and ethnic data are noted.

Some of the data needed to investigate impaired fertility are of a sensitive, personal nature. Obtaining these data may be viewed as an invasion of privacy. The tests and examinations are occasionally painful and intrusive and can take the romance out of lovemaking. A high level of motivation is needed to endure the investigation.

Many couples have already visited various physicians and have read extensively on the subject. Their previous experiences are recorded. The depth and breadth of their knowledge base is explored.

Nursing Diagnoses

Following are examples of nursing diagnoses that may become apparent from the data base.

Knowledge deficit related to
- Anatomy and physiology of reproduction
- Investigation of impaired fertility
- Cause, course, management, and expected prognosis of condition

Potential impaired individual/family coping or altered sexuality patterns related to
- Need for and methods used in the investigation of impaired fertility

Self-esteem disturbance related to
- Impaired fertility

Potential social isolation or spiritual distress or dysfunctional grieving related to
- Impaired fertility, its investigation and management

Decisional conflict related to
- Therapies for impaired fertility
- Alternatives to therapy: childlessness or adoption

Planning

Planning requires sensitivity to the client's needs. Based on knowledge of impaired fertility, the nurse is equipped to assist with the development of a plan of care for the couple with impaired fertility. The plan is developed in collaboration with the physician in light of the nurse's level of expertise and with other members of the health team and the couple to achieve certain mutually determined goals. The ***goals*** are phrased in client-centered terms and may include the following:

1. Couple is educated in the anatomy and physiology of the reproductive system
2. Any abnormalities identified through various tests and examinations are treated (e.g., infections, blocked uterine tubes, sperm allergy, varicocele)
3. Couple receives an estimate of their chances to conceive
4. Couple resolves guilt feelings and does not need to focus blame
5. Couple conceives or, failing to conceive, decides on an alternative acceptable to both of them (e.g., childlessness, adoption)
6. Couple finds acceptable methods for handling pressures they may feel from peers and relatives regarding their childless state

Implementation

Nursing actions vary with the nurse's level of education, position held, and policies of the agency. Basic to all nursing actions is knowledge of those factors that are essential to or contribute to fertility, of assessment strategies (history, examinations, and tests), and of management and therapy. The nurse acts on the client's readiness to learn and her or his level of understanding of impaired fertility. Although primary responsibility for teaching the client or clients rests with the physician, the nurse assists in the identification of the client's gaps in knowledge, clarifies information, and reinforces the physician's explanations and instructions. Occasionally the nurse acts as the client's advocate by helping the client state a concern or question or request further explanation from the physician or technician.

The nurse's nonverbal behavior before and during the procedure can reassure and support the client. Often the client feels inadequate because of the necessity for testing and the intimidating nature of the tests.

Written and verbal instructions for specific preparation for tests will increase the client's feeling of adequacy. Supportive nursing actions include providing privacy while giving instructions for obtaining specimens and changing clothes, draping, creating a comfortable physical environment, padding the stirrups of the examination table, efficiency in use of equipment, warming the speculum, and coaching for relaxation.

In addition to discussing the specifics of common tests for impaired fertility, nurses can provide sensory information about these future tests. To acquire descriptions of commonly used tests, nurses can interview current clients and ask them to describe their tests in sensory terms. Then nurses can share the most commonly occurring descriptions with future clients. Providing preparatory information can help clients form a mental image of what an experience will include and thus help make the testing experience more tolerable and less distressing.

Women often experience anxiety when undergoing a pelvic examination (Chapter 10). After any procedure, after the client is fully dressed and comfortably seated (at the same level as the nurse and physician), she or he benefits from an opportunity to talk about the experience in an unhurried manner. Not only do these behaviors help the client relax, but also they indicate that the recipient of such care is worthy and thus helps build self-esteem. The goal of nursing-medical *care* is to encourage the client to become an active partner in care as well as to establish rapport to ensure that therapy and eventual counseling are facilitated.

The nurse needs to know the correct method for obtaining, labeling, and transporting specimens to the laboratory. A mishandled specimen may lead to misdiagnosis or the need to obtain another specimen. These errors create added expense and stress to the client as well as significant time delays before therapy can be instituted.

Nurses can help clients express and talk about their feelings as honestly as possible. Ventilation may help couples unburden themselves of negative feelings. Professional referral may be necessary.

The myriad of psychologic responses to a diagnosis of impaired fertility may tax a couple's giving and receiving of physical and sexual closeness. The prescriptions and proscriptions for achieving conception may add tension to a couple's sexual functioning. Couples are instructed about frequency and timing of intercourse as well as use of certain coital positions. It is no wonder that these couples complain of decreased desire for intercourse, orgasmic dysfunction, or midcycle erectile disorders. A once spontaneous act of expressing love has become a mechanical act for creating a baby.

During evaluation of impaired fertility, the previously private act of intercourse becomes a topic of discussion. Even in the sexually liberated culture of the 1990s, few people eagerly share the frequency of coitus and positions used during intercourse.

To be able to deal comfortably with a couple's sexuality, nurses must be comfortable with their own sexuality. Nurses need to resolve their sexual identity, have up-to-date factual knowledge about human sexual practices, be able to accept the preferences and activities of others without being judgmental, acquire skill in interviewing and in therapeutic use of self, develop sensitivity to the nonverbal cues of others, and be knowledgeable of the couple's sociocultural and religious tenets. Once nurses are comfortable with their own sexuality, they can better help couples understand why the private act of lovemaking needs to be shared with health care professionals.

Because of the interference with the spontaneity of coitus, many infertility specialists limit the period of investigation. These specialists have found that the shorter the diagnostic period, the less the disruption of a couple's sexual life-style.

The woman or couple facing impaired fertility exhibits behaviors that resemble the *grieving process* that is associated with loss (Chapter 29). The loss of one's genetic continuity with the generations to come leads to loss of self-esteem, of a sense of adequacy as a woman (or man), of control over one's destiny, and of a sense of self. The investigative process leads to a loss of spontaneity and control over the couple's marital relationship and sometimes over one's progress toward career and life goals. All people do not experience every one of the reactions described below nor can the length of time be predicted that any one reaction will last for an individual.

The nurse may feel at a loss in knowing how to assist. Table 6-2 presents characteristic behaviors of people experiencing the psychologic impact of impaired fertility along with some suggestions for nursing (or other health professionals') actions.

The support systems of the couple with impaired fertility need to be explored. This exploration should include persons available to assist, their relationship to the couple, their ages, their availability, and the cultural or religious support that is available. This type of assessment is suitable for a health team conference where representatives of several disciplines can share ideas and work cooperatively in developing a plan for management.

If the couple conceives, nurses need to be aware that

Table 6-2 Nursing Actions in Response to Behavior Associated with Impaired Fertility

Behavioral Characteristic	Nursing Actions
Surprise: each person assumes she or he is fertile and that pregnancy is an option.	Point out resemblance to grieving process—a normal, expected reaction to loss (Chapter 29). Refer to support group.* Prepare them for length of time it may take to grieve, types of feelings (psychologic, somatic) to expect. Encourage and allow time to talk of past and present feelings of sexuality, self-image, and self-esteem.
Denial: "It can't happen to me!"	Allow time for denial because it gives the body and mind time to adjust a little at a time. Do not feed into the client's denial; instead say, "It must be hard to believe such a devastating report."
Anger: toward others (perhaps even at the nurse) or themselves.	Explain that the reaction to loss of control and to a feeling of helplessness is often anger, which can easily be projected onto another person. Without release, anger can lead to chronic depression. Anger is a natural feeling. Allow time to express anger at losing their sense of control over their bodies and destinies; identify and direct energy directly at the problem. Airing one's own anger often eases the intensity of the emotion. A helpful approach may be, "It's OK to be angry . . . at those who are pregnant, at people who want abortions, at self, at mate, at caregivers, and so forth."
Bargaining: "If I get pregnant, I'll dedicate the child to God.	Accept bargaining statements without comment.
Depression:	
Isolation: personal.	Allow time for both woman and man to talk about how it feels whenever a sight, event, or word serves as a reminder of own state of impaired fertility. Develop role playing situations to practice interactions with others under various circumstances to increase the couple's ability to cope and to problem solve (increases their self-confidence). The nurse may say, "You must feel so terribly alone sometimes."
Guilt/unworthiness.	Allow time to identify feelings that may be based on earlier behaviors (e.g., abortion, premarital sex, contact with sexually transmitted disease [STD]). Goal: couple or person comes to the realization that "unworthiness" and impaired fertility are unrelated.
Acceptance (resolution).	Clients need to know that grief feelings are never laid away forever; they may be activated by special reminders (e.g., anniversaries).

*RESOLVE, Inc, PO Box 474, Boston, Mass, 02178 and 5 Water Street, Arlington, Mass, 02174.

the concerns and problems of the previously infertile couple may not be over. Many couples are overjoyed with the pregnancy. However, some are not. Some couples rearrange their lives, sense of self, and personal goals within their acceptance of their infertile state. The couple may feel that those who worked with them to identify and treat impaired fertility expect them to be happy with the pregnancy. The couple may be shocked to find that they themselves feel resentment because the pregnancy, once a cherished dream, now necessitates another change in goals, aspirations, and identities. The normal ambivalence toward pregnancy (Chapter 9) may be perceived as reneging on the original choice to become parents. The couple may choose to abort the pregnancy at this time (see p. 149). Other couples worry about spontaneous abortion. If the couple wishes to continue with the pregnancy, they will need the care other pregnant couples need (see Unit II). The couple may need extra preparation for the realities of pregnancy, labor, and parenthood, because they have developed fantasies about childbearing when they thought it was beyond their reach. *A history of impaired fertility is considered to be a risk factor for pregnancy.* The couple who has a history of impaired fertility before this pregnancy faces another label, that of being at high risk for this pregnancy (see Chapter 22).

The couple too may desire information about contraception after the birth of this baby. If the previously infertile couple desires additional children, the couple is advised about those contraceptive methods that are least likely to cause damage and impair fertility.

If the couple does not conceive, they are assessed regarding their desire to be referred for help with adoption, therapeutic intrauterine insemination, or with choosing childlessness. The couple would find a list of such agencies within their particular community helpful.

Evaluation

The nurse can be reasonably assured that care was effective when the client-centered goals have been achieved:

1. Couple increases their knowledge of anatomy and physiology of reproduction.
2. Couple collaborates with the investigation of impaired fertility.
3. Any abnormalities identified through various tests and examinations are treated successfully.
4. Couple resolves guilt feelings and does not need to focus blame.
5. If the couple conceives, the couple accepts their responses to pregnancy; realigns their goals, aspirations, and identities; and is comfortable with their decisions regarding the pregnancy.
6. If the couple does not conceive, they decide on an acceptable alternative and seek support as necessary. They find acceptable methods for handling pressures they may feel from peers and relatives regarding their childless state, and they receive a list of community agencies that assist with adoptions or provide appropriate support.

Reproductive Alternatives

There have been remarkable developments in reproductive medicine (Evans et al, 1989). Alternative birth technologies, heralded by involuntarily childless couples, are creating ethical and legal issues (Chapter 3). Several alternatives are presented here in some detail: in vitro fertilization and embryo transfer (IVF-ET), gamete intrafallopian tube transfer (GIFT), and zygote intrafallopian transfer (ZIFT). Other alternatives, including surrogate motherhood, are mentioned.

In Vitro Fertilization and Embryo Transfer. The first successful term delivery of an infant conceived by in vitro fertilization (test-tube pregnancy) in 1978 was the culmination of years of study and experimentation by Robert Edwards and Patrick Steptoe in England. Since then several other "laboratory conceived" and normal-appearing newborns have been delivered.

Many women whose uterine tubes either are obstructed or have been removed are not potential candidates for similar treatment. However, because of the complexity and cost of the procedure, the likelihood is that this approach to impaired fertility must remain limited for the near future. The following steps, ultrasimplified, are necessary for **in vitro fertilization-embryo transplant.**

1. Ovulation is induced by gonadotropin therapy (e.g., clomiphene or menotropin) to ensure as many mature follicles as possible.
2. Mature follicles are identified by laparoscopy, pelvic ultrasound, or transvaginal ultrasound. Needle aspiration may be through the laparoscope, transvaginally, or transurethrally (Seibel, 1988).
3. Ova are examined through a microscope to verify maturity and then transferred to tissue culture media.
4. Before laparoscopy, semen is collected. Freshly ejaculated sperm cannot fertilize an ovum; they must be capacitated. A simple process in humans, capacitation involves only a short incubation period in a culture medium. After capacitation, sperm are added to the ova (Pernoll and Benson, 1987).

5. After fertilization a second tissue culture transfer allows division to approximately a 12-cell blastocyst (3 to 6 days) when it is returned to the uterus.
6. Progesterone therapy in the interval induces a late secretory type of endometrium, whereupon the blastocyst is transferred to the uterus, where the implantation (nidation) of the zygote occurs and embryonic development proceeds. The efficacy of progesterone therapy has not been established but most centers administer it anyway (Seibel, 1988).

Within an 18-month period, overall success rates for in vitro fertilization worldwide have risen from 1% to 8% to 20% to 30%, depending on the clinical facility. This vast improvement is attributable to increased precision in predicting ovulation and in retrieving the ovum. The conventional methods of predicting ovulation—calendar, BBT, cervical mucus, fertility awareness, and laboratory tests such as vaginal cytology and serum hormone determination—can only approximate the moment of ovulation. The more precise methods are beyond the scope of this text but are mentioned here for interest. These methods are (1) stimulating ovulation with clomiphene or menotropin given at a precise time during the cycle, (2) monitoring ovulatory function with realtime ultrasound, and (3) performing rapid radioimmunoassay for estrogen level. Through a laparoscope or transvaginally, the ovum is retrieved by inserting an aspiration needle into the ripened follicle and removing the ovum. Semen is collected and treated before its use for fertilization of the ovum. The complete procedure is described by Marrs (1982). In vitro fertilization cost from $5000 to $8000 per treatment in 1989.

Human experimentation and manipulation of this type have been sanctioned by the U.S. Department of Health and Human Services. The Roman Catholic Church is strongly opposed to in vitro fertilization. Legal aspects of in vitro fertilization are discussed in Chapter 3.

Gamete Intrafallopian Tube Transfer. Gamete intrafallopian (uterine) tube transfer (GIFT) is similar to IVF-ET. Ovulation is induced as in IVF-ET; a menotropin injection is given; and the oocytes are aspirated from follicles via laparoscopy (Fig. 6-7, *A*) or minilaparotomy (Pernoll and Benson, 1987). A newer approach is the use of ultrasonographic transvaginal ovum retrieval (Rabar et al, 1988; Chapter 22). Before laparoscopy, semen is collected. Sperm are capacitated using the same technique as for IVF-ET. The eggs are identified in the laboratory. Capacitated sperm are then mixed with the ova and drawn up into a catheter. The ova and sperm are then transferred to the uterine tubes (Fig. 6-7, *B*) permitting natural fertilization and cleavage, with subsequent successful pregnancies. A 20% to

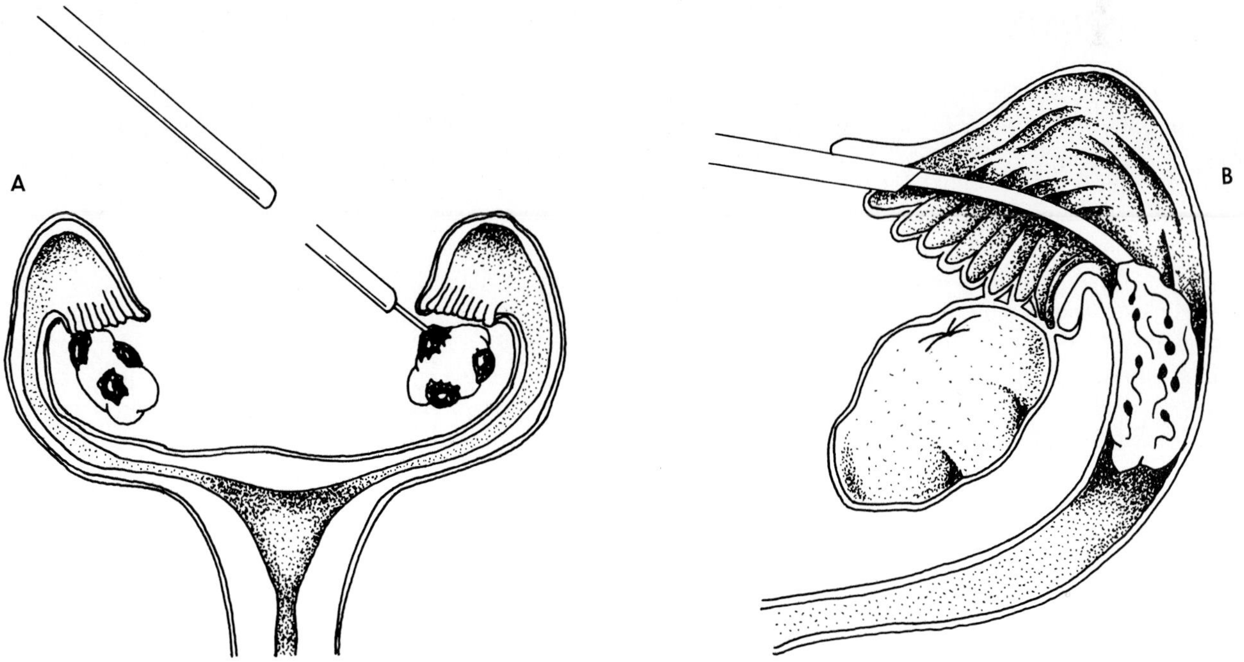

Fig. 6-7 **A,** Via laparoscope, a ripe follicle is located and the fluid containing the egg is removed. **B,** The separated sperm and egg are placed into the uterine tubes where fertilization occurs.

30% pregnancy rate per cycle has been reported for this technique.

GIFT is only useful for women who have normal tubal function. The success of this technique has not been compared with the less complicated technique of simple induced ovulation combined with therapeutic intrauterine insemination. GIFT is more expensive to perform than IVF-ET using ultrasound egg aspiration.

Zygote Intrafallopian Transfer. A third technique, zygote intrafallopian transfer (ZIFT), combines the advantages of IVF-ET and GIFT (Hamori et al, 1988). Ovulation is induced, the mature follicles are aspirated, and the semen is prepared as with IVF-ET and GIFT. The follicles are inseminated in a petri dish. They are examined 18 hours later for pronuclei (evidence that fertilization has occurred). The zygotes are then transferred back to the uterus via laparoscopy into the fimbriated end of the fallopian tubes. No more than two zygotes are implanted on either side. This technique is possible only for women with at least one patent fallopian tube.

ZIFT appears to have certain advantages: abnormally fertilized eggs can be rejected, and the zygote follows as close to "natural" a path as possible. However, the success rate is still low (12.1%).

For IVF-ET, GIFT, and ZIFT procedures, the protocols vary from center to center. In any of these procedures, donated sperm, ova, or even embryos may be used.

Care of Recipients. Most of these procedures are done on an out-of-hospital basis. However, a woman may be admitted to the hospital for a few hours to recover after a follicular retrieval or an implantation. These women are generally in good health and have little or no pain. However, they need supportive nursing care. The nurse should remember that the woman may already have a sense of failure because of her inability to get pregnant without intervention. The couple has an enormous financial and emotional investment in this child. The woman may be tense, irritable, and afraid to urinate or even move. The nurse may feel that because the woman is not ill, may not have been anesthetized, and has voluntarily undergone this procedure, she does not need much nursing care. Actually, the woman would benefit from the nurse sitting with her for a few minutes and talking calmly. After any of these procedures, the woman must be able to walk and urinate before leaving the hospital.

Therapeutic Insemination. During a 12-month interval from 1986 to 1987, 11,000 physicians performed artificial insemination with spousal or donor semen on 172,000 women in the United States (U.S. Congress, 1988). Approximately 30,000 births occurred during that year as a result of therapeutic donor insemination (TDI), previously referred to as artificial insemination donor (AID) (Ory, 1989). Donor semen is subjected to laboratory testing to reduce the possibility of life-threatening illnesses for the recipient and her fetus, as well as for factors that could jeopardize the woman's future fertility or compromise the chance of the success of the procedure (Ory, 1989). Donor semen is tested for serology, serum hepatitis B antigen, *Neisseria gonorrhoeae, Chlamydia trachomatis,* cytomegalovirus (CMV) antibodies, and human immunodeficiency virus (HIV) antibodies (Ory, 1989).

When the husband's sperm has poor quality or motility, several semen samples are collected from him. The samples consist of split ejaculates, that is, the sperm-rich *first portion* only is collected for freezing and later pooling for **therapeutic intrauterine insemination.** Rapid freezing with liquid nitrogen and subsequent thawing do not cause genetic damage even after 10 years' storage using glycerol. Pooling should increase the sperm count and improve the placement of a portion of the total semen specimen at the cervical os.

Assuming normal female fertility, therapeutic intrauterine insemination (husband) at or about the time of ovulation has resulted in pregnancy in as many as 70% of cases. Numerous inseminations may be necessary to ensure proper timing of ovulation. Ovulation detection kits using urinary LH or serial ultrasound offer more reliable evidence of impending ovulation than do BBT charts (Ory, 1989). Approximately 50% of pregnancies with therapeutic intrauterine insemination (donor) will occur within 2 months; almost 90% occur within 6 months.

Insemination directly into the uterine cavity should be avoided because of severe cramping (prostaglandin effect) and possible infection. The recommended procedure is the instillation of about 0.5 ml of the specimen into the cervical canal with the remainder deposited in a cleanly washed contraceptive diaphragm to be worn by the woman for about 1 hour.

Insemination with the husband's semen presents no legal problems, but insemination with donor sperm may involve many legal, ethical, and emotional aspects (Ory, 1989; Chapter 3). The couple must know there is no guarantee of pregnancy and that in either case the spontaneous abortion rate is approximately the same as in a control population. There is no increase in maternal or perinatal complications; the same frequency of anomalies (about 5%) and obstetric complications (between 5% and 10%) that accompanies normal insemination applies also to therapeutic insemination.

Other Techniques. *Ovum or embryo transfer* involves inseminating a donor female with semen from the husband of an infertile woman (Bustillo et al, 1984). After 4 days, when the fertilized (or unfertilized) egg reaches the uterus, it is lavaged out of the donor female and placed into the uterus of the infertile wife. The infertile woman carries the pregnancy. Term pregnancy rate is only 3%.

Embryos have been *donated* from one woman to another with resultant live births. These women are not candidates for IVF-ET because of severe pelvic adhesions or absence of functional ovaries. In the latter case, the endometrium must be primed with estrogen and progesterone before transfer to the donated embryo. Progesterone supplementation must be maintained for 10 weeks.

Freezing and preservation of the embryo for thawing and transfer in a later cycle have been successful in cattle but have had limited success in humans. Oocyte cryopreservation has not been successful in any species. No one advocates the discarding of embryos (see ethical issues, Chapter 3).

These, as well as the other procedures, have enormous future potential but create many ethical and legal concerns.

Complications. Other than the established risks associated with laparoscopy and general anesthesia, few risks are associated with IVF-ET, GIFT, or other techniques. Transvaginal needle aspiration requires no anesthesia. Congenital anomalies occur no more frequently than in normally conceived embryos. Ectopic pregnancies, however, do occur, and these carry a significant maternal risk.

Surrogate Motherhood. Surrogate motherhood can be achieved by two methods. One way is to have the surrogate mother inseminated with semen from the infertile woman's husband and carry the baby to delivery. Then the baby is formally adopted by the infertile couple. A less common method is to retrieve an ovum from the infertile woman, fertilize it with her husband's sperm, and place it into the uterus of the surrogate mother-to-be. These newer interventions cause some legal and ethical problems (Chapter 3).

Adoption. For couples who can give up the quest for biologic parenthood, adoption is also an option (Adoption, 1989). However, with increasing numbers of single mothers keeping their babies, the achievement of this option may take 3 or more years.

The decision to adopt should be mutual. The clients' attitudes and feelings must be examined before they can assume the responsibility for an adopted child. Most adults assume that they will be able to have children of their own. To discover that they are unable to do so is often accompanied by feelings of inferiority, doubts about masculinity or femininity, and feelings of guilt or blame in relation to the spouse. These feelings and frustrations, superimposed on the anxious waiting for pregnancies, feelings of loss, and the endless medical procedures to investigate impaired fertility, provide an adoptive couple with their own unique needs in preparing for parenthood (Whaley and Wong, 1991).

Whatever motivates a couple to seek adoption, the decision needs to be based on emotionally healthy needs. The welfare of the child should be the primary consideration in her or his placement. Motives such as the need to strengthen an unstable marriage, to treat emotional problems (including grief over death of a child), or to treat psychogenic sterility should be carefully explored. Also, when adoption satisfies the needs of only one of the two parents, the outcome is questionable (Whaley and Wong, 1991).

❑ CONTROL OF FERTILITY

Contraception is the voluntary prevention of pregnancy having both individual and social implications. It has been established that more than 90% of couples in the United States have used or intend to use some method of contraception (birth control).

Religious Considerations. Family planning is accepted in principle by all religions. Some strict protestant denominations, Hasidic Jews, and Roman Catholics believe that family planning can be achieved by periodic abstinence alone. Religion, however, may not be as great a barrier as once believed. Ostling (1987) reported that according to the National Center for Health Statistics many women under age 45 have used contraceptive methods not approved by their religions. Samoans represent a variety of religions, but for them contraceptive practices are not highly valued (Clark and Howland, 1978). Rather, priority is placed on demonstration of male and female fertility through childbirth. In some religious and cultural groups, attitudes regarding menstruation might appear to present a barrier to the use of any agent that alters menstrual function (Kaunitz, 1989).

Cultural Considerations. Cross-cultural information about contraceptive practices is limited. Before modern times, probably the most effective contraception resulted from sexual taboos. Postpartum taboos were generally effective. Kay (1982) points out that the Mexican-Americans she studied continued to place a 40-day restriction on sexual intercourse after childbirth.

In the past, American Indians used herbs as oral contraceptives (Vogel, 1973). Information about these herbs was useful in the development of today's oral contraceptives. Some American Indian groups today favor the use of contraceptives, but others believe that contraceptives are against God's will. Although the Japanese were one of the earliest cultural groups to accept the use of birth control and abortion (Okamoto, 1978), Japanese couples are reluctant to use contraception until they have borne one child (Bernstein and Kidd, 1982).

Fertility management has posed numerous problems

for nurses working with persons whose belief systems place a high value on having children. Nevertheless, many persons with these belief systems are interested in learning about contraception and will listen to explanations if they include respect for another's values. Health care innovations are accepted or rejected depending on how they fit into the client's cultural pattern.

Assessment

A history, physical examination, and laboratory tests precede the initiation of some forms of contraception. A complete gynecologic examination is performed. Menstrual, contraceptive, and obstetric histories are taken. The woman's knowledge about contraception and her sexual partner's commitment to any particular method are determined. Data are required about the frequency of coitus (once every so often or several times per week), whether the woman has one sexual partner or several, the level of involvement the woman wishes to assume, and her (their) objections to any methods. The woman's level of comfort and willingness to touch her genitals and cervical mucus are assessed. Myths are identified. Religious and cultural factors are determined. The woman's verbal and nonverbal responses to hearing about the various available methods are carefully noted. An individual's reproductive-life plan needs to be considered. Individuals need to consider the following questions. How sad would they be if they could never become biologic parents? How concerned would they be if they were to become pregnant before they were ready to biologically childbear? If they became pregnant before they wanted to be, would abortion be an alternative?

Nursing Diagnoses

Nursing diagnoses reflect the assessment findings. Following are examples of nursing diagnoses that may emerge.

Knowledge deficit related to
- The number and nature of options available
- The advantages, disadvantages, modes of action, and effectiveness of methods
- Responsibility of woman and partner for a chosen method
- Side effects to report to health care provider

Potential for decisional conflict related to
- Unplanned pregnancy

Potential for infection or injury related to
- Inappropriate use of contraceptive method

Potential for altered sexuality patterns related to
- Inappropriate method of contraception
- Inappropriate use of chosen method of contraception

Planning

Planning is a collaborative effort among the woman, her sexual partner (when appropriate), the physician, and the nurse. The ***goals*** are determined and stated in client-centered terms, and may include the following:

1. The woman learns accurate information about contraceptive methods
2. The woman is comfortable and satisfied with the chosen method
3. If further childbearing is desired, the couple achieves pregnancy at the time planned
4. The couple experiences no adverse sequelae as a result of the chosen method of contraception

Implementation

Client teaching (Chapter 1) is fundamental to initiating and maintaining any form of contraception. A care-provider relationship based on trust is an important facet in client compliance. The nurse counters myths with facts, clarifies misinformation, and fills in gaps of knowledge (see guidelines for client teaching). There are various contraceptive techniques used in North America. The ideal contraceptive should be safe, easily available, economical, acceptable, simple to use, and promptly reversible. Although no means or method may ever achieve all these objectives, impressive progress has been made recently. The woman or couple must be fully informed of the risks, effectiveness, reversibility, and alternatives (see discussion of informed consent, Chapter 3).

Contraception failure rate refers to the percentage of contraceptive users expected to experience an accidental pregnancy during the first year, even when they use a method consistently and correctly. Failure rates decrease over time either because a user will gain experience with and use a method more appropriately or because the less effective users will drop out of the study.

Contraception employs one or more of the following methods:

1. Methods available to people without prescription
   a. Biologic periodic abstinence: natural family planning
   b. Chemical barriers: spermicidal creams, gels, or vaginal suppositories and sponges
   c. Mechanical barrier: condoms or sheaths

Guidelines for Client Teaching
GENERAL CONTRACEPTIVE METHODS

ASSESSMENT

1. Complete physical assessment and history.
2. Assessment of woman's (couple's) knowledge of method selected.
3. Assessment of body image.
4. Assessment of motivation needed for method selected.
5. Assessment of life-style and discussion whether method selected fits into daily life.

NURSING DIAGNOSES

Knowledge deficit related to method selected.

Potential for pregnancy or injury related to knowledge deficit or ignorance of method selected.

Potential for infection related to not adhering to proper guidelines of method selected.

Altered nutrition: less than body requirements related to side effects of oral contraceptives.

GOALS

Short-term

Nurse identifies myths, clarifies information, and dispells misinformation.

Woman (couple) becomes comfortable in the use of the method.

Woman learns relevant information regarding the method being used (i.e., use, action, advantages, disadvantages, side effects, and effectiveness).

Intermediate

Woman (couple) confers with care provider when questions arise regarding use or desire to change to another method.

Women reports side effects or complications or suspected pregnancy immediately.

Woman returns to care provider for periodic checkups or when a change in the method is warranted.

Long-term

Woman remains in good health while using chosen method.

Woman achieves desired objective for contraception.

Woman indicates satisfaction with chosen method and care received.

REFERENCES AND TEACHING AIDS

Inserts from packages of chosen method.

Hospital or clinic teaching pamphlets or booklets.

Flip chart showing anatomy of pelvic structures or total body plastic medical model.

Audiovisuals or films for teaching.

Samples of contraceptive device (i.e., BBT charts and thermometer).

Fresh egg white for teaching about cervical mucus.

Mirror.

Handouts of printed material.

RATIONALE/CONTENT	TEACHING ACTION
Knowledge provides a basis for decision-making.	*Encourage general discussion through use of the following:*
Provide general discussion about selected method, its mode of action, and reasons for choosing it. Teach at the client's level without being condescending.	Provide time, privacy, and assurance regarding confidentiality. Create a receptive, nonjudgmental atmosphere. Consider appropriate cultural/ethnic, intellectual/educational, and developmental factors. *Using references and equipment listed above, implement the following:*
Supply information about action, advantages, disadvantages, side effects, and effectiveness.	Discuss information about method selected.
Discuss method, its placement, locus of action.	Indicate on illustration or medical model the placement of the device (IUD, diaphragm, cervical cap or sponge, condom), and describe the loci of action (hormonal contraceptive versus diaphragm).
Competence and confidence increase with practice.	Demonstrate appliance (diaphragm with spermicide), characteristics of "fertile" cervical mucus (egg white), entering temperature on BBT graph, calculating fertile times.
Reinforce content in a variety of ways.	Supervise client's return demonstration and practice.
Provide time and hands-on experience with chosen method.	Assess client's recall of content taught or its availability on printed material provided.
Review the material presented.	Ascertain that client has appropriate phone numbers for questions and suggest client call back, prn, after implementing method at home.

EVALUATION Woman (couple) demonstrates competence and asks appropriate questions regarding method of choice: goals are met within an appropriate time frame.

2. Methods that require periodic medical examination and prescription*
   a. Hormonal therapy: estrogen or progestogen preparations or a combination of these compounds
   b. Mechanical barrier: cervical uterine occlusion by diaphragms or caps
   c. Intrauterine contraceptive devices
3. Methods that require surgical intervention
   a. Female sterilization
   b. Male sterilization

The nurse supervises return demonstrations and practice to assess client understanding. The client is given written instructions and phone numbers for questions. If the client has difficulty with written instructions, the woman (couple) is offered graphic material and a phone number to call as necessary, or an offer to return for further instruction.

Evaluation

The nurse can be reasonably assured that care was effective if the goals of care have been achieved: the woman (couple) learns about the various methods of contraception; the couple achieves pregnancy only when it has been planned; and they experience no adverse sequelae as a result of the chosen method of contraception.

NONPRESCRIPTION METHODS FOR CONTROL OF FERTILITY

Several nonprescription methods for control of fertility are practiced. Prescription and supervision are unnecessary for barrier methods, that is, condom, foam, spermicide, and vaginal sponges, as well as for periodic abstinence. In 1987, among women aged 15 to 44 years exposed to the risk of unwanted pregnancy, 92% used some form of contraception (Mishell, 1989). Oral contraception was used by 32%, 17% used the condom, 6% used spermicide, 4% used the diaphragm, 4% used periodic abstinence (i.e., "natural family planning"), and 3% had an intrauterine device (IUD). Two methods were practiced that are *not* recommended: 6% used withdrawal (coitus interruptus),† and 1% used douching. The percentages do not add up because some women used more than one method (Mishell, 1989).

Periodic Abstinence

The term **periodic abstinence** is preferred over "natural family planning" for contraceptive methods that rely on avoidance of intercourse during presumed fertile days of the menstrual cycle. Many couples find abstinence for 7 to 18 or more consecutive days of each menstrual cycle to be unnatural (Klaus, 1982).

Periodic abstinence methods employ a combination of the following:

1. Rhythm or calendar method
2. BBT method
3. Cervical mucus (Billings, ovulation) method
4. Sympto-thermal method
5. Fertility awareness method
6. Predictor test for ovulation

These methods depend on the continuous observation and recording of events of the menstrual cycle. The woman or couple must be able to assess hormone-induced signs and symptoms that indicate whether she is in the fertile or infertile part of the menstrual cycle. While teaching a woman about fertility awareness, the nurse uses this opportunity for helping the woman or couple learn a great deal about their bodies.

The *mode of action* for these methods of contraception is the avoidance of intercourse during the presumed fertile period of the menstrual cycle.*

The human ovum can be fertilized no later than 16 to 24 hours after ovulation. Motile sperm have been recovered from the uterus and the oviducts as long as 60 hours after coitus. However, their ability to fertilize the ovum probably lasts no longer than 24 to 48 hours. Pregnancy is unlikely to occur if a couple abstains from intercourse for 4 days before and for 3 or 4 days after ovulation (**fertile period**). Unprotected intercourse on the other days of the cycle (**safe period**) should not result in pregnancy. There are two principal problems with this method: the exact time of ovulation cannot be predicted accurately, and couples may find it difficult to exercise restraint for several days before and after ovulation. Women with irregular menstrual periods have the greatest risk of failure with this form of con-

*Certified nurse-midwives and some certified nurse-practitioners may be educated to provide this service.

†NOTE: Coitus interruptus, a method practiced for centuries, requires the man to withdraw before ejaculation. Extreme self-discipline is needed, and the sexual relationship may be strained. The danger of pregnancy from sperm in the pre-ejaculatory drops is ever present. No advantages are given for this method, which has the lowest rate of effectiveness, comparable to the use of no contraceptive method.

*The World Health Organization (Liskin and Fox, 1981) concluded in 1979 that the cervical mucus and sympto-thermal methods "had very limited application, particularly in developing countries, and recommended that the World Health Organization Programme devote no further research to measuring their effectiveness." Similarly, the International Planned Parenthood Federation concluded in 1982 that "couples electing to use periodic abstinence should, however, be clearly informed that the method is not considered an effective method of family planning."

traception (Medical Letter, 1988). The typical failure rate is 20% during the first year of use (Hatcher et al, 1988).

Ovulation usually occurs about 14 days before the onset of menstruation. Therefore variations in the length of menstrual cycles are usually a result of differences in the length of the preovulatory phases. The fertile period can be anticipated by the following:

1. Calculating the time at which ovulation is likely to occur based on the lengths of previous menstrual cycles *(calendar method)*
2. Recording the rise in basal body temperature (BBT), a result of the thermogenic effect of progesterone *(temperature method)*
3. Recognizing the changes in cervical mucus at different phases of the menstrual cycle *(ovulation or Billings method)*
4. Using a predictor test for ovulation
5. Utilizing a combination of several methods

Unique developments of monoclonal antibody technology have added the *predictor test* for ovulation. This type of test is a major addition to the periodic abstinence methods to help women who want to plan the time of their pregnancies and those who are trying to conceive.

Calendar Method. Practice of the **calendar method** is based on a count of the number of days in each cycle counting from the first day of menses (Labbok and Queenan, 1989). With the calendar method the fertile period is determined after accurately recording the lengths of menstrual cycles for 1 year. The first unsafe day (beginning of the fertile period) can be determined by subtracting 18 days from the length of the shortest cycle. The last unsafe day (beginning of postovulatory safe period) can be calculated by subtracting 11 days from the length of the longest cycle. If the shortest cycle is 24 days and the longest is 30 days, application of the formula is as follows:

Shortest Cycle	Longest Cycle
24	30
−18	−11
6th day	19th day

To avoid conception the couple would abstain during the "fertile" period, days 6 through 19.

If the woman has very regular cycles of 28 days each, the formula indicates the fertile days to be:

Shortest Cycle	Longest Cycle
28	28
−18	−11
10th day	17th day

To avoid pregnancy, the couple abstains from day 10 through 17 because ovulation occurs on day 14 ±2 days. A major drawback of the calendar method is that one is trying to predict future events with past data. The predictability of the menstrual cycle to be unpredictable is also not taken into consideration.

The method is most useful as an adjunct to the BBT or cervical mucus method. It is *not* useful in the postpartum period, during lactation, or at extremes of reproductive age when cycles are most variable (Labbok and Queenan, 1989).

Basal Body Temperature. The **basal body temperature (BBT)** during the menses and for approximately 5 to 7 days thereafter usually varies from 36.2° to 36.3° C (97.2° to 97.4° F) (see Table 4-1, p. 69). If ovulation fails to occur, this pattern of lower body temperature continues throughout the cycle. Infection, fatigue, less than 3 hours of sleep per night, awakening late, and anxiety may cause temperature fluctuations, altering the expected pattern. If a new BBT thermometer is purchased, this fact is noted on the chart because the readings may vary slightly. Jet lag, alcohol taken the evening before, or sleeping in a heated water bed must also be noted on the chart because each will affect the BBT (see guidelines for client teaching, p. 130).

About the time of ovulation, a slight drop in temperature (about 0.05° C [0.1° F]) may be seen; after ovulation, in concert with the increasing progesterone levels of the early luteal phase of the cycle, the BBT rises slightly (about 0.2° to 0.4° C, [0.4° to 0.8° F]) (Fig. 6-8; Table 4-1) (Labbok and Quenan, 1989). The temperature remains on an elevated plateau until 2 to 4 days before menstruation. Then it drops to the low levels recorded during the previous cycle.

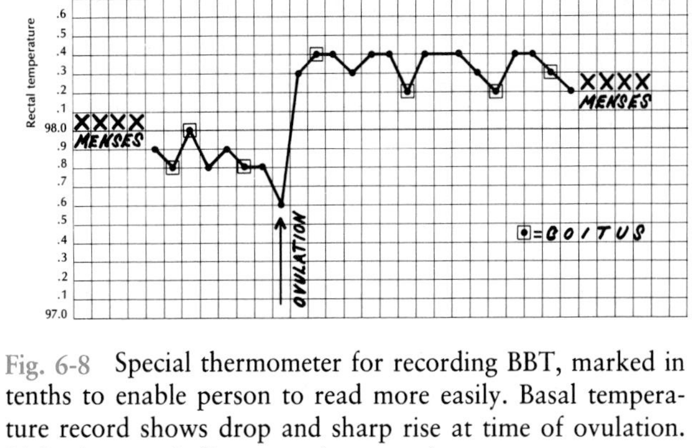

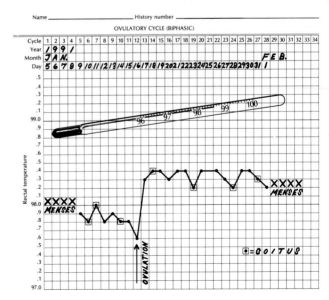

Fig. 6-8 Special thermometer for recording BBT, marked in tenths to enable person to read more easily. Basal temperature record shows drop and sharp rise at time of ovulation. Biphasic curve indicates ovulatory cycle.

The drop and subsequent rise in temperature are referred to as the **thermal shift.** When the entire month's temperatures are recorded on a graph, the pattern described above is more apparent. It is more difficult to perceive day-to-day variations without the entire picture (Fig. 6-8). The BBT alone is not a reliable method to predict ovulation (Labbok and Queenan, 1989). To determine if a rise in temperature is indeed the thermal shift, the woman must be aware of other signs approaching ovulation while she continues to assess the BBT. See discussion of sympto-thermal method for other indicators of ovulation.

Most counselors advise the couple who wish to prevent conception to avoid unprotected intercourse from

Guidelines for Client Teaching

BASAL ("RESTING") BODY TEMPERATURE

ASSESSMENT

1. Woman having trouble conceiving for pregnancy.
2. Need for presumptive evidence of ovulation and an adequate luteal (progesterone) phase.
3. Woman interested in learning how to determine her ovulation time.

NURSING DIAGNOSES

Knowledge deficit related to BBT, the procedure to take it and keep a graph.

Potential self-esteem disturbance related to the inability to conceive a child.

Sexual dysfunction related to possible infertility and anovulation.

GOALS

Short-term

Woman learns what BBT is and how to take and record it.

Intermediate

Woman maintains a record of BBT, fever, stress, cervical mucus characteristics.

Long-term

Woman is motivated enough to obtain and maintain BBT graph for several months.

REFERENCES AND TEACHING AIDS

Pamphlets, booklets, diagrams, any printed material depicting the taking and recording of the BBT.

BBT thermometer and graphs.

RATIONALE/CONTENT	TEACHING ACTION
Knowledge provides a basis for developing competence and confidence.	Discuss BBT with the woman.
In an ovulating woman, there is a variation in the BBT during the course of her menstrual cycle because of hormones working in her body (p. 67). If fertilization of the ovum takes place, the BBT remains elevated. However, if fertilization does not take place, the corpus luteum deteriorates and the BBT falls to the lower level again, until the next ovulation occurs.	Show woman a diagram depicting the phases of the menstrual cycle (Fig. 4-21). Discuss the different hormones in the woman's body that are responsible for her menstrual cycle and ovulation. Leave time for questions. Show woman a sample BBT graph (Fig. 6-8) and the biphasic line seen in ovulatory cycles.
The BBT thermometer is calibrated in tenths rather than fifths. If woman does not want to buy a BBT thermometer, a regular oral thermometer may be used, but it must be left under the tongue for 5 minutes.	Show the client the BBT thermometer, and how it is calibrated.
Discuss the procedure woman will follow every day: Before going to bed, the woman will shake the thermometer down and leave it on the bedside table. On awakening the following morning, the woman will put the BBT thermometer under her tongue and not move any more. After 3 minutes she will take the thermometer out of her mouth and replace it on the night stand. On arising, the woman will read the thermometer and record the temperature on the graph.	Provide a demonstration. Encourage woman to demonstrate taking and reading the thermometer and how she will graph the temperature while nurse watches. Encourage woman to start a log at the same time that keeps track of any other activity that might interfere with her true BBT (see Fig. 6-9).

EVALUATION Woman verbalizes understanding of the instructions given, provides a return demonstration, asks appropriate questions, and meets all goals mutually set. When woman returns after 2 or 3 cycles, she brings a completed log and graph and can identify phases of her menstrual cycle by using these data.

the day of the drop in the BBT and for 3 days of elevated temperature (Labbok and Queenan, 1989). Others require the woman to abstain for the entire preovulatory period, starting with day 1 of menses until the third consecutive day of elevated BBT (Mishell, 1989).

Cervical Mucus Method. The **cervical mucus method** also called the *Billings method* or the *ovulation method,* requires that the woman recognize and interpret the characteristic cyclic changes in the amount and consistency of cervical mucus (see Table 4-1 and Figs. 4-22 and 4-23). The cervical mucus that accompanies ovulation is necessary for viability and motility of sperm. Without adequate cervical mucus, coitus will not result in conception. These changes are easily learned by most couples (see guidelines for client teaching). To ensure learning accurate assessment of changes, the cervical mucus should be free of semen, contraceptive gels or foams, and blood or discharge from vaginal infections for at least one full cycle. Other factors that create difficulty in identifying mucus changes include douches and vaginal deodorants, being in the sexually aroused state (which thins the mucus),

Guidelines for Client Teaching

CERVICAL MUCUS CHARACTERISTICS

ASSESSMENT

1. Woman (couple) wants to know how cervical mucus changes with the menstrual cycle.
2. Woman (couple) wants to know how to tell period of maximum fertility by using the changes in cervical mucus.

NURSING DIAGNOSIS

Knowledge deficit related to the changes in cervical mucus during the menstrual cycle and how changes affect fertility.

GOALS

Short-term

Woman learns how to assess for peak mucus sign.

Intermediate

Woman learns to check for mucus several times per day.

Woman learns to record observations daily as to quantity, consistency, color, and sensation starting from last day of menstrual flow.

Long-term

Woman records findings along with BBT for several menstrual cycles.

Woman (couple) knows when peak mucus sign occurs for maximum fertility.

REFERENCES AND TEACHING AIDS

Pamphlets and booklets distributed by hospitals, clinics, or physicians.

Raw egg white.

RATIONALE/CONTENT	TEACHING ACTION
Knowledge provides a basis for developing competence and confidence. Explain to woman (couple) how cervical mucus changes throughout the menstrual cycle. Right before ovulation, the watery, thin, clear mucus becomes more abundant and thick. It feels like a lubricant and can be stretched 5+ cm; this is called **spinnbarkheit.** This indicates the period of maximum fertility. Sperm deposited in this type of mucus can survive until ovulation occurs.	Show charts of menstrual cycle along with changes in the cervical mucus. Have woman practice with raw egg white. Show findings favorable to fertility (see Figs. 4-22 and 4-23). Fertile days begin from the appearance of the slippery, fertile mucus until 72 hours after the progesterone-induced changes.
Explain to woman (couple) that assessment of cervical mucus characteristics is best learned when mucus not mixed with semen, contraceptive jellies or foams, or discharge from infections.	Couple asked to refrain from ejaculation of semen into or near vaginal opening for at least one infection-free cycle.
Woman is to assess cervical mucus several times a day for several cycles. Mucus can be obtained from vaginal introitus; there is no need to reach into vagina to cervix. Woman records her findings on the same record on which her BBT is entered. Woman records any other events also.	**Good hand washing is imperative** to begin and end all self-assessment. From last day of menstrual flow the woman starts her observations. Supply woman with a BBT log and graph, if she does not already have one.

EVALUATION Woman (couple) follows your directions, asks appropriate questions, and all goals are met. When woman returns after two or three cycles, she can describe the changes in her cervical mucus during each phase.

and medications such as antihistamines, which dry up the mucus.

It is difficult to evaluate the mucus in the presence of semen or discharge from vaginal infection. Therefore the woman double checks for fertility by assessing her BBT record and other symptoms of fertility. (NOTE: Each woman has her own unique pattern of mucus changes.)

Whether or not the individual wants to use this method for contraception, it is to the woman's advantage to learn to recognize mucus characteristics at ovulation. Assessing changes in cervical mucus can be useful diagnostically for any of the following purposes:

1. To alert the couple to the reestablishment of ovulation while breastfeeding and after discontinuation of oral contraception
2. To note anovulatory cycles at any time and at the commencement of menopause
3. To assist couples in planning a pregnancy

Sympto-thermal Method. The sympto-thermal

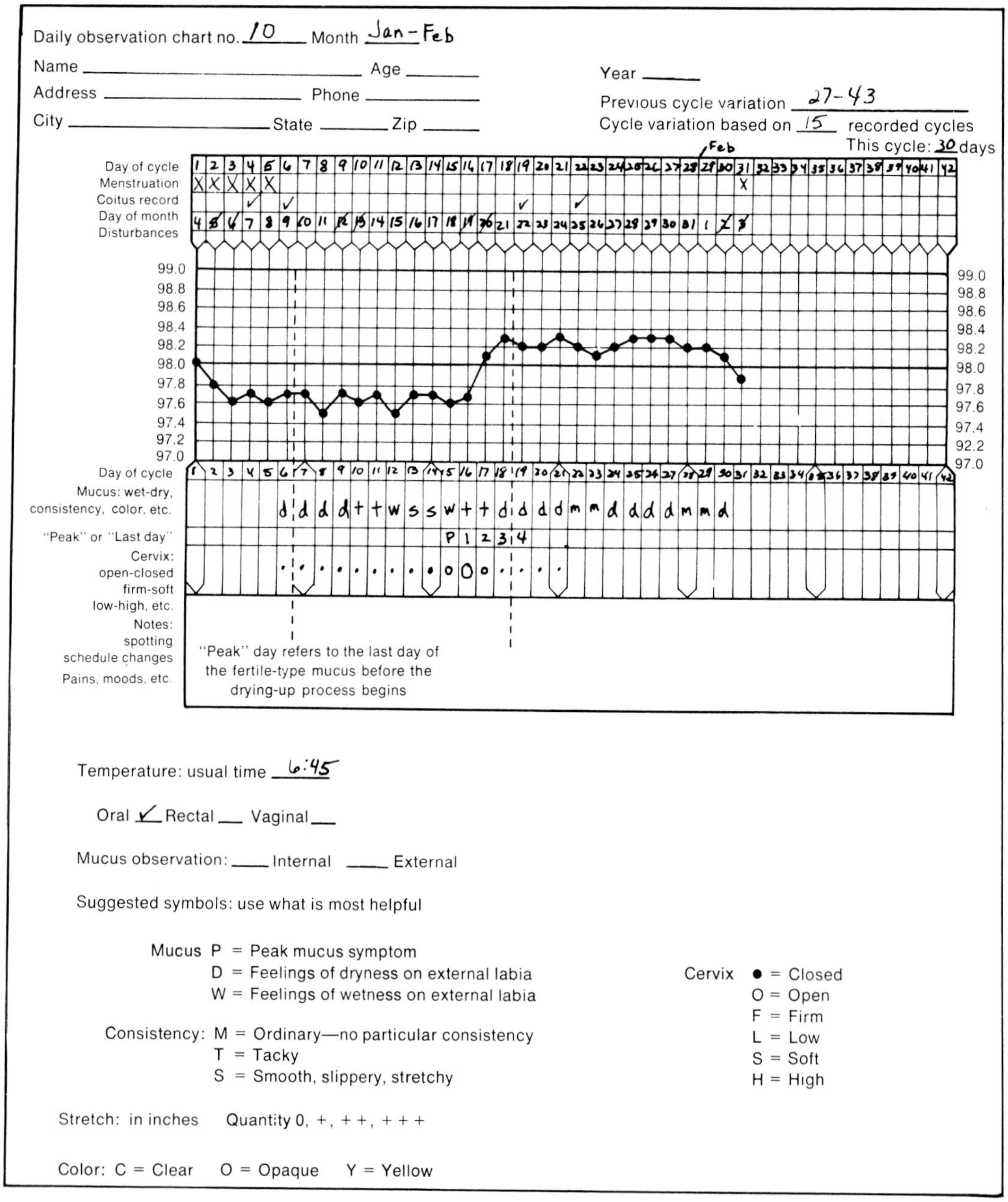

Fig. 6-9 Example of completed sympto-thermal contraceptive method chart. (From Fogel CI and Woods, NF: Health care of women, St Louis, 1981, The CV Mosby Co.)

method combines the BBT and cervical mucus methods with awareness of secondary, cycle phase–related symptoms (see Table 4-1). Both partners take responsibility for assessments, recordings, and evaluation of their findings. Together they determine the days for abstinence. Couples who use the sympto-thermal method commonly report an improvement in their sexual relationship.

The couple gains fertility awareness as they learn the woman's individual psychologic and physiologic symptoms that mark the phases of her cycle. Secondary symptoms (see Table 4-1) include increased libido, midcycle spotting, mittelschmerz, pelvic fullness, or tenderness, and vulvar fullness. The couple, perhaps using a speculum, looks at the cervix to assess for changes indicating ovulation: that is, the os dilates slightly, the cervix softens and rises in the vagina, and cervical mucus is copious and slippery. To complete their records, the couple notes days on which coitus, changes in routine, illness, and so on have occurred (Fig. 6-9). Calendar calculations and cervical mucus changes are used to estimate the onset of the fertile period, changes in cervical mucus or the BBT are used to estimate its end.

Effectiveness of the sympto-thermal method with abstinence during the fertile period ranges between 73% and 97%.

Fertility Awareness Method. The fertility awareness method is a combination of the sympto-thermal method and barrier contraception. During the fertile period the couple has the choice of abstinence from genital-genital contact or the use of barrier contraception. After ovulation the couple may enjoy freedom from contraception for the remaining nonfertile days of the menstrual cycle.

Predictor Test for Ovulation. All of the preceding discussion is about assessments that are indicative of but do not prove the occurrence and exact timing of ovulation. The **predictor test** for ovulation detects the sudden surge of LH that occurs approximately 12 to 24 hours *before* ovulation. Unlike BBT, the test is not affected by illness, emotional upset, or physical activity. Available for home use, a test kit contains sufficient material for several days' testing during each cycle. A positive response indicative of an LH surge is noted by color change that is easy to read. Directions for use of this home test kit vary with the manufacturer. This test is often used to predict ovulation to achieve a pregnancy.

Chemical Barriers

A vaginal **spermicide** is a physical barrier to sperm penetration that also has a chemical action on sperm. *Nonoxynol 9* (N-9) and octoxynol 9 are the most commonly used spermicidal chemicals. Intravaginal spermicides are marketed as aerosol foams, foaming tablets, suppositories, creams and gels (Fig. 6-10). Preloaded, single-dose applicators small enough to be carried in a small purse are available (Grimes, 1986). This form of contraceptive must be placed deeply in the vagina in contact with the cervix before each coitus. Special precautions must be taken. The can of foam must be shaken to distribute the spermicide before use. Tablets and suppositories take from 10 to 30 minutes to dissolve. *Maximum spermicidal effectiveness lasts usually no longer than 1 hour.* If intercourse is to be repeated, reapplication of additional spermicide must precede it. Douching must be avoided for at least 6 hours after coitus (Grimes, 1986).

Spermicides provide a physical and chemical barrier that prevents viable sperm from entering the cervix. The effect is local, within the vagina.

Ease of application, safety, low cost, and ready availability without prescription or previous medical examination characterize this method. The delicate vaginal mucosa is not harmed unless the woman is allergic to a particular preparation. Spermicides aid in lubrication of the vagina. Because their effect is local, spermicides offer an alternative to hormonal contraception (e.g., for the nursing mother [to avoid interfering with lactation], for the premenopausal woman [to prevent masking symptoms of onset of the climacterium], and as a backup for the woman who forgets to take her oral contraceptive). There is evidence that *nonoxynol 9 plus a barrier method provide some protection against sexually transmitted disease* through bacteriostatic action (North, 1988; Louv et al, 1988). In the laboratory, it has been shown to have both bac-

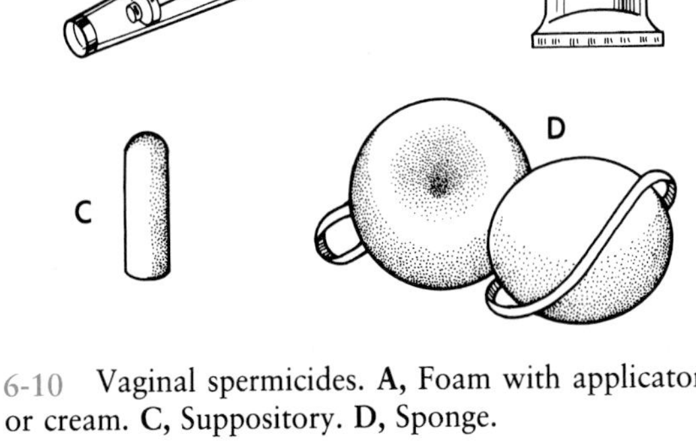

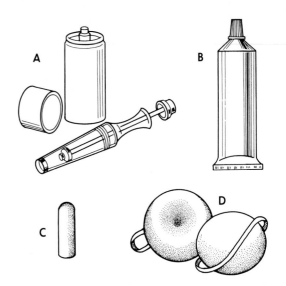

Fig. 6-10 Vaginal spermicides. **A**, Foam with applicator. **B**, Gel or cream. **C**, Suppository. **D**, Sponge.

tericidal and virucidal activity (Connell, 1989). The addition of spermicides increases the effectiveness of the other forms of contraception (e.g., condoms, diaphragms).

Users of this method may complain of its "messiness," unpleasant "fizz," stickiness, or unpleasant taste. Allergic response or irritation of vaginal or penile tissue may occur. Some users experience decreased tactile sensation. The need to wait 10 minutes to 30 minutes before coitus initially and to reapply additional spermicide before repeated intercourse is not acceptable to all people.

According to Cunningham, MacDonald, and Gant (1989), the high pregnancy rate seen with this method is probably the result of inconsistent use of the spermicide. A typical failure rate is 21% (accidental pregnancy rate during the first year of use).

The nurse encourages open communication between the sexual partners to discuss intravaginal contraception. Clients are offered the opportunity to see and handle a variety of samples. To maximize learning, the woman is given the opportunity to insert one application into a medical model of the vagina. The male partner sometimes indicates an interest in learning how to insert the spermicide into his female partner. The nurse needs to feel comfortable teaching him as well.

Vaginal Sponge

The polyurethane **vaginal sponge** was approved by the Food and Drug Administration (FDA) in 1983 (see Fig. 6-10). Water is needed to activate the spermicide (nonoxynol 9) and facilitate insertion. Spermicide is released continuously for 24 hours. A woven loop is used for retrieval from the vagina. It is recommended that at least 6 hours lapse between last intercourse and removal (Grimes, 1986). Therefore the sponge has a total allowable wear-time of 30 hours (Connell, 1989). The sponge should be discarded after removal. It must not be washed and reused. Washing removes the spermicide.

The mode of action is the same as that for the spermicides.

Like the other spermicides, the sponge is an over-the-counter (OTC) product. It offers spontaneity and is less "messy" than other spermicide delivery systems. Furthermore, use of the sponge has been found to reduce the risk of chlamydial infection by one third and that of gonorrhea by two thirds (Hatcher et al, 1988). In vitro studies suggest it is effective against *Staphylococcus aureus,* which causes toxic shock syndrome (TSS) (Connell, 1989). Reapplication of spermicide during the 24 hours the sponge is in place is unnecessary.

The only reported effects were allergic reactions (2% to 3%) or irritation (2% to 3%) that typically occur with all nonoxynol 9 products. There is an increased risk for candidiasis (Rosenberg et al, 1987). Six percent of users reported difficulty in removing the sponge (Grimes, 1986). Water must be available to activate the nonoxynol 9. To decrease the risk of TSS, no obstructive vaginal barrier (i.e., sponge, diaphragm) should be used during menses or soon after childbirth (Connell, 1989).

The first-year failure rates reported for sponge users range from 17 to 24.5 pregnancies per 100 women. Parous users (women who have borne children) were twice as likely as nulliparous users (women who have not borne children) to become pregnant (Hatcher et al, 1988; Grimes, 1986).

Nursing actions are similar to those for other spermicides. Clients are reminded that each sponge is to be used once, for 24 hours only. It is left in place for 6 hours after coitus, and discarded. The woman is coached to "bear down" to facilitate removal of the sponge.

Condom

The **condom** is a thin, stretchable sheath to cover the penis (Fig. 6-11). In addition to three available sizes, four basic features differ among condoms marketed in the United States. These features are material, shape, lubricants, and spermicides. Ninety-nine percent

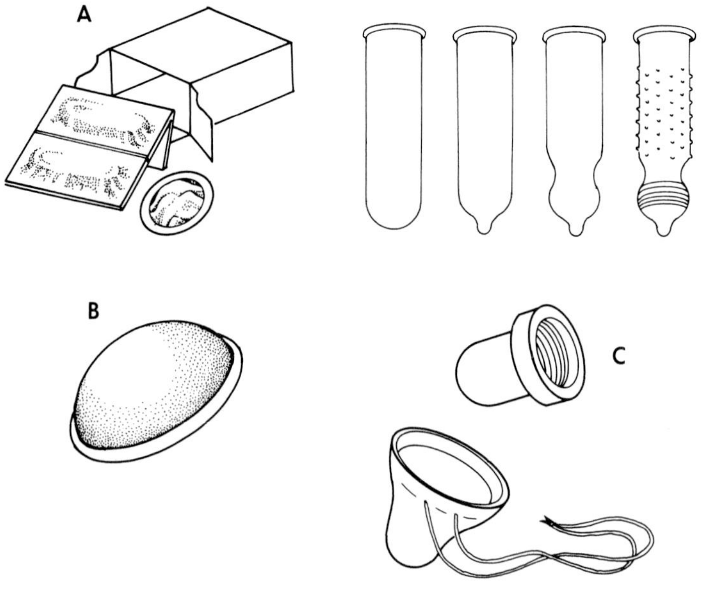

Fig. 6-11 Mechanical barriers. **A,** Condoms (no prescription required); types of condoms. **B,** Diaphragm. **C,** Cervical caps.

are made of latex rubber. A functional difference in condom shape is the presence or absence of a sperm reservoir tip. To enhance vaginal stimulation, some condoms are contoured and rippled or have ribbed or roughened surfaces. Thinner construction increases heat transmission and sensitivity; a variety of colors increase their acceptability and attractiveness (Connell, 1989). A wet jelly or dry powder lubricates some condoms. Since 1982, spermicide (0.5 g of nonoxynol 9) has been added to the interior or exterior surfaces of some condoms. The addition of nonoxynol 9 to latex condoms not only increases contraceptive effectiveness, it also increases protection against HIV transmission (Hatcher et al, 1988). No viable HIV organisms were found, even after rupture, in an in vitro study (Rietmeijer et al, 1987; Connell, 1989).

The sheath is applied over the erect penis before insertion or loss of preejaculatory drops of semen. Conception is made possible even if preejaculatory drops fall around the external vaginal opening because sperm are contained in these drops.

Used correctly, condoms prevent sperm from entering the cervix. Spermicide-coated condoms cause ejaculated sperm to be immobilized rapidly, thus increasing contraceptive effectiveness.

Condoms are safe, without side effects, and are readily available. Premalignant changes in the cervix can be prevented or ameliorated in women whose partners use condoms (Cunningham, MacDonald, and Gant, 1989). If the condom is used throughout the act of intercourse and there is no unprotected contact with female genitals, a latex rubber condom, which is impermeable to viruses, can act as a protective measure against spread of sexually transmitted diseases (STDs). The STDs include gonorrhea, syphilis, herpes, chlamydia, acquired immunodeficiency syndrome (AIDS), human papillomavirus (HPV), and trichomoniasis (Morbidity Mortality Weekly Report, 1988; Hatcher et al, 1988; Mishell, 1989). The unique feature of this method is **male contraception** (Grimes, 1986).

Some couples object to interrupting lovemaking to apply the sheath or complain that sensation is blunted. If condoms are used improperly, spillage of sperm can result in pregnancy. On occasion, condoms have torn during intercourse (Consumer Reports, 1989).

The pregnancy rate can be as low as 2% among correct and consistent users and about 12% among typical users (Hatcher et al, 1988). Condoms with spermicide are highly effective at killing sperm within the condom. The effectiveness of the spermicides on the outside of the condom in cases where the condom breaks has not been evaluated (Hatcher et al, 1986).

For years, health care providers assumed that everyone knew how to use condoms, so proper instruction was not provided. To prevent spread of STDs, it is essential that condoms be used correctly. To this end, the FDA has recently suggested instructions for protection against STDs (Connell, 1989) (see guidelines for client teaching, next page).

❑ METHODS REQUIRING PRESCRIPTION

Several methods for the control of fertility require prescription and supervision. Interview, physical examination, and occasionally laboratory tests are prerequisites for some forms of contraception. These methods of contraception include hormonal therapy, use of diaphragms or cervical caps, and IUDs.

Hormonal Contraception

Steroidal contraceptives are available in several dosage forms. General classes are described in Table 6-3, p. 137. Because of the wide variety of preparations available, the woman and nurse need to read the package insert for information about specific products prescribed. Formulations include combined estrogen-progestin steroidal medications, progestational agents, and an estrogenic agent. The formulations are administered orally, subdermally, or by implantation. Combined estrogen-progestin steroidal medications are discussed first.

Mode of Action. The normal menstrual cycle is maintained by a feedback mechanism (Chapter 4). Follicle-stimulating hormone (FSH) and luteinizing hormone (LH) are secreted in response to *fluctuating* levels of ovarian estrogen and progesterone. Regular ingestion of combined estrogen-progestin steroidal medication suppresses the action of the hypothalamus and anterior pituitary leading to inappropriate secretion of FSH and LH. Therefore follicles do not mature; ovulation is inhibited.

Other contraceptive effects are induced by the combined steroids. Maturation of the endometrium is altered, making it a less favorable site for implantation should ovulation and conception occur. It also has a direct effect on the endometrium, so that from 1 to 4 days after the last steroid tablet is taken, the endometrium sloughs and bleeds as a result of hormone withdrawal. The **withdrawal bleeding** usually is less profuse than that of normal menstruation and may last only 2 to 3 days. Some women have no bleeding at all.

The cervical mucus remains thick as a result of the effect of the progestin. Cervical mucus under the effect of progesterone does not provide as suitable an environment for sperm penetration as does the thin, watery mucus at ovulation (Willson and Carrington, 1987).

The possible role, if any, of altered tubal and uterine motility induced by the steroidal hormones is not clear (Cunningham, MacDonald, and Gant, 1989). As a consequence of these actions, **oral hormonal contraceptives,** if taken daily for 3 weeks of every 4, provide virtually absolute protection against conception (Cunningham, MacDonald, and Gant, 1989).

Phasic pills (e.g., triphasic oral contraceptives) are those in which the amount of progestin, and sometimes the amount of estrogen, varies within each cycle. These preparations reduce the total dosage of steroid hormones in a single cycle without sacrificing contraceptive efficacy or cycle control (Cunningham, MacDonald, and Gant, 1989). The theoretic advantage is a re-

Guidelines for Client Teaching

USE OF CONDOMS

ASSESSMENT

1. Client (couple) needs to know how to use condoms.

NURSING DIAGNOSES

Potential for infection related to improper use of condom.
Potential for pregnancy related to improper use of condom.
Knowledge deficit related to proper use of condoms.

GOALS

Short-term

Client verbalizes proper way to use condom.
Client learns how to apply condom.

Intermediate and Long-term

Client continues proper use of condoms.

REFERENCES AND TEACHING AIDS

Pamphlets and booklets distributed by hospitals, clinics, or physicians.
Inserts from packages.
Price list.
Variety of condoms.
Plastic anatomic model.

RATIONALE/CONTENT	TEACHING ACTION
Knowledge provides a basis for decision-making. Review mode of action, advantages, disadvantages, and effectiveness.	Facilitate discussion of woman's (couple's) feelings concerning use of condoms. Answer questions.
FDA instructions foster clear understanding and skill in proper use (Connell, 1989). Use a new condom for each act of sexual intercourse or other acts between partners that involve contact with the penis.	Decreases risk of using a damaged condom.
Place condom after penis is erect and before intimate contact.	Decreases risk of possible pregnancy and transmission of STD organisms that may be present in lesions, preejaculate secretions, semen, vaginal secretions, saliva, urine, and feces.
Place condom on head of penis and unroll it all the way to the base.	Provides maximum barrier to sperm and organisms.
Leave an empty space at the tip; remove any air remaining in the tip by gently pressing air out towards the base of the penis.	Provides reservoir to collect sperm.
If a lubricant is desired, use water-based products such as K-Y jelly.	Prevents rapid damage and leakage of sperm and organisms (leakage noted within 3 min) seen with oil-based products (petrolatum jelly, mineral or vegetable oil, or cold cream).
After ejaculation, carefully withdraw still erect penis, holding onto condom rim; discard.	Prevents spillage of sperm and possible contact between genital structures of the partners.
Store unused condoms in cool, dry place.	Safeguards against the rapid deterioration that occurs with heat and humidity.
Do not use condoms that are sticky, brittle, or obviously damaged.	Avoids use of ineffective barrier.

EVALUATION The woman (couple) does not experience pregnancy or the transmission of STDs as a result of improper use of a condom.

Table 6-3 **Hormonal Contraception**

Composition	Route of Administration	Duration of Effect
Combination of an estrogen and a progestin	Oral	24 hours
Minipill: progestin (norethindrone, 0.35 mg) only	Oral	24 hours
Morning-after pill: estrogen (diethylstilbestrol [DES]) in very high doses—25 mg	Oral	Taken within 72 hours of unprotected coitus during fertile period; because of DES effect on fetus, abortion advised if method fails
Depo-Provera: progestin only (medroxyprogesterone acetate), 150 mg	Intramuscular injection	From 3 to 6 months
Norplant system: progestin (Levonorgestrel) in silastic containers	Implant, subdermal	Up to 5 years

duction in progestin-related metabolic changes and the adverse effects attributed to those metabolic changes. The estrogen dose is also kept low with only 30 to 40 μg of ethinyl estradiol; no tablet sold in the United States contains more than 50 μg (FDA Bulletin, 1988; Cunningham, MacDonald, and Gant, 1989).

Advantages. For motivated women it is easy to take an oral contraceptive (OC) at about the same time each day. Taking the pill does not relate directly to the sexual act; this fact increases its acceptability to some women. Commonly, there is an improvement in sexual response once the possibility of pregnancy is not an issue. For some, it is convenient to know when to expect the next "menstrual" flow.

There has been little publicity about the advantages of hormonal contraceptives. Mishell (1989) and Cunningham, MacDonald, and Gant (1989) list the noncontraceptive health benefits of oral contraceptives. The benefits include decreased menstrual blood loss and resultant decreased iron-deficiency anemia, regulation of menorrhagia and irregular cycles, lowered incidence of dysmenorrhea (menstrual cramps) and premenstrual syndrome (PMS), protection against endometrial adenocarcinoma, reduced incidence of benign breast disease and possibly breast cancer, protection against the development of functional ovarian cysts, protection against acute salpingitis* and pelvic inflammatory disease (PID) caused by gonorrhea, and possible protection against ovarian cancer and postmenopausal osteoporosis. However, there is biologic and epidemiologic evidence that PID caused by *Chlamydia* is enhanced by oral contraceptives (Washington et al, 1985). Combination oral contraceptives have been used to treat such medical conditions as idiopathic thrombocytopenia purpura and endometriosis.

Since ovulation is suppressed, the risk for ectopic pregnancy is about one tenth that of women not using contraceptives. This form of contraception is associated with minimum risk for women aged 15 to 29 years. The mortality is 1.2 and 1.4/100,000 for nonsmoking and smoking women, respectively.

Women taking steroidal contraceptives are examined before the medication is prescribed and yearly thereafter. The examination includes medical and family history, weight, blood pressure, general physical and pelvic examination, screening cervical cytologic analysis (Pap smear), and hemoglobin determination. Consistent medical surveillance is valuable in the detection of noncontraception-related disorders as well, so that timely treatment can be initiated.

Use of oral hormonal contraceptives is initiated on one of the first 7 days of the menstrual cycle (day 1 of the cycle is the first day of menses). Other women start their use after delivery or abortion. If contraceptives are to be started at any time other than during normal menses, or within 3 weeks after delivery or abortion, another method of contraception should be used throughout the first week to avoid the risk of ovulation (Cunningham, MacDonald, and Gant, 1989).

Disadvantages and Side Effects. Since hormonal contraceptives have come into use, the amount of estrogen and progestational agent contained in each tablet has been reduced considerably (Cunningham, MacDonald, and Gant, 1989). This is of importance, because adverse effects are, to a degree, dose-related.

Women must be screened for conditions that present absolute or relative contraindications to oral contraceptive use. *Absolute contraindications* include a history of thromboembolic disorders, cerebrovascular or coronary artery disease, breast cancer, estrogenic-dependent tumors, undiagnosed abnormal genital bleeding, known or suspected pregnancy, liver tumor, sickle

*Wolner-Hanssen et al (1985) suggest that this protection may apply to both gonococcal and chlamydial salpingitis. Oral contraceptives provide no protection against HIV transmission.

cell disease, or migraine headaches (Grimes, 1986; Hatcher et al, 1988). *Relative contraindications* include age of 40 years or older, diabetes mellitus, hypertension, heavy smoking (more than 15 cigarettes per day), gallbladder disease, gestational cholestasis, history of renal disease, impaired liver function, and hyperlipidemia (Grimes, 1986). The main causes of hospitalization and death are cardiovascular problems (e.g., myocardial infarction [heart attack], cerebrovascular accident [stroke], and thromboembolism) (Grimes, 1986).

The risk of dying as a consequence of using this method of contraception is very low if the woman is less than 35 years of age, has no systemic illness, and is a nonsmoker. The risk of death secondary to use of oral contraceptives is less than that from pregnancy, and the risk of dying with pregnancy is quite low (Cunningham, MacDonald, and Gant, 1989; Porter, Jick, and Walker, 1987).

Certain side effects of anovulatory drugs are attributable to estrogen and progestin or both. Side effects of *estrogen excess* include nausea and vomiting, dizziness, edema, leg cramps, increase in breast size, chloasma (mask of pregnancy), visual changes, hypertension, and vascular headache. Side effects of *estrogen deficiency* include early spotting (days 1 to 14), hypomenorrhea, nervousness, and atrophic vaginitis leading to painful intercourse (dyspareunia). Side effects of *progestin excess* include increased appetite, tiredness, depression, breast tenderness, vaginal yeast infection, oily skin and scalp, hirsutism, and postpill amenorrhea. Side effects of *progestin deficiency* include late spotting and breakthrough bleeding (days 15 to 21), heavy flow with clots, and decreased breast size.

The risk of *deep vein thrombosis* and *pulmonary embolism* has been estimated to be 3 to 11 times greater in women who use oral contraceptives than in otherwise apparently similar women who do not (Peterson and Lee, 1989). The risk of postoperative thromboembolism is increased if the woman uses oral hormone contraceptives during the month before the operative procedure. There is a smaller increase in risk for women taking preparations containing less estrogen (Cunningham, MacDonald, and Gant, 1989).

In the presence of side effects, especially those that are bothersome to the woman, a different product, a different drug content, or another method of contraception may be required. The "right" product for a woman contains the lowest dose of sex steroid hormones that prevents ovulation and that has the fewest and least harmful side effects. There is no way to predict the "right" dose* for any particular woman; trial and error is the main method for prescribing OCs, starting with the lowest possible estrogen dose.

The *changes in glucose tolerance* that occur in some women taking OCs are similar to those changes that occur during pregnancy. The dose, type, and potency of progestin (not estrogen) produce some deterioration of glucose tolerance in normal women, as well as in those with a history of gestational diabetes (Mishell, 1989).

The changes in levels of *nutrients* that have been described for some women who use oral contraceptives are similar to changes induced by normal pregnancy. Some investigators have described lower plasma levels in users compared with nonusers, for ascorbic acid, folic acid, vitamin B_{12}, niacin, riboflavin, and zinc (Cunningham, MacDonald, and Gant, 1989). Combined estrogen-progestin oral contraceptives conserve a woman's iron by reducing the amount of blood lost during menstruation.

Women who discontinue oral contraception for a planned pregnancy commonly ask whether they should wait before attempting to conceive. Although data are controversial, studies indicate that these infants have no greater chance of being born with any type of birth defect than infants born to women in the general population, even if conception occurred in the first month after the medication was discontinued (Lammer and Cordero, 1986; Mishell, 1989).

After discontinuing oral contraception there is usually a delay before ovulation and menstrual cycles recur, similar to that experienced by a newly delivered mother. However, *postpill amenorrhea* exceeding 6 months should be investigated.

It is unclear whether oral hormonal contraceptives contribute to the development of breast cancer. Four recently published studies fail to clarify the controversy (Meirik et al, 1986; and Peterson and Lee, 1989).

Uncommonly *hypertension* is first noted after the woman begins oral contraception, especially if she is 30 years of age or older. In some women, higher blood levels of angiotensinogen and plasma renin have been found. It is thought that these factors play a part in the hypertension experienced by some women (Mishell, 1989). After discontinuing oral contraception, hypertension subsides.

Some women complain of *edema,* which is associated with administration of estrogens; however, if the dose of estrogen is sufficiently low, fluid retention is not likely to occur or can be compensated for by decreasing the oral intake of sodium compounds.

Some conditions are aggravated by fluid retention. Women susceptible to *migraine headaches* may notice an increase in headaches when taking the pill. Since headaches are also symptomatic of cerebral thrombo-

*Warn women, young and old, that using another woman's OCs may not prevent ovulation if the dose is not correct for them.

sis, there may be confusion with correct diagnosis. Therefore women who experience migraine headaches are counseled to use other forms of contraception. Although many women with *epilepsy* tolerate OCs well, others tend to have an increased incidence of seizures.

More serious *neuroocular lesions* are associated with use of OCs. Optic neuritis, or retinal thrombosis, although rare, has been reported. Symptoms such as sudden or gradual and partial or complete loss of vision and double vision require immediate diagnosis and treatment. *Women must stop taking OCs at the first sign of visual disorders.*

A somewhat increased risk of gallstones and gallbladder disease has been reported. One study (Royal College, 1982) suggests that oral contraceptives may only accelerate the development of gallbladder disease in women who are susceptible; there is no overall increased long-term risk.

The effectiveness of OCs is decreased along with an increased possibility of break-through bleeding if the woman is receiving any of the following drugs:

- Barbiturates (for sedation)
- Phenytoin sodium (for seizure disorders)
- Ampicillin (for infections)

Long-term use of OCs slows diazepam (Valium) clearance by the liver; therefore higher blood levels of the drug increase the risk of an overdose of diazepam. Planned Parenthood facilities keep current information about newly identified drug interactions as it becomes available.

Effectiveness. The combined estrogen-progestin pill taken daily 3 weeks out of every 4 is the most effective reversible form of contraception available (Cunningham, MacDonald, and Gant, 1989). Taken exactly as directed, OCs prevent ovulation, and pregnancy cannot occur; the overall effectiveness rate is almost 100%. Almost all failures (i.e., pregnancy occurs) are caused by omission of one or more pills during the regimen.

Nursing Actions. There are many different preparations of oral hormonal contraceptives. The nurse needs to review the prescribing information in the package insert with the client. Because of the wide variations, each woman must be clear about the unique dosage regimen for the preparation prescribed for her. Directions for care after missing one or two tablets also vary. Recent findings indicate that if one or two tablets are missed, another form of contraception needs to be used until the required regimen is reestablished. Typical counseling regarding missed doses follows:

The woman needs to take the pill at the same time each day to maintain constant blood levels of estrogen and progesterone for 21 days. If one pill is missed, the woman takes that pill as soon as she remembers it. She takes the next pill at the regularly scheduled time. If the woman misses two pills, she takes both as soon as she remembers to do so. A second form of contraception (e.g., diaphragm with spermicide) for the rest of that cycle is advised. If three pills are missed, the remainder of the pills in that packet are discarded and use of a back-up type of contraceptive is advised. A new packet of pills is begun on about the fifth day of the next cycle (bleeding should begin within 2 to 3 days after she misses the pills; day 1 of the new cycle is the first day of bleeding.)

Withdrawal bleeding ("periods") tends to be short and scanty when some combination OCs are taken. A woman may see no fresh blood at all. Some women may have only a drop of blood or a brown smudge on their tampon or underwear. This counts as a period. This fact may explain why some women have difficulty remembering the first day of their last period.

No more than 50% to 70% of women who start taking OCs are still taking them after 1 year. It is therefore important that nurses recommend that all women choosing to use the OC also be provided with a second method of birth control and that women be instructed and comfortable with this backup method. Most women stop taking OC's for nonmedical reasons; that is, they *choose* to stop; not because they develop a complication or a serious side effect.

Before OCs are prescribed and periodically throughout hormone therapy, the woman is alerted to stop taking the pill and to report any of the following symptoms to the physician immediately. The word *aches* helps in retention of this list:

A—Abdominal pain: may indicate a problem with the liver or gallbladder
C—Chest pain or shortness of breath: may indicate possible clot problem within lungs or heart
H—Headaches (sudden or persistent): may be caused by cardiovascular accident or hypertension
E—Eye problems: may indicate vascular accident or hypertension
S—Severe leg pain: may indicate a thromboembolic process

A general teaching tool for contraceptive methods is presented in the guidelines for client teaching, p. 127.

Progestational Agents

Oral Progestins ("Mini-pill"). The mini-pill of 0.5 mg or less of a progestational agent daily presumably impairs fertility. Ovulation may occur. Progestational impact on cervical mucus decreases sperm penetration and alters endometrial maturation to discourage implantation should conception occur. Users report a higher incidence of irregular bleeding.

Injectable Progestins. The advantages of depo medroxyprogesterone (DMPA, Depo-Provera) include a contraceptive effectiveness comparable to combined oral contraceptives, long-lasting effects, the requirement of injections only 2 to 4 times a year, and lactation not likely to be impaired (Cunningham, MacDonald, and Gant, 1989). The modes of action are several and include inhibition of ovulation and alteration in endometrial maturation and cervical mucus. Disadvantages are prolonged amenorrhea or uterine bleeding and increased risk of venous thrombosis and thromboembolism. Medroxyprogesterone is used by millions of women world-wide, but not in the United States. FDA approval has not been granted as yet. "Newer injectable and implantable progestin-only methods should, by the 1990s, expand the selection of these convenient and effective and popular methods of contraception for women world-wide" (Kaunitz, 1989).

Implantable Progestins. Norplant consists of six nonbiodegradable silastic capsules. They contain progestin for 5 years of contraception. Insertion and removal of the capsules are minor surgical procedures involving a small incision and a local anesthetic. The capsules are placed subdermally on the inner aspects of the upper or lower arm. The progestin prevents some, but not all, ovulatory cycles and alters cervical mucus and endometrium maturation.

Irregular bleeding is the most common side effect; other side effects are rare (Kaunitz, 1989). Other products are biodegradable or pellets; these provide effective contraception for 1½ years and 1 year respectively. Norplant is approved for use in 7 countries, with applications pending in 31 other countries, including the United States (Cunningham, MacDonald, and Gant, 1989; Kaunitz, 1989).

Estrogen Agent. Diethylstilbestrol (DES) provides postcoital contraception (see Table 6-3). It is also known as the "morning-after" pill. This preparation must be started within 3 days after intercourse. DES, 25 mg, is taken twice daily for 5 days. The mechanism of action is not understood (Cunningham, MacDonald, and Gant, 1989). Nausea and vomiting are common effects. DES' teratogenic effects must be considered should pregnancy occur and continue despite therapy; elective abortion by cervical **dilatation and curettage** (**D&C**) may be considered.

Diaphragm with Spermicide

The vaginal **diaphragm** is a shallow, dome-shaped rubber device with a flexible wire rim that covers the cervix. There are three main styles of diaphragms available in a wide range of diameters (50 to 95 mm). Diaphragms differ in the inner construction of the circular rim. The three types of rims are flat spring, coil spring, and arching spring.

The diaphragm should feel comfortable. It should be the largest size the woman can wear without her being aware of its presence. The use of a contraceptive gel or cream with the diaphragm offers both mechanical and chemical barriers to pregnancy.

The diaphragm is a mechanical barrier preventing the meeting of the sperm with the ovum. The diaphragm holds the spermicide in place against the cervix for the 6 hours it takes to destroy the sperm.

Except for occasional allergic responses to the diaphragm or spermicide, there are no side effects from a well-fitted device. The diaphragm can be inserted as long as 6 hours before intercourse to increase spontaneity, but spermicide must be added each time intercourse is repeated (Medical Letter, 1988). The woman who engages in intercourse infrequently may choose this barrier method. The spermicide does offer additional lubrication if it is needed. A decreased incidence of vaginitis, cervicitis (including cervicitis caused by *Chlamydia* and *Gonorrhea*), PID, and cervical intraepithelial neoplasia is noted among women who use contraceptive creams, foams, and gels with the diaphragm.

This method is contraindicated for the woman with relaxation of her pelvic support (uterine prolapse) or a large cystocele. It is also not advised for the woman who is "uninformed."

Disadvantages include the reluctance of some women to insert and remove the diaphragm. A cold diaphragm and a cold gel temporarily reduce vaginal response to sexual stimulation if insertion of the diaphragm occurs immediately before intercourse. Some women or couples object to the "messiness" of the spermicide. These annoyances of diaphragm usage, along with failure to insert the device once foreplay has begun, are the most common reasons for failures of this method. Side effects may include irritation of tissues related to contact with spermicides. Urethritis and recurrent cystitis (Strom, 1987) caused by upward pressure of the diaphragm rim against the urethra may be increased by the use of the contraceptive diaphragm.

The *effectiveness* of this combined method is approximately 83% to 90%. Highly motivated women may achieve rates of 99%.

Nursing Actions. The woman is informed that she needs an annual gynecologic examination. The device may need to be refitted after 2 years, the loss or gain of 9 kg (20 lb) or more, term delivery, or second trimester abortion (Kugel and Verson, 1986; Connell, 1989). Since there are various types of diaphragms on the market, the nurse uses the package insert for teaching the woman how to use and care for the diaphragm. The directions for one product are given on p. 141.

Toxic shock syndrome (TSS) (Chapter 23), although reported in very small numbers, can occur in association with the use of the contraceptive diaphragm (Connell, 1989). The nurse should instruct the woman

USE AND CARE OF THE DIAPHRAGM

POSITIONS FOR INSERTION OF DIAPHRAGM

Squatting

This is the most commonly used position and most women find this position satisfactory.

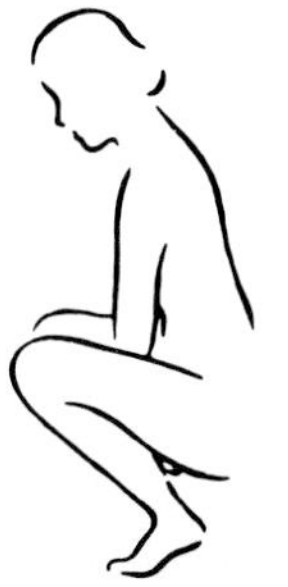

Leg Up Method

A position to suit the convenience of particular women is to raise the left foot (if right hand is used for insertion) on a low stool, and in a bending position the diaphragm is inserted.

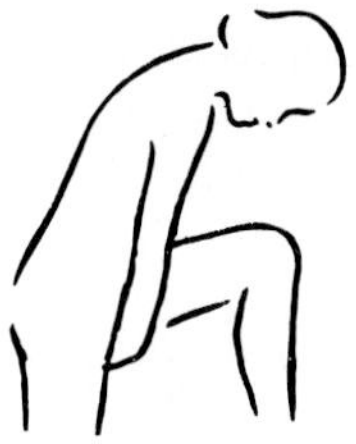

Chair Method

A practical method for diaphragm insertion is for the woman to sit far forward on the edge of a chair.

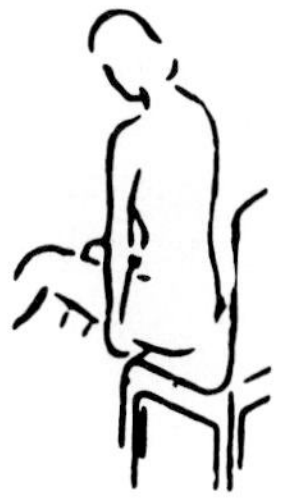

Reclining

In some instances, certain women prefer to insert the diaphragm while in a semi-reclining position in bed.

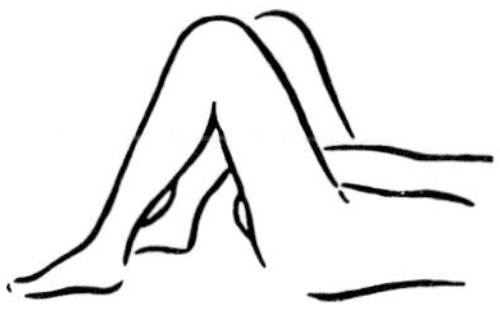

INSPECTION OF DIAPHRAGM

Your diaphragm must be inspected carefully before each use. The best way to do this is:

Hold the diaphragm up to a light source. Carefully stretch the diaphragm at the area of the rim, on all sides, to make sure there are no holes. Remember, it is possible to puncture the diaphragm with sharp fingernails.

Another way to check for pinholes is to carefully fill the diaphragm with water. If there is any problem, it will be seen immediately.

If your diaphragm is "puckered," especially near the rim, this could mean thin spots.

The diaphragm should not be used if you see any of the above . . . consult your physician.

PREPARATION OF DIAPHRAGM

Your diaphragm must always be used with a spermicidal lubricant to be effective. Pregnancy cannot be prevented effectively by the diaphragm alone.

Always empty your bladder before inserting the diaphragm. Place about 2 teaspoonsful of contraceptive gel, contraceptive jelly, or contraceptive cream on the side of the diaphragm that will rest against the cervix (or whichever way you have been instructed). Spread it around to coat the surface and the rim. This aids in insertion and offers a more complete seal. Many women also spread some gel (jelly) or cream on the other side of the diaphragm. (See Fig. A.)

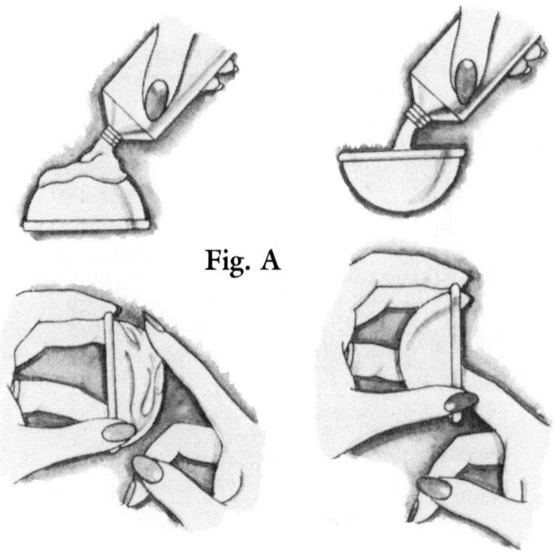

Fig. A

INSERTION OF DIAPHRAGM

The diaphragm can be inserted as much as 6 hours before intercourse. Hold the diaphragm between your thumb and fingers. The dome can either be up or down, as directed by your physician. Place your index finger on the outer rim of the compressed diaphragm. (See Fig. B.) Use the fingers of the other hand to spread the labia (lips of the vagina). This will assist in guiding the diaphragm into place.

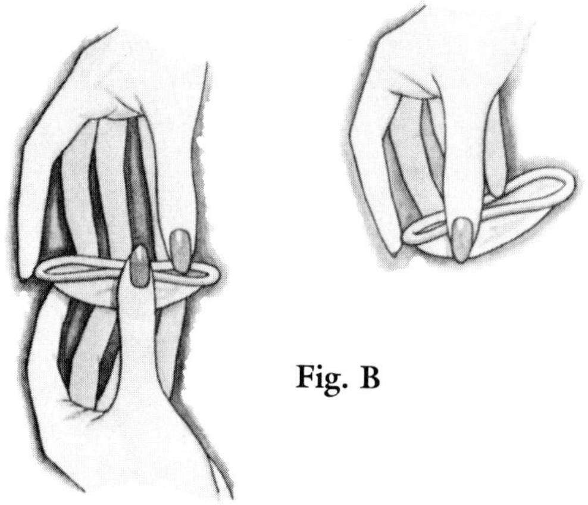

Fig. B

Continued.

USE AND CARE OF THE DIAPHRAGM—cont'd

Insert the diaphragm into the vagina. Direct it inward and downward as far as it will go to the space behind and below the cervix. (See Fig. C.)

Fig. C

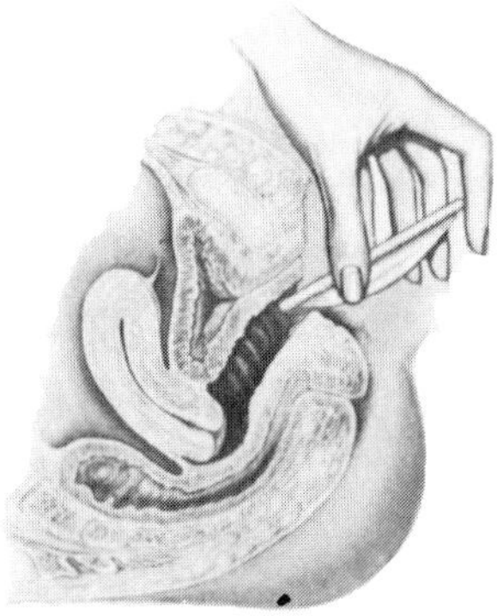

Tuck the front of the rim of the diaphragm behind the pelvic bone so that the rubber hugs the front wall of the vagina. (See Fig. D.)

Fig. D

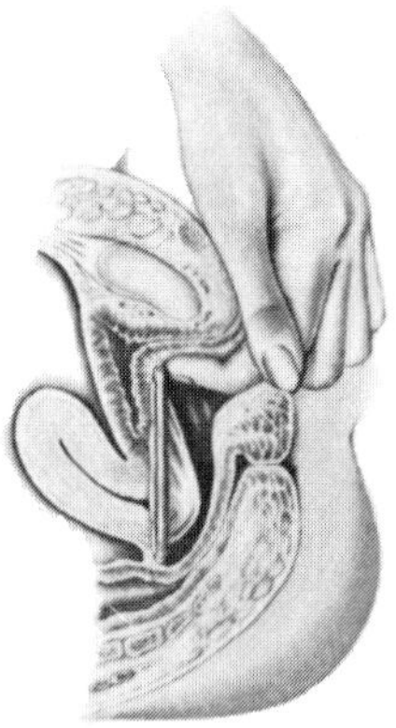

DIRECTIONS FOR INSERTION WITH DIAPHRAGM INTRODUCER

Hold the introducer in either hand. Compress the diaphragm, dome up, with the fingers of your other hand. Place one end of the rim in the grooved end of the introducer. (See Fig. E.)

Fig. E

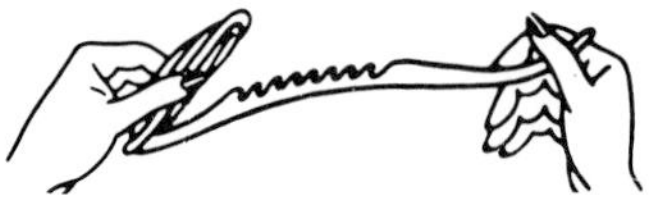

Fit the other end of the diaphragm over the notch corresponding to the diaphragm size. (See Fig. F.) Squeeze approximately 1 tablespoonful of gel, jelly, or cream into the folds of the diaphragm. Spread a small amount around the rim.

Fig. F

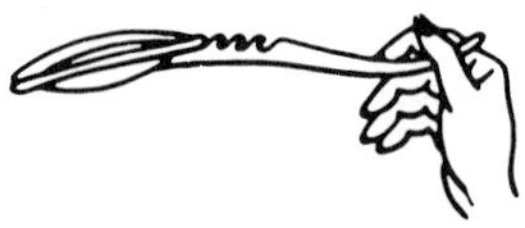

The diaphragm may be inserted while you are lying flat with your legs drawn up. However, any position may be used if more convenient. See positions for insertion of diaphragm.

Insert the diaphragm in a downward direction as far back as it will comfortably go . . . past the cervix. (See Fig. G.)

Fig. G

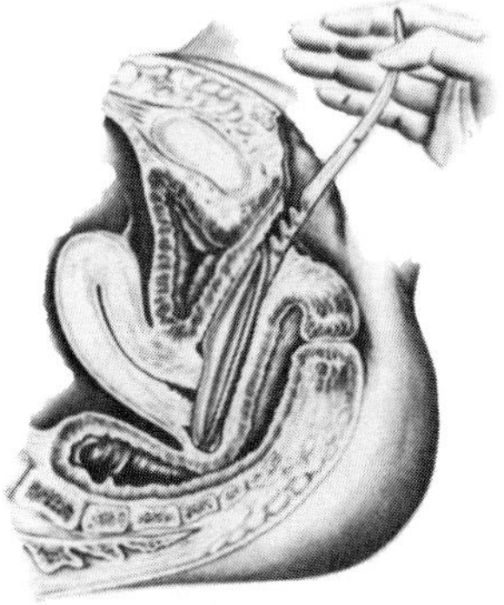

To release the diaphragm, rotate the introducer to the right or left and gently withdraw it. (See Fig. H.) After the introducer is removed, tuck the front rim of the diaphragm behind the pelvic bone. (See Fig. D.)

Fig. H

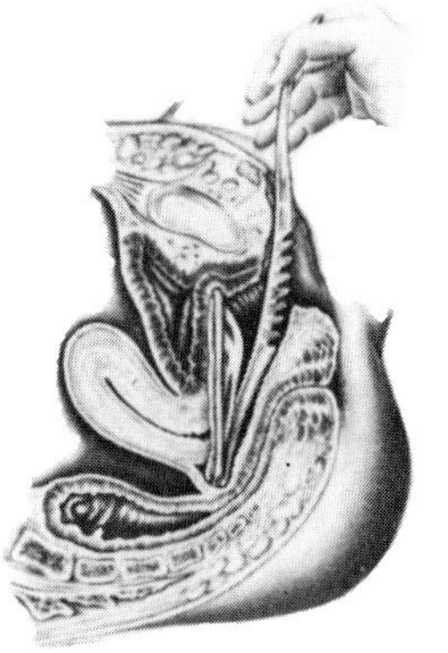

Feel for your cervix through the diaphragm to be certain it is properly placed and securely covered by the rubber dome. See Fig. I.)

Fig. I

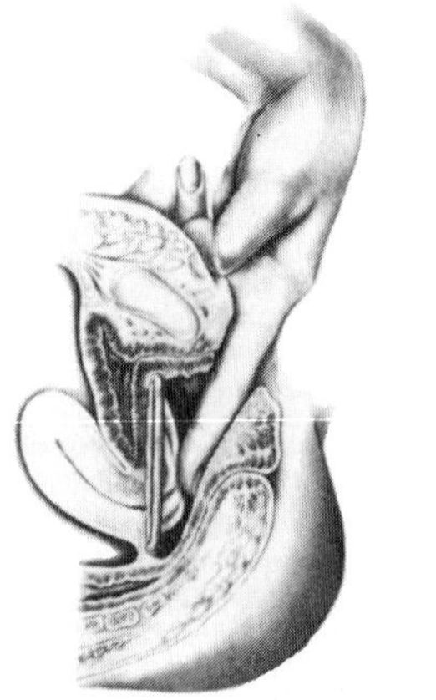

To clean the introducer, wash with mild soap and warm water, rinse and dry thoroughly.

USE AND CARE OF THE DIAPHRAGM—cont'd

FINAL CHECKING

Whether the diaphragm is inserted manually or with the introducer, the finger test must always be made to see that the outer rim of the diaphragm is tucked firmly behind the pelvic bone (see Fig. D). At the same time, you must check to see that the small round knob of the cervix (mouth of the womb) is securely covered by the rubber dome of the diaphragm. (See Fig. I.)

REPEATED INTERCOURSE

Without removing the diaphragm, an additional applicatorful of gel (jelly) or cream must be used if intercourse takes place more than 6 hours after the diaphragm has been inserted or for each repeated intercourse. The diaphragm must remain in place for at least 6 hours after the last intercourse.

Fig. J

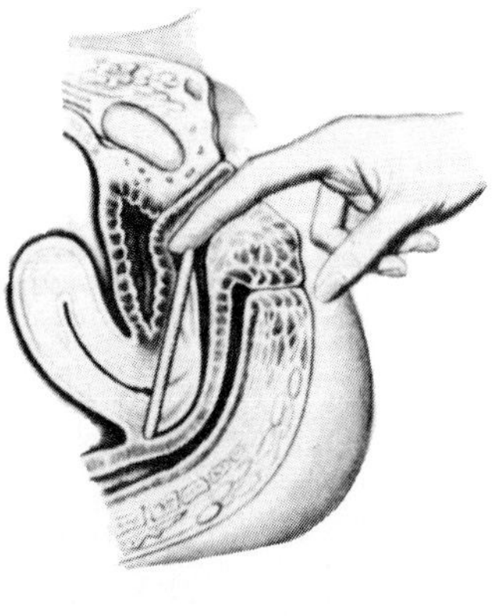

GENERAL INFORMATION

Regardless of the time of the month, this method of contraception must be used each and every time intercourse takes place. Your diaphragm must be left in place for at least 6 hours after the last intercourse. If you remove your diaphragm before the 6-hour time period, your chance of becoming pregnant could be greatly increased. You should not leave your diaphragm in place for more than 24 hours; to do so may encourage growth of bacteria that could result in infection or toxic shock syndrome.

Douching is not necessary after the use of the diaphragm. However, if desired or recommended by your physician, you must wait the full 6 hours after the last intercourse.

REMOVAL OF DIAPHRAGM

The only proper way to remove the diaphragm is to insert your forefinger up and over the top side of the diaphragm, and slightly to the side.

Next, turn the palm of your hand downward and backward hooking the forefinger firmly on top of the inside of the upper rim of the diaphragm, *breaking the suction.*

Pull the diaphragm down and out. This avoids the possibility of tearing the diaphragm with the fingernails. The diaphragm *should not* be removed by trying to catch the rim from *below* the dome. (See Fig. J.)

CARE OF DIAPHRAGM

When using a vaginal diaphragm, avoid using products that may contain petroleum, such as certain body lubricants, vaginal lubricants, or vaginitis preparations. These products can weaken rubber.

A little care means longer wear for your diaphragm. After each use the diaphragm should be washed in warm water and Ivory soap. Do not use detergent soaps, cold cream soaps, deodorant soaps, and soaps containing petroleum, since they can weaken the rubber. *Ivory soap should be the only soap used.*

After washing, the diaphragm should be dried thoroughly. All water and moisture should be removed with your towel. The diaphragm should then be dusted with *cornstarch.* Scented talc, body powder, baby powder, and the like should not be used because they can weaken the rubber. Remember, only *cornstarch* for dusting.

The diaphragm should then be placed back in the plastic case for storage. It should not be stored near a radiator or heat source, or exposed to light for an extended period.

about ways to reduce her risk for TSS. These measures include prompt removal 6 to 8 hours after intercourse; not using the diaphragm during menses; and learning and watching for danger signs of TSS. These danger signs include temperature of 38.4° C (101° F), diarrhea, vomiting, muscle aches, and sunburn-like rash.

Cervical Cap

The Prentif cavity-rim **cervical cap** was approved in the late 1980s for use in the United States (Brokaw, Vaker, and Haney, 1988; Women's Health, 1989; Mishell, 1989). The cap has a 1¼- to 1½-inch soft natural rubber dome with a firm but pliable rim (see Fig. 6-11, C). It fits snugly around the base of the cervix close to the junction of the cervix and vaginal fornices (Hatcher et al, 1988). The device is available in four sizes. It is recommended that the cap remain in place no less than 8 hours and not more than 48 hours at a time (NAACOG 1988; Mishell, 1989). It is left in place 6 to 8 hours after the last act of intercourse. The seal provides a physical barrier to sperm; spermicide inside the cap adds a chemical barrier.

The extended period of wear is an added convenience for women who previously used the diaphragm. Instructions for the actual insertion and use of the cervical cap closely resemble the instructions for use of the contraceptive diaphragm. Some of the differences are that the cervical cap can be inserted hours before sexual intercourse without a need for additional spermicide later, no additional spermicide is required for repeated acts of intercourse when the cap is used, and the cervical cap requires less spermicide than the diaphragm when initially inserted (NAACOG, 1988).

Some women are not good candidates for wearing the cervical cap. They include women with abnormal Pap test results, women who cannot be fitted properly with the existing cap sizes, women who find the insertion and removal of the device too difficult, women with a history of TSS, women with vaginal or cervical infections (NAACOG, 1988), and women who experience allergic responses to the cap or spermicide.

The angle of the uterus, the vaginal muscle tone, and the shape of the cervix may interfere with ease of fitting and use. Correct fitting requires time, effort, and skill from both the client and the clinician (Brokaw, Vaker, and Haney, 1988). The woman must check the cap's position before and after each act of intercourse.

After 3 months of use, cervical cap users had a higher rate of conversion from class I (no abnormal cells present) to class III (suspicious abnormal cells present) Pap tests when compared with diaphragm users (NAACOG, 1988; Mishell, 1989). These conversions may be manifestations of the human papillomavirus (HPV). Women using the cap should have a Pap test at least every year. If the cap is left in place more than 48 hours, it will produce an odor.

Whereas no link has been discovered between TSS and the use of the cervical cap, such an association remains possible (NAACOG, 1988).

The package insert recommends that another form of birth control be used during menstrual bleeding and up to at least 6 postpartum weeks.

The cap should be refitted after any gynecologic surgery or delivery, and after major weight losses or gains. Otherwise, the size should be checked at least once a year (Women's Health, 1989).

Strong client motivation is the most important criterion for successful cap use. First-year failure rates range from 8 to 27 pregnancies per 100 women who initiate the use of this method (Hatcher et al, 1988; Mishell, 1989; Women's Health, 1989). That failure rating is similar to the one given the diaphragm.

The client must be given the information available for this product as presented above. The nurse needs to assess the woman's understanding and skill in the use of the cervical cap.

Vaginal Sheath (Female Condom)

The vaginal sheath of natural latex rubber has flexible rings at both ends (Connell, 1989) (Fig. 6-12). Basically this device is a combination of a diaphragm and a condom. The closed end of the pouch is inserted into the vagina and is anchored around the cervix; the open ring covers the labia. It can be applied well in advance of intercourse so that spontaneity is unaffected. Before intercourse, a spermicide is added. Since it is a relatively loose sheath, it tends to heighten sensation for the man. Both women and men report that intercourse with the sheath is generally about as satisfying as intercourse without the sheath. Application of this disposable barrier requires no special training. This device may provide more protection against STDs than do condoms.

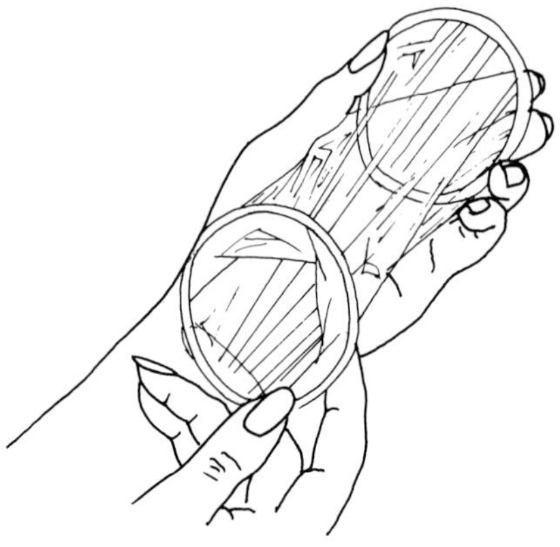

Fig. 6-12 WPC-333 soft polymer vaginal sheath.

Intrauterine Devices

An **intrauterine device (IUD)** is a small, T-shaped device inserted into the uterine cavity. Medicated IUDs have taken the place of nonmedicated IUDs (Grimes, 1986).* Medicated IUDs are loaded with either copper† (Fig. 6-13) or a progestational agent. These chemically active substances are released continuously; for example, copper-bearing devices for 4 years (at present) and progesterone devices for 1 year. IUDs are impregnated with barium sulfate for radiopacity.

The mechanism of action is not precisely known. Previously, it was thought that the IUD caused pronounced foreign body reaction that made the endometrium unsuitable for the implantation of fertilized ova. This has been found to be incorrect (Grimes, 1989). The copper-bearing IUD damages sperm in transit to the uterine tubes and "interferes with the reproductive process anatomically and temporally before ova reach the uterus" (WHO, 1987; Ortiz and Croxatto, 1987; Grimes, 1989). The progesterone-bearing IUD causes progestin-related effects on cervical mucus and endometrial maturation. Because the effect is local,

*The last nonmedicated plastic IUD (the Lippes loop) was discontinued by its manufacturer in 1985.

†Searle and Company removed CU-7 and TATUM-7 from the United States market on February 1, 1986.

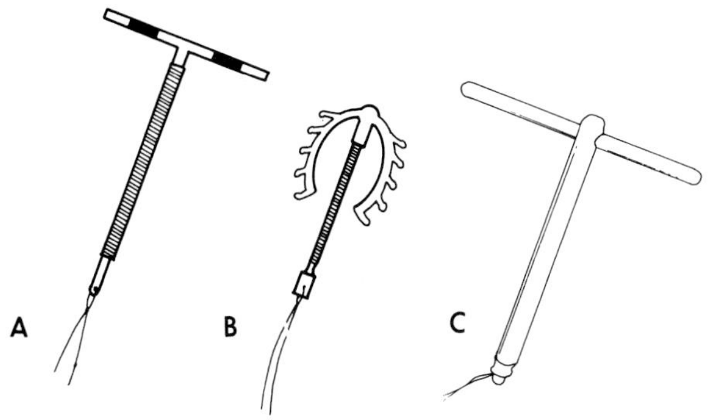

Fig. 6-13 Intrauterine devices. **A,** Copper-T 380A. The "380" signifies the total of 380 mm^2 of copper (mounted on polyethylene) exposed to the endometrium; the "A" refers to the copper on the arms (approved by FDA). **B,** Multiload devices come in different sizes and are prepared with different loads of copper. Not yet available in the United States, they are widely available outside of the United States. C, Progestasert.

there is no disruption of the woman's ovulatory pattern.

The IUD offers constant contraception without the need to remember to take pills each day or engage in other manipulation before or between coital acts. If pregnancy can be excluded, an IUD may be placed at any time during the menstrual cycle. An IUD may be inserted immediately after abortion (Liskin and Fox, 1982).

The absence of interference with hormonal regulation of menstrual cycles makes the IUD more appropriate than hormonal contraception for heavy smokers, women over 35, women who have hypertension, or those with a history of vascular disease or familial diabetes. Contraceptive effects are reversible. When pregnancy is desired, the IUD may be removed by the physician.

The Progestasert offers two important noncontraceptive progesterone-related advantages: less blood loss during menstruation and decreased primary dysmenorrhea. The mean blood loss is increased for the copper IUD. This blood loss may be clinically significant in undernourished populations. Because the IUD reduces the absolute number of pregnancies overall, current IUD wearers have only 40% the risk for ectopic pregnancy experienced by women not using contraception (Grimes, 1989). The copper device protects better than the progesterone device.

The use of an IUD is contraindicated for women with a history of PID, known or suspected pregnancy, undiagnosed genital bleeding, suspected genital malignancy, or a distorted intrauterine cavity.

When compared with contraceptive methods that protect against PID, the risk of infection with an IUD seems high. Earlier studies did not take into consideration the number of sex partners and exposure to STDs (Grimes, 1989). There is no increased risk of PID among IUD users who reported having only one sex partner (Cramer et al, 1985; Lee, Rubin, and Borucki, 1988; Grimes, 1989). The risk of IUD-related PID clusters around the time of insertion. The endometrium is contaminated with bacteria during insertion and rids itself of these bacteria soon thereafter. Women may benefit from prophylactic antimicrobial medication taken 1 hour before insertion (Grimes, 1989). The two monofilament tails on contemporary IUDs are *not* associated with an increased risk of PID.

The presence of the IUD thread must be checked after menstruation and at the time of ovulation as well as before coitus to rule out expulsion of the device. If pregnancy occurs with IUD in place, it should be removed immediately, if possible (Grimes, 1986). Retention of the IUD during pregnancy increases the risk of septic spontaneous abortion and other obstetric problems (Liskin and Fox, 1982). Some women allergic to copper develop a rash, necessitating the removal of the copper-bearing IUD.

The use of medical diathermy (shortwave and microwave) in a woman with a metal-containing IUD may cause heat injury to surrounding tissue. Therefore medical diathermy to the abdominal and sacral areas should not be used on women using copper-bearing IUDs.

Because of the litigious nature of American contemporary society, most health care providers are requiring lengthy detailed consent forms to be signed by any woman requesting an IUD. In 1988 a new copper IUD was released on the U.S. market (see Fig. 6-13, *A*). Family planning experts recommend that only women who are involved in stable, monogamous relationships and who have at least one child are appropriate candidates for IUDs. The manufacturer does not recommend women using the Copper-T 380A if they are either under 25, have never had children, or are involved in anything but an exclusive, monogamous relationship (ParaGard, 1988; Medical Letter, 1988; Mishell, 1989).

According to Hatcher et al (1988), of 100 users who start out the year using an IUD and who use it correctly and consistently, the lowest observed failure rate will be 0.5 pregnancies.

Contemporary IUDs provide highly effective contraception that is superior to use-effectiveness of combined oral hormonal contraceptives (Grimes, 1989). The efficacy of the Copper-T 380A is greater than the Progesterone-T.

The nursing actions related to the IUD are presented in the form of teaching tools. A general teaching tool for contraceptive methods is given on p. 127.

Vaccine to Block Pregnancy. An experimental birth control vaccine shows promise for blocking pregnancy for 6 months without significant side effects, a preliminary study suggests. The vaccine was designed to spur the immune system into making antibodies that block the action of human chorionic gonadotropin, which is produced during pregnancy.

Sterilization

Sterilization refers to surgical procedures intended to render the person infertile. Most procedures involve the occlusion of the passageways for the ova and sperm (Fig. 6-14). For the female the oviducts (uterine tubes) are occluded; for the male the sperm ducts (vas deferens) are occluded. Only surgical removal of the ovaries (oophorectomy) or uterus (hysterectomy) or both will result in absolute sterility for the woman. All other operations have a small but definite failure rate; that is, pregnancy may result.

Since 1950, voluntary sterilization has grown rapidly in acceptance and is currently the most prevalent method of contraception in the world. In the United States, voluntary sterilization is the most common choice of contraception for couples who are 30 years of age or older.

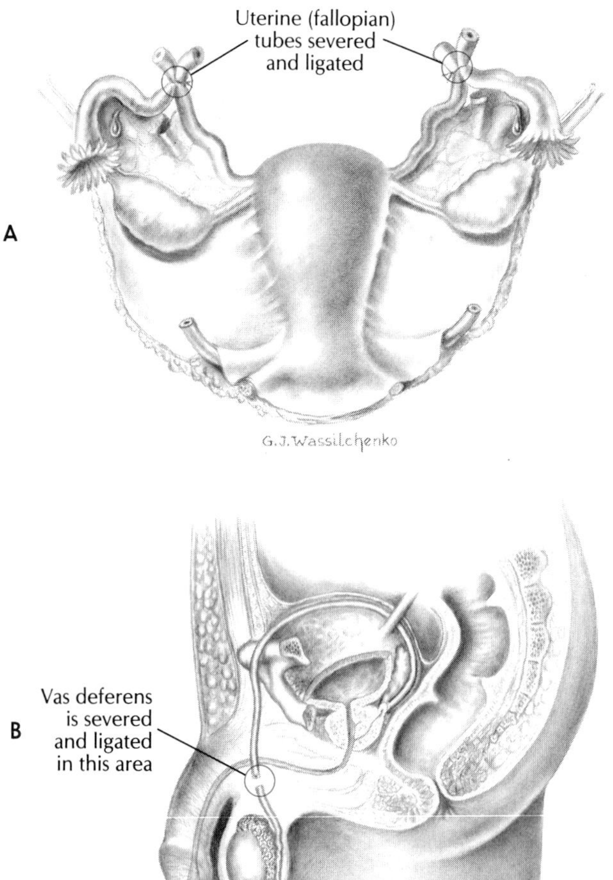

Fig. 6-14 Sterilization. **A,** Oviduct ligated and severed (tubal ligation). **B,** Sperm duct severed (and ligated) (vasectomy).

Motivation for Sterilization. Motivation for elective sterilization includes personal preference; obstetric reasons, such as multiparity; medical reasons such as hypertensive, cardiovascular, or renal disease in the woman or recurrent acute epididymitis in the man; and diagnosis of inheritable disease.

Sterilization as a means of contraception may be requested by couples who have almost come to the end of their childbearing years and have the desired number of children. It is also chosen by young adults who have decided not to bear children. Persons in the first group are generally acceptive of the procedure even though there may be some feelings of regret because one of life's phases is over. Persons in the second group need the opportunity to explore the consequences of their choice. See surgical interruption of pregnancy (p. 149) for values clarification and counseling techniques helpful in implementing the nursing process with clients seeking sterilization.

Laws and Regulations. All states have strict regulations for informed consent (see Chapter 3). Many states in the United States permit voluntary sterilization of any mature, rational woman without reference to her marital or pregnancy status. Although the partner's consent is not required, the client is encouraged to discuss the situation with her or his partner.

Sterilization of minors or mentally incompetent females is restricted by most states. The operation often requires the approval of a board of eugenicists or other court-appointed individuals.

If federal funds are used, the person must be at least 21 years of age and mentally competent. Some state and federal regulations govern Medicaid funds for elective sterilization; for example, counseling and a waiting period after the decision is made are mandatory.

Assessment

Motivation for sterilization and the result of exploration of alternatives are explored. The client's knowledge of the sterilization methods and of the chosen method is assessed. Gaps in knowledge and misinformation are noted.

History, physical examination, and laboratory data are collected. The record is reviewed for the signed informed consent, and the client's understanding is verified. General preoperative, operative, and postoperative assessments are performed.

Nursing Diagnoses

Examples of nursing diagnoses for the woman undergoing surgical sterilization include the following:

Decisional conflict related to
- Alternatives
- Readiness for permanent termination of fertility

Knowledge deficit related to
- Alternatives
- Method chosen
- Preoperative and postoperative events

Pain related to
- Postoperative period

Potential spiritual distress related to
- Reason for choosing sterilization

Planning

Planning is a collaborative effort among the woman, her sexual partner (where appropriate), the physician, and the nurse. Depending on the motivation for sterilization, other physicians may need to be part of the health care team. ***Goals*** are determined and stated in client-centered terms and may include the following:

1. Client has received and understood all information necessary to give informed consent
2. Client experiences a successful procedure and uneventful recovery
3. Client continues to be satisfied with the decision for sterilization, the procedure, and the experience with the health care team

Implementation

The nurse plays an important role in assisting people with decision making so that all requirements for informed consent are met. People seek information about the various methods of sterilization. Clinical information about the various procedures follows the evaluation section. The nurse also provides information about alternatives to sterilization, for example, contraception.

The nurse acts as a sounding board for people who are exploring the possibility of choosing sterilization and their feelings about and motivation for this choice. The nurse records this information, which may be the basis for referral to a family planning clinic, a psychiatric social worker, or another professional health care provider.

Information about what is entailed in various procedures, how much discomfort or pain can be expected, and what type of care is needed must be given. Many individuals fear sterilization procedures because of the imagined effect on their sexual life. They need reassurance concerning the hormonal and psychologic basis for sexual function and the fact that uterine tube occlusion or vasectomy has no biologic sequelae in terms of sexual adequacy.

Preoperative Preparation. Printed instructions are usually available for clients from the physician. The physician performs the preoperative health assessment, which includes a psychologic assessment, physical examination, and laboratory test. The nurse assists with the health assessment, answers questions, and confirms the client's understanding of printed instructions (e.g., NPO [nothing by mouth] after midnight). Ambivalence and extreme fear of the procedure are reported to the physician.

Postoperative Care. Postoperative care depends on the procedure performed, for example, laparoscopy (p. 110) or laparotomy for tubal occlusion, or vasectomy. General care includes postanesthesia recovery, vital signs, fluid-electrolyte balance (intake and output, laboratory values), prevention of or early identification and treatment for infection or hemorrhage, control of discomfort, and assessment of emotional response to the procedure and recovery.

Discharge Planning. Discharge planning depends on the type of procedure performed. In general, the client is given written instructions about observing for and reporting symptoms and signs of complications, the type of recovery to be expected, and the date and time for a follow-up appointment.

Personnel who function in infertility and birth control clinics or in hospitals must be carefully selected. Studies indicate that attitudes of personnel significantly affect the client's perception of the quality of care received. This consideration is important in planning for the overall delivery of health services. Seeking help for infertility and fertility control is often the only contact some people have with the health care system. Positive perceptions of the interest, concern, and technical skill of health workers in this instance may induce wider use of health facilities and care in the future.

Evaluation

The nurse can be assured that care was effective when the goals of care are achieved: the client has received and understood all information necessary to give informed consent; the procedure was successful and recovery was uneventful; and the client continues to be satisfied with the decision for sterilization, the procedure, and the experience with the health care team.

Female Sterilization

Female sterilization may be done immediately after delivery (within 24 to 48 hours), concomitantly with abortion, or as an interval procedure (during any phase of the menstrual cycle). Most sterilization procedures are performed immediately after a pregnancy, probably because of heightened motivation or increased practicality. Usually the woman is already in the hospital and all preoperative preparations (blood work, physical examination, etc.) have been completed.

However, all sterilization procedures have the lowest morbidity and failure rates when accomplished at a time other than immediately after a pregnancy. Tissue edema continues during the early postpartum period, which may permit the sutures to cut through the tubal wall and leave an opening into the uterine tube.

Tubal Occlusion. The operation used commonly is the laparoscopic tubal fulguration (destruction of tissue by means of an electric current [electrocoagulation]). See p. 110 for laparoscopy examination, a procedure of entering the abdomen for access to the uterine tubes. A minilaparotomy may be used for tubal ligation (Fig. 6-15) or for the application of bands or clips. Bands (e.g., Falope ring) and clips (e.g., Hulka-Clemens) are placed around the tubes to block them (Cunningham, MacDonald, and Gant, 1989). Fulguration and ligation are considered to be permanent methods. Use of the bands or clips have the theoretic advantage of possible removal and return of tubal patency.

For the minilaparotomy approach the woman is admitted the morning of surgery, having received nothing by mouth (NPO) since midnight. Preoperative sedation is given. The procedure may be carried out with local

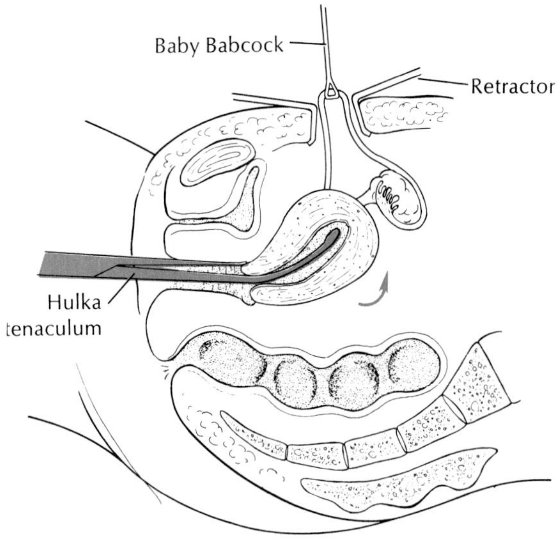

Fig. 6-15 Use of minilaparotomy to gain access to oviducts for tubal occlusion procedures. Tenaculum is used to lift uterus upward *(arrow)* toward incision.

anesthesia. A small vertical incision is made in the abdominal wall below the umbilicus. The woman may experience sensations of tugging but no pain, and the operation is completed within 20 minutes. She may be discharged 4 hours later if she has recovered from anesthesia. Any abdominal discomfort usually can be controlled with a mild analgesic (e.g., aspirin). Within 10 days the scar is almost invisible.

Major medical complications after elective sterilization are rare. Dysfunctional uterine bleeding or ovarian cyst formation may occur after tubal surgery, presumably because of disturbance of the utero-ovarian circulation. As occurs with any surgery, there is always a possibility of complications of anesthesia, infection, hemorrhage, and trauma to other organs. Psychologic trauma is seen in some women.

Tubal Reconstruction. Restoration of tubal continuity (reanastomosis) and function is technically feasible except after laparoscopic tubal fulguration. Sterilization reversal, however, is costly, difficult (requiring microsurgery), and uncertain (Cunningham, MacDonald, and Gant, 1989). The success rate varies with the extent of tubal destruction and removal. The incidence of successful pregnancy after reanastomosis is only about 15%. The loss of a segment of tube necessary for sperm capacitation and fertilization is the probable cause.

Male Sterilization

Vasectomy is the easiest and most commonly employed operation for male sterilization. In the United States one-half million men undergo vasectomy each year (Cunningham, MacDonald, and Gant, 1989). Vasectomy can be carried out with local anesthesia and on an out-of-hospital basis.

In vasectomy, short right and left incisions are made into the anterior aspect of the scrotum above and lateral to each testis over the spermatic cord (Fig. 6-14). Each vas deferens is identified and doubly ligated with fine nonabsorbable sutures. Then each vas deferens is incised between the ligatures. Occasionally the surgeon fulgurates the cut stumps of the sperm ducts. Many surgeons bury the cut ends into scrotal fascia to lessen the chance of reunion. Then the skin incisions are closed. Usually one nonabsorbable suture is used for closure of each skin incision. A dressing is applied.

The man is instructed in self-care to promote a safe return to routine activities. To reduce swelling and relieve discomfort, ice packs are applied to the scrotum intermittently for a few hours postoperatively. A suspensory, or bandage, is applied to decrease discomfort by supporting the scrotum. Moderate inactivity for about 2 days is advisable because of local scrotal tenderness. The skin suture can be removed 5 to 7 days postoperatively. Sexual intercourse may be resumed as desired.

Sterility is not immediate. Some sperm will remain in the proximal portions of the sperm ducts after vasectomy. One week to several months are required to clear the ducts of sperm. Therefore some form of contraception is needed until the sperm count in the ejaculate on two consecutive tests is down to zero (Cunningham, MacDonald, and Gant, 1989).

Vasectomy has no effect on potency (ability to achieve and maintain an erection) or volume of ejaculate. Endocrine production of testosterone continues so that secondary sex characteristics are not affected. Sperm production continues. Men occasionally may develop a hematoma, discharge, or infection. Less common are painful granulomas from accumulation of sperm. Sperm unable to leave the epididymis are lyzed by the immune system.

Complications after bilateral vasectomy are uncommon and usually not serious. They include bleeding (usually external), suture reaction, and reaction to anesthetic agent. Sterilization failures, usually caused by a recanalization, are rare, occurring in about 2 per 1000 men.

Tubal Reconstruction. Microsurgery to reanastomose (restoration of tubal continuity) the sperm ducts can be accomplished successfully in 90% of cases (i.e., sperm in the ejaculate) (Jarow, 1987). However, the fertility (pregnancies) rate is much lower, 40% to 60% in most series. The rate of success decreases as the time since the procedure increases. The vasectomy may result in permanent changes in the testes that leave men unable to father children. The changes are those ordinarily seen only in the elderly (e.g., interstitial fibrosis [scar tissue between the seminiferous tubules]). Some men develop antibodies against their own sperm (autoimmunization). The role of antisperm antibodies in fertility after vasectomy reversal has not been completely determined.

❏ SURGICAL INTERRUPTION OF PREGNANCY

Elective abortion is the purposeful interruption of a previable pregnancy. Indications for elective abortion are as follows:

1. Preservation of the life or health of the mother (e.g., class III or IV heart disease)
2. Avoidance of the birth of an offspring with a serious developmental or hereditary disorder (e.g., Tay-Sachs disease)
3. Elective abortion (e.g., because of inability of the parents to support or care for the child, rape, mental incompetence, or because of severe emotional problems)

The control of birth, dealing as it does with human sexuality and the question of life and death, is one of the most emotionalized components of health care. Abortion as one of the surgical alternatives to contraception is regulated in most countries. Regulations exist presumably to protect the mother from the complications of abortion or because of religious constraints. The U.S. Supreme Court set aside previous antiabortion laws in January 1973, holding that first-trimester abortion is permissible inasmuch as the mortality from interruption of early gestation is now less than the mortality after normal term delivery. Second-trimester abortion was left to the discretion of the individual states. Roman Catholic hospitals and some of those maintained by strict fundamentalists forbid abortion (and often sterilization) despite legal challenge.

Before the legalization of abortion, many illegal abortions took place, with little-documented sequelae other than death from infection or hemorrhage or both. Although studies indicate that biologic sequelae do occur after abortion, rates of biologic complications tend to be low, especially if the woman aborts during the first trimester. Studies related to psychologic sequelae reveal that they are short lived. Sequelae are related to circumstances surrounding the abortion, such as rape or the attitudes reflected by friends, family, and health workers. It must be remembered that the woman facing an abortion is pregnant and will exhibit the emotional responses shared by all pregnant women, including postdelivery depression.

In an attempt to regulate the conflict between professional responsibilities and personal ethics the Nurses' Association of the American College of Obstetricians and Gynecologists (NAACOG) published a position paper on the nurse's role with the abortion client in December 1989, in which the simultaneous rights of each are described (NAACOG, 1989). Women have the right to expect and receive supportive, nonjudgmental care. Nurses have the right to refuse to assist with abortions or sterilizations in keeping with their own moral or religious beliefs, unless the woman's life is in danger.

The values and moral convictions of the nurse are involved to the same extent as those of the pregnant woman. The conflicts and doubts of the nurse can be readily communicated to women who are already anxious and overly sensitive. Health professionals need assistance to identify and come to terms with their own feelings. It is not uncommon for confusion to arise as beliefs are challenged by the reality of care. A nursing student reacted to learning experiences associated with in-hospital abortions in the following manner:

> I really feel I believe in the rightness of elective abortion, but when I watched the physician insert the needle and then

inject the dose of prostaglandin, I felt an unreasoning rage sweep over me. I could have attacked him. Funny, I felt no anger toward the woman at all. I really need to rethink my beliefs.

Responses can also change with life experiences. A nurse who before her marriage had worked as counselor in a municipal clinic established a reputation as a supportive and concerned counselor of young persons with regard to birth control. Four years later she remarked:

I've been trying to get pregnant for the past 3 years. I didn't realize how important it would be to me. You know I can't counsel about abortion any more. I can't be objective. I keep feeling, "Have your baby and please give it to me." I am more concerned about myself now, not them [the pregnant women], and counseling won't work that way.

Assessment

A thorough assessment is conducted through history, physical examination, and laboratory tests. If the woman is Rh negative and the pregnancy is greater than 8 weeks' gestation, she is a candidate for prophylaxis against Rh isoimmunization (p. 99). She receives Rh_o (D) immune globulin within 72 hours after the abortion if she is D^u negative and Coombs negative (unsensitized or has not developed isoimmunization). Compelling medical, surgical, or psychiatric indications for elective abortion, though not numerous, are possible factors. The following conditions probably would qualify: class III coronary heart disease; fulminating (pelvic) Hodgkin's disease; stage 1B carcinoma of the cervix; and Marfan's syndrome with early aortic aneurysm. The length of pregnancy and the condition of the woman need to be determined to select the appropriate type of abortion procedure.

The woman's understanding of alternatives, the types of abortions, and expected recovery is assessed. Misinformation and gaps in knowledge are identified. The record is reviewed for the signed informed consent and the client's understanding is verified. General preoperative, operative, and postoperative assessments are performed.

Nursing Diagnoses

Following are examples of nursing diagnoses for the woman undergoing interruption of pregnancy.

Knowledge deficit or decisional conflict related to
- Alternatives to abortion
- Types of abortion
- Preoperative and postoperative events

Potential for infection related to
- The procedure itself
- Lack of understanding of preoperative and postoperative self-care

Potential pain related to
- The procedure

Potential self-esteem disturbance related to
- The procedure

Planning

Planning is a collaborative effort among the woman, her sexual partner (as appropriate), the physician, and the nurse. Depending on the motivation for elective abortion, other physicians may need to be part of the health care team. ***Goals*** are established collaboratively, should be stated in client-centered terms, and may include the following:

1. Client has received and understood all information necessary to give informed consent
2. Client experiences a successful procedure and recovery is uneventful
3. Client continues to be satisfied with the decision for elective abortion, the procedure, and the experience with the health care team

Implementation

Counseling about abortion includes help for the woman in identifying how she perceives the pregnancy; information about the choices available, that is, having an abortion or carrying the pregnancy to term and then either keeping the child or giving it up for adoption; and information about types of abortion procedures. *The goal is to assist the woman in coming to a decision that is her own.*

Second and third trimester procedures include hysterotomy (a cesarean incision) and hysterectomy. *Hysterotomy* is the preferred method if the woman wishes tubal ligation or hysterectomy to follow. *Hysterectomy* may be performed at or before 24 weeks gestation without first emptying the uterus. Possible complications are those seen after major surgery: hemorrhage and infection. The fetus may be born alive, opening ethical, moral, religious, and legal problems. The mortality risk is 10% greater than with D&C.

The woman will need help to explore the meaning of the various alternatives and consequences to herself and her significant others. It is often difficult for a woman to express her true feelings (e.g., what abortion means to her now and in the future, and what support or regret her friends and peers may demonstrate). A calm, matter-of-fact approach on the part of the nurse can be helpful (e.g.: "Yes, I know you are pregnant, I am here to help. Let's talk about alternatives.") Listening to what the woman has to say and encouraging her to speak are essential. Neutral responses such as "Oh," "Uh-huh," and "Umm" and nonverbal encouragement such as nodding, maintaining eye contact, and use of touch are helpful in setting an open, accepting environment. Clarifying, restating, and reflecting statements, use of open-ended questions, and giving feedback are communication techniques that can be used to maintain a reality focus on the situation and bring the woman's problems into the open. Once a decision has been made, the woman must be assured of continued support. Information about what is entailed in various procedures, how much discomfort or pain can be expected, and what type of care is needed must be given. If family or friends cannot be involved, scheduling time for the nursing personnel to give the necessary support is an essential component of the care plan.

Preoperative preparation, postoperative care, and discharge planning parallel the methods used for sterilization.

Evaluation

The nurse can be reasonably assured that care was effective when the goals of care have been met: the client has received and understood all information necessary to give informed consent; the procedure is successful, recovery is uneventful, and the client continues to be satisfied with the decision for elective abortion, the procedure, and the experience with the health care team.

First Trimester Abortion

Methods for performing early **elective abortion** (EAB) (sometimes called therapeutic abortion [TAB]) include the following:

1. Menstrual extraction—early aspiration of the endometrium in women who have not yet missed a period
2. Surgical D&C when newer aspiration equipment is unavailable
3. Uterine aspiration after one or two missed periods

Surgical D&C refers to cervical dilatation (D) followed by curettage (C) of the uterine endometrium. Curettage is the scraping of the uterine lining with a metal curette or a flexible aspiration tip to remove the products of conception implanted in the endometrium. The procedure is similar to that of uterine aspiration. Cervical trauma and uterine perforation, infection, or hemorrhage are possible though rare complications.

Uterine aspiration (vacuum or suction) abortion is the most common procedure. The insertion of a small laminaria tent retained by a vaginal tampon for 4 to 24 hours usually will facilitate the purposeful interruption of a first-trimester pregnancy by dilating the cervix atraumatically (see Fig. 6-1). On removal of the moist, expanded laminaria, the cervix will have dilated two or three times its original (dry) diameter. Rarely will further mechanical dilatation of the cervix be required. The insertion of an adequate-sized aspiration cannula (8.5 to 10.5 mm) is almost always possible. Cervical laceration and bleeding are reduced by the use of laminaria. A disadvantage is the delay necessary and the need for an additional visit to the physician's office or clinic.

The woman comes to the clinic or physician's office the day before the abortion procedure. An antiseptic solution is used to prepare the pelvic area. A vaginal speculum is inserted, and the vaginal canal and cervix are cleansed. Injection of a local anesthetic agent into the cervix may follow (see paracervical block, Chapter 13, p. 345). Again the area is cleansed, and the laminaria tent is inserted into the endocervical canal. Prophylactic use of an antibiotic is usually begun. Some women experience a mild cramping or have light spotting from the anesthetic injection. Discomfort can usually be controlled with analgesics.

Aspiration abortion may be performed in the physician's office or in the hospital setting. If the woman chooses a hospital setting, she is admitted the day after insertion of the laminaria tent and is given preoperative sedation. The vaginal area is cleansed (shaving is not necessary). The suction procedure for accomplishing an early elective abortion (ideal time is 8 to 10 weeks since last menstrual period) usually requires less than 5 minutes and can easily be effected under paracervical block anesthesia and single sedation. During the procedure the nurse or physician keeps the woman informed as to what to expect next, for example, menstrual-like cramping, sounds of suction machine. The nurse assesses the woman's vital signs. The aspirated uterine contents must be carefully inspected to ascertain whether all fetal parts and adequate placental tissue have been evacuated. A single dose of oxytocin is usually sufficient to control bleeding. The woman may remain in the hospital 3 or 4 hours for detection of excessive cramping or excessive bleeding and then is discharged. If the procedure is done in the physician's office, preoperative sedation is usually not given, and the anesthetic of choice is usually paracervical block. After the abortion the woman rests on the table until she is ready to get up. Then she remains in the waiting room until she feels she can travel. She may be discharged in the company of a relative or friend.

Bleeding after the operation normally is about the

equivalent of a heavy menstrual period, and cramps are rarely severe. Infection such as endometritis or salpingitis occurs in about 8% of women. Subsequently a D&C procedure for bleeding or sepsis caused by retained placental tissue is necessary in about 2% of women. Serious depression or other psychiatric problems are rare.

Postabortal instructions differ with the institution (e.g., use of tampons may be denied for only 3 days or for up to 6 weeks, and resumption of sexual intercourse may be permitted within 1 week or discouraged for 6 weeks). The woman may bathe or shower daily. Instruction is given to watch for excessive bleeding, cramps, or fever and to avoid douches of any type. The woman may expect her menstrual period to resume 4 to 6 weeks from the day of the procedure. The nurse offers information about the birth control method the woman prefers if this has not been done previously during the counseling interview that usually precedes the decision to have an abortion. The woman must be strongly encouraged to return for her follow-up visit so that complications can be avoided and an acceptable contraceptive method prescribed.

Second- and Third-trimester Abortions

There are four types of techniques used for second- and third-trimester abortions:

1. *Transabdominal intrauterine injection of hypertonic sodium chloride.* The woman is admitted to the hospital for this procedure. Amniocentesis is performed. The physician determines where the needle (an 18-gauge, 7.5 cm [3 in] spinal needle) will be inserted. The area is cleansed, and if desired, a local anesthetic agent is given. Approximately 200 ml of amniotic fluid is withdrawn, and a similar amount of sterile 20% sodium chloride is injected. The woman is instructed to report when uterine contractions begin—generally, within 8 to 48 hours. In most cases augmentation with oxytocin is necessary to effect uterine evacuation in a reasonable time. Occasionally reinjection is required. Labor begins, in theory at least, because the hypertonic saline solution releases the placental uterine progesterone blockade that normally prevents the onset of labor. The same careful monitoring of uterine contractions is as necessary as for a term delivery. Instruction in relaxation and breathing techniques is indicated, and analgesia can be administered for discomfort. The assistance of a supportive person at the time of birth of the dead fetus is essential. If the woman wishes to see the fetus, emotional support should be provided before and after the procedure. Many woman are relieved to find the fetus normal and commonly inquire as to its sex. After the delivery the standard observations and postpartum care are carried out (see Chapter 21). Contraceptive counseling is given before discharge. The woman is advised to return should excessive bleeding occur.

Complications of hypertonic saline injection for second-trimester abortion may occur. Complications with the approximate frequency of their occurrence include infection (10%), need for D&C to remove retained tissue (15%), failure to abort (10%), and excessive bleeding, necessitating transfusion (2%). Symptomatology to saline solution (hypernatremia) includes tinnitus, tachycardia, and headache; that of water intoxication, edema, oliguria (≤200 mg/8 hours), dyspnea, thirst, and restlessness. Rarely, disseminated intravascular coagulation (DIC) or expulsion of the fetus through the uterine isthmus occurs.

2. *Injection of urea solution after amniocentesis.* After the removal of about 200 ml of amniotic fluid, 200 ml of 30% solution of urea in 5% dextrose in water is introduced into the uterus by gravity drip. After 1 hour a solution of 5 units of oxytocin in 500 ml of 5% dextrose in water is started intravenously. Fetal death occurs, and delivery ensues in most cases within 12 hours. Complications are less common and are less serious than with hypertonic saline solution.

3. *Transabdominal intrauterine injection of 40 to 45 mg of prostaglandins $PGF_2\alpha$, E_2.* The undesirable side effects of hypertonic saline solution, such as hypernatremia or DIC, do not occur with prostaglandins; therefore it has become the treatment of choice. However, nausea and vomiting are common problems. Abortion usually takes place within 18 to 24 hours after injection. If it does not occur, the procedure is repeated, but only half the dosage is used.

4. *Abdominal or vaginal hysterotomy.* Hysterotomy may be chosen after more than 14 to 16 weeks of pregnancy, after failure of intrauterine injection of saline solution or $PGF_{2\alpha}$, and when sterilization is desired. The vaginal approach is employed when transabdominal surgery should be avoided. The management is comparable to that of cesarean delivery.

RU 486 (Mifepristone)

Progesterone is essential for the maintenance of pregnancy. RU 486 (mifepristone) is a progesterone antagonist that prevents implantation of a fertilized egg. It is most effective in early gestation, during the luteal phase, within 10 days of the expected onset of what would be the first missed period after conception. It can be taken up to 5 weeks after conception. The effectiveness of RU 486 is inversely related to gestational age as determined by β-hCG levels and duration of amenorrhea (Grimes et al, 1988). However, it is considered to be an effective and safe method for termination of early pregnancy. The medication should be used only under close medical supervision (Couzinet et al, 1986).

Uterine bleeding begins within 4 days of administration of the first dose. Usually a period of painless heavy bleeding is reported. Termination of pregnancy occurs for most women. For the woman in whom abortion does not occur, evacuation of the uterus by aspiration is facilitated by the softening of the uterine cervix. RU 486 is responsible for cervical softening. Some women experience slight nausea and fatigue during the period of bleeding.

The present results are similar to those reported in investigations in which prostaglandin analogs were used to terminate early pregnancy. Although the success rate with prostaglandins also approaches 85%, this method is associated with painful uterine contractions and gastrointestinal side effects in approximately 50% of subjects. In contrast, RU 486 is well tolerated. Supporters of this method feel that even with known disadvantages, RU 486 offers a reasonable alternative to surgical abortion, which carries the risks of anesthesia, surgical complications, infertility, and psychologic sequelae (Couzinet et al, 1986; Debate 1987a). Others have taken a strong stand against the use of RU 486 (Debate, 1987b). Other possible roles are emerging for RU 486 (Hodgen, 1988; Spitz and Bardin, 1989): it opens, softens, and dilates the cervix; suppresses breast tumors; opposes proliferation of endometrial tissue (as seen in endometriosis); and blocks ovulation. It may have a future application for uterine evacuation following fetal death. RU 486 may be considered as a "transitional" contraceptive pill for women aged 35 to 50.

Anesthesia for Gynecologic Procedures. Paracervical block anesthesia is used for a variety of obstetric (Chapter 13) and gynecologic procedures (see Fig. 13-8). Tests for infertility such as endometrial biopsy and aspiration abortion are two such procedures. Complications may include vasovagal syncope and intravascular injection.

The procedure is explained to the woman. She is asked to void if her bladder is full. Her vital signs are checked and recorded. The sight of the long needle used to inject the anesthesia may be frightening (see Fig. 13-8). The woman can be reassured that only the tip of the needle will be inserted. For this sterile procedure the physician or anesthesiologist will need the nurse's assistance in positioning the woman (dorsal recumbent position with knees flexed), handling supplies, and helping the woman remain immobile while the injection is made.

SUMMARY

The roles of the nurse vary in the care of clients requiring treatment for impaired fertility, control of fertility, termination of fertility, and interruption of pregnancy. A solid knowledge base of anatomy and physiology, mastery of nursing skills, and the nurse's self-awareness are all essential factors in meeting client needs. Professional satisfaction is the reward for the nurse who is able to assist clients coping with reproductive issues. Seeking help for impaired fertility and fertility control is commonly the only contact some people have with the health care system. Positive perceptions of the interest, concern, and technical skill of health care providers may induce wider use of health facilities and care in the future.

KEY CONCEPTS

- Impaired fertility is the inability to conceive and carry a child to term gestation at a time the couple has chosen to do so.
- Impaired fertility affects between 15% to 20% of otherwise healthy adults.
- Male and female factors each separately account for 40% of impaired fertility. Factors from both partners are responsible for the remaining 20%.
- Common etiologic factors of impaired fertility include decreased sperm production, interference with hypothalamic-pituitary-ovarian axis, tubal occlusion, and varicocele.
- It is estimated that 40% to 50% of couples with impaired fertility who seek assistance will be able to become pregnant and carry the child to viability.
- Reproductive alternatives to achieve parenthood include IVF-ET, GIFT, ZIFT, therapeutic insemination, surrogate motherhood, and adoption.
- There are a variety of contraceptive methods and various effectiveness ratings, advantages, and disadvantages.
- Nurses need to help couples choose the contraceptive method or methods best suited to them.
- Proper concurrent use of spermicides and latex condoms provides protection against AIDS.
- Tubal ligations and vasectomies are permanent sterilization methods used by increasing numbers of women and men.
- Elective abortion accomplished in the first trimester is 10 times safer than carrying a pregnancy to term.

LEARNING ACTIVITIES

1. Discuss three ways a nurse can help a couple cope with a diagnosis of impaired infertility.
2. In a small group (2 to 6 students) prepare a peer counseling class on periodic abstinence methods of contraception. Consider the following:
   a. Calendar method
   b. Cervical mucus (ovulation) method
   c. Sympto-thermal method
   d. Fertility awareness
3. In a small group (2 to 6 students) prepare a teaching plan for a couple who wishes to conceive. Consider 2, a to d above.
4. Practice application of contraceptive devices using medical models. Role-play teaching application to clients.
   a. Condom
   b. Vaginal diaphragm
5. Discuss the ethical issues resulting from therapeutic intrauterine insemination, in vitro fertilization-embryo transplant, GIFT, or surrogate motherhood.

References

Adoption services for your pregnant patient, Contemp OB/GYN 33(3):114, 1989.

Bernstein JL and Kidd YA: Childbearing in Japan. In Kay MA, editor: Anthropology of human birth, Philadelphia, 1982, FA Davis Co.

Brokaw AK, Vaker NN, and Haney SL: Fitting the cervical cap, Nurse Pract 13(7):49, 1988.

Brownlee AT: Community, culture, and care: a cross-cultural guide for health workers, St Louis, 1978, The CV Mosby Co.

Bustillo M et al: Nonsurgical ovum (embryo) transfer as a treatment in infertile women: preliminary experience, JAMA 251:1171, 1984.

Can you rely on condoms? Consumer Reports 54(3):135, 1989.

Clark AL and Howland IH: The American Samoan. In Clark AL, editor: Culture/childbearing/health professionals, Philadelphia, 1978, FA Davis Co.

Clark M: Health in the Mexican-American culture: a community study, Berkeley, 1970, University of California Press.

Connell, EB: Barrier contraceptives, Clin Obstet Gynecol 32(2):377, 1989.

Coughlin R: Pregnancy and birth in Vietnam. In Hart D et al, editors: Southeast Asian birth customs: three studies in human reproduction, New Haven, Conn, 1965, Human Relations Area Files.

Couzinet B et al: Termination of early pregnancy by the progesterone antagonist RU 486 (mifepristone), N Engl J Med 315(25):1565, 1986.

Cramer DW et al: Tubal infertility and the intrauterine device, N Engl J Med 312:941, 1985.

Cunningham FG, MacDonald PC, and Gant NF: Williams obstetrics, ed 18, Norwalk, Conn, 1989, Appleton & Lange.

The debate: Abortion pill (RU 486): we should test this drug in the USA, USA Today, p 10A, Jan 15, 1987a.

The debate: Abortion pill: keep this chemical killer out of the USA (an opposing view), USA Today, p 10A, Jan 15, 1987b.

Evans MI et al, editors: Fetal diagnosis and therapy: science, ethics and the law, Philadelphia, 1989, JB Lippincott Co.

Food and Drug Administration: Data inconclusive on birth control pills and ovarian cysts, FDA Talk Paper, June 15, 1988.

Grimes DA: Reversible contraception for the 1980s, JAMA 255(1):69, 1986.

Grimes, DA: Whither the uterine device? Clin Obstet Gynecol 32(2):369, 1989.

Grimes DA et al: Early abortion with a single dose of the antiprogestin RU-486, Am J Obstet Gynecol, 138(6):1307, 1988.

Hamori MH et al: Zygote intrafallopian transfer (ZIFT): evaluation of 42 cases, Fertil Steril 50(3):519, 1988.

Hatcher RA et al: Contraceptive technology, ed 13, New York, 1986, Irvington Publishers, Inc.

Hatcher, RA, et al: Contraceptive technology: 1988-1989, ed 14, New York, 1988, Irvington Publishers, Inc.

Hodgen GD: Progesterone antagonists (RU 486), Contemp OB/GYN 32(special issue):65, Sept, 1988.

Jarow JP: Vasectomy: autoimmunity and reversal, JAMA 257(15):2087, 1987.

Kaunitz AM: Injectable contraception, Clin Obstet Gynecol 32(2):356, 1989.

Kay MA, editor: Anthropology of human birth, Philadelphia, 1982, FA Davis Co.

Klaus H: Natural family planning: a review, Obstet Gynecol Surv 37:128, 1982.

Kugel C and Verson H: Relationship between weight change and diaphragm size change, JOGN Nurs 15:123, March/April, 1986.

Labbok M and Queenan JT: The use of periodic abstinence for family planning, Clin Obstet Gynecol 32(2):387, 1989.

Lee NC, Rubin GL, and Borucki R: The intrauterine device and pelvic inflammatory disease revisited: new results from the Women's Health Study, Obstet Gynecol, 72:1, 1988.

Liskin LS and Fox G: Periodic abstinence: how well do new approaches work, Popul Rep (I), no 3, 1981.

Liskin LS and Fox G: IUDs: an appropriate contraceptive for many women, Popul Rep (B), no 4, 1982.

Louv WC et al: J Infect Dis, 158:518, Sept, 1988.

Marrs RP: In vitro fertilization's future looks bright, Contemp OB/GYN 20:135, 1982.

Mattison DR et al: Effects of drugs and chemicals on the fetus, Contemp OB/GYN 33(3):164, 1989.

Medical Letter: Choice of contraceptives, Med Lett 30(779): whole issue, Nov 18, 1988.

Meirik O et al: Oral contraceptive use and breast cancer in young women: a joint national case—control study in Sweden and Norway, Lancet 1:650, 1986.

Menning B: Infertility: a guide for the childless couple, Englewood Cliffs, NJ, 1977, Prentice-Hall, Inc.

Mishell DR: Contraceptions, N Engl J Med 320 (12):777, 1989.

Morbidity, Mortality Weekly Report: Sexually transmitted diseases, MMWR 37:133, 1988.

NAACOG: Cervical cap enters North American market, NAACOG Newsletter, 15(9):1, 1988.

NAACOG: Statement: abortion, The Organization, 1989.

North, BB: Spermicides, J Reprod Med, 33:307, 1988.

Okamoto NJ: The Japanese American. In Clark A, editor: Culture—childbearing/health professionals, Philadelphia, 1978, FA Davis Co.

Ortiz ME and Croxatto HB: The mode of action of IUDs, Contraception, 36:37, 1987.
Ory SJ: Keeping up to date on donor insemination, Contemp OB/GYN 33(3):88, 1989.
Ostling RN: A bold stand on birth control. In Haas K and Haas A: Understanding sexuality, St Louis, 1987, Times Mirror/Mosby College Publishing.
ParaGard Intrauterine Copper Contraceptive model T-3804, Somerville, NJ, 1988, Gyno Pharm, Inc.
Pernoll ML and Benson RC, editors: Current obstetric and gynecologic diagnosis and treatment, ed 6, Los Altos, Calif, 1987, Appleton & Lange.
Peterson HB and Lee NC: The health effects of oral contraceptives: misperceptions, controversies, and continuing good news, Clin Obstet Gynecol 32(2):309, 1989.
Porter JB, Jick H, and Walker AM: Mortality among oral contraceptive users, Obstet Gynecol, 70:29, 1987.
Rabar FG et al: Ultrasonographic transvaginal ovum retrieval: a new approach to in vitro fertilization, AORN J 48(1):36, 1988.
Rietmeijer CAM et al: Condoms as physical and chemical barriers against human immunodeficiency virus, JAMA 257(17):2308, 1987.
Rock J et al: Effects of adoption on infertility, Fertil Steril 16:305, 1965.
Rosenberg MJ et al: Effect of the contraceptive sponge on chlamydial infection, gonorrhea, and candidiasis, JAMA 257(17):2308, 1987.
Royal College of General Practitioners' Oral Contraceptive Study: Oral contraceptives and gallbladder disease, Lancet 2:957, 1982.
Scott JR et al: Danforth's obstetrics and gynecology, ed 6, Philadelphia, 1990, JB Lippincott Co.
Seibel MM: A new era in reproductive technology: in vitro fertilization, gamete intrafallopian transfer, and donated gametes and embryos, N Engl J Med 318(13):828, 1988.
Speroff L et al: Clinical gynecologic endocrinology and infertility, Baltimore, 1983, Williams & Wilkins.
Spitz IM and Bardin CW: Progesterone antagonists on the horizon, Clin Obstet Gynecol 32(2):403, 1989.
Strom BL et al: Diaphragms, Ann Intern Med 107:816, 1987.
US Congress, Office of Technology Assessment, Artificial Insemination: Practice in the United States: Summary of a 1987 survey—background paper, OTA-BP-BA-48, Washington, DC, 1988, US Government Printing Office.
Veevers JE: The social meaning of parenthood, Psychiatry 36:291, 1973.
Vogel G: American Indian medicine, New York, 1973, Ballantine Books, Inc.
Washington AE et al: Oral contraceptives: *Chlamydia trachomatis'* infection, and pelvic inflammatory disease, JAMA 253:2246; 1985.
Whaley LF and Wong DL: Nursing care of infants and children, ed 4, St Louis, 1991, The CV Mosby Co.
Willson JR and Carrington ER: Obstetrics and gynecology, ed 8, St Louis, 1987, The CV Mosby Co.
Wolner-Hanssen P et al: Laparoscopic findings and contraceptive use in women with signs and symptoms suggestive of acute salpingitis, Obstet Gynecol 66:233, 1985.
Women's Health: Cervical cap approved for marketing, Am J Nurs AJN 89(2):165, 1989.
World Health Organization: Mechanism of action, safety, and efficacy of intrauterine devices, Technical Report Series 753, Geneva, 1987, World Health Organization.

Bibliography

Clinical News: Cervical cap approved for marketing, Am J Nurs 89(2):165, 1989.
Darney PD: Long-acting hormonal contraception, Contemp OB/GYN (special issue) 32:90, 1988.
Davis DC: A conceptual framework for infertility, JOGN Nurs 16(1):30, 1987.
DeMoya D and DeMoya A: Best contraceptive for paraplegic women, RN 48:56, Dec, 1985.
Dirubbo NE: The condom barrier, Am J Nurs 87(10):1306, 1987.
Few BJ: Treating endometriosis with naferekin, MCN 13(5):323, 1988.
Francis G and Nosek J: Ethical considerations in contemporary reproductive technologies, J Perinat Neonat Nurs 1(3):37, 1988.
Grimes DA: Contraception, Clin Obstet Gynecol 32(2):305, 1988.
Hirsch AM and Hirsch SM: The effect of infertility on marriage and self concept, JOGN Nurs 18(1):13, 1989.
Horsley JE: Can you refuse to assist in abortions? RN, p 65, May, 1987.
Itskovitz, J et al: Transvaginal ultrasonography-guided aspiration of gestational sacs for selective abortion in multiple pregnancy, Am J Obstet Gynecol 160(1):215, 1989.
Lethbridge DJ: The use of breastfeeding as a contraceptive, JOGN Nurs 18(1):31, 1989.
Lutwak RA, Ney AM, and White JE: Maternity nursing and Jewish law, MCN 13(1):44, 1988.
McBarnette L: Women and poverty: the effects on reproductive status, Women Health 12(3/4):55, 1987.
Milne BJ: Couples' experiences with in vitro fertilization, JOGN Nurs 17(5):347, 1988.
Nero FA: When couples ask about infertility, RN: p 26, Nov, 1988.
Nichol C: The birth control clinic: helping teens and young adults deal with sexuality, Can Nurse: p 24, Feb, 1989.
Panzarine S and Gould CL: Knowledge about contraceptive use and conception among a group of urban, black adolescent mothers, JOGN Nurs 17(4):279, 1988.
Peterson NF and Rhoe J: Endometriosis, AORN J 48(4):700, 1988.
Ponzetti NF and Hoefler S: Natural family planning: a review and assessment, Fam Community Health 11(2):36, 1988.
Research: Childbearing Cambodian refugee women, Can Nurse: p 46, June, 1988.
Rubin LN and Borucki R: The intrauterine device and pelvic inflammatory disease revisited: new results from the women's health study, Obstet Gynecol 72(1):1, 1988.
Sherrod RA: Coping with infertility: a personal perspective turned professional, MCN 13(3):191, 1988.
Sise BC: Maternal rights versus fetal interests: an ethical issue with nursing implications, J Prof Nurs 4(4):262, 1988.
Stubblefield PG: Choosing the best oral contraceptive, Clin Obstet Gynecol 32(2):316, 1989.
Tyrer LG and Salas JE: Contraceptive problems unique to the United States, Clin Obstet Gynecol 32(2):307, 1989.
Ullman K: A GIFT for infertile couples, Am J Nurs 87(9):1130, 1987.
Youngkin EQ and Miller LG: The triphasics: insights for effective clinical use, Nurse Pract 12(2):17, 1987.
Zion AB: Resources for infertile couples, JOGN Nurs 17(4):255, 1988.

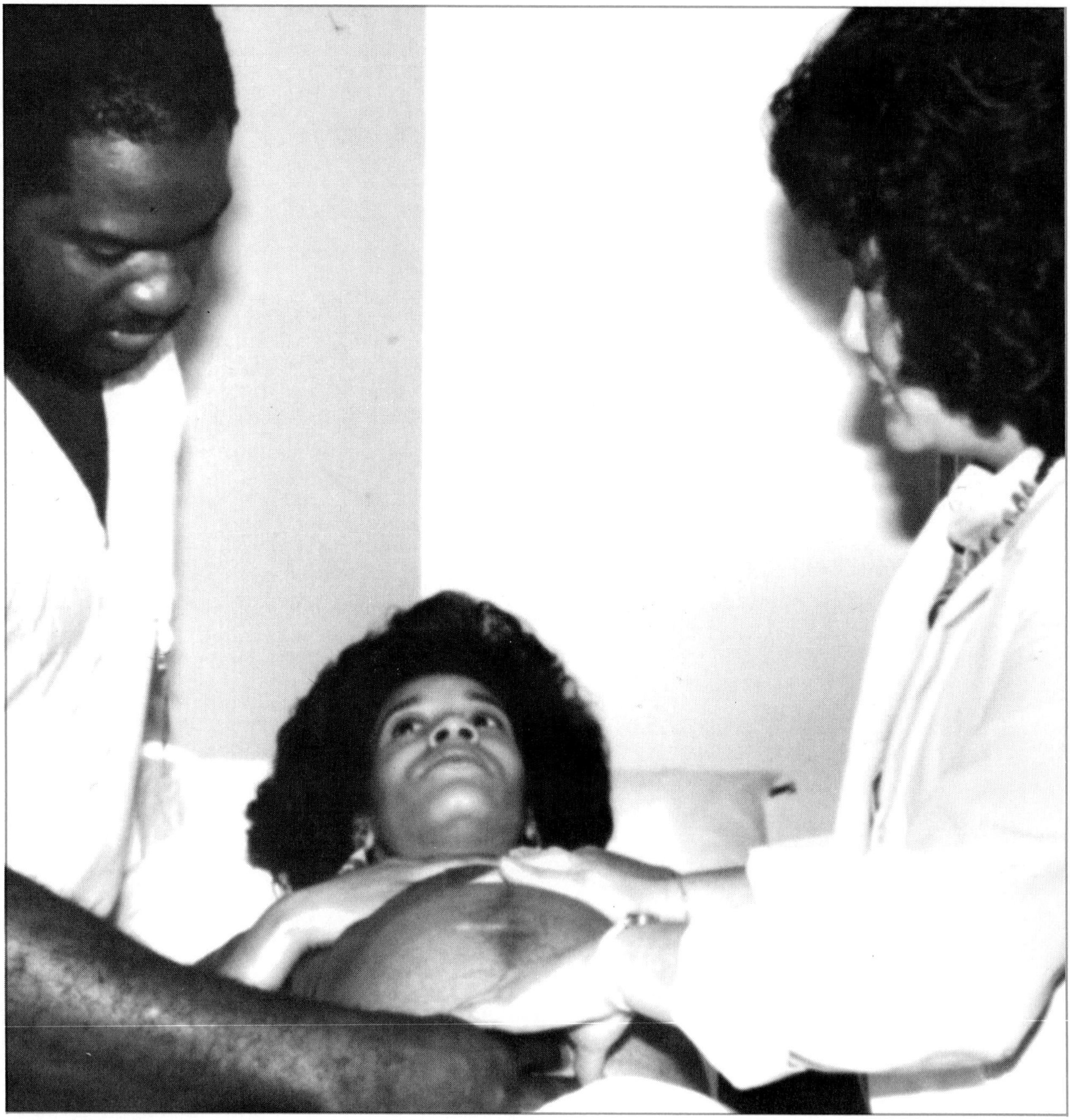

UNIT

II

NORMAL PREGNANCY

CHAPTER

7 Genetics, Conception, and Fetal Development

Irene M. Bobak

Learning Objectives

Correctly define the key terms listed.

Summarize the process of fertilization.

Explain the fundamental principles of genetics.

Discuss the functions of the placenta and amniotic fluid.

Identify at least three organs and tissues arising from each of the three primary germ layers.

Explain the importance of pulmonary surfactant and the L/S ratio.

Explore the potential effects of teratogens on the embryo and fetus week by week during gestation.

Key Terms

amniotic fluid
chorionic villi
chromosomes
decidua
ductus arteriosus
embryo
fertilization (conception)
fetal circulation
fetal heart rate (FHR)
fetal membranes
fetus
foramen ovale
gametogenesis
genes
gestational age
hematopoiesis
human chorionic gonadotropin (hCG)
implantation
karyotype
lanugo
last menstrual period (LMP)
lecithin/sphingomyelin (L/S) ratio
meconium
Mendel's laws
neural tube
placenta
placental barrier
quickening
surfactants
viability
zygote

The maternity nurse is in the unique position of providing nursing care to the unborn. Gravidas and their families have many questions about fetal development, such as "When is our baby due?" "How big is my baby now?" "My friend had a baby with blue eyes, but both of them have brown eyes. Is that possible?" These questions commonly crop up in childbirth classes and private conversations with the woman or her partner. The wide media coverage of substances that affect the unborn can be disturbing to parents. The knowledgeable nurse can advise parents based on understanding of conception and normal fetal development. This chapter is designed to help nurses answer these questions. It gives a brief overview of the genetic basis of inheritance and normal embryonic and fetal development from conception to full-term gestation.

❑ GENETIC BASIS OF INHERITANCE

The biologic and behavioral characteristics of each human being are determined by the action of thousands of minute particles of hereditary material contained within the nuclei of all living cells. Each of these particles or **genes,** has a specific function in the control or regulation of cellular activity. Alone or in combination with other genes, they are responsible for all human traits or characteristics, for the orderly pattern and timing of development from conception to death, and for continuity of the species through consistent transmission of these traits from generation to generation.

The genes are composed of tiny segments of *deoxyribonucleic acid* (DNA), which enables them to duplicate themselves exactly during cell division. Each body cell contains two sets of genes arranged in a line to form larger structures, the **chromosomes,** within the cell nucleus. Each cell nucleus contains two sets of chromosomes consisting of two matching sets of genes, one set obtained from each parent during the process of fertilization. When members of a pair of genes are alike and produce the same effect they are called *homozygous;* when they are not alike and produce different effects, they are said to be *heterozygous.*

Chromosomes cannot be seen except under a microscope. For analysis they are stained, magnified, and photographed. Then each individual chromosome is cut out and arranged in a **karyotype** (profile of an individual's chromosomes: their number, form, and size) according to size and shape. They appear as structures with either an X or a Y shape. Fig. 7-1 illustrates the chromosomes in a body cell.

Somatic cells (all the cells in the body except gametes) divide by the process of *mitosis,* in which the cell components, including the genetic material, divide and are distributed equally to the two newly formed cells. Each new cell contains the same composition and genetic potential as the original cell.

Gametogenesis

By the third week of development, primitive germ cells have formed in the human embryo. This is called **gametogenesis.** As early as the fifth week, these primitive germ cells may have migrated from the yolk sac to the developing gonads (Cunningham, MacDonald, and Gant, 1989). Oogenesis (formation of ova [singular, ovum]) and spermatogenesis (formation of sperm) share a basic process of maturation limited to germ cells. This process is a special cellular division known as meiosis (Fig. 7-2). During meiosis, the number of chromosomes in primary oocytes (oo = egg; cyte = cell) and spermatocytes is reduced by one half. Each cell usually contains 22 *pairs* of autosomes (non-sex–determining chromosomes) and one *pair* of sex-determining chromosomes. Collectively, these 46 chromosomes constitute the *diploid* number. Normal females (46,XX) have a total of 46 chromosomes: 44 autosomes and two sex-determining chromosomes, XX. Normal males (46,XY) have a total of 46 chromosomes: 44 autosomes and two sex-determining chromosomes, XY. After meiotic division, only 22 *single* autosomes and one sex-chromosome remain; this is known as the *haploid* number of chromosomes. The diploid number is restored at fertilization with the union of an X-bearing ovum and either an X-bearing or a Y-bearing sperm.

If the mature ovum (23,X) is fertilized by a sperm with a Y chromosome, the result will be a male zygote (46,XY); if the ovum is fertilized by a sperm bearing an X-chromosome, a female zygote (46,XX) will be produced. Thus the male supplies the genetic material (an X or a Y chromosome) that determines the sex of the child.

Spermatogenesis in the male gonad is a continuous process that begins about the time of puberty and lasts until senescence (see Fig. 7-2). Unlike spermatogenesis,

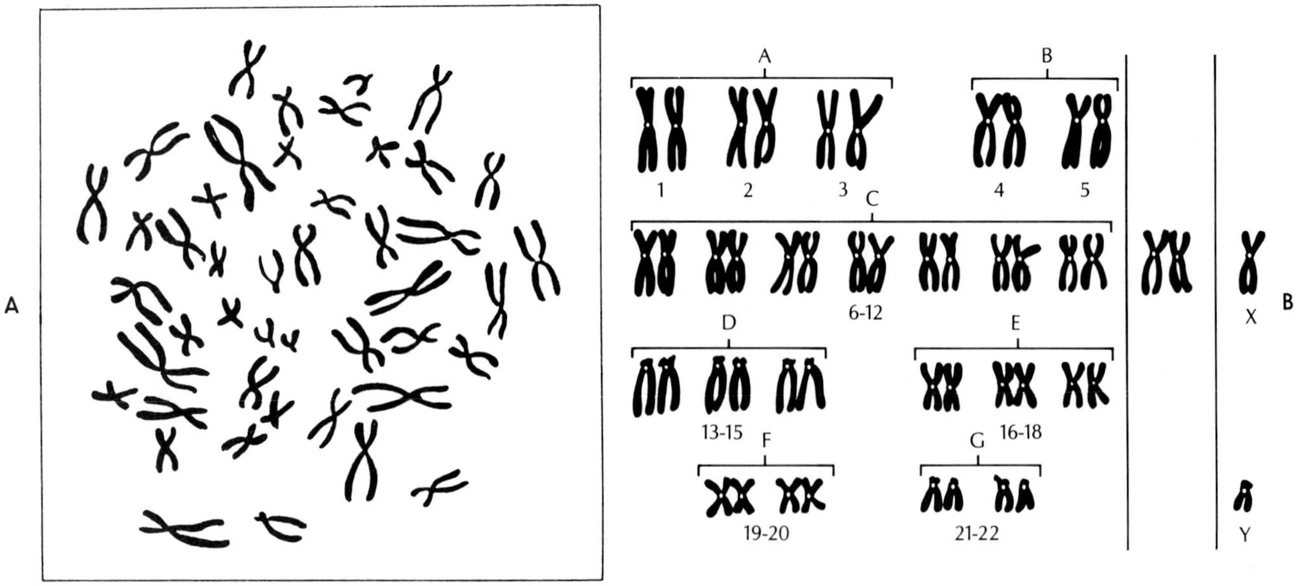

Fig. 7-1 Chromosomes during cell division. **A,** Example of photomicrograph. **B,** Chromosomes arranged in karyotype; female and male sex-determining chromosomes.

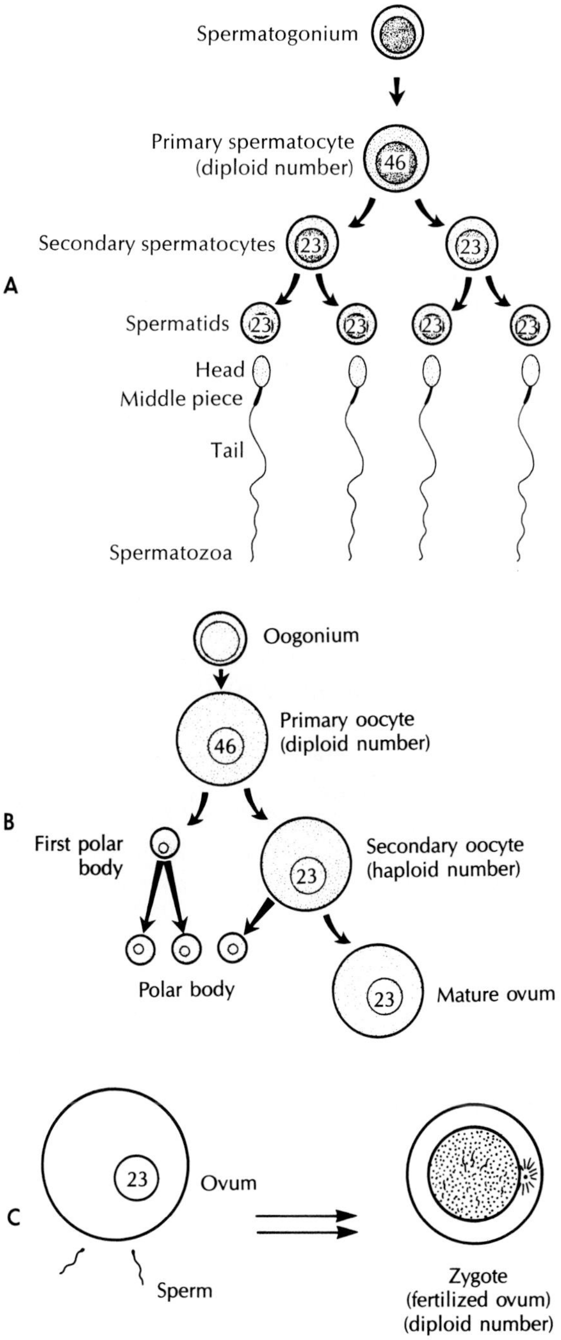

Fig. 7-2 **A,** Spermatogenesis. Gametogenesis of the male produces four mature gametes, the sperm. **B,** Oogenesis. Gametogenesis in the female produces one mature ovum and three polar bodies. Note the relative difference in overall size between the ovum and sperm. **C,** Fertilization results in the single-cell zygote and the restoration of the diploid number of chromosomes.

the process of oogenesis in the ovaries is not a continuous process. Oogenesis begins during intrauterine life. The female gametes have already enlarged and developed into primary oocytes at the time of birth (see Fig. 7-2). There may be an estimated 2 million primary oocytes present at birth, but only about 300,000 are found in prepubertal girls (Baker, 1978, as cited by Cunningham, MacDonald, and Gant, 1989). These primary oocytes have begun the first meiotic (reduction) division but remain suspended at this stage until, one at a time (usually) they are stimulated to complete meiosis. The ovum (Fig. 7-3) does not complete the second meiotic division until triggered by the entrance of the sperm at fertilization. At the moment when the sperm and the ovum meet and form a zygote (fertilized ovum) (see Fig. 7-2, C), the sex of the new human is determined, and the blueprints for the growth, development, and maturation of a new individual are laid down.

Genetic Transmission

Mendel's Laws. Mendel's laws of gene activity during gamete formation and fertilization are the foundation of the science of genetics. Generally, the nurse will not be the one who does in-depth genetic counseling, but a general knowledge of Mendel's laws in the transmission of heritable characteristics is an essential tool for health workers.

Mendel's laws are the basic principles of inheritance based on the breeding experiments of garden peas by the nineteenth century Austrian monk Gregor Mendel. These are usually stated as two laws, commonly called the *law of segregation* and the *law of independent assortment.* According to the first, each characteristic of a species is represented in the somatic cells by a pair of genes that separate during meiosis so that each gamete receives only one gene for each trait. According to the second law, the members of a gene pair on different chromosomes segregate independently from other pairs during meiosis, so that the gametes show all possible combinations of factors. Genes on the same chromosome are affected by linkage and segregate in blocks according to the amount of crossing over that occurs; a discovery made after Mendel.

Linkage refers to the location of two or more genes on the same chromosome so that they do not segregate independently during meiosis but tend to be transmitted together as a unit. The concept of linkage, which opposes the independent assortment theory of mendelian genetics, led to the foundation of the modern chromosome theory of genetics. Crossing over refers to the exchange of sections of chromosomes between homologous pairs of chromosomes during the prophase stage of the first meiotic division. The process results in the recombination of genes.

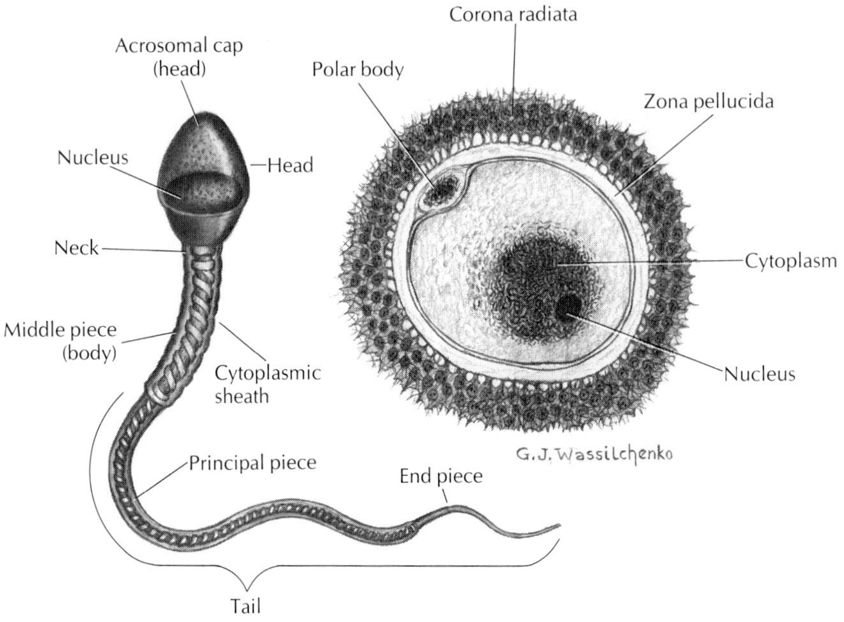

Fig. 7-3 Sperm and ovum.

Dominance is a basic principle stating that not all genes determining a given trait operate with equal vigor. If two genes at a given locus produce a different effect, as eye color, they compete for expression. The gene that is manifest is dominant; it masks the effect of the other gene, which is recessive. Recessive describes a gene the effect of which is masked or hidden if there is a dominant gene at the same locus. If both genes are recessive and produce the same trait, the trait is expressed in the individual. A recessive trait is a genetically determined characteristic that is expressed only when present in the homozygotic state. In the example in Fig. 7-4, brown eye color (shaded area) is dominant over blue (white area); blue eye color is recessive. One recessive gene comes from each parent carrier who may not show the trait. The line between the circles is the mating bar. The vertical line from the marriage bar identifies the offspring and the genetic combinations possible.

Chromosomal abnormalities may occur during either mitotic or meiotic division, resulting in too much genetic material in some cells or too little in others. Abnormalities in chromosomal structure or number occur in both autosomal and sex chromosomes.

Autosomal Defects. *Down's syndrome* (mongolism) is the most commonly occurring autosomal defect. In 95% of cases of mongolism, nondysjunction occurs during meiosis (usually in the female germ cell) of chromosome number 21. This results in germ cells carrying 24 or 22 chromosomes. Cells with 22 chromosomes are nonviable. When the ovum with 24 chromosomes is fertilized, an individual with 47 chromosomes results. Trisomy 21 (three of chromosome number 21) carries the clinical characteristics of Down's syndrome (Fig. 7-5): small, round head with flattened occiput; large fat pads at nape of short neck; protruding tongue; small mouth and high palate; epicanthal folds with slanting palpebral fissures (mongoloid slant of eyes); hypotonic muscles with hypermobility of joints; short, broad hands with inward curved little finger and wide separation between thumb and index finger; transverse simian palmar crease; and mental retardation. Feeding problems arise from poor sucking ability, and there is a greater risk for upper respiratory tract infections.

The incidence of this type of chromosomal aberration increases with maternal age: in young mothers, 1 per 1000 to 2000 births; in women from 35 to 40 years of age, 1 per 300 births; and in mothers over 45 years of age, 1 per every 30 to 35 births.

In about 5% of cases, Down's syndrome is the result of translocation of a portion of a chromosome or mosaicism. Translocation Down's syndrome is more common in younger mothers. In this circumstance, there are 46 total chromosomes but part of chromosome number 21 is added to another chromosome, usually number 14. Such a child exhibits the same clinical features as in trisomy 21. Mothers of these babies are at greater risk for the recurrence of the disorder in subsequent pregnancies.

Mosaicism is a condition in which some somatic cells are normal, whereas others have trisomy 21. The

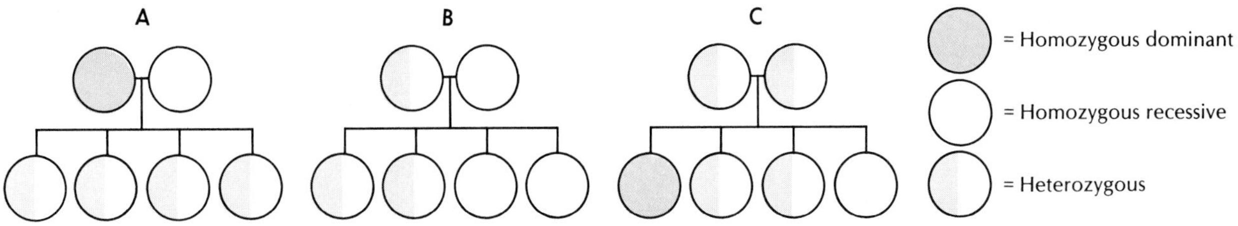

Fig. 7-4 Possible offspring in three types of matings. **A,** Homozygous-dominant parent and homozygous-recessive parent. Children all heterozygous, displaying dominant trait. **B,** Heterozygous parent and homozygous-recessive parent. Children 50% heterozygous display dominant trait; 50% homozygous display recessive trait. **C,** Both parents heterozygous. Children 25% homozygous display dominant trait; 25% homozygous display recessive trait; 50% heterozygous display dominant trait.

number of abnormal cells determines the degree to which characteristic clinical features of Down's syndrome are expressed.

It should be noted that children with Down's syndrome and their siblings are more prone to develop leukemia. The basis for this fact is unknown.

Cri du chat syndrome is the result of partial deletion of a portion of chromosome number 5. An infant with this disorder can easily be identified by his unique cry. *Cri du chat* is a French phrase meaning "cry of a cat," which aptly describes the child's weak, high-pitched, "meow-like" cry. These children have small heads with widely spaced eyes, are profoundly retarded mentally, and fail to thrive.

Sex Chromosome Defects. Deletion of a sex chromosome may go unnoticed until adolescence or later when the individual seeks counseling for infertility. In Turner's syndrome, the dwarfed female has only 45 chromosomes (44 + X). This defect results in stunted growth, "streak ovaries," and occasionally perceptual problems. A zygote with 45 chromosomes and a single Y chromosome is nonviable.

Males with 47 chromosomes (44 + XXY **karyotype**) (Klinefelter's syndrome) can appear to be normal, but others are mentally retarded and infertile.

Individuals with 48 chromosomes (karotypes: female, 44 + XXXX; male, 44 + XXXY) generally have severe mental and physical abnormalities.

Individuals with 45 chromosomes, that is, lacking the second X chromosome or the Y chromosome (44 + XO), are hermaphrodites. They may possess genital organs of both sexes, and the diagnosis may be difficult or impossible by examination of external genitals alone (see Fig. 28-50).

Recessive Trait Transmission. Some diseases that are recessive in nature may be carried in the heterozygous state by persons who may seem clinically normal (e.g., cystic fibrosis). In instances of recessive trait transmission, the probability of appearance of the trait

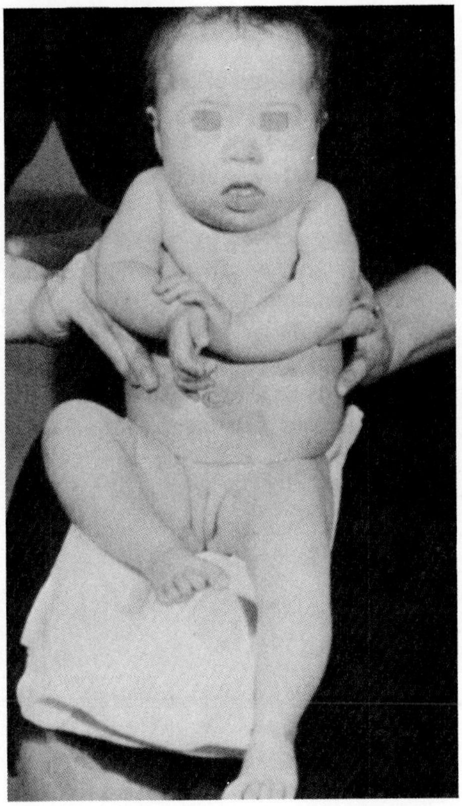

Fig. 7-5 Infant with Down's syndrome. (Courtesy Frederick Hecht, MD.)

in each offspring is only 1:4 or 25%. Despite this favorable risk factor, it is possible for each offspring of a couple to be homozygous for the recessive trait.

Most structural disorders of the infant result from dominant genes, whereas inborn errors of metabolism are primarily the expression of recessive genes (see below).

Some autosomal recessive genes do exert their influence in the heterozygous carrier. The carrier of a recessive gene for *cystic fibrosis* may be more prone to respiratory problems throughout his life. Persons with *sickle cell trait* may have less stamina and resilience to physiologic stress such as excessive physical exertion, infection, and high altitude. Women with *sickle cell disease* may have more pregnancy complications and should never receive general anesthetic agents. Women with the disease or the trait should be cautioned against the use of oral contraceptives because the risk of complications is greatly increased.

Sex-linked Transmission. A trait that is carried on a sex chromosome (usually the X chromosome) is known as sex linked (or X linked) and may be dominant or recessive. Mendelian laws prevail in the patterns of transmission. However, unlike autosomes, sex chromosomes are dissimilar in morphology and gene complement (Fig. 7-6). Therefore the pattern of transmission will be affected depending on the sex of the individual. The female sex chromosomes (XX) are homologous, that is, females are heterozygous or homozygous for genes at all loci (or sites) on the X chromosomes. The male sex chromosomes, one X and one Y, are not homologous. Males with only one X chromosome are hemizygous (having only one gene) with no counterpart on the Y chromosome (see Fig. 7-6). The single genes on the male's X chromosome are therefore always expressed. One indication for an X-linked (sex-linked) trait is a pedigree that shows no father-to-son transmission of that trait.

Inborn Errors of Metabolism. Disorders of protein, fat, or carbohydrate metabolism reflecting absent or defective enzymes generally follow a recessive pattern of inheritance. Enzymes, the actions of which are genetically determined, are essential for all the physical and chemical processes that sustain body systems. Defective enzyme action interrupts the normal series of chemical reactions from the affected point onward. The result may be an accumulation of a damaging product such as phenylalanine or the absence of a necessary product such as thyroxin or melanin. (See Appendix G for screening tests for inborn errors of metabolism.)

Phenylketonuria (PKU) is an uncommon disorder caused by autosomal recessive genes. Heterozygous carriers and affected infants may be identified by genetic screening methods. A deficiency in the liver enzyme phenylalanine hydroxylase results in failure to metabolize the amino acid phenylalanine, allowing its metabolites to accumulate in the blood. The incidence of this disorder is 1 per every 10,000 to 20,000 births. The highest incidence is found in whites (from northern Europe and the United States). It is rarely seen in Jewish, African, or Japanese populations.

Tay-Sachs disease, inherited as an autosomal recessive trait, results from a deficiency of hexosaminidase.

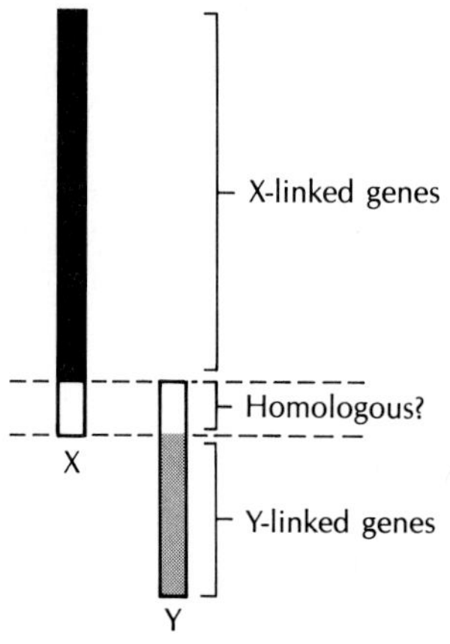

Fig. 7-6 X and Y chromosomes.

It occurs primarily in Jewish families. Until 4 to 6 months of age, infants appear normal; in fact, these infants are considered very beautiful. Then the clinical symptoms appear: apathy and regression in motor and social development and decreased vision. Death occurs between 3 and 4 years of age. There is as yet no known treatment for Tay-Sachs disease. In subsequent pregnancies amniocentesis may be performed on women who have delivered infants with this condition.

Cystic fibrosis (mucoviscidosis or fibrocystic disease of the pancreas) is inherited as an autosomal recessive trait characterized by generalized involvement of exocrine glands. Clinical features are related to the altered viscosity of mucus-secreting glands throughout the body. It is a serious chronic disease occurring primarily in whites but can appear in those of mixed ancestry. Overall incidence is 1 per every 2000 births. It is thought that the carrier state is 1:20 to 25. Advances in diagnosis and treatment have improved the prognosis so that now many affected individuals live to adulthood. Some affected women have borne children, but men generally are sterile.

Meconium ileus occurs in about 10% of newborns with cystic fibrosis. Although an initial stool may be passed from the rectum with none thereafter, no meconium is usually passed during the first 24 to 48 hours, the abdomen becomes increasingly distended, and eventually the newborn requires a laparotomy for diagnosis and treatment of the condition.

Polygenic Trait Transmission. The inheritance pattern for many congenital abnormalities is not clear, but they often cluster in families. The abnormalities may be the result of additive effects of aberrant genes at separate loci on several chromosomes. The recurrence risk varies with the number of members of a family who have the disorder. Some congenital abnormalities in this category are cleft lip, cleft palate, spina bifida and other neural tube defects, and pyloric stenosis.

❑ FERTILIZATION (CONCEPTION)

During sexual intercourse, 2.5 to 3.5 ml (range: 1 to 10 ml) of semen, usually containing approximately 70 sperm per ml is ejaculated into the female vagina. Sperm reach the site of fertilization shortly (often only 5 minutes) after ejaculation, but on the average, a time of 4 to 6 hours seems more reasonable. Of the millions of sperm ejaculated only about 200 reach the ampulla (Cunningham, MacDonald, and Gant, 1989). By flagellar movement the sperm make their way through the fluids of the cervical mucus (if the mucus is receptive), across the endometrium, and into the uterine tube to meet the descending ovum in the ampulla of the tube (see Chapter 4 for further discussion).

Before fertilization the sperm undergo a physiologic change called *capacitation* and a structural change called *acrosome reaction.* Capacitation refers to the removal of a protective coating from the sperm. Enzymes produced by the lining of the uterine tubes assist in capacitation of the sperm. The acrosome reaction refers to the small perforations that form in the anterior head of the sperm. Enzymes (e.g., hyaluronidase) escape through these perforations and digest a path for the sperm through the corona radiata and zona pellucida of the ovum. Only one sperm is required for actual fertilization, but the presence of many increases the chances for one to penetrate.

Fertilization (conception), the fusion of a *sperm* and an *ovum* (oocyte), is a process that requires about 24 hours. To fertilize an egg the sperm must pass through the *corona radiata* and *zona pellucida* and enter the egg; then female and male pronuclei undergo changes that result in a **zygote** (see Fig. 7-2, **C**).

In general, the process of fertilization takes place as follows. The cells of the corona radiata are dispersed by enzyme action of tubal mucosa and sperm. With the aid of its tail movements, the sperm can pass through this outermost covering of the egg. The acrosomes of several sperm release enzymes that digest a pathway through the zona pellucida. One sperm (usually) attaches to and fuses with the egg's plasma membrane, which then breaks down at the point of contact. At the moment that a sperm makes contact with the egg's plasma membrane, the oocyte reacts in two ways: a "zona reaction" (as yet not understood) occurs, preventing the entry of more sperm, and the oocyte matures (its nucleus is now known as the female pronucleus). The head and tail of the sperm enter the egg, leaving the sperm's plasma membrane (cytoplasmic sheath) attached to that of the oocyte. The tail of the sperm degenerates rapidly; its head enlarges to form the male pronucleus. The female and male pronuclei come together in the center of the oocyte and lose their cell membranes.

The fertilized ovum begins to divide, differentiate, and grow into a person, a replica of humanity's continuing generations and yet a unique individual. The growth that takes place from conception to birth is more rapid than at any other time in a person's life. The zygote weighs 15 ten-millionths of a gram; a 7-pound term baby weighs about 3175 g. In those 9 months the zygote increases in size by more than 200 billion times.

Multifetal Pregnancy

Twins. Twins most commonly result from the fertilization of two ova. The dizygotic (di = two; zygote = fertilized ovum) fertilization yields "fraternal" twins. One third as often, twins develop from a single fertilized ovum. Subsequently this zygote divides into two similar individuals called monozygotic (*mono* = one) or "identical" twins.

Dizygotic or fraternal twins are not true twins. They are the result of the maturation of two ova during one ovulatory menstrual cycle. Two ova are fertilized at the same time or within hours of each other. The resulting twins may be of the same sex or of different sexes. They are no more alike genetically than brothers or sisters born at different times. Dizygotic twins always have two amnions and two chorions, but the chorions and placentas may be fused (Fig. 7-7).

Monozygotic or identical twins are true twins since they result from the division of one zygote into two equivalent or more or less separate individuals. Identi-

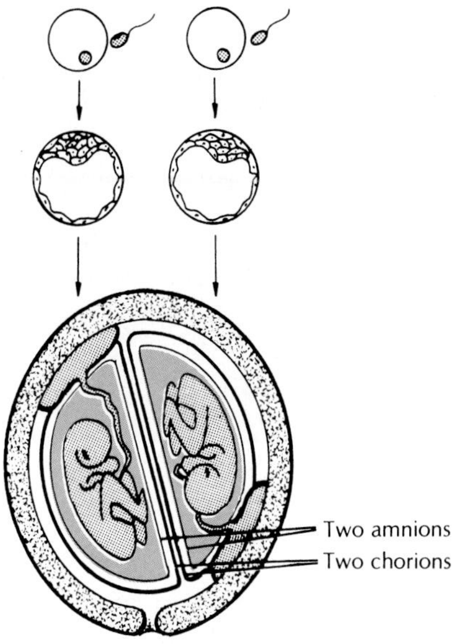

Fig. 7-7 Formation of dizygotic twins. There is fertilization of two ova, two implantations, two placentas, two chorions, and two amnions. (From Whaley LF: Understanding inherited disorders, St Louis, 1974, The CV Mosby Co.)

cal (monozygotic) twins are not always identical. The division of one zygote does not necessarily result in equal sharing of protoplasmic materials. However, there is an equal sharing of chromosomes.

A fertilized ovum may divide at various stages of development (Fig. 7-8). If it divides within 72 hours after fertilization, two embryos, two amnions, and two chorions will result. There may be two distinct placentas or one fused placenta. If division occurs between the fourth and eighth days after fertilization, the two embryos and two amnions will be covered by a single chorion. Division that occurs after about eight days results in two embryos within one amnion and chorion. Such twins are rarely delivered alive because the umbilical cords are commonly entangled so that circulation ceases and one or both fetuses die. Later division results in an incomplete cleavage (separation or division) of the embryonic disk and conjoined (united) twins are formed. In the United States, united or conjoined twins are commonly referred to as Siamese twins.

The frequency of dizygotic twins is related to race, heredity, maternal age and parity, and the use of fertility drugs. The incidence of monozygotic twinning remains relatively constant worldwide at about 1 set per 250 births (Cunningham, MacDonald, and Gant, 1989). Monozygotic twinning is largely independent of race, heredity, and maternal age and parity. Use of ovulation induction for impaired infertility (Chapter 6) almost doubles the incidence of monozygotic twinning (Derom et al, 1987).

The true frequency of twinning is not known, however. The use of ultrasound in early pregnancy has revealed an incidence of multifetal pregnancies much higher than figures based on the birth of two fetuses. Robinson and Coines (1977) identified twin pregnancies in 30 women. Of these, only 14 eventually gave birth to twins. It may be that some women who are diagnosed with threatened abortion early in their pregnancies may be experiencing an actual abortion of one embryo from an unrecognized twin gestation (Cun-

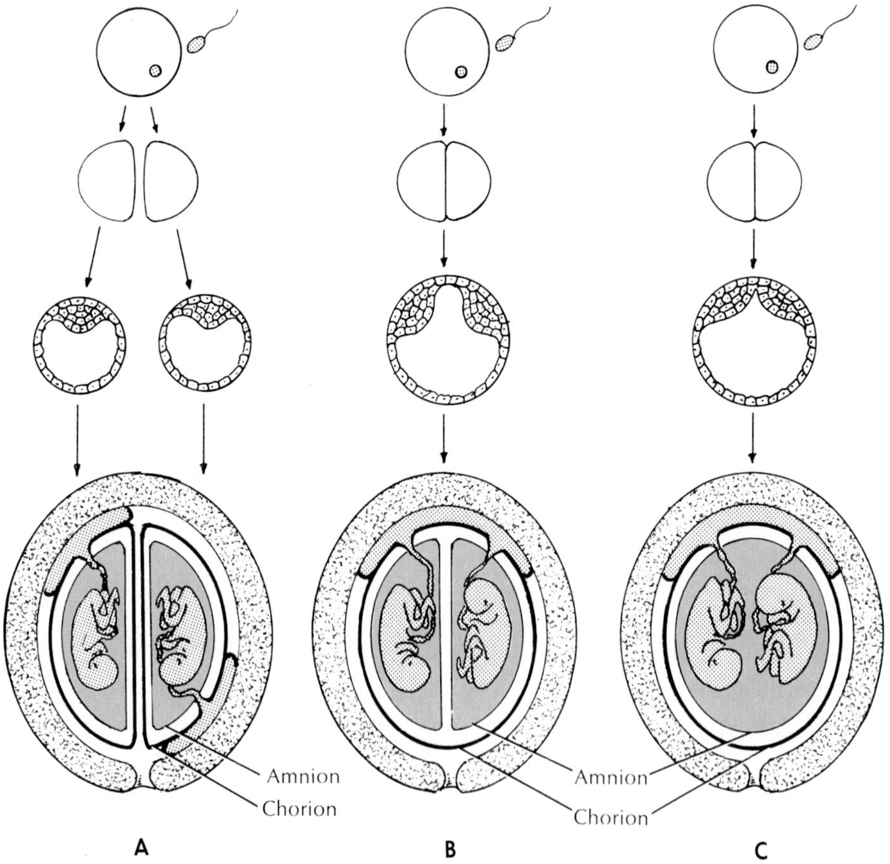

Fig. 7-8 Formation of monozygotic twins. **A,** One fertilization: blastomeres separate, resulting in two implantations, two placentas, and two sets of membranes. **B,** One blastomere with two inner cell masses, one fused placenta, one chorion, and separate amnions. **C,** Later separation of inner cell masses, with fused placenta, and single amnion and chorion. (From Whaley LF: Understanding inherited disorders, St Louis, 1974, The CV Mosby Co.)

ningham, MacDonald, and Gant, 1989). Fetal death even as late as the end of the first trimester (first 3 months) of pregnancy may be followed by a complete resorption of the fetus leaving no evidence of its existence at the time of the birth of the remaining twin (Cunningham, MacDonald, and Gant, 1989).

The incidence of multifetal pregnancies varies among different *races*. White women experience the birth of twins in 1 out of every 100 pregnancies; and for black women, 1 out of every 79 pregnancies results in the birth of twins. Twinning is less common among Asian women, occurring only once in every 155 births (Cunningham, MacDonald, and Gant, 1989). The *heredity* (genotype) *of the mother* is more important than that of the father. In one study, women who were dizygotic twins gave birth to twins at a rate of 1 set per 58 births; if the father was a dizygotic twin the rate was 1 set per 126 pregnancies (race and age were not specified) (Cunningham, MacDonald, and Gant, 1989). *Maternal age* and *parity* also affect the incidence of twinning. For any increase in age up to about 40, or parity up to 7, the frequency of twinning increased (Waterhouse 1950, as cited in Cunningham, MacDonald, and Gant, 1989). *Maternal size* seems to be related to the rate of twinning. MacGillivray (1986) found that dizygotic twinning is more common in large and tall women than in small women. Nutrition rather than body size may be the underlying factor. *Ovulation induction* (e.g., clomiphene) is likely to increase both monozygotic and dizygotic twinning.

Other Multifetal Pregnancies. *Triplets* occur once in about 7600 pregnancies and may be derived from (1) one zygote and be identical, (2) two zygotes and consist of identical twins and a single infant, or (3) three zygotes and be of the same sex or of different sexes. In the last case, the infants are no more similar than those from three separate pregnancies. Similar possible combinations occur in *quadruplets, quintuplets, sextuplets, septuplets,* and so forth. Types of multifetal births higher than triplets are rare. They have occurred more often in recent years following ovulation induction or in vitro fertilization (Chapter 6).

Implantation (Nidation)

The ovum is released from the ovary at ovulation and passes into the uterine tube where it is met and fertilized by a sperm. After conception the zygote, propelled by ciliary action and irregular peristaltic contractions, starts to move through the uterine tube into the uterine cavity (Fig. 7-9). During the 3- to 4-day period it takes to travel down the uterine tube, the zygote begins a process of rapid cell division called *mitosis,* or *cleavage.* The initial division of the zygote results in two *blastomeres* which subsequently divide into progressively smaller blastomeres. At the end of 3 to 4 days, the developing individual comprises about 16 blastomeres arranged in a ball-like structure called a *morula.* After the morula enters the uterus, a cavity forms within the dividing cells, changing the morula into a *blastocyst.* The blastocyst remains free in the uterus for 1 or 2 days, and then the exposed cells of the *trophoblast* (cellular wall of the blastocyst) implant, generally in the endometrium of the anterior or posterior fundal region. A common attachment site is the posterior uterine wall.

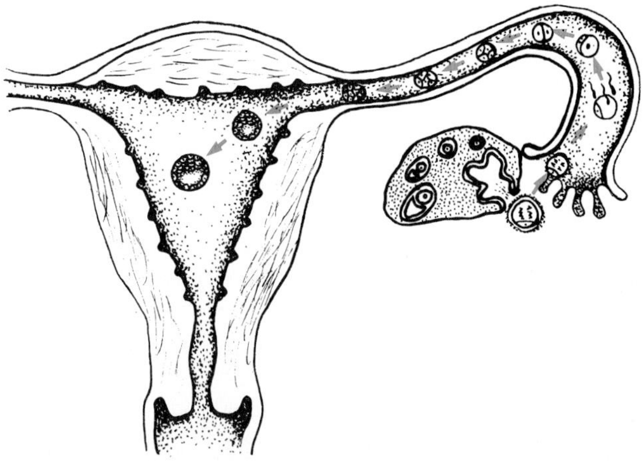

Fig. 7-9 Diagrammatic summary of the ovarian cycle, fertilization and development during the first week. (See Fig. 7-11, day 14 since LMP, and week 1.)

Cells of the attaching portion of the trophoblast secrete proteolytic (causing breakdown of proteins) and cytolytic (causing breakdown of cells) enzymes to help them burrow their way into the compact layer of the endometrium. This burrowing into the endometrium is called **implantation,** or *nidation.* Slight bleeding, called *implantation bleeding,* occurs in some women. Trophoblastic burrowing usually stops before it reaches the myometrium. About 7 to 10 days elapse between fertilization and the completion of implantation.

During the first few weeks after implantation, trophoblasts (primary villi) appear over the entire blastodermic vesicle. Trophoblasts are vascular processes that have the power of cytolysis and are able to tap maternal blood vessels as sources of nourishment and oxygen for the embryo. These villi are the first stage of the developing **chorionic villi** (fingerlike projections) that secrete the **human chorionic gonadotropin hormone** (**hCG**) and synthesize proteins and glucose for approximately 12 weeks. By 12 weeks, the fetal liver can supply its own glucose and insulin. The hCG stimulates continued secretion of progesterone and estrogen by the corpus luteum, thus preventing ovulation and menstruation during pregnancy.

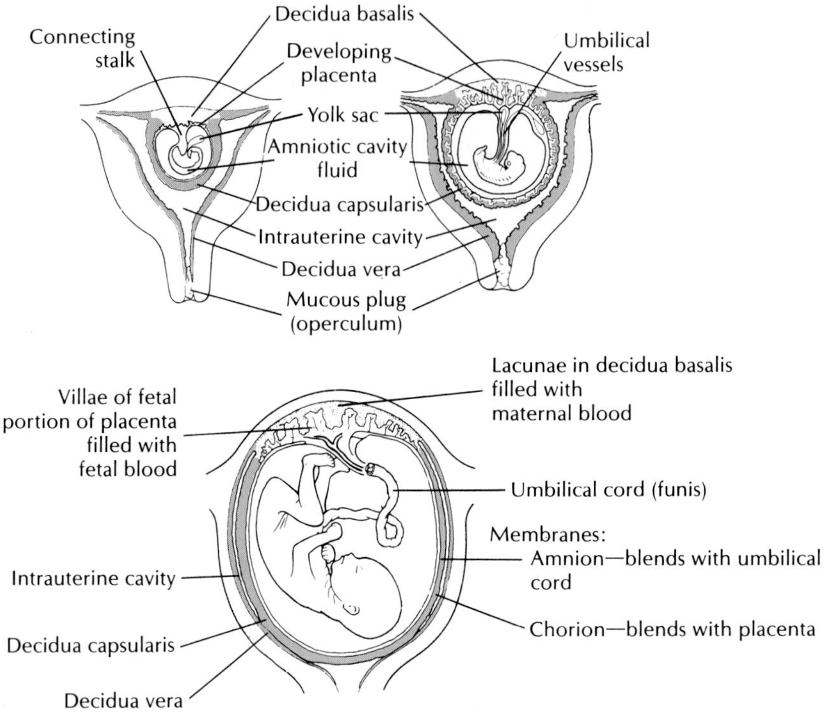

Fig. 7-10 Development of fetal membranes. Note gradual obliteration of intrauterine cavity as decidua capsularis and decidua vera meet. Also note thinning of uterine wall. Chorionic and amnionic membranes are in apposition to each other but may be peeled apart.

Chorionic villi invasion of the endometrium by enzyme action occasionally opens a maternal vein and artery causing lacunae (small blood lakes) in the decidua basalis. This rich blood supply causes the adjacent villi to multiply rapidly. These villi become the *chorion frondosum,* or fetal portion, of the future placenta.

Decidua. As part of the morphologic changes in the endometrium during the secretory phase (phase of the corpus luteum) of the menstrual cycle (see Fig. 7-11, week 1), the blood vessels enlarge and the entire lining becomes more succulent and richer in glycogen. After conception the vascularity of the uterine wall increases greatly under the influence of the ovarian hormones, principally progesterone. After implantation, the endometrium is called the **decidua,** which means "to cast off," or "to discard," since this lining of the endometrium *is* cast off in a vaginal discharge called lochia (Chapter 19).

The decidua is divided into three areas (Fig. 7-10): vera (parietalis), capsularis, and basalis. The *decidua basalis* is the portion of the decidua vera where nidation takes place; that is, the area where chorionic villi invade the maternal blood vessels and develop into the placenta, usually in the posterior uterine wall.

❑ GESTATION

Time Units

The chronology of pregnancy may be referred to in several ways, for example, 10 lunar months (of 4 weeks each), 40 weeks of gestation, or 9 calendar months (3 trimesters of 3 months each). *In this chapter, conceptional age in weeks refers to the time since fertilization.* In clinical practice however, the term **gestational age,** or menstrual age, refers to the time since the first day of the **last menstrual period (LMP).**

There is a difference of 2 weeks in calculating the duration of pregnancy, depending on the reference point used (Table 7-1). Calculation from the LMP (for a 28-day cycle) is 2 weeks longer than that from the time of fertilization. A graphic representation of the differences is seen in Fig. 7-11. The first square is "day 1 of menses" or day 1 of LMP. Note that 2 weeks pass before fertilization. These 2 weeks are added when discussing menstrual age of the pregnancy. The third row of squares identifies the onset of development after fertilization on the first day of the third week of the menstrual cycle.

The date of birth is calculated as about 266 days after fertilization, or 280 days after the onset of the last

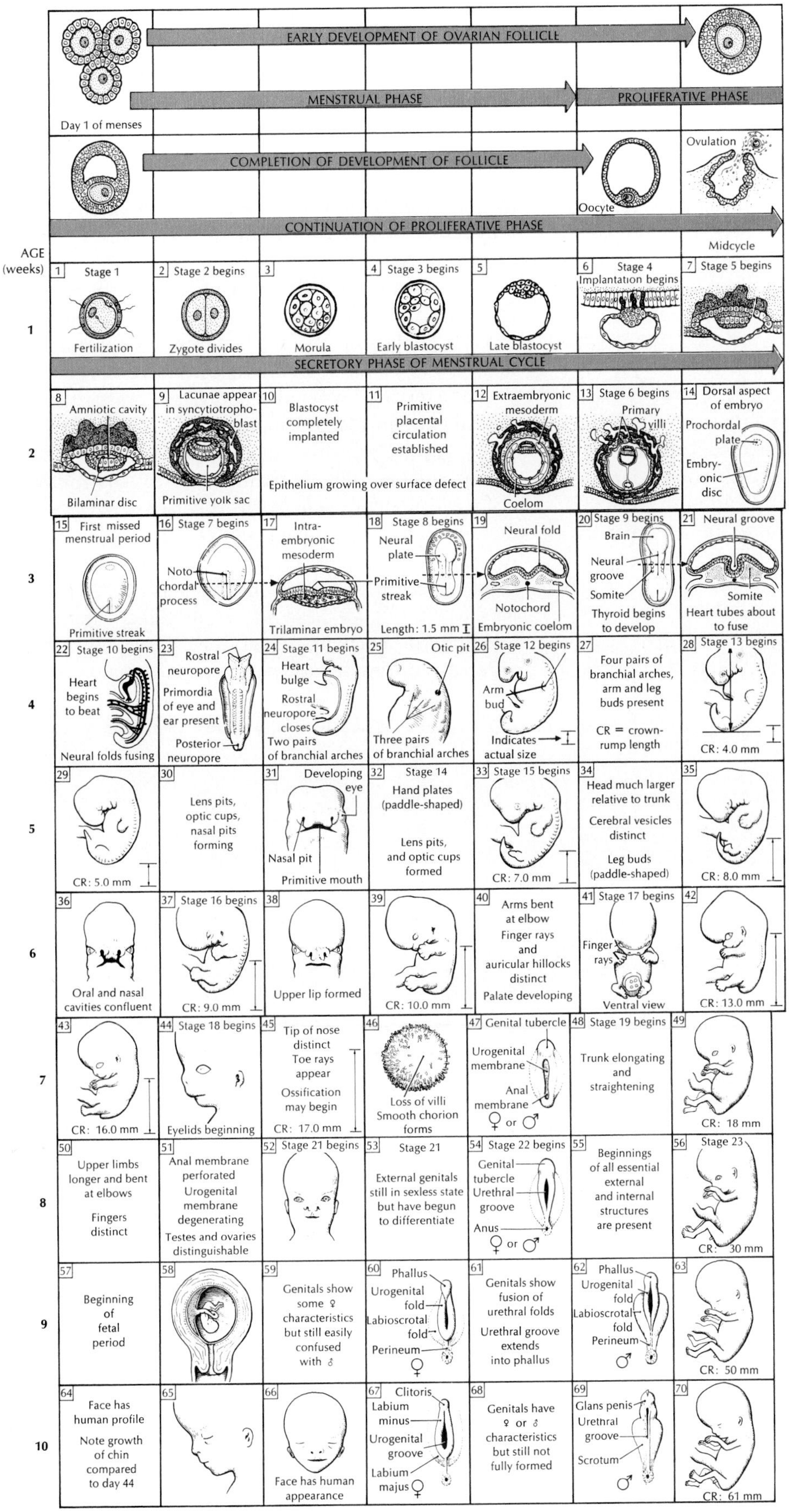

Fig. 7-11 Timetable of human prenatal development from LMP and weeks 1 to 10 following fertilization. Within large boxes are small boxes with numbers in upper left corner. These numbers refer to days since fertilization. (From Moore KL: The developing human: clinically oriented embryology, ed 2, Philadelphia, 1977, WB Saunders Co.)

Table 7-1 Comparison of Gestational Time Units

	Reference Point	
	Fertilization	Last Menstrual Period (LMP)
Days	266	280
Weeks	38	40
Calendar months	8¾	9
Lunar months	9½	10

From Moore KL: Before we are born: basic embryology and birth defects, Philadelphia, 1974, WB Saunders Co.

normal menstrual period (LNMP). From fertilization to the end of the embryonic period, age is best expressed in days. Thereafter age is commonly given in weeks. Because ovulation and fertilization are usually separated by not more than 12 hours, these events are more or less interchangeable in expressing prenatal age.

Developmental Stages

The fusion of the nuclei of the two gametes is called conception or fertilization. Fusion initiates the first of the three stages of human prenatal development: ovum, embryo, and fetus.

The conceptus is called an *ovum* during the period from conception until primary villi appear. Villi appear approximately 12 to 14 days after fertilization or about 4 weeks since LMP (see "primary villi" in Fig. 7-11, week 2, day 13). By the end of this period, implantation (nidation) is complete. The conceptus is totally within the endometrium and is covered by surface epithelium.

The organism is called an **embryo** during the period from the end of the ovum stage until it measures approximately 3 cm (2.5 in) from crown to rump, normally 54 to 56 days (10 weeks since LMP). This period is characterized by rapid cell division and is the most critical time in the development of an individual (Fig. 7-12). All the principal organ systems are being established and are highly vulnerable to environmental agents (e.g., teratogens such as viruses, drugs, radiation, or infection). There are at least two means by which malformations of embryos and fetuses can result from exposure to teratogenic agents. Such teratogens may cause cellular necrosis, or they may destroy cell function by biochemical paralysis. Developmental interference during this time can result in major congenital (existing before birth) abnormalities (Chapters 23, 24, 28, and Appendix F). By the end of this period the

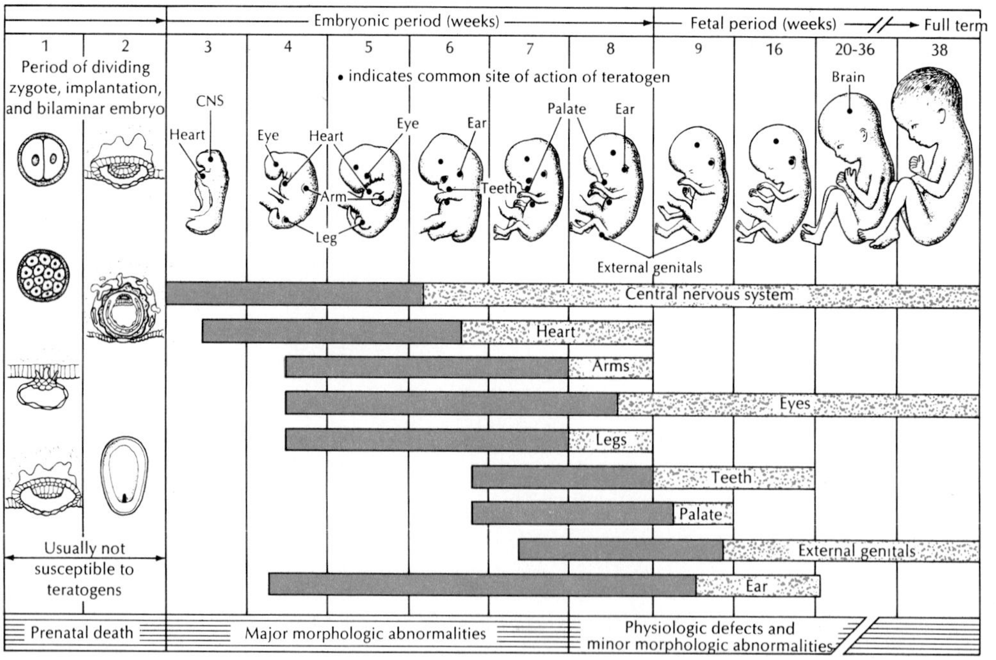

Fig. 7-12 Sensitive or critical periods in human development. Solid color denotes highly sensitive periods; stippled color indicates stages that are less sensitive to teratogens. (From Moore KL: The developing human: clinically oriented embryology, ed 2, Philadelphia, 1977, WB Saunders Co.)

beginnings of all the main systems have been established. The embryo attains characteristics that establish it as unquestionably human and is then referred to as a **fetus,** a Latin word meaning *offspring.*

The embryo becomes a fetus at the end of the embryo stage and remains a fetus until the pregnancy is terminated (see Fig. 7-11, week 9, day 57). Changes occurring during the fetal period, although important, are not as dramatic as those in the preceding period, because the fetus is less vulnerable to the teratogenic effects of drugs, viruses, or radiation—*malformations.* However, these noxious agents may interrupt normal *functional development* of organs, especially the central nervous system (Fig. 7-12).

Viability

The capability of a fetus to survive outside the uterus at the earliest gestational age is called **viability.** Until recently it was believed that viability was reached when the fetus weighed more than 1000 g and had reached at least 28 weeks' gestational age. Improvement in maternal and neonatal care now suggests that a new standard of viability must be established. On the basis of the limits of available clinical technology, current published literature about fetal lung development, and the age at which the respiratory system is capable of supporting satisfactory gas exchange, fetal viability can be first expected at approximately 20 to 22 weeks' gestation since fertilization (22 to 24 weeks since LMP). Since there is a problem with accuracy in estimating gestational age, it is difficult to establish definite criteria.

Survival outside the uterus depends on two factors: (1) the maturity of the fetal central nervous system (CNS) for directing rhythmic respirations and controlling body temperature and (2) the maturity of the lungs.

❑ EMBRYONIC DEVELOPMENT

Placenta

The maturing **placenta** (Greek for "flat cake") develops into 15 or 20 subdivisions called *cotyledons.* Each of these is partially separated from other cotyledons by fenestrated septa (windowed partitions); thus in essence each cotyledon is a functioning unit.

The placenta develops after the third week of gestation. Growth of the thickness of the placenta continues until 16 to 20 weeks' gestation. The placental circumference continues growing until later pregnancy. The fully developed placenta *(afterbirth)* is a reddish, discoid organ 15 to 20 cm (6 to 10 in) in diameter and 2.5 to 3 cm (about 1 in) thick (Fig. 7-13). The weight of a term placenta is 400 to 600 g (1 lb to 1 lb, 5 oz) or approximately one sixth the weight of the newborn. About four fifths of the placenta by weight is of fetal origin; the remainder is maternal.

The maternal surface of the placenta, the area originally adherent to the decidua basalis of the uterus, is rough and beefy red. The cotyledons stand out as segments with shallow clefts between. The fetal surface of the placenta is shiny and slightly grayish. The umbilical vessels that enter the cord can be seen as a branching system just beneath the membranes (Fig. 7-13). The fetal membranes cover the fetal surface of the placenta and extend from the placental margins to envelop the fetus and its amniotic fluid.

In multifetal pregnancy, one or more placentas will be present. The number depends on the number of fertilized ova and the manner of ovum segmentation (see discussion of multifetal pregnancy).

Functions. The placenta has many unique properties. Most of these properties—endocrine, metabolic, and immunologic—are derived from the trophoblasts. Understanding placental functions gives insight into prenatal life and is helpful in providing nursing care to the unborn and the newborn.

Placental function depends almost entirely on maternal circulation. Maternal circulation depends on the woman's blood pressure, condition of her blood vessels, maternal position, and uterine contractions. *Optimum circulation to the placenta and fetus is possible when the woman is lying on her left side* (see Fig. 15-9).

During pregnancy a new group of *protein* hormones of placental origin is seen. One of these, hCG, is the basis for pregnancy tests.

The hCG also prevents the corpus luteum from involuting at the end of the menstrual cycle. It causes the corpus luteum to secrete estrogen and progesterone that is needed to maintain the pregnancy until the placenta begins production of these hormones. The hCG reaches maximum levels approximately 50 to 70 days after fertilization.

Steroid hormones include estrogens and progesterone. Among the actions of placental hormones are the maintenance of pregnancy and the initiation of labor.

The intervillous space serves as the depot from which materials are transferred actively or passively through the chorionic epithelium to the fetal vessels. In this space substances from the fetus enter the maternal circulation. Because this process of transfer supplies the fetus with oxygen, as well as nutrients, and provides for elimination of metabolic waste products, the chorionic villi and the intervillous space function as a lung, gastrointestinal tract, and kidney for the fetus.

"The placenta and fetus appear to defy the laws of transplantation immunology" (Cunningham, MacDonald, and Gant, 1989). "The placenta corresponds to a natural homograft in that it is a transplant of living tissue within the same species, yet it does not normally evoke the usual immune response reaction to homografts, resulting in destruction and rejection of the graft" (Willson and Carrington, 1987). This quality of the placenta is of major interest. If the "secret" of the placenta can be unlocked, the problem of rejection in organ transplants and other immune phenomena may be eliminated.

Two layers of cells separate maternal and fetal circulation for the first 12 weeks of gestation. During the second and third trimesters, only one cell layer separates the two blood streams. This so-called **placental barrier** is a partial (semipermeable) barrier; it provides only limited protection to the fetus. Throughout pregnancy it either actively or passively permits, facilitates, and adjusts the amount and rate of transfer of a wide range of substances to the fetus.

Placental Transfer. The placenta is a complex organ of transfer. Its major function is to transfer oxygen and a great variety of nutrients from the mother to the fetus. Conversely, it conveys carbon dioxide and other

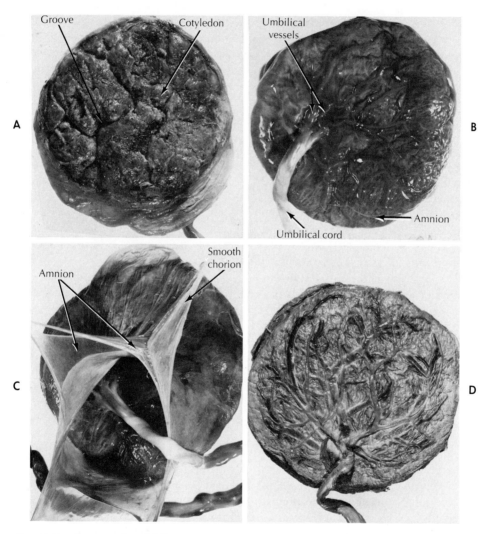

Fig. 7-13 Photographs of full-term placenta. **A,** Maternal (or uterine) surface, showing cotyledons and grooves. **B,** Fetal (or amniotic) surface showing blood vessels running under amnion and converging to form umbilical vessels at attachment of umbilical cord. **C,** Amnion and smooth chorion are arranged to show that they are (1) fused and (2) continuous with margins of placenta. **D,** Placenta with a marginal attachment of the cord, often called a *battledore placenta* because of its resemblance to bat used in medieval game of battledore and shuttlecock. (From Moore KL: The developing human: clinically oriented embryology, ed 2, Philadelphia, 1977, WB Saunders Co.)

metabolic wastes from the fetus to the mother. The placenta, and to a limited extent the attached membranes, supply all material for fetal growth and energy production while removing all products of fetal catabolism.

There is no continuous direct communication between the fetal blood in the vessels of the chorionic villi and the maternal blood in the intervillous space. Although maternal and fetal circulations are independent, development of occasional breaks in the chorionic villi permits the escape of varying numbers of fetal erythrocytes into the maternal circulation. This *leakage* is the clinically significant mechanism by which some Rh-negative women become sensitized by the erythrocytes of their Rh-positive fetus (see Chapter 28). The transfer of substances from mother to fetus and from fetus to mother depends on a variety of conditions (e.g., maternal blood saturation, rate of maternal-fetal-placental blood flow, lipid solubility, electrical charge, molecular size, and placental mass).

Most substances with a molecular weight less than 500 can diffuse readily through the placental tissue. Molecular weight clearly has a bearing on the rate of transfer by diffusion; generally the smaller the molecule, the more rapid is the rate. Diffusion, however, is not the only mechanism of transfer of compounds with a low molecular weight. The placenta actually facilitates the transfer of a variety of such compounds, especially those that are in low concentration in maternal plasma but that are essential for the rapid growth of the fetus.

Simple diffusion appears to be the mechanism involved in the transfer of oxygen, carbon dioxide, water, and most but not all electrolytes. Anesthetic gases are highly lipid soluble and pass through the placenta within minutes of administration by simple diffusion, according to the concentration gradient.

Steroid hormones from the adrenal glands and hormones from the thyroid may cross the placenta but do so at slow rates. Substances of high molecular weight do not usually traverse the placenta, but there are pronounced exceptions, such as immune γ-globulin G (IgG) with a molecular weight of about 160,000. IgG crosses the placenta with considerable efficiency. All four major subclasses of IgG appear to cross the placenta from mother to fetus but whether by the same or different transport systems is not clear. Near term, the immunoglobulin IgG is present in approximately the same concentrations in cord and maternal sera. IgA and IgM of maternal origin are effectively excluded from the fetus.

Although diffusion is an important method of placental transfer, the chorionic villus exhibits enormous selectivity in transfer, maintaining different concentrations of a variety of metabolites on the two sides of the villus.

Selectivity may occur by *active transport* and *pinocytosis*. Active transport results in the transfer of glucose, amino acids, calcium, iron, and other substances of higher molecular weight. Pinocytosis is a mechanism by which minute particles, including free fatty acids, may be engulfed and carried across the cell. Albumin and γ-globulin are transported by pinocytosis.

The concentrations of a number of substances that are not synthesized by the fetus are several times higher in fetal blood than in maternal blood. *Ascorbic acid* is one example of this phenomenon. The concentration of ascorbic acid is two to four times higher in fetal plasma than in maternal plasma.

The unidirectional transfer of *iron* across the placenta provides another example of the unique capabilities of the human placenta for transport. Iron is transported actively from maternal to fetal plasma, and in the human fetus the amount transferred appears to be independent of maternal iron status (Cunningham, MacDonald, and Gant, 1989).

Because of their small size, some viruses traverse the placenta with ease; the larger bacteria rarely involve the fetus except when inflammation of the placenta develops.

Many viruses, including those responsible for rubella, chickenpox, measles, mumps, vaccinia, poliomyelitis, cytomegalic inclusion disease, coxsackie virus disease, parvovirus B19, and western equine encephalitis, may cross the placenta and infect the fetus. *Treponema pallidum*, Lyme disease (a spirochete, *Borrelia burgdorferi*), *Toxoplasma* and *Plasmodium* species, and *Mycobacterium tuberculosis* may similarly produce intrauterine infection. With protozoal and bacterial, but not necessarily viral, infections, there is almost always histologic evidence of involvement of the placenta (Cunningham, MacDonald, and Gant, 1989).

Many drugs cross the placenta readily (e.g., caffeine, alcohol, nicotine, carbon monoxide, pesticides, the over 1000 other toxic substances and gases* inhaled from cigarette smoke, antibiotics, antihistamines, sedatives, analgesics, narcotics, and anesthetics). Most drugs promptly cross the placenta, and many are harmful to the human fetus. Examples of these drugs are given in Appendix F. *Because medications, as well as vaccines and excessive amounts of certain vitamins, may contain elements harmful to the fetus, all but essential medications should be avoided, particularly during the first trimester.*

*Hydrogen cyanide is present in cigarette smoke. This is the same gas used to execute prisoners in gas chambers.

Fetal Membranes

Two closely applied but separate membranes line the uterine cavity and surround the developing embryo-fetus (Fig. 7-14). Both **fetal membranes,** the *amnion* (inner membrane) and the *chorion* (outer membrane), arise from the zygote. As the chorion develops, it blends with the fetal portion of the placenta; the amnion blends with the fetal umbilical cord, or *funis*. These deceptively strong, translucent membranes contain not only the fetus but also the amniotic fluid, and they are continuous with the margins of the placenta.

The outer membrane, the chorion, forms a large portion of the connective tissue thickness of the placenta on its fetal side. It is the structure in and through which the major branching umbilical vessels travel on the surface of the placenta. Ordinarily the chorion does not have a fetal blood supply except in the case of velamentous insertion of the cord. Its vascular support is primarily provided by blood vessels arising from the decidua. On its fetal surface it is juxtaposed to the outer layer of amnion.

The inner avascular membrane, the amnion, is bathed by amniotic fluid on one side and on the other side is contiguous with the chorion laeve. The umbilical cord originates from the amnion. Direct communication between the fetus and avascular amnion is established by way of the amniotic fluid. There is some evidence to support the formation of large quantities of prostaglandins by amnion cells. Fetal urine appears to stimulate PGE_2 production by amnion cells. Thus the fetal kidney and fetal urine appear to be important components of a fetal signal in the initiation and maintenance of labor in women (Cunningham, MacDonald, and Gant, 1989).

Amniotic Fluid

During pregnancy the **amniotic fluid** volume increases at an average rate of 25 ml per week during the first trimester, and 50 ml per week during the second trimester. The full-term fetus is immersed in about 1000 ml (range of 800 to 1200 ml) of clear, slightly yellowish liquid that has a faint characteristic (not foul) odor. The specific gravity of amniotic fluid is 1.007 to 1.025, and the pH is neutral to slightly alkaline (7.0 to 7.25). It contains albumin, urea, uric acid, creatinine, lecithin, sphingomyelin, bilirubin, fat, fructose, inorganic salts, epithelial cells, a few leukocytes, various enzymes, and lanugo hairs. Amniotic fluid, *replaced every 3 hours,* is thought to have multiple origins and a composition that changes during pregnancy. Early in pregnancy it probably originates from maternal serum, but as pregnancy proceeds, a greater proportion of it is derived from fetal urine.

Amniotic fluid accomplishes numerous functions for the fetus, including the following:

1. Protects the fetus from direct trauma by distributing and equalizing any impact the mother may receive
2. Separates the fetus from the fetal membranes
3. Allows freedom of fetal movement and permits musculoskeletal development
4. Facilitates symmetric growth and development of the fetus
5. Protects the fetus from the loss of heat and maintains a relatively constant fetal body temperature
6. Serves as a source of oral fluid for the fetus (the fetus swallows up to 400 ml/day)
7. Acts as an excretion-collection repository for substances from the fetal urinary, respiratory, and alimentary tracts

There is still much to be learned about amniotic fluid. However, study of its components has provided a great deal of knowledge about the sex, state of health, and maturity of the fetus. Amniocentesis (Chapter 22) has made it possible to detect diseases and abnormalities that may suggest the options of therapeutic abortion or intrauterine treatment.

There is great variation within the normal volume; however, more than 2 L (hydramnios) or less than 300 ml (oligohydramnios) is usually associated with fetal disease or abnormality (see Chapter 22).

Umbilical Cord

The umbilical cord (funis) is the lifeline that links the embryo and the placenta. It extends from the umbilicus to the fetal portion of the placenta and is attached either centrally or eccentrically. At term this light gray, smooth, vascular attachment is 50 to 55 cm long, slightly longer than the fetus, and is approximately 2 cm in diameter.

The surface of the cord is composed of thin squamous epithelium and is an extension of the skin of the fetus; however, *it contains no pain receptors.* The cord normally contains two umbilical arteries and one umbilical vein. The vein carries oxygenated blood to the fetus, and the arteries return deoxygenated blood to the placenta. Commonly these vessels are longer than the cord and consequently become coiled on themselves, giving the cord a lumpy appearance. They are supported by a loose connective tissue containing a cushioning mucoid material called Wharton's jelly. This jelly prevents kinking of the cord in utero and interference with circulation to the fetus.

Approximately 400 ml of blood flows through the cord every minute. The pressure exerted by this rapid flow makes the cord relatively stiff and not flexible as it

Text continued on p. 180.

Fig. 7-14 Summary of fetal development, maternal events, common discomforts, examples of remedies, and drug substances to avoid. (From Safe passage: A woman's guide to a healthier pregnancy, McNeil Consumer Products Co., Fort Washington, Pennsylvania.)

Week 1	Week 2	Week 3	Week 4	Week 5	Week 6	Week 7	Week 8
Baby's Development The ovum becomes fertilized, divides and burrows into the uterus.	The embryonic disk (ectoderm, entoderm, mesoderm) is formed. These three primitive germ layers will generate every organ and tissue in your baby's body.	The first body segments appear, which will eventually form the primitive spine, brain and spinal cord.	Heart, blood circulation and digestive tract take shape. The embryo is now one-fifth of an inch long, the head one-third of its total length.	The heart starts to pump blood; limb buds appear. Major divisions of the brain can now be discerned.	Eyes begin to take shape; external ears develop from skin folds.	Development is proceeding rapidly. The face is now complete with eyes, nose, lips and tongue — even primitive milk teeth. Tiny bones and muscles appear beneath the thin skin.	The embryo is now a little more than an inch long, its tiny heart beating at about 40-80 times a minute.

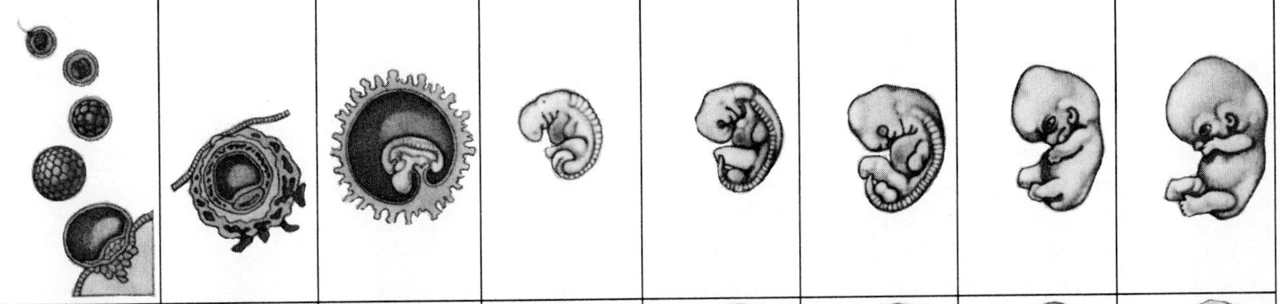

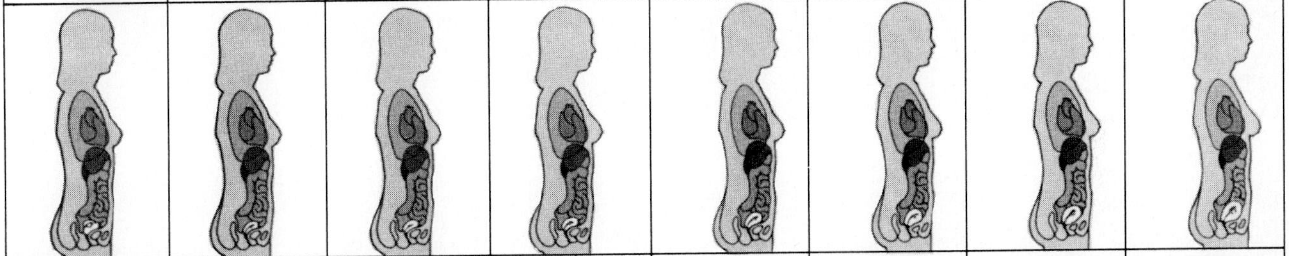

	Week 1	Week 2	Week 3	Week 4	Week 5	Week 6	Week 7	Week 8
Maternal Events	Ovaries increase production of "pregnancy maintaining" hormone, progesterone.	First missed period	Placenta grows to cover one-fifteenth of the uterine interior. Breast may begin to feel tender. No weight gain.			Exchange of fetal and maternal metabolites begins across the placenta, yet the two circulations are completely separate.	No noticeable weight gain.	The placenta now covers about one-third of the uterus lining.
Common Discomforts			**Morning sickness** occurs because increased hormonal activity slows down your digestive system, apparently to enhance the absorption of nutrients for your baby.	**Fatigue** is thought to be caused by a change in ovarian hormone production (progesterone and relaxin), the purpose of which is to relax pelvic ligaments, stimulate breast growth, and soften the cervix.		**Urinary frequency** is caused by the uterus compressing the bladder against the pelvic bones, thus reducing its capacity. Also by hormonal changes which affect the water balance in your body.		
Remedies			Eat a few dry crackers before arising. Frequent, small, low-fat meals during the day should also help. Drink liquids between meals.	Exercise regularly, get plenty of sleep with frequent naps during the day		You can decrease pressure on the bladder at night by sleeping on your side. Also, drink no fluids after 6 p.m.		
Drug Substances to Avoid			**Antiemetics** • cyclizine (Migral® Marezine®) • meclizine (Antivert®, Bonine®) • trimethobenzamide (Tigan®) (Avoid throughout pregnancy)	**Stimulants** • amphetamines • excessive caffine (Avoid throughout pregnancy)				
Acceptable Alternatives	None: Avoid all drugs not prescribed by a physician for a specific condition. Avoid X-rays.							

Fig. 7-14—cont'd. Summary of fetal development, maternal events, common discomforts, examples of remedies, and drug substances to avoid. (From Safe passage: A woman's guide to a healthier pregnancy, McNeil Consumer Products Co., Fort Washington, Pennsylvania.)

	Week 9	Week 10	Week 11	Week 12	Week 13	Week 14	Week 15	Week 16
Baby's Development	Genitalia is now well defined; the baby's sex is determined. Eyelids finish forming and seal shut. The embryo has become a fetus.	The fetus assumes a more human shape as the lower body rapidly develops. Blood and bone cells form. The first movements begin.	Organs begin to function. The pancreas is producing insulin; the kidneys, urine.	The lungs have taken shape; primitive breathing motions begin. The swallowing reflex has been mastered as the fetus sucks its thumb while floating weightlessly in the amniotic fluid.		The musculoskeletal system has matured. The nervous system begins to exercise some control over the body; blood vessels rapidly develop.	With hands ready to grasp, the fetus — now weighing about 7 ounces — kicks restlessly against the amniotic sac.	All organs and structures have been formed and a period of simple growth begins.

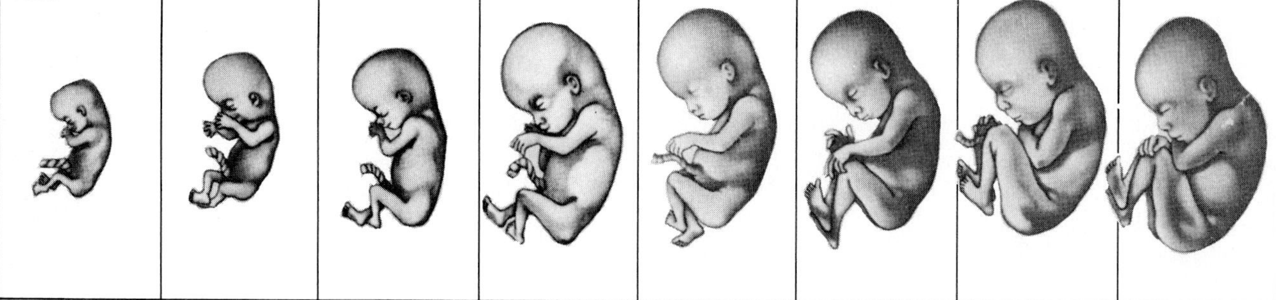

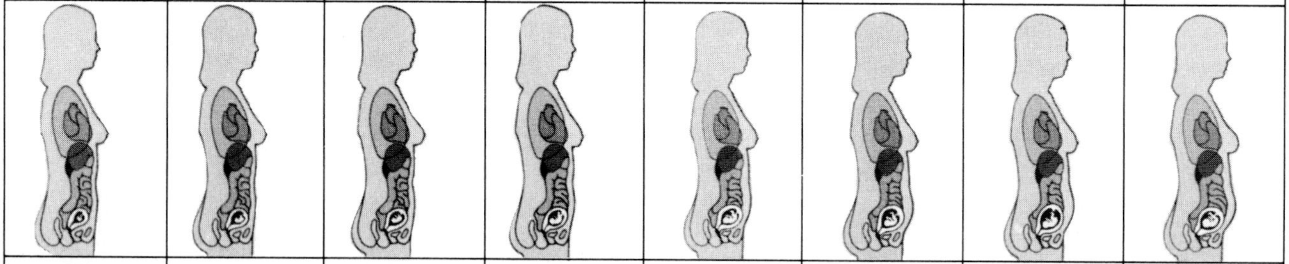

	Week 9	Week 10	Week 11	Week 12	Week 13	Week 14	Week 15	Week 16
Maternal Events	Maternal blood volume has increased 30-40%.	The sensation of these first movements has been described by some women as if something were blowing bubbles through a straw in their stomachs.	2-3 lb weight gain. Possible increase in perspiration.	The placenta has reached complete functional maturity, acting as the baby's lungs, kidneys, liver, digestive and immune systems.		3-4 lb weight gain. Belly beginning to show.		The fetal heartbeart can now be heard with an amplified stethoscope. Placenta begins producing the estrogen hormone.
Common Discomforts		**Sleeplessness** may result from the discomfort or anxieties of pregnancy.				Vaginal secretions are the result of an increased supply of blood and glucose to the vaginal mucosa. Severe itching, irritation and malodor suggest an infection is present.		**Headaches** may occur while your body becomes adjusted to changes in blood volume and vascular tone. Emotional tension may also be a factor.
Remedies		A glass of warm milk before bedtime can work wonders. It's also good for your baby!				If infection is suspected, consult a health professional. Otherwise, cleanse daily with warm water, keeping the area dry to prevent chafing. Apply yogurt for vulvar itch.		Change body positions slowly. Resting with a damp cloth on the forehead helps some women. Drinking milk and/or eating a small snack also produces relief in some.
Drug Substances to Avoid		• tranquilizers • narcotics • antihistamines • alcohol • barbiturates (Avoid throughout pregnancy)				Vaginal Anti-infectives • metronidazole (Flagyl®) (Avoid throughout pregnancy)		**Analgesics** • salicylates (aspirin) • phenacetin/caffeine • propoxyphene (Darvon®) • Indomethacin (Indocrin®) **Tranquilizers** (Avoid throughout pregnancy)
Acceptable Alternatives	None: Avoid all drugs not prescribed by a physician for a specific condition. Avoid X-rays.					• AVC™ Cream • Nystatin vaginal tablets (Mycostatin®) • Miconazole vaginal cream (Monistat®)		**TYLENOL®** brand acetaminophen

	Week 17	Week 18	Week 19	Week 20	Week 21	Week 22	Week 23	Week 24
Baby's Development		An oily coating protects the fetus. Fine hair covers the body and keeps the oil on the skin.	Eyebrows, eyelashes and head hair develop.	The fetus is now following a regular schedule of sleeping, turning, sucking and kicking—and has settled upon a favorite position within the uterus.		The skeleton is developing rapidly as the bone-forming cells increase their activity.	Eyelids begin to open and close.	The fetus now weighs about 27 ounces.
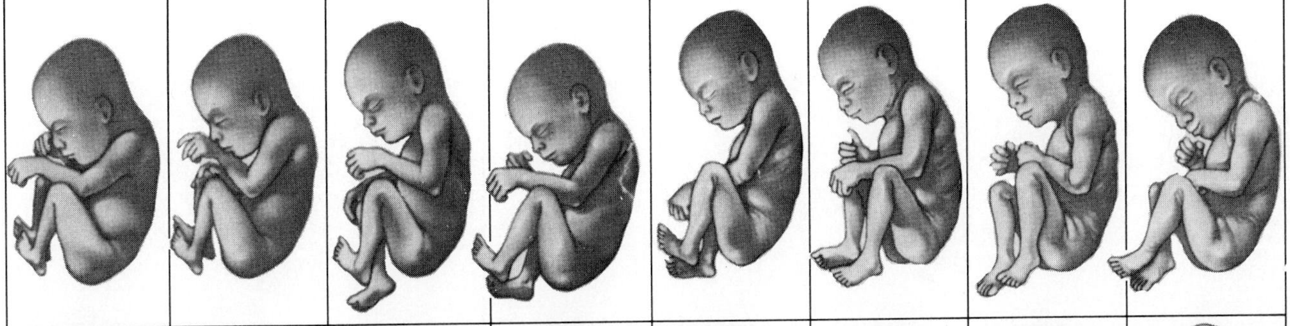								
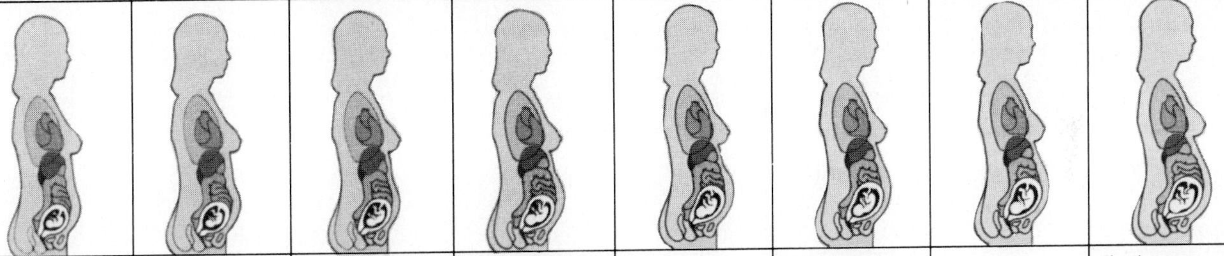								
Maternal Events		3-4 lb weight gain.	Breasts begin secreting colostrum in preparation for nursing.	The placenta reaches its largest size relative to the fetus, covering one-half of the uterine lining. There is 400 ml of fluid now present in the amniotic sac.		3-4 lb weight gain.		The placenta becomes thicker rather than wider. Mother can now sense when baby's awake.
Common Discomforts		**Faintness or dizziness** when standing suddenly. This is caused by reduced blood flow to the brain as your body adjusts to new circulatory patterns. Possible shortness of breath.	**Varicose veins** are often the result of rising blood pressure in the lower extremities. This is caused by the enlarged uterus cutting off blood flow back from the legs to the heart.	**Allergies,** such as hay fever, are a common problem for some people.		**Skin changes** such as darkened nipples, stretch marks, splotches on cheeks and forehead, acne, redness on palms of hands and soles of feet are mainly due to increased hormone levels in your blood.		**Nosebleeds** sometime occur because of increased blood volume and nasal congestion.
Remedies		Try to sit with your feet up whenever possible; rise slowly and support yourself.	Whenever sitting, rest legs on footstool with feet elevated; avoid pressure on lower thighs. Many women find support stockings helpful.	Air conditioning (with a clean filter) often helps, and a pollen mask can be worn to screen out allergens.		Be patient. Virtually all of these effects will subside soon after childbirth.		Apply a little petroleum jelly in each nostril; that should stop the bleeding. A humidifier may also help. Do not irritate nasal mucosa.
Drug Substances to Avoid		• tranquilizers • alcohol (Avoid throughout pregnancy)		**Most antihistamines** • hydroxyzine (Atarax®) • trimeprazine (Temaril®) (Avoid throughout pregnancy)		Tetracycline (for acne) (Avoid throughout pregnancy)		
Acceptable Alternatives (occasional use)		• smelling salts • aromotic spirits of ammonia		Chlorpheniramine for congestions; nasal spray for stuffy nose, occasionally. Calamine Lotion for rashes.		If nipples or abdomen itch, a lanolin-based cream or baby oil can provide relief. A mild soap can remove the excessive facial oil produced by acne.		Pseudoephedrine or nasal spray may be used occasionally for stuffy nose, if necessary.

Continued.

Fig. 7-14—cont'd. Summary of fetal development, maternal events, common discomforts, examples of remedies, and drug substances to avoid. (From Safe passage: A woman's guide to a healthier pregnancy, McNeil Consumer Products Co., Fort Washington, Pennsylvania.)

Week 25	Week 26	Week 27	Week 28	Week 29	Week 30	Week 31	Week 32
Baby's Development	To a certain extent, the baby can now breathe, swallow and regulate its body temperature, but still depends greatly upon maternal support.	A substance called *surfactant* forms in the lungs, preparing them to function independently at birth.	Baby is two-thirds grown.	Fat deposits are building up beneath the skin to insulate the baby against the abrupt change in temperature at birth.	The digestive tract and the lungs are now nearly fully matured and the skin becomes less red and wrinkled.	The baby has grown to about 14 inches.	
	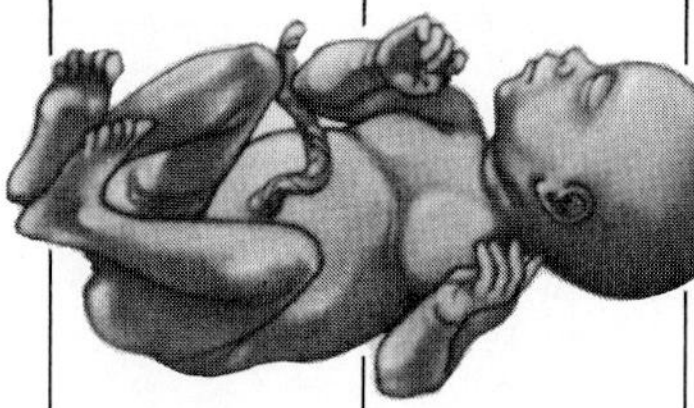				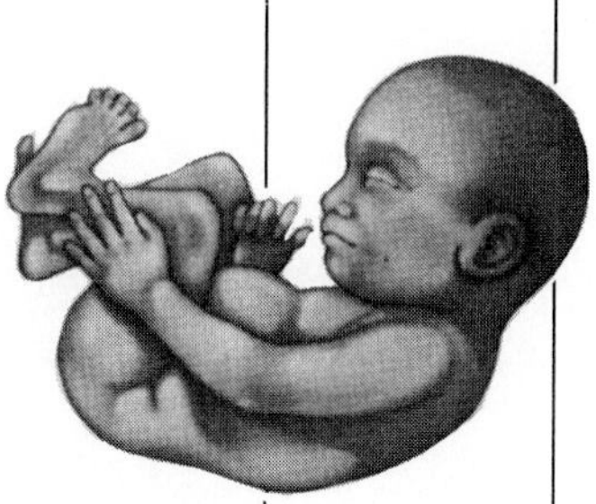		
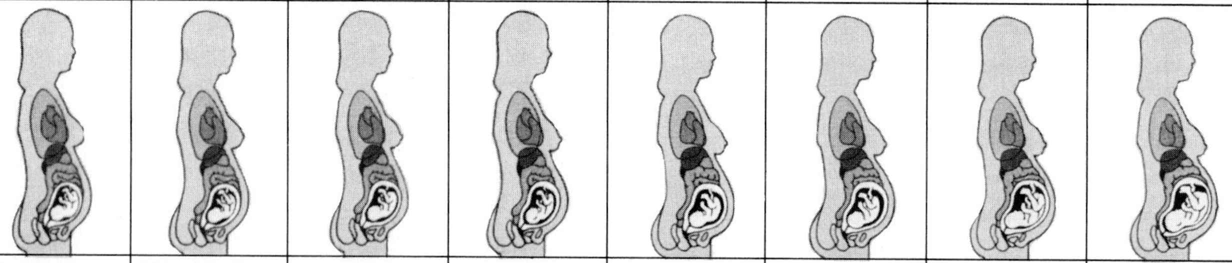							
Maternal Events	3-4 lb weight gain.	Respiratory movements can be detected by ultrasound. Mother sometimes feels baby's breathing as "hiccups."	The volume of amniotic fluid decreases to make room for growing fetus.		3-5 lb weight gain.		Mother may have trouble sleeping because of baby's activity.
Common Discomforts		**Leg and muscle cramps** may be caused by fatigue, by pressure exerted on the nerves by the uterus, or by too little calcium/too much phosphorus in the diet.	**Heartburn** often occurs as the stomach emptying time is delayed, causing a burning sensation in the throat.		**Swollen ankles.** The pressure of the uterus on the large veins returning blood to the heart may induce water retention.	**Constipation** is another result of the decelerated digestive process. As food moves slowly through your intestines, more water is extracted, leaving the stool drier and harder.	**Hemorrhoids** may also develop.
Remedies		Exercise regularly, walking especially. Elevate legs and flex toes when resting. Increase milk consumption.	Drink milk between small, frequent meals. This problem will disappear soon after your baby's birth.		Elevate legs—once or twice a day for an hour or so—level with your hips. Sleep on your left side.	Eat foods containing roughage, such as raw fruits, vegetables, cereals with bran. Drink liquids and exercise frequently.	Soaking in a warm bath or sitting on soft pillows should soothe the symptoms of hemorrhoids.
Drug Substances to Avoid		• salicylates (aspirin) • tranquilizers (Avoid throughout pregnancy)	**Antacids** • calcium carbonate • magnesium trisillicate (Gaviscon®) • sodium bicarbonate (Baking Soda) • cimetideine (Tagamet®) (Avoid throughout pregnancy)		**Most diuretics** ("water pills") (Avoid throughout pregnancy)	**Laxatives** • mineral oil • castor oil (Avoid throughout pregnancy)	
Acceptable Alternatives (occasional use)		Calcium supplements with little or no phosphorus.	• Maalox® • Mylanta® (also for "gas")			For Constipation: • Metamucil® • Senokot® • teaspoon of milk of magnesia at bedtime	For Hemorrhoids: • Nupercainal® suppositories or cream • Anusol® • Medicone®

Week 33			To Term
Baby's Development	Virtually the entire uterus is now occupied by the baby and its activity is restricted.	Maternal antibodies against measles, mumps, rubella, whooping cough and scarlet fever are transferred to the baby, providing protection for about 6 months until the infant's own immune system can take over.	
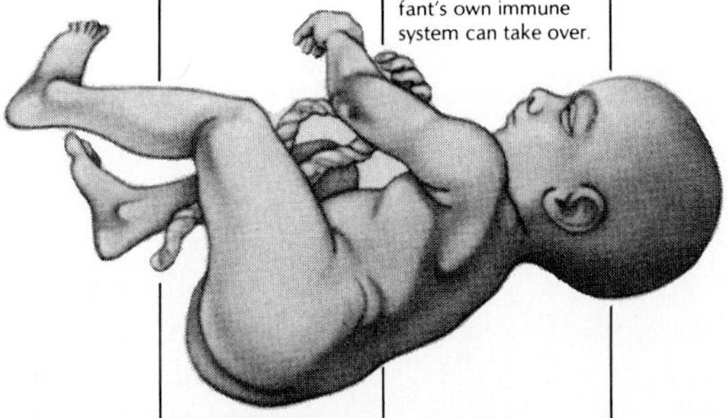			
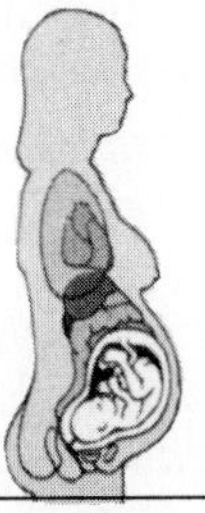	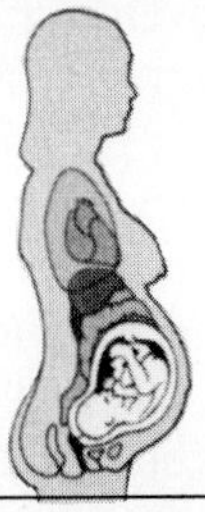	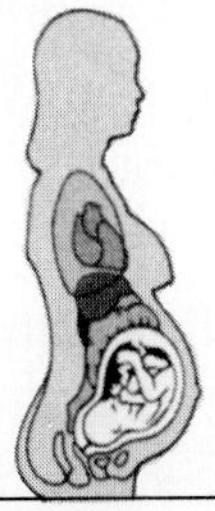	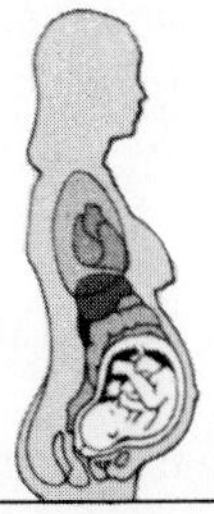
Maternal Events	The placenta is nearly 4 times as thick as it was 20 weeks ago, and weighs about 20 ounces.	Preparing for birth, the baby descends deeper into the mother's pelvis. 3-5 lb weight gain.	In 9 short months, the miracle is complete: you have transformed a single, microscopic fertilized cell into a six thousand billion celled human being.
Common Discomforts	**Backaches** are often caused by muscles and ligaments relaxing in preparation for the stretching required in delivery. Also by the added off-center weight of the enlarged uterus.	**Urinary frequency** is caused—for the second time in your pregnancy—by the uterus compressing the bladder against the pelvic bones, thus reducing its capacity.	**Uterine contractions** become perceptible as the cervix and lower uterine segment prepare for labor.
Remedies	Back exercises, such as the "pelvic tilt", can help strengthen back and abdominal muscles. Wear low-heeled shoes or flats; avoid heavy lifting.	You can decrease pressure on the bladder at night by sleeping on your side. Urinate frequently.	
Drug Substances to Avoid	**Analgesics** • Salicylates (aspirin) • propoxyphene (Darvon®) • phenacetin/caffeine • indomethacin (Indocin®) • codeine (Avoid throughout pregnancy)		
Acceptable Alternatives (occasional use)	**TYLENOL®** brand acetaminophen		

is after birth. If fetal movements cause the cord to loop, its stiffness prevents the loops from kinking and from knotting tightly. The higher water content of Wharton's jelly causes the cord to shrink quickly after birth. In addition, several naturally occurring prostaglandins in Wharton's jelly have a vasoconstrictive effect that inhibits bleeding from the umbilical cord stump when it is cut after birth.

Yolk Sac

By 9 weeks, the yolk sac has shrunk to a pear-shaped remnant, about 5 mm in diameter, which is connected to the midgut by the narrow yolk stalk (see Fig. 7-14). Although the yolk sac and allantois (not discussed here) are vestigial structures, their formation is essential for normal embryonic development. Both are important early sites of blood formation, and part of the yolk sac is incorporated into the embryo as the primitive gut.

The yolk sac shrinks as pregnancy advances and eventually becomes very small. The yolk stalk usually detaches from the gut by the end of the fifth week. In about 2% of adults, the intraabdominal part of the yolk stalk persists as a diverticulum of the ileum known as *Meckel's diverticulum* (Moore, 1977a).

❑ FETAL MATURATION

Fetal maturation takes place in an orderly and predictable pattern (see Fig. 7-14). There is steady increase in overall growth, and organ systems develop from the three primary germ layers: the ectoderm (ecto = outside), the entoderm (ento = inner), and the mesoderm (meso = middle). The *ectodermal* germ layer gives rise to such tissues as the skin and nails, the nervous system, and tooth enamel. The *entodermal* germ layer develops into such tissues as epithelial inner linings of the gastrointestinal and respiratory tracts, endocrine glands, and auditory canal. The *mesodermal* germ layer forms tissues such as the connective tissue, teeth (except for the enamel), muscles, and blood and vascular systems.

Cardiovascular System

The first system to function in the developing human is the cardiovascular system. Blood vessel formation begins early in the third week; it follows the first missed menstrual period of the mother. The cardiovascular system must form early to bring nourishment and oxygen from the mother to the embryo. The cardiovascular system is functional (heart is beating) before the mother's menstrual period is 1 week late. At this time (3 weeks since conception), circulation of blood begins the fetomaternal exchange of oxygen, nutrients, and waste products. This exchange is necessary because the fetal lungs and digestive system are not functional until after birth.

Fetal Circulation. In **fetal circulation,** the single umbilical vein carries oxygen-enriched blood from the placenta (Fig. 16-1). Upon entering the liver, the vein gives off a number of branches and then enters the ductus venosus. About half the oxygenated blood bypasses the liver through the ductus venosus into the inferior vena cava. There it mixes with deoxygenated blood from the fetal lower extremities, abdomen, and pelvis. Most of this blood then enters the right atrium and is pumped through the **foramen ovale** into the left atrium, where it mixes with a small amount of deoxygenated blood returning from the lungs through the pulmonary veins. The blood then flows into the left ventricle and exits through the ascending aorta. *As a result, the vessels leading to the heart, head, neck, and upper limbs receive well-oxygenated blood.* This circulatory pattern is the reason for the embryo's cephalocaudal (head-to-tail) development, which persists in subsequent motor development, making it possible for the infant to manipulate his or her hands long before being able to walk.

A small quantity of oxygenated blood from the inferior vena cava remains in the right atrium and mixes with deoxygenated blood from the superior vena cava and coronary sinus. It then flows into the right ventricle and pulmonary artery, passing through the ductus arteriosus into the aorta; a small amount is diverted to the nonfunctional lungs.

The paired umbilical arteries return most of the mixed blood from the descending aorta to the placenta. There the fetal blood simultaneously gives up carbon dioxide and waste materials and takes up oxygen and nutrients from the maternal blood. The remaining blood circulates through the lower part of the fetal body and ultimately enters the inferior vena cava.

The pattern of blood flow* is as follows (Fig. 16-1):

1. Placenta
   ↓
   Umbilical vein ↗ Liver, sinusoids, hepatic veins ↘ Inferior vena cava
   ↘ Ductus venosus→
2. Inferior vena cava→Right atrium→**Foramen ovale**→ Left atrium→Left ventricle→Aorta
3. Superior vena cava→Right atrium→Right ventricle→ Pulmonary artery→Small amount to nonfunctional lungs but most of it through **Ductus arteriosus**→ Aorta→Hypogastric arteries→**Umbilical arteries**→Placenta

*The four structures that differentiate fetal circulation from extrauterine circulation are shown in bold type. The foramen ovale and ductus arteriosus allow fetal blood to bypass the fetal lungs.

Fetal Heart Rate and Fetal Hemoglobin. Following are a number of compensatory circulatory factors that benefit the fetus (these values are those of the fetus near term):

1. The **fetal heart rate (FHR)** is 120 to 160 beats per minute (bpm), and the fetal cardiac output is approximately 350 to 500 ml/kg/min, or about that of the adult at rest.
2. The hemoglobin of the fetus is primarily fetal hemoglobin (HgF), a type synthesized before birth. HgF is capable of maintaining a high oxygen saturation at a lower pressure (P_{O_2}). It has been estimated that HgF can carry as much as 20% to 30% more oxygen than can maternal hemoglobin.
3. The hemoglobin concentration of the fetus is about 50% higher than that of the mother.

As a result of these compensatory circulatory factors, greater amounts of oxygen can be transported to the fetal tissues.

Hematopoietic System

Hematopoiesis (formation and development of blood cells) occurs in the yolk sac between weeks 3 and 6. Hematopoietic activity begins in the liver about the sixth week of gestation, when vascular channels have been formed. Later, blood formation occurs in the spleen, bone marrow, and lymph nodes.

Platelets are present in the circulation by the eleventh week of gestation. The isoagglutinogens (e.g., the Rh factor) that determine blood grouping are present in the red blood cells soon after the sixth week. Because of the early appearance of red blood cells, the *Rh-negative woman needs to be protected against isoimmunization after each pregnancy that lasts longer than 6 weeks after fertilization, as well as after the birth of each child who is Rh positive* (for extensive discussion, see Chapters 5 and 28).

Respiratory System

As previously mentioned the fetal lungs do not function until after delivery. Simple diffusion (passing from higher to lower concentration across a semipermeable membrane) across the placenta explains the exchange of oxygen and carbon dioxide in the fetus (see p. 172).

Development of human lungs occurs in four overlapping phases (from conception):

1. *Pseudoglandular period* (5 to 17 weeks' gestation): formation of bronchi and terminal bronchi
2. *Canalicular period* (13 to 25 weeks' gestation): enlargement of lumens of bronchi and terminal bronchioles, development of respiratory bronchioles and alveolar ducts, increased vascularity of lung tissue
3. *Terminal sac period* (24 weeks gestation to birth): growth of primitive alveoli (terminal air sacs) from alveolar ducts; *fetuses younger than 24 weeks are not likely to survive* if born before the terminal sac period begins
4. *Alveolar period* (late fetal period to approximately 8 years of age): formation of characteristic pulmonary alveoli as the lining of the terminal air sacs thins, with the number of alveoli increasing 6 to 8 times between birth and age 8 years.

Pulmonary Surfactants. During the terminal sac period *pulmonary surfactants* are produced in increasing amounts by the alveolar cells. **Surfactants** are substances that act as wetting agents that prevent alveolaral walls from sticking together (ie, atelectasis). Of this group, *lecithin* (phosphatidylcholine) may be the crucial factor responsible for lubricating alveolar surfaces so that they can remain open on expiration following birth. In extrauterine life, lungs must remain partially expanded at all times.

The effect of decreased surface tension, caused by the presence of lecithin in the lining layer of alveoli, can be compared to powdering rubber gloves so that they do not stick together and to the Teflon coating on cooking utensils. The active ingredient in sprays used to keep foods from sticking to frying pans is lecithin. If insufficient surfactants are present, the lungs cannot be properly inflated, and respiratory distress syndrome (RDS) may develop.*

Pulmonary surfactants migrate from the lung fluid and mix with amniotic fluid in the upper respiratory tract and then flow into the amniotic fluid. The presence of surfactants in the amniotic fluid is used as a biochemical marker for determining the degree of fetal lung maturity. Lung maturity is the capacity of lungs to accommodate to normal ventilation after birth. Lecithin builds up in the amniotic fluid from about the twenty-fourth week, while sphingomyelin, another pulmonary phospholipid, remains unchanged. Hence, by determining the amount of lecithin present in relation to sphingomyelin, or the **lecithin/sphingomyelin (L/S) ratio,** an appraisal of fetal lung maturity is possible (Table 7-2).

Following is a list of maternal diseases that have been shown to alter the normal developmental schedule of pulmonary maturity; that is, the attainment of an L/S ratio of 2 or more was either accelerated (pulmonary maturity before 35 weeks) or delayed (pulmonary maturity after 35 weeks). Maternal conditions associated with accelerated development of pulmonary maturity are generally those that cause diminished maternal blood flow to the placenta and therefore an in-

*Some diseases in adults result in decreased lecithin production and the development of adult respiratory distress syndrome (ARDS).

Table 7-2 Secretion of Pulmonary Surfactant since LMP

Gestation Age (weeks)	L/S Ratio*	Lung Maturity
26-27	Secretion into alveolar space begins	Viability attained
30-32	1.2 to 1	
35	2 to 1	Maturity attained†

*Lecithin/sphingomyelin ratio.
†May not indicate maturity in some newborn infants of pregnancies complicated by diabetes mellitus (Chapter 24).

sufficiency or impairment, to a varying extent, of oxygen transport to the fetus (Korones, 1986). The resultant fetal distress apparently increases the blood level of corticosteroid, which triggers production of surfactant in alveolar cells.

The following disorders are associated with alteration from normal time of appearance of mature L/S ratio*:

Accelerated maturity can be expected in the presence of the following:

1. Maternal conditions
   a. Hypertension, regardless of origin (preeclampsia, other hypertensive states)
   b. Sickle cell disease
   c. Narcotic addiction
   d. Diabetes mellitus with vascular involvement
   e. Chronic retroplacental hemorrhage (e.g., partial premature separation of placenta [abruptio placentae])
   f. Hyperthyroidism
   g. Corticosteroids,† aminophylline
   h. Maternal infections (see Chapter 23)
2. Fetal conditions such as prolonged rupture of fetal membranes (48 to 72 or more hours before delivery), intrauterine infection, or both

Decelerated maturity can be anticipated in the presence of the following:

1. Maternal conditions
   a. Diabetes mellitus (e.g., gestational diabetes) (Chapter 24)
   b. Chronic glomerulonephritis
2. Fetal conditions
   a. Rh disease, particularly with hydrops fetalis (Chapter 28)
   b. Smaller of identical twins (nonparasitic)

*Adapted from Korones, SB: High-risk newborn infants: the basis for intensive nursing care, ed 4, St Louis, 1986, The CV Mosby Co.
†This finding was the basis for corticosteroidal (β-methasone) therapy to stimulate fetal lung maturity when preterm delivery is anticipated (Chapter 26).

Numerous other variables may affect the outcome of predictions of pulmonary maturity based on the L/S ratio. For example, the presence of maternal blood in amniotic fluid tends to lower the L/S ratio. Thus a mature ratio in bloody fluid is a valid result; an immature ratio may be incorrect. The presence of meconium in amniotic fluid affects results in an unpredictable way; it may either raise or lower the L/S ratio from its true value by a mechanism that is not understood. In some instances a ratio of 2 or more may be associated with postnatal RDS caused by events that transpire after collection of the sample. As data accumulate, new insights will evolve regarding accuracy and error in the predictive value of the L/S ratio (Cunningham, MacDonald, and Gant, 1989).

Maternal Oxygenation. A reduction in the rate and depth of maternal respiration may be reflected in fetal oxygenation. Excessive amounts of barbiturate, narcotic analgesia, or maternal hypoxia during anesthesia may reduce the fetal P_{O_2}. Moreover, heavy maternal sedation by those drugs that readily cross the placenta may depress the fetal CNS respiratory center to further jeopardize the baby at birth. Breathing of pure oxygen (10 to 12 L/min) by the mother before delivery and again before cessation of pulsation in the cord after delivery may aid the infant.

Respiratory Movement. *Periodic fetal hiccup* can be seen and palpated, and rhythmic fetal respiratory movements can be demonstrated by ultrasonography in advanced pregnancy. Fetal cellular wastes (squamae) and **lanugo** fragments are commonly found in the fetal respiratory passages. Hence respirations at birth appear to be an extension of intrauterine respiratory movement.

Renal System

The placenta is the major fetal excretory organ and effectively eliminates waste products from fetal blood. The placenta, in collaboration with maternal lungs and kidneys, maintains fetal water, electrolyte, and acid-base balance. Kidneys are *not* necessary for fetal growth and development but are important in the control of the composition and volume of amniotic fluid. An infant may be born alive without kidneys. However, renal excretory and regulatory functions must begin immediately after delivery to maintain life and health.

In preparation for extrauterine existence the fetal kidneys develop rapidly. They appear in the fifth week and begin to function during the eighth week. Urine is excreted into and mixes with the amniotic fluid that the fetus swallows.

Neurologic System

The *neural plate* (a thickened area of embryonic ectoderm), from which the infant's nervous system develops, appears during the third week of gestation. The **neural tube*** and *neural crest* evolve from this structure, the first differentiating into the CNS (the brain and cord) and the second into the peripheral nervous system.

Development of the Brain. The brain, which is formed at the cranial end of the neural tube, consists of the forebrain, midbrain, and hindbrain. The longest part of the neural tube ultimately becomes the spinal cord.

The human brain is only partially developed and functional at birth. It grows in three stages: first, prenatally by hyperplasia (an increase in cell number); second, during the first 6 months of life by a combination of hyperplasia and hypertrophy (an increase in size of existing cells); and third, thereafter until puberty by hypertrophy. An adequate supply of protein and calories is required for this process, particularly during the first and second stages. Prenatal maternal anemia and malnutrition compromise fetal brain development: if the fetus does not receive adequate nutrition early in development, there is a smaller number of cells developed; if the fetus continues to receive inadequate nutrition, the existing cells are smaller in size.

The late fetal and early neonatal phases of maturation are especially critical to later achievement. Disease, trauma, or unfavorable environmental factors may irreparably alter the development of the CNS (see Fig. 7-12).

Hypoxia attributable to maternal causes (e.g., premature separation of the placenta), fetal causes (e.g., cord entanglement), or iatrogenic causes (e.g., maternal hypotension after being given spinal anesthesia) may be critical to the infant. Many of the survivors of severe asphyxia develop cerebral palsy, mental retardation, or other neurologic deficits. Newborns of 36 weeks' gestational age or younger are less sensitive to hypoxia but are more sensitive to birth trauma than mature newborns. Fortunately, however, the infant has remarkable powers of recuperation, and many depressed babies appear to recover satisfactorily. See Chapter 16 for more information on newborn neurologic function.

Neuromuscular Behavior. Fundamental to the successive development of behavior patterns is the development of neuromuscular structure and functioning. Behavior advances through five stages: (1) myogenic (originating in the muscle) response, (2) neuromotor (muscle movement stimulated by nerves) response, (3) reflex response, (4) integration of simple reflexes, and (5) integration and control from higher centers. Fetal development of the nervous system parallels fetal behavior.

Studies revealed that before the middle of the seventh week since LMP, "the human embryo appears incapable of any type of reflex activity" in response to stimulation (Hooker, 1952). During the next 6½ weeks increasing sensitivity was evidenced. By 13½ weeks all areas of the body except the top and back of the head appeared to be sensitive. Stimulation of parts of the body were found to cause a response. For example, lips were pressed together when stroked, the tongue moved when the inside of the mouth was touched, and stimulation of the palm resulted in finger closing and wrist flexion.

At 9 weeks since LMP the whole fetus moves in a jerky, rather convulsive manner, but between 10 and 12 weeks, periods of quiet or resting can be noted (Van Dongen and Goudie, 1980); and "instead of the mechanical, stereotyped movement seen earlier, the various activities are graceful and flowing—the fetus is very active" (Hooker, 1952). In one study using ultrasonography the fetus was seen to propel himself around in the amniotic fluid by using paddling movements with the feet, to roll over, turn somersaults, place his hands behind his head and over his ears, suck his thumb, and grasp the umbilical cord (Freud, 1983). Respiratory efforts have been visualized at 18½ weeks, swallowing with tongue movements by 12½ weeks, and sucking by 29 weeks. By 16 weeks fetal muscle movement is strong enough to activate receptors on the maternal abdominal wall; the mother usually interprets this as "the baby moving" and professionals refer to it as **quickening.**

Behavioral States. Active and inactive periods noted first between 10 and 12 weeks since LMP develop a sequential pattern by 28 weeks. Stainton (1983a, 1985) identifies three behavioral states—active, quiet, and sleeping—from data acquired from 23 expectant parents during interviews about their knowledge of their unborn child in the last trimester of pregnancy. Both mothers and fathers described times when the fetus was responsive to their voices or to rubbing of the mother's abdomen by kicking and moving. Parents noted times when the fetus was quiet but awake and aware. At other times parents said that calling in a loud voice or shaking the abdomen did not result in more than a brief movement. In those pregnancies in which the father's style was expressive (May, 1980), the father's descriptions validated the mother's. Brazelton (1982) notes that most mothers can delineate three behavioral states in the fetus: active "alert," deep sleep with little or no movement, and intermediate sleep with irregular startlelike movement.

*The nurse may need to explain to parents about neural tube defects, one of several malformations that can be identified in utero through amniocentesis (see test for α-fetoprotein).

Sensory Awareness. Most pregnant women can verify that the fetus touches the uterine wall during pregnancy. In doing so the fetus experiences *touch*. Fetal response to touch through the uterine wall has not been studied through ultrasonic observation, but parental reports of its effect are consistent. Pregnant women are often seen to be rubbing their abdomens and describe success in assisting their unborn infant to "calm down" or "settle down" when upset (Stainton, 1983b). Prospective fathers also have reported being able to "calm" a restless fetus by patting or rubbing the mother's abdomen (Stainton, 1983a).

Fetal response to painful stimuli can be demonstrated. A fetoscope placed on the mother's abdomen with pressure will usually result in fetal movement away from the site, thus requiring someone to hold the fetus in position to ensure accurate assessment. The insertion of an amniocentesis needle near or touching the fetus will also provoke a moving away movement (Liley, 1972).

If procedures recognized as painful to a newborn or adult are being considered for the fetus (e.g., intrauterine correction of a defect), fetal anesthesia is warranted. Anesthesia is administered to the mother, and by placental transfer the fetus is anesthetized. Anesthesia is provided during intrauterine transfusions requiring puncture of the fetal abdominal wall and during insertion of catheters to drain urine from the fetus with urinary tract anomalies (Harrison, 1981).

The fetus is able to *hear* both internal and external sounds by the fifth month of pregnancy (Liley, 1972). The fetus lives in an environment bombarded with sound. Pulsations of maternal blood flow through the large abdominal vessels supplying the lower body areas, placenta, and uterus and the noise emanating from the mother's digestive tract has been measured to be as high as 85 decibels (Walker et al, 1971; Henshall, 1972). Clements (1977) found that 4- to 5-month-old fetuses discriminated between musical sounds by kicking and moving violently when the music of Beethoven, Brahms, or rock groups was played and quieting with Vivaldi or Mozart.

The sensitive hearing of the fetus has prompted researchers to investigate to what extent the fetus, while in utero, can hear, learn to recognize, and record sounds that contribute to its later social responses, particularly with its mother. Numerous studies (Condon, 1977; Eisenberg, 1979) point to a selective listening to the mother's voice sounds and rhythms during intrauterine life that prepares the newborn for recognition and interaction with her or his primary caregiver. Parents have reported feeling gentle movements in response to talking or singing to their fetus (Stainton, 1983a). One mother reported that her baby began "irritable jerky movements" when she changed from vacuuming a carpet to moving the vacuum over a hardwood floor (Stainton, 1983a).

Taste buds are well developed in the fetus. The fetus has a larger number of taste buds than either a child or an adult and they are more widely distributed (Liley, 1972). Apparently the fetus can distinguish between sweet and sour tastes. In addition, cold solutions, introduced into the amniotic fluid, can induce hiccups in the fetus.

Until recently, newborns were thought to be only slightly light sensitive and unable to *see*. It is now known that light enters the uterus, especially in late pregnancy when the tissues are thin, and that both rods and cones are present at birth. Fetal movement has been elicited through the use of bright light directed on the uterus (Grimwade et al, 1971). Als et al (1979) found that during the last trimester the fetus would startle when a bright light was directed on the mother's abdomen near the head and turned actively but smoothly toward a soft light. These findings were based on reports by mothers and confirmed with ultrasound.

The fetus is well equipped with sensory devices to assist in the accumulation of information to promote continued development. The human newborn is not inexperienced at birth—she or he possesses a repertoire of behaviors that meet needs and provide protection. The behavioral state at birth is derived from a gradual development during the fetal period of life. Awareness of fetal response is stimulating research into the concept of prebirth parenting and the effects that mother-father-fetus interactions may have on subsequent parent-child relationships.

Gastrointestinal System

The digestive system forms during the fourth week. The middle portion of the intestine projects out into the umbilical cord during the fifth week of development because there is not enough room in the abdomen (the liver and kidneys are taking up considerable space at this time). The intestines return to the abdomen during the tenth week. Failure of the intestines to return to the abdomen results in a condition known as *omphalocele*.

Intrauterine nutrition and elimination occur through the placenta, making it unnecessary for the slowly developing gastrointestinal system to function before birth. During the second trimester the fetus begins to swallow amniotic fluid.

While in utero the fetus exists in a nondemanding physical environment. Constant ambient temperature, minimum physical activity, depressed muscle tone, and effective insulation against heat loss all contribute to a relatively low metabolic rate. The fetus maintains a temperature about 0.4° C (0.7° F) above maternal temperature. Oxygen consumption is about one third that of the neonate. Most of the caloric intake is used to accomplish growth and development.

The fetus receives its glucose, its main source of energy, from the mother. *Maternal insulin does not pass to the fetus; the fetus secretes insulin.* The fetus synthesizes glycogen and anabolizes (forms) his or her own fat rather than receiving these nutrients in these forms from the mother.

As term approaches, increasing amounts of **meconium** (the end product of fetal metabolism) are found in the fetal intestinal tract. Normal meconium is a sterile, dark, greenish brown, semisolid residue of bile and embryonic secretions, plus cellular waste (squamous epithelial cells) and hair swallowed in utero. The presence of meconium in amniotic fluid before delivery usually, but not always, indicates fetal hypoxia (Chapter 22).

Hepatic System

Liver function begins at about the fourth week after conception. Hematopoiesis starts at about the sixth week of intrauterine life; this activity is primarily responsible for the rapid growth and relatively large size of the liver during the second month of gestation.

The fetal liver at term is proportionately much larger than the liver of the 1-year-old infant. It is a metabolic and glycogen storage organ that also secretes bile and acts as a depot for iron. Full liver function is not achieved until well after delivery, however. For example, coagulation factors contributed to or produced by the liver and fibrinogen are low at the time of delivery but adjust in early infancy. The production of fetal liver enzymes is limited, especially in the fetus of less than 36 weeks' since conception (38 weeks since LMP).

Endocrine System

The fetal *adrenal cortex,* or outer part of the gland, produces cortisol. Increasing amounts of cortisol may be important in the initiation of labor.

The *thyroid* gland is the first endocrine gland to develop in the fetus. By the fourth week the thyroid can synthesize thyroxine.

By the twelfth week insulin may be extracted from the beta cells of the fetal *pancreas.* The fetus must supply whatever is needed for its metabolism of glucose. Insulin is the primary hormone regulating the rate of fetal growth. If the mother is diabetic, the response of the beta cells of the fetal pancreas to repeated stimuli of *hyperglycemia* (caused by high levels of maternal glucose) will be hyperplasia (increased amount of tissue) of all body structures except the brain. This is thought to account for the large size of the infants of diabetic mothers and the hyperinsulinism found in these newborns immediately after birth.

Reproductive System

Until the end of the ninth week, female and male external genitals appear somewhat similar (see Fig. 4-1). It is not until the twelfth week that external genitals are well enough developed to be easily distinguishable.

The fetal ovary (see Fig. 4-4) has many primordial (primitive) follicles and produces small but increasing amounts of estrogen. It is the high level of maternal estrogen that stimulates the fetal endometrium; the rapid drop in maternal estrogens in fetal circulation following birth is followed by withdrawal bleeding. *Withdrawal bleeding* accounts for the brief mucoid vaginal discharge and even slight bloody spotting that may be noted in female neonates.

During childhood a small but continuing secretion of estrogen occurs. Before puberty a much greater production of estrogen accounts for the development of female secondary sex characteristics.

Early in embryonic development, the gonads of the genetically male fetus (fetus with a Y chromosome) play a critical role in the formation of the genital tract. As the gonads evolve in the testicular pattern, presumably under the influence of maternal hCG, luteinizing hormone (LH), and fetal adrenal hormones, the testes produce androgenic hormones that result in growth and differentiation of male genitals.

After delivery a slow increase in the production of androgen and traces of estrogen continue until just before puberty, when much larger amounts of testosterone, in particular, are secreted. This increase causes development of the male secondary sex characteristics.

Immune System

Near term, the fetus passively acquires natural immunity of IgG antibodies via placental transfer (p. 172). The fetus will develop IgM antibodies in response to maternal bacterial or viral infection. An indepth discussion of the immune defense system across the life span is presented in Chapter 5. See Chapter 16 for discussion of the immune system in the newborn.

SUMMARY

Nurses need to understand basic genetic concepts and the ways hereditary factors interact with the constantly changing environment. This includes knowledge about the genetic basis of inheritance and normal development from conception through full-term gestation. Fig. 7-14 summarizes fetal development, maternal events, common discomforts, examples of remedies, and drug substances to avoid. It was taken from a brochure prepared for coaching parents through pregnancy.

LEARNING ACTIVITIES

1. Visit a biology lab to examine specimens of human embryos. Compare the differing stages of development.
2. Obtain a placenta with membranes from the delivery area, examine carefully; explain the structures and their development. (Remember to wear gloves and follow with handwashing.)
3. Visit local pharmacies and other stores to find what over-the-counter drugs are available to pregnant women (including alcohol and tobacco). List at least three different preparations that might affect the embryo or fetus and describe both their effects and the method of transport of the drug to the fetus.
4. Visit a prenatal clinic and conduct a class on the effects of over-the-counter drugs on the fetus. Prepare handouts for the clients. Include stages of fetal development in your discussion.

KEY CONCEPTS

- Genes are responsible for all human traits, for the orderly pattern and timing of development from conception to death, and for continuity of the species through consistent transmission of these traits from generation to generation.
- At fertilization, a zygote is formed, the sex of the new human is determined, and the blueprints for the growth, development, and maturation of a new individual are laid down.
- Genes act in predictable fashion during gamete formation and fertilization (Mendel's laws).
- Human gestation is approximately 280 days since last menstrual period; 266 days after fertilization.
- The placenta is the most accurate record of the infant's prenatal experience.
- Fetal maturation takes place in an orderly and predictable pattern.
- There are sensitive, or critical, periods in human development during which tissues are highly vulnerable to environmental agents, for example, teratogens.
- The L/S ratio provides one method of assessing for fetal lung maturity in most instances.
- The fetus is well equipped with sensory devices to assist in the accumulation of information to promote continued development. The human newborn possesses a repertoire of behaviors that meet needs and provide protection.

References

Als H et al: Dynamics of the behavioral organization of the premature infant: a theoretical perspective. In Field TM et al, editors: Infants born at risk, New York, 1979, Spectrum Press.

Brazelton TB: Joint regulation of neonate-parent behavior. In Tronick EZ: Social interchange in infancy: affect, cognition, and communication, Baltimore, 1982, University Park Press.

Clements M: Observations on certain aspects of neonatal behavior in response to auditory stimuli. Paper presented at the Fifth International Congress of Psychosomatic Obstetrics and Gynecology, Rome, 1977.

Condon WS: A primary phase in the organization of infant responding behavior. In Schaffer HR, editor: Studies in mother-infant interaction, New York, 1977, Academic Press, Inc.

Cunningham FG, MacDonald PC, and Gant NF: Williams obstetrics, ed 18, Norwalk, Conn, 1989, Appleton & Lange.

Derom C et al: Increased monozygotic twinning rate after ovulation induction, Lancet 1:1237, 1987.

Eisenberg RB: Stimulus significance as a determinant of infant responses to sound. In Thoman EB, editor: Origins of the infant's social responsiveness, The Johnson & Johnson Baby Products Co, Pediatric Round Table, 2, Skillman, New Jersey, 1979.

Freud E: Prenatal attachment and bonding, Paper presented to the First International Congress on Pre- and Peri-natal Psychology, Toronto, July 8, 1983.

Grimwade JC et al: Human fetal heart rate change and movement in response to sound and vibration, Am J Obstet Gynecol 109:86, 1971.

Harrison, MR: Management of the fetus with a correctable congenital defect, JAMA 246:774, 1981.

Henshall WR: Intrauterine sound levels, Am J Obstet Gynecol 112:576, 1972.

Hooker D: The prenatal origin of behavior, Lawrence, 1952, University of Kansas Press.

Korones SB: High-risk newborn infants: the basis for intensive nursing care, ed 4, St Louis, 1986, The CV Mosby Co.

Liley AW: The foetus as a personality, Aust NZ J Psychiatry 6:99, 1972.

MacGillivray I: Epidemiology, Semin Perinatol 10:4, 1986.

May KA: A typology of detachment/involvement styles adopted during pregnancy by first-time expectant fathers, West J Nurs Res 2:445, 1980.

Moore KL: Before we are born: basic embryology and birth defects, rev ed, Philadelphia, 1977a, WB Saunders Co.

Moore KL: The developing human, ed 2, Philadelphia, 1977b, WB Saunders Co.

Stainton MC: A comparison of pre-natal and post-natal perceptions of their babies by parents, Paper presented to the First International Congress on Pre- and Peri-natal Psychology, Toronto, July 8, 1983a.

Stainton MC: The fetus: a growing member of the family, Fam Relations 34(7):321, 1985.

Stainton MC: Interview data, 1983b.

Van Dongen LG and Goudie EG: Fetal movement patterns in the first trimester of pregnancy, Br J Obstet Gynaecol 87:191, 1980.

Walker D et al: Intrauterine noise: a component of the fetal environment, Am J Obstet Gynecol 109:91, 1971.

Willson JR and Carrington ER: Obstetrics and gynecology, ed 8, St Louis, 1987, The CV Mosby Co.

Bibliography

Bernhardt J: Sensory capabilities of the fetus, MCN 12(1):44, 1987.

England MA: Color atlas of life before birth: normal fetal development 1983. Distributed in North America and Canada by Year Book Medical Publishers, Inc, by arrangement with Wolfe Medical Publications, Ltd.

Ericson AJ: What is a teratogen? Childbirth Education: 44, Winter 1986/1987.

Fanaroff AA and Martin RJ, editors: Neonatal-perinatal medicine: diseases of the fetus and infant, ed 4, St Louis, 1987, The CV Mosby Co.

Lowrey GH: Growth and development of children, ed 8, Chicago, 1986, Year Book Medical Publishers, Inc.

Whaley LF: Understanding inherited disorders, St Louis, 1974, The CV Mosby Co.

Williams SR: Basic nutrition and diet therapy, ed 8, St Louis, 1988, The CV Mosby Co.

CHAPTER

8 Anatomy and Physiology of Pregnancy

Irene M. Bobak

Learning Objectives

Correctly define the key terms listed.

Describe various pregnancy tests.

Explain the expected maternal anatomic and physiologic adaptations to pregnancy.

Identify the maternal hormones produced during pregnancy, as well as their target organs. Relate their major effects on pregnancy.

List signs and symptoms of pregnancy.

Describe gravidity and parity using the 5-digit, 4-digit, and 2-digit systems.

Compare and contrast the abdomen, vulva, and cervix of the nullipara and multipara.

Key Terms

amenorrhea
ballottement
Braxton Hicks' sign
Chadwick's sign
diastasis recti abdominis
chloasma
epulis
ferning
friability
funic souffle
Goodell's sign
gravidity
  gravida
  multigravida
  nulligravida
  primigravida
Hegar's sign
hirsutism
hyperplasia
hypertrophy
leukorrhea
lightening
linea nigra
mean arterial pressure (MAP)
monoclonal antibody
Montgomery's tubercles
operculum
palmar erythema
parity
  multipara
  nullipara
  primipara
parturient
pyrosis
quickening
radioimmunoassay
striae gravidarum
telangiectasias
uterine souffle

A healthy pregnancy with a physically safe and emotionally satisfying outcome for both mother and infant is the goal of maternity care. Consistent health supervision and surveillance are of utmost importance. Many maternal adaptations are unfamiliar to pregnant women and their families. The knowledgeable maternity nurse can help the pregnant woman recognize the relationship between her physical status and the plan for her care. Sharing information encourages the pregnant woman to participate in her own care, depending on her interest, need to know, and readiness to learn.

Essential to the study of maternity care is an understanding of the following terms used to describe the pregnant woman:

gravida A woman who is pregnant.

parturient A woman in labor.

gravidity Pregnancy.

parity The number of *pregnancies* in which the fetus or fetuses have reached viability, not the number of fetuses delivered. Whether the fetus is born alive or is stillborn after viability is reached does not affect parity.

nulligravida A woman who has never been pregnant.

primigravida A woman who is pregnant for the first time.

multigravida A woman who has had two or more pregnancies.

nullipara A woman who has *not* completed a pregnancy with a fetus or fetuses who have reached the stage of fetal viability (i.e., capacity to live outside the uterus; about 22 to 24 weeks since last menstrual period).

primipara A woman who has completed one pregnancy with a fetus or fetuses who have reached the stage of fetal viability.

multipara A woman who has completed two or more pregnancies to the stage of fetal viability.

This information is abbreviated as gravidity/parity. For example, "I/O" means that a woman is pregnant for the first time (primigravida) and has not carried a pregnancy to viability (nullipara).

Another abbreviation commonly employed in maternity centers is even more detailed. It consists of five digits with hyphens for separation. The first digit represents the total number of pregnancies, including the present one; the second digit represents the total number of deliveries; the third indicates the number of preterm babies; the fourth identifies the number of abortions, and the fifth is the number of children currently living. If a woman pregnant only once with twins delivers at the thirty-fifth week and the babies survive, the abbreviation that represents this information is "1-0-1-0-2." During her next pregnancy the abbreviation is "2-0-1-0-2." Additional examples are given in Table 8-1.

Others prefer a 4-digit system. The first digit (see Table 10-1, A) of the 5-digit system, which signifies gravidity, is dropped. The 4 remaining digits are defined in Table 8-1, B to E.

❑ PREGNANCY TESTS

All tests that are in current use detect the presence of human chorionic gonadotropin (hCG) (Chapter 7, p. 167). Early detection of pregnancy allows early initiation of care. Human chorionic gonadotropin can be measured by radioimmunoassay and detected in the blood as early as 6 days after conception, or about 20 days since the last menstrual period (LMP). Its presence in the urine in early pregnancy is the basis of the various laboratory tests for pregnancy, and it can sometimes be detected in the urine as early as 14 days after conception (Ganong, 1989). Less specific tests may not be accurate until 4 to 10 days after the missed menstrual period or 3 weeks after conception.

A first-voided morning urine specimen contains levels of hCG approximately the same as those in serum, whose levels increase exponentially between days 21 and 70 (counting from the first day of the LMP). Random urine samples usually have lower levels. The ability to recognize the beta subunit of hCG is the newest innovation in the evolution of endocrine tests for pregnancy. The wide variety of tests precludes discussion of each, however, several categories of tests are described here. The nurse should read the manufacturer's directions for the test to be used.

Latex agglutination inhibition (LAI) tests are easy to do and give results in 2 minutes. They are accurate from 4 to 10 days following missed menses. Examples of this type of test include the Gravindex slide, Pregnosticon slide, and UCG Beta slide.

Hemagglutination inhibition (HAI) tests are more sensitive than LAI tests but require 1 to 2 hours to obtain results. Except for one test, Neocept, which gives accurate results at or before missed menses, all HAI tests are accurate about 4 days following missed menses. Also on the market is e.p.t. (early pregnancy test), an HAI in-home test available for consumer purchase (Doshi, 1986).

The *radioreceptor assay* is one of the newest categories of pregnancy tests. This 1-hour serum test requires fairly sophisticated equipment. Radioreceptor assays are usually accurate at time of missed menses (14 days after conception) (Brucker and MacMullen, 1985). Biocept G is an example of this type of test.

Radioimmunoassay pregnancy tests for the beta subunit of hCG use radioactively labeled markers, which require the testing to be done in a laboratory. Depending on the degree of sensitivity required, the test time

Table 8-1 Gravidity and Parity Using Five-Digit and Two-Digit Systems

	Five-digit System					Two-digit System
Condition	A*	B	C	D	E	F
Judith is pregnant for the first time.	1	-0	-0	-0	-0	I/0
She carries the pregnancy to term and the neonate survives.	1	-1	-0	-0	-1	I/I
She is pregnant again.	2	-1	-0	-0	-1	II/I
Her second pregnancy ends in abortion.	2	-1	-0	-1	-1	II/I
During her third pregnancy, she delivers viable twins.	3	-2	-0	-1	-3	III/II

*A, Times uterus has been pregnant (gradivity); B, number of deliveries (parity); C, number of preterm deliveries; D, number of abortions (spontaneous or elective); E, number of living children; F, gravidity/parity; corresponds to A and B of the 5-digit system.

ranges from 1 to 48 hours. Radioimmunoassays are the most sensitive pregnancy tests available today (Brucker and MacMullen, 1985). Pregnancy can be diagnosed 8 days after ovulation or 6 days before missed menses.

Enzyme immunoassays use complex monoclonal anti-hCG with enzymes.* A visible color change makes the results easy to read. This new test holds promise for the future. Confidot is an immunoenzymatic assay home pregnancy test. The manufacturers of Confidot claim that this self-administered test confirms pregnancy approximately 10 days after fertilization, about 4 days before missed menses.

Enzyme-linked immunosorbent assay (ELISA) testing is the most popular testing procedure for pregnancy (Batzer, 1985; Scott et al, 1990). It uses a specific **monoclonal antibody** produced by hybrid cell-line technology (News, 1985). An enzyme rather than a radioactive compound identifies the antigen of the substance to be measured. The enzyme induces a simple color-change reaction. The endpoint of the test can be read with either the eye or a spectrometer.

ELISA testing has many advantages. The antigen enzyme conjugate and test reagents are stable, the equipment needs are simple, and there are no nuclear waste products. As an office or home procedure it requires minimum time and offers results in 5 minutes coupled with sensitivities from 25 to 50 mIU/ml of hCG in the specimen. ELISA technology is the basis for the new over-the-counter tests. The manufacturer provides directions for collection of specimen (serum, plasma, or urine), care of specimen, testing procedure, and reading of results.

Interpretation of the results of pregnancy tests requires some judgment. The type of pregnancy test and its degree of *sensitivity* (ability to detect low levels of a substance) and *specificity* (ability to discern the absence of a substance) are interpreted in conjunction with the woman's history, which includes the date of the last normal menstrual period (LNMP), usual cycle length, and results of previous pregnancy tests. It is important to know if the woman is a substance abuser. Interactions with other drugs can give false results. Improper collection of the specimen, hormone-producing tumors, and laboratory errors may be responsible for false reports (Doshi, 1986). Where there is any question, serial testing may be the answer (Batzer, 1985). Speed and convenience need to be weighed against sensitivity and specificity.

*Read package inserts for a description of "monoclonal anti-hCG with enzymes."

❑ ADAPTATIONS TO PREGNANCY

This chapter provides the basis for preventive, curative, and rehabilitative maternity care. Maternal adaptations are attributed to the *hormones* of pregnancy and to *mechanical pressures* arising from the enlarging uterus and other tissues. These adaptations protect the woman's normal physiologic functioning, meet the metabolic demands pregnancy imposes on her body, and provide for fetal developmental and growth needs. Although pregnancy is a normal phenomenon, problems can occur. The nurse needs an adequate foundation in normal maternal physiology to accomplish the following:

1. Identify potential or actual deviation from normal adaptation to initiate remedial care
2. Help the mother understand the anatomic and physiologic changes during pregnancy.
3. Allay the mother's (and family's) anxiety, which may result from lack of knowledge
4. Teach the mother (and family) signs and symptoms that must be reported to the physician

Among the expected adjustments to pregnancy are changes that are found in some disease states; for example, low hemoglobin levels, a high erythrocyte sedimentation rate, dyspnea at rest, and alterations in cardiac function and endocrine balance. These changes reflect the body's effort to protect the mother and the fetus. An understanding of these changes is necessary for anyone who participates in the care of the mother and the fetus.

Some of the adaptations are recognized as signs and symptoms of pregnancy. These signs and symptoms appear in **bold print** throughout the chapter. A summary of the signs and symptoms of pregnancy and their order of appearance are presented in Chapter 10.

❑ REPRODUCTIVE SYSTEM AND BREASTS

Hypothalamus-Pituitary-Ovarian Axis

During pregnancy, elevated levels of estrogen and progesterone suppress secretion of follicle-stimulating hormone (FSH) and luteinizing hormone (LH). The maturation of a follicle and ovulation of an ovum do not occur. Menstrual cycles cease. Although the majority of women experience **amenorrhea** (absence of menses), at least 20% have some slight, painless spotting during early gestation for unexplained reasons. A great majority of these women continue to term and have normal infants.

After implantation, the fertilized ovum and the chorionic villi produce hCG, which maintains the corpus luteum's production of estrogen and progesterone for the first 8 to 10 weeks of pregnancy until the placenta takes over their production (Scott et al, 1990).

Uterus

The phenomenal uterine growth in the first trimester occurs in response to the hormonal stimulus of high levels of estrogen and progesterone. Enlargement results from (1) increased vascularity and dilatation of blood vessels, (2) hyperplasia (production of new muscle fibers and fibroelastic tissue) and hypertrophy (enlargement of preexisting muscle fibers and fibroelastic tissue), and (3) development of the decidua (Fig. 8-1). By 7 weeks the uterus is the size of a large hen's egg; by 10 weeks, the size of an orange (twice its nonpregnant size); by 12 weeks, the size of a grapefruit. Table 8-2 compares uterine measurements for the nonpregnant and pregnant uterus at 40 weeks' gestation. After the third month uterine enlargement is primarily the result of mechanical pressure of the growing fetus (Seidel et al, 1987).

As the uterus increases in size, it also changes in weight, shape, and position. The muscular walls strengthen and become more elastic. At conception the uterus is shaped like an upside-down pear. During the second trimester it is spheric or globular. Later, as the fetus lengthens, the uterus becomes larger and more ovoid, and it rises out of the pelvis into the abdominal cavity. In the nonpregnant woman, the uterine cavity holds about 10 ml of fluid; during pregnancy, its capacity increases to 5 to 10 L or more (Cunningham, MacDonald, and Gant, 1989).

A reasonably accurate correlation of **uterine enlargement** and the duration of amenorrhea in weeks counting from the sixth week to term is possible in most normal pregnant women. Variation in the positions of the fundus or the fetus, variations in the amount of amniotic fluid present, or the presence of more than one fetus reduces the accuracy of this estimation of the duration of pregnancy.

The pregnancy may "show" after the fourteenth week, although this depends to some degree on the woman's height and weight. **Abdominal enlargement** may be less apparent in the primigravida with good abdominal muscle tone (Fig. 8-2). Posture also influences the type and degree of abdominal enlargement seen.

During the early weeks of pregnancy an increase in uterine blood flow and lymph causes pelvic congestion and edema. As a result, the uterus, cervix, and isthmus soften perceptibly and progressively, and the cervix takes on a bluish color (**Chadwick's sign**).

At about the seventh to eighth week the following patterns of uterine softening are noted: isthmic softening and compressibility (**Hegar's sign**; Fig. 8-3), cervical softening (**Goodell's sign**), easy flexion of the fundus on the cervix (**McDonald's sign**), softening and slight fullness of the fundus near the area of implantation (**Braun von Fernwald's sign**), or a soft lateral bulge with cornual implantation (**Piskacek's sign**). After the eighth week, general enlargement and softening of the uterine corpus and cervix are likely.

Some believe that the nonsteroid ovarian hormone, relaxin, may act synergistically with progesterone (Cunningham, MacDonald, and Gant, 1989; Scott et

Table 8-2 Comparison of Measurements for Nonpregnant and Pregnant Uterus at 40 Weeks*

Measurement	Nonpregnant	Pregnant (40 Weeks)
Length	6.5 cm (2½ in)	32 cm (12½ in)
Width	4 cm (1½ in)	24 cm (9½ in)
Depth	2.5 cm (1 in)	22 cm (8½ in)
Weight	60-70 g (2½ oz)	1100-1200 g (2½ lb)
Volume	≤10 ml	5000 ml

*Note that references vary as to the exact values but all references agree on the magnitude of the growth the uterus undergoes during pregnancy.

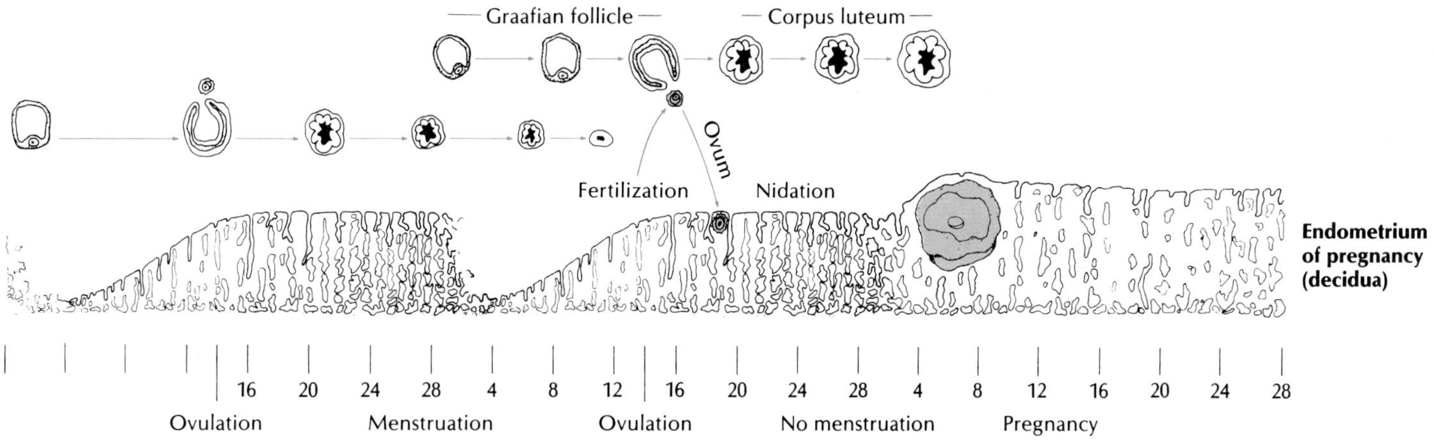

Fig. 8-1 Changes in endometrium and corpus luteum if pregnancy occurs (in days).

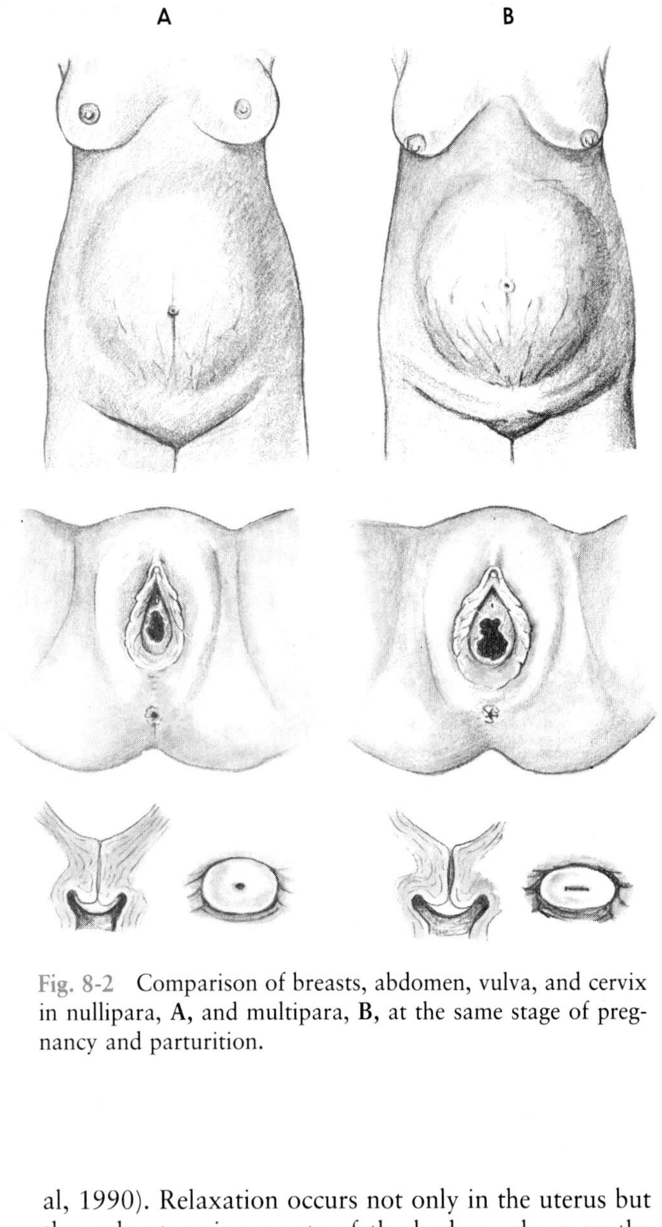

Fig. 8-2 Comparison of breasts, abdomen, vulva, and cervix in nullipara, **A,** and multipara, **B,** at the same stage of pregnancy and parturition.

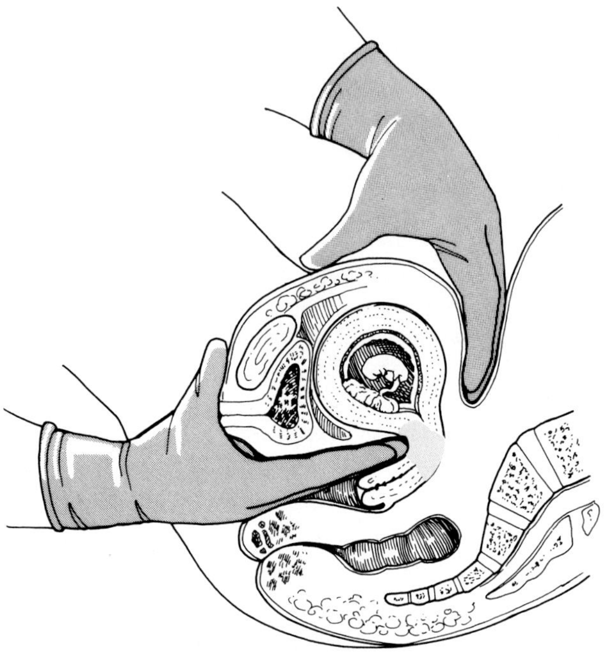

Fig. 8-3 Hegar's sign. Bimanual examination for assessing softening of isthmus while the cervix is still firm.

al, 1990). Relaxation occurs not only in the uterus but throughout various parts of the body, such as on the joints and walls of blood vessels.

As the uterus grows it is elevated out of the pelvic area and may be palpated above the symphysis pubis sometime between the twelfth and fourteenth weeks of pregnancy (Fig. 8-4). The softness of the isthmus results in exaggerated uterine anteflexion during the first 3 months of pregnancy. The fundus presses on the urinary bladder, which along with edema of the bladder wall, causes the woman to experience urinary frequency. The uterus rises gradually to the level of the umbilicus at about 22 to 24 weeks and nearly reaches the xiphoid process at term. Between weeks 38 and 40, fundal height drops as the fetus begins to engage in the pelvis (**lightening**).

Generally the uterus is rotated to the right as it ele-

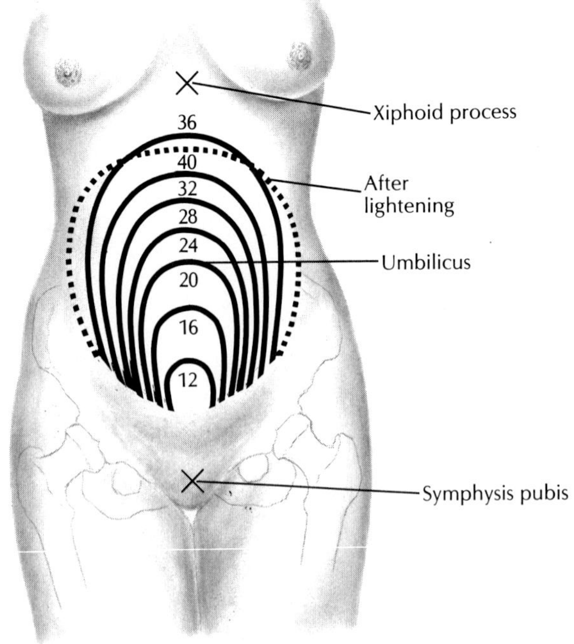

Fig. 8-4 Height of fundus by weeks of normal gestation with a single fetus. Dotted line indicates height after lightening. (Adapted from Malasanos L et al: Health assessment, ed 3, St Louis, 1985, The CV Mosby Co.)

vates, probably because of the presence of the rectosigmoid colon on the left side. However, the extensive **hypertrophy** (enlargement) of the round ligaments keeps the uterus in line. Eventually the growing uterus touches the anterior abdominal wall and displaces the intestines to either side of the abdomen. When a pregnant woman stands, the major part of her uterus rests against the anterior abdominal wall and contributes to altering her center of gravity.

Soon after the fourth month of pregnancy, uterine contractions can be felt through the abdominal wall. These contractions are referred to as the **Braxton Hicks' sign,** a probable sign of pregnancy. Braxton Hicks' contractions are a continuation of the irregular, painless contractions that occur intermittently throughout each menstrual cycle. The contractions are felt as uterine firmness through the abdominal wall or are evident because they raise and push the uterus forward. Contractions facilitate uterine blood flow and thereby promote oxygen delivery to the uterus. Although Braxton Hicks' contractions are not ordinarily painful, some women do complain they are annoying. After the twenty-eighth week, contractions become much more definite, especially in slender women. Generally these contractions cease with walking or exercise. Rarely they may be perceived as painful. They may become strong enough during the last few weeks to be confused with the contractions of beginning labor.

Blood flow increases rapidly as the uterus increases in size. Although uterine blood flow increases twentyfold, the size of the conceptus grows more rapidly. Consequently, more oxygen is extracted from the uterine blood during the latter part of pregnancy (Ganong, 1989). In a normal term pregnancy, one sixth of the total maternal blood volume is within the uterine vascular system. The rate of blood flow through the uterus averages 500 ml/min, and oxygen consumption of the gravid uterus averages 25 ml/min. Maternal arterial pressure, contractions of the uterus, and maternal position are three factors known to influence blood flow. Estrogens also play a role in uterine blood flow.

Using an ultrasound device or a fetal stethoscope, the physician or nurse may hear (1) the **uterine souffle** or bruit, a rushing sound of maternal blood going to the placenta that is synchronous with the maternal pulse, (2) the **funic souffle,** which is synchronous with the fetal heart rate and caused by fetal blood coursing through the umbilical cord, and (3) the **fetal heart rate (FHR).** For further discussion, see Chapter 16.

Passive movement of the unengaged fetus is called **ballottement.** Ballottement can be identified generally between the sixteenth and eighteenth week. Ballottement is a technique of palpating a floating structure by bouncing it gently and feeling it rebound. The examiner's finger within the vagina taps gently upward; the fetus rises. Then the fetus sinks, and a gentle tap is felt on the finger (Fig. 8-5). Internal ballottement of a fetus within a uterus is a probable objective sign of pregnancy.

The first recognition of fetal movements, or "feeling life," by the multiparous woman may occur as early as the fourteenth to sixteenth week. The nulliparous woman may not notice these sensations until the eighteenth week or later. **Quickening** is commonly described as a flutter and is difficult to distinguish from peristalsis. Noting the week in which quickening occurs provides a tentative clue in dating the duration of gestation.

A softening of the cervical tip may be observed about the beginning of the sixth week in a normal, unscarred cervix. The softening of the cervix during pregnancy (Goodell's sign) is brought about by increased vascularity, slight hypertrophy, and **hyperplasia** of the muscle and its collagen-rich connective tissue, which becomes loose, edematous, highly elastic, and increased in volume. The glands near the external os proliferate beneath the stratified squamous epithelium, giving the cervix the velvety consistency characteristic of preg-

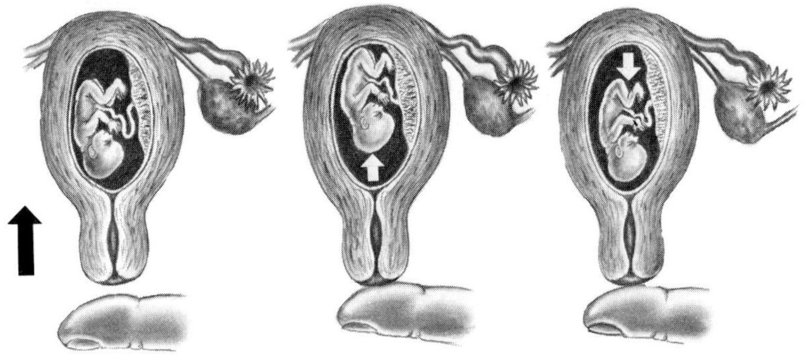

Fig. 8-5 Internal ballottement (18 weeks).

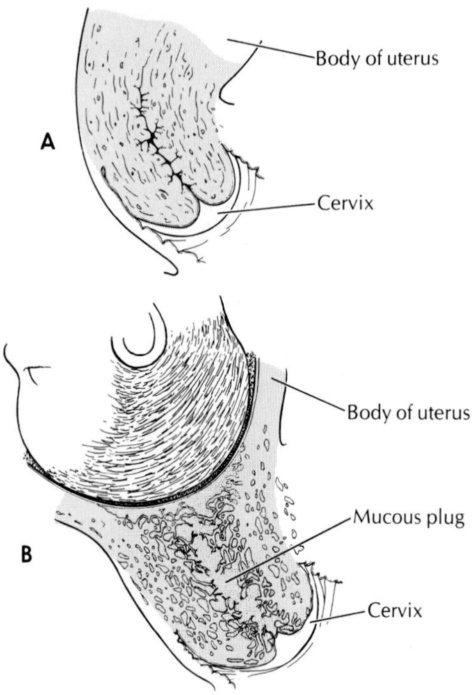

Fig. 8-6 **A,** Cervix in nonpregnant woman. **B,** Changes in cervix during pregnancy.

nancy. The changes in the cervix, as well as those of the vagina, help prepare the birth canal for the fetus's passage through it (Fig. 8-6). **Friability** is increased; that is, the cervix bleeds easily when scraped or touched. Increased friability is the cause of the few drops of blood seen after coitus with deep penetration or vaginal examination. These few drops are usually within normal limits.

The cervix of the nullipara is rounded. Lacerations of the cervix almost always occur during the birth process. With or without lacerations, following childbirth the cervix becomes more oval in the horizontal plane, and the external os appears as a transverse slit (see Fig. 8-2).

Vagina and Vulva

Pregnancy hormones prepare the vagina for distension during labor by producing a thickened vaginal mucosa, loosened connective tissue, hypertrophied smooth muscle, and an increase in the length of the vaginal vault. Increased vascularity results in a violet-bluish color to the vaginal mucosa and cervix. The deepened color, termed *Chadwick's sign* or *Jacquemier's sign,* may be evident as early as the sixth week, but is easily noted at the eighth week of pregnancy. Desquamation (or exfoliation) of the vaginal, glycogen-rich cells occurs under estrogen stimulation. The cells that are shed contribute to the thick, whitish vaginal discharge, leukorrhea.

During pregnancy the pH of vaginal secretions becomes less acidic. The pH changes from 4 to 5 to about 5.5 to 6.5. *The rise in pH makes the pregnant woman more vulnerable to vaginal infections,* especially yeast infections. A diet of large quantities of sugars can make the vaginal environment even more suitable for a yeast infection.

The increased vascularity of the vagina and other pelvic viscera results in a marked increase in sensitivity. The *increased sensitivity may lead to a high degree of sexual interest and arousal,* especially during the second trimester of pregnancy. The increased congestion plus the relaxed walls of the blood vessels and the heavy uterus may result in edema and varicosities of the vulva. The edema and varicosities usually resolve during the postpartum period.

External structures of the *perineum* are enlarged during pregnancy because of an increase in vasculature, hypertrophy of the perineal body, and deposition of fat (Fig. 8-7). The labia majora of the nullipara approximate and obscure the vaginal introitus; those of the parous woman separate and gape after childbirth and perineal or vaginal injury. Torn residual tags of the hymen remain after the use of tampons, coitus, and vaginal delivery. Fig. 8-2 compares the nullipara and the multipara in relation to several characteristics: pregnant abdomen, vulva, and cervix.

Leukorrhea is a white or slightly gray mucoid discharge with a faint musty odor. Increased estrogen and progesterone stimulation of the cervix produces copious mucoid fluid. The fluid is whitish because of the presence of many exfoliated vaginal epithelial cells caused by normal pregnancy hyperplasia. This vaginal discharge is never pruritic or blood stained. Because of the progesterone effect, **ferning** (see Fig. 4-23) does *not* occur in the dried cervical mucous smear. The mucus fills the endocervical canal, resulting in the formation of the mucous plug (**operculum**) (Fig. 8-6). The operculum acts as a barrier against bacterial invasion during pregnancy.

Breasts

Fullness, heightened sensitivity, tingling, and **heaviness** of the breasts begin as early as the sixth week of gestation. Breast sensitivity varies from mild tingling to frank pain (mastodynia). **Nipples** and **areolae** become more **pigmented,** a **secondary pinkish areola** develops, and nipples become more erectile. Hypertrophy of the sebaceous (oil) glands embedded in the primary areola, called **Montgomery's tubercles** (see Fig. 4-18, *B*), may be seen around the nipples. These sebaceous glands

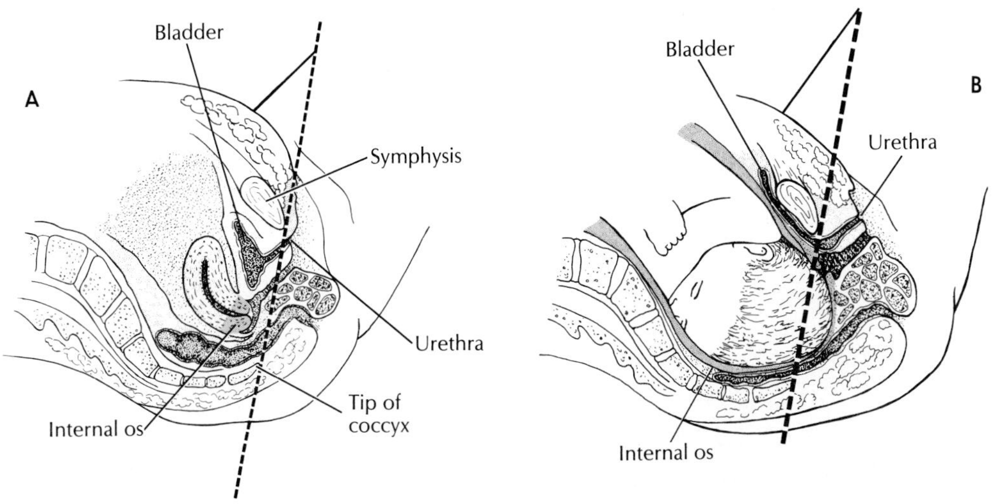

Fig. 8-7 **A,** Pelvic floor in nonpregnant woman. **B,** Pelvic floor at end of pregnancy. Note marked projection (growth of tissue) below line joining tip of coccyx and inferior margin of symphysis. Note elongation of bladder and urethra as a result of compression. Fat deposits are increased.

may have a protective role in that they keep the nipples lubricated. Suppleness of the nipples is jeopardized if the protective oils are washed off with soap.

The richer blood supply dilates the vessels beneath the skin. Once barely noticeable, the blood vessels now become visible, often appearing in an intertwining blue network beneath the surface of the skin. Venous congestion in the breasts is more obvious in primigravidas. Striae may appear at the outer aspects of the breasts.

During the second and third trimesters, growth of the mammary glands accounts for the progressive increase in breast size. The high levels of luteal and placental hormones in pregnancy promote proliferation of the lactiferous ducts and lobule-alveolar tissue, so that the palpation of the breasts reveals a generalized, coarse nodularity. The increase in glandular tissue displaces connective tissue, and as a result the tissue becomes softer and looser. Overstretching of the fibrous suspensory Cooper's ligaments (Fig. 4-18, *A*) supporting the breasts may be prevented with a well-fitted maternity brassiere.

Although development of the mammary glands is functionally complete by midpregnancy, lactation is inhibited until a drop in estrogen level occurs after delivery of the fetus and placenta. A thin, clear, viscous precolostrum secretion, however, may be expressed from the nipples by the end of the sixth week (Seidel et al, 1987).* This secretion thickens as term approaches and is then known as **colostrum.** Colostrum, the creamy, white to yellowish premilk fluid, may be expressed from the nipples during the third trimester. See discussion of pituitary prolactin in this chapter.

*References differ as to the gestational week during which precolostrum can be expressed. Some references cite week 16 as the earliest time at which fluid may be expressed from the breasts.

GENERAL BODY SYSTEMS

Cardiovascular System

Maternal adjustments to pregnancy involve extensive changes in the cardiovascular system, both anatomic and physiologic. Cardiovascular adaptations protect the woman's normal physiologic functioning, meet the metabolic demands pregnancy imposes on her body, and provide for fetal developmental and growth needs.

Slight cardiac hypertrophy (enlargement) or dilatation is probably secondary to increased blood volume and cardiac output. As the diaphragm is displaced upward, the heart is elevated upward and rotated forward to the left (Fig. 8-8). The apical impulse (PMI) is shifted upward and laterally about 1 to 1.5 cm (½ in). The degree of shift depends on the duration of pregnancy and the size and position of the uterus.

Auscultatory changes accompany the changes in heart size and position. Increases in blood volume and cardiac output also contribute to auscultatory changes common in pregnancy. There is more audible splitting of S_1 and S_2, and S_3 may be readily heard after 20 weeks of gestation. Additionally, grade II systolic ejection murmurs may be heard over the pulmonic area.

Between 14 and 20 weeks, the *pulse* increases slowly up to 10 to 15 beats per minute, which then persists to term. Palpitations may occur.

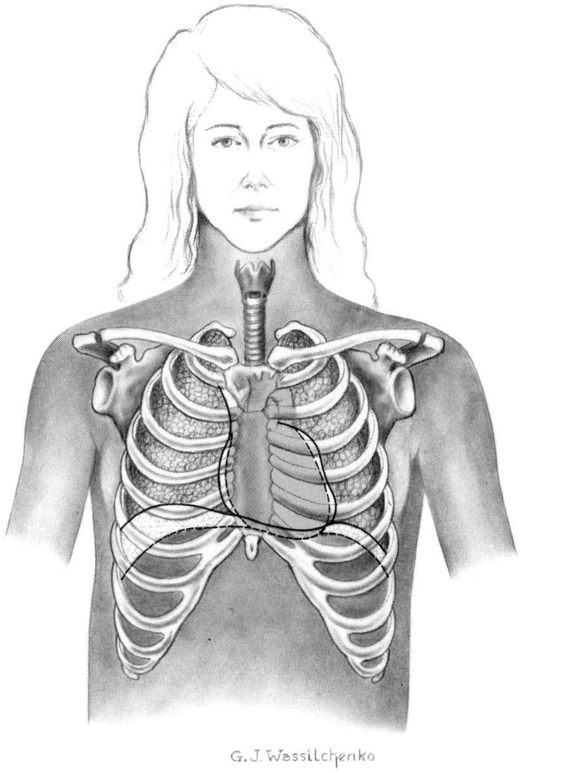

Fig. 8-8 Changes in position of heart, lungs, and thoracic cage in pregnancy. *Broken line,* Nonpregnant. *Solid line,* Change that occurs in pregnancy.

Blood Pressure. *Arterial blood pressure* (brachial artery) varies with age. Additional factors must be considered. These factors include maternal position, maternal anxiety, and size of cuff. **Maternal position** affects readings. Brachial blood pressure is highest when the woman is sitting, lowest when she is lying in the left lateral recumbent position, and intermediate when she is supine. Therefore the same maternal position and the same arm are used at each visit. The position and arm used are noted along with the reading. During the first half of pregnancy, there is a decrease in both systolic and diastolic pressure of 5 to 10 mm Hg. The decrease in blood pressure is probably the result of peripheral vasodilatation from hormonal changes during pregnancy. During the third trimester, maternal blood pressure should return to the values obtained during the first trimester.

The mean arterial pressure (MAP) increases the diagnostic value of the findings. The MAP is estimated by adding one third of the *pulse pressure* to the diastolic pressure. Pulse pressure is the difference between the systolic and diastolic values.

Example

Blood pressure: 106/70 at 22 weeks
Pulse pressure (106 − 70): 36 ÷ 3 = 12
MAP: (diastolic) 70 + 12 = 82

MAP readings of 82 at 22 weeks are within the normal range for the length of gestation.

Some degree of compression of the vena cava occurs in all women who lie on their back during the second half of pregnancy. Some women experience a fall of ≥30 mm Hg systolic. After 4 to 5 minutes a reflex bradycardia is seen, cardiac output is reduced by half, and the woman feels faint (see *hypotensive syndrome*, p. 199; and Fig. 15-9).

Edema of the lower extremities and varicosities results from obstruction of the iliac veins and inferior vena cava by the uterus and causes increased *venous pressure*.

Blood Volume and Composition. The degree of blood volume expansion varies considerably (Cunningham, MacDonald, and Gant, 1989). Blood volume increases by approximately 1500 ml* (normal value: 8.5% to 9% of body weight). The increase is made up of 1000 ml *plasma* plus 450 ml *red blood cells* (RBCs). The increase in volume starts about the tenth to twelfth week, peaks at about 25% to 45% above the nonpregnant levels at the thirty-second to thirty-fourth week, then decreases slightly to the fortieth week. The increased volume is a protective mechanism. It is essential for (1) the hypertrophied vascular system of the enlarged uterus, (2) adequate hydration of fetal and maternal tissues when the woman assumes an erect or supine position, and (3) fluid reserve for blood loss during the delivery and puerperium. Peripheral vasodilatation maintains a normal blood pressure despite the increased blood volume in pregnancy.

During pregnancy there is an accelerated production of RBCs (normal 4 to 5.5 million/mm^3). The percentage of increase depends on the amount of iron available. The RBC mass increases by 30% to 33% by term if an iron supplement is taken. It increases by only 17% in some women if no supplement is taken. For the discussion of iron therapy, see Nutrition, Chapter 11.

Despite an increase in RBC production, there is an apparent decrease in normal *hemoglobin* values (12 to 16 g/dl blood) and *hematocrit* values (37% to 47%). This condition is referred to as *physiologic anemia.* The decrease is more noticeable during the second trimester, when rapid expansion of blood volume takes place. If the hemoglobin value drops to 10 g/dl or less, or if the hematocrit drops to 35% or less, the woman is considered anemic.

*Expansion of blood volume: primigravidas, 1250 ml; multigravidas, 1500 ml; twin pregnancies, 2000 ml.

The total *white cell count* increases during the second trimester and peaks during the third trimester. This increase is primarily in the granulocytes; the lymphocyte count stays about the same throughout pregnancy. See Appendix E for laboratory values during pregnancy.

Cardiac Output. Cardiac output increases from 30% to 50% by the thirty-second week of pregnancy; it declines to about a 20% increase at 40 weeks. The elevated cardiac output is largely a result of increased stroke volume and in response to increased tissue demands for oxygen (normal value is 5 to 5.5 L/min) (Fig. 8-9). Cardiac output in late pregnancy is appreciably higher when the woman is in the lateral recumbent position than when she is supine. In the supine position, the large heavy uterus often impedes venous return to the heart (Chapter 10). Cardiac output increases with any exertion such as labor and delivery.

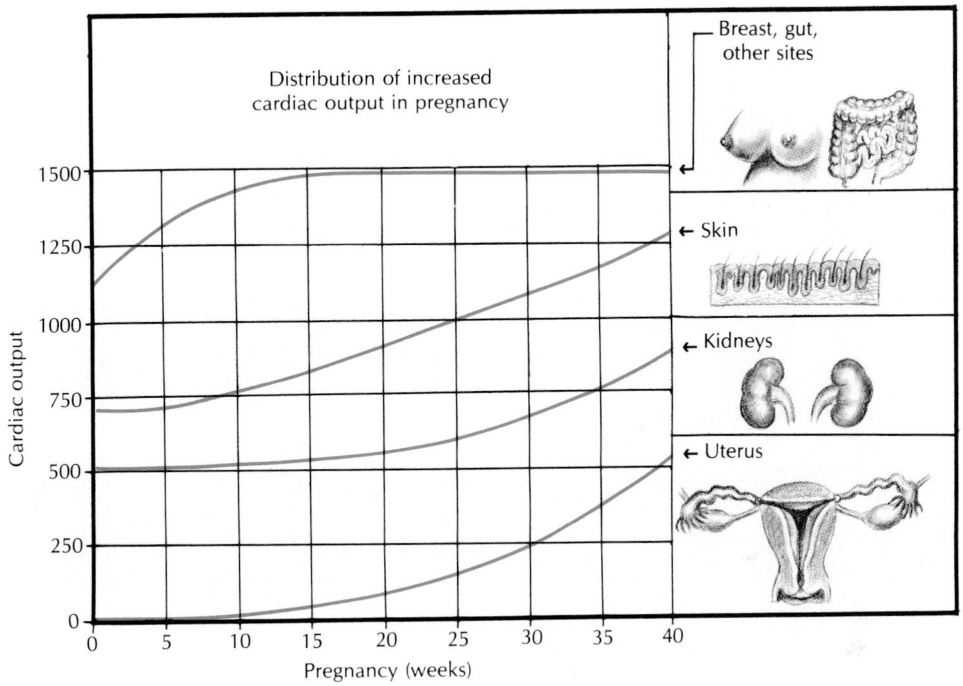

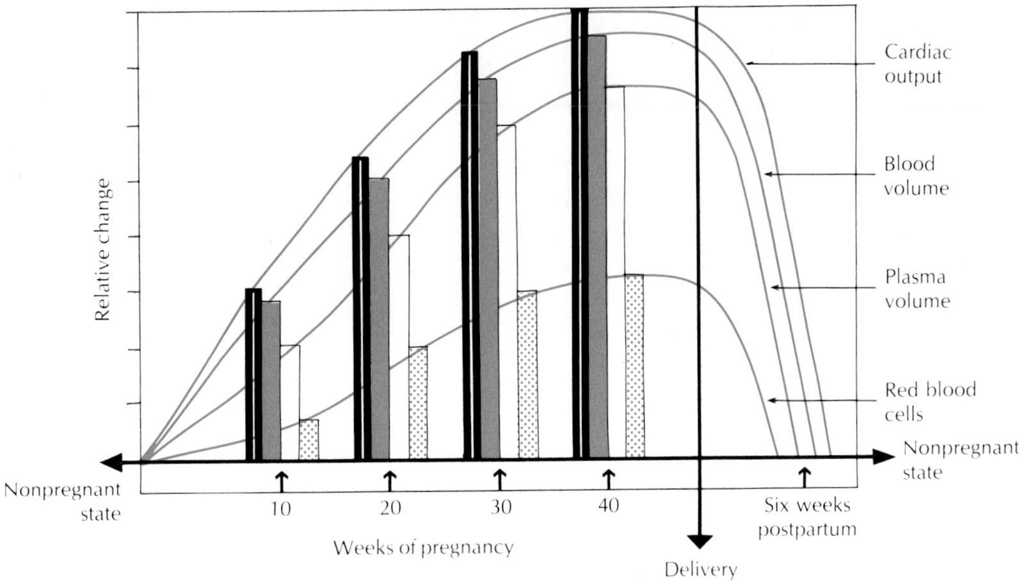

Fig. 8-9 Distribution of increased cardiac output in pregnancy.

Circulation and Coagulation Times. The circulation time decreases slightly by week 32. It returns to near normal near term.

There is a greater *tendency to coagulation* during pregnancy because of increases in various clotting factors. Fibrinolytic activity (the splitting up or the dissolving of a clot) is depressed during pregnancy. During the postpartum period, fibrinolytic activity is depressed, and the woman is again more vulnerable to thrombosis.

Respiratory System

Structural and ventilatory adaptations occur during pregnancy to provide for both maternal and fetal needs. Maternal oxygen requirements increase in response to the acceleration in metabolic rate and the need to add to the tissue mass in the uterus and breasts. The conceptus requires oxygen and a way to eliminate carbon dioxide.

Elevated levels of estrogen cause the ligaments of the rib cage to relax, permitting increased chest expansion (see Fig. 8-8). In preparation for the enlarging uterus, the length of the lungs decreases. The transverse diameter of the thoracic cage increases by about 2 cm (¾ in), and the circumference increases by 5 to 7 cm (2 to 2¾ in) (Cunningham, MacDonald, and Gant, 1989). The costal angle of approximately 68 degrees before pregnancy increases to about 103 degrees in the third trimester. The lower rib cage appears to flare out. After delivery, the chest may not return to its prepregnant state (Seidel et al, 1987).

The level of the diaphragm is displaced by as much as 4 cm (1½ in) during pregnancy. With advancing pregnancy, thoracic breathing replaces abdominal breathing, and descent of the diaphragm with inspiration becomes less possible.

Increased vascularization in response to elevated levels of estrogen also occurs in the upper respiratory tract. As the capillaries become engorged, edema and hyperemia develop within the nose, pharynx, larynx, trachea, and bronchi. This congestion within the tissues of the respiratory tract gives rise to several conditions commonly seen during pregnancy. These conditions include nasal and sinus stuffiness, epistaxis (nosebleed), changes in the voice, and marked inflammatory response to even a mild upper respiratory infection.

Increased vascularity also swells tympanic membranes and eustachian tubes, giving rise to symptoms of impaired hearing, earaches, or a sense of fullness in the ears.

Pulmonary Function. The pregnant woman breathes deeper (increases *tidal volume,* the volume of gas moved into or out of the respiratory tract with each breath) but increases her respiratory rate only slightly (about two breaths per minute). The increase in respiratory tidal volume associated with the normal respiratory rate results in an increase in respiratory minute volume by approximately 26%. The increase in the respiratory minute volume is the *hyperventilation of pregnancy,* which is responsible for a decreased concentration of carbon dioxide in alveoli. The hyperventilation of pregnancy is apparently caused by the increased levels of progesterone, since it has been mimicked in males given progesterone (Scott et al, 1990).

During pregnancy, changes in the respiratory center result in a lowered threshold for carbon dioxide. Progesterone and estrogen are presumed to be responsible for the increased sensitivity of the respiratory center to carbon dioxide. In addition, pregnant women experience increased awareness of the need to breathe; some may complain of dyspnea at rest.

Although pulmonary function is not impaired by pregnancy, diseases of the respiratory tract may be more serious during gestation (Cunningham, MacDonald, and Gant, 1989). One important factor may be the increased oxygen requirements.

Basal Metabolism Rate. The basal metabolism rate (BMR) usually rises by the fourth month of gestation. It is increased by 15% to 20% by term. The BMR returns to nonpregnant levels by 5 to 6 days postpartum. The elevation in BMR reflects increased oxygen demands of the uterine-placental-fetal unit, as well as oxygen consumption from increased maternal cardiac work. Peripheral vasodilatation and acceleration of sweat gland activity assist in dissipating the excess heat resulting from the increased metabolism during pregnancy. Gravidas may experience heat intolerance, which is annoying to some women. **Lassitude** and **fatigability** after only slight exertion are described by many women in early pregnancy. These feelings may persist, along with a greater need for sleep. Lassitude and fatigability may be caused in part by the increased metabolic activity (see discussion of thyroid gland later in this chapter).

Acid-base Balance. By about the tenth week of pregnancy, there is a decrease of about 5 mm Hg in P_{CO_2}. Progesterone may be responsible for increasing the sensitivity of the respiratory center receptors so that tidal volume is increased and P_{CO_2} falls, the base excess (HCO_3, or bicarbonate) falls, and pH rises (becomes more basic). These alterations in acid-base balance indicate that *pregnancy is a state of respiratory alkalosis* compensated by mild metabolic acidosis.

Renal System

The kidneys are vital excretory organs. Their purpose is to maintain the body's internal environment in the relatively constant homeostatic state necessary for the efficient functioning of the body at the cellular level. The kidneys are responsible for maintenance of electrolyte and acid-base balance, regulation of extracellular fluid volume, excretion of waste products, and the conservation of essential nutrients.

Anatomic Changes. Changes in renal structure result from hormonal activity (estrogen and progesterone), pressure from an enlarging uterus, and an increase in blood volume. As early as the tenth week of pregnancy, the renal pelvis and the ureters dilate. Dilatation of the ureters is more pronounced above the pelvic brim, in part because they are compressed between the uterus and the pelvic brim. Dilatation above the pelvic brim is more marked on the right side. In most women the ureters below the pelvic brim are of normal size. The smooth muscle walls of the ureters undergo hyperplasia and hypertrophy and relaxed muscle tone. The ureters elongate, become tortuous, and form single or double curves. In the latter part of pregnancy, the right renal pelvis and ureter dilate more than on the left as a result of the displacement of the heavy uterus to the right by the sigmoid colon.

Because of these changes, a larger volume of urine is held in the pelves and ureters and urine flow rate is slowed. Urinary stasis or stagnation has several consequences:

1. There is a lag between the time urine is formed and when it reaches the bladder. Therefore clearance test results may reflect substances contained in glomerular filtrate several hours before.
2. Stagnated urine is an excellent medium for the growth of microorganisms. In addition, the urine of pregnant women contains greater amounts of nutrients, including glucose. Therefore during pregnancy, women are more susceptible to urinary tract infection.

Bladder irritability, nocturia, and **urinary frequency** and **urgency** (without dysuria) commonly are reported in early pregnancy. Near term, bladder symptoms may return.

Urinary frequency results from increased bladder sensitivity and later from compression of the bladder (see Fig. 8-7). In the second trimester the bladder is pulled up out of the true pelvis into the abdomen. The urethra lengthens to 7.5 cm (3 in) as the bladder is displaced upward. The pelvic congestion of pregnancy is reflected in hyperemia of the bladder and urethra. This increased vascularity causes the bladder mucosa to be traumatized and bleed easily. There may be a decrease in bladder tone, which permits distension of the bladder to approximately 1500 ml. At the same time the bladder is compressed by the enlarging uterus, resulting in the urge to void even if the bladder contains only a small amount of urine.

Renal Function Changes. In normal pregnancy, renal function is altered considerably. Glomerular filtration rate (GFR) and renal plasma flow (RPF) increase early in pregnancy (Cunningham, MacDonald, and Gant, 1989). The woman's kidneys must manage the increased metabolic and circulatory demands of the maternal body and also excretion of fetal waste products. Changes in renal function are caused by pregnancy hormones, an increase in blood volume, the woman's posture, physical activity, and nutritional intake.

Renal function is most efficient when the woman lies in the left lateral recumbent position and least efficient when the woman assumes a supine position. When the pregnant woman is lying supine, the heavy uterus compresses the vena cava and the aorta, and cardiac output decreases. The result is a drop in maternal blood pressure and fetal heart rate (vena cava or *hypotensive syndrome*) and a drop in the volume of blood to the kidneys (see Fig. 8-9). When cardiac output drops, blood flow to the brain and heart is continued at the expense of other organs, including the kidneys and uterus.

Fluid and Electrolyte Balance. Selective renal tubular reabsorption maintains sodium and water balance regardless of changes in dietary intake and losses through sweat, vomitus, or diarrhea. From 500 to 900 mEq of sodium is normally retained during pregnancy to meet fetal needs. The need for increased maternal intravascular and extracellular fluid volume requires additional sodium to expand fluid volume and to maintain an isotonic state. To prevent excessive sodium depletion, the maternal kidneys undergo a significant adaptation by increasing tubular reabsorption. As efficient as the renal system is, it can be overstressed by excessive dietary sodium intake or restriction or by use of diuretics. *Severe hypovolemia and reduced placental perfusion are two consequences.*

The capacity of the kidneys to excrete water during the early weeks of pregnancy is more efficient than later in pregnancy. Occasionally in early pregnancy the extent of water loss may cause some women to feel thirsty. The pooling of fluid in the legs in the latter part of pregnancy decreases renal blood flow and GFR. The diuretic response to the water load is triggered when the woman lies down, preferrably on her left side, and the pooled fluid reenters general circulation. This pooling of blood in the lower legs is sometimes referred to as **physiologic edema,** which requires no treatment.

Normally the kidney reabsorbs almost all of the glucose and other nutrients from the plasma filtrate. In pregnant women tubular reabsorption of glucose is impaired so that *glucosuria* does occur at varying times and to varying degrees. Normal values are 0 to 20 mg/dl. That is, during any one day the urine is sometimes positive and sometimes negative. When it is positive, the amount of glucose varies from 1+ to 4+.

In nonpregnant women, blood glucose levels must be at 160 to 180 mg/dl before glucose is "spilled" into the urine (not reabsorbed). During pregnancy, glucosuria occurs when maternal glucose levels are lower than 160 mg/dl. Why glucose, as well as other nutrients such as amino acids, is wasted during pregnancy is not understood, nor has the exact mechanism been discovered. Although glucosuria may be found in normal pregnancies (indeed 1+ levels may be seen with increased anxiety states), the possibility of diabetes mellitus must be kept in mind (Chapter 24).

Albumin and globulin are proteins that are not normal constituents of urine at any time. Small (trace) amounts of protein may occasionally be found in concentrated urine or in first-voided urine following sleep. However, a measurable amount (over 150 mg in 24 hours) of protein in the urine is a significant sign of renal disease at any time.

Integumentary System

Alterations in hormonal balance and mechanical stretching are responsible for several changes in the integumentary system during pregnancy. General changes include increases in skin thickness and subdermal fat, hyperpigmentation, hair and nail growth, accelerated sweat and sebaceous gland activity, and increased circulation and vasomotor activity. There is greater fragility of cutaneous elastic tissues, resulting in striae gravidarum, or stretch marks. Cutaneous allergic responses are enhanced.

Pigmentation is caused by the anterior pituitary hormone melanotropin, which is increased during pregnancy (Chapter 10). Facial melasma, also called **chloasma** or **mask of pregnancy,** is a blotchy, brownish hyperpigmentation of the skin over the malar prominences and the forehead, especially in dark-complexioned expectant women. Chloasma appears in 50% to 70% of pregnant women, beginning after the sixteenth week and increasing gradually to delivery. The sun intensifies this pigmentation in susceptible women. Chloasma caused by normal pregnancy usually fades after delivery. Darkening of the nipples, areolae, axillae, and vulva occurs at about the same time.

The **linea nigra** is a pigmented line extending from the symphysis pubis to the top of the fundus in the midline; this line is known as the linea alba before hormone-induced pigmentation. In primigravidas the extension of the linea nigra, beginning in the third month, keeps pace with the rising height of the fundus; in multigravidas the entire line often appears earlier than the third month.

Striae gravidarum, or stretch marks (seen over lower abdomen in Fig. 8-2), which appear in 50% to 90% of gravidas during the second half of pregnancy, may be caused by action of adrenocorticosteroids. Striae reflect separation within the underlying connective (collagen) tissue of the skin. These slightly depressed streaks tend to occur over areas of maximum stretch (i.e., abdomen, thighs, and breasts). The stretching sometimes causes a sensation that resembles itching. Tendency to the development of striae may be familial. After delivery they usually fade, although they never disappear completely. In the multipara, in addition to the reddish striae of the present pregnancy, glistening silvery lines representing the cicatrices (scars) of previous striae are commonly seen.

Angiomas or **telangiectasias** are commonly referred to as **vascular spiders.** They are tiny, stellate or branched, slightly raised and pulsating end-arterioles. The spiders, a result of elevated levels of circulating estrogen, are usually found on the neck, thorax, face, and arms. They are also described as focal networks of dilated arterioles radiating about a central core. The spiders are bluish in color and do not blanch with pressure. Striae may be evident on the breasts as a result of stretching as they increase in size. Vascular spiders appear during the second to the fifth month of pregnancy in 65% of white women and 10% of black women. The spiders usually disappear after delivery.

Pinkish red, diffuse mottling or well-defined blotches are seen over the palmar surfaces of the hands in about 60% of white women and 35% of black women during pregnancy (Cunningham, MacDonald, and Gant, 1989). These pigmentation changes and **palmar erythema** may also be seen in women taking oral hormonal contraceptives.

Epulis (gingival granuloma gravidarum) is a red, raised nodule on the gums that bleeds easily. This lesion may develop around the third month and usually continues to enlarge as pregnancy progresses. Treatment by excision is initiated only if it becomes excessive in size, causes pain, or bleeds excessively.

By the sixth week some women notice **thinning and softening of the fingernails and toenails.** Nail polish and nail polish remover may need to be discontinued and the nails kept short to prevent breakage. **Oily skin** and **acne vulgaris** may occur during pregnancy. For other women the skin clears and looks radiant. **Hirsutism** is commonly reported. An increase in fine hair growth may occur. The fine hair tends to disappear after pregnancy. Growth of coarse or bristly hair does not usually disappear after pregnancy. Some women comment that their hair is thickest and most abundant during pregnancy.

Musculoskeletal System

The gradually changing body and increasing weight of the pregnant woman cause marked alterations in

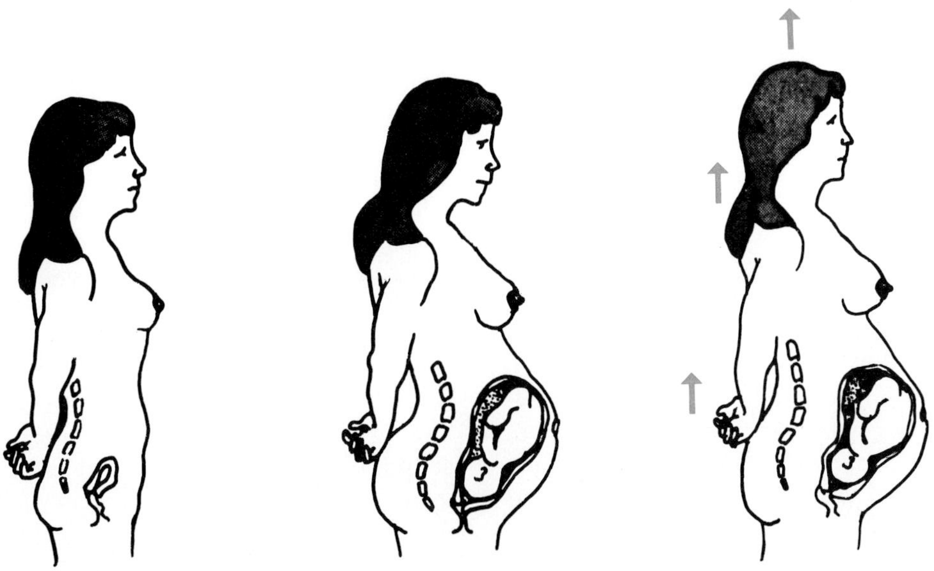

Fig. 8-10 Postural changes during pregnancy. **A,** Nonpregnant. **B,** Incorrect posture. **C,** Correct posture.

posture (Fig. 8-10) and walking. The great abdominal distension that gives the pelvis a forward tilt, decreased abdominal muscle tone, and increased weight bearing in late pregnancy require a realignment of the spinal curvatures. The woman's center of gravity shifts forward. An increase in the normal lumbosacral curve develops, and a compensatory curvature in the cervicodorsal region (exaggerated anterior flexion of the head) is required to maintain balance. Large breasts and a stoop-shouldered stance will further accentuate the lumbar and dorsal curves. Locomotion is more difficult, and the waddling gait of the gravid woman, called "the proud walk of pregnancy" by Shakespeare, is well known. The ligamentous and muscular structures of the mid and lower spine may be severely stressed. These and related changes often cause musculoskeletal discomfort.

The young, well-muscled woman may tolerate these changes without complaint. However, older women or those with a back disorder or a faulty sense of balance may have a considerable amount of back pain during and just after pregnancy.

Slight relaxation and increased mobility of the pelvic joints are normal during pregnancy. This is secondary to exaggerated elasticity and softening of connective and collagen tissue, and the result of increased circulating steroid sex hormones. These adaptations permit enlargement of pelvic dimensions. The degree of relaxation varies, but considerable separation of the symphysis pubis and the instability of the sacroiliac joints may cause pain and difficulty in walking. Obesity and multifetal pregnancy tend to increase the pelvic disability.

The muscles of the abdominal wall stretch and ultimately lose some tone. During the third trimester the rectus abdominis muscles may separate (Fig. 8-11), allowing abdominal contents to protrude at the midline. The umbilicus flattens or protrudes. After delivery, the muscles gradually regain tone. However, separation of the muscles (**diastasis recti abdominis**) may persist. The maternal pelvis is discussed in detail in Chapter 12.

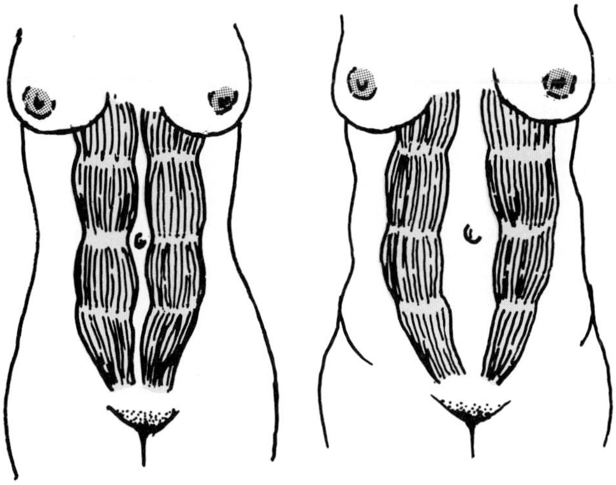

Fig. 8-11 Possible change in rectus abdominis muscles during pregnancy. **A,** Normal position in nonpregnant woman. **B,** Diastasis recti in pregnant woman.

Neurologic System

Little is known regarding specific alterations in function of the neurologic system during pregnancy, aside from hypothalamic-pituitary neurohormonal changes. Specific physiologic alterations resulting from pregnancy may cause the following neurologic or neuromuscular symptomatology:

1. Compression of pelvic nerves or vascular stasis caused by enlargement of the uterus may result in sensory changes in the legs.
2. Dorsolumbar lordosis may cause pain because of traction on nerves or compression of nerve roots.
3. Edema involving the peripheral nerves may result in *carpal tunnel syndrome* during the last trimester. The edema compresses the median nerve beneath the carpal ligament of the wrist. The syndrome is characterized by paresthesia (abnormal sensation such as burning or tingling because of a disorder of the sensory nervous system) and pain in the hand, radiating to the elbow. The dominant hand is usually affected most.
4. Acroesthesia (numbness and tingling of the hands) is caused by the stoop-shouldered stance (see Fig. 8-10, *B*) assumed by some women during pregnancy. The condition is associated with traction on segments of the brachial plexus.
5. Tension headache is common when anxiety or uncertainty complicates gestation. However, vision problems such as refractive errors, sinusitis, or migraine may also be responsible for headaches.
6. "Lightheadedness," faintness, and even syncope (fainting) are common during early pregnancy. Vasomotor instability, postural hypotension, or hypoglycemia may be responsible.
7. Hypocalcemia may cause neuromuscular problems such as muscle cramps or tetany.

Gastrointestinal System

The functioning of the gastrointestinal tract during pregnancy presents a curiously interesting picture. The appetite increases. Intestinal secretion is reduced. Liver function is altered, and absorption of nutrients is enhanced. The colon is displaced laterally upward and posteriorly. Peristaltic activity (motility) decreases. As a result bowel sounds are diminished, and constipation, nausea, and vomiting are common. Blood flow to the pelvis increases as does venous pressure, contributing to hemorrhoid formation in later pregnancy.

Mouth. The gums are hyperemic, spongy, and swollen. They tend to bleed easily because the rising levels of estrogen cause selective increased vascularity and connective tissue proliferation (a nonspecific gingivitis). There is no increase in secretion of saliva. Women do complain of **ptylism** (excessive salivation). This perceived increase is thought to be caused by the decrease in unconscious swallowing by the woman when nauseated. Epulis and bleeding gums are discussed under Integumentary System.

Teeth. The pregnant woman requires about 1.2 g of calcium and approximately the same amount of phosphorus every day during pregnancy. This is an increase of about 0.4 g of each of these elements over nonpregnant needs. With a well-balanced diet (Chapter 11), these requirements are satisfied. Serious dietary deficiency, however, may deplete the mother's osseous stores of these elements but does not draw on calcium in her teeth. Demineralization of teeth does not occur during pregnancy. Hence the old adage "for every child a tooth" is untrue. Poor dental hygiene during pregnancy or anytime and gingivitis may contribute to dental caries, which could result in the loss of a tooth.

Esophagus, Stomach, and Intestine. Herniation of the upper portion of the stomach *(hiatal hernia)* occurs after the seventh or eighth month of pregnancy in about 15% to 20% of gravidas. This condition results from upward displacement of the stomach, which causes a widening of the hiatus of the diaphragm. It occurs more often in multiparas and older or obese women.

Increased estrogen production causes decreased secretion of hydrochloric acid. Therefore peptic ulcer formation or flare-up of existing peptic ulcers is uncommon during pregnancy.

Increased progesterone production causes decreased tone and motility of smooth muscles, so that there is esophageal regurgitation, decreased emptying time of the stomach, and reverse peristalsis. As a result the woman may experience "acid indigestion" or *heartburn* (**pyrosis**).

In response to increased needs during pregnancy, iron is absorbed more readily in the small intestine. In general, if the individual is deficient in iron, iron absorption is increased.

Increased progesterone (causing loss of muscle tone and decreased peristalsis) results in an increase in water absorption from the colon. **Constipation** may result. In addition, constipation is secondary to hypoperistalsis (sluggishness of the bowel), unusual food choice, lack of fluids, abdominal distension by the pregnant uterus, and displacement of intestines with some compression. *Hemorrhoids* (varicose veins of the rectum and anus) may be everted or may bleed during straining at stool. Bowel habits and a characteristic type of stool are established early in life. Variations will be noted with concern and may be perceived as a disease process. A mild ileus (sluggishness, lack of movement) that follows delivery, as well as postdelivery fluid loss and perineal discomfort, contribute to continuing constipation.

Gallbladder and Liver. The gallbladder is quite often distended because of its decreased muscle tone during pregnancy. Decreased emptying time and thickening of bile are typical. These features, together with slight hypercholesterolemia from increased progesterone levels, may account for the common development of *gallstones* during pregnancy.

Hepatic function is difficult to appraise during gestation. However, only minor changes in liver function develop during pregnancy. Occasionally, intrahepatic cholestasis (retention and accumulation of bile in the liver, caused by factors within the liver) in response to placental steroids, occurs late in pregnancy and may result in *pruritus gravidarum* (severe itching) with or without jaundice. Oatmeal baths and lotions help ease the itching. These distressing symptoms subside promptly after delivery.

Abdominal Discomfort. Intraabdominal alterations that can cause discomfort include pelvic heaviness or pressure, round ligament tension, flatulence, distension and bowel cramping, and uterine contractions. In addition to displacement of intestines, pressure from the expanding uterus increases venous pressure in the pelvic organs. Although most abdominal discomfort is a consequence of normal maternal alterations, the physician is constantly alert to the possibility of disorders such as bowel obstruction or an inflammatory process.

Appendicitis may be difficult to diagnose. The *appendix* is displaced upward and laterally, high and to the right, away from McBurney's point.

Endocrine System

Profound endocrine changes occur that are essential for pregnancy maintenance, normal fetal growth, and postpartum recovery. Metabolic changes and weight gain are discussed in detail in Chapter 11.

Thyroid Gland. During pregnancy there is moderate enlargement of the thyroid gland caused by hyperplasia of the glandular tissue and increased vascularity (Cunningham, MacDonald, and Gant, 1989; Scott et al, 1990). Oxygen consumption and BMR increase secondary to the metabolic activity of the products of conception. For a discussion of changes in thyroid hormone production see Cunningham, MacDonald, and Gant (1989); and Scott et al (1990).

Parathyroid Gland. Pregnancy induces a slight secondary hyperparathyroidism, a reflection of increased requirements for calcium and vitamin D. When the needs for growth of the fetal skeleton are greatest (during the last half of pregnancy), plasma parathormone levels are elevated; that is, the peak level occurs between 15 and 35 weeks' gestation.

Pancreas. The fetus requires significant amounts of glucose for its growth and development. To meet its need for fuel, the fetus not only depletes the store of maternal glucose but also decreases the mother's ability to synthesize glucose by siphoning off her amino acids. Maternal blood glucose levels fall. Maternal insulin does *not* cross the placenta to the fetus. As a result, in early pregnancy, the pancreas decreases its production of insulin.

However, as pregnancy continues, the placenta grows and produces progressively larger amounts of hormones (i.e., human placental lactogen [hPL], estrogen, and progesterone). Cortisol production by the adrenals also increases. Estrogen, progesterone, hPL, and cortisol collectively decrease the mother's ability to utilize insulin. Cortisol stimulates increased production of insulin but also increases the mother's peripheral resistance to insulin (i.e., the tissues cannot use the insulin). Insulinase is an enzyme produced by the placenta to deactivate maternal insulin. Decreasing the mother's ability to utilize her own insulin is a protective mechanism that ensures an ample supply of glucose for the needs of the fetoplacental unit.

The result is an added demand for insulin by the gravida. The normal beta cells of the islets of Langerhans in the pancreas can meet the demand for insulin that continues to increase at a steady rate until term (see Chapter 24).

Pituitary Prolactin. In pregnancy, serum prolactin begins to rise in the first trimester and increases progressively to term. It is generally believed that although all the hormonal elements (estrogen, progesterone, thyroid, insulin, and free cortisol) necessary for breast growth and milk production are present in elevated concentrations during pregnancy, the high levels of estrogen inhibit active alveolar secretion by blocking the binding of prolactin to breast tissue, thus inhibiting the milk-producing effect of prolactin on the target epithelium (Scott et al, 1990).

Endocrine System and Maternal Nutrition. *Progesterone* causes the deposit of fat in subcutaneous tissues over the abdomen, back, and upper thighs. The fat serves as an energy reserve for both pregnancy and lactation. Several other hormones affect nutrition. *Aldosterone* conserves sodium. *Thyroxin* regulates metabolism. *Parathyroid hormone* controls calcium and magnesium metabolism. *Human placental lactogen (hPL)* acts as a growth hormone. *Human chorionic gonadotropin (hCG)* induces nausea and vomiting in some women in early pregnancy.

SUMMARY

The intimate union of mother and fetus is referred to as the fetoplacental maternal unit. Because the maternal organism responds as a total unit to the developing fetus, the intrauterine environment of the fetus is maintained at an optimum level only to the extent that the mother's systems can adjust to the developing organism.

Adaptation to pregnancy involves all of a woman's body systems. The mother's physical response is assessed in relation to normal expected alterations. Subjective symptoms and objective signs arising from these changes serve as a basis for diagnosis of pregnancy.

LEARNING ACTIVITIES

1. Spend several hours observing and participating at a prenatal clinic.
   a. What anatomic adaptations to pregnancy did you observe or assess?
   b. Were any physiologic adaptations to pregnancy apparent? If so, what?
   c. What complaints or questions were asked by clients related to anatomic or physiologic changes?
2. Interview three pregnant women (and spouse, or other, if present) at different stages of their pregnancy:
   a. How does each feel about changes in her body related to anatomic and physiologic adaptations?
   b. Which changes do they find pleasant?
   c. Which changes do they find uncomfortable?
   d. What is their level of understanding of these adaptations?
   e. Does the nurse in the clinic function as a teacher?
3. Prepare a class for expectant mothers (parents) in which they discuss adaptations.
4. Explore own emotions and attitudes regarding the changes a woman's body undergoes during pregnancy.

KEY CONCEPTS

- The biochemical, physiologic, and anatomic adaptations that occur during pregnancy are profound and return almost completely to the nonpregnant state following delivery and lactation.
- Maternal adaptations are attributed to the hormones of pregnancy and to mechanical pressures arising from the enlarging uterus and other tissues.
- The understanding of these adaptations to pregnancy remains a major goal, for without such knowledge it is difficult, if not impossible, to understand the disease processes—pregnancy-induced or coincidental—that can threaten women during pregnancy and the puerperium.
- The ability to recognize the beta subunit of hCG through monoclonal antibody technology has revolutionized endocrine tests for pregnancy.
- Adaptations to pregnancy protect the woman's normal physiologic functioning, meet the metabolic demands pregnancy imposes, and provide for fetal developmental and growth needs.
- The rise in pH of the pregnant woman's vaginal secretions makes her more vulnerable to vaginal infections.
- Increased vascularity and sensitivity of the vagina and other pelvic viscera may lead to a high degree of sexual interest and arousal.
- Some adaptations to pregnancy result in discomforts such as fatigue, urinary frequency, nausea, and breast sensitivity.
- Balance and coordination are affected by changes in joints and the woman's center of gravity as pregnancy progresses.

References

Batzer FR: Guidelines for choosing a pregnancy test, Contemp OB/GYN 26:37, Oct 1985 (special issue).
Brucker MC and MacMullen NJ: What's new in pregnancy tests? JOGN Nurs 14:353, Sept-Oct 1985.
Cunningham FG, MacDonald PC, and Gant NF: Williams obstetrics, ed 18, Norwalk, Conn, 1989, Appleton & Lange.
Doshi ML: Accuracy of consumer performed in-home tests for early pregnancy detection, Am J Public Health, 76:512, 1986.
Ganong WF: Review of medical physiology, ed 13, Norwalk, Conn, 1989, Appleton & Lange.
News: Monoclonals: new frontiers in reproductive medicine in Technology 1986 Contemp OB/GYN 26:75, Oct 1985.
Scott JR et al: Danforth's obstetrics and gynecology, ed 6, Philadelphia, 1990, JB Lippincott Co.
Seidel HM et al: Mosby's guide to physical examination, St Louis, 1987, The CV Mosby Co.

Bibliography

Gibbs CE: Sudden sensorium derangement during pregnancy, Contemp OB/GYN 20:39, 1982.
Goodlin RC et al: Clinical signs of normal plasma volume expansion during pregnancy, Am J Obstet Gynecol 145:1001, 1983.
Malasanos L et al: Health assessment, ed 4, St Louis, 1989, The CV Mosby Co.
Miller BK: How to spot . . . and treat . . . carpal tunnel syndrome . . . early, Nurs '80 10:50, 1980.
Rosen T and Mills J: Tattletale lesions: could this be a "stretchmark"? RN 46(2):49, 1983.
Samples JT et al: The dynamic characteristics of the circumvaginal muscles, JOGN Nurs 17(3):194, 1988.
Stauffer RA et al: Gallbladder disease in pregnancy, Am J Obstet Gynecol 144:661, 1982.
Willson JR and Carrington ER: Obstetrics and gynecology, ed 8, St Louis, 1987, The CV Mosby Co.

CHAPTER

9 Family Dynamics of Pregnancy and Preparation for Childbirth

Edna Quinn

Learning Objectives

Correctly define the key terms listed.

Examine maternal adaptation to pregnancy in regard to acceptance, identification with motherhood role, family relationships, and anticipation of labor.

Examine paternal adaptation to pregnancy in regard to acceptance, identification with fatherhood role, family relationships, and anticipation of labor.

Discuss sibling adaptation to pregnancy.

Discuss grandparent adaptation to pregnancy.

Evaluate pregnancy after age 35.

Determine appropriate content for classes designed for the first, second, third, and "fourth" trimesters of pregnancy.

Review "Education for choice."

Explain parent preparation for cesarean birth.

Outline prebirth education for gravidas, siblings, and, grandparents during this period.

Discuss the advantages of childbirth education.

Compare and contrast childbirth preparation methods.

Outline the advantages and disadvantages of birth-setting choices.

Key Terms

alternative birth center
announcement phase
ASPO
attachment
birthing room
birth-setting choices
body boundaries
body image
couvade
developmental tasks
educational diagnosis
emotional lability
expressive style
fantasy child
focusing phase
husband-coached childbirth
ICEA
informed choice
instrumental style
maturational crisis
mitleiden
monitrice
moratorium phase
natural childbirth
observer style
rite of passage
safe passage

Pregnancy involves all family members. Because "conception is the beginning, not only of a growing fetus but also of the family in a new form with an additional member and with changed relationships," each family member must adapt to the pregnancy and interpret its meaning in light of his or her own needs (Grossman, 1980).

This process of family adaptation to pregnancy takes place within a cultural environment. There have been dramatic changes in the fabric of Western society in recent years, and the nurse must be prepared to support single-parent families, reconstituted families, and dual-career families in the childbirth experience. Because much of the research on family dynamics in pregnancy and childbirth preparation in the United States and Canada has been done with white, middle-class families, findings may not apply to subcultures, minorities, or families who do not fit the traditional American model. The terms "spouse" or "husband" and "wife" are used consistently in the literature. The nurse may have to adapt these terms to apply to corresponding roles in many families. The reality of today's family may differ significantly from the image of the ideal family perpetuated by research on self-selected families.

The role of women has changed. In most families, women have moved out of the home and participate actively in the economic, social, and political life of their communities. This has resulted in a corresponding role change for many men—the role of father now includes more direct participation in childbirth preparation, the birth process, and in caring for the child. More research is needed to assess the impact of this involvement on the family, but it has been reported that more involvement of fathers fosters positive attitudes and behaviors toward the mother and child (Jones, 1986; Westney, Cole, and Munford, 1988).

Another trend related to the changing role of women is the tendency to postpone childbearing. The number of primigravidas 35 to 40 years of age has increased by 40%. Births in this age group have increased by 37% over the last 10 years. It is no longer uncommon to see primigravidas in their late 30s or even their early 40s. Reasons include advanced education, career priorities, and better contraceptive measures.

These women choose parenthood over a child-free life-style. They often are successfully established in a career and have a life-style with a partner that includes time for self-attention, establishment of a home with accumulated possessions, and freedom to travel. When questioned as to why they chose pregnancy late in life, many reply, "because time is running out." Age 35 brings a biologic boundary, a "closing of the gates," into view (Deutch, 1945; Sheehy, 1977). Older primigravidas and their partners share in planning for a family-centered birth and the desire to be loving and competent parents. If isolation with her infant and the reality of child care prove difficult for the mother who is accustomed to the stimulation of other adults, anger and resentment toward the father (or infant) can result, even if they "prepare" themselves for these aspects of parenting.

In a recent study of the psychologic dimension of older primigravidas, Winslow (1987) reported that women in this group approached pregnancy as a "project" and took a more conscious, active role in planning for childbirth and anticipating the future demands of parenting than did young mothers. They were very aware of movement from one role and life-style to another. They expressed concern about meeting the demands of parenting, fitting a new role into the established role as working woman, meeting the need to alter their relationships with their husbands, and restructuring their lives to include care of the baby.

Older multiparas may be women who have never used contraceptives because of personal choice, religious belief, or lack of knowledge about contraceptives. Or they may be women who used contraception successfully, but ceased to menstruate regularly as menopause approached, stopped using contraceptives, and consequently became pregnant. The older multipara often experiences displacement, feeling that pregnancy alienates her from her peers and that her age interferes with close associations with young mothers (Hogan, 1979). Other parents may welcome the unexpected infant as evidence of continuing parental roles.

During pregnancy, both mother and father explore the possibilities and responsibilities of changing identities and new roles. They must prepare a safe and nurturing environment during pregnancy and after birth. They must also integrate the child into an established family system and negotiate new roles (parent roles, sibling roles, grandparent roles) for family members.

❑ MATERNAL ADAPTATION

Women, from teenagers to women in their 40s, use the 9 months of pregnancy to adapt to the maternal role. This is a complex social and cognitive process that is not intuitive but learned (Rubin, 1967a). In becoming a mother, the teenager must shift from being mothered to mothering. The adult must move from "well-established routines to the unpredictable context created by an infant" (Mercer, 1981). The nullipara "the woman without child," becomes "the woman with child" and the multipara, "the woman with child," becomes the "woman with children" (Lederman, 1984).

Rubin (1984) proposes that the subjective experience of time and space changes during pregnancy as plans and commitments become regulated by the expected date of delivery (EDD). Early in pregnancy nothing seems to be happening, and there may be a resistance to giving up the full days of social demands and activities for a "burdensome, empty time." A lot of time is spent sleeping. With quickening in the second trimester, there is a reduction of time and space, both geographic and social, as the woman turns her attention inward to her pregnancy and to relationships with her mother and other women who have been or are pregnant. With the third trimester there is a slower pace and a sense that time is running out as the woman's activities are curtailed (Rubin, 1984).

Pregnancy is a **maturational crisis** that can be stressful but rewarding as the woman prepares for a new level of caring and responsibility. Her self-concept must change in readiness for parenthood as the dynamic interaction between intrapsychic and biologic processes cause her to reassess her "self-image, beliefs, values, priorities, behavior patterns, relationships with others, and problem-solving skills" (Lederman, 1984). Gradually, she moves from being self-contained and independent to being committed to a lifelong concern for another human being. This growth requires mastering certain developmental tasks: accepting the pregnancy, identifying the role of mother, reordering the relationships between mother and daughter and between husband and wife, establishing a relationship with the unborn child, and preparing for the birth experience (Caplan, 1959; Deutch, 1945; Lederman, 1984; Rubin, 1967a; Stainton, 1985a, 1985b). Studies indicate that the husband's emotional support is an important factor in the successful accomplishment of these developmental tasks (Ballou, 1978; Leifer, 1980; Entwistle and Doering, 1981; Mercer, 1981). Even unwed adolescent fathers may provide significant support to young mothers who must master the developmental tasks of pregnancy superimposed on those of adolescence (Westney, Cole, and Munford, 1988).

Acceptance of Pregnancy

The first step in adapting to the maternal role is acceptance of the idea of pregnancy and assimilation of the pregnant state into the woman's way of life (Lederman, 1984). The degree of acceptance is reflected in the woman's readiness for pregnancy and her emotional responses.

Readiness for Pregnancy. The availability of birth control means that pregnancy for many women is a joint commitment between responsible partners. Planning a pregnancy, however, does not necessarily ensure acceptance of the pregnancy (Entwistle and Doering, 1981). Other women view pregnancy as a natural outcome of the marital relationship that may or may not be desired, depending on circumstances. For the adolescent, pregnancy can result from sexual experimentation using no contraception.

Women prepared to accept a pregnancy are prompted by early symptoms to seek medical validation of the pregnancy, but some women who have strong feelings of "not me," "not now," and "not sure," may postpone seeking supervision and care (Rubin, 1970). Examples of conversational cues to acceptance or denial are given in Table 9-1.

Once pregnancy is confirmed, a woman's emotional response may range from great delight to shock, disbelief, and despair. The reaction of many women is the "someday but not now" response:

> There is a real pleasure in finding oneself functionally capable of becoming pregnant. There is pleasure in learning that others are pleased with the promise of having, and being given, a child. But these feelings exist independently of the question of time. Personally and privately she is not ready, not now (Rubin 1970).

Caplan (1959) reports that the majority of his clients were dismayed initially at finding themselves pregnant. However, eventual acceptance of pregnancy paralleled the growing acceptance of the reality of a child. He cautions against equating nonacceptance of the pregnancy with rejection of the child. A woman may dislike being pregnant but feel love for the child to be born.

Emotional Responses. Women who are happy and pleased about their pregnancies often view pregnancy as biologic fulfillment and part of their life plan. They have high self-esteem and tend to be confident about

Table 9-1 **Conversational Cues Regarding Possible Pregnancy**

Symptom	Acceptance	Denial
Amenorrhea	"I'll wait one more time; the doctor will think I'm crazy if I go in right away."	"This has happened before. My periods are always irregular. When I went away to college I didn't menstruate for nearly a year."
Tingling and tenderness of breasts	"This is always the second symptom I have. Then I'm pretty sure I'm pregnant."	"My breasts always hurt just before I menstruate." "I am gaining weight. I need a new bra." "My breasts are finally developing. I thought they never would."
Nausea and vomiting	"I didn't think I'd be one who gets sick, but you never know."	"I must have the flu—that's what I'll say if old Smith (teacher) says anything. I've had to go out of the room three mornings in a row."
Urinary frequency	"I have to go at the worst times, but now I don't care. I just say, 'Jane take over the class' and go."	"I'm so nervous all the time it makes me want to go to the bathroom constantly. It is so hard to explain to your teacher."
Feeling of fatigue	"When I'm first pregnant I could just sleep all the time."	"Mother asks how come I'm so tired. She doesn't know how hard I work at tennis."

outcomes for themselves, their babies, and other family members. Even though a general state of well-being predominates, an **emotional lability** expressed as rapid mood changes is commonly encountered in pregnant women.

Rapid mood changes and an increased sensitivity to others are disconcerting to the mother-to-be and those around her. Increased irritability, explosions of tears and anger, and feelings of great joy and cheerfulness alternate, apparently with little or no provocation. According to one father-to-be:

> ■ I sometimes think she is crazy—we're going somewhere she wants to go, out to dinner or a concert. She goes upstairs happy as a lark and in 2 minutes is down again in a regular temper, won't go, and shouts at me. I really feel bewildered by it all.

Many reasons, such as sexual concerns or fear of pain during delivery, have been postulated to explain this seemingly erratic behavior. Profound hormonal changes that are part of the maternal response to pregnancy may also be responsible for mood changes, much as they are before menstruation or during menopause.

As pregnancy progresses, the woman becomes more open about her feelings toward herself and others (Caplan, 1959). She is willing to talk about matters previously not discussed or discussed only within the family and seems to believe that her thoughts and symptoms will be of interest to the listener whom she deems protective. This openness, coupled with a readiness for learning, makes working with pregnant women a delight and increases the likelihood of supportive care being therapeutically effective.

When the child is wanted, the discomforts associated with pregnancy tend to be considered as irritations, and measures taken to relieve them are usually successful. Pleasure derived from thinking about the unborn child and a feeling of closeness to the child helps the mother adjust to these discomforts.

In some instances the woman who commonly complains about physical discomforts may be asking for help with conflicts regarding the mothering role and its responsibilities. Further assessment of coping measures and tolerance is indicated (Lederman, 1984).

Response to Changes in Body Image. The physiologic changes of pregnancy result in rapid and profound changes in body contour. During the first trimester body shape changes little, but by the second trimester obvious bulging of the abdomen, thickening of the waist, and enlargement of the breasts proclaim the state of pregnancy. The woman develops a feeling of an overall increase in the size of her body and of occupying more space. This feeling intensifies as pregnancy advances (Jessner, 1970). There is a gradual loss of definite **body boundaries** that serve to separate the self from the nonself and provide a feeling of safety: "I looked in the mirror and wondered if it were really me. I had a sudden feeling that I was ballooning outward, there was no end, and I did not know how to bring it together and be myself again." Fawcett (1978) describes this feeling as an awareness of the "perceived zone of separation between self and nonself."

Men respond in a variety of ways to their wife's changing shape. Some say their wife is most beautiful when pregnant, whereas others make derisive comments.

Negative feelings may be countered by a "Mother Earth" feeling, one of being a protective shield for the fetus (Deutch, 1945; Colman, 1969; Rubin, 1970), or by exercise. Research on exercise in pregnancy is relatively new and should be examined critically, but it indicates that moderate exercise seems to be beneficial in combating a negative **body image** and reducing anxiety (Reich, 1987). For most women the feeling of liking or not liking their bodies in the pregnant state is temporary and does not cause significant changes in their perception of themselves.

Ambivalence During Pregnancy. Ambivalence is defined as simultaneous conflicting feelings, such as love and hate toward a person, thing, or state of being. Ambivalence is a normal response experienced by persons preparing for a new role. Most women have some ambivalent feelings during pregnancy.

Even women who are pleased to be pregnant may experience feelings of hostility toward the pregnancy or unborn child from time to time. Such things as a husband's chance remark about the attractiveness of a slim, nonpregnant woman or hearing about a colleague's promotion when the decision to have a child means relinquishing a job can give rise to ambivalent feelings. Body sensations, feelings of dependence, or realization of the responsibilities associated with child care can trigger such feelings.

Intense feelings of ambivalence that persist through the third trimester may indicate unresolved conflict with the motherhood role (Lederman, 1984). If the birth of a healthy child ensues, memories of these ambivalent feelings are dismissed. If a child with a defect is born, a woman may look back at the times of not wanting the child and feel intensely guilty. She may believe that her ambivalence caused the defect in her child.

Being a self-reliant person, someone in control of her own destiny, has become part of the mother's expectations of herself. Pregnancy alters this state: her baby is always with her as part of her body consciousness. She needs nurturing and support from others through birth and child rearing. Adaptation to dependency requires a change in self-image as one moves from independence to dependency.

Adult Responsibilities. Pregnancy functions as a **rite of passage** indicative of reaching maturity in a society that has no other obvious rituals. In many states the pregnant woman is legally an adult regardless of her age and may give personal consent for any type of care for herself or for her newborn. She is entitled to financial and other aid from a government source if needed and, if unwed, is considered to be the sole legal guardian of her child. As such she has the right to care for the child herself, place the child in a foster home, or give the child up for adoption.

Identification with Motherhood Role

The process of identifying with the motherhood role begins early in each woman's life, with the memories she has of being mothered as a child. Her social group's perception of what constitutes the feminine role can also make her lean more toward motherhood or a career, toward being married or single, or toward being independent rather than interdependent. Stepping-stone roles, such as playing with dolls, baby-sitting, or taking care of siblings, may increase her understanding of what being a mother entails.

Many women have always wanted a baby, liked children, and looked forward to motherhood. They are highly motivated to become parents, which affects acceptance of pregnancy and eventual prenatal and parental adaptation (Grossman, 1980; Lederman, 1984). Other women apparently have not considered in any detail what motherhood means to them. During pregnancy conflicts such as not wanting the pregnancy or child or career-related decisions need to be resolved.

Mother-Daughter Relationship

The woman's relationship to her mother has proved significant in adaptation to pregnancy and motherhood (Deutch, 1945; Caplan, 1959; Rubin, 1967a, b; Ballou, 1978; Mercer, Hackley, and Bostrom, 1982). Lederman (1984) noted the importance of four components in the gravida's relationship with her mother: the mother's availability (past and present), her reactions to the daughter's pregnancy, respect for her daughter's autonomy, and the willingness to reminisce.

During childhood the availability of the mother was perceived as her being there, loving and supportive. Women with such mothers used them as role models. Other women in the study perceived that their mothers were not available. However, when some of these mothers became available to their daughters during the pregnancy, they were emotionally supportive. "With the common bond of motherhood and mutual availability, subjects often described a closeness that appeared to facilitate the development and adaptation of both individuals" (Lederman, 1984).

The mother's reaction to the daughter's pregnancy signified her acceptance of the grandchild and of her daughter. If the mother was supportive, the daughter had an opportunity to discuss pregnancy and labor and her feelings of joy or ambivalence with a knowledgeable and accepting woman. Rubin (1975) noted that if the gravida's mother is not pleased with the pregnancy, the daughter begins to have doubts about her self-worth and the eventual acceptance of her child by others.

Mothers who respected their daughters' autonomy prompted feelings of self-confidence in their daughters. The coming child helped the grandmother-to-be move toward a grandmother role. Some grandmothers used the birth of their grandchildren as a second chance at mothering. Grandparents who had helped their children become independent were seen as being willing to help rather than interfere or dominate.

Reminiscing about the gravida's early childhood and sharing the grandmother-to-be's account of her childbirth experience helped the daughter anticipate and prepare for labor and delivery (Levy and McGee, 1975). Hearing about themselves as young children made the gravidas feel loved and wanted. They drew closer to their parents and began to feel that in spite of the errors they might make in their own mothering experiences, they would continue to be loved by their children.

Wife-Husband Relationship

The most important person to the pregnant woman is usually the father of her child (Richardson, 1983). There is increasing evidence that the woman who is nurtured by her male partner during pregnancy has fewer emotional and physical symptoms, fewer labor and childbirth complications, and an easier postpartum adjustment (Lederman et al., 1979; Grossman, 1980; May, 1982b). Women have expressed two major needs within the wife-husband relationship during pregnancy (Richardson, 1983). The first need relates to the wife's securing indications that she is loved and valued. The second need relates to securing her husband's acceptance of the child and assimilating the child into the family. Rubin (1975) states that "as the childbearer, it devolves on the pregnant woman to ensure the necessary social and physical accommodation within the family and within the household for a new member."

The marital relationship is not static but evolves

over time. The addition of a child changes forever the nature of the bond between wife and husband. Lederman (1984) reported that wives and husbands grew closer during pregnancy. In this study pregnancy had a maturing effect on the wife-husband relationship as the partners assumed new roles and discovered new aspects of one another. Partners who trusted and supported each other were able to share mutual dependency needs. Women expressed a need for the fathers' active involvement in preparation for birth. The husband was seen as a stabilizing influence, a good listener to expressions of doubts and fears, and a source of physical and emotional reassurance (Grossman, Eichler, and Winckoff, 1980). Most women were aware of the developmental needs of their husbands during pregnancy. They were sympathetic toward the husband's need for reassurance as to his importance to the wife and recognized that he could feel jealous of the unborn baby.

Concerns about Sexual Relationship. Sexual expression is a concern for many couples during pregnancy (Zalar, 1976; Ellis, 1980; Swanson, 1980; Lederman, 1984). It is affected by physical, emotional, and interactional factors, including myths about sex during pregnancy, sexual dysfunction problems, and physical changes in the woman.

Myths about body functions and fantasies about the influence of the fetus as a third party in lovemaking are frequently expressed. Anomalies, mental retardation, and other injuries to the mother and fetus are often attributed to sexual relations during pregnancy. Many couples fear that the woman's genitals will be drastically changed by the birth process. Embarrassment or not wanting to appear foolish often prevents couples from expressing their concerns to the health professional.

Dyspareunia (painful intercourse), differing sexual drives, and erectile problems (impotence) are the three major problems reported. Dyspareunia may be caused by pressure on the woman's abdomen and deep penile thrusting. Postcoital cramping, backache, and even breast tenderness during the first trimester have also been reported.

As pregnancy progresses, changes in body shape, body image, and levels of discomfort influence both partners' desire for sexual expression. During the first trimester the woman is frequently plagued by nausea, fatigue, and sleepiness. As she progresses into the second trimester, her combined sense of well-being and increased pelvic congestion may profoundly increase her desire for sexual release. In the third trimester, fatigue, fetal demands, and physical bulkiness increase her physical discomfort and lower her libido.

Both husband and wife need to feel free to discuss their sexual responses during pregnancy. Sensitivity to each other and a willingness to share concerns can strengthen their sexual relationship. Communication between the couple is important. Partners who do not understand the seemingly rapid physiologic and emotional changes of pregnancy can become confused by the other's behavior. By talking to each other about the changes they are experiencing, couples are able to define problems and offer the needed support.

Concerns About the Fetus. Parental concern for the health of the child seems to vary during the course of pregnancy (Leifer, 1980). The first concern appears in the first trimester and relates to abortion. One woman expressed her feelings as follows: "I spotted [blood] off and on. The doctor said, 'If you are going to hold it, you will; if you abort it, it is probably just as well.' How could he say 'it'? He was talking about my baby." As the child becomes more of a reality, with movement and an audible heartbeat, parental anxiety focuses on possible defects in the child. Parents talk openly about these anxieties and press for confirmation that the child will be all right. In the later stages of pregnancy fear about the death of the child is less identifiable; this possibility is evidently remote for parents.

Mother-Child Relationship

Emotional **attachment** to the child begins during the prenatal period as women use fantasizing and daydreaming to prepare themselves for motherhood (Rubin, 1975; Leifer, 1977; Cranley 1981a, b; Stainton, 1983, 1985b). They think of themselves as mothers and imagine mother qualities they would like to possess. Expectant parents desire to be warm, loving, and close to their child. They try to anticipate changes in their lives the child will bring and wonder how they will react to noise, disorder, less freedom, and caregiving activities. They question their ability to share their love for other children with the unborn child. Rubin (1967a, b) found that women "try on" and test the motherhood role by taking their own mothers or substitute mothers as role models who serve as confidantes, support persons, or sources of information and experience.

The mother-child relationship progresses through pregnancy as a developmental process (Shereshefsky and Yarrow, 1973; Rubin, 1975; Leifer, 1980). Three developmental tasks in the evolution of the relationship have been identified by theorists:

1. To accept the biologic fact of pregnancy. The woman needs to be able to state, "I am pregnant" and incorporate the idea of a child into her body and self image.

Early in pregnancy the mother's thoughts center around herself and the immediate reality of the pregnancy itself. The child is viewed as "part of one's self" and the majority of women think of their fetus as "unreal" during the early period of pregnancy (Ballou, 1978; Lumley, 1980a, b, 1982a).

2. To accept the growing fetus as distinct from the self and as a person to nurture. The woman can now say, "I am going to have a baby."

During the second trimester, usually by the fifth month, there is a growing awareness of the child as a separate being. This differentiation of the child from the woman's self permits the beginning of the mother-child relationship that involves not only *caring* but also *responsibility*. Researchers have noted that women who planned the pregnancy are pleased with their pregnancy and develop attachment to the child earlier than other women (Leifer, 1980; Cranley, 1981a, b; Lumley, 1982b; Koniak-Griffin, 1988). Robson and Kumar (1980) noted a delayed onset of *maternal attachment* in women who do not perceive the fetus as an individual by 36 weeks of gestation.

With acceptance of the reality of the child (hearing the heartbeat and feeling the child move) and the subsidence of early symptoms, the woman enters a quiet period, and becomes more introspective. A **fantasy,** or dream, **child** becomes precious to the woman. As she seems to withdraw and to concentrate her interest on the unborn child, her husband sometimes feels "left out," and other children in the family become more demanding in their efforts to redirect the mother's attention to themselves.

3. To prepare realistically for the birth and parenting of the child. The woman expresses the thought, "I am going to be a mother" and defines the nature and characteristics of the child.

In the last months of pregnancy the mother becomes more realistic about her maternal role and about her child. Although the mother alone experiences "the child within," both parents and siblings believe the unborn child responds in a very individualized, personal manner. Family members may interact a great deal with the unborn child by talking to the fetus and stroking the mother's abdomen, especially when the fetus shifts position (Fig. 9-1).

Most of our ideas about maternal-fetal attachment are based on clinical impressions and theoretical notions rather than empirical data. There seems to be support for the theory that attachment is a gradual prenatal developmental process (Gaffney, 1988). However, the growing body of research relating psychologic variables to prenatal attachment has produced "counter-intuitive" or conflicting findings. Gaffney (1988) has summarized selected studies that fail to show consistent significant correlations between factors believed to effect maternal-fetal attachment.

Koniak-Griffin's 1988 study of 90 pregnant adolescents representing a variety of ethnic backgrounds failed to show that maternal attachment was related to self-esteem and social support. Although maternal attachment is believed to develop over time, length of pregnancy was not a significant predictor of prenatal attachment (Koniak-Griffin, 1988). Kemp and Page (1986) found no significant relationship between attachment and maternal age, race, whether the pregnancy was planned, or whether the woman had a sonogram. In a study by Carson and Virden (1984), teaching prenatal palpation had no significant influence on maternal-fetal attachment. Concepts from theoretical models, such as anxiety, early relationships with the mother, and self-esteem, appear to be only a few of the many factors that shape parental attitudes (Mercer et al, 1988).

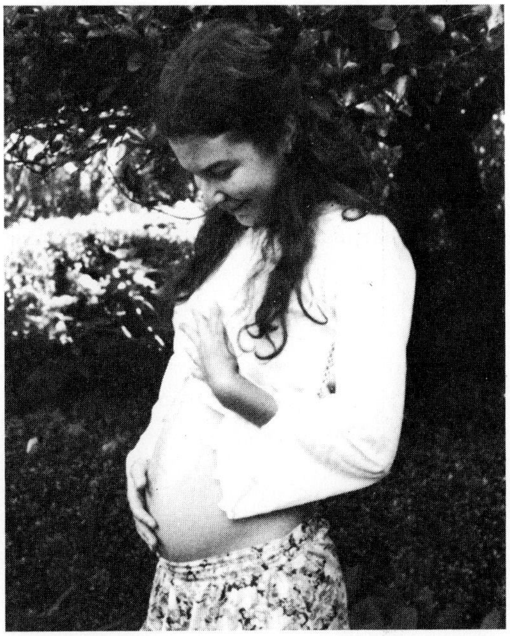

Fig. 9-1 Mother talks to her baby: "How are you doing in there?"

Theories may be useful even in the absence of solid empirical support; and in spite of methodologic flaws, studies of maternal-fetal attachment are useful. Nurses become better observers when they test theory and question the assumptions on which their practice is based. They must continue to seek to understand and foster attitudes and behaviors that promote early attachment and reduce the risk of negative long-term sequelae such as child neglect and abuse. More research relating psychologic variables to prenatal attachment and maternal-fetal interaction with maternal-infant interaction is needed.

Nature and Characteristics of the Child. Stainton (1985a) found that expectant parents usually agreed on the nature and characteristics of the unborn child, as expressed in five categories: appearance, communication, gender, sleep-wake cycles, and temperament.

The description of *appearance* of the child included features such as color of hair, size and shape of eyes, and size of the infant. For races other than Caucasian, color of hair and eyes were taken for granted.

Both fathers and mothers believed there was *communication* with the fetus. The unborn child responded to quiet talking, music, or massage by "settling down," and to loud voices or music by moving or kicking excessively.

Cultural conditioning may color the couple's preference for the *gender* of children. Women frequently defer to their husbands' stated preference. If the sex of the child was known by sonogram, the child might be named and referred to by name. If the sex was not known, it was ascribed by the parents because of the size of the baby or type of movement (Stainton, 1985a). Regular movement is associated with fetal well-being (Cohen, 1985).

The *sleep-wake cycles* of the child are described as (1) sleeping: when the unborn child is still and unresponsive to noise, talking, or touch; (2) a quiet but calm state: the child gently rocks or rolls slightly; and (3) an upset or alert state: the child responds readily to touch or noise by kicking, stretching, and, until past 30 weeks gestation, rolling over (Stainton, 1985a).

The *temperament* of the child was described variously as "calm, cooperative" or "having a temper just like mine." Movements of the child are interpreted as indicating pleasure, discomfort, or playfulness. Some parents reported their newborn's activity, responsiveness, and sleep-wake patterns at 2 months of age to be remarkably similar to their description of the unborn child's behavior at 8 months' gestation (Stainton, 1983).

Preparation for Childbirth

Many women prepare actively for birth. They read books, view films, attend parenting classes, and talk to other women (mothers, sisters, friends, strangers). Other women tend to recount problems they experienced with deliveries and may frighten nulliparas. The multipara has her own history of labor and delivery that can either comfort her or make her fearful.

Anxiety can arise from concern about a **safe passage** for herself and her child during the birth process (Rubin, 1975). This may not be expressed overtly, but cues are given as the nurse listens to plans women make for care of the new baby and other children in case "anything should happen." These feelings persist despite statistical evidence about the safe outcome of pregnancy for the mother. Many women fear the pain of delivery or mutilation because they do not understand anatomy and the birth process. Women express concern over what behaviors will be appropriate during the birth process and how the persons who will be caring for them will accept them and their actions. Lederman (1984) found women fear loss of control and concomitant loss of self-esteem in labor.

Loss of control was related to the loss of physical control and also to medical decisions regarding care made without the woman's knowledge (Highley and Mercer, 1978). Women worried about emotional control—crying or becoming hysterical or hostile to their husbands or the staff. Possible loss of control in labor affected the women's plans for use of analgesics and anesthesia during labor, varying from complete rejection to acceptance. The use of drugs during labor was also related to concern about the safety of the child.

Reaching the hospital in time for the birth, arranging for the care of children at home, and being unable to plan specific dates for outside help or the partner's vacation were concerns that made the last few weeks a time of tension; the tension was compounded by a lack of adequate rest. The ability to participate wholeheartedly in situations that result in growth, joy, and pleasure and, conversely, the ability to face pain, separation, disability, or death adequately come in part from the feelings one has about the ability to maintain control, in part from sharing these critical periods with those who care, and in part from the nurturing provided by others. The best preparation for labor was found to be "a healthy sense of the realistic—an awareness of work, pain, and risk balanced by a sense of excitement and expectation of the final reward" (Lederman, 1984).

Readiness for Childbirth. Toward the end of the third trimester breathing is difficult and movements of the fetus become vigorous enough to disturb the mother's sleep. Backaches, frequency and urgency of urination, constipation, and varicose veins can become troublesome. The bulkiness and awkwardness of her body interfere with the woman's ability to care for other children, perform routine housekeeping duties, and assume a comfortable position for sleep and rest.

By this time most women become impatient for labor to begin, whether the birth is anticipated with joy, dread, or a mixture of both. A strong desire to see the end of pregnancy, "to be over and done with it," make women at this stage ready to move on to childbirth.

Second-time Mothers. Mothers expecting their second child have different concerns in pregnancy (Merilo, 1988). They may have unresolved feelings about their first labor. They may be so focused on their first child that they are less excited and think less about the second baby than they did about the first. They are concerned about the first child's reaction to separation at the sibling's birth and aware that a change in their relationship with the first child will occur after the new baby is born. These concerns may lead to a sense of loss and sadness. Friends and family, assured of the mother's ability to care for an infant, may offer less attention and help.

The nurse needs to recognize that there are dependency needs with every pregnancy. She can help second-time mothers meet their dependency needs by encouraging them to take time out to focus on the second child and their own needs. They need to set realistic expectations for themselves, arranging for household help and child care and reducing outside commitments. Prenatal classes in which second-time mothers are able to share concerns and experiences can help these women recognize that their needs are legitimate and will promote a positive adaptation to the many demands of their new role (Merilo, 1988).

❑ PATERNAL ADAPTATION

Expectant fathers, like expectant mothers, have been preparing for parenthood throughout their lives (Sherwen, 1987). Subconsciously or consciously men think about having a wife and children. During courtship and early marriage discussion of future plans may even include the number, spacing, and names of their children-to-be (Bobak, 1968).

The father's beliefs and feelings about the ideal mother and father and his cultural expectation of appropriate behavior during pregnancy will affect his response to his partner's need for him.

One man may engage in nurturing behavior. Another may feel lonely and alienated as the woman becomes physically and emotionally engrossed in the unborn child. He may seek comfort and understanding outside the home or become interested in a new hobby or involved with his work. Some men view pregnancy as a proof of their masculinity and their dominant role. To others, pregnancy has no meaning in terms of responsibility to either mother or child. However, for most men pregnancy is a time of preparation for the parental role, of fantasy, of great pleasure, and of intense learning.

How fathers adjust to the parental role is the subject of increasing contemporary research. In older societies the man is expected to subject himself to various behaviors and taboos associated with pregnancy and giving birth (Bobak, 1968; May, 1982b). These practices are known as ***couvade*** (French, "to hatch"). By enacting the *couvade,* the man's responses are channeled into acceptable modes of expression and this new status is recognized and endorsed. His behavior acknowledges his psychosocial and biologic relationship to the mother and child. In Western societies participation of fathers in childbirth has risen dramatically over the last 20 years, and the father in the role of labor coach is now well established (May, 1982b).

The man's emotional responses to becoming a father, his concerns, and informational needs change during the course of pregnancy. Phases of the developmental pattern become apparent. May (1982c) describes three phases characterizing the three developmental tasks experienced by the expectant father: the announcement phase, the moratorium phase, and the focusing phase.

The early period, the **announcement phase,** may last from a few hours to a few weeks. The developmental task is to accept the biologic fact of pregnancy. The man needs to be able to state, "She is pregnant and I am the father." Men react to the confirmation of pregnancy with joy or dismay depending on whether the pregnancy is desired or unplanned or unwanted. Realization of the reality of the pregnant state seems to come more slowly for the father who does not experience the early symptoms of pregnancy and sees little physical change in his wife in the first trimester of pregnancy. On seeing a sonograph of his son at 12 weeks, one man remarked, "Until I saw his picture, it was all unreal. I knew intellectually my wife was pregnant, but it didn't mean anything to me. It was amazing—in a few minutes I became a father."

The second phase, the **moratorium phase,** is the period of adjusting to the reality of pregnancy. The developmental task is to accept the pregnancy and to be able to state, "We are going to have a baby, and we are changing." Men appear to put conscious thought of the pregnancy aside for a time. They become more introspective and engage in many discussions about their philosophy of life, religion, childbearing, and child-rearing practices and their relationships with family members and friends. Depending on the man's readiness for the pregnancy, this phase may be relatively short or persist until the last trimester (May, 1982c).

The third phase, the **focusing phase,** begins in the last trimester and is characterized by the father's active involvement in both the pregnancy and his relationship with his child. The developmental task is to negotiate with his partner the role he is to play in labor and to prepare for parenthood. He needs to be able to state, "I know my role during the birth process, and I am going to be a parent." In this phase the man concentrates on "his own experience of pregnancy, and in doing so he feels more in tune with his wife. He begins to redefine himself as a father and the world around him in terms of his future fatherhood" (May, 1982c).

Acceptance of Pregnancy

Readiness for Pregnancy. May (1982c) found that fathers' readiness for pregnancy was reflected in three areas: "(1) a sense of relative financial security, (2) stability in the couple relationship, and (3) a sense of closure to the childless period in their relationship."

Many men express concern for the family's *economic security.* Today the majority of young married women as well as men are employed outside the home. Although pregnant women and mothers with young children may be employed in a work setting, many childbearing and child-rearing women have a phase of unemployment. Length of leave from employment is determined by a combination of factors, such as the couple's economic status, the policies of the employer, and the couple's value system. Some men attempt to compensate for anticipated needs by keeping their current jobs even though they had planned a change. They may put more effort into earning rapid promotions by working overtime or by taking on extra work. Some men acquire new or additional insurance at this time (Bobak, 1968).

Those couples who have a *stable relationship* before pregnancy tend to draw closer as a result of their coming parental roles (Lederman, 1984).

Their wives' pregnancies bring *to closure the childless period* in men's lives. Many men view having children and being a father as an integral part of their life plan. Couples who plan for pregnancy are more accepting of pregnancy (Lederman, 1984). If pregnancy is unplanned or unwanted, some men find the alterations in life plans and life-styles difficult to accept and do not necessarily become reconciled to the pregnancy (May, 1982c).

Emotional Responses. *Styles of involvement* in pregnancy refers to the "general patterns of feelings and behaviors that reflect the way men see themselves in relation to pregnancy" (May, 1980). Their basic personality structure is reflected in the style in which they project themselves. May (1980, 1982a) describes three styles characteristic of men studied during their wives' first-time pregnancy: the observer style, the expressive style, and the instrumental style.

Observer style was defined as a detached approach to involvement in the pregnancy. The fathers in this category fell into two major groupings, those who wanted the pregnancy and those who did not. Those who were happy about the pregnancy were supportive of their wives and wanted to be good fathers. However, because of cultural values or shyness, they needed to distance themselves from such activities as prenatal classes, decisions about breastfeeding, or choosing professional care. By nature unemotional and matter-of-fact, they appeared to need an "emotional buffer zone" and the pregnancy did not change them (May, 1982a).

The other group who were not happy about the pregnancy reported feelings of ambivalence about pregnancy and the role of father (May, 1982c). These men needed time to adjust to the idea of pregnancy and fatherhood and responded to the feelings of ambivalence by becoming involved in careers and resisting their wives' attempts to involve them in preparations for the coming child. "Men established an emotional distance from the pregnancy in relation to the amount of ambivalence they experienced. Women often sensed this distance and attempted to involve their partners more closely. Often the man responded by withdrawing more" (May, 1982c).

Expressive style was defined as a strong emotional response to pregnancy and a desire to be a full partner in the project (Fig. 9-2). These husbands showed awareness of their wives' needs for support and were conscious of the times when they were not able to give their wives the support needed. They experienced the same emotional lability and ambivalence that characterizes pregnant women. They were excited and pleased about the baby, but also worried about their ability to be good fathers. These fathers may experience the discomforts usually associated with women in pregnancy, such as nausea, lassitude, and various aches and pains. ***Mitleiden*** (suffering along), or psychosomatic symptoms of expectant fathers, has long been recognized as a phenomenon of expectant fatherhood. In 1627 Bacon observed, "That loving and kinde Husbands, have a Sense of their Wives Breeding Childe, by some Accident in their owne Body." And another au-

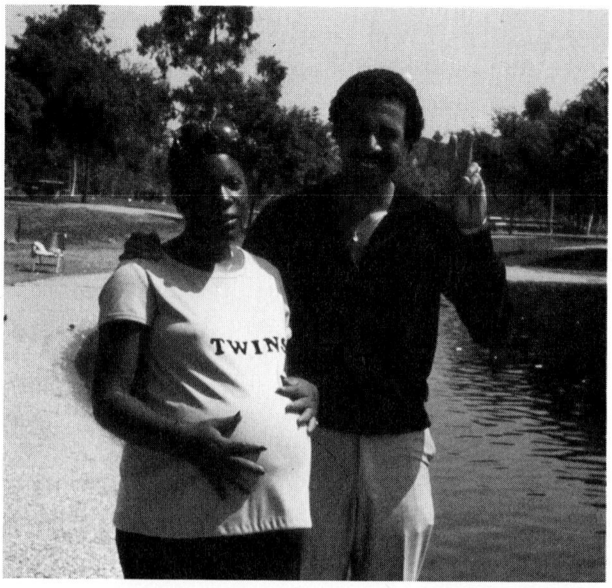

Fig. 9-2 Mother and father walk together. Women respond positively to their spouse's interest and concern. (Courtesy Marjorie Pyle, RNC, Lifecircle, Costa Mesa, Calif.)

thor in the 1600s commented, "It often falls out, that when the woman is in good health, the husband is sick, yea sometimes being many miles off" (Hunter and Macalpine, 1963). The husband alone may suffer these discomforts. The symptoms can bring the couple closer together and help the father in becoming more caring.

The **instrumental style** was adopted by men who emphasized tasks to be accomplished and saw themselves as "caretakers or managers of the pregnancy" (May, 1980). They asked questions, became interested in the role of labor coach, and planned for photographs during pregnancy, birth, and the neonatal period. They felt responsible for the outcome of pregnancy and were protective and supportive of their wives.

The three styles of involvement emphasize the different ways men can experience pregnancy. Each needs to feel free to define his role in pregnancy just as the woman does. Not all men are able or willing to attend childbirth classes or act as labor coaches because of cultural conditioning or a different supportive style. More research is needed to determine if similar styles of involvement occur in partners of multiparous women.

Identification with Fatherhood Role

Every father brings to pregnancy attitudes that affect the manner in which he adjusts to pregnancy and the parental role (Cronenwett and Kunst-Wilson, 1981; Kunst-Wilson and Cronenwett, 1981; Lederman, 1984).

The father's memories of fathering by his own father, the experiences he has had with child care, and the perceptions of the male and father role within his social group will guide his selection of the tasks and responsibilities he will assume. Some men are highly motivated to nurture and love a child. They may be excited and pleased about the anticipated role of father. Men who have reasonable self-esteem and control of financial resources and working conditions seem more able to incorporate fatherhood into their life plans. Identification with the fatherhood role is a crucial developmental step: "It can temporarily reactivate conflicts with his own parents, intensify feelings of separation, heighten dependency needs, and rekindle feelings of sibling rivalry. The husband who can look at these temporary regressions honestly is more likely to effect attachment and bonding with his newborn" (Lederman, 1984).

House (1981) outlined four types of support necessary for preparing for fatherhood:

1. *Emotional support.* The man's primary source of support is his spouse (Lein, 1979). This support has to be modified to permit nurturing of the baby and the additional nurturing his wife needs. Therefore the father needs to seek support from family and friends.
2. *Instrumental support.* The father needs to know that he can depend on family or friends for help if necessary.
3. *Informational support.* The father needs to know who is available (e.g., professionals or relatives) to provide "tips" on how to solve immediate problems.
4. *Appraisal support.* The father needs to find others to provide criteria against which he can measure his performance.

Husband-Wife Relationship

Ballou (1978) found the husband's role in pregnancy to be one of nurturance, responding to his wife's feelings of vulnerability in both her biologic state and in her relationship with her own mother. The husband's support indicates to his wife his involvement in the pregnancy and his preparation for attachment to their child (Caplan, 1959; Grossman, Eichler, and Winckoff, 1980; Leifer, 1980; Lederman, 1984).

In psychoanalytic literature some aspects of the father's behavior indicates rivalry. Rivalry between the expectant father and his pregnant wife is not new. In Greek legend, Zeus, angered by his wife's superior wisdom after she conceived, swallowed her and later gave birth to Athena, who emerged full grown from his forehead. In the same instant he both punished and replaced his wife. Direct rivalry with the fetus may be evident, especially during sexual activity. Husbands may protest that fetal movements prevent sexual gratification, making comments such as, "We can't have sex with 'that' kicking around in there" (Bobak, 1968).

The wife's increased introspection may cause her husband to experience a sense of uneasiness as she becomes preoccupied with thoughts of the child and of her mother, with her growing dependence on her male physician, and with her reevaluation of their relationship. He may sense that his wife's support—his key support—is being withdrawn.

Deciding on the infant's feeding method is of concern when the partners' preferences differ or when one partner has intense reactions. Recognized benefits and disadvantages of one method over another appear to be irrelevant. Some men insist that the wife breastfeed; others are adamantly set against breastfeeding. When the husband refuses to voice an opinion, the wife experiences uneasiness. Inwardly, she may accuse him of disinterest or feel uncertain about choosing the right way. The wife seems to ask for his support for whatever choice is made.

Father-Child Relationship

The father-child attachment can be as strong as the mother-child relationship and fathers can be as competent as mothers in nurturing their infants (Greenberg and Morris, 1974; Parke and Sawin, 1976; Jones, 1981; Cronenwett, 1982). Paternal behavior toward children does not differ significantly from maternal behavior, with the exception of play with the infants (Field, 1978).

Men prepare for fatherhood in many of the same ways as women do for motherhood—reading, fantasizing, and daydreaming about the baby. They may adjust work commitments to include new responsibilities or plan vacations to enable them to spend time with their new families.

Daydreaming is a form of role playing or anticipatory psychologic preparation for the infant most common in the last weeks before delivery. Rarely do men confide their daydreams unless they are reassured that daydreams are normal and fairly common. Questions such as the following help the nurse and the parent in identifying concerns and allow for reality testing:

1. What do you expect the child to look and act like?
2. What do you think being a father will be like?
3. Have you thought about the baby's crying? Changing diapers? Burping the baby? Being awakened at night? Sharing your wife with the baby?

The father may not wish to share his answers with the nurse at the moment, but may need time to think them through or discuss them with his spouse.

If an expectant father can imagine only an older child and has difficulty visualizing or talking about the infant, this area needs to be explored. The nurse can give information about the unborn child's ability to respond to light, sound, and touch and encourage the father to feel and talk to the fetus. Plans for seeing, holding, and examining his newly born child can be made.

As the birth day approaches, questions regarding fetal and newborn behaviors increase. "What do they do in there (in utero)?" "Is he hiccuping?" "Does he suck his thumb?" "How is he breathing?" "What does a newborn baby look like?" Some fathers express shock or amazement about the small size of clothes and furniture for the baby. Other fathers protest, "He'll only be real to me when I can hold him in my arms."

Some fathers become involved by picking the child's name and anticipating the child's sex. As early as the first month, the name of the child may be selected. Family tradition, religious mandate, and continuation of one's own name or names of relatives and friends are important in the selection process. The names chosen are tried on for fit; for example, the father might emphatically state, "I just can't picture myself as being a father to a boy named John." Armed with several names, one husband said he would decide on his final choice only after he saw the baby, pointing out that "to be named Eric, he *must* be blue-eyed and blond" (Bobak, 1968).

At the time of birth, most parents are able to accept the sex of the child born to them, but occasionally disappointment is evident and voiced. The parents may experience a grief reaction and a sense of loss at birth as they release the fantasized child and begin to accept the real child.

Anticipation of Labor

The days and weeks immediately preceding the expected day of delivery are characterized by anticipation and anxiety. Boredom and restlessness are common as the couple focuses on the birth process.

During the last 2 months of pregnancy, many expectant fathers experience a surge of creative energy, both at home and on the job. Dissatisfaction with present living space increases, and the need to alter the environment is acted on wherever possible. This may be tangible evidence of sharing in the childbearing experience while channeling the anxiety or other feelings of the final weeks before birth. This behavior earns recognition and compliments from friends, relatives, and the wife.

The father's anxieties may be expressed by refusal to think about the birth, by planning other activities during his wife's labor, or by sleeping and resting to the exclusion of all else. The expectant mother may become concerned about the possibility of being deserted physically or emotionally at a time when she is feeling most vulnerable.

The father's major concerns are getting the mother to a medical facility in time for the birth and not appearing ignorant. Many fathers want to be able to recognize labor and to determine when it is appropriate to leave for the hospital or call the physician or midwife. They may fantasize several ridiculously humorous situations and plan what they will do or rehearse the routes to the hospital, timing each route at different times of the day. Suitcase, car, and essential telephone numbers are readied.

Many fathers have questions about the labor suite's furniture, nursing staff, location, and availability of physician and anesthesiologist. Others want to know what is expected of them when their wives are in labor. The father has fears of mutilation and death for his wife and child. While he harbors these fears within, he cannot help his mate with her unspoken or overt apprehension. Words such as "dropped," "rupture of bag of waters," "bloody show," "tears and stitches," and "labor pains" have violent overtones (Bobak, 1968).

With the exception of parent education classes, a father has few opportunities to learn how to be an involved and active partner in this rite of passage into parenthood. Tensions and apprehensions of the unprepared, unsupportive father are readily transmitted and may increase the mother's fears. His own self-doubts and fear of inadequacy may be realized if he is not supported. Self-confidence comes from achieving realistic goals and earning the approval of others.

❑ SIBLING ADAPTATION

The mother with other children must devote much time and energy to reorganizing her relationships with existing children. She needs to prepare siblings for the birth of the child and to begin the process of role transition in the family by including the children in the pregnancy and being sympathetic to older children's protests against losing their places in the family hierarchy. No child willingly gives up a familiar position (Richardson, 1983).

Siblings' responses to pregnancy vary with age and dependency needs. The 1-year-old infant seems largely unaware of the process, but the 2-year-old child notices the change in mother's appearance and may comment, "Mommy's fat." The 2-year-old child's need for sameness in the environment makes the child aware of any change. Toddlers may exhibit more "clinging" behavior and revert to dependent behaviors in toilet training or eating.

By the third or fourth year of age children like to be told the story of their own beginning and accept its being compared to the present pregnancy. They like to listen to heartbeats and feel the baby moving in utero. Sometimes they worry about how the baby is being fed and what it wears. Parents often take older children with them to antepartal visits, particularly in the last few weeks (Fig. 9-3). One mother reported, "Near the end [of the pregnancy] he began to kiss my belly. I was surprised by that" (Walz and Rich, 1983). Interference with established routines can cause anger. One 4-year-old boy resented not being able to fit on his mother's lap anymore; his father resolved the issue by making the child a small ski he could slide down his mother's bosom and over her abdomen ("over the hump"). He could still sit close by, touch her, and accept her abdomen as part of his life. Sharing possessions with the unborn child is often short-lived and cribs or toys donated to the coming child are mostly reclaimed.

School-age children take a more clinical interest in their mother's pregnancy. They may want to know in more detail, "How did the baby get in there?" and "How will it get out?" Children in this age group notice pregnant women in stores, churches, and schools and sometimes seem shy if they need to approach a

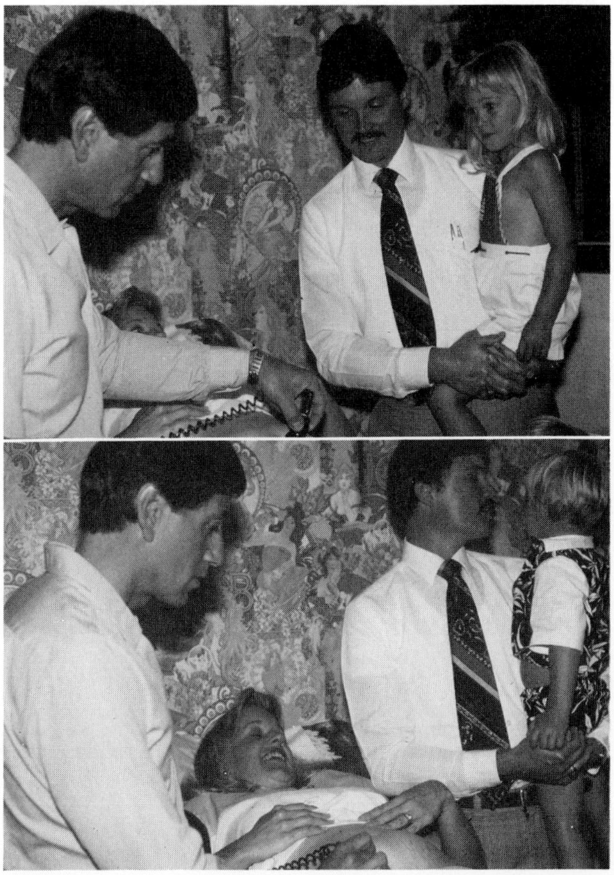

A

B

Fig. 9-3 Father and siblings accompany mother on prenatal visit. **A,** Daughter's attention is focused on nurse listening to baby's heart. **B,** Son is reluctant to watch as fetal heart rate is assessed.

pregnant woman directly. On the whole they look forward to the new baby, see themselves as "mothers" or "fathers," and enjoy buying baby supplies and readying a place for the baby. Because they still think in concrete terms and base judgments on the here and now, they respond positively to their mother's current good health and do not seem to be anxious about a future injury to her or to the unborn child. They need help to cope with any adverse change in the status of the parent or newborn, since they do not anticipate such a change.

Early and middle adolescents preoccupied with the establishment of their own sexual identity may have difficulty accepting the overwhelming evidence of the sexual activity of their parents. They reason that if they are "too young" for such activity, certainly their parents are "too old." They seem to take on a critical parental role and may ask, "What will people think?" or "How can you let yourself get so fat?" Many pregnant women with teenage children will confess that their teenagers are the most difficult factor in their current pregnancy.

On the positive side, parents-to-be may be suddenly confronted by a warm, sensitive person who is able to restore the mother's self-esteem, as illustrated by the following example.

> I came home one day feeling very pregnant, tired, and heavy and dreading the idea of making dinner and being helpful—you know—the mother bit! Mary [age 15 years] was cooking some hamburger, had the table set for dinner, and even had a flower centerpiece. For some reason I just started to cry. She came to me and hugged me and said, 'I think you're doing the loveliest thing in the world, having a baby.' I'll always remember that—she was really *my* mother for the moment.

Late adolescents do not appear to be unduly disturbed. They think that they soon will be gone from home. Parents usually report they are comforting and act more as other adults than as children. One mother delivering her tenth baby remarked, "The only complaint my oldest daughter made was, 'Mother, I'm getting married in August, so don't you dare be too pregnant to come to the wedding.' "

GRANDPARENT ADAPTATION

Some grandparents-to-be do not welcome the new role for their daughters or sons. It may make them aware of their own aging or represent the victory of the ex-child in obtaining an equal role with the parent. Some grandparents-to-be not only are nonsupportive but also use subtle means to decrease the self-esteem of the young parents-to-be. Mothers may talk about their terrible pregnancies; fathers may discuss the endless cost of rearing children; and mothers-in-law may describe the neglect of their son as the concern of others is directed toward the pregnant daughter-in-law.

However, most grandparents are delighted with the prospect of a new baby in the family. It reawakens their feelings of their own youth, the excitement of giving birth, and their delight in the behavior of the parents-to-be when they were infants. They set up a memory store of first smiles, first words, and first steps, which can be used later for "claiming" the newborn as a member of the family. Satisfaction comes with the realization that continuity between past and present is guaranteed.

Recent research indicates the importance of the grandparent-grandchild relationship. Grandparents act as a potential resource for families. Their support can strengthen family systems by widening the circle of support and nurturance (Barranti, 1985). The parent acts as negotiator in establishing the grandparent-grandchild relationship (Greene and Polivka, 1985). Many women report that their pregnancies bridged the final gap between them and their own mothers. The estrangement that began in adolescence disappeared as the now-pregnant daughter experienced joys, concerns, and anxieties similar to those her mother had felt before her.

PREBIRTH EDUCATION

The Nurses' Association of the American College of Obstetricians and Gynecologists (NAACOG) published its definition of *childbirth education* in 1981 as follows:

> The process designed to assist parents in making the transition from the role of expectant parents to the role and responsibilities of parents of a new baby which includes the period from the time of conception to approximately three months after birth.

This statement implies that childbirth education is *preparation for parenting,* not just preparation for labor and delivery, which has traditionally been the focus of childbirth education. It is now being advocated that preparation for parenting begin as preconception counseling included in routine women's health care (Barron, Brown, and Ganong, 1987). Earlier education regarding exercise, nutrition, alcohol, smoking, and drugs in pregnancy, as well as reproductive choices, may lead to healthier and more satisfying outcomes.

Most childbirth educators would agree that expectant parents need a comprehensive education program to prepare them for the role and responsibilities of parenthood, but there are philosophic disagreements on when and how different topics should be taught. For example, Bliss-Holtz (1988), in a study of primiparas' learning needs ($N = 189$), found that interest in learning infant care was low, even in the third trimester, and suggested that this content be taught postpartum:

> Currently, pregnant women have more decisions to make about their antepartal health care and selection of coping strategies for labor and delivery than their counterparts 25 years ago. With the shift in responsibility from health care provider to client, concerns for learning have changed from concern about infant care to more immediate concerns about maintaining maternal health and learning about the labor process.

Many childbirth educators will continue to focus almost exclusively on preparation for labor and delivery in the third trimester because this seems to be the major concern of parents (Bliss-Holtz, 1988).

Education for birth and parenting has traditionally occurred in formal classes in the United States and Canada, but education is a lifelong process that occurs in many ways. Formal education may be ineffective for people who do not find the classroom stimulating. Nurses have limitless opportunities to teach parents, not only in formal classes, but also in small group sessions, in office and clinic waiting rooms, and at home.

Teaching is a deliberate intentional action taken to help another person learn to do what that person cannot presently do. *Learning* involves measurable behavior change resulting from practice and experience. Like the nursing process, teaching is a process involving assessment, formulation of diagnoses (educational) planning, implementation, and evaluation (Fig. 9-4).

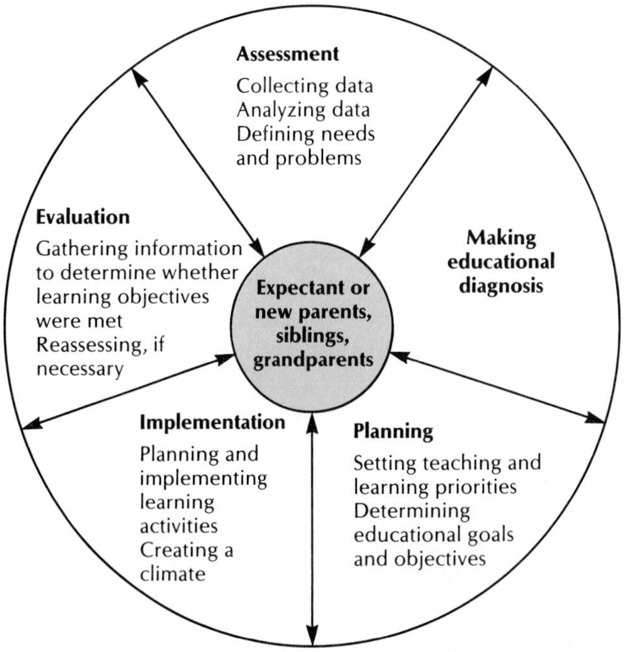

Fig. 9-4 The teaching process parallels the nursing process. Arrows indicate direction of communication.

Assessment

Assessment involves data collection to identify client needs. Pertinent data include the ages of the learners, their culture or ethnicity, and their readiness to learn. Data gathering is a continuous collection of information from a variety of valid and reliable sources. Examples of sources include group discussion, observation, and formal pen-and-pencil assessment of learning needs; personal interviews (Winslow, 1987); client health records; other health-care team members; family members; and review of pertinent literature.

Educational Diagnosis

An **educational diagnosis** can be formulated after the collected data have been analyzed. It identifies the client's learning needs and suggests a plan of action. For example, a second-time mother expresses concern about the impact the new baby will have on her older child. An educational diagnosis would be "knowledge deficit regarding management of sibling rivalry." Related objectives would be "the mother will set clear limits for the child" and "the mother will suggest acceptable outlets for the child's feelings."

The special needs of all pregnant women must be met (Mercer, 1979). For example, those experiencing first pregnancy after age 35 who have had successful careers require more sophisticated childbirth courses than younger primigravidas. Winslow (1987) found that a population of primigravidas, 35 to 44 years of age, felt out of place and did not receive the caliber or quality of information they had hoped for in the classes they attended.

Planning

Nurses establish teaching and learning priorities for the identified needs using their personal philosophy of childbirth and parent education as a guide. Educational goals and objectives are established. Objectives are statements related to the goal that are specific, measurable, attainable, and agreed on by the family and the nurse.

Implementation

Implementation involves carrying out the learning activities designed to meet the learning objectives. It encompasses selecting instructional methods such as discussion, role playing, repetition, testing, rewards, the use of audiovisual materials, and demonstration. Learning is enhanced when the instructor creates a climate of friendliness and acceptance.

Evaluation

Evaluation methods commonly used to evaluate client learning are direct observation, client records, reports, tests, interviews and questionnaires with clients and their families, interviews and questionnaires with staff, and research using statistical comparisons.

Parent Education Programs

Expectant parents and their families have different interests and information needs as the pregnancy progresses. A typical program is designed to meet the information needs of parents at the three major stages of pregnancy and after birth.

Early pregnancy ("early bird") classes provide fundamental information. Classes are developed around the following areas: (1) early fetal development, (2) physiologic and emotional changes of pregnancy, (3) human sexuality, and (4) the nutritional needs of the mother and fetus. Environmental and workplace hazards have become important concerns in recent years. Even though pregnancy is considered a normal process, exercises, danger signs, drugs, and self-medication are topics of interest and concern.

Midpregnancy classes emphasize the woman's participation in self-care. Classes provide information on preparation for breastfeeding and formula-feeding, basic hygiene, common complaints and simple, safe remedies, infant health, and parenting.

Late pregnancy classes are designed to meet the needs of the entire family: (1) couple discussion groups, (2) expectant father discussion groups, (3) sibling classes, (4) grandparents' classes, and (5) newborn care classes. Special classes are developed for teenage parents, for parents expecting a cesarean delivery (Hart, 1980), and for parents of twins. Refresher courses for those who feel they are prepared through previous childbirth experience but would like to review a few things are also available (Mercer, 1979).

Throughout the series of classes there is discussion of support systems that people can use during pregnancy and after birth; such support systems help parents function independently and effectively. During all the classes the open expression of feelings and concerns about any aspect of pregnancy, birth, and parenting is welcomed.

After-birth classes help parents meet the tasks and responsibilities of their new roles. Topics for discussion can include coping mechanisms for the reality of parenting, use of support systems, and infant care and growth and development. Birth control methods and adapting to new roles (wife-lover ⇌ mother and husband-lover ⇌ father) are explored.

Childbirth Methods

Women have always shared information on childbirth with other women, and until the late nineteenth century, childbirth was "women's work." Most babies in America were delivered at home by midwives. Then, instead of training midwives in the newly acquired medical science, physicians brought birth into the hospital and exerted pressure in state after state to ban midwives and give physicians a monopoly on obstetric care.

A concern for public health led to the first formal classes in childbirth education in the United States by the American Red Cross in 1913 and by The Maternity Center Association in New York in 1919. It was much later before formal classes in childbirth education would become available to most couples in this country.

The earliest classes were led by individuals or groups that were not affiliated with the "establishment." They were consumer-oriented and encouraged women to help themselves in labor and to avoid analgesia and anesthesia. The popular trend toward prepared childbirth education that began in the 1960s paralleled advances in the women's movement, the consumers' movement, and the increased use of nurse-midwives in the delivery of maternity care.

Childbirth educators see themselves as parents' advocates. They evaluate hospital practices from the parents' perspective, help parents question procedures that do not conform to their expectations, and suggest alternatives. Nurses should be on the cutting edge of this movement. Preparation for childbirth is an integral part of the nursing process, and nurses must help parents make informed decisions.

Today most physicians and hospitals recommend or offer childbirth classes to expectant parents. Major methods taught in the United States are (1) the Dick-Read or **"natural childbirth"** method, (2) the Lamaze or psychoprophylactic method (PPM), and (3) the Bradley method or **"husband-coached childbirth."**

Dick-Read Method. Grantly Dick-Read was an English physician who published two books, *Natural Childbirth* (1933) and *Childbirth Without Fear* (1944), in which he theorized that pain in childbirth was the result of social conditioning and a fear-tension-pain syndrome.

According to Dick-Read (1959):

> Fear, tension, and pain are three veils opposed to the natural design which have been concerned with preparation for and attendance at childbirth. If fear, tension, and pain go hand in hand, then it must be necessary to relieve tension and to overcome fear in order to eliminate pain. The implementation of my theory demonstrates methods by which fear can be overcome, tension may be eliminated and replaced by physical and mental relaxation.

Dick-Read's work became the foundation for organized programs of childbirth preparation and teacher training throughout the United States, Canada, Great Britain, and South Africa. Nurses prepared in this method established the International Childbirth Education Association (**ICEA**) in 1960.

To replace fear of the unknown with understanding and confidence, Dick-Read's program includes information on labor and birth, as well as nutrition, hygiene, and exercise. Classes include practice in three techniques: physical exercise to prepare the body for labor; conscious relaxation; and breathing patterns.

Conscious relaxation involves progressive relaxation of muscle groups in the entire body. With practice, many women are able to relax on command, both during and between contractions. Some women actually sleep between contractions.

Breathing patterns include deep abdominal respirations for most of labor, shallow breathing toward the end of the first stage, and, until recently, breath holding for the second stage of labor. Teachers of the Dick-Read method contend that the weight of the abdominal musculature on the contracting uterus increases pain. The woman is taught to force her abdominal muscles to rise as the uterus rises forward during a contraction, thus lifting the abdominal muscles off the contracting uterus.

The Dick-Read method has been adapted to ensure that labor support provided in the past by the nursing staff is now provided by the father or a support person chosen by the mother.

Lamaze Method. During the 1960s the *Lamaze method* gained popularity in the United States after Marjorie Karmel introduced the psychoprophylaxis method (PPM) in her book, *Thank You, Dr. Lamaze.* The American Society for Psychoprophylaxis in Obstetrics (ASPO) was formed in 1960 and the National Association of Childbirth Education, Inc. (NACE) was formed in 1970 to promote the Lamaze method and prepare teachers in the method. In 1971 the national Council of Childbirth Education Specialists, Inc. (CCES) was founded to offer teacher training seminars.

The Lamaze method grew out of Pavlov's work on classical conditioning. According to Lamaze, pain is a conditioned response. Women can also be conditioned not to experience pain in labor; the Lamaze method conditions women to respond to "mock" uterine contractions with controlled muscular relaxation and breathing patterns instead of crying out and losing control (Lamaze, 1970.) Coping strategies also include focusing on a "focal point," such as a favorite picture or pattern, to keep nerve pathways occupied so they cannot respond to painful stimuli.

The woman is taught to relax uninvolved muscle groups while she contracts a specific muscle group. She applies this in labor by relaxing uninvolved muscles while her uterus contracts. Women who attended Lamaze-type childbirth preparation classes maintained a significantly higher level of neuromuscular control during the first stage of labor than women who were self-prepared (Bernardini, Maloni, and Stegman, 1983). The perception of maintaining control is closely associated with satisfaction, according to studies by Cronenwett (1980) and Cronenwett and Brickman (1983).

Lamaze teachers believe that chest breathing lifts the diaphragm off the contracting uterus, thus giving it more room to expand. Chest breathing patterns vary according to the intensity of the contractions and the progress of labor. Teachers also seek to eliminate fear by increasing the understanding of how the body functions and the neurophysiology of pain. Support in labor is provided by the woman's husband or other support person or by a specially trained labor attendant termed a ***monitrice.***

Bradley Method. Robert Bradley, a Denver obstetrician, published *Husband-Coached Childbirth* in 1965, advocating what he calls true "natural childbirth," without anesthesia or analgesia and with a husband-coach and use of labor breathing techniques. The American Academy of Husband-Coached Childbirth (AAHCC) was founded to prepare teachers and make the method available.

The Bradley method is based on observations of animal behavior during birth and emphasizes working in harmony with the body, using breath control, abdominal breathing, and general body relaxation (Bradley, 1965). The technique stresses environmental factors such as darkness, solitude, and quiet to make childbirth a more natural experience. Women using the Bradley method often appear to be sleeping in labor, but they are actually in a state of deep mental relaxation.

Although the father's presence during labor seems to be very important to most women, the concept of the father as "coach" has been criticized by some (Klein et al, 1981). Some men are not comfortable with this role but can still be supportive of their wives during pregnancy and childbirth.

Comparison of Childbirth Methods. Most proponents of prepared childbirth agree that the major causes of pain in labor are fear and tension. All methods attempt to reduce these two factors and eliminate pain by increasing the woman's knowledge of what to expect in labor and delivery, enhancing her self-confidence and sense of control, preparing a support person (usually her husband), and training her in physical conditioning and relaxation breathing.

There are a few fine differences in approach. For example, Bradley teachers discourage the use of medication, encouraging the woman to focus inwardly and to take direction from her own body. Lamaze teachers believe that the judicious use of pain medication can be an appropriate adjunct to relaxation techniques and stress external focusing and distraction. In reality few instructors adhere strictly to one particular method but, instead, incorporate a variety of strategies aimed at increasing the woman's ability to cope with labor and minimize her need for medication (Fig. 9-5).

Studies indicate that women who attend prepared childbirth classes and have support in labor need less pain medication (Beck and Hall, 1978; Cogan, 1980).

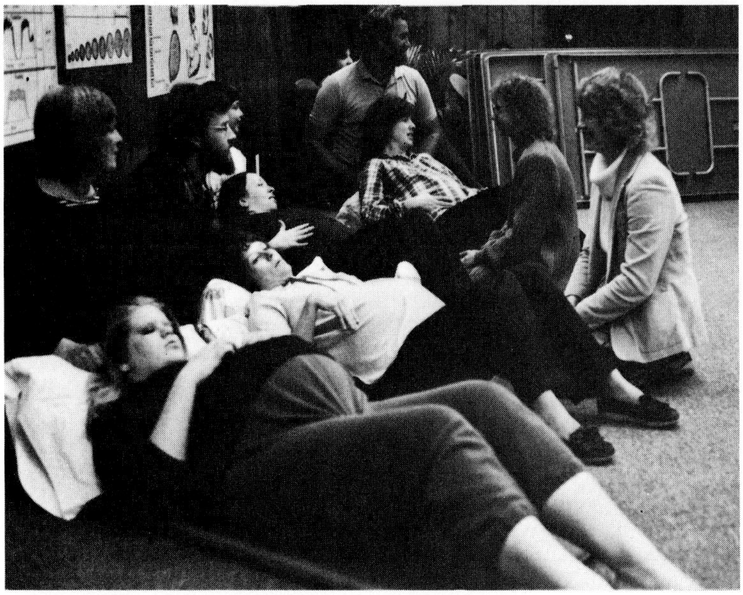

Fig. 9-5 Teaching relaxation. Women are exhaling slowly and performing effleurage. Coaches are watching a clock and counting off the seconds of this "contraction." (Courtesy Lisa Livingston, R.N., B.S.N., director, Maternal Child Health Education, Community Birth Center, Community Hospital, Santa Cruz, Calif.)

However, several extensive reviews of childbirth education research have yielded conflicting and inconsistent findings about the ability of childbirth preparation methods to reduce physical pain (Velvovsky, 1960; Chertok, 1967; Huttel et al, 1972; Coussens and Coussens, 1984). Either the methods do not produce reliable results or poorly controlled research fails to demonstrate their effectiveness.

Research on the psychologic effects of childbirth preparation continues to be overwhelmingly in agreement that women who attend classes have a more positive self-image (Coussens and Coussens, 1984) and express more satisfaction with their birth experience (Cronenwett, 1980; Cronenwett and Brickman, 1983) (Fig. 9-5). They also have a greater sense of control, and as Roberts (1983) points out:

> The distress associated with pain during labor seems to be caused not only by the pain but also by the feelings of helplessness and lack of control . . . pain reduction techniques are really coping measures that diminish distress by enabling the person to stay in control of the painful experience.

The mechanism by which preparation for childbirth classes benefit those who participate is still unclear, but it is clear that they increase satisfaction and play an important role in helping couples take a more active role in managing their labor.

Recent Trends. Childbirth education has grown from a small consumer movement to a significant force in maternity care in the United States. Hospital programs are proliferating and have been accused of "indoctrinating" parents about specific approaches of the sponsoring institution instead of equipping them to make real choices about the management of childbirth.

There is a widening gap between the "medical" model of childbirth and the "physiologic" model. DeVries (1984) notes:

> It *appears* as if the trend toward 'medicalization' of birth, marked by increased numbers of surgical deliveries and new technological capabilities for intervening and controlling the birth process, has been slowed—if not halted—by a desire on the part of both consumers and professionals to 'humanize' the care given to childbearing women and their families.

However, there is still too much professional control over childbearing to suit many consumers.

Within the original childbirth education movement the validity of certain techniques (such as breath-holding while pushing) has been questioned (Lindell and Rossi, 1986; Roberts et al, 1987). Women are being encouraged to *tune into their own body cues* and to incorporate natural responses. Techniques include vocalization or "sounding" to relieve tension, effleurage, imagery-assisted relaxation (IAR), or visualization to guide women into positive spaces ("seeing" the vagina open up around the baby), hot compresses to the perineum, perineal massage, warm showers or bathing during labor, and relaxing music and subdued lighting. Biofeedback, yoga, and acupressure may also be employed (Lindberg and Lawlis, 1988).

Obstetrics is becoming more and more complex. Changes are occurring so rapidly that it is difficult for childbirth educators to keep current. The demands have become so great that there is a trend toward specialization (e.g., teaching only exercise, or cesarean and vaginal birth after cesarean classes) and group practices (Shearer and Bunnin, 1983).

Clients are also changing. According to Shearer and Bunnin (1983):

> We are seeing a dramatic increase in the ages of parents, in the proportion who have had infertility investigations and treatments, and in the number who have gone through a series of genetic tests. More and more women in childbirth classes have had a sonogram at each prenatal visit, and perhaps antepartum fetal monitoring procedures as well. These experiences set today's parents apart from those in prenatal classes 5 years ago. The precise ways these parents differ, and the needed changes in childbirth educators, have not yet been addressed. The number of adolescent parents has also increased dramatically.

Care must be individualized for each woman or couple. *Each woman has a right to labor and give birth in whatever way she chooses, provided the way is safe for both mother and baby.*

Parent Preparation for Cesarean Birth

Concerned professional and lay groups in the community have established councils for cesarean birth in an attempt to meet the needs of women and their families. Such groups advocate including preparation for cesarean birth in all parenthood preparation classes (Fawcett and Henklein, 1987). No woman can be guaranteed a vaginal delivery, even if she is in good health and there is no indication of danger to the fetus before the onset of labor. Every woman needs to be prepared for this possibility. The unknown and unexpected is ego weakening; accurate data to build new coping abilities or to strengthen old ones before a crisis increases one's sense of control and serves to minimize the sense of loss experienced.

Childbirth educators emphasize the similarities as well as differences between cesarean and vaginal births. Many hospitals have changed policies to permit fathers to share in cesarean births as they have in vaginal ones (see Chapter 26). The presence and support of their partners have helped many women undergoing cesarean birth to have a positive experience.

> ■ Knowing that he would be there and that he would be among the first to hold and nurture our baby made a tremendous difference to me. Even though "I" as the woman couldn't participate as directly as I had anticipated, "we" as the family could. I felt a sense of control, not a sense of being a passive . . . well . . . organ.

In many hospitals today care of parents experiencing a cesarean birth is family centered rather than surgery centered. As education on cesarean birth is being incorporated into prenatal classes, couples are becoming aware of options available to them if a cesarean delivery is necessary. Some of the alternatives available include the following:

1. Cesarean delivery in the labor and delivery area, rather than in the general surgery area
2. The choice of regional instead of general anesthesia, whenever possible
3. The option of having a support person (preferably father) present during the birth
4. The opportunity for skin-to-skin contact with baby and parents immediately after birth
5. Initiation of early rooming-in with help from staff until mother is able to assume responsibility for baby care
6. Encouragement of breastfeeding
7. Extended and unlimited visiting privileges for the immediate family members

Cesarean delivery can be a positive birth experience when parents, physicians, and hospital personnel collaborate.

Sibling Preparation

Sharing the spotlight with a new brother or sister may be the first major crisis for a child. The older child often experiences a sense of loss or feels jealous on being "replaced" by the new baby (Kuhn and Kopcinski, 1984; MacLaughlin and Johnston, 1984). See also Chapters 2 and 20. Some of the variables that influence the child's response are age, the parents' attitudes, the role of the father, the length of separation from the mother, the hospital's visitation policy, and how the child has been prepared for the change (Honig, 1986).

Professionals are developing classes to prepare children for the birth of a new brother or sister (Fig. 9-6). A general teaching plan used for young children is found in the guidelines for client teaching: sibling preparation for childbirth. The general plan can be modified to fit needs of children of different ages and the needs of children who will be present during the birth.

Guidelines For Client Teaching
SIBLING PREPARATION

ASSESSMENT

1. Couple expecting second child in 3 months. Four-year-old son asking many questions about the baby in "mommy's tummy."
2. Parents express desire for preparation of older sibling.

NURSING DIAGNOSES

Knowledge deficit related to older sibling's capabilities and needs.

Impaired verbal communication related to older child's development level.

Altered family process related to addition of new family member.

GOALS

Short-term

Child and parents feel less anxious about the mother's impending hospitalization.

Child begins to develop realistic expectations of newborn.

Parents begin to develop strategies to prepare the older child for the mother's hospitalization and newborn sibling.

Intermediate

Child begins to prepare for role transition to be brother.

Parents begin to develop strategies for caring for older sibling and new child.

Parents begin to prepare for role transition.

Long-term

Child develops realistic expectations of newborn.

Child and parents learn new coping skills.

Parents successfully make role transition.

REFERENCES AND TEACHING AIDS

Audiovisual materials: films, slides, doll, cassette recordings, materials with which to draw pictures.

See bibliography for list of references.

Enroll and attend a sibling class.

Sibling visitation while mother is hospitalized.

RATIONALE/CONTENT	TEACHING ACTION
Familiarity with a new environment helps allay anxiety: Have older sibling: Visit hospital classroom. Dress up in hospital clothing. Learn hospital "rules," such as walk slowly, and talk quietly. Tour maternity area, see and touch telephone that he can use to talk to his mother. See naked newborn.	Prepare a room to convey warmth and friendliness. Explain hospital clothing, then change to scrub outfit worn by fathers and nurses. Help child try on hospital gowns, masks, and caps. During tour, answer questions and expect child to abide by hospital "rules."
Realistic expectations help in accepting the newborn's behavior: Have older sibling practice in new role: By listening to stories about what newborns can do and how older children react to newborn babies. By holding a doll with care to support the head. By exploring what he can do when the baby cries.	Read stories and employ role-playing. Ask open-ended or leading questions. Help child with holding the doll. Demonstrate ways to console a crying baby. Caution against picking up baby and touching baby's head. Play cassette of baby sounds and encourage questions and discussion.
Children need assistance in substituting acceptable behavior for unacceptable behavior: Have older sibling practice through role-playing: When parent spends time with the newborn. When the child gets angry with the newborn.	Role-play situation demonstrating positive responses to newborn in selected situations. Involve child with problem-solving in selected situations.
Recognizing one's feelings can increase one's ability to cope: Have older sibling: Watch a film depicting jealousy, anger, and being left out (Johnsen and Gaspard, 1985).	Show film and encourage discussion.
Participate in discussion of film and how to ask for help when needed.	Lead discussion; encourage comments.
Participate in drawing a picture to show how he feels and what he understands of his mother's pregnancy and the coming baby.	Provide equipment, space and directions for drawing, such as "draw a picture of your family." Ask child to tell a story about his picture.

EVALUATION The nurse can be reasonably assured that the teaching plan has been effective when all goals have been met. Older sibling demonstrates realistic expectations of the newborn and remains reassured about parental love. Child and parents learn new coping skills. Parents and sibling successfully make the role transition necessitated by addition of a new family member.

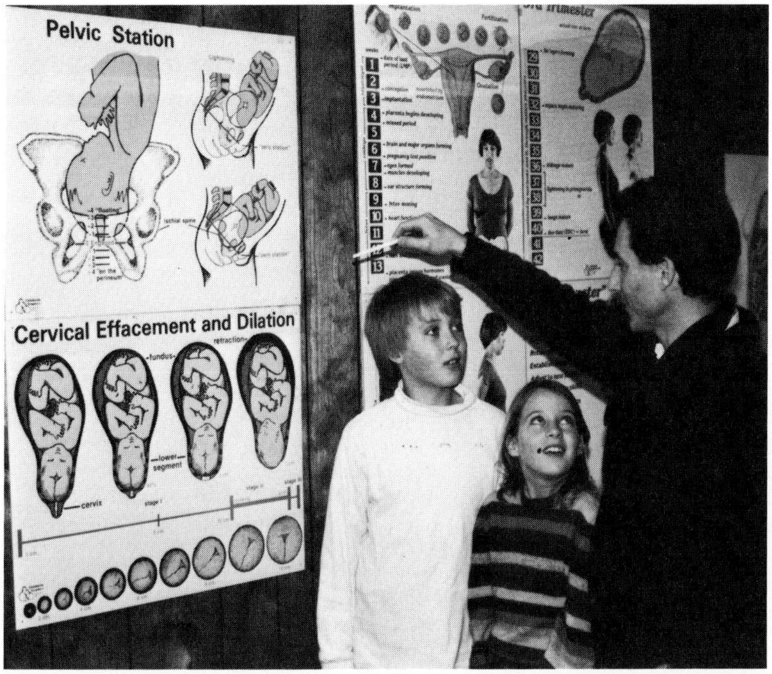

Fig. 9-6 Sibling preparation class. (Community Birth Center, Community Hospital, Santa Cruz, Calif.)

Grandparent Preparation

Childbirth educators are becoming more aware of the unique role of the grandparent and are forming classes for grandparents (Hassid, 1984; McKay and Phillips, 1984; Horn and Manion, 1985). The grandparent is the historian who transmits the history of the family and provides continuity with the present, a resource person who shares knowledge based on experience, a role model, and a support person. Other sources of information cannot replace the unique contribution that grandparents make.

To be truly *family-oriented,* maternity care must consider the grandparent when implementing the nursing process with childbearing families. (See also Chapter 20). Grandparents' classes represent one method of facilitating the adjustment to the grandparenting role, of incorporating the grandparents into the family system, and of encouraging communication between the generations (Maloni, McIndoe, and Rubenstein, 1987).

Grandparents' anxieties and concerns and their relationships with expectant parents and with grandchildren should be opened to discussion during courses for expectant parents as well (see guidelines for client teaching: grandparent preparation, p. 226). The expectant parents may use this opportunity to begin to resolve conflicts and perceived differences with their parents, a task that can enhance their ability to relate to their own children.

Education for Choice

In June 1978 a joint statement, "The Development of Family-Centered Maternity/Newborn Care in Hospitals" was prepared by the Interprofessional Task Force on Health Care of Women and Children, which included representatives from the American Academy of Pediatrics (AAP), the American College of Nurse-Midwives (ACNM), the American Nurses' Association (ANA), ACOG, and the Nurses' Association of the American College of Obstetricians and Gynecologists (NAACOG). These five organizations endorsed the concept of family-centered childbirth and supported efforts to develop alternative childbirth centers along the lines described in the statement. The American Hospital Association added its support. The definition of family-centered care in the joint statement follows:

> Family-centered maternity/newborn care can be defined as the delivery of safe, quality health care while recognizing, focusing on, and adapting to both the physical and psychological needs of the client-patient, the family, and the newly born. The emphasis is on the provision of maternity/newborn health care which fosters family unity while maintaining physical safety.

The statement recommends significant changes in hospital maternity care, including the following:

1. The option of a homelike **birthing room** where woman remains (with her family if desired)

Guidelines For Client Teaching
GRANDPARENT PREPARATION

ASSESSMENT

1. Expectant parents voice concerns about role of grandparents and request assistance (depends on grandparent's readiness to learn).
2. Expectant grandparents request information about hospital policies and procedures, modern childbirth methods, new parents' needs, and their own roles.
3. Expectant grandparents would like to provide support to expectant parents before and after the birth of the baby.

NURSING DIAGNOSES

Knowledge deficit related to hospital policies, childbirth methods, and how to provide support to expectant parents.

Altered family processes related to addition of a new family member.

Potential for ineffective individual coping related to need for role change.

GOALS

Short-term

Grandparents are oriented to hospital routines and policies.

Grandparents are oriented to childbirth method and experience expected by their children.

Grandparents learn current techniques of infant care.

Intermediate

Grandparents prepare for role change from parents to grandparents.

Grandparents begin to define mutually acceptable role-relationship with their children.

Grandparents relive and come to terms with own childbirth experience.

Long-term

Grandparents develop and maintain mutually satisfying role-relationship with children and new grandchild.

Grandparents become effective and supportive grandparents and parents.

REFERENCES AND TEACHING AIDS

Audiovisual materials: films, slides, charts.

List of references available to the general public.

Tour of maternity unit; introduction to gowns, shoe covers, and caps.

Values clarification or attitude awareness exercise (Horn and Manion, 1985).

RATIONALE/CONTENT	TEACHING ACTION
Exploring one's values and attitudes facilitates individual coping, therefore the nurse will teach: Values-clarification, attitude awareness exercise: When I think about myself as a grandparent, I feel _____. Children bring a couple _____. During their child's labor and delivery, grandparents should _____. The happiest (most satisfying) memory of my (my wife's) labor and childbirth was _____. The unhappiest (least satisfying) memory of my (my wife's) labor and childbirth was _____.	Develop and administer values and attitudes exercise. Use exercise as a basis for starting small-group discussion. Encourage members of group to compare and contrast own experiences, values, and attitudes.
Knowledge provides a basis for decision making: Conduct grandparents class. Use prioritized list of topics they wish to discuss as focus. Conduct tour of unit. Provide hands-on experience with equipment and supplies. Introduce personnel. Describe personnel's services and responsibilities. Bring closure to class. Review the grandparent's questions. Discuss their comparisons. Summarize the experience.	Elicit topics the grandparents wish to discuss, write on a chalkboard, and ask group to prioritize list; encourage questions. Use appropriate audiovisual materials: charts, films, slides. Offer or conduct a tour of the maternity area including restrooms, waiting room, telephones, cafeteria, and selected supplies (gowns, shoe-covers) and equipment (fetoscope). Introduce the grandparents to available personnel and review their roles. Return group to classroom. Encourage questions. Encourage the grandparent's to compare and contrast their own experiences with the class content. Provide printed material. Thank the group for their interest.

EVALUATION Teaching has been effective when grandparents develop and maintain a mutually satisfying role-relationship with their children and grandchildren. Goals have been met when grandparents become effective and supportive to their children and grandchildren.

2. Flexible rooming-in with maximum mother-child contact during the first 24 hours
3. Breastfeeding and handling of the baby immediately after delivery
4. Allowing the father or other support persons to be present throughout the labor, delivery, and recovery periods
5. Allowing siblings to visit in a special family room
6. Optional early discharge from the hospital with careful follow-up after discharge
7. Childbirth preparation classes offered by the hospital

The alternative birth movement is the practical application of the family-centered concept of maternity-newborn care. The attitude of the health care providers is the most important aspect of family-centered care. Family-centered care recognizes birth as a vital life event and not a surgical procedure. It gives people the right to make informed choices regarding their childbirth experiences.

Organizations such as ICEA and ASPO and the National Association of Parents and Professionals for Safe Alternatives in Childbirth (NAPSAC) have increased the public's knowledge of prepared childbirth techniques and their impact on birth outcomes. The prepared childbirth movement has fostered greater acceptance of birth as a normal, rather than a pathologic, event and has encouraged expectant parents to become more knowledgeable about and accountable for their participation. As women began to experience childbirth awake and aware, they began to feel greater self-esteem and control over their lives. Also, the social significance of the birth experience became very clear to many women and their mates.

Consumer response has been varied, demonstrating the intensely personal quality of every birth experience and the need for safe, sensible choices in care during this important life event (Periscope, 1987). The key element in optimal care of the childbearing family is **informed choice** about the place of birth, the plan of care, and the people present. In fact, the ICEA has always subscribed to the motto, "Freedom of choice based on knowledge of alternatives."

Choice and the Nurse. Understanding why families choose alternatives to traditional hospital birth is imperative. Cohen (1982) compared women who chose two different childbirth alternatives: a hospital or a freestanding **alternative birth center** (ABC). Women choosing the birth center planned to emphasize autonomy and independence rather than intimacy in their child rearing. Their closest relationships were much more supportive and involved in the birth than those women choosing hospital births. Women delivering at the Childbearing Childrearing Center (CCC) at the University of Minnesota, Minneapolis (Rising and Lindell, 1982) reported three major reasons they chose the center: (1) to have control over their experience, (2) to have family-centered care, and (3) to have no routine procedures administered. Kieffer (1980) compared the attitudes of 109 women before and after experiencing birth using the birthing room. The four highest ranking reasons for choice of the birthing room were (1) philosophy, (2) no separation of mother and baby, (3) personal involvement in the birth, and (4) freedom to make choices regarding labor and birth. These studies seem to indicate that attitudes toward issues of choice in the childbirth experience are related to the degree of control that families expect to exert over the birth event (Fullerton, 1982).

Most people who choose home birth are concerned about their own safety and the health and safety of their unborn child (Searles, 1981). There are many sincere and well-considered reasons for choosing home birth. For many birth is a very special, intensely personal event to be shared only with family and friends, and not with assorted hospital personnel who are strangers. For others, birth is an intensely spiritual experience for which a hospital setting is totally inappropriate. Still others refuse to give up responsibility for their children's births to hospital personnel; these people want to control their own experience. Most people choosing home birth understand fully the risk involved but also believe that there are risks in hospital birth.

The nurse's concern is to encourage expectant couples to explore the birth alternatives available to them so they can make a responsible, informed decision. It is the nurse's responsibility to become actively involved in ensuring that a variety of options for safe childbirth are available in communities.

Birth-setting Choices

More **birth-setting choices** are available now than in the past. Family-centered maternity care is implemented in birthing rooms or alternative birth centers (ABCs) in the hospital. Hospital ABCs, as well as freestanding birth centers, are an alternative to home birth, a compromise between traditional hospital births and home birth. More and more, consumers and professionals are accepting and using birthing rooms and ABCs that have been shown to be safe alternatives to birth in a traditional hospital delivery setting (Mann, 1981; Marieskind, 1980).

Birthing Rooms. Unlike ABCs in hospitals, there are very few admission or risk criteria for the use of hospital birthing rooms. Birthing rooms offer families a comfortable, private space for childbirth (Rosen, 1980; Sumner and Phillips, 1981). Fig. 15-18 shows a bed that has the ability to "break," so the woman can quickly be put into stirrups if an episiotomy is deemed necessary or laceration occurs. Even in the unbroken mode a simple push of a button will cause the upper half of the bed to rise approximately 25 cm (10 inches) and allow the easy management of an unanticipated shoulder dystocia.

Giving birth in a birthing room rather than moving from labor room to delivery room has the advantage of not interfering with the progress of labor. The woman can concentrate on pushing her baby out without moving to a stretcher and then moving again to the delivery table. Her vital signs may be taken continuously if necessary, and the fetal monitor may remain in place until the baby is born. The father is able to provide continuous support. If rapid delivery is necessary, the woman's legs may be placed in the leg supports and the baby born quickly without time being wasted in transport to a delivery room. Other advantages of a birthing room include the following:

1. The nursing staff does not have to decide when to move the mother to the delivery room
2. Only one room for each woman needs to be set up
3. Costs may be reduced, since fewer rooms and less laundry and equipment are used, and hospital space is better utilized

Hospital birthing rooms humanize the birth experience, minimize intervention, and afford continuity of care. These facilities offer a two-tiered model of care (low risk and high risk) and emphasize individualizing the birth experience. When deemed appropriate, local anesthesia, forceps, fetal monitoring, and so on are used to facilitate a safe birth.

Alternative Birth Centers. Alternative birth centers (ABCs) usually are in hospital suites away from the traditional obstetrics department but close to the delivery and operating rooms in case serious problems arise. ABCs have homelike accommodations, including a double bed for the couple and a crib for the newborn. Emergency equipment and drugs are discreetly stored out of view but are easily accessible. Private bathroom facilities, some with jacuzzis, are incorporated into each birth center. There may be an early labor lounge or living room and small kitchen. Only low-risk and prepared women or couples are accepted.

Ideally the ABC becomes the private space for one childbearing family, including older siblings and friends, throughout their birth experience and often until they are ready to go home. It is a warm, private, friendly space within a complex, fully equipped medical constellation. Although emphasizing normalcy, self-help, and family participation, ABCs are fully supported by the presence of a maternity nurse or nurse-midwife and by the availability of obstetric and pediatric house staff at all times, with attending staff backup.

If a situation that could threaten the safety of the mother or baby should arise at any time during labor, the mother would be moved to the standard labor and delivery area. Her nurse and her partner or other family member would go with her.

Early discharge from the center, often during the day of delivery, must meet medical criteria. Many centers arrange for the mother and infant to be seen within 24 hours of discharge by a nurse-midwife or perinatal nurse specialist.

Freestanding Alternative Birth Centers. Freestanding alternative birth centers are outside the hospital but are often close to a major hospital so that quick transfer to that institution is possible if necessary.

Most freestanding birth centers are staffed by physicians who have privileges at the local hospital and also certified nurse-midwives. Ambulance service and emergency procedures are readily available. Fees vary with the services provided and the ability of the family to pay (reduced-fee sliding scale). Several insurance companies, as well as Medicaid, recognize and reimburse these clinics.

Services provided by the freestanding birth centers include those necessary for safe management during the childbearing cycle. There are some significant additions, however:

1. Attendance at childbirth and parenting classes is required of all clients. Prenatal supervision of the woman in good nutritional and health status must begin in the first trimester. All clients must be familiar with situations requiring transfer to a hospital.
2. Each expectant family identifies its *"birth plan"* (Arms, 1978), an explanation of practices and procedures they would like to include in or exclude from their childbirth experience. A sampling of choices follows:
   a. *Preparation:* enema, "miniprep," hospital gown instead of own clothing?
   b. *Labor:* electronic monitor or fetoscope, freedom to choose positions and activity in labor (walking, squatting), analgesia, presence of siblings, translator?
   c. *Birth:* presence of mate or chosen person, presence of siblings, draping, mirror, dimmed lights, Leboyer bath?
   d. *Recovery:* recovery with or without baby or mate or chosen person?
   e. *After recovery:* rooming-in, sibling visitation, vitamin K for baby, circumcision, demand feeding—breast or bottle?

Birth centers usually have available a lending library, reference files on related topics, recycled maternity clothes and baby clothes, and equipment, supplies, and reference materials for childbirth educators. The centers have referral files for community resources that offer services relating to childbirth and early parenting, including support groups (such as single parents, post-delivery support group, parents of twins), genetic counseling, women's issues, and consumer action.

The concept of the birthing center remains controversial, particularly among physicians. However, many consumers are happy with this alternative to hospital delivery. Since the Maternity Center Association (MCA) in New York City opened its first demonstration project in out-of-hospital maternity care in 1975, more than 153 centers in 38 states have replicated the unit (Lubic, 1989). Profound changes in obstetrical care in New York City have been attributed to this competing service for low-risk mothers: hospitals have introduced birthing rooms, length of stay has been shortened, and the trend toward family-centered maternity care has been strengthened.

Home Birth. Home birth has always been popular in certain advanced countries, such as Great Britain, Sweden, and the Netherlands. In developing countries, hospitals or adequate lying-in facilities often are unavailable to most pregnant women, and home birth is a necessity. In North America home birth is gaining popularity.

National groups supporting home birth are HOME (Home Oriented Maternity Experience) and NAPSAC (National Association of Parents for Safe Alternatives in Childbirth). These groups support changes toward more humane childbearing practices at all levels. The literature on childbirth contains excellent statistics on medically directed home birth services with skilled nurse-midwives and medical backup. Two examples of such services are the Chicago Maternity Center with 12,000 home births from 1950 to 1960 without a single maternal death and the home delivery statistics of the Frontier Nursing Service in Appalachia with 23 years without a single maternal death. In the United States there are reports of very low-risk home delivery populations who have very low levels of difficulty and consequently have excellent statistics. However, there is danger in taking these data on very select populations and applying them to the total population. It must be recognized that even though labor and delivery are normal physiologic events, they do present potential hazards to the mother and fetus both before and after birth. These hazards require provisions for emergency intervention and medical backups that are available only in hospitals and some birthing homes or in independent birth centers.

Selective home birth in uncomplicated pregnancies is feasible, provided those women at high risk can be identified during the prenatal period and referred for hospital delivery and assuming that a transport system is available for transfer of women with suddenly complicated labors to a nearby adequate medical facility. Collaboration with and supervision of midwives are the obstetrician's duty in many countries. Nurse specialists, general practitioners, and obstetric specialist consultants have become incorporated into home delivery units. A midwife or general practitioner can call on or refer women or infants to essential backup services for study or specialty care during pregnancy and the early puerperium. When a woman is to be assisted by a midwife, it is the practice in most areas for the general practitioner to supervise her; meanwhile, both are under the direction of the obstetric specialist.

Although some physicians and nurses are proponents of home births that use good medical and emergency backup systems, many regard this practice as exposing the mother and the fetus to unnecessary danger.

One advantage of home birth is that delivery may be more natural or physiologic in familiar surroundings. The mother may be more relaxed and less tense than she might be in the impersonal, sterile environment of a hospital. The family can assist in and be a part of the happy event, and mother-father-infant (and sibling-infant) contact is sustained and immediate. In addition, home birth may be less expensive than a hospital confinement. Serious infection may be less likely, assuming strict aseptic principles are followed. People generally are relatively immune to their own home bacteria.

Because home births are not generally accepted by the medical community, a family may have difficulty finding a qualified health care professional to give prenatal care and to attend the delivery. Also, backup emergency care by a physician in a hospital may be difficult to arrange in advance. And, emergency transfer to a hospital may be life-threatening if the hospital is more than a 10-minute distance from the home or if emergency care is not available during the transfer from home to hospital.

Hospital, not home, birth is indicated for the following:

1. High-risk women (fetal or maternal jeopardy) (see Chapter 22)
2. Women who cannot be transferred easily to a hospital should the need arise unexpectedly
3. Women who are opposed to home birth
4. Women with inadequate home facilities

Facilities and supplies can approximate those available in hospitals. The family works closely with the physician, nurse, or midwife to complete preparations well in advance of delivery. Attendance by both parents-to-be at childbirth classes adds to the competence and pleasure of the parents and other family members. Classes for siblings and grandparents are recommended.

Detailed descriptions for preparation are required and may be obtained from either the physician's office or from local health agencies. The agencies may provide some of the equipment and supplies. A visit to the home by the community health nurse is recommended well before the expected date of birth.

Home birth is a selected alternative to hospital birth for some women and couples and a necessity for many. A safe outcome can be anticipated for most women and their infants, if they are prepared and have adequate health care support.

Prebirth Preparation

Not all gravidas and support persons attend formal classes in preparation for childbirth. For those who do attend, extensive preparation is possible. Many do not take advantage of classes for a variety of reasons: employment; inaccessibility because of time, cultural/ethnic/religious orientation; cost; lack of knowledge regarding choices in prenatal education classes; lack of readiness. Therefore clinicians need to provide information that includes the following:

1. Process of labor: admission, examination, care in labor
2. Plans to get to hospital (when to go and where); care of other children
3. Methods to control pain (e.g., analgesia and anesthesia, breathing-relaxing techniques) (see Chapter 13)
4. Supplies to have in a suitcase ready for the trip to the hospital: personal items for grooming, items for labor as desired (i.e., warm socks, focal point), supportive bra, nightgowns, slippers
5. Responsibilities of the spouse, family member, or friend who will be accompanying the woman through labor and delivery
6. Care of the newborn (i.e., clothing, feeding, daily hygienic care), and postnatal care (see Chapters 17 and 18)
7. Emergency arrangements (e.g., precipitate delivery) (see Chapter 15)

A nurse needs to be ready to teach when the woman is ready to learn as shown by the following example. One nurse described her intervention with a gravid woman as follows:

> I tried to teach her about relaxation and breathing techniques during childbirth, but she was not interested. When she phoned to tell me she was at the hospital in labor, she said, "What was all that stuff you were saying about breathing?" In between the next few contractions I repeated the salient points.

Even if the woman (couple) has attended prebirth classes, the nurse discusses preparation for childbirth. The following topics are discussed:

- Symptoms of impending labor (see box below) and what information to report
- Breathing and relaxation techniques
- Involvement of husband or significant other
- Provision for needs of other children
- Plans to get to hospital
- Plans of labor, terminology, and what care to expect
- Preparation for baby
- Preparation of grandparents and siblings

If a hospital delivery is planned, the woman registers at the hospital of choice. Most hospitals provide information such as where to report when labor begins and policies pertaining to visitors. Many facilities also conduct tours.

Counseling is provided to relieve emotional tensions. (e.g., anxiety about pain or possible delivery of the child before reaching the hospital). Nursing strategies include discussing the woman's specific fears or anxieties, helping her plan what she will do when labor starts, repeating instructions, and having "sharing sessions" with mothers who have recently delivered. If possible, involve significant others in preparation for the birth. Arrange to have them participate in a supportive way during labor. Most men whose wives are approaching labor may have their anxieties decreased through activities such as the following:

1. A hospital tour of the labor room and waiting areas (This will allow him to familiarize himself with the area and determine his role)
2. A demonstration of supportive measures to comfort his wife during labor
3. A brief review of what to expect from his wife during labor (e.g., irritability, breathing, grunting)
4. A description of what to expect of the staff during labor

SYMPTOMS OF IMPENDING LABOR

1. Uterine contractions: The woman is instructed to report the frequency, duration, and intensity of uterine contractions. Nulliparas are usually counseled to remain at home until contractions are regular and 5 minutes apart. Parous women are counseled to remain at home until contractions are regular and 10 minutes apart. If the woman lives more than 20 minutes from the hospital or has a history of rapid labors, these instructions are modified accordingly.
2. Rupture of the membranes (see Chapter 15).
3. Bloody "show": The "show" is scant, pink in color, and sticky (contains mucus).

A realistic discussion of all known factors helps the father plan for the event. Such discussions are ego strengthening because they help focus energies toward more appropriate coping strategies by decreasing anxieties about the unknown. Today many men elect to participate actively during labor and delivery. However, some men through personal or cultural concepts of the father role neither wish to nor intend to participate. *The important concept is that the partners agree on the other's roles.* For nurses to advocate any changes in these roles may cause confusion or feelings of guilt.

SUMMARY

Pregnancy represents a maturational crisis that requires changes in outlook, role responsibilities, and everyday living of all family members. The ability to respond to changes with new behaviors and new self-concepts is fostered not only by intrinsic strengths but also by extrinsic strengths, such as the love and support of outsiders.

Nurses can act as one source of extrinsic strength. The knowledge they possess of the responses of all family members to a pregnancy enables them to use their responses as the cornerstones of nursing-care plans. The long-term contact nurses have with clients and their families provides unique opportunities for informed supportive nursing that may have a long-term effect on family life. The nurse encourages the childbearing family to participate in prenatal classes. Attendance at such classes permits sharing of experiences with other couples and families. The couple is reassured by knowing that their thoughts, feelings, and concerns are common to others. Classes can increase confidence and self-assurance and help parents develop new coping skills.

Consumers learn about birth-setting choices from a variety of sources. The knowledgeable nurse serves as a valuable resource for couples who want to individualize their childbirth experience.

LEARNING ACTIVITIES

1. Develop a table or chart outlining characteristics of adaptation to pregnancy—maternal, paternal, sibling, and grandparental. Interview prospective parents and other family members, comparing and contrasting their adjustments with expected adaptation.
2. Compare the concerns in pregnancy of a first-time mother with those of a second-time mother.
3. Through discussion with an expectant couple, identify ambivalent feelings experienced throughout the pregnancy.
4. Focus discussion of students and peers who have experienced childbirth on emotional responses, body image, and realization of role changes.
5. Check libraries and bookstores for popularized accounts of pregnancy and childbirth processes (the "how-to" approach). Choose one book to critique for the class in terms of its accuracy compared with the discussion of the possible effect such books might have on the pregnant woman and her husband.
6. Role-play one or more of the following; then critique the interactions in a group session:
   a. Marital support.
   b. Assisting an expectant couple in choosing a birth setting; that is, ABC or home birth.

References

Arms S: Five women, five births, Film, 1978, Davidson Films, Inc.

American College of Obstetricians and Gynecologists: The development of family-centered maternity/newborn care in hospitals, Washington, DC, 1978, The College.

Ballou JW: The psychology of pregnancy, Lexington, Mass, 1978, DC Heath & Co.

Barranti C: The grandparent/grandchild relationship: family resource in an era of voluntary bonds, Fam Relat 34:3, July 1985.

Barron ML, Brown MC, and Ganong LH: Prepared for pregnancy: a counseling guide, Clin Nurs Specialist, 1(3):111, 1987.

Beck NC and Hall D: Natural childbirth: a review and analysis, Obstet Gynecol 52:371, Sept 1978.

Bernardini JY, Maloni JA, and Stegman CE: Neuromuscular control of childbirth-prepared women during the first stage of labor, JOGN Nurs 2:105, March/April 1983.

Bliss-Holtz J: Primiparas' prenatal concern for learning infant care, Nurs Res 37:20, Jan/Feb 1988.

Bobak I: Fathers, Unpublished research, 1968.

Bradley R: Husband-coached childbirth, New York, 1965, Harper & Row, Publishers Inc.

Brown MA: Marital support during pregnancy, JOGN Nurs 15(6):475, 1986.

Caplan G: Concepts of mental health and consultation, Washington, DC, 1959, US Department of Health, Education, and Welfare.

Carson K and Virden S: Can prenatal teaching promote maternal attachment? Practicing nurses test Carter-Jessop's prenatal attachment intervention, Health Care for Women International 5:355, 1984.

Close S: Sex during pregnancy and after childbirth, San Bernardino, Calif, 1986, Borgo Press.

Cogan R: Effects of childbirth preparation, Clin Obstet Gynecol 23:1, March 1980.

Cohen A: Movement as a yardstick for fetal wellbeing, Contemp OB/Gyn 26:61, Aug 1985.

Cohen RL: A comparative study of women choosing two different birth alternatives, Birth 9:1, Spring 1982.

Colman AD: Psychological state during the first pregnancy, Am J Orthopsych 39:778, 1969.

Coussens WR and Coussens PD: Maximizing preparation for childbirth, Health Care for Women International, 5:335, 1984.

KEY CONCEPTS

- Pregnancy involves all family members, who react to pregnancy and interpret its meaning in light of their own needs and the needs of the others affected.
- The process of family adaptation to pregnancy takes place within a cultural environment.
- Pregnancy presents several developmental tasks to the mother- and father-to-be as they prepare for new levels of caring and responsibility.
- Since pregnancy is a developmental crisis, it is a time of emotional upheaval for both the man and the woman, necessitating adequate communication between them.
- The parent-child, sibling-child, and grandparent-child relationships start during the pregnancy.
- Maternal and familial adaptations to pregnancy generate needs that the nurse-clinician can anticipate and meet by providing support, and teaching/counseling/advocacy.
- The psychosocial aspects of care are of paramount importance and may well affect the whole course of pregnancy, childbirth, and the adjustment of the new family.
- Childbirth education is a process designed to help parents make the transition from the role of expectant parents to the role and responsibilities of parents of a new baby.
- Regardless of the gravida's readiness to learn, attention to prebirth preparation is a necessary component of prenatal care.
- The nursing process and the teaching process are parallel.
- Maternity care should be family-centered regardless of the method of birth and the place of birth.
- The goal of preparation for childbirth and parenting is "education for choice."

Cranley MS: Development of a tool for the measurement of maternal attachment during pregnancy, Nurs Res 30:281, 1981a.
Cranley MS: Roots of attachment: the relationship of parents with their unborn, Birth Defects 17(6):59, 1981b.
Cronenwett LR: Elements and outcomes of a postpartum support group program, Res Nurs Health 3(3):33, 1980.
Cronenwett LR: Father participation in child care: a critical review, Res Nurs Health 5:63, 1982.
Cronenwett LR and Brickman P: Models of helping and coping in childbirth, Nurs Res 32:84, March/April 1983.
Cronenwett LR and Kunst-Wilson W: Stress, social support, and the transition of fatherhood, Nurs Res 30:196, 1981.
Deutch H: The psychology of women, vol 2, New York, 1945, Bantam Books.
DeVries RG: "Humanizing" childbirth: the discovery and implementation of bonding theory, Int J Health Serv 14(1):89, 1984.
Dick-Read G: Childbirth without fear, ed 2, New York, 1959, Harper & Row, Publishers Inc.
Ellis D: Sexual needs and concerns of expectant parents, JOGN Nurs vol 9, Sept/Oct 1980.
Entwistle DR and Doering SG: The first birth: a family turning point, Baltimore, 1981, Johns Hopkins University Press.
Fawcett J: Body image and the pregnant couple, MCN 3:227, 1978.
Fawcett J and Henklein JC: Antenatal education for cesarean birth: extension of a field test, JOGN Nurs 16(1):61, 1987.
Field T: The three Rs of infant-adult interactions: rhythms, repertoires, and responsitivity, J Pediatr Psychol 3:131, 1978.
Fullerton JDT: The choice of in-hospital or alternative birth environment as related to the concept of control, J Nurse Midwife 27:2, March/April 1982.
Gaffney KF: New directions in maternal attachment research, J Pediatr Health Care 2:181, 1988.
Greenberg M and Morris N: Engrossment: the newborn's impact upon the father, Am J Orthopsych 44:520, 1974.
Greene R and Polivka J: The meaning of grandparent day cards: an analysis of the intergenerational network, Fam Relat 34:2, April 1985.
Grossman FK, Eichler LS, and Winckoff SA: Pregnancy, birth, parenthood, San Francisco, 1980, Jossey-Bass Inc, Publishers.
Hart G: Maternal attitudes in prepared and unprepared cesarean deliveries, JOGN Nurs 9:243, 1980.
Hassid P: Textbook for childbirth educators, ed 3, New York, 1984, JB Lippincott Co.
Highley BL and Mercer RT: Safeguarding the laboring woman's sense of control, Matern Child Nurs J 3(1):39, 1978.
Hogan LR: Pregnant again—at 41, Matern Child Nurs J 4:174, 1979.
Honig JC: Preparing preschool-aged children to be siblings, MCN 11(1):37, 1986.
Horn M and Manion J: Creative grandparenting: bonding the generations, JOGN Nurs 14:233, May/June 1985.
House JS: Work, stress and social support, Reading, Mass, 1981, Addison-Wesley Publishing Co, Inc.
Hunter R and Macalpine I, editors: Three hundred years of psychiatry: 1535-1860, London, 1963, Oxford University Press.
Huttell FA et al: A quantitative evaluation of psychoprophylaxis in childbirth, J Psychosom Res 16:81, 1972.
Johnsen NM and Gaspard ME: Theoretical foundations of a prepared sibling class, JOGN Nurs 14:237, May/June 1985.
Jones C: Father to infant attachment, effects of early contact and characteristics of the infant, Res Nurs Health 4:193, 1981.

Jones LC: A meta-analytic study of the effects of childbirth education on the parent-infant relationship, Health Care for Women International, 7:357, 1986.

Karmel M: Thank you, Dr. Lamaze, New York, 1965, Doubleday & Co, Inc.

Kemp VH and Page CK: Maternal prenatal attachment in normal and high-risk pregnancies, JOGN Nurs 16(3):179, 1987.

Kieffer MJ: The birthing room concept at Phoenix Memorial Hospital. II. Consumer satisfaction during one year, JOGN Nurs 9:158, May/June 1980.

Klein RN et al: A study of father and nurse support during labor, Birth 8:161, 1981.

Koniak-Griffin D: The relationship between social support, self-esteem, and maternal-fetal attachment in adolescents, Res Nurs Health 11:269, 1988.

Kuhn J and Kopcinski E: Siblings at birth: professional philosophy and preparation, Health Care Women Int 5:223, 1984.

Kunst-Wilson W and Cronenwett L: Nursing care for the emerging family: promoting paternal behavior, Res Nurs Health 4:201, 1981.

Lamaze F: Painless childbirth: the Lamaze method, Chicago, 1970, Regnery Books.

Lederman RP: Psychosocial adaptation in pregnancy: assessment of seven dimensions of maternal development, Englewood Cliffs, NJ, 1984, Prentice-Hall, Inc.

Lederman R et al: Relationship of psychological factors in pregnancy to progress in labor, Nurs Res 28:2, 1979.

Lederman RP, Weingarten CT, and Lederman E: Postpartum self-evaluation questionnaire: measures of maternal adaptation. In Lederman R, Raff B, and Carroll P, editors: Perinatal parental behavior: nursing research and implications for newborn health, New York, 1981, Alan R Liss Inc.

Leifer M: Psychological effects of motherhood: a study of first pregnancy, New York, 1980, Praeger Publishers.

Leifer M: Psychological changes accompanying pregnancy and motherhood, Genet Psychol Monogr 95:57, 1977.

Lieberman A: Giving birth, New York, 1987, St Martin's Press Inc.

Lein L: Male participation in home life: impact of social supports and breadwinner responsibility on the allocation of tasks, Fam Coord 28:489, 1979.

Levy JM and McGee RK: Childbirth as a crisis, J Pers Soc Psychol 31:171, 1975.

Lindberg C and Lawlis GF: The effectiveness of imagery as a childbirth preparatory technique. J Ment Imagery 12(1):103, 1988.

Lindell SG and Rossi MA: Compliance with childbirth education classes in second stage labor, Birth 13(2):96, 1986.

Lubic RW: Personal communication, April 28, 1989.

Lumley J: The development of maternal-fetal bonding in first pregnancy. In Zichella LJ, editor: Emotions and reproduction, New York, 1980a, Academic Press.

Lumley J: The image of the fetus in the first trimester, Birth Fam J 7:5, 1980b.

Lumley J: Attitudes to the fetus among primigravidas, Aust Pediatr J 18:106, 1982a.

Lumley J: Maternal-fetal bonding. II. Implications for the next three months, unpublished manuscript, Melbourne, 1982b, Monash University.

MacLaughlin SM and Johnston KB: The preparation of young children for the birth of a sibling, J Nurse Midwife 29:371, Nov/Dec 1984.

Maloni JA, McIndoe JE, and Rubenstein G: Expectant grandparents class, JOGN Nurs 16(1):26, 1987.

Mann RJ: San Francisco General Hospital Nurse-midwifery practice: the first thousand births, Am J Obstet Gynecol 140:6, July 1981.

Marieskind HI: Women in the health system: patients, providers, and programs, St Louis, 1980, The CV Mosby Co.

May KA: A typology of detachment and involvement styles adopted during pregnancy by first-time expectant fathers, West J Nurs Res 2:445, 1980.

May KA: The father as observer, MCN 7:319, 1982a.

May KA: Father participation in birth: fact and fiction, J Calif Perinat Assoc 2:41, Fall 1982b.

May KA: Three phases of father involvement in pregnancy, Nurs Res 31:337, 1982c.

McKay S and Phillips CR: Family-centered maternity care: implementation strategies, Rockville, Md, 1984, Aspen Systems Corp.

Mercer RT: "She's a multip . . . she knows the ropes," MCN 4:301, Sept/Oct 1979.

Mercer RT: A theoretical framework for studying factors that impact on the maternal role, Nurs Res 30:2, March/April 1981.

Mercer RT et al: Further exploration of maternal and paternal fetal attachment, Res Nurs Health, 11:83, 1988.

Merilo KF: Is it better the second time around? MCN 13:200, 1988.

Nurses' Association of the American College of Obstetricians and Gynecologists: Guidelines for childbirth education, Washington, DC, 1981, The Association.

Parke RD and Sawin DB: The father's role in infancy: a reevaluation, Fam Coord 25:365, 1976.

Periscope: Alternative birthing study publishes findings, Calif Perinatal Assn, p 4, Winter 1987.

Reich CL: Exercise in pregnancy: a review for nurse practitioners, Health Care for Women International 8:349, 1987.

Richardson P: Women's perceptions of change in relationships shared with children during pregnancy, Matern Child Nurs J 12:2, Summer 1983.

Rising SS and Lindell SG: The Childbearing Childrearing Center: a nursing model, Nurs Clin North Am 17:1, March 1982.

Roberts JE: Factors influencing distress from pain during labor, MCN 8:62, 1983.

Roberts JE et al: A descriptive analysis of involuntary bearing-down efforts during the expulsive phase of labor, JOGN Nurs 16:48, 1987.

Rubin R: Attainment of the maternal role. I. Processes, Nurs Res 240:237, 1967a.

Rubin R: Attainment of the maternal role. II. Models and referents, Nurs Res 16:342, 1967b.

Rubin R: Cognitive style in pregnancy, Am J Nurs 70:502, 1970.

Rubin R: Maternal tasks in pregnancy, Matern Child Nurs J 4: Spring, 1975.

Rubin R: Maternal identity and the maternal experience, New York, 1984, Springer Publishing Co.

Searles C: The impetus toward home birth, J Nurse Midwife 26:3, May/June 1981.

Shearer MH and Bunnin N: Childbirth educators in the 1980's: a survey of 25 veterans, Birth 10(4):251, 1983.

Sheehy G: Passages: predictable crises of adult life, New York, 1977, Bantam Books, Inc.

Shereshefsky PM and Yarrow LJ, editors: Psychological aspects of a first pregnancy and early postnatal adaptation, New York, 1973, Raven Press.

Sherwen LN: Psychosocial dimensions of the pregnant family, New York, 1987, Springer Publishing Co, Inc.
Stainton MC: A comparison of prenatal and postnatal perceptions of their babies by parents, paper presented to the First International Congress on Pre- and Peri-natal Psychology, Toronto, July 8, 1983.
Stainton MC: The fetus: a growing member of the family, Fam Relations 34:321, 1985a.
Stainton MC: Origins of attachment: culture and cue sensitivity. Dissertation Abstracts International, *46*, 3786-B. (University Microfilms No. 8600606), 1985b.
Sumner P and Phillips C: Birthing rooms: concept and reality, St Louis, 1981, The CV Mosby Co.
Swanson J: The marital sexual relationship during pregnancy, JOGN Nurs vol 9: Sept/Oct, 1980.
Walz B and Rich O: Maternal tasks of taking on a second child in the postpartum period, Matern Child Nurs J 12:3, Fall 1983.
Westney OE, Cole OJ, and Munford TL: The effects of prenatal education intervention on unwed prospective adolescent fathers, J Adolesc Health Care 9:214, 1988.
Winslow W: First pregnancy after 35: what is the experience? MCN 12(2):92, 1987.
Zalar MK: Sexual counseling for pregnant couples, Matern Child Nurs J 1(3):176, 1976.

Bibliography

Austin SE: Childbirth classes for couples desiring VBAC (vaginal birth after cesarean), MCN 11(4):250, 1986.
Avant KC: Stressors on the childbearing family, JOGN Nurs 17(3):179, 1988.
Bennett A et al: Antenatal preparation and labor support in relation to birth outcomes, Birth 12(1):9, 1985.
Brown MA: Social support, stress, and health: a comparison of expectant mothers and fathers, Nurs Res 35(2):72, 1986.
Carter ER: Quality maternity care for the medically indigent, MCN 11(2):85, 1986.
Clinton J: Couvade patterns, predictors, and nursing management, West J Nurs Res 7:221, 1985.
Clinton JF: Expectant fathers at risk for couvade, Nurs Res 35(5):290, 1986.
Clinton JF: Physical and emotional responses of expectant fathers throughout pregnancy and the early postpartum period, Int J Nurs Stud 24(1):59, 1987.
DelGiudice GT: The relationship between sibling jealousy and presence at a sibling's birth, Birth 13(4):250, 1986.
Durham L and Collins M: The effect of music as a conditioning aid in prepared childbirth education, JOGN Nurs 15(3):268, 1986.
Fawcett J and York R: Spouses' physical and psychological symptoms during pregnancy and the postpartum, Nurs Res 35(4):144, 1986.
Fawcett J et al: Spouses' body image changes during and after pregnancy: a replication and extension, Nurs Res 35(4):220, 1986.
Gill PJ and Katz M: Early detection of preterm labor: ambulatory home monitoring of uterine activity, JOGN Nurs 15(6):439, 1986.
Griffin S: Childbearing and the concept of culture, JOGN Nurs 11:181, 1982.
Humenick SS: Pregnant adult learners, NAACOG Update Series 1:lesson 24, 1984.
Jordan B: Birth in four cultures, Montreal, 1983, Eden Press.
Josselyn IM: Psychology of fatherliness, Smith College Studies Social Work 26:1, Feb 1956.
Maeder EC: Effects of sports and exercise in pregnancy, Postgrad Med 77(2):112, Feb 1, 1985.
Mercer RT: First-time motherhood: experiences from teens to forties, New York, 1986, Springer Publishing Co.
Mercer RT et al: Theoretical models for studying the effect of antepartum stress on the family, Nurs Res 35(6):339, 1986.
Moore L et al: Self-assessment: a personalized approach to nursing during pregnancy, JOGN Nurs 15(4):311, 1986.
Mueller LS: Pregnancy and sexuality, JOGN Nurs 14(4):289, 1985.
Nichols F and Humenick SS: Childbirth education, practice, research, and theory, Philadelphia, 1988, WB Saunders Co.
Norton SF and Nichols CW: Champions of choice, Am J Nurs 85(4):380, 1985.
Oehler J: The frog family books: color the pictures "sad" or "glad," MCN 6:281, 1981.
Olson ML: Fitting grandparents into new families, MCN 6(6):419, 1981.
Redman BK: The process of patient education, ed 6, St Louis, 1988, The CV Mosby Co.
Roberts JE et al: A descriptive analysis of involuntary bearing-down efforts during the expulsive phase of labor, JOGN Nurs, p 48, Jan/Feb 1987.
Stephany T: Supporting the mother of a patient in labor, JOGN Nurs 12(5):345, 1983.
Strang VR and Sullivan PL: Body image attitudes during pregnancy and the postpartum period, JOGN Nurs 14(4):332, 1985.
Strickland OL: The occurrence of symptoms in expectant fathers, Nurs Res 36(3):184, 1987.
Waller MM: Siblings in the childbearing experience, NAACOG Update Series 1:lesson 17, 1984.
Waryas FS and Leubbers MG: A cluster system for maternity care, MCN 11(2):98, 1986.

CHAPTER

10 Nursing Care During Pregnancy

Irene M. Bobak

Learning Objectives

Correctly define the key terms listed.

Summarize health assessment of the gravida and fetus.

Assess the presumptive, probable, and positive manifestations of pregnancy.

Outline the schedule of visits for a woman with a normal pregnancy.

Evaluate cultural influences of the woman's (family's) response to pregnancy and the use of the health care system.

List the 11 physical danger signs of the prenatal period.

Evaluate emotional appraisal and marital support during pregnancy.

Discuss physiology and treatment of discomforts related to maternal adaptations.

Explain counseling for prenatal danger signs.

Discuss client teaching for recognizing preterm labor, and identify six warning signs and symptoms of preterm labor.

Delineate guidelines for client teaching for prevention of urinary tract infections, breast self-examination, and Kegel's exercises.

Explore and give the rationale for standards for maternity care and employment.

Review the risks and care for the woman with a multifetal pregnancy.

Key Terms

ankle edema
body mechanics
breast fullness
carpal tunnel syndrome
conscious relaxation
constipation
cultural variations
dyspnea
effleurage
estimated date of delivery (EDD)
fetal gestational age
fetal health status
fetal heart rate (FHR)
fundal height
gestational age
gingivitis and epulis
hemorrhoids
imitative magic
insomnia
Kegel's exercises
last menstrual period (LMP)
leg cramps
leg edema
lithotomy position
morning sickness
Nägele's rule
nipple cup
Papanicolaou smear
pelvic tilt (rock)
perineal discomfort
pinch test
proscription
roll-over test
round ligament pain
supine hypotension
taboos
tailor sitting position
urinary frequency
varicosities

The prenatal period is a preparatory one, both physically, in terms of fetal growth and maternal adaptations, and psychologically, in terms of anticipation of parenthood. Becoming a parent represents one of the maturational crises of our lives and as such can represent a time of growth in responsibility and concern for others. It is a time of intense learning for the parents and for those close to them, as well as a time for development of family unity.

During a woman's life, pregnancy is unique because only then does the healthy woman seek ongoing health care. Regular prenatal visits, ideally beginning soon after the first missed menstrual period, offer opportunities to ensure the health of the expectant mother and her infant. Prenatal health supervision permits diagnosis and treatment of maternal disorders that may have preexisted or may develop during the pregnancy. It is designed to follow the growth and development of the fetus and to identify abnormalities that may interfere with the course of normal labor. The woman and her family can seek support for stress and learn parenting skills.

❑ FIRST TRIMESTER

The initial visit of the woman to either the physician's office or an obstetric clinic is important in setting the tone for her care. The woman needs to feel welcomed and important. The initial visit may include diagnosing the pregnancy and establishing the data base, depending on the duration of gestation. If pregnancy is too early and cannot be verified, her next appointment is scheduled in 2 weeks.

Pregnancy spans 9 months, approximately 40 weeks. Pregnancy is divided into three 3-month periods or trimesters. The first trimester covers week 1 through 13; the second, weeks 14 through 26; the third, weeks 27 through term gestation (38 to 40 weeks).

Once pregnancy is diagnosed, prenatal care is instituted. Nursing care follows the nursing process: assessment, analysis and formulation of nursing diagnoses, planning, implementation, and evaluation.

Diagnosis of Pregnancy

The clinical diagnosis of pregnancy before the second missed period may be difficult in at least 25% to 30% of women. Physical variability, lack of relaxation, obesity, or tumors, for example, may confound even the experienced obstetrician or midwife. Accuracy is most important, however, because emotional, social, medical, or legal consequences of an inaccurate diagnosis, either positive or negative, can be extremely serious. A correct date for the **last menstrual period (LMP)**, the date of intercourse, or the basal body temperature (BBT) record may be of great value in the accurate diagnosis of pregnancy. Reexamination in 2 to 4 weeks may be required for verifying the diagnosis.

Great variability is possible in the subjective and objective symptoms of pregnancy. The diagnosis of pregnancy is classified as follows: presumptive, probable, and positive. The ***positive signs*** of pregnancy are demonstration of a fetal heart distinct from that of the mother, appreciation of fetal movement by someone other than the mother, and visualization of the fetus with a technique such as ultrasound (Scott et al, 1990). The positive signs used to confirm the diagnosis of pregnancy include certain pregnancy tests (Chapter 8).

The nurse is referred to Chapter 8 for an in-depth discussion of the symptoms reflecting maternal adaptations to pregnancy. Many of the signs and symptoms of pregnancy are clinically useful in the diagnosis of pregnancy. The ***presumptive signs and symptoms*** of pregnancy can be caused by conditions other than gestation. Therefore no one manifestation can be relied on for a final impression, nor are combinations of manifestations diagnostic. For example, amenorrhea may be caused by an endocrine disorder; lassitude and fatigue may signify anemia or infection; and nausea or vomiting may be caused by a gastrointestinal upset or allergy.

Presumptive findings include subjective symptoms and objective signs. Subjective symptoms may include amenorrhea, nausea and vomiting (**morning sickness**), **breast fullness** and sensitivity, **urinary frequency**, lassitude or fatigue, weight gain, and mood swings. "Quickening" may be noted between weeks 16 and 20. Objective signs include a variety of demonstrable anatomic and physiologic changes (Chapter 8), elevation of BBT; skin changes such as striae gravidarum, deeper pigmentation (chloasma, linea nigra); breast changes; abdominal enlargement; and changes in the uterus and vagina.

Probable subjective symptoms are the same as presumptive symptoms. When combined with probable objective signs, they strongly suggest pregnancy. Objective signs include uterine enlargement, Braxton Hicks contractions and souffle, ballottement, and positive pregnancy test results from less sophisticated tests.

Estimated Date of Delivery

Following the diagnosis of pregnancy the woman's first question usually concerns when she will deliver. This date has traditionally been termed the estimated date of confinement (EDC). To promote a more positive perception of both pregnancy and delivery, however, the term **estimated date of delivery (EDD)** is usually used. Because the precise date of conception generally must remain conjectural, many formulas or rules of thumb have been suggested for calculating the EDD. None of these rules of thumb are infallable, but Nägele's rule is reasonably accurate and is the method usually used.

Nägele's Rule. Nägele's rule is as follows: add 7 days to the first day of the LMP, subtract 3 months, and add 1 year. The formula becomes EDD + ([LMP + 7 days] − 3 months) + 1 year. For example, if the first day of the LMP was July 10, 1990, the EDD is April 17, 1991. In simple terms, add 7 days to the LMP and count forward 9 months.

Nägele's rule assumes that the woman has a 28-day cycle and that the pregnancy occurred on the fourteenth day. An adjustment is in order if the cycle is longer or shorter than 28 days. With the use of Nägele's rule, only about 4% to 10% of gravidas will deliver spontaneously on the EDD. Most women will deliver during the period extending from 7 days before to 7 days after the EDD.

Assessment

The process of assessment continues throughout the prenatal period. It begins when a woman makes contact with health professionals because she suspects she is pregnant. Assessment techniques include the interview, physical examination, and laboratory tests.

A checklist of care needs spanning pregnancy is a valuable tool. It provides the team of care providers with a communication tool to prevent gaps and identify areas of repeated concern for clients. When shared with clients, the checklist items validate their universality among gravidas and their families. Knowledge that items are common to many offers some reassurance. Reading the checklist also reminds clients of otherwise forgotten data. A checklist for the first trimester follows below. Checklists for the second and third trimesters can be found on p. 261 and p. 275.

Interview

The initial assessment interview establishes the therapeutic relationship between nurse and client. It is planned, purposeful communication that focuses on specific content. Two sources are usually used in collecting data: the client's subjective interpretation of health status and the nurse's objective observations. During the interview the nurse observes the client's affect, posture, body language, skin color, and other physical and emotional signs. These observations become important data in the assessment.

Often the client will be accompanied by a family member or members. The nurse builds a relationship with these persons as part of the social context of the client. They also are helpful in recalling and validating information related to the client's health problem. With the client's permission, those accompanying her can be included in the initial prenatal interview. Wright and Leahey (1984) offer excellent guidance to the nurse in developing skills for interviewing families and assessing the interaction between family members. Observations and information about the client's family are part of the interview. For example, if the client is accompanied by small children, the nurse can inquire about her plans for child care during the forthcoming labor and delivery.

FIRST TRIMESTER CHECKLIST

- Diagnosis and expected date of delivery
- Schedule and events of visits
- Counseling for self-care:
  - Adaptations/discomforts
    - Breast changes
    - Urinary frequency
    - Nausea and vomiting
    - Fatigue
    - Psychosocial responses and family dynamics
- Exercise and rest
- Relaxation
- Nutrition
- Sexuality
- Danger signs
- Resources
  - Education
  - Dental evaluation
  - Medical service
  - Social service
  - Emergency room
- Diagnostic tests
  - Specify
- Other

The interview provides information about the client's biopsychosocial status. Although the format for interviewing or recording the client's health history may differ, the information obtained is universal.

Reason for Seeking Care. The client's description of the purpose for the request for care is quoted verbatim in the record. For example, "I think I am pregnant," or "My legs get so swollen I can hardly walk." This statement does not constitute a diagnosis, because the client's condition needs to be confirmed by the nurse or physician before any care is instituted. Recording the chief purpose of a visit in the client's own words alerts other personnel to the "priority of need" as seen by the client.

Medical History. The interviewer will record such information as the woman's menstrual history, sexual activity, and previous pregnancies and their outcomes. The conduct of the *present pregnancy* is predicated on the reports of previous pregnancies.

The medical history describes medical or surgical conditions that may affect the course of pregnancy or that may be affected by the pregnancy. For example, the pregnant woman who has diabetes or epilepsy will require special care. Because most clients are anxious during the initial interview, reference to cues such as a Medic Alert bracelet will help the client explain allergies, chronic diseases, or medications being used (e.g., cortisone, insulin, or anticonvulsants). If the woman is using any medication, she is asked to list them and describe their use.

Previous surgeries are described. Abortion may predispose the woman to incompetent cervix; uterine surgery or extensive repair of the pelvic floor may necessitate cesarean birth; appendectomy rules out appendicitis as cause of right lower quadrant pain; spinal surgery contraindicates spinal or epidural anesthesia. Any *injury* involving the pelvis is noted particularly.

Often clients who have adapted well to chronic or handicapping conditions forget to mention them because they are so integrated into their life-style. Special shoes or a limp may indicate a pelvic structural defect, which is an important consideration in pregnancy. The nurse who observes these special characteristics and can inquire about them sensitively obtains individualized data that will provide the basis for a comprehensive nursing care plan. Observations are vital components of the interview process because they prompt the nurse and the client to focus on the specific needs of the client and her family.

Family History. The family history provides information about the client's immediate family, including parents, siblings, and children. This helps identify familial or genetic disorders or conditions that could affect the present health status of the woman. A description of a detailed family history is presented in Chapter 2.

Social and Experiential History. *Situational factors* such as the family's ethnic and cultural background and socioeconomic status are determined in the social and experiential history. *Perception of this pregnancy* is explored. Is this pregnancy wanted or not, planned or not? Is the woman (couple) pleased, displeased, accepting, or nonaccepting? Is the pregnancy "hers" or "theirs"? What problems arise because of the pregnancy: financial, career, and living accommodations? The *family support* system is determined (see Chapter 2). What primary support is available to the mother? Are there changes needed to promote adequate support for the mother? What are the existing relationships between mother, father, siblings, and in-laws? What preparations are being made for the care of the woman and dependent family members during labor and for the care of the infant after birth? Is community support needed, for example, financial, educational? What are the woman's (couple's) ideas about childbearing, expectations of infant's behavior, and outlook on life and the female role? Questions that need to be asked include, What will it be like to have a baby in the home? How is your life going to change by having a baby? What plans do having a baby interrupt? During interviews throughout the pregnancy the nurse remains alert for potential parenting disorders such as depression, lack of family support, and inadequate living conditions. What is the woman's (couple's) attitude toward health care, particularly during childbearing? What is expected of the physician, and how is the relationship between the woman (couple) and nurse viewed?

Coping mechanisms and patterns of interacting are identified (see Chapters 2 and 9). Early in the pregnancy the nurse determines the woman's (couple's) knowledge of pregnancy, maternal changes, fetal growth, care of self, and care of the newborn, including feeding. It is important to ask about attitudes toward unmedicated or medicated childbirth, and about parental knowledge of availability of parenting skills classes. Before planning for nursing care, the nurse needs information about the woman's (couple's) decision-making abilities and living habits (e.g., exercise, sleep, diet, diversional interests, personal hygiene, clothing).

Attitudes concerning the range of *acceptable sexual behavior* during pregnancy are explored. Questions such as the following could be asked: What has your family (partner, friends) told you about sex during pregnancy? or What are your feelings about sex during pregnancy? *Sexual self-concept* is given more emphasis by employing questions such as, How do you feel about the changes in your appearance? How does your partner feel about your body now? Do maternity clothes make pregnant women attractive?

Review of Systems. During this portion of the interview, symptoms indicative of pregnancy are elicited. In addition, preexisting or concurrent problems are identified and described for all body systems and mental status. The woman is questioned about physical symptoms she has experienced such as shortness of breath or pain. Pregnancy affects and is affected by all body systems (see Chapter 8); therefore knowledge of the present status of body systems is important in planning care. For each sign or symptom expressed, the following additional data should be obtained: body location, quality, quantity, chronology, setting, aggravating or alleviating factors, and associated manifestations (onset, character, course) (Seidel et al, 1987).

Woman With a Disability. Clients with serious and handicapping physical or emotional disorders—the deaf, the blind, the depressed, the physically disabled, the mentally retarded, the brain injured—must all be respected and the assessment approach adapted to their needs. Clients who are emotionally restricted may not be able to give an effective history, but they must be respected, and the history should be obtained from *them* to the extent possible. Their points of view and their attitudes matter. Still, when necessary, the family, other health professionals involved in care, and the client's record must be queried to get the complete story. Each client must be fully respected and fully involved to the limit of emotion, cognitive capacity, or physical handicap.

Physical Examination

The initial physical examination provides the baseline for assessing subsequent changes. The examiner needs to determine the client's needs for basic information regarding the structure of the genital organs and provide this information, along with a demonstration of the equipment that may be used and an explanation of the procedure itself. The interaction requires an unhurried, sensitive, and gentle approach with a matter-of-fact attitude.

It is important that the examiner ensure the cleanliness of the facilities, equipment, supplies, and hands. All equipment necessary for the procedure should be in place to avoid interrupting the examination (Fig. 10-1).

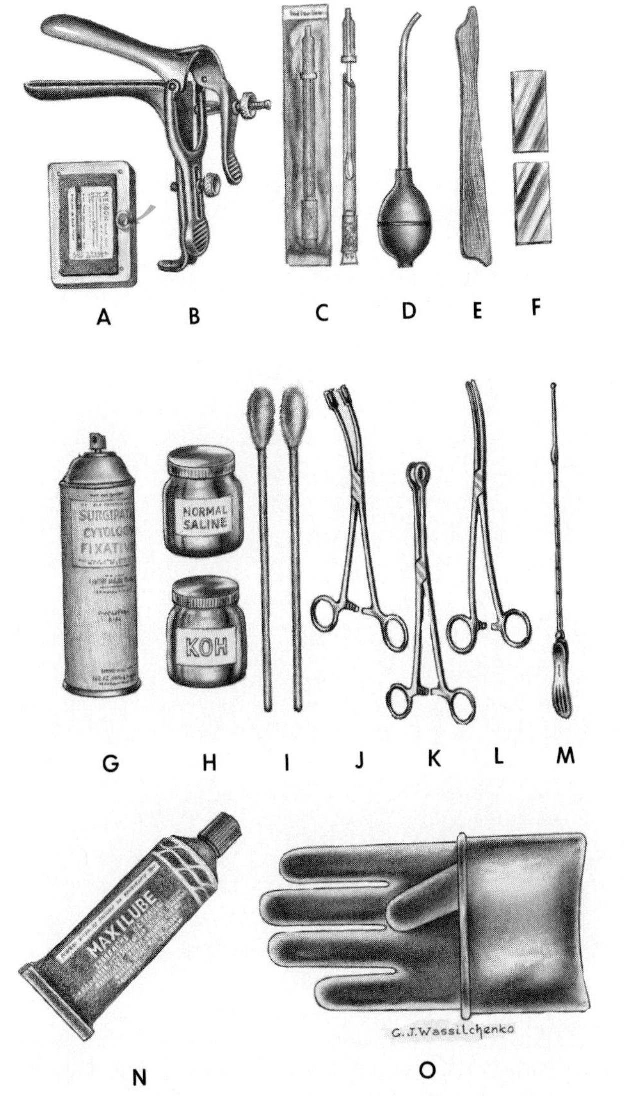

Fig. 10-1 Equipment used for pelvic examination. **A,** Thayer-Martin medium for isolation of *Neisseria gonorrhoeae.* Cylindrical container *(arrow)* is for pellet that releases carbon dioxide; medium and specimen are refrigerated until transport to laboratory. **B,** Vaginal speculum. **C,** Culturette, modified Stuart's bacterial transport medium with self-contained sterile swab. **D,** Vaginal pipette with rubber bulb. **E,** Plastic spatula for Papanicolaou smear and cytology specimens. **F,** Slides for cytology specimens (Pap smear) or for wet mounts for diagnosing cause of vaginitis. **G,** Spray can of fixative for slide specimens. When dry, slides are packaged in cardboard for transport to laboratory. **H,** Normal saline and 10% potassium hydroxide (KOH) for wet mounts of vaginal fluids. **I,** Cotton pledget stick. **J,** Tenaculum. **K,** Ring (sponge or stick) forceps. **L,** Tissue forceps. **M,** Uterine sound (slightly curved for insertion). **N,** Sterile lubricant; may be antiseptic. **O,** Glove for vaginal and rectal examinations (sterile for vaginal, clean for rectal).

The woman is assured of privacy for the examination without unexpected intrusions. She is given a cover gown and drape for modesty. The environment is comfortably warm and pleasant.

The physical examination begins with assessment of vital signs, height and weight, and blood pressure. Because the bladder must be empty before pelvic examination, the urine specimen is obtained.

Each examiner has developed a routine for proceeding with the physical examination; most choose the head-to-toe progression. Heart and breath sounds are evaluated, and extremities are examined. Distribution, amount, and quality of body hair is of particular importance because the findings reflect nutritional status, endocrine function, and general emphasis on hygiene. The thyroid gland is assessed carefully. The typical basic examination is usually completed without much difficulty for the healthy woman.

The examiner needs to remain alert to the woman's clues that give direction to the remainder of the assessment and that indicate imminent untoward response such as supine hypotension.

Thyroid Gland. The thyroid gland is the largest endocrine gland in the body and the only one accessible to direct physical examination. Assessment of thyroid function or possible dysfunction includes more than observation and palpation of the area where the thyroid gland is located. Metabolic rates and rhythms, including menstrual regularity in the woman of childbearing age, are governed by the thyroid gland. The effects of thyroid activity are widespread. Therefore observations of behavior, appearance, skin, eyes, hair, and cardiovascular status are important. Several findings require further attention (e.g., enlargement, coarse and gritty consistency, nodules).

Breasts. The gynecologic examination includes an evaluation of the breasts primarily to establish a data base of normal findings. However, the practitioner needs to be alert to the possibility of carcinoma at all times. Early detection of potential malignancies has been and continues to be the single most important factor in the successful treatment of this disease. Since professional assessment is done only periodically, each woman is advised to do a breast self-examination (BSE) on a monthly basis at the time when the breast is least affected by menstrual changes, 4 to 10 days after the last menstrual period (Fig. 4-20) (women who no longer menstruate can use the first of every month for BSE).

Anatomy and physiology of the breast are presented in several sections of this text.* As the examiner pro-

*Anatomy, physiology, growth, development across the life span, Chapter 4; maternal adaptation to pregnancy, Chapter 8; during the post-delivery period, Chapter 19; during lactation, Chapter 18.

ceeds through the examination, the woman is taught about BSE, or if she already follows a routine for BSE, her knowledge and technique are refreshed.

At the start of the examination, the breasts are observed for symmetry, contour, color, size, and surface characteristics such as vascularity, moles, and nevi. The nipples are checked for areolar pigmentation and discharge and for response to stimulation (i.e., erection, flattening, or inversion). The woman then presses her hands against her waist to cause pectoral contraction and repeats the assessment above.

When the woman raises her arms above her head, the position of the nipple and any dimpling (localized skin retraction) of the surface are noted. Breast may appear symmetric at rest, but elevating the breast may reveal lesions. If the woman's breasts are pendulous, and problems exist, leaning forward to allow the breast to hang loose may reveal dimpling or other irregularities.

For the next part of the examination, the woman lies flat with her arm abducted and her hand under her head to help flatten breast tissue evenly over the chest wall, facilitating inspection and palpation. A pillow placed under the shoulder of the breast to be examined helps position breast tissue. Each breast is examined separately. The examiner can use both hands; however, in self-examination, the woman uses the hand opposite the side being examined. The fingers are held flat against the breast, and the tissue is palpated gently against the chest wall. The examination may be done either by using a circular method, quadrant by quadrant, or a spoke-wheel pattern (Fig. 10-2). The presence of regions of tenderness are distinguished, as are thickened or firm zones. Any masses are noted for location, size, consistency, and mobility or fixation to the skin or chest wall. Palpation of the breast includes glandular tissue, areolar areas, and the nipples. Normally breast tissue is slightly lobular; hard fixed masses are abnormal. The nipple should be palpated then compressed to reveal any drainage. No examination is complete without assessing those parts of the breast known as the tail of Spence and the axillary lymph nodes. The lymph nodes are palpated while the client is in a sitting position. Easy access is gained to the axillary nodes with the client's arms at her sides and muscles relaxed. To gain the necessary muscle relaxation, the examiner supports the client's arm. The lymph nodes are assessed by using a rotary motion with two or three fingertips. Although malignancy may occur anywhere in the breast, the most common site is the upper outer quadrant.

Abdomen. The examination of the abdomen is done carefully and systematically. The skin is assessed for general condition, color, rashes, lesions, scars,

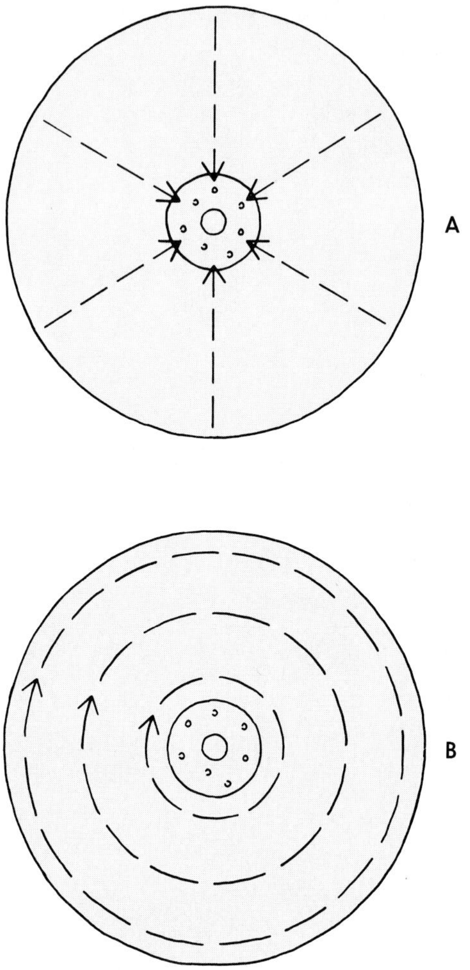

Fig. 10-2 Two methods of systematic breast palpation. **A,** Palpation in wedge sections (spoke-wheel fashion) from breast periphery to center. **B,** Palpation along concentric circles from periphery to center. It usually takes three circles to cover all breast tissue. (From Malasanos L et al: Health assessment, ed 3, St Louis, 1986, The CV Mosby Co.)

striae, dilated veins, turgor, texture, and hair distribution. Contour, symmetry, and presence of hernias are noted. Bowel sounds are auscultated.

Pelvic Examination

The pelvic examination may be deferred to the next prenatal visit if the woman is anxious, tense, or refuses to have one at this visit. The vagina enlarges, and supporting structures are more relaxed as pregnancy advances. When the examination is performed, the tone of the pelvic musculature and need for and knowledge of **Kegel's exercises** (p. 251) are assessed. During the pelvic examination the nurse remains alert for symptoms of supine hypotension (p. 241).

Many women are intimidated by the gynecologic portion of the physical examination. The nurse in this instance can take an advocacy approach that supports a partnership relationship between the client and the care provider.

The woman is assisted into the **lithotomy position** (see Fig 10-10, *A*) for the pelvic examination (see Procedure 10-1). When she is in the lithotomy position, the woman's hips and knees are flexed with the buttocks at the edge of the table and her feet supported by heel or knee stirrups. Some women prefer to keep their shoes or socks on, especially if the stirrups are not padded.

Many women express feelings of vulnerability and strangeness when in the lithotomy position. During the procedure the nurse assists the woman with relaxation techniques—the physician's and nurse's behavior toward her to this point adds to her ability to relax. One method of helping the woman relax is to have her place her hands on her chest at about the level of the diaphragm, breathe deeply and slowly (in through her nose and out through her O-shaped mouth), concentrate on the rhythm of breathing, and relax all body muscles with each exhalation (Malasanos et al., 1990; Chapter 9). This breathing technique is particularly helpful for the adolescent or the woman whose introitus may be especially tight, or for whom the experience may be new and may provoke tension.

Some women relax when they are encouraged to become involved with the examination with a mirror placed so that the area being examined can be seen by the client. This type of participation helps with health teaching as well. Distraction is another technique that can be used effectively. For example, placement of interesting pictures or mobiles on the ceiling over the head of the table.

The nurse is reminded that the woman *must not squeeze her eyes closed or clench her fists;* tightening these muscles permits the tightening of the perineal muscles.

Many women find it distressing to attempt to converse in the lithotomy position. Most clients appreciate an explanation of the procedure as it unfolds as well as coaching for the type of sensations they may expect. But in general women prefer not to have to respond to questions until they are again upright and at eye level with the examiner. Questioning during the procedure, especially if they cannot see their questioner's eyes, may make women tense.

Supine Hypotension. When a woman is lying in the lithotomy position (Fig 10-3, *A*), the weight of abdominal contents may compress the vena cava and aorta, resulting in a drop in blood pressure (**supine hypotension**). Pallor, breathlessness and clammy skin are other objective signs. Symptoms include *a fall in blood pressure, pallor, breathlessness,* and *clammy skin.* Nursing actions include *positioning the woman on her side until her signs and symptoms subside.* If the woman is unable to tolerate the lithotomy position, the left lateral position may be used for genital examination (Fig. 10-3, *B*).

External Inspection. The examiner sits at the foot of the table for the inspection of the external genitals and for the speculum examination. To facilitate open communication and to help the woman relax, the woman's head is raised on a pillow and the drape is arranged so that eye-to-eye contact can be maintained. In good lighting, external genitals are inspected for sexual maturity, clitoris, labia, and perineum. After childbirth or other trauma there may be healed scars. Normal findings are discussed in Chapter 4.

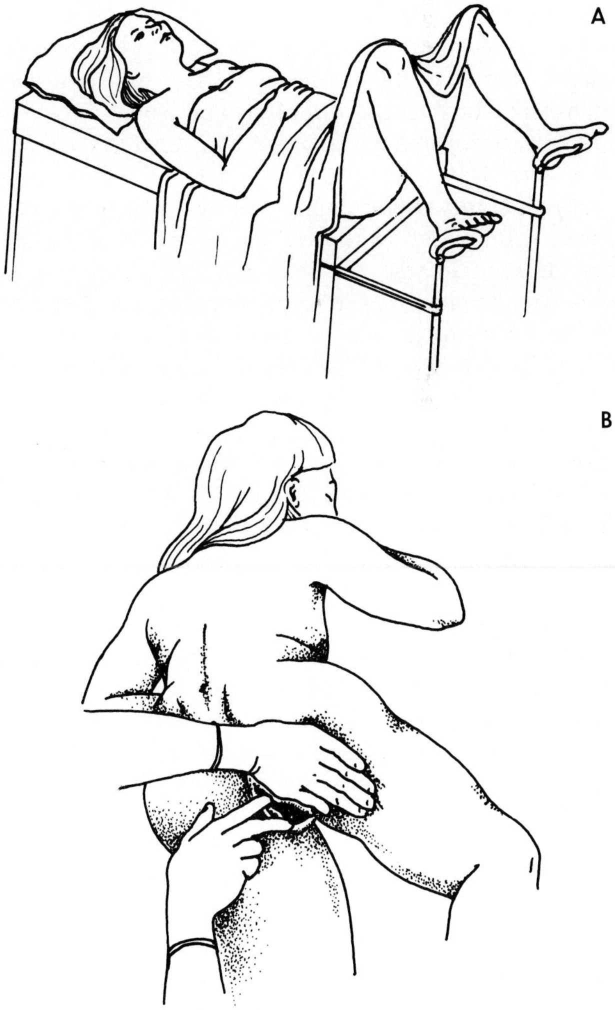

Fig. 10-3 **A,** Lithotomy position. **B,** Alternate position for examination of genitals, left lateral position.

External Palpation. The examiner proceeds with the examination using palpation* and inspection. The examiner wears gloves for this portion of the assessment. The labia are spread apart to expose the structures in the vestibule: urinary meatus, Skene's glands, vaginal orifice, and Bartholin's glands. To assess the Skene's glands, the examiner inserts one finger into the vagina and "milks" the area of the urethra. Any exudate from the *urethra* or the *Skene's glands* is cultured. Masses and erythema of either structure are assessed further. Ordinarily, the openings to the Skene's glands are not visible; prominent openings may be seen if the glands are infected (e.g., with gonorrhea). During the examination, the examiner keeps in mind the findings from the review of systems, such as history of burning on urination.

The *vaginal orifice* is examined. Carunculae myrtiformes (hymenal tags) are normal findings. With one finger still in the vagina, the examiner repositions the index finger near the posterior part of the orifice. With the thumb outside the posterior part of the labia majora, the examiner compresses the area of *Bartholin's glands* located at the 8 o'clock and 4 o'clock positions and looks for swelling, discharge, and pain.

The *support* of the anterior and posterior *vaginal wall* is assessed. The examiner spreads the labia with the index and middle finger and asks the woman to strain down. Any bulge from the anterior wall (urethrocele or cystocele) or posterior wall (rectocele) is noted and compared with the history, such as difficulty to start the stream of urine or constipation.

The *perineum* (area between the vagina and anus) is assessed for scars from old lacerations or episiotomies, for thinning, fistulas, masses, lesions, and inflammation. The *anus* is assessed for **hemorrhoids,** hemorrhoidal tags, and integrity of the anal sphincter. Occasionally, following traumatic delivery with lacerations that extended into the anal sphincter, the muscle may not have been correctly repaired; for example, the examiner will see a "dimple" over two ends of separated muscle and the "wink" reflex is incomplete. If the anal sphincter was not repaired correctly, the woman may have given a history of incontinence. The anal area is also assessed for lesions, masses, abscesses, tumors. If there is a history of sexually transmitted disease, the examiner may want to culture the anal canal at this time.

Throughout the genital examination, the examiner notes the odor. Odor may indicate infection and poor hygienic practices.

Internal Examination. When the woman made the appointment for her examination, she was asked to refrain from douching or using vaginal medications for the previous 24 hours. (NOTE: Douching is *not* recommended during pregnancy.) These actions cloud diagnosis based on secretions, cells, and odor. In addition, douching removes vaginal secretions, making insertion of the vaginal speculum more difficult. Some women have a hard time complying with this request; they cannot go to the doctor feeling unclean in the genital region.

Vaginal specula consist of two blades and a handle. Specula come in a variety of types and styles (Fig. 10-4). Vaginal specula are used to view the vaginal vault and cervix. The pelvic examination is detailed in Procedure 10-1.

The speculum blades are opened to reveal the cervix and are locked into the open position. The cervix is inspected: position and appearance of os, position, color, lesions, bleeding, and discharge. Cervical findings not within normal limits (for example, ulcerations, masses, inflammation, excessive protrusion into the vaginal vault), anomalies (for example, cock's comb [protrusion over cervix that looks like a rooster's comb], hooded, or collared cervix [seen in DES daughters]), and polyps are noted.

Collection of Specimens

Collection of specimens for cytologic examination is an important part of the gynecologic examination. *Infection* can be diagnosed through examination of specimens collected during the pelvic examination. These infections include gonorrhea, *Chlamydia trachomatis,* and herpes simplex types 1 and 2. Once the diagnoses have been made, treatment can be instituted.

Papanicolaou Smear. *Carcinogenic conditions,* potential or actual, can be determined by examination of cells from the cervix collected during the pelvic examination. The woman needs to know the purpose of the test and what sensations she will feel as the specimen is obtained (i.e., pressure, not pain). The woman is counseled to avoid douching, using any vaginal medications, or engaging in intercourse at least 24 hours before the procedure. In addition, no lubricant is used before obtaining the specimen. These precautions are taken to avoid cell distortion.

The specimen for the **Papanicolau smear** is obtained by placing the S-shaped end of the cervical spatula just within the cervical canal at the external os. The blade is rotated 360 degrees so that the surface at the squamocolumnar junction is uniformly scraped. If the

*As a sign of caring and to assist the woman to feel more at ease, the woman should receive a verbal cue and a cue through touch on a nonemotionally charged body part (e.g., knee) before experiencing touch on her genitals. The back of the hand, lightly touching the inner aspect of the thigh, often works well.

PROCEDURE 10-1

PELVIC EXAMINATION

DEFINITION

Inspection and palpation of the internal and external structures comprising the female reproductive system. Examination may be done manually or with aid of instrumentation.

PURPOSE

To provide a data base for medical diagnoses, medical therapy, nursing diagnoses, and nursing care. To involve the woman as an active participant in her own health supervision, maintenance, and care.

To obtain specimens for screening potential problems.

EQUIPMENT

Gynecologic table and drapes.

Supplies as necessary (see Fig. 10-1).

NURSING ACTIONS	RATIONALE
Wash hands.	Minimizes chance for nosocomial infection.
Ask client to empty her bladder before the examination (obtain clean-catch urine specimen as needed)	Increases woman's comfort and facilitates accurate assessment.
Instruct woman to remove her clothing (from the waist down if only the pelvic exam is to be done) and put on a cover gown; provide privacy for this.	Provides adequate exposure for thorough gynecologic examination. Shows respect.
Explain purpose of the procedure and how it is done. Describe sensations to expect. Inform the client who will do the procedure and about how long it will take. Ask her if she wishes a mirror to watch.	Reduces anxiety related to knowledge deficit. Provides woman with chance to have more control over situation and to learn more about her body.
Assist the woman into the lithotomy position (the woman's hips and knees are flexed with the buttocks at the edge of the table with her feet supported by heel or knee stirrups), and drape appropriately.	Increases her comfort and facilitates examination; however, other positions can be used (Fig. 10-3). Meets her need for modesty and provides warmth.
Adjust pillow under client's head.	Increases her comfort and helps relax her abdominal musculature.
Lubricate examiner's fingers with water or water-soluble lubricant before bimanual examination	Reduces friction and discomfort and avoids other types of lubricant that can distort findings.
Warm speculum in warm water.	Increases client's comfort because warm metal is less shocking to the mucous membrane.
During the examination, support client. Explain the procedure during inspection of external genitals, insertion of speculum for examination of vagina and cervix, and bimanual examination of internal organs.	Reduces her anxiety by keeping her informed. Increases her knowledge about her body.
Refrain from questioning the woman extensively. Hold questions until she is sitting up and at eye level with the examiner.	Prevents tension that can develop if she is questioned, especially if she cannot see the questioner's eyes.
Assist with relaxation techniques. Have the woman place her hands on her chest at about the level of the diaphragm, breathe deeply and slowly (in through her nose and out through her O-shaped mouth), concentrate on the rhythm of breathing, and relax all body muscles with each exhalation (Malasanos et al, 1990).	Decreases common feelings of vulnerability and strangeness when in lithotomy position. Helps her relax perineum during the examination. NOTE: This breathing technique is particularly helpful for the adolescent or the woman whose introitus may be especially tight. Others for whom the experience may be new or tension provoking can also benefit from using this technique.
Encourage woman to become involved with the examination if she shows interest. For example, a mirror can be placed so that the area being examined can be seen by the woman.	Assists the interested woman and motivates other women to be participants in their own care. Provides health teaching.
Distract the attention of the tense woman by placing interesting mobiles or pictures on the ceiling or wall near her head.	Provides distraction, which is an effective method of reducing tension.
Remind the woman not to squeeze her eyes closed, clench her fists, or squeeze the nurse's hand.	Helps her relax her perineum, because tightening these muscles encourages tightening of the perineal muscles.

Continued.

PROCEDURE 10-1—cont'd

NURSING ACTIONS	RATIONALE
Assess woman for and treat imminent untoward responses such as supine hypotension, p. 241.	Ensures the safety and health of the woman.
Instruct woman to bear down when speculum is being inserted	Opens the vaginal introitus and relaxes perineal muscles for easier insertion of the speculum.
Apply gloves and assist examiner with collection of specimens for cytology such as Papanicolaou smear. After handling specimens, remove gloves and wash hands.	Implements universal precautions when handling body fluids (see Chapter 23). Reduces possibility of contamination of specimens. Minimizes nosocomial infections.
Assist woman at completion of examination to a sitting position and then a standing position.	Attains a sitting position comfortably without strain. Reduces possibility of transient or orthostatic hypotension that may occur if position is changed rapidly.
Provide tissues to wipe lubricant from perineum.	Provides comfort and promotes cleanliness.
Provide privacy for woman while she is dressing.	Shows respect and promotes feelings of security and worth.
Inform woman as to the next step in the assessment protocol.	Supplies information to reduce tension that arises from facing the unknown.
Record findings on the appropriate forms.	Provides permanent record of data base to foster continuity of care.

A

B

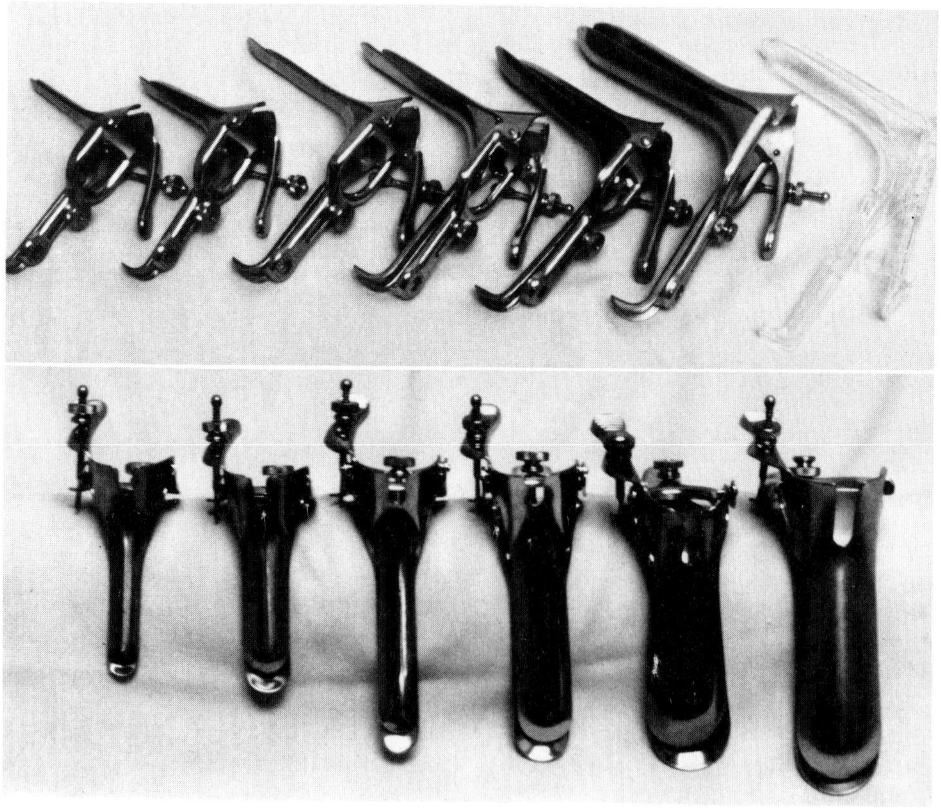

Fig. 10-4 Vaginal specula. From left to right: **A,** Short-billed pediatric, pediatric, small Pederson, Pederson, small Graves, large Graves, plastic Graves. **B,** Short-billed pediatric, pediatric, small Pederson, Pederson, small Graves, large Graves. (From Seidel H et al: Mosby's guide to physical examination, St Louis, 1987, The CV Mosby Co.)

junction is inside the cervical canal, a swab may be used to obtain cells. If gross exudate is present, the excess is gently pushed away from the os with the end of the spatula. The specimen is spread on a slide without rubbing or drying, sprayed lightly with fixative, and allowed to dry. Some mucus is obtained from the posterior fornix (vaginal pool) with the rounded end of the spatula, spread on another slide, sprayed, and dried. The specimens are sent to the pathology laboratory promptly for staining, evaluation, and a written report, with special reference to abnormal elements, including cancer cells.

Gonorrheal Culture. A culture for gonorrhea is done to screen women for gonorrheal infection that could compromise the woman, her fetus if she is pregnant, and her partner. The woman is told the reason for the test (e.g., test for vaginal infection). If she is pregnant, the test is done routinely at the first prenatal visit and repeated toward the end of pregnancy (week 36).

The specimen is obtained at the same time as the Papanicolaou smear, and the same precautions regarding use of digital examinations and lubricant are followed. A specimen is obtained from the endocervical canal using a sterile cotton-tipped applicator. The applicator is rolled on a culture plate with a special medium (Thayer-Martin). The plate is then incubated.

***Chlamydia Trachomatis* Smear.** Smears of urethral or cervical secretions are collected during the pelvic examination, following the same precautions used for the Papanicolaou smear. A fluorescein-conjugated monoclonal antibody test system for the detection of *Chlamydia* antigen is available. Slides containing the smears are incubated for 30 minutes with fluorescein-labeled antibodies. The physician, nurse practitioner, or midwife then examines the slides using a fluorescent microscope.

Tissue cultures are still sometimes used, although they are more expensive and it takes longer to obtain results with them than with the monoclonal tests.

Herpes Simplex, Types 1 and 2 Culture*. If an open lesion is present at the time of the initial pelvic examination, a viral culture is obtained from the lesion and is repeated at intervals. A positive Papanicolaou smear may be caused by the presence of herpes simplex, type 2.

Vaginal Examination

For assessing vaginal discharges other than blood, see Chapters 8 and 23. After the specimens are obtained, the vagina around the cervix is viewed by rotating the speculum. The speculum blades are unlocked and partially closed. As the speculum is withdrawn, it is rotated and the vaginal walls inspected for color, lesions, rugae, fistulas, and bulging.

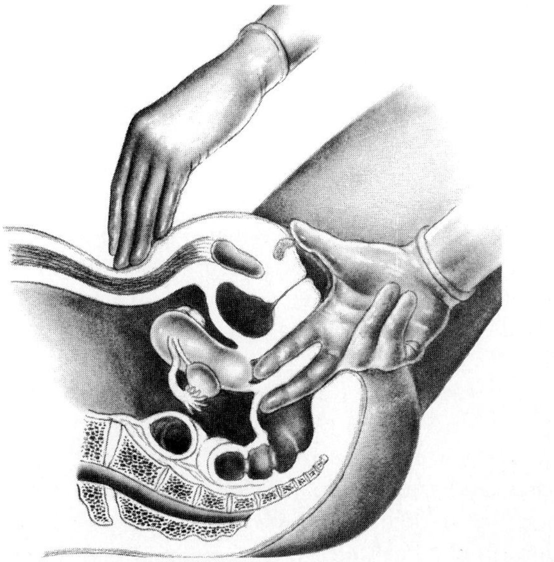

Fig. 10-5 Rectovaginal palpation. (From Seidel H et al: Mosby's guide to physical examination, St Louis, 1987, The CV Mosby Co.)

Incontinence of urine during straining is not a normal finding and is noted. A variety of factors can cause incontinence, including pubococcygeal muscles that are weak from lack of exercise (Kegel's) or trauma from childbirth (see Kegel's exercises, p. 251).

Bimanual Palpation. The examiner stands for this part of the examination. A small amount of lubricant is dropped* onto the fingers of the gloved hand for the internal examination. To avoid tissue trauma and contamination, the thumb is abducted and the ring and little fingers are flexed into the palm (Fig. 10-5).

The vagina is palpated for distensibility, lesions, and tenderness. The cervix is examined for position, shape, consistency, motility, and lesions. The fornix around the cervix is palpated.

The other hand is placed on the abdomen halfway between the umbilicus and symphysis pubis and exerts pressure downward toward the pelvic hand. Upward pressure from the pelvic hand traps reproductive structures for assessment by palpation. The uterus is as-

*See also Chapter 23.

*If the contaminated glove touches the tube, the tube is discarded.

sessed for position (see Fig. 4-7), size, shape, consistency, regularity, motility, masses, and tenderness.

Moving the abdominal hand to the right lower quadrant and the fingers of the pelvic hand in the right lateral fornix, the adnexa is assessed for position, size, tenderness, and masses. The examination is repeated on her left side.

Just before the intravaginal fingers are withdrawn, the woman is asked to tighten her vagina around the fingers as much as she can. If the muscle response is weak, the woman is assessed for her knowledge about Kegel's exercises (see Kegel's exercises, p. 251).

Rectovaginal Palpation. To prevent contamination of the rectum from organisms in the vagina (e.g., gonorrhea) it is best to change gloves, add fresh lubricant, and then reinsert the index finger into the vagina and the middle finger into the rectum (see Fig. 10-5). Insertion is facilitated if the woman strains down. The maneuvers of the abdominovaginal examination are repeated. The rectovaginal examination permits assessment of the rectovaginal septum, the posterior surface of the uterus, and the region behind the cervix.

After the pelvic examination, the woman is assisted into a sitting position, given tissues or wipes to cleanse herself, and privacy to dress. The woman often returns to the examiner's office for a discussion of findings, prescriptions for therapy, and counseling.

Laboratory Tests

The data obtained from laboratory examination of specimens add important information concerning the symptoms of pregnancy and health status. Both nursing and medical diagnoses stem from such information.

Specimens are collected at the initial visit so that results of their examination will be ready for the next scheduled visit (Table 10-1). A clean-catch urine specimen is tested. Tine or purified protein derivative of tuberculin (PPD) tests are administered for exposure to tuberculosis. During the pelvic examination cervical and vaginal smears for cytology (Papanicolaou smear and herpes simplex type 2) and for infection (*Chlamydia* organisms, gonorrhea) are obtained. Blood is drawn to test for a variety of conditions: venereal disease research laboratory (VDRL) test for syphilis; complete blood count (CBC) with hematocrit, hemoglobin, and differential values; blood type and Rh factor; antibody screen (Kell, Duffy, rubella, toxoplasmosis, and anti-Rh); sickle cell anemia; level of folacin when indicated. Urine is tested for glucose, protein, and acetone; culture and sensitivity tests are ordered as necessary.

Fetal Development

A summary of the development of the fetus is presented in the box on p. 247.

Table 10-1 Laboratory Tests in Prenatal Period

Laboratory Test	Purpose
Hemoglobin/hematocrit, WBC, differential	To detect anemia
Hemoglobin electrophoresis	To identify women with hemoglobinopathies (e.g., sickle cell anemia)
Blood type, Rh, and irregular antibody	To identify those fetuses at risk for developing erythroblastosis fetalis or hyperbilirubinemia in neonatal period
Rubella titer	To determine immunity to rubella
VDRL/FTA-ABS*	To identify women with untreated syphilis
AIDS antibody, hepatitis	To screen high-risk population
Urinalysis, including microscopic examination of urinary sediment; pH, specific gravity, color, glucose, albumin/protein, RBC, WBC, casts, acetone; hCG	To identify women with unsuspected diabetes mellitus, renal disease, hypertensive disease of pregnancy; infection; pregnancy
Urine culture	To identify women with asymptomatic bacteriuria
Renal function tests: BUN,† creatinine, electrolytes, creatinine clearance, total protein excretion	To evaluate level of possible renal compromise in women with a history of diabetes, hypertension, or renal disease
Papanicolaou smear	To screen for cervical intraepithelial neoplasia and herpes simplex type 2
Vaginal or rectal smear for *Neisseria gonorrhoeae, Chlamydia*	To screen high-risk population for asymptomatic infection
Tuberculin skin testing	To screen high-risk population
Cardiac evaluation: ECG, chest x-ray film, and echocardiogram	To evaluate cardiac function in women with a history of hypertension or cardiac disease

*FTA-ABS, fluorescent treponemal antibody absorption test.
†BUN, blood urea nitrogen.

FETAL DEVELOPMENT AT 13 WEEKS

Differentiation of tissues complete as period of organogenesis ends
Human appearance
Sex distinguishable
Skeleton ossifying
Tooth buds forming
Respiratory activity evident
Insulin secreted (since eighth week)
Kidneys secreting
Intestine returns to abdomen
Head is one third of total length
Length: 9 cm (3½ in)
Weight: 15 g (½ oz)
Fetus less susceptible to malformation from teratogenic agents

Early in pregnancy, before the uterus is an abdominal organ, the fetal heart tones (FHTs) can be heard with an ultrasound fetoscope or an ultrasound stethoscope (Fig. 14-4, *C, D*). The instrument is placed in the midline just anterior to the symphysis pubis. Firm pressure is needed as the scope is used. The woman and her family can be offered the opportunity to listen to the FHTs.

Nursing Diagnoses

Each client and family will have a unique set of responses to pregnancy. To attend to these responses the nurse begins by formulating appropriate nursing diagnoses (Chapter 1). Following are examples of nursing diagnoses arising from analysis of assessment findings during the first trimester:

Anxiety, potential, related to
- Concern about herself
- Physical changes with pregnancy
- Her (or other's) feelings about the pregnancy

Pain, related to
- Early discomforts of pregnancy

Altered family processes related to
- Family's response to diagnosis of pregnancy

Knowledge deficit, related to
- Maternal and familial adaptations to pregnancy
- Maternal and familial adaptations to EDD

Altered nutrition: less than body requirements, related to
- Morning sickness

Altered sexuality patterns, related to
- Discomforts of early pregnancy

See nursing care plans in this chapter, pp. 248-250.

Planning

Planning care for clients during the first trimester is based on the biopsychosocial assessment of the client and her family. For each client a plan is developed that relates specifically to her clinical and nursing problems. The information in this chapter is general; that is, not all women will experience all problems discussed or require all facets of the care described. The nurse selects those aspects of care relevant to the client and the client's family based on the following goals:

Goals related to physiologic care:

1. Client's pregnancy is diagnosed and EDD determined.
2. Client will have pertinent knowledge of the adaptation of the maternal body to a developing fetus as a basis for understanding the rationale and necessity for modalities of care.
3. Client will have information and counseling, including those relating to nutritional needs, sexual needs, activities of daily living, and discomforts of pregnancy.
4. Client's risk factors are identified and therapy initiated promptly.
5. Client is alerted to symptoms that indicate deviations from normal progress and protocols for reporting them.

Goals related to psychosocial care:

1. Client's information needs/readiness for learning are identified.
2. Clients and their families become active participants in their care during the first trimester of pregnancy.

The general nursing care plan, p. 248, provides general guidelines for students participating in or observing a nurse during a client's first prenatal visit. The specific nursing care plan for a gravida with morning sickness and fatigue, p. 250, demonstrates how the general care plan is adapted for the individual client.

Implementation

Nurses assume many caregiving roles during the prenatal period. The clinician's role can be categorized as both supportive and teacher/counselor/advocate.

Supportive Activities

The nurse-client relationship is critical in setting the tone for further interactions (see Chapter 1). The techniques of listening with an attentive expression, touching, and using eye contact have their place, as does recognition of the client's feelings and her right to express

General Nursing Care Plan

INITIAL PRENATAL VISIT

ASSESSMENT	NURSING DIAGNOSIS (ND), PLAN/GOAL (P/G)	RATIONALE/ IMPLEMENTATION	EVALUATION
Woman suspects pregnancy; needs confirmation of diagnosis. Sexual intercourse without contraception. Missed menstrual period(s).	ND: Knowledge deficit related to diagnosis of pregnancy. P/G: The woman will become knowledgeable about diagnosis of pregnancy and her status (pregnant or not).	*Client's diagnosis must be confirmed:* Establish a client data base. Take a nursing history. Obtain laboratory data per physician order. Provide time to discuss physician's diagnosis and explanations.	Woman verbalizes understanding of diagnostic measures. Woman learns whether she is pregnant.
Woman asks when she will have the baby.	ND: Knowledge deficit related to estimated date of delivery (EDD). P/G: The woman will become knowledgeable about her EDD.	*Client's EDD must be confirmed:* Calculate EDD based on: Information from the client data base and nursing history. Naegle's rule. Ultrasound. Fundal height measurements.	Woman verbalizes understanding of the EDD and asks relevant questions.
		Knowledge provides gravida with a sense of control: Explain how the EDD is determined and that it is not 100% accurate.	Woman understands that she may give birth just before or after the EDD.
Woman needs a schedule for subsequent prenatal visits.	ND: Knowledge deficit related to schedule of prenatal visits throughout pregnancy. P/G: The woman will schedule appointments throughout pregnancy P/G: The woman will keep scheduled appointments. P/G: The woman understands the importance of regular visits	*Knowledge provides gravida opportunity to collaborate in her care:* Inform the woman of the schedule for prenatal visits. Discuss the importance of adhering to the schedule unless otherwise informed.	Woman schedules appointments as per plan. Woman keeps scheduled appointments. Woman understands and verbalizes rationale of appointment schedule.
Woman asks what she should do differently and how her body will change now that she is pregnant.	ND: Knowledge deficit related to the psychologic and physiologic adaptations to pregnancy. ND: Knowledge deficit related to self-care behavior. P/G: The woman will be able to identify her body's physiologic and psychologic adaptations to pregnancy. P/G: The woman will use self-care behaviors to maintain an optimum level of wellness for herself and the fetus.	*Learning occurs when woman is ready to learn, and teaching is based on her perceived needs and level of understanding:* Interview woman and gain the information for the prenatal health assessment. Explain normal psychologic and physiologic adaptations to pregnancy. Inform the woman of self-care techniques. Explain the purpose and importance of each technique.	Woman verbalizes understanding of physiologic and psychologic adaptations to pregnancy. Woman asks appropriate questions regarding physiologic and psychologic adaptations to pregnancy. Woman verbalizes that she feels well. Physical assessment confirms that woman and fetus are healthy.

General Nursing Care Plan—cont'd

ASSESSMENT	NURSING DIAGNOSIS (ND), PLAN/GOAL (P/G)	RATIONALE/ IMPLEMENTATION	EVALUATION
Woman says that making love has become uncomfortable.	ND: Altered sexuality patterns related to discomforts of early pregnancy. P/G: Woman will understand how physiology of pregnancy affects intercourse.	*Physiologic effects of pregnancy on intercourse concern many women:* Discuss sexuality and sexual behaviors during pregnancy. Discuss those symptoms the woman is experiencing that affect intercourse and foreplay.	The woman will ask appropriate questions and verbalize understanding of information discussed.
Woman indicates she is unaware of signs and symptoms that could signal danger to her and her fetus during pregnancy.	ND: Knowledge deficit of signs and symptoms, potential for danger to mother and fetus. P/G: The woman will gain knowledge about danger signs during pregnancy.	*Medical conditions compromising mother or fetus must be identified and treated promptly:* Obtain information about preexisting or concurrent medical conditions. Discuss danger signs with the woman. Inform the woman of signs and symptoms she should consider abnormal. Provide the woman with a printed paper with danger signs of pregnancy and phone number of physician, hospital, and clinic.	The woman verbalizes understanding of problems or danger signs that should be reported.

them. The intervention may occur in various formal or informal settings. For certain persons, involvement in goal-directed health groups is neither feasible nor acceptable. Encounters in hallways or clinic examining rooms, home visits, or telephone conversations may provide the only opportunities for contact and can be used effectively. Sometimes women seek information about a particular problem repeatedly, not so much for the advice given, but to direct the nurse's attention toward themselves. The nurse can help these women by asking for a client-generated solution and a report of its effectiveness.

In supporting a client one must remember that both the nurse and the client are contributing to the relationship. The nurse has to accept the client's responses as a factor in trying to be of help. An example of one nurse-client relationship follows:

■ Mrs. ________________ had been very forthright in saying that this pregnancy was unplanned but had countered this statement with comments such as "All things happen for the best," "We always wanted the boys to have a family to turn to," and "Children bring their own love."

Over a period of time, as our relationship developed to one of *mutual* trust, she complained increasingly of her fear of pain, her hating to wear maternity clothes, and her having to give up helping the family. Finally I ventured to say, "Sometimes when a pregnancy is unplanned, women resent it very much and are angry about it." Her relief was evident. She said, "Oh, you don't know how angry I've been."

As a result the whole tenor of support being offered changed, and the plan was adjusted to meet her real needs.

Specific Nursing Care Plan

NAUSEA (MORNING SICKNESS) AND FATIGUE

Ruth Piper has just been diagnosed as being 8 weeks pregnant. During her initial prenatal visit she tells the nurse that she is experiencing nausea and dry heaves in the morning on awakening. She states that this is interfering with her morning routine and sometimes making her late to work. Ruth also reports that at 4 PM, when she gets home from work, she is so tired that she can't fix dinner for herself and her husband; all she wants to do is go to bed for the night. This break in her routine is upsetting her and she asks for help.

ASSESSMENT	NURSING DIAGNOSIS (ND), PLAN/GOAL (P/G)	RATIONALE/ IMPLEMENTATION	EVALUATION
Ruth says she is experiencing nausea and dry heaves on awakening.	ND: Pain related to change in hormone levels and the body's adaptation to pregnancy. ND: Sleep pattern disturbance related to nausea (morning sickness) of pregnancy. P/G: Ruth will be free of nausea and dry heaves. P/G: Ruth will resume normal sleep-rest pattern.	*Measures can be used to reduce nausea:* Take a 24-hour diet history. Advise Ruth to keep unsalted crackers or other dry carbohydrates at her bedside, and to eat some on awakening, before getting out of bed. Caution Ruth to avoid eating fried or greasy foods, especially before bed. Discuss eating small, frequent meals instead of three large ones to avoid having an empty stomach.	Ruth verbalizes understanding of instructions. Nausea lessens or stops; dry heaves stop. Ruth resumes normal sleep-rest pattern.
Ruth states she is extremely fatigued.	ND: Fatigue related to early pregnancy. ND: Activity tolerance, decreased, related to fatigue. ND: Knowledge deficit related to common discomforts of pregnancy. P/G: Ruth will learn how to deal with the fatigue of early pregnancy. P/G: Ruth will be able to increase her activity level and resume activities of daily living without undue fatigue.	*Knowledge provides woman opportunity to increase ability to cope through self-help:* Discuss ways to deal with the fatigue of pregnancy. Suggest ways to help Ruth assume activities of daily living.	Ruth verbalizes understanding of instructions. Ruth will be able to resume activities of daily living. Ruth will resume self-care. Ruth will increase activity level.

The nurse also needs to accept the fact that the woman must be a willing partner in a purely voluntary relationship. As such, the relationship can be refused or terminated at any time by the pregnant woman or her family.

Supportive care involves developing, augmenting, or changing the mechanisms used by women and families in coping with stress. An effort is made to promote active participation by the individuals in the process of solving their own problems. Clients are helped to gather pertinent information, explore alternative actions, make decisions as to choice of action, and assume responsibility for the outcomes. These outcomes may be any or all of the following: living with a problem as it is; mitigating effects of a problem so that it can be accepted more readily; or eliminating the problem through effecting change.

Expectations of success in the area of emotional supportive care must of necessity be flexible. It is not within the province of any outsider to ensure another person a rewarding, satisfying experience. The mother and persons significant to her are crucial elements in this process. Many of their problems are beyond the scope or capabilities of any professional worker. In describing her work with young and poor persons, Edwards (1973) notes: "They did not usually change their living situation and I was not instrumental in modifying home or drug problems." However, this did not deter her from encouraging clients to use the decision-making process as a means of coping with problems rather than merely complaining about injustice.

At other times a successful outcome can be readily documented. A woman who early in her pregnancy had predicted a severe depressive state in the postdelivery period was elated when such a state did not materialize. She remarked to the nurse who had provided support during the pregnancy and birth, "You're the best nerve medicine I've ever had!"

Teacher/Counselor/Advocate

Health maintenance is an important aspect of prenatal care. Client participation in the care ensures prompt reporting of untoward responses to pregnancy. Client assumption of responsibility of health maintenance is prompted by understanding of maternal adaptations to the growth of the unborn child and a readiness to learn. Nurses in their roles of teacher/counselor/advocate provide clients with the information necessary for compliance with health care measures.

The expectant mother needs information about many subjects. During the initial health assessment, the woman may have indicated a need to learn self-care activities such as breast self-examination, prevention of urinary tract infection, and Kegel's exercises. Guidelines for client teaching for breast self-examination are on p. 252.

Prevention of Urinary Tract Infection. Urinary tract infections may be asymptomatic. Whether symptomatic or not, urinary tract infections present a risk to both mother and fetus. Prevention of these infections is essential. The woman's understanding and use of general hygiene measures is assessed. Before developing a plan of care, the nurse needs to elicit feelings or ideas concerning cultural, ethnic, religious, or other factors affecting health practices.

The woman may need to learn that every woman should always wipe from front to back after urinating or moving bowels and use a clean piece of toilet paper for each wipe. Wiping from back to front may carry bacteria from the rectal area to the urethral opening and increase risk of infection. Soft, absorbent toilet tissue, preferably white and unscented, should be used because harsh, scented, or printed toilet paper may cause irritation. Women need to change tampons, panty shields, or sanitary napkins often. Bacteria can multiply in menstrual blood or on soiled napkins. Women need to wear underpants and panty hose with a cotton crotch. They should avoid wearing tight-fitting slacks or jeans or panty shields for long periods. A buildup of heat and moisture in the genital area may contribute to the growth of bacteria.

Some women do not have an adequate fluid and food intake. After eliciting her food preferences, the nurse should advise the woman to drink 2 to 3 quarts (8 to 12 glasses) of liquid a day. Eight to 10 ounces of cranberry juice may be included because cranberry juice is more acidic than other fluids and can lower the pH of the urinary tract, making it less hospitable to developing bacteria. Yogurt and acidophilus milk may also help prevent urinary tract and vaginal infections.

The nurse should review with the woman healthy urination practices. Women should urinate frequently. They need to maintain fluid intake to ensure urination and not limit fluids to reduce frequency of urination. They should not ignore signals that indicate the need to urinate. Holding urine increases the time bacteria are in the bladder and allows them to multiply. Women should plan ahead when entering situations where urination must be delayed (e.g., a long car ride). They should always urinate before going to bed at night. Bacteria can be introduced during intercourse. Therefore women are advised to urinate before and after intercourse, then drink a large glass of water to promote additional urination.

The nurse can be reasonably assured that teaching was effective if the woman does not develop a urinary tract infection.

Kegel's Exercises. Kegel's exercises (exercises for the pelvic floor) strengthen the muscles around the reproductive organs and improve muscle tone.

Many women are not aware of the muscles of the pelvic floor (see Figs. 4-13 and 4-14) until it is pointed out that these are the muscles used when urinating and during sexual intercourse and are therefore consciously controlled. Since pelvic floor muscles encircle the outlet through which the baby must pass, it is important that they be exercised, because an exercised muscle can stretch and contract readily at the time of birth.

To help the pelvic floor muscles return to normal functioning, Kegel's exercises should be started immediately after delivery. Kegel's exercises can strengthen these muscles and improve muscle tone. If practiced on a regular basis, the exercises help prevent prolapsed uterus and stress incontinence later in life.

The exercise:

A. The muscles that stop the flow of urine are the pubococcygeal muscles. Doing Kegel's exercises during

Guidelines for Client Teaching
BREAST SELF-EXAMINATION

ASSESSMENT

1. Woman states she does not know how to examine her breasts.

NURSING DIAGNOSIS

Knowledge deficit related to self-care: breast self-examination (BSE).

GOALS

Short-term

Woman will verbalize reasons why BSE is important.
Woman will verbalize steps of BSE and rationale for each step.
Woman will demonstrate BSE procedure correctly.

Intermediate (By first postpartum check-up or by next gynecologic examination)

Woman verbalizes steps of BSE and rationale.
Woman states she has examined her breasts once.
After weaning: woman will be familiar with the normal feel and appearance of her breasts.

Long-term

Woman performs BSE every month.

REFERENCES AND TEACHING AIDS.

American Cancer Society's pamphlet, *How to examine your breasts.*
Mirror.
Model for practicing palpation and recognition of masses.

RATIONALE/CONTENT	TEACHING ACTION
Knowledge provides a basis for decision making regarding self-care. *Practice increases self-confidence and competence in observation:* Review content and rationale for BSE during the menstrual cycle. Perform observation: Woman sits in front of mirror and observes her breasts while assuming four positions. 1. Arms relaxed at her sides. 2. Hands pressed against her waist. 3. Arms over head. 4. Leaning forward. Review normal and suspicious characteristics.	Encourage questions to uncover anxieties, concerns, and knowledge gaps about BSE. Review content and rationale, as needed. Encourage questions. Demonstrate for woman. Help woman assume postures correctly. Review, compare with woman's breasts and with pamphlet. Assist woman with verbalization of her observations of herself.
Practice increases self-confidence and competence in palpation; therefore the nurse will teach that: Palpation is performed with the woman in the supine position and a pillow under the shoulder on the side of the breast to be examined. Examination is performed in a systematic manner and includes the nipple. Palpation of axillary lymph nodes is most easily done by the practitioner. However, the woman can learn too. *Accuracy and timeliness in recording and reporting findings helps caregivers develop diagnoses; therefore the nurse will teach that:* Findings are described by their characteristics (e.g., color, discharge) and by their location. When woman notes reportable signs or symptoms, she needs to note the phase of her menstrual cycle (after pregnancy).	Using a teaching model or illustration, demonstrate methods of systematic breast palpation. Demonstrate palpation on model and on woman's breast; observe return demonstration. Assist woman to supine position with pillow under shoulder on side to be examined. Assist woman through self-examination and verbal description of her findings. Encourage and answer questions. Review characteristics while referring to pamphlet or other printed matter. Show woman how to locate lesion.

EVALUATION Teaching of the cognitive and motor aspects of BSE is considered effective when the woman verbalizes and demonstrates the steps of the procedure. Teaching related to the affective/psychologic aspect of BSE may be considered effective if the woman performs BSE routinely *and* reports any findings immediately.

urination helps the woman know whether she is doing them correctly. If she can stop the stream of urine, her tone is good.

B. After a woman has located the correct muscles, Kegel's exercises can be done in the following ways:
   1. *Slow:* Tighten the muscle, hold it for the count of three, and relax it.
   2. *Quick:* Tighten the muscle, and relax it as rapidly as possible.
   3. *Push out–pull in:* Pull up the entire pelvic floor as though trying to suck up water into the vagina. Then bear down as if trying to push the imaginary water out. This uses abdominal muscles also.

Practice: This exercise needs to be practiced several times a day to be effective. It must be done every day for the rest of the woman's life.

This exercise can be done 10 times in a row at least 3 times or more a day. Although some people recommend doing this exercise as many as 100 times in a row, this only fatigues the pelvic floor muscles.

A good time to practice is during trips to the bathroom, but additional practice at other times is even more beneficial.

The nurse can be reasonably assured that teaching was effective if the woman reports increased muscle tone to control urine flow and during sexual intercourse.

Additional Teaching. Other subjects about which clients need information include diet, exercise, sleep, bowel habits, smoking, alcohol ingestion, medication usage, and sexual relations. It is impossible to impart at one visit all of the information the woman and her family may need at the time her pregnancy is diagnosed. She can be given printed information* at this time, either in the form of notes that are prepared by the obstetrician or as a listing of the books pertaining to pregnancy that have been written for lay persons. If the latter, the obstetrician, nurse, or nurse-midwife should have read the books carefully to be certain they supply the kind of information desired.

Nutritional intake is an important factor in the maintenance of maternal health during pregnancy and in the provision of adequate nutrients for embryonic/fetal development. Assessing nutritional status and providing nutritional information are part of the nurse's responsibilities in prenatal care. For detailed information concerning maternal and fetal nutritional needs, see Chapter 11.

Formal classes in childbirth and parenthood education have proved successful for some women and families. "Early bird" classes provide fundamental information to meet the needs of most expectant parents during the first trimester (Chapter 9). Allowing the expectant mother or family the opportunity to ask questions and express any anxieties or fears she or they may have is also important.

*The nurse must determine, in a sensitive manner, that the woman can read the material given to her. Some women do not use reading as a means of coping, so that other means may be more appropriate (e.g., videotapes or audio-cassettes).

DANGER SIGNS

Potential Complications of Pregnancy

- Visual disturbances—blurring, double vision, or spots
- Swelling of face, fingers or over sacrum
- Headaches—severe, frequent, or continuous
- Muscular irritability or convulsions
- Epigastric pain (perceived as severe stomachache)
- Persistent vomiting—beyond first trimester, severe vomiting at any time
- Fluid discharge from vagina—bleeding or amniotic fluid (anything other than leukorrhea)
- Signs of infections—chills, fever, burning on urination, diarrhea
- Pain in abdomen—severe or unusual
- Change in fetal movements—absence of fetal movements after quickening, any unusual change in pattern or amount

Schedule for Care. During the initial visit, women appreciate knowing the schedule for return prenatal visits. Most women can expect to return every 4 weeks until the twenty-eighth week of pregnancy, every 2 weeks until the thirty-sixth week of pregnancy, and then every week from week 37 until delivery. More frequent visits may be needed to accommodate the woman's individual needs. The initial prenatal visit is usually lengthy. Women can be reassured by knowing what to expect on subsequent visits (pp. 261 and 274).

Danger Signs. One of the first responsibilities of persons involved in the care of the pregnant woman is to alert her to signs and symptoms that indicate a potential complication of pregnancy. The client needs to know how to report such danger signs (see box, above). When one is stressed by a disturbing symptom, it is difficult to remember specifics. Therefore the gravida and her family are reassured if they receive a printed form listing the signs and symptoms that warrant an investigation and the phone numbers to call in an emergency.

Discomforts of Pregnancy. Women pregnant for the first time are confronted with symptoms that would be considered abnormal in the nonpregnant state. Much of prenatal care requested by such women relates to explanations of the causes of the discomforts and what measures can be taken to relieve them. The discomforts are fairly specific to each trimester of pregnancy. Information about the physiology, prevention, and treatment of discomforts experienced during the first trimester are given in Table 10-2.

Nurses can anticipate these symptoms and provide anticipatory guidance for women. Women who have a knowledge of the physical basis for the discomforts of pregnancy are less apt to become overly anxious concerning their health. An understanding of the rationale for treatment promotes their participation in their own care. Nurses need to use terminology the woman (or couple) can understand.

Employment. Many women continue to work during pregnancy. Whether the expectant mother can work and for how long depends on the physical activity involved, industrial hazards, and medical or obstetric complications. A prime consideration is the avoidance of a fetotoxic environment (e.g., chemical dust particles or gases such as inhalation anesthesia). Em-

Table 10-2 Discomforts During the First Trimester

Discomfort	Physiology	Treatment
Breast changes, new sensations: pain, tingling	Hypertrophy of mammary glandular tissue and increased vascularization, pigmentation, and size and prominence of nipples and areolae caused by hormone stimulation	Supportive maternity brassiere with pads to absorb discharge may be worn at night; wash with warm water and keep dry; see Maternal physiology and sexual counseling
Urgency and frequency of urination	Vascular engorgement and altered bladder function caused by hormones; bladder capacity reduced by enlarging uterus and fetal presenting part	Kegel's exercises; limit fluid intake before bedtime; reassurance; wear perineal pad; refer to physician for pain or burning sensation
Languor and malaise; fatigue (early pregnancy, usually)	Unexplained, may be caused by increasing levels of estrogen, progesterone, and hCG or to elevated BBT; psychologic response to pregnancy and its required physical/psychologic adaptations	Reassurance; rest as needed; well-balanced diet to prevent anemia
Nausea and vomiting, morning sickness—occurs in 50% to 75% of pregnant women; starts between first and second missed periods and lasts until about fourth missed period; may occur any time during day; if mother does not have symptoms, expectant father may; may be accompanied by "bad taste" in mouth	Cause unknown (may result from hormonal changes, possibly hCG; may be partly emotional, reflecting pride in, ambivalence about, or rejection of pregnant state)	Avoid empty or overloaded stomach; maintain good posture—give stomach ample room; stop or decrease smoking; eat dry carbohydrate on awakening; remain in bed until feeling subsides, or alternate dry carbohydrate 1 hour with fluids such as hot tea, milk, or clear coffee the next hour until feeling subsides; eat five to six small meals per day; avoid fried, odorous, spicy, greasy, or gas-forming foods; consult physician if intractable vomiting occurs; reassurance
Ptyalism (excessive saliva)—may occur starting 2 to 3 weeks after first missed period	Possibly caused by elevated estrogen levels; may be related to reluctance to swallow because of nausea	Astringent mouth wash; chewing gum; support
Psychosocial dynamics (Chapter 9): mood swings, mixed feelings	Hormonal and metabolic adaptations; plus feelings about female role, sexuality, timing of pregnancy, and resultant changes in one's life and lifestyle	Treatment same as prevention; both partners need reassurance and support; support significant other who can reassure woman about her attractiveness, etc.; improved communication with her partner, family, and others; refer to social worker, if needed, or supportive services (financial assistance, food stamps)

ployment during later pregnancy is discussed later in this chapter.

Physical Activity. A number of researchers have recommended moderate exercise during pregnancy (Bullard, 1981; Dean, 1981; Hutchinson et al, 1981; Jopke, 1983) (see box below). However, activities continued to the point of exhaustion or fatigue compromise uterine perfusion and fetoplacental oxygenation (Dale et al, 1982). If the woman is accustomed to jogging, she may continue; however, she should not reach the point of fatigue. Heat stress may also endanger the fetus. Furthermore, as gestation advances the woman's center of gravity changes, her bony pelvic support loosens, her coordination usually decreases, and she notices a sensation of awkwardness. Awkwardness may cause her to lose balance and fall, injuring herself.

Exercises such as those depicted in Fig. 10-6 are taught either at prenatal classes or by the nurse in the clinic or the physician's office. The exercises promote comfort and help prepare the woman for labor. Posture and how to lift and move objects safely also are discussed and demonstrated to counteract the awk-

EXERCISE TIPS FOR PREGNANT WOMEN

Consult your health-care provider when you know or suspect you are pregnant. Discuss your medical and obstetric history, your current regimen, and the exercises you would like to continue throughout pregnancy.

Seek help in determining an exercise routine that is well within your limit of tolerance, especially if you have not been exercising regularly.

Consider decreasing weight-bearing exercises (jogging, running) and concentrate on non-weight-bearing activities such as swimming, cycling, or stretching. If you are a runner, you may wish to walk instead, starting in your seventh month.

Because strenuous exercise during the last few weeks of pregnancy increases the risk of low birthweight, stillbirth, and infant death, reduce exercise sharply 4 weeks before your due date.

Avoid risky activities such as surfing, mountain-climbing, sky-diving, and racquetball. Activities requiring precise balance and coordination may be dangerous.

Exercise regularly at least three times a week, as long as you are healthy, to improve muscle tone and increase or maintain your stamina. Sporadic exercises may put undue strain on your muscles.

Limit activity to shorter intervals. Exercise for 10 to 15 minutes, rest for 2 to 3 minutes, then exercise for another 10 to 15 minutes.

Decrease your exercise level as your pregnancy progresses. The normal alterations of advancing pregnancy, such as decreased cardiac reserve and increased respiratory effort, may produce physiologic stress if you exercise strenuously for a long time.

Take your pulse every 10 to 15 minutes while you are exercising. If it's more than 140 beats per minute, slow down until it returns to a maximum of 90.

Avoid becoming overheated for extended periods. It's best not to exercise for more than 35 minutes, especially in hot, humid weather. As your body temperature rises, the heat is transmitted to your fetus. Prolonged or repeated fetal temperature elevation may result in birth defects, especially during the first 3 months.

Limit the time you spend in hot tubs, saunas, or hot baths. Here are some guidelines:

- Hot tub: water temperature 39.0° C (102.2° F) for less than 15 minutes or 41.0° C (105.8° F) for less than 10 minutes
- Sauna: room temperature 81.4° C (178.5° F) for less than 5 minutes.
- Hot bath: water temperature 39.0° C (102.2° F) for less than 15 minutes.

Warmup and stretching exercises prepare your joints for more strenuous exercise and lessen the likelihood of strain or injury to your joints.

A cool-down period of mild activity after exercising will help bring your respiration, heart, and metabolic rates back to normal and avoid pooling of blood in the exercise muscles.

Rest for 10 minutes after exercising, lying on your left side. As the uterus grows, it puts pressure on a major vein carrying blood to your heart on the right side of your abdomen. Lying on your left side takes the pressure off and promotes return circulation from your extremities and muscles to your heart, increasing blood flow to your placenta and fetus.

Drink two or three 8-ounce glasses of water after you exercise, to replace the body fluids you lost through perspiration. While exercising, drink water whenever you feel the need.

Increase your caloric intake to replace the calories burned during exercise. Choose such high-protein foods as fish, cheese, eggs, or meat.

Take your time. This is not the time to be competitive or train for activities requiring long endurance.

Wear a supportive bra. Your increased breast weight may cause changes in posture and put pressure on the ulnar nerve.

Wear supportive shoes. As your uterus grows, your center of gravity shifts and you compensate by arching your back. These natural changes may make you feel off balance and more likely to fall.

Stop exercising immediately if you experience shortness of breath, dizziness, numbness, tingling, abdominal pain, or vaginal bleeding, and consult your health care provider.

Modified from Paglone A and Worthington S: Cautions and advice on exercise during pregnancy, Contemp OB/GYN 25:160, May, 1985 (special issue).

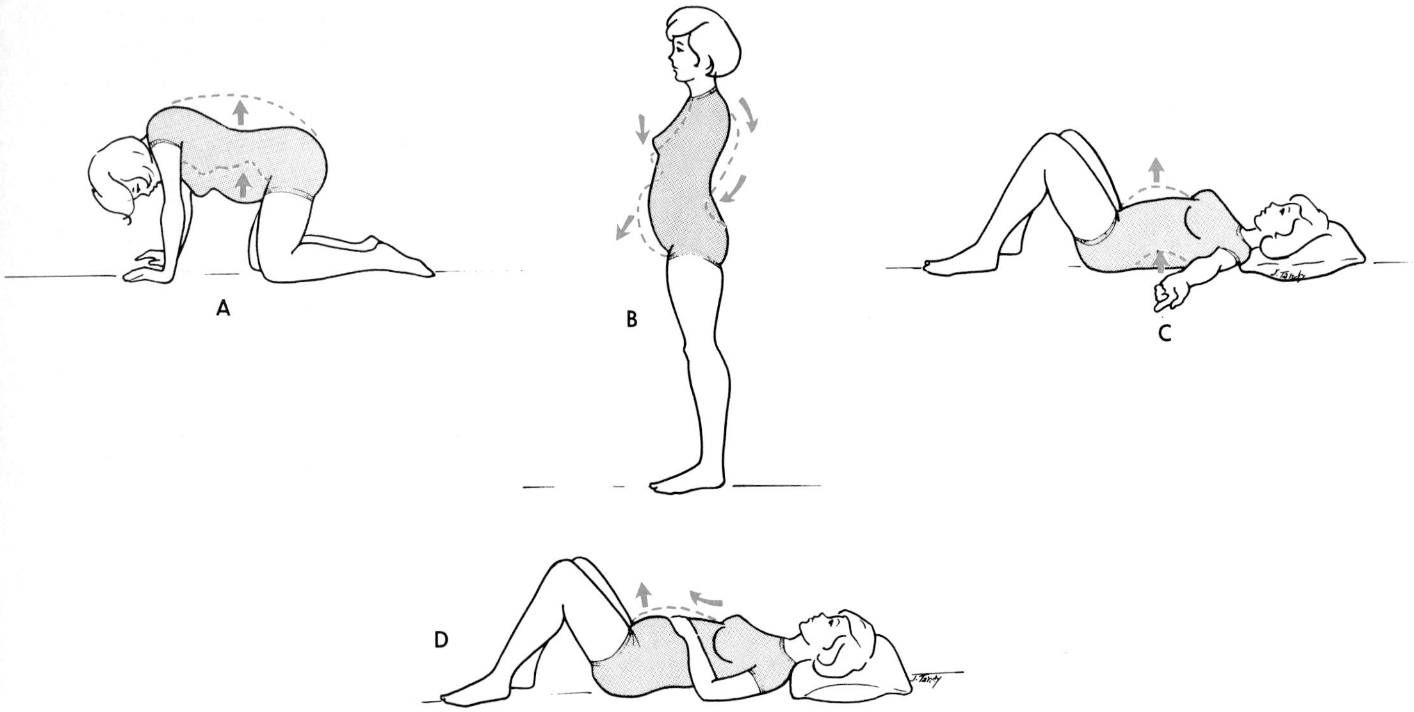

Fig. 10-6 Exercises. **A** to **C**, Pelvic rocking relieves low backache (excellent for relief of menstrual cramps as well). **D**, Abdominal breathing aids relaxation and lifts abdominal wall off uterus.

wardness and prevent the discomfort experienced starting in the second trimester of pregnancy.

Dental Health. Dental care during pregnancy is especially important. Nausea during pregnancy may lead to poor oral hygiene, and dental caries may develop. No physiologic alteration during gestation can cause dental caries. Calcium and phosphorus in the teeth are fixed in enamel. Therefore the old adage "for every child a tooth" need not be true.

There is no scientific evidence that filling teeth or even dental extraction with the use of local or nitrous oxide–oxygen anesthesia causes abortion or premature labor. Antibacterial therapy should be considered for sepsis, however, especially in gravidas who have had rheumatic heart disease or nephritis. Extensive dental surgery is postponed until after delivery for the woman's comfort, if possible (Martin and Reeb, 1982, 1983).

Medications. Although much has been learned in recent years about fetal drug toxicity (Appendix F), the possible teratogenicity of many drugs, both prescription and over-the-counter (OTC), is still unknown. This is especially true for new medications and combinations of drugs. Moreover, certain subclinical errors or deficiencies in intermediate metabolism in the fetus may convert an otherwise harmless drug into a hazardous one. The greatest danger of causing developmental defects in the fetus from drugs exists from fertilization through the first trimester. Self-treatment must be discouraged. All drugs, including aspirin, should be limited, and a careful record of therapeutic agents used should be kept (Howard and Hill, 1979; McKay, 1980; Luke, 1982).

Immunization. There has been some concern over the safety of various immunization techniques during pregnancy (Barry and Bia, 1989; Cunningham, MacDonald, and Gant, 1989). Immunization with live or attenuated live viruses is contraindicated during pregnancy because of potential teratogenicity. Vaccines with killed viruses may be used. Live virus vaccines include measles (rubeola and rubella) and mumps. Some women may need immunization against influenza. For immediate protection following exposure, inactivated polio vaccine (IPV) may be used. Immunization against cholera, thyphoid, and poliomyelitis may be needed if the woman must travel to endemic areas. Tetanus toxoid or varicella immune globulin may be given when necessary.

Substance Abuse. Although occasional alcoholic beverages *may* not be harmful to the mother or her infant, complete abstinence is strongly advised. The period of greatest susceptibility of the embryo/fetus and the dose-response relationship are not known (Beckman and Brent, 1986). Excesses must be avoided. Regular drinkers or those who drink heavily during pregnancy have infants who demonstrate fetal alcohol syndrome (see Chapter 28; Appendix F).

Cigarette smoking or continued exposure to a smoke-filled environment (even if the mother does not smoke) is associated with fetal growth retardation and an increase in perinatal and infant morbidity and mortality. Smoking also increases the frequency of preterm labor, premature rupture of membranes (PROM), abruptio placentae, placenta previa, and fetal death (Main, 1988). Laboratory studies indicate a lowered Po_2 level in both mother and fetus during exposure to cigarette smoke. Smoking may result in a lessened supply of milk during lactation, and harmful substances may be transferred to the infant in the milk.

If the woman is a smoker, the nurse needs to discuss the options she has regarding methods designed to help her quit. If she is resistant to the idea of quitting, the nurse can try to offer ways in which she can cut down.

Most studies of human pregnancy report no association between caffeine consumption and birth defects or low birth weight (Leviton, 1988; Cunningham, MacDonald, and Gant, 1989). Other effects are unknown; therefore pregnant women are advised to limit caffeine intake. Possible hazards of a commonly used artificial sweetener are discussed in Chapter 24.

Any mind-altering substance has a deleterious effect on the fetus and should not be used (see Chapter 25 and Appendix F). Marijuana, heroin, and cocaine are well-known examples of such substances.

Sexual Counseling During Pregnancy

Sexual counseling includes countering misinformation, providing reassurance of normalcy, and suggesting alternative behaviors. The uniqueness of each couple is considered within a biopsychosocial framework.

Counseling couples concerning sexual adjustment during pregnancy demands self-assessment by the nurse as well as a knowledge of the physical, social, and emotional responses to sex during pregnancy (Zalar, 1976). Not all maternity nurses are comfortable dealing with the sexual concerns of their clients. Nurses who are aware of their personal strengths and limitations in dealing with sexual content are in a better position to make referrals when necessary.

A significant number of clients merely need *permission* to be sexual during pregnancy. Many other clients need *information* about the physiologic changes that occur during pregnancy and to have myths associated with sex during pregnancy debunked. Giving permission and providing information are within the purview of the maternity nurse and should be an integral component of providing health care. See guidelines for client teaching, p. 258.

A few couples must be referred for either *sex therapy* or *family therapy*. Couples with sexual dysfunction problems of long standing that are intensified by pregnancy are referred for sex therapy. When a sexual problem is a symptom of a more serious interactional problem, the couple would benefit from family therapy.

Obtaining a History. The history provides a baseline for sexual counseling. History taking is an ongoing process. Receptivity to changes in attitudes, body image, marital relationships, and physical status is relevant throughout pregnancy. When changes occur, unexpected problems may develop that require intervention. The history reveals the client's knowledge of female anatomy and physiology, attitudes about sex during pregnancy, as well as perceptions of the pregnancy, the health status of the couple, and the quality of their marital relationship. Identification of the couple's subjective experience provides the direction and focus of sexual counseling.

Countering Misinformation. Many myths and much of the misinformation related to sex and pregnancy are masked behind seemingly unrelated issues. For example, a question about the baby's ability to hear and see in utero may be related to the baby's role as an observer in lovemaking. The counselor must be extremely sensitive to questions behind the question when counseling in this highly charged emotional area.

Fetal heart rate (**FHR**) decreases during orgasm; however, fetal distress has not been noted. Although it has been suggested that preterm delivery may be induced by the effect of oxytocin released during maternal response, by orgasmic contractions, or by prostaglandins in the male ejaculate, researchers have not validated these hypotheses. When possible, the couple is counseled together. Expectant parent education classes can also be an effective way to explore these kinds of concerns because of the support and sharing offered by the group.

Providing Reassurance of Normalcy. Couples are relieved to learn that their fears and concerns do not make them "weird" or "crazy." A breast-feeding mother may welcome the knowledge that her erotic response to suckling is normal. At the same time the father may be relieved to know that many fathers are jealous of their suckling infants.

It is important for the counselor to view sexuality in its broadest sense. Kissing, hugging, massaging, petting, and increased gentleness and sensitivity are valid forms of sexual expression and signs of affection. Each of these behaviors is pleasurable in itself and is not always a preliminary behavior leading to intercourse. When a couple cannot have, or chooses not to have, penile-vaginal intercourse, the need for closeness and intimacy can be expressed in many other ways.

Guidelines for Client Teaching
SEXUAL COUNSELING DURING PREGNANCY

ASSESSMENT

1. Woman experiencing adaptations to pregnancy (fatigue, nausea).
2. Woman indicates breasts hurt when touched.
3. Woman and husband request information.
4. This is woman's first pregnancy, with no history of vaginal bleeding or uterine cramping.

NURSING DIAGNOSES

Knowledge deficit, alternative positions.
Altered sexuality patterns.
Potential for anxiety if reactions are perceived as abnormal.
Potential for ineffective individual coping.

GOALS

Short-term

To validate and assure the universality of their responses.
To meet information needs.
To problem-solve regarding solutions and needed changes.

Intermediate

To continue to make adjustments regarding sexuality throughout pregnancy.
To verbalize mutual satisfaction with their choices.

Long-term

To continue to make mutually acceptable adjustments regarding sexuality across the life span.

REFERENCES AND TEACHING AIDS

Bing E and Colman L: Making love during pregnancy, New York, 1982, FA Davis Co.
Rakowitz E and Rubin GS: Lovemaking in pregnancy. Lamaze Parents' Magazine, 1985 edition, ASPO Lamaze, 55 Northern Blvd, Greenvale, LI, NY, 11548-1390.
Plastic learning models, illustrations.

RATIONALE/CONTENT	TEACHING ACTION
A broad knowledge base regarding sexuality and sexual expression during pregnancy provides a basis for decision-making regarding self-care: Discuss maternal physiologic adaptations to pregnancy: breasts, nausea, fatigue, abdominal changes, perineal enlargement, leukorrhea, pelvic vasocongestion, and orgasmic responses. Discuss maternal and paternal responses to pregnancy. Identify clients' cultural prescriptions and proscriptions. Discuss responses to interview questions. Inform couple that, although her libido may be depressed during first trimester, it increases during the second and third trimesters. In subsequent visits and postpartum, discuss: Breastfeeding and father's responses, mother's fantasies and sexual feelings during breast-feeding, milk spurt during orgasm. Resumption of sexual relationship after delivery. Discuss: Alternative behaviors (e.g., mutual masturbation, foot massage, cuddling). Alternative positions (e.g., female-superior, side-lying).	Provide a safe, open, nonjudgmental atmosphere. Remain alert to personal beliefs and values to avoid decreasing one's effectiveness in providing sexual counseling. Validate feelings; give permission. Ask about things they have heard, read; what they want to discuss. Time the discussions to clients' phase in childbearing cycle and readiness to learn. Provide comfortable environment, offer alternatives, show illustrations.
Knowledge helps decrease the potential for infection and reduce anxiety about injury to the fetus; Inform that intercourse is safe as long as it is not uncomfortable for the woman and the membranes have not ruptured. Review signs of ruptured membranes.	Show illustrations of fetus in utero with closed cervix and intact membranes.

EVALUATION The nurse can be assured that teaching was effective when the woman (couple) verbalizes increased knowledge and uses it to make mutually accepted adjustments regarding sexuality throughout pregnancy.

*For alterations in sexual practice if she or her sexual partner has tested positive for AIDS virus (HIV) see Chapter 23.

Suggesting Alternative Behaviors. To date research has not proved conclusively that coitus and orgasm are contraindicated before the last 4 weeks or so of pregnancy for the obstetrically and medically healthy woman (Cunningham, MacDonald, and Gant, 1989). However, a history of more than one spontaneous abortion or a threatened abortion in the first trimester, impending miscarriage in the second trimester, or premature rupture of membranes, bleeding, or abdominal pain during the third trimester warrant precaution against coitus and orgasm. Naeye (1979) suggests that improved genital hygiene and perhaps other actions may reduce the risk of intrauterine infection. Until we have more data, "a reasonable policy might be to recommend the avoidance of intercourse and orgasm in the third trimester in women with a poor reproductive history or in those who, on pelvic examination, have premature ripening of the cervix." In an interview Naeye commented further that he "was not prepared to recommend prolonged abstinence during pregnancy, since this can cause serious marital discord."

Solitary and mutual masturbation and oral-genital intercourse may be used by couples as *alternatives to penile-vaginal intercourse.* Men who enjoy cunnilingus may feel "turned off" by the normal increase in amount and odor of vaginal discharges during pregnancy. Couples who practice cunnilingus should be cautioned concerning the blowing of air into the vagina, particularly during the last few weeks of pregnancy. There have been cases reported of maternal death and near-fatal cases from air emboli caused by forceful blowing of air into the vagina (Bernhardt et al, 1988). If the cervix is slightly open (as it may be near term), there is the possibility that air will be forced between the membranes and the uterine wall. Some air may enter the maternal placental lakes, thus gaining entrance into the maternal vascular bed.

The woman or couple should also be cautioned against masturbatory activities when orgasmic contractions are contraindicated. Studies have shown that orgasm is often more intense when induced by masturbation. After being cautioned against orgasm, some women require reassurance if they experience erotic dreams.

Pictures of possible variations of *coital position* are often helpful. The female-superior, side-by-side, and rear-entry positions are possible alternative positions to the traditional male-superior position. The woman astride (superior position) allows her to control the angle and depth of penile penetration as well as to protect her breasts and abdomen. The side-by-side position is the one of choice, especially during the third trimester, since it requires reduced energy and pressure on the pregnant abdomen. For other positions, the reader is referred to Bing and Colman (1977) and McCary (1982).

Multiparous women have reported severe *breast tenderness* in the first trimester. A coital position that avoids direct pressure on the woman's breasts and decreased breast fondling during love play can be recommended. The woman should also be reassured that this condition is normal and temporary. *Lactating mothers* lose milk in uncontrolled spurts in response to sexual stimulation. The couple that is forewarned can be prepared for this eventuality.

Some women complain of lower abdominal cramping and backache after orgasm during the first and third trimesters. A back rub can often relieve some of the discomfort, as well as provide a pleasant experience. A tonic contraction, often lasting up to a minute, replaces the rhythmic contractions of orgasm during the third trimester. Changes in FHRs without fetal distress have been reported.

The National Family Planning and Reproductive Health Association, Washington, DC, suggests that for some women, *use of the contraceptive condom should be continued* throughout the pregnancy. The objective is prophylaxis against the acquisition and transmission of sexually transmitted diseases (e.g., herpes simplex virus [HSV], gonorrhea, acquired immunodeficiency syndrome [AIDS]) (Goldsmith, 1989). The entire policy statement is given in Chapter 23.

Well-informed nurses who are comfortable with their own sexuality and the sexual counseling needs of pregnant couples can offer counseling in a valuable but often neglected area. They can establish an open environment in which couples can feel free to introduce their concerns about sexual adjustment and seek support and guidance (Mueller, 1985).

Cultural Variation in Prenatal Care

Prenatal care as we know it is a phenomenon of Western medicine. The Western biomedical model of care encourages women to seek prenatal care as early as possible in their pregnancy by visiting a physician or clinic. Visits are usually routine and follow a systematic sequence, with the initial visit followed by a monthly and then weekly visits. Monitoring weight and blood pressure; testing blood and urine; teaching specific information about diet, rest, and activity; and preparing for childbirth are common components of prenatal care.

This model not only is unfamiliar but commonly seems strange to many groups (NPA, 1988; Lee, 1988, 1989). Many **cultural variations** in prenatal care exist. Even when the prenatal care described is familiar, some practices may conflict with a subcultural group's beliefs and practices. Because of these and other factors, such as lack of money, lack of transportation, and poor communication on the part of health care providers, many groups do not participate in the prenatal care system. Their behavior may be misinterpreted by nurses as uncaring, lazy, or ignorant.

A concern for *modesty* is also a deterrent for prenatal care for many persons. Exposing one's body parts, especially to a man, is a major violation of modesty. For many women invasive procedures such as vaginal examination may be so threatening that they cannot be discussed, even with one's own husband. Thus many women prefer a midwife over a male physician. Too often health care providers assume women lose this modesty during pregnancy and labor. Most women value and appreciate efforts to maintain modesty.

For numerous cultural groups a physician is deemed appropriate only in times of illness. A physician is considered inappropriate when pregnancy is considered a normal process and the woman is in a state of health. Even when problems with pregnancy develop according to beliefs of Western medicine, they may not be perceived as problems but may be considered normal.

Although pregnancy is considered normal by many, certain practices are expected of women of all cultures to ensure a good outcome. *Prescriptions* tell women what to do, and **proscriptions** establish **taboos.** The purposes of these practices are to prevent maternal illness from a pregnancy-induced imbalanced state and protect the vulnerable fetus. Prescriptions and proscriptions are related to emotional response, clothing, activity and rest, sexual activity, and dietary practices.

Emotional Response. Virtually all cultures emphasize the importance of a socially harmonious and agreeable environment. Absence of stressful relationships is important for a successful outcome for mother and baby. Harmony with other persons must be fostered. Visits from extended family members may be required to demonstrate continued pleasant and noncontroversial relationships. If dissonance exists in any relationship with others, it is usually dealt with in culturally prescribed ways.

Imitative magic functions in other proscriptions in addition to food. Mexicans advise against pregnant women witnessing an eclipse of the moon because they believe it may cause a cleft palate in the infant. Exposures to an earthquake may result in preterm delivery or miscarriage. A breech presentation may occur if the earthquake was exceptionally strong (Clark, 1970). Snow (1974) notes that among blacks a pregnant woman must not ridicule someone with an affliction for fear her child might be born with the same handicap. A mother should not hate a person lest her child resemble that person, and dental work should not be done during pregnancy because it may cause a baby to have a harelip. Carrington (1978) describes a widely held folk belief in many cultures that includes refraining from raising one's arm above one's head and refraining from tying knots, so that the umbilical cord does not wrap around the baby's neck and become knotted.

Clothing. Although most cultural groups do not prescribe specific clothing for pregnancy, modesty is an expectation for many (Clark, 1970; Meleis and Sorrell, 1981). Spanish-speaking people of the Southwest wear a cord beneath the breast and knotted over the umbilicus. This cord, called a *muneco,* is thought to prevent morning sickness and ensure a safe delivery (Brown, 1976). Amulets, medals, and beads may be worn to ward off evil spirits.

Physical Activity and Rest. Norms that regulate physical activity of mothers during pregnancy vary tremendously. Many groups (Carrington, 1978; Stringfellow, 1978; Horn, 1982; Lee, 1989). encourage women to be active, to walk, and to engage in normal although not strenuous activities to ensure that the baby is healthy and not too large. On the other hand, the Filipino woman is cautioned that any activity is dangerous, and others willingly take over work (Affonso, 1978; Stern, 1981). The belief among Filipinos is that inactivity constitutes a protection for mother and child. The mother is encouraged to simply produce the succeeding generation. Health care providers could misinterpret this behavior as laziness or noncompliance with the health regimen desired in prenatal care. Again it is important for the nurse to find out the meaning of activity and rest for each culture.

Sexual Activity. In most cultures sexual activity is not prohibited until the end of pregnancy. Among blacks sexual relations are viewed as natural because pregnancy is a state of health (Carrington, 1978). Mexican-Americans view sexual activity as necessary to keep the birth canal lubricated (Kay, 1982). On the other hand, Vietnamese have definite proscriptions about sexual intercourse, requiring abstinence as early as the sixth month (Stringfellow, 1978; Hollingsworth et al, 1980; Lee, 1989). Sexual taboos are more common after delivery.

Diet. Nutritional information given by Western health care providers may be a source of conflict for many cultural groups. The conflict is commonly not known by the health care providers unless they have an understanding of dietary beliefs and practices of the persons for whom they are caring (see Chapter 11).

Evaluation

Maternal and fetal goals are continuously evaluated according to measurable, established criteria. The clinical findings that represent normal response are presented as plans/goals in the nursing care plans for each client. These criteria are used as a basis for selecting appropriate nursing actions and evaluating their effectiveness.

SECOND TRIMESTER

By the second trimester the pregnancy usually has been positively diagnosed. The woman and her family have had time to adjust to the pregnancy, and the initial visit or two have been completed. For many women, discomforts common to the first trimester are resolving, but it is still too early to focus intently on the labor and birth.

For most women no apparent major problems are identified. For them, a common pattern for return visits is scheduled. Throughout the second trimester, monthly visits are sufficient, although additional visits may be warranted should the need arise.

SECOND TRIMESTER CHECKLIST

- Schedule and events of visits
- Counseling for self-care:
  - Adaptations/discomforts
    - Skin changes
    - Palpitations
    - Faintness
    - GI distress
    - Varicosities
    - Neuromuscular and skeletal distress
  - Safety (seat belts)
  - Exercise and rest
  - Relaxation
  - Nutrition
  - Sexuality
  - Personal hygiene
  - Danger signs
  - Preparation for childbirth and parenthood classes
- Fetal growth and development
- Diagnostic tests
  - Specify
- Other

Assessment

Maternal Assessment

Interview. Follow-up visits are less extensive than the initial prenatal visit (see general nursing care plan, p. 264). At each visit, the woman is asked for a summary of events since the previous visit. She is asked about her general well-being, complaints or problems, or questions she may have. The interviewer can reinforce teaching about danger signs by inquiring about them at each visit. Personal and family needs are identified and explored (see Chapter 9). Success or failure of self-care measures is discussed; and learning needs and readiness for learning are assessed.

Careful, precise, and concise recording of client responses and laboratory results contribute to the continuous supervision vital to the mother and fetus. A checklist of care needs during the second trimester of pregnancy is a valuable tool. It provides the team of care providers with a communication tool to prevent gaps and identify areas of repeated concern for clients. A sample checklist for the second trimester is shown in the box , above, right.

Physical Examination. Reevaluation is constant. Each woman reacts differently to pregnancy. Careful monitoring of pregnancy and reactions to care is vital. A data base updated at each contact with a client reveals patterns in movement and content.

At each visit temperature, pulse, and respirations are measured; blood pressure (right arm, woman sitting) is taken; weight and the determination of whether weight gain (or loss) is compatible with overall plan for weight gain are evaluated (see Chapter 11); and presence and degree of edema are noted. These findings reflect the status of maternal adaptations. When the interview or physical examination findings are suspicious, an in-depth examination is performed.

Careful interpretation of blood pressure is important in risk-factor analysis for all gravidas. Blood pressure is evaluated on the basis of absolute values and length of gestation and is interpreted in the light of modifying factors.

Absolute values of a systolic blood pressure $\geq$ 140 mm Hg and a diastolic blood pressure $\geq$90 mm Hg are suggestive of hypertension. A rise in systolic blood pressure $\geq$30 mm Hg over baseline and in diastolic blood pressure $\geq$15 mm Hg over baseline are also significant regardless of whether absolute values are less than 140/90. For example, if a woman's blood pressure normally is 105/60, a change to 120/75 must be viewed as potential for hypertension.

The *mean arterial pressure* (MAP) reaches its lowest point in the second trimester at about 22 weeks, then rises slowly to term (Page, Villee, and Villee, 1981). A MAP of $\geq$90 in the second trimester is associated with an increase in the incidence of pregnancy-induced hypertension (PIH) in the third trimester.

Maternal anxiety can elevate readings. If an elevated reading is found, the gravida is given time to rest, and the reading is repeated.

Laboratory Tests. Routine laboratory tests during the second trimester are limited. A clean-catch urine specimen is used to detect glucose, acetone, and albumin/protein. Pregnant women may experience glycosuria (see nutrient excretion, p. 199). Urine for culture and sensitivity and blood samples are obtained only if signs and symptoms warrant. Hematocrit (HCT) or packed cell volume (PCV) may be done at each visit in some offices.

Fetal Assessment

Fundal Height. During the second trimester the uterus becomes an abdominal organ. Measurement of the height of the uterus above the symphysis pubis is used as one indicator of the progress of fetal growth. It also provides a gross estimate of the duration of pregnancy.

A pliable (not stretchable) tape measure or a pelvimeter may be used to measure **fundal height.** The height of the fundus is measured from the notch of the pubic symphysis over the top of the fundus without tipping the corpus back.

To increase measurement reliability and facilitate management, the same person examines the gravida at each of her prenatal visits, and one protocol is established for use by all examiners providing care to a group of gravidas. The protocol must include the gravida's position on the table and the measuring device and method used. The gravida's position is supine with the knees slightly bent and the head and shoulders slightly elevated. Early in pregnancy, her bladder should be empty. If a pliable measuring tape is used, it should be specified whether the measurement is taken with the tape held in contact with the skin from the uterus to the fundus or whether the measurement is read with the palm of the hand at the fundus and the tape elevated between the forefinger and middle finger (Fig. 10-7). *McDonald's rule* adds precision to the measurement of fundal height during the second and third trimesters. It is calculated as follows:

Height of fundus (cm) × 2/7 (or + 3.5) = Duration of pregnancy in lunar months

Height of fundus (cm) × 8/7 = Duration of pregnancy in weeks

Measurement of fundal height may aid in identification of high-risk factors. A stable or decreased fundal height may indicate intrauterine growth retardation; an excessive increase could mean multifetal gestation or hydramnios (see Unit VI). Among the factors that affect the accuracy of measurement are obesity (subtract 1 cm from the measurement if the gravida weighs 90 kg [200 pounds] or more), the amount of amniotic fluid, multifetal gestation, the fetal size and attitude, and the tilt of the uterus.

Gestational Age. In a normal pregnancy, **fetal gestational age** is estimated by determining the duration of pregnancy and the date of delivery. Fetal gestational

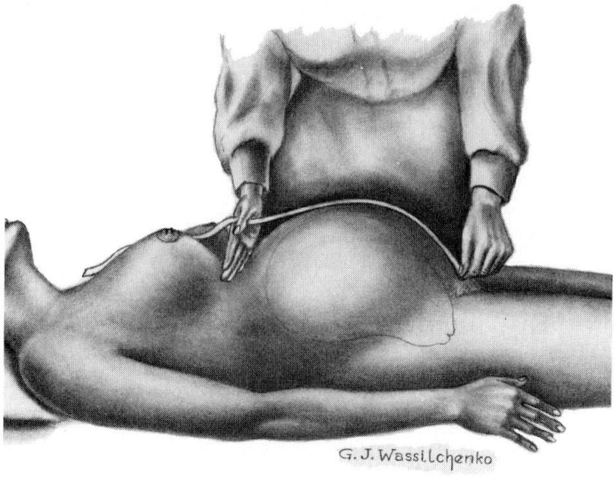

Fig. 10-7 Measurement of fundal height from symphysis.

age is correlated from the menstrual history, contraceptive history, pregnancy test, and clinical evaluation:

- Menstrual History
  - LNMP*: Date, duration, amount
  - LMP: Date, duration, amount
  - PMP†: Date, duration, amount
  - Menarche: Date, interval, duration
  - History of menstrual irregularity
- Contraceptive History
  - Type of contraceptive
  - When stopped
- Pregnancy Test
  - Date:
  - Type:
  - Result:
- Clinical Evaluation
  - First uterine size estimate: Date, size
  - FHT first heard: Date, Dopptone, fetoscope
  - Date of quickening
  - Current fundal height, EFW‡
  - Current week of gestation
  - Ultrasound: Date, Week of gestation, BPD§
  - Reliability of dates

In some centers ultrasonography is used with all pregnancies, and a more exact estimation of **gestational age** can be made. Ultrasonography may be used to establish the duration of pregnancy if the woman is unable to give a precise date for her LMP or if the size of the uterus does not conform to the stated date of the

*Last normal menstrual period.
†Previous menstrual period (before LMP).
‡Estimated fetal weight.
§Biparietal diameter.

LMP (see Chapter 22). Ultrasonography is not, however, a universally recommended procedure (see Chapter 22).

Health Status. Assessment of **fetal health status** includes consideration of fetal movement, fetal heart rate (FHR), and abnormal maternal or fetal symptoms.

The mother is instructed to note the extent and timing of fetal movements and to report immediately if the pattern changes or if movement ceases. Regular movement has been found to be a reliable determinant of fetal health (Cohen, 1985).

The FHR is checked on routine visits once it has been heard (Fig. 10-8). Early in this trimester, the FHR may be heard with the ultrasound stethoscope (Fig. 10-8, C) or the ultrasound fetoscope (see Fig. 15-3). Before the fetus can be palpated by Leopold's maneuvers (see p. 374), the scope is moved around the abdomen until the FHR is heard. Each nurse develops a set pattern for searching the abdomen, for example, starting first in the midline about 2 to 3 cm (1 in) above the symphysis followed by the left lower quadrant, and so on. The FHR is counted and the quality and rhythm noted (see Chapter 14). Later in the second trimester, the FHR can be determined with the fetoscope or stethoscope (Fig. 10-8, *A* and *B*). Normal rate and rhythm are other good indicators of fetal health. Absence of FHR, once noted, requires immediate investigation.

The second trimester is a period of rapid growth. The box above, right, summarizes fetal development.

Intensive investigation of fetal health status is initiated if any maternal or fetal complications arise (e.g., maternal hypertension, growth lag, premature rupture of membranes, or irregular or absent FHR). (For a discussion of electronic fetal monitoring, see Chapter 14; for other monitoring techniques of the fetus at risk, see Chapter 22).

FETAL DEVELOPMENT AT 26 WEEKS

Viable at week 24
Fetal movements obvious
FHR readily heard
Scalp hair, eyebrows, eyelashes, fine downy lanugo and vernix cover the skin
Eyelids still fused
Skin is red, shiny, and thin
Face is wrinkled, giving an "old man appearance"
Length is 30 cm (12 in)
Weight is 600 g (1¼ lb)
Uterus at or just above level of umbilicus

Nursing Diagnoses

Each individual is affected differently by pregnancy. Careful monitoring of the pregnancy and responses to care is of utmost importance. It is particularly difficult to distinguish discomforts of the second and third trimesters. Multiparous women tend to demonstrate

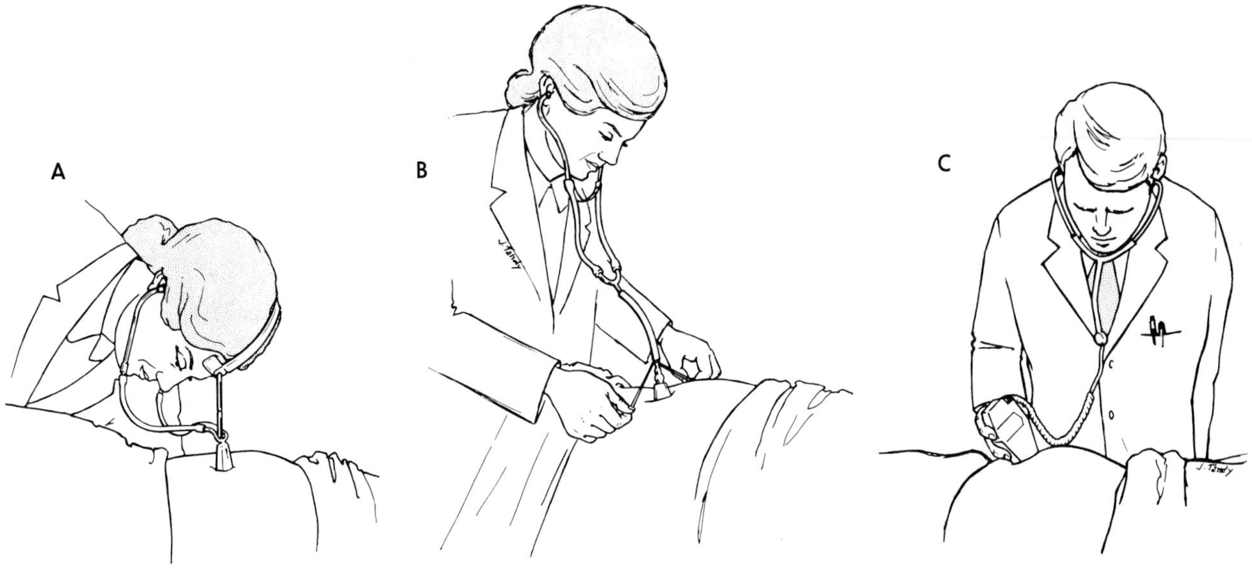

Fig. 10-8 Detecting fetal heartbeat. **A**, Fetoscope. **B**, Stethoscope with rubber band. **C**, Ultrasound stethoscope.

some discomforts in pregnancy earlier than nulliparous women do. Continuous assessment, analysis, and formulation of diagnosis is imperative. The following are only a few examples of nursing diagnoses that can emerge from the data base.

Anxiety, potential for, related to
- Discomforts of pregnancy
- Changing family dynamics
- Fetal well-being

Pain, potential for, related to
- Discomforts of pregnancy

Knowledge deficit, related to
- Self-care measures for rest and relaxation
- Personal hygiene (increased sweating, oily skin, leukorrhea)
- Preparation for parenthood

Altered family processes related to
- Lack of understanding of second trimester changes
- Changing sexual relationship or marital support

Potential for injury related to
- Nonuse of safety harness in automobiles

Planning

Planning care for clients during the second trimester of pregnancy is given direction from the nursing diagnosis. A plan is developed mutually with each client to the extent possible. The plan is individualized, relating specifically to her needs. The information in this chapter is general; not all women will experience all problems discussed or require all facets of care described. The general nursing care plan below serves as a guide for students developing a plan of care.

The nurse continues to foster the growing relationship between care provider and client. Goals are the same as those for the mother, fetus, and family given for the first trimester.

Implementation

Nurses assume many caregiving roles during the second trimester of the prenatal period. The clinician's roles can be categorized as both supportive and as teacher/counselor/advocate. Midpregnancy classes focus on parental needs during this time (see Chapter 9).

Supportive Role

The same guidelines as those discussed for the first trimester are pertinent in the second trimester as well. The manner in which the nurse implements the roles of teacher/counselor/advocate and the consideration shown the mother while technical tasks are performed also support and reassure the gravida and her family.

Teacher/Counselor/Advocate

Several new discomforts or changes are experienced by women as maternal adaptations continue in the second trimester. Clear separation of discomforts and changes by trimester is impossible. Check pp. 254 and 278 if a discomfort or change is not found in Table 10-3.

Clothing. Comfortable, loose clothing is best. Washable fabrics (e.g., absorbent cottons) are often preferred. Since maternity clothes are expensive and

General Nursing Care Plan

SUBSEQUENT PRENATAL VISITS: SECOND TRIMESTER

ASSESSMENT	NURSING DIAGNOSIS (ND), PLAN/GOAL (P/G)	RATIONALE/ IMPLEMENTATION	EVALUATION
Woman making subsequent office or clinic visit.	ND: Knowledge deficit related to second trimester of pregnancy. P/G: The woman will become knowledgable about the second trimester of pregnancy.	*Ongoing assessment of general well-being provides a basis for care:* Interview woman regarding events, complaints, or problems since previous visit. Identify personal and family needs. Assess learning needs. Answer any questions woman may ask.	Woman understands and verbalizes rationale for sharing any relevant information with the nurse. Woman exhibits a readiness to learn by verbalizing and asking appropriate questions.

General Nursing Care Plan—cont'd

ASSESSMENT	NURSING DIAGNOSIS (ND), PLAN/GOAL (P/G)	RATIONALE/ IMPLEMENTATION	EVALUATION
Physical evaluation of gravida.	ND: Altered body systems related to second trimester of pregnancy. P/G: The woman will maintain physical well-being during pregnancy by gaining knowledge about normal physical alterations during this time.	*Ongoing assessment of physical well-being provides a basis for care:* Monitor the gravida's weight gain and blood pressure. Measure fundal height. Listen to fetal heart tones. Test urine for sugar and protein.	Woman understands and verbalizes rationale for observation of these parameters. Woman cooperates by bringing urine specimen with her.
Gravida needs education regarding self-care activities.	ND: Knowledge deficit related to self-care activities during second trimester of pregnancy. P/G: Woman will learn self-care activities.	*Knowledge enables the woman to collaborate in her care:* Discuss importance of keeping scheduled appointments. Discuss good nutrition, eating habits, and a favorable weight gain. Explain importance of maintaining an exercise program. Discuss safety hazards relevant to work and travel. Explain importance of wearing nonrestrictive and flattering clothes to help woman with her self-image.	Woman keeps scheduled appointments. Woman reports eating habits and maintains a favorable weight gain. Woman verbalizes an understanding of a safe exercise program and safety hazards associated with work and travel. Woman refrains from wearing regular girdles, garters, or other restrictive clothes.
Lack of knowledge regarding danger signs.	ND: Knowledge deficit related to danger signs during second trimester. P/G: Woman will learn to recognize those signs and symptoms that signal danger for her and her fetus.	*Early identification and prompt therapy for risk factors are essential; therefore the nurse will discuss the following signs and symptoms with the client:* Absence of fetal movement or change in pattern of fetal movement. Swollen feet, ankles, hands; puffy eyes. Rapid gain in weight. Headaches, blurred vision, dizziness. Premature rupture of membranes. Vaginal bleeding. Sudden, sharp pains in abdomen. Provide gravida with phone numbers of physician or hospital.	Woman verbalizes understanding of these danger signs and asks relevant questions. Woman knows where to call if she should experience any of these signs or symptoms.

Table 10-3 Problems Related to Maternal Adaptations to Pregnancy

Discomfort	Physiology	Prevention/Treatment
Pigmentation deepens, acne, oily skin	Melanocyte-stimulating hormone (from anterior pituitary)	Not preventable; usually resolved during puerperium; reassurance given to women and their families
Spider nevi (telangiectasias)—appear during trimesters 2 or 3 over neck, thorax, face, and arms	Focal networks of dilated arterioles (end-arteries) from increased concentration of estrogens	Not preventable; reassurance that they fade slowly during late puerperium; rarely disappear completely
Palmar erythema occurs in 50% of pregnant women; may accompany spider nevi	Diffuse reddish mottling over palms and suffused skin over thenar eminences and fingertips may be caused by genetic predisposition or hyperestrogenism	Not preventable; reassurance that condition will fade within 1 week after giving birth
Pruritus (noninflammatory)	Unknown cause; various types as follows:	Keep fingernails short and clean; refer to physician for diagnosis of cause
	Nonpapular; closely aggregated pruritic papules	Not preventable; symptomatic: Keri baths; mild sedation
	Increased excretory function of skin and stretching of skin possible factors	Distraction; tepid baths with sodium bicarbonate or oatmeal added to water; lotions and oils; change of soaps or reduction in use of soap; loose clothing
Palpitations	Unknown; should not be accompanied by persistent cardiac irregularity	Not preventable; reassurance; refer to physician if accompanied by symptoms of cardiac decompensation
Supine hypotension (vena cava syndrome) and bradycardia	Posture induced by pressure of gravid uterus on ascending vena cava when woman is supine; reduces uterine-placental and renal perfusion	Side-lying position or semisitting posture, with knees slightly flexed (see supine hypotension, p. 241)
Faintness and, rarely, syncope (orthostatic hypotension): may persist throughout pregnancy	Vasomotor lability or postural hypotension from hormones; in late pregnancy may be caused by venous stasis in lower extremities	Moderate exercise, deep breathing, vigorous leg movement; avoid sudden changes in position* and warm crowded areas; move slowly and deliberately; keep environment cool; avoid hypoglycemia by eating 5 to 6 small meals per day; elastic hose; sit as necessary; if symptoms are serious, refer to physician
Food cravings (see Chapter 11)	Cause unknown; cravings determined by culture or geographic area	Not preventable; satisfy craving unless it interferes with well-balanced diet; report unusual cravings to physician
Heartburn (pyrosis, or acid indigestion): burning sensation in lower chest or upper abdomen, occasionally with burping and raising of a little sour-tasting fluid	Progesterone slows GI tract motility and digestion, reverses peristalsis, relaxes cardiac sphincter, and delays emptying time of stomach; stomach displaced upward and compressed by enlarging uterus	Limit or avoid gas-producing or fatty foods and large meals; maintain good posture; sips of milk for temporary relief; hot tea, chewing gum; physician may prescribe antacid between meals, refer to physician for persistent symptoms

*Caution woman to rise slowly and sit on edge of bed or to assume hands-and-knees posture before rising, and to get up slowly after sitting or squatting.

Table 10-3 Problems Related to Maternal Adaptations to Pregnancy—cont'd

Discomfort	Physiology	Prevention/Treatment
Constipation	GI tract motility slowed because of progesterone, resulting in increased resorption of water and drying of stool; intestines compressed by enlarging uterus; predisposition to constipation because of oral iron supplementation	Six glasses of water per day; roughage in diet; moderate exercise; regular schedule for bowel movements; use relaxation techniques and deep breathing; *do not* take stool softener, laxatives, other drugs, or enemas without first consulting physician; *never* ingest mineral oil
Flatulence with bloating and belching	Reduced GI motility because of hormones, allowing time for bacterial action that produces gas; swallowing air	Chew foods slowly and thoroughly; avoid gas-producing foods, fatty foods, large meals; exercise; regular bowel habits
Varicose veins, may be associated with aching legs and tenderness; may be present in legs and vulva; hemorrhoids are varicosities in the perianal area	Hereditary predisposition; relaxation of smooth muscle walls of veins because of hormones, causing pelvic vasocongestion; condition aggravated by enlarging uterus, gravity, and bearing down for bowel movements; thrombi from leg varices rare but may be produced by hemorrhoids	Avoidance of obesity, lengthy standing or sitting, constrictive clothing, and constipation and bearing down with bowel movements; moderate exercises; rest with legs and hips elevated (Fig. 10-9); support stockings; thrombosed hemorrhoid may be evacuated; relieve swelling and pain with warm sitz baths, local application of astringent compresses
Leukorrhea: often noted throughout pregnancy	Hormonally stimulated cervix becomes hypertrophic and hyperactive, producing abundant amount of mucus	Not preventable; *do not douche;* hygiene; perineal pads; reassurance; refer to physician if accompanied by pruritus, foul odor, or change in character or color
Headaches (through week 26)	Emotional tension (more common than vascular migraine headache); eye strain (refractory errors); vascular engorgement and congestion of sinuses from hormone stimulation	Emotional support; prenatal teaching; conscious relaxation; refer to physician for constant "splitting" headache, after assessing for pregnancy-induced hypertension (PIH)
Carpal tunnel syndrome (involves thumb, second and third fingers, lateral side of little finger)	Compression of median nerve from changes in surrounding tissues: pain, numbness, tingling, burning; loss of skilled movements (typing); dropping of objects	Not preventable; elevation of affected arms, splinting of affected hand may help; surgery is curative
Periodic numbness, tingling of fingers (acrodysesthesia): occurs in 5% of pregnant women	Brachial plexus traction syndrome from drooping of shoulders during pregnancy (occurs especially at night and early morning)	Maintain good posture; wear supportive maternity brassiere; reassurance that condition will disappear if lifting and carrying baby does not aggravate it
Round ligament pain (tenderness)	Stretching of ligament caused by enlarging uterus	Not preventable; reassurance, rest, good body mechanics to avoid overstretching ligament; relieve cramping by squatting or bringing knees to chest
Joint pain, backache, and pelvic pressure; hypermobility of joints	Relaxation of symphyseal and sacroiliac joints because of hormones, resulting in unstable pelvis; exaggerated lumbar and cervicothoracic curves caused by change in center of gravity from enlarging abdomen	Maternity girdle; good posture and body mechanics; avoid fatigue; wear low-heeled shoes; conscious relaxation; firm mattress; local heat and back rubs; pelvic rock exercise; rest; reassure that condition will disappear 6 to 8 weeks after delivery

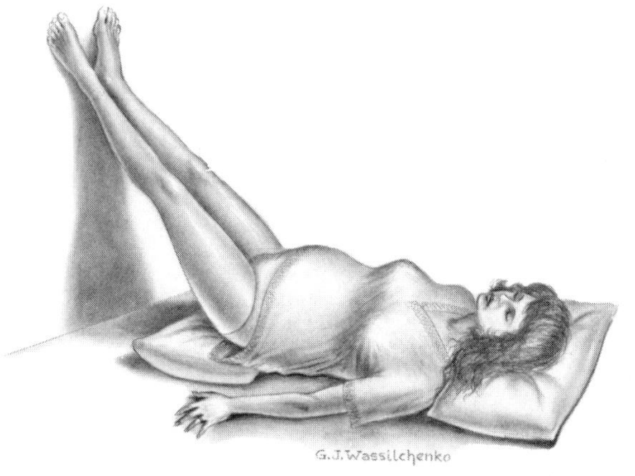

Fig. 10-9 Position for resting legs and reducing swelling, edema, and varicosities. Encourage woman with vulvar varicosities to include pillow under her hips.

rarely wear out, hand-me-downs or used clothes from garage sales can suffice. Tight brassieres and belts, stretch pants, garters, tight-top knee socks, panty girdles, and other constrictive clothing should be avoided. Tight clothing over the perineum encourages vaginitis and miliaria (heat rash). Impaired circulation in the lower extremities favors varices.

A well-fitted maternity girdle, frequently readjusted, may be used for backache by obese women or those with a multifetal pregnancy. The woman should be cautioned to begin fastening the girdle from the pubic symphysis upward to support the uterus from below. An old, even large, girdle meant for the nonpregnant woman is unsuitable during pregnancy because it pushes the abdomen (uterus) inward. A nonmaternity girdle may also aggravate backache and leg ache.

Maternity brassieres are constructed to accommodate the increased breast weight, chest circumference, and size of breast tail tissue (under the arm). These brassieres have drop flaps over the nipples to facilitate breastfeeding. A good brassiere can help prevent neckache and backache.

Elastic hose or leotards may give considerable comfort to women with large varicose veins or swelling of the legs. Comfortable shoes that provide firm support and promote good posture and balance are advisable. Very high heels and platform shoes are not recommended because of the woman's changed center of gravity. She has a tendency to lose her balance. In the third trimester her pelvis tilts forward and her lumbar curve increases. Leg aches and **leg cramps** (p. 278) are aggravated by nonsupportive shoes.

Posture and Body Mechanics. Many maternal adaptations predispose the woman to backache and possible injury. The pregnant woman's center of gravity changes (see Fig. 8-10). Pelvic joints soften and relax. Stress is placed on abdominal musculature (see Figs. 8-10 and 8-11). Posture and **body mechanics** contribute to discomfort and potential for injury.

Women can acquire a kinesthetic sense for good body posture. In addition to fostering good posture (see Figs. 8-10 and 10-10), the following activities can be used to prevent or relieve backache:

- **Pelvic tilt (rock)** in standing position against a wall, or lying on floor (see Fig. 10-6, *B* and *C*).
- Pelvic tilt (rock) on hands and knees, and while sitting in straight-back chair (see Fig. 10-6, *A*).
- Abdominal muscle contractions during pelvic tilt while standing, lying, or sitting helps strengthen rectus abdominis muscle (see Fig. 10-6, *D*).

To restrict the lumbar curve, the woman can be instructed to:

- Wear a maternity girdle to support weak abdominal muscles.
- For prolonged standing (e.g., ironing, out-of-home employment), place one foot on low footstool or box; change positions often.
- Move car seat forward so that knees are bent and higher than hips. If needed, use a small pillow to support low back area.
- Sit in chairs low enough to allow both feet on floor and preferably, with knees higher than hips.

Good body mechanics can also be implemented. Some suggestions the nurse can offer are:

- Use leg muscles to reach objects on or near floor. Bend at the knees, not the back. Knees are bent to lower body to squatting position. Feet are kept 12 to 18 inches apart for a solid base to maintain balance (see Fig. 10-10, *B*).
- Lift with the legs. To lift heavy object (young child), one foot is placed slightly in front of the other and kept flat as woman lowers herself on one knee. She lifts the weight holding it close to her body, and never higher than chest high. To stand up or sit down, one leg is placed slightly behind the other as she raises or lowers herself.

Implement suggestions to prevent **round ligament pain** and strain on abdominal muscles given in Table 10-3.

Bathing and Swimming. Tub bathing is permitted even in late pregnancy, because water does not enter the vagina unless under pressure. However, tub bathing is contraindicated after rupture of the membranes. Baths and warm showers can be therapeutic because they relax tense tired muscles, help counter insomnia, and make the pregnant woman feel fresh. Physical maneuverability presents a problem (increased chance of falling) late in pregnancy. Swimming is also permitted during normal pregnancy, although diving is discouraged because of possible traumatic injury.

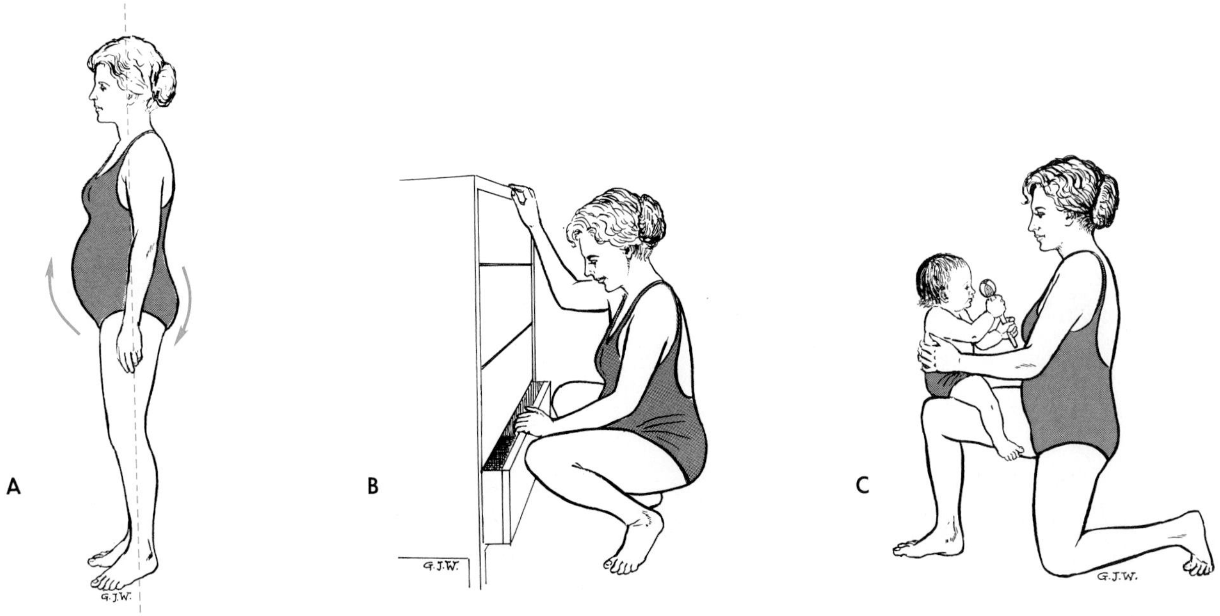

Fig. 10-10 Correct body mechanics. **A,** Standing. **B,** Stooping. **C,** Lifting.

Physical Activity. Physical activity promotes a feeling of well-being in the pregnant woman. It improves circulation, assists relaxation and rest, and counteracts boredom as it does in the nonpregnant woman. Exercise tips for pregnancy are presented in detail on p. 255. Suggestions for client teaching of Kegel's exercises to strengthen the muscles around the reproductive organs and improve muscle tone are found on p. 251.

Rest and Relaxation. The pregnant woman is encouraged to plan regular rest periods particularly as pregnancy advances (Fig. 10-11). The side-lying position is recommended to promote uterine perfusion and fetoplacental oxygenation by eliminating pressure on the ascending vena cava (supine hypotension). During shorter rest periods, the woman can assume the position in Fig. 10-9 to promote venous drainage from the legs and relieve **leg edema** and varicose veins. The mother is shown how to rise slowly from a side-lying position to avoid strain on the back and minimize the hypotension caused by changes in position common in the latter part of pregnancy. To stretch and rest back muscles at home or at work, the nurse can instruct the woman to:

Stand behind a chair. Support and balance self using the back of the chair (Fig. 10-12). Squat for 30 seconds; stand for 15 seconds. Repeat six times, several times per day, as needed.

While sitting in chair, lower head to knees for 30 seconds. Raise up. Repeat six times, several times per day, as needed.

Relaxation is the release of the mind and body from tension through conscious effort and practice. The abil-

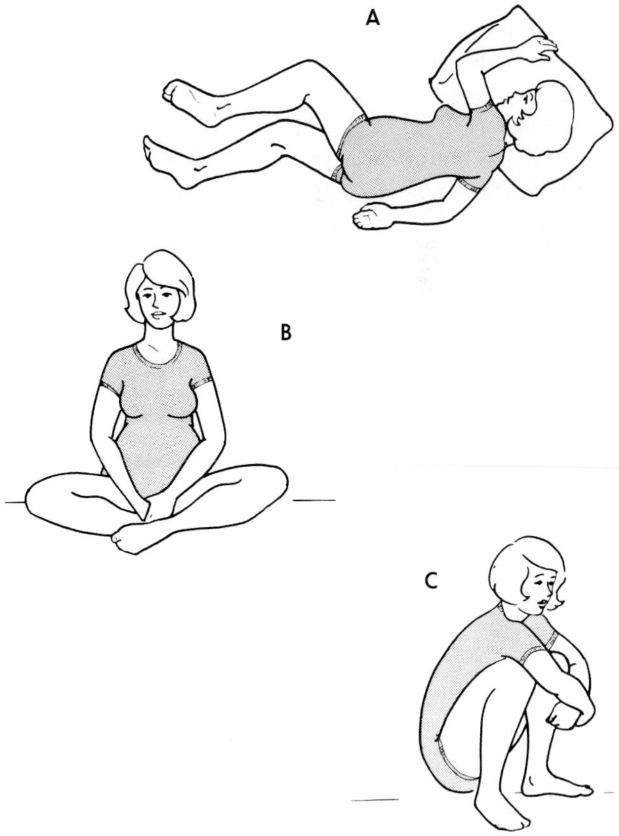

Fig. 10-11 Positions for rest and relaxation. **A,** Side-lying position. Some women prefer to support upper leg with pillows. **B, Tailor sitting position** aids in relaxing muscles of pelvic floor. **C,** Squatting helps relax the pelvic floor. All these positions can be assumed during labor.

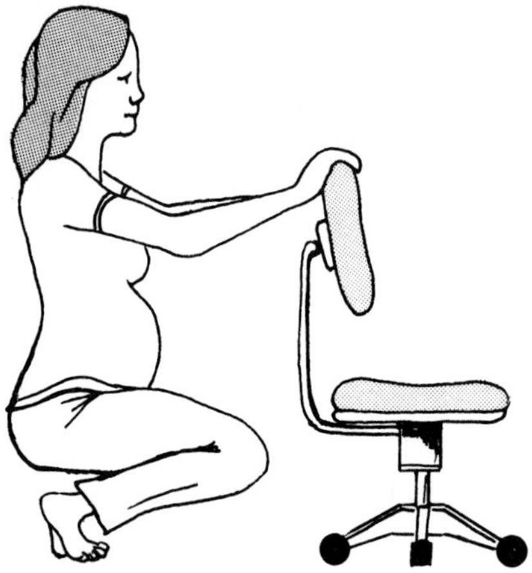

Fig. 10-12 Squatting for muscle relaxation and strengthening and for keeping leg and hip joints flexible.

ity to relax consciously and intentionally can be beneficial for the following reasons:

Relief of normal discomforts related to pregnancy

Reduction of stress and therefore diminished pain perception during the childbearing cycle

Heightened self-awareness and trust in own ability to control one's responses and functions

Coping with stress in everyday life situations, pregnant or not

The techniques for **conscious relaxation** are numerous and varied. The following guidelines can be used by anyone:

Preparation: Loosen clothing, assume a comfortable sitting (Fig. 10-11, *B*) or side-lying position with all parts of body well-supported with pillows.

Beginning: Allow self to feel warm and comfortable. Inhale and exhale slowly, and imagine peaceful relaxation coming over each part of the body starting with the neck and working down to the toes. Often persons who learn conscious relaxation speak of feeling relaxed even if some discomfort is present.

Maintenance: Imagine (fantasize or daydream) to maintain the state of relaxation. With *active imagery* the person imagines herself as moving or doing some activity and experiencing its sensations. With *passive imagery,* one imagines watching a scene, such as a lovely sunset.

Awakening: The return to the wakeful state is gradual. The person begins slowly to take in the stimuli from the surrounding environment.

Further retention and development of the skill: Regular practice for regular periods of time each day, for example, at the same hour for 10 to 15 minutes each day, is refreshing, revitalizing, and invigorating.

Employment. Continued assessment during the prenatal period is necessary to determine if working is causing undue fatigue or stress. It may be possible for the woman to change the type of work being done with a recommendation from her physician (Bryant, 1985). Some women may lose interest in work as they become more introverted during the second trimester of pregnancy. This response may be difficult to accept for the woman who has always been competent and independent before pregnancy.

Activities that depend on a good sense of balance should be discouraged, especially during the last half of pregnancy. Commonly, excessive fatigue is the deciding factor in the termination of employment. Women in sedentary jobs need to walk around at intervals and should neither sit nor stand in one position for long periods. Activity is necessary to counter the usual sluggish, dependent circulation that potentiates development of varices and thrombophlebitis. The pregnant woman's chair should provide adequate back support. A footstool can prevent pressure on veins, relieve strain on varices, and minimize swelling of feet. Work breaks are best spent resting in the left lateral side-lying position. It is recommended that employers have an area where women can lie down. Standards for maternity care and employment of mothers in industry have been recommended by the United States Children's Bureau to safeguard the interests of expectant mothers employed in industry.

The nurse can encourage each woman to consider the effects of working postnatally on herself and her newborn. Flexible scheduling of working hours, if possible, can allow for breastfeeding. Also, women who plan to return to work after giving birth may appreciate information about daycare centers.

Travel. If traveling for long distances, periods of activity and rest should be scheduled. While sitting, the woman can practice deep breathing, foot circling, and alternating contracting and relaxing different muscle groups. Fatigue should be avoided.

Although travel in itself is not a cause of either abortion or preterm labor, certain precautions are recommended. A woman who does not wear automobile restraints risks injury to herself and her fetus (Krozy et al, 1985). Maternal death as a result of injury is the most common cause of fetal death (Crosby, 1983). The next most common cause is placental separation. Body contours change in reaction to the force of a collision. The uterus as a muscular organ can adapt its shape to that of the body. The placenta lacks the resiliency to change, and placental separation can occur (Crosby, 1983). A combination lap belt and shoulder harness is the most effective automobile restraint (Fig. 10-13) (Chang, 1985). Both shoulder and lap belts should be used. The lap belt should be worn low across the hip

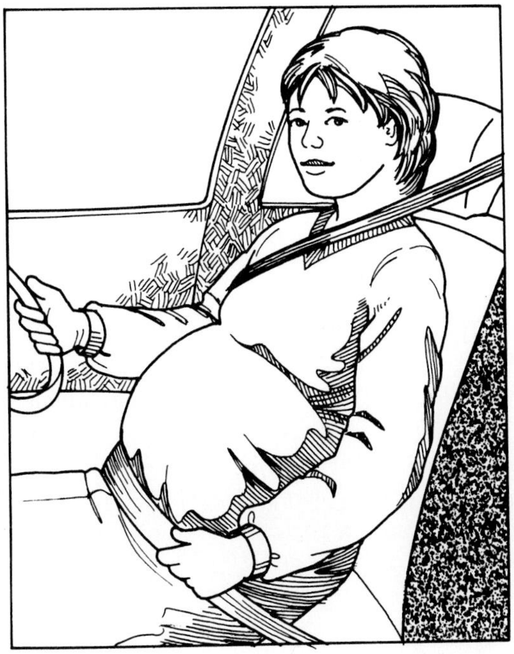

Fig. 10-13 Proper use of seat belt and head rest.

bones and as snug as is comfortable. The shoulder belt should be worn above the gravid uterus and below the neck to avoid chafing. The pregnant woman should sit upright. The headrest should be used to avoid a whiplash injury.

In high-altitude regions, lowered oxygen levels may cause fetal hypoxia, especially if the gravida is anemic (Barry and Bia, 1989). Women who travel extensively expose themselves to the risk of serious accident and may find themselves far removed from good maternity care. In addition, fatigue or tension, as well as altered regular personal habits and diet during arduous travel, may be detrimental.

If long-distance travel is necessary, the trip should be made by air. Perhaps fortuitously, U.S. flight regulations do not permit pregnant women aboard during the last month without a statement from an obstetrician. Most foreign airlines have a cutoff of 35 weeks' gestation. Many health insurance carriers do not cover delivery in a foreign setting or even hospitalization for preterm labor (Barry and Bia, 1989). Air travel itself carries little risk. Magnetometers used at airport security checkpoints are not harmful to the fetus. The 8% humidity at which cabins are maintained in commercial airlines may result in some water loss; hydration (with *water*) should be maintained under these conditions (Barry and Bia, 1989). Sitting in a cramped seat of an airliner for prolonged periods may increase the risk of superficial and deep thrombophlebitis. A 15-minute walk around the aircraft for every hour of travel is recommended to minimize this risk. A seat in the nonsmoking section of flights where smoking is permitted is advised to prevent elevated carboxyhemoglobin levels.

Many women experience a sense of uneasiness when traveling by any vehicle. They describe feelings of fear for the safety of their unborn baby. Guidelines for client teaching: safety, are found on p. 272.

Preparation for Feeding the Newborn. Pregnant women are usually eager to discuss their plans for feeding the newborn. Breast milk is the food of choice, and breastfeeding is associated with a decreased incidence in perinatal morbidity and mortality. However, immaturity of the infant, deep-seated aversion to breastfeeding by mother or father, and certain medical complications, such as pulmonary tuberculosis, are contraindications to breastfeeding. The woman and her partner are encouraged to decide which method of feeding is suitable for them. Once the couple has been given information about the advantages and disadvantages of bottle-feeding and breastfeeding, they are in a position to make an informed choice. Nurses need only to support their decisions.

Most women are motivated by the sixth or seventh month of pregnancy to learn about breast preparation and breastfeeding. Each woman is first assessed for risk of preterm labor. Anticipatory guidance during pregnancy contributes to later success in breastfeeding (Nicholson, 1985).

The **pinch test** determines whether the nipple is erectile or retractile (Fig. 10-14). The nurse guides the woman through the pinch test. The woman places her

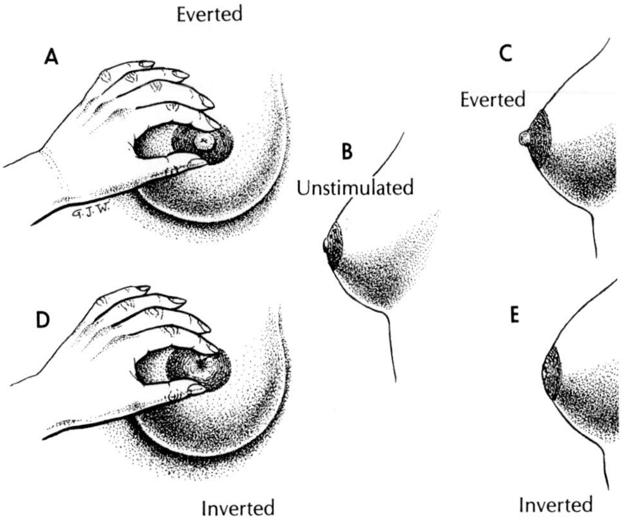

Fig. 10-14 **A** and **C**, When stimulated, nipples evert (protract or erect). **B**, Unstimulated, nipples look the same. **D** and **E**, When stimulated, nipples invert (retract).

Guidelines for Client Teaching
SAFETY

ASSESSMENT

1. Pregnant woman works within or outside the home, in the yard, drives or rides in a car.

NURSING DIAGNOSES

Knowledge deficit related to source of safety hazards and safety measures.

Potential for injury to mother and fetus related to possible hazards in the environment and workplace.

GOALS

Short-term

Woman is alerted to sources of safety hazards.

Woman is alerted to self-care related to safety measures.

Intermediate

Woman will eliminate exposure to chemicals and fumes.

Long-term

Woman will persist in use of safety measures throughout life span.

REFERENCES AND TEACHING AIDS

Printed instructions and information from sources such as clinic, doctor, safety councils.

RATIONALE/CONTENT	TEACHING ACTION
Safety awareness and measures are critical during pregnancy; therefore the nurse will teach that:	
Maternal adaptations to pregnancy involve relaxation of joints, alteration in center of gravity, faintness, and discomforts. Problems with coordination and balance are common. Embryonic and fetal development is vulnerable to environmental teratogens.	Encourage and answer questions regarding maternal changes and body mechanics during pregnancy. Exercise caution to avoid causing anxiety. Review precautions for drug use.
Sources of safety hazards must be explained so the woman will know how to avoid them; therefore the nurse will teach that:	
Many potentially dangerous chemicals are present in the home, yard, and workplace: cleaning agents, paints, sprays, herbicides, and pesticides. The soil and water supply may be unsafe. Many activities require coordination and balance. High altitudes (not in pressurized aircraft) could jeopardize oxygen intake.	Learn status of local area from community health agencies. Review questions regarding employment and body mechanics. Encourage and answer questions regarding which changes the woman is able to implement.
Self-care can be enhanced through consistent use of safety measures; therefore the nurse will teach the woman to:	
Read all labels for ingredients and proper use of product. Ensure adequate ventilation with "clean" air. Dispose of wastes appropriately. Wear gloves when handling chemicals. Change job assignments or workplace as necessary. Use good body mechanics. Use safety features on tools/vehicles; safety seat belts and head rests, goggles, helmets, as specified. Avoid activities requiring coordination, balance, and concentration.	Present alternatives and problem-solve solutions together. Explore with woman what she does during the course of a typical day. Make a list of potential/actual hazards and mutually problem-solve solutions (e.g., avoid use, provide substitutions, ensure ventilation and proper disposal, use safety equipment, make changes in sports and recreation, and schedule rest periods).
Take rest periods, reschedule daily activities to meet rest and relaxation needs.	Show illustrations (Figs. 10-9 and 10-11) and discuss.

EVALUATION The woman can verbalize knowledge of hazards and problem-solve solutions. The woman consistently implements self-care safety measures. She and fetus experience no harm from safety-related causes.

thumb and forefinger on her areola and presses inward gently. This will cause her nipple to stand erect or to retract (invert). Most nipples will stand erect. Inverted nipples need more preparation time. Nipple preparation for these women can start during the last 2 months of pregnancy.

The woman learns that nipples are cleansed with warm water to prevent blocking of the ducts with dried colostrum. They are dried with a rough towel. Soap is not used because it removes protective oils that keep nipples supple.

Toughening of nipples can be accomplished in a variety of ways. Following a bath or shower, the woman can towel dry nipples well, but not so hard as to cause irritation or soreness. The woman can grasp the nipple between the thumb and forefinger and roll each nipple gently for a short time each day (Fig. 10-15). Since this procedure may cause uterine contractions, it may be contraindicated for those women at risk for preterm labor. Exposing nipples to air and sunlight for short periods of time each day can also toughen nipples, but sunburn must be avoided.

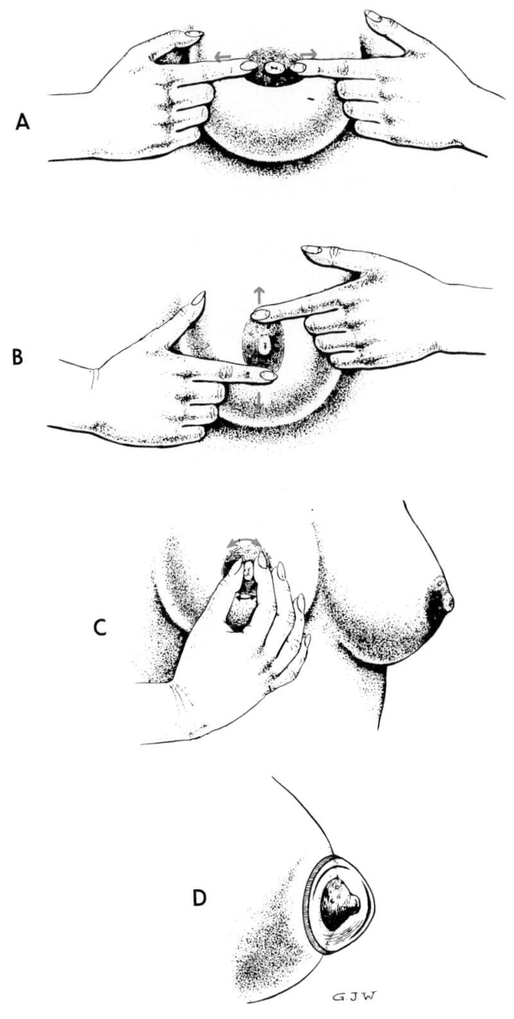

Fig. 10-15 **A** and **B**, Nipple stretching. **C**, Nipple rolling. **D**, Nipple cup in place. (Some concern has been expressed regarding nipple stimulation and potential for preterm labor.)

Other techniques can be employed to encourage protraction of inverted nipples. The woman can place four fingers close to the inverted nipple, pressing firmly into the breast tissue, and gradually pull away from areola. Massage is done vertically and horizontally, about five times each day.

Some women obtain **nipple cups** designed specifically for correcting inverted nipples. Plastic doughnut-shaped cups are available for correcting inversions or retractions (Fig. 10-15, *D*). A continuous, gentle pressure exerted around the areola pushes the nipple through a central opening in the inner shield. Nipple cups should be worn during the last two trimesters of pregnancy for 1 to 2 hours daily. The time for wearing them should be increased gradually. Brand names for these cups include Woolwich, Netsy, La Leche League Cups, Nurse-Dri, Free and Dry, and Hobbit Shields. These cups can also be worn after childbirth. However, because body warmth can foster rapid bacterial growth and contamination, milk that collects in the cup should be discarded and not fed to the infant (Riordan, 1983).

Breast stimulation may also produce uterine activity and should be avoided in women at risk for preterm labor if contractions are noted (Iams, Johnson, and Creasy, 1988). However, the assumption that nipple stimulation causes the release of exogenous oxytocin has not been proved. Ross et al (1984) were unable to detect a surge of oxytocin into the plasma of women whose uterus contracted in association with nipple stimulation (Cunningham, MacDonald, and Gant, 1989).

The possibility of contaminants in breast milk concerns many women, both consumers and professionals (Doucette, 1978). Breast milk can be potentially hazardous as illustrated in the following examples. The mother harboring *Salmonella kottbus* transmits this organism through her milk. Environmental pollutants tend to concentrate in humans. The long-term effects of contamination of breast milk with pollutants such as polybrominated biphenyl (PBB) is as yet unknown. Medications that pass through the mother's milk are listed in Appendix H.

Evaluation

Maternal and fetal goals are continuously evaluated according to measurable, established criteria. The clinical findings that represent normal response are presented as plans/goals in the nursing care plans for each client. These criteria are used as a basis for selecting appropriate nursing actions and evaluating their effectiveness.

THIRD TRIMESTER

The quiet period of the second trimester gives way to an active period, a trimester more oriented in reality for the expectant parents. Parental attachment to the fetus grows in the third trimester. Mixed among the daydreams about the "coming baby" are parental anxieties that focus on possible defects in mental and physical abilities of the child. The expectant mother's attention turns to thoughts of a "safe passage" for herself and her child. Fears of pain and mutilation and concerns about her behavior and possible loss of control during labor are important issues.

Physical discomforts and fetal movements often interrupt the expectant mother's rest. **Dyspnea,** return of urinary frequency, backache, constipation, and **varicosities** are experienced by most gravidas in late pregnancy. Increased bulkiness and awkwardness affect the gravida's ability to perform activities of daily living. Positions of comfort are more difficult to achieve. Increasingly, the gravida becomes more impatient to "get this over with."

For the expectant father, the moratorium phase of the second trimester passes into the focusing phase (see p. 213). Activity and energy to create and achieve characterize this phase. Styles of involvement differ according to the man's perception of the male and fathering roles within his social group. Many expectant fathers become more involved with the pregnancy. They begin to redefine their relationship to the fetus and themselves as fathers. Role playing through daydreaming is common. The expectant father feels some of the same concerns as the expectant mother. Often, however, he does not share these concerns with anyone.

Expectant families approaching childbirth have many needs. Siblings and grandparents must be considered, too. Clearly the nurse is in a pivotal position within the team of health care providers to assist parents with these needs during the third trimester of pregnancy. The schedule of care reflects the increased need. Starting with week 28, visits are scheduled every 2 weeks until week 36, and then every week until delivery.

Assessment

During the third trimester current family occurrences and their effect on the mother are assessed; for example, siblings' and grandparents' responses to the pregnancy and the coming child. In addition, the following questions are addressed:

- What anticipatory planning is in progress concerning new parenting responsibilities, sibling rivalry, recuperation from pregnancy and birth, and fertility management?
- What successes or frustrations is the mother experiencing with diet, rest and relaxation, sexuality, and emotional support?
- What is the mother's understanding of her family's needs in relation to the pregnancy and child?
- How well prepared are the parents in the event of emergency? That is, does the mother know and understand danger signs and how and to whom to report them?
- Does the mother know the signs of preterm and term labor?
- What is the mother's understanding of the labor process, expectations of herself and others during labor, and what to bring to the hospital?
- What plans has the mother and her family made for labor (see education for choice, p. 229)?
- What anxieties is the mother or her family experiencing regarding labor or child?
- What does the mother wish to know about control of discomfort during labor?
- Is the mother planning to attend any prebirth classes?
- Does the mother have questions about fetal development and methods to assess fetal well-being?

A checklist for third trimester assessment should be used to ensure that important areas are addressed (see box, p. 275).

Maternal Assessment

Interview. The initial question in the third-trimester interview is asked with the intent to identify the *gravida's* main concern for the moment. Focusing on the woman takes advantage of her readiness to learn and affirms the caregiver's interest in her as a person. Based on the client's expressed needs, her status to date, and generally accepted needs of most women in late pregnancy, the nurse's clinical judgment guides the content and direction of the interview.

A review of physical systems is appropriate at each meeting. Any suspicious signs or symptoms are assessed in depth. Discomforts reflecting pregnancy adaptations are identified. Special inquires are made about possible infections (e.g., genitourinary tract, respiratory tract). Knowledge of and success with self-care measures and prescribed therapy are assessed. Psychosocial responses to the pregnancy and approaching parenthood are assessed.

Physical Examination. During the third-trimester physical examination, temperature, pulse, respirations, blood pressure, and weight are assessed and noted. Suspicious signs and symptoms uncovered during the interview are assessed. Presence, location, and degree of edema are documented carefully. Gestational age is confirmed. Weekly pelvic examinations are begun at

THIRD TRIMESTER CHECKLIST

Schedule and events of visits
Counseling for self-care:
- Adaptations/discomforts
  - Dyspnea
  - Insomnia
  - Psychosocial responses and family dynamics
  - Gingivitis and epulis
  - Urinary frequency
  - Perineal discomfort and pressure
  - Braxton Hicks' contractions
  - Leg cramps
  - Ankle edema
- Safety (balance)
- Exercise and rest
- Relaxation
- Nutrition
- Sexuality
- Danger signs—general
- Danger signs—preterm labor

Fetal growth and development
Preparation for baby
- Feeding method
- Nipple preparation

Preparation for labor
- Recognition: false versus true
- Prenatal classes
- Control of discomfort
- Hospital tour
- Provision for other family members
- Preparation for homecoming

Diagnostic tests
- Specify

Other

weeks 36 to 38 and are continued until term, primarily to confirm presenting part, corroborate station, and determine cervical dilation and effacement. Risk assessment continues throughout pregnancy (see Chapter 22).

The **roll-over test** is sometimes used as one predictor of a potential hypertensive problem in the third trimester. This test may be done at each visit after the twentieth week of gestation. The roll-over test can be done as follows (Zuspan and Quilligan, 1982; Fanaroff and Martin, 1987; Cunningham, MacDonald, and Gant, 1989): position the woman on her side. Determine the blood pressure (BP) level in the upper arm once it is stable. "Roll" her over onto her back, checking the pressure again. Wait 5 minutes and check the BP level once again. An increase of 20 mm Hg in diastolic blood pressure from the side position to the back position indicates a *positive roll test*. The significance of a roll test is that if negative, the chances are less than 1 in 100 that the gravida will develop preeclampsia. If the test is positive, even though the BP level is within normal limits and the gravida has no signs of fluid retention, full-blown pregnancy-induced hypertension (PIH) will develop at least 60% of the time. If the roll test is positive, it is imperative that home self-care measures be instituted. The woman should spend more time in bed in the lateral recumbent position, stress in the home should be reduced, and her diet should be reviewed (see Chapter 23).

Laboratory Tests. At each visit urine is tested for glucose (to assess for diabetes) and albumin protein (to assess for hypertension). A urine culture and sensitivity test is done as necessary. Hematocrit determination by finger stick is made at each visit in some facilities. Blood tests are repeated as necessary: Venereal Disease Research Laboratory (VDRL) test for syphilis; complete blood count (CBC) with hematocrit, hemoglobin, and differential values; antibody screen (Kell, Duffy, rubella, toxoplasmosis, anti-Rh, AIDS); sickle cell; and level of folacin when indicated. If not done earlier in pregnancy, a glucose screen for women over 25 years of age is performed. Glucose challenge is usually done between 24 and 48 weeks (see Chapter 24). Cervical and vaginal smears are repeated at 32 weeks or as necessary: for *Chlamydia* organisms, gonorrhea, and herpes simplex, types 1 and 2.

Fetal Assessment

Beginning at the thirty-second week, identification of fetal presentation, position, and station (engagement), with the aid of Leopold's maneuvers (see Chapter 15), is done weekly. This period of rapid fetal growth is summarized in the box below.

Fundal height is measured at each visit. The method described on p. 262 is used. Uterine measurements and size (weight) of fetus are compared with supposed duration of pregnancy. Although some clinicians can esti-

FETAL DEVELOPMENT AT 40 WEEKS

Nutrients and maternal immunoglobulins are stored
Subcutaneous fat deposited
Dramatic storage of iron, nitrogen, and calcium
In male: testes are within well-wrinkled scrotum
In female: labia are well-developed and cover vestibule
Lanugo shed, except for shoulders, generally
Body contours plump
Decreased vernix
Scalp hair 2 to 3 cm (1 in) long
Cartilage in nose and ears well developed
45 to 55 cm (18 to 22 in) in length
Weighs 3400 g (7½ lb) (average)
Fundal height below xiphoid after lightening

mate fetal weight with unbelievable accuracy, estimations are generally inconsistent and unreliable. Accuracy in estimating fetal weight improves with ultrasound determination of biparietal diameter (BPD). Possible growth retardation of fetus, multifetal pregnancy, or inaccuracy of the estimated date of delivery (EDD) may be disclosed by ultrasound (see Chapter 22).

Fetal health status is evaluated at each visit. The mother is requested to describe fetal movements. She is asked if she has danger signs (see p. 253) to report, for example, change in fetal movements, rupture of membranes. (For a discussion of electronic monitoring, see Chapter 14; for other monitoring techniques, see Chapter 22).

Nursing Diagnoses

Each gravida and her family respond to and are affected by pregnancy in different ways. Careful monitoring of the pregnancy and responses to care is of the utmost importance. The following are representative of nursing diagnoses that can be formulated in the third trimester from the data base of a "normal" pregnancy.

Anxiety, potential, related to
- Discomforts of pregnancy
- Approaching labor

Knowledge deficit related to
- Assessment for risks such as preterm labor
- Recognizing onset of true versus false labor
- Self-care measures
- Emergency arrangements

Altered family processes related to
- Inadequate understanding of third-trimester changes and needs
- Increased concern about labor
- Insomnia or sleep deficit

Sleep pattern disturbance related to
- Discomforts of late pregnancy
- Anxiety about approaching labor

Potential for injury to mother and fetus related to
- Labor
- Mother's altered balance and coordination

Activity intolerance related to
- Increased weight and change in center of gravity
- Anxiety
- Sleep disturbances

Planning

Planning care for clients and their families during the third trimester of pregnancy is given direction from identified nursing diagnoses and from a comprehensive view of the expectant family. A plan is developed mutually with the client to the extent possible. The plan is individualized, relating specifically to the client's needs and the needs of her family. The information in this chapter is general; not all women will experience all problems discussed or require all facets of care described. The nurse and client select those aspects of care that are relevant to the client and the client's family. The general and specific nursing care plans provide guidelines for students.

Implementation

Nurses assume many caregiving roles during the third trimester of pregnancy. The nurse-clinician's roles can be categorized as both supportive, and teacher/counselor/advocate.

Supportive Activities

In this trimester, House's (1981) categorization of social support (see Chapter 9) serves as a guide in providing comprehensive support. This categorization of support includes emotional, appraisal, informational (see teacher/counselor/advocate section), and instrumental.

Esteem, affection, trust, concern, consideration of cultural and religious responses, and listening are components of emotional support. The woman's feelings of satisfaction with her relationships and support, and of competence and sense of being in control are important issues to address in the third trimester. A discussion of parental awareness of the unborn child's responses to stimuli, such as sound, light, maternal posture or tension, and patterns of sleeping and waking can be helpful. Opportunities are also provided to discuss probable emotional tensions related to the following: childbirth experience such as fear of pain, loss of control, and possible delivery of child before reaching hospital; responsibilities and tasks of parenthood; mutual parental concerns arising from anxiety for safety of mother and unborn child; mutual parental concerns related to siblings and their acceptance of new baby; mutual parental concerns about social and economic responsibilities; and mutual parental concerns for cognitive dissonance arising from conflicts in cultural, religious, or personal value systems.

The father's commitment to the pregnancy, the couple's relationship, and their concerns about sexuality and sexual expression emerge as concerns for many expectant parents. An important support measure is to validate normalcy of their responses (if they fall within normal limits). Validation, feedback, and social comparison characterize appraisal support.

Providing opportunity to discuss concerns, providing a listening ear, and validating the normalcy of responses will meet the gravida's needs to varying degrees. Nurses also need to implement specific "interventions targeted at improving expectant parents' partner support satisfaction, because this support constitutes the majority of their total support" (Brown, 1986).

Nurses need to recognize the increased vulnerability of men during pregnancy and implement anticipatory guidance and health promotion strategies to help them with their concerns. Nursing intervention may directly help fathers with concerns such as the need to share intimate feelings or may do so indirectly by education of mothers. Health care providers can stimulate and encourage open dialogue between the couple.

Nursing students especially are cautioned that, despite their knowledge, skill, concern, and caring, there will be clients who will be unable to benefit from their interventions. It is equally important for the nurse to maintain self-esteem and a positive self-concept in the face of a less than optimum client outcome.

Teacher/Counselor/Advocate

Not only are some new discomforts seen in the third trimester, but others seen previously in the first trimester (e.g., fatigue) also recur. Women experiencing pregnancies later in life may experience an aggravation of varicose veins or severe backache from postural changes associated with a heavy, pendulous abdomen and relaxed joints. Such symptoms are frightening and uncomfortable.

In Table 10-4, the physiology, prevention, and treatment of several discomforts are discussed. Relaxation, exercises, body mechanics, safety, and employment issues are described and discussed earlier in this chapter. Nutrition is covered in Chapter 11.

Review of Danger Signs. The nurse needs to answer questions honestly as they arise during pregnancy. It is often difficult for the gravida to know when to report signs and symptoms. The mother is encouraged to refer to a printed list of danger signs (see p. 253) and to listen to her body. If she senses that "something is wrong," she should call her care provider. Several signs and symptoms need to be discussed more extensively. These include vaginal bleeding, alteration in fetal movements, symptoms of PIH, rupture of membranes, and preterm labor.

If *vaginal bleeding* occurs in the third trimester, it is important to rule out brownish spotting occurring 48 hours after vaginal examination and to rule out "show" of pinkish mucus. The woman is to come to the hospital's emergency area immediately for diagnosis and treatment if bleeding is other than one of the preceding types.

Should the gravida notice cessation, noticeable diminution, or acceleration in the amount of *fetal movement,* she is to come to the clinic or the physician's office for evaluation.

Appearance of *edema* of the hands and around the eyes, severe *headaches, visual changes,* or feelings of *jitteriness* require immediate evaluation for PIH.

A gush or trickle of clear *watery discharge* that appears to come from the vagina may indicate rupture of membranes. The diagnosis requires a visit to the clinic or hospital for evaluation.

Recognizing Preterm Labor. Teaching gravidas to recognize preterm labor is necessary for each woman (Herron, 1988; Johnson, 1989). Hospitals have developed pamphlets to help mothers remember what they learn. Guidelines for client teaching: preterm labor recognition follow on p. 280.

Occasionally, birth occurs before the gravida has access to professional attendants. Emergency childbirth is outlined in Chapter 15.

Prebirth Preparation

Not all gravidas and support persons attend formal classes in preparation for childbirth. For those who do attend, extensive preparation is possible (see Fig. 9-5). Many do not take advantage of classes for a variety of reasons: employment; inaccessibility because of time, cultural/ethnic/religious orientation; cost; lack of knowledge regarding choices in prenatal education classes; lack of readiness. Therefore clinicians need to provide information that includes the following:

- Process of labor: admission, examination, care in labor
- Plans to get to hospital (when to go and where); care of other children
- Methods to control pain (e.g., analgesia and anesthesia, breathing-relaxing techniques) (see Chapter 13)
- Supplies to have in a suitcase ready for the trip to the hospital: personal items for grooming, items for labor as desired (i.e., warm socks, focal point), supportive bra, nightgowns, slippers
- Responsibilities of the spouse, family member, or friend who will be accompanying the woman through labor and delivery
- Care of the newborn (i.e., clothing, feeding, daily hygienic care), and postnatal care (see Chapter 17)
- Emergency arrangements (e.g., precipitate delivery) (see Chapter 15)

Table 10-4 Problems Related to Maternal Adaptations During the Third Trimester

Problem	Physiology	Treatment
Shortness of breath and dyspnea—occur in 60% of pregnant women	Expansion of diaphragm limited by enlarging uterus; diaphragm is elevated about 4 cm (1½ in); some relief after lightening	Good posture; flying exercise; sleep with extra pillows; avoid overloading stomach; stop smoking; refer to physician if symptoms worsen to rule out anemia, emphysema, and asthma
Insomnia (later weeks of pregnancy)	Fetal movements, muscular cramping, urinary frequency, shortness of breath, or other discomforts	Reassurance; conscious relaxation; back massage or **effleurage** (Fig. 10-16); support of body parts with pillows; warm milk or warm shower before retiring
Psychosocial responses (Chapter 9): mood swings, mixed feelings, increased anxiety	Hormonal and metabolic adaptations; feelings about impending labor, delivery, and parenthood	Reassurance and support from significant other and nurse; improved communication with partner, family, and others
Gingivitis and epulis (hyperemia, hypertrophy, bleeding, tenderness): condition will disappear spontaneously 1 to 2 months after delivery	Increased vascularity and proliferation of connective tissue from estrogen stimulation	Well-balanced diet with adequate protein and fresh fruits and vegetables; gentle brushing and good dental hygiene; avoid infection
Urinary frequency and urgency return	Vascular engorgement and altered bladder function caused by hormones; bladder capacity reduced by enlarging uterus and fetal presenting part	Kegel's exercises; limit fluid intake before bedtime; reassurance; wear perineal pad; refer to physician for pain or burning sensation
Perineal discomfort and pressure	Pressure from enlarging uterus, especially when standing or walking; multifetal gestation	Rest, conscious relaxation and good posture; maternity girdle; refer to physician for assessment and treatment if pain is present; rule out labor
Braxton Hicks contractions	Intensification of uterine contractions in preparation for work of labor	Reassurance; rest; change of position; practice breathing techniques when contractions are bothersome; effleurage; *rule out labor*
Leg cramps (gastrocnemius spasm)—especially when reclining	Compression of nerves supplying lower extremities because of enlarging uterus; reduced level of diffusible serum calcium or elevation of serum phosphorus; aggravating factors: fatigue, poor peripheral circulation, pointing toes when stretching legs or when walking, drinking more than 1 L (1 qt) of milk per day	Rule out blood clot by checking for Homans' sign; use massage and heat over affected muscle; stretch affected muscle until spasm relaxes (Fig. 10-17); stand on cold surface; oral supplementation with calcium carbonate or calcium lactate tablets; aluminum hydroxide gel, 1 oz, with each meal removes phosphorus by absorbing it
Ankle edema (nonpitting) to lower extremities	Edema aggravated by prolonged standing, sitting, poor posture, lack of exercise, constrictive clothing (e.g., garters), or by hot weather	Ample fluid intake for "natural" diuretic effect; put on support stockings before arising; rest periodically with legs and hips elevated (Fig. 10-9), exercise moderately; refer to physician if generalized edema develops; *diuretics are contraindicated*

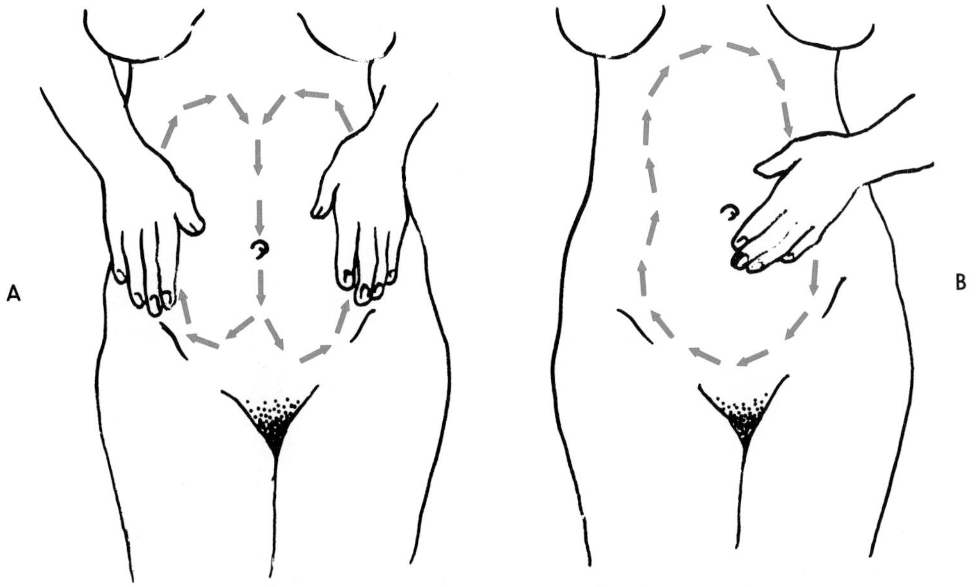

Fig. 10-16 Pattern for effleurage, a light, rhythmic stroking useful for inducing relaxation. **A**, Self-effleurage. **B**, Effleurage by another.

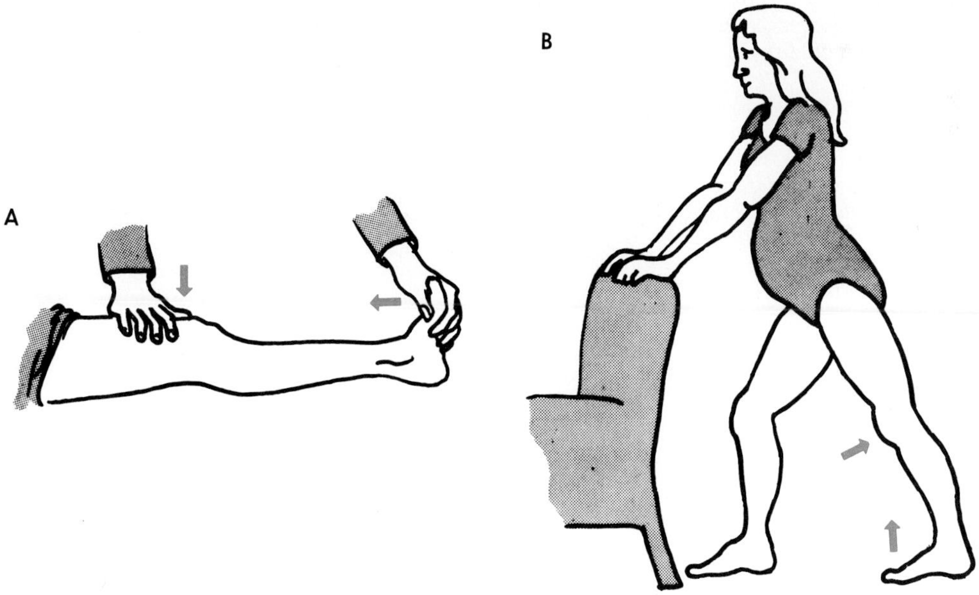

Fig. 10-17 Relief of muscle spasm (leg cramps). **A**, Another person dorsiflexes the foot with the knee extended. **B**, Woman stands and leans forward, thereby dorsiflexing foot of affected leg.

Guidelines for Client Teaching
PRETERM LABOR RECOGNITION

ASSESSMENT

1. Pregnancy after the twentieth week but before the thirty-seventh week.
2. Gravida has no signs or symptoms of preterm labor at present.

NURSING DIAGNOSES

Knowledge deficit related to the warning signs of preterm labor.
Potential for injury to fetus related to preterm birth.
Potential for body image disturbance: situational low self-esteem related to preterm delivery.
Potential for spiritual distress related to preterm labor.

GOALS

Short-term

Woman begins to learn the warning signs and symptoms of preterm labor.

Intermediate

Woman remains alert for preterm labor without undue anxiety.
Woman definitely recognizes warning signs and symptoms and can self-detect uterine contractions.

Long-term

Woman knows what to do if she should exhibit any of the warning signs and symptoms of preterm labor.
Regardless of outcome of pregnancy, woman will maintain or enhance her self-concept and supportive family processes, and spiritual distress is avoided or minimized.

REFERENCES AND TEACHING AIDS

Printed instructions outlining warning signs and symptoms, steps to take if woman has problems, and the doctor's phone number; videotapes
Illustrations or charts.

RATIONALE/CONTENT	TEACHING ACTION
Knowledge provides the basis for decision making about self-care; gravida needs to understand the definition of preterm labor:	
Preterm labor occurs after the twentieth week but before the thirty-seventh week of pregnancy. It is a condition in which uterine contractions cause the cervix to open earlier than normal. It could result in the birth of a preterm baby.	Read through pamphlet with woman or group of women. Women can use group for support.
Gravida needs to understand the cause of preterm labor:	
Although certain factors may increase a woman's chances of having preterm labor, such as carrying twins, the specific cause or causes are not known.	Encourage discussion of this information, and clarify or answer any questions woman may have. Discuss the woman's risk factors, if she has any.
Gravida needs to understand importance of early recognition:	
It may be possible to prevent a preterm birth by knowing the warning signs and symptoms of preterm labor and by seeking care early if warning signs and symptoms should occur.	Reassure woman that she is not responsible if preterm labor proceeds despite her efforts.
The gravida must be able to differentiate between normal and preterm labor uterine contractions:	
It is *normal* to have some uterine contractions throughout the day. They usually occur when a woman changes positions. These usually irregular and mild contractions are called Braxton-Hicks contractions. They help with uterine tone and uteroplacental perfusion. It is *not normal* to have frequent uterine contractions (every 10 minutes or more often for 1 hour).	Instruct woman in self-detection of uterine contractions: Since the onset of preterm labor is subtle and often hard to recognize, it is important to know how to feel your abdomen for uterine contractions. You can feel for contractions this way: While lying down, place your fingertips on the top of your uterus. A contraction is the periodic "tightening" or "hardening" of your uterus. If your uterus is contracting, you will actually feel your abdomen get tight or hard, and then feel it relax or soften when the contraction is over.
Contractions of labor are regular, frequent, and hard. They may also be felt as a tightening of the abdomen or a backache. This type of contraction causes the cervix to efface and dilate.	Discuss and answer questions. Demonstrate. Watch return demonstration. Praise accomplishments appropriately.

Guidelines for Client Teaching—cont'd

RATIONALE/CONTENT	TEACHING ACTION
PRETERM LABOR RECOGNITION **Warning signs and symptoms include:** **Uterine contractions** that occur every 10 minutes or more with or without other signs. **Menstruallike cramps** felt in lower abdomen constantly or intermittently. **Low dull backache** felt below the waistline constantly or intermittently. **Pelvic pressure** that feels like baby is pushing down constantly or intermittently. **Abdominal cramping** with or without diarrhea. **Increase or change in vaginal discharge;** more than usual or change in consistency or color.	Read through warning signs and symptoms with the client. Instruct the woman to begin assessment as follows: If you think you are having any of the other signs and symptoms of preterm labor, lie down tilted toward your side, and place a pillow at your back for support. Check for contractions for 1 hour. To tell how often contractions are occurring, check the minutes that elapse from the beginning of one contraction to the beginning of the next.
A caring environment and encouragement to participate in self-care and decision making increases the likelihood of compliance: It is often difficult to identify preterm labor. Accurate diagnosis requires assessment by the care provider usually in the hospital or clinic.	Assist the woman with decision-making by providing written instructions such as the following: Call your doctor, clinic, or delivery room, or go to the hospital if: You have uterine contractions every 10 minutes or more often for 1 hour *or* You have any of the other signs and symptoms for 1 hour *or* You have any spotting or leaking of fluid from your vagina. Suggest posting these instructions where they can be seen by everyone.

EVALUATION Teaching has been effective when all goals have been met. Woman verbalizes knowledge of the warning signs and symptoms and knows how to contact her physician. If preterm labor occurs, she recognizes it and informs her physician immediately. Regardless of the outcome of pregnancy, woman will maintain or enhance her self-concept and supportive family processes, and spiritual distress is avoided or minimized.

A nurse needs to be ready to teach when the woman is ready to learn as shown by the following example. One nurse described her intervention with a gravid woman as follows:

- I tried to teach her about relaxation and breathing techniques during childbirth, but she was not interested. When she phoned to tell me she was at the hospital in labor, she said, "What was all that stuff you were saying about breathing?" In between the next few contractions I repeated the salient points.

Even if the woman (couple) has attended prebirth classes, the nurse discusses preparation for childbirth. The following topics are discussed:

Symptoms of impending labor (see box at right) and what information to report
Breathing and relaxation techniques
Involvement of husband or significant other
Provision for needs of other children
Plans to get to hospital
Plans of labor, terminology, and what care to expect
Preparation for baby
Preparation of grandparents and siblings (see Chapter 9)

SYMPTOMS OF IMPENDING LABOR

Uterine contractions: The woman is instructed to report the frequency, duration, and intensity of uterine contractions. Nulliparas are usually counseled to remain at home until contractions are regular and 5 minutes apart. Parous women are counseled to remain at home until contractions are regular and 10 minutes apart. If the woman lives more than 20 minutes from the hospital or has a history of rapid labors, these instructions are modified accordingly.
Rupture of the membranes (see Chapter 15).
Bloody "show": The "show" is scant, pink, and sticky (contains mucus).

If a hospital delivery is planned, the woman is required to register at the hospital of choice. Most hospitals now provide pamphlets containing information such as where to report when labor begins and policies pertaining to visitors and visiting hours. Many facilities also conduct tours.

Counseling is provided to relieve emotional tensions, which often relate directly to the childbirth experience (e.g., anxiety about pain or possible delivery of the child before reaching the hospital). Nursing strategies include providing an opportunity for discussing the woman's specific fears or anxieties, helping her make definite plans concerning what she will do when labor starts, repeating instructions willingly, and having "sharing sessions" with mothers who have recently delivered. If possible, involve significant others in preparation for the birth. Arrange to have them participate in a supportive way during labor and delivery. These techniques may be effective in allaying or diffusing anxiety.

Most men whose wives are approaching labor may have their anxieties decreased through intervention before the event. Fantasies can be replaced by knowledge gained through activities such as the following:

- A hospital tour to enable visualization of the labor room and waiting areas
- A demonstration of helping and supportive measures to comfort his wife during labor
- A brief review of what to expect from his wife during the labor process
- A description of what to expect of the staff during his wife's labor

A realistic discussion of all known factors helps the father problem-solve more rationally and plan for the event. Such discussions are ego strengthening because they help focus the father's energies toward more appropriate coping strategies by helping alleviate anxieties about the unknown. Today many men elect to participate actively during labor and the delivery of their child. However, some men through personal or cultural concepts of the father role neither wish nor intend to participate. *The important concept is that the partners agree on the other's roles.* For nurses to advocate any changes in these roles may cause confusion or feelings of guilt.

Evaluation

Evaluation is a continuous process. To be effective, evaluation needs to be based on measurable outcome criteria. The criteria reflect the parameters used to measure the goals for care. The maternal and fetal areas consistently assessed as indicators of maternal and fetal well-being and the clinical findings that represent normal response are presented as plans/goals in the general nursing care plan, pp. 283-285. These plans/goals are used as a basis for selecting appropriate nursing actions and evaluating their effectiveness.

❑ MULTIFETAL PREGNANCY

A pregnancy with more than one fetus places the mother and fetuses at risk. Maternal blood volume is increased in multiple gestations resulting in an increased strain on the maternal cardiovascular system. Anemia often develops because of a greater demand for iron by the fetuses. Marked uterine distension and increased pressure on the adjacent viscera and pelvic vasculature occur in multifetal pregnancies. Diastasis of the two recti abdominis muscles (in the midline) may occur. Placenta previa develops more commonly in multifetal pregnancies because of the large size or placement of the placentas (see Fig. 7-8, *A;* note placement of placentas). Premature separation of the placenta may occur before the second and subsequent fetuses are born.

The weights of each twin and her or his placenta usually are less than an infant and placenta of a singleton pregnancy after the thirtieth week. However, the aggregate weight is almost twice that of a singleton near term. The mean weight of twins in the United States is more than 2270 g (5 lb). Congenital malformations are twice as common in monozygotic twins as in singletons. There is no increase in the incidence of congenital anomalies in dizygotic twins. Two-vessel cords, that is, cords with a single umbilical artery, occur more often in twins than in singletons. This abnormality is most common in monozygotic twins. The most serious problem for the fetus is the local shunting of blood between placentas (twin-to-twin transfusion) (see Fig. 7-8, *B* and *C*). The *recipient* twin is larger. However, this twin may develop congenital heart failure during the first 24 hours after birth. The *donor* twin will be small, pallid, dehydrated, malnourished, and hypovolemic. Prematurity is a serious problem for the newborns.

Clinical diagnosis of multifetal pregnancy is accurate in only about three fourths of cases. A correct diagnosis of twins may be possible by the twenty-fourth to twenty-sixth week based on the following:

- History of dizygous twins in the female lineage
- Abnormally large maternal weight gain (inconsistent with diet or edema)
- Hydramnios
- Palpation of excessive number of small or large parts
- Asynchronous fetal heart beats or more than one fetal electrocardiographic (ECG) tracing
- Radiographic or ultrasonographic evidence of more than one fetus (Chapter 22)

General Nursing Care Plan

THIRD TRIMESTER

ASSESSMENT	NURSING DIAGNOSIS (ND), PLAN/GOAL (P/G)	RATIONALE/ IMPLEMENTATION	EVALUATION
Woman in third trimester. Teaching needs: danger signs and recognition of preterm labor.	ND: Knowledge deficit related to signs and symptoms of preterm labor. ND: Anxiety related to development of preterm labor. P/G: Woman will learn signs and symptoms of preterm labor. P/G: Woman will remain calm and alert and report signs and symptoms promptly if they occur.	*Knowledge permits the woman to collaborate in her care:* Provide written materials defining signs and symptoms of preterm labor; nurse will read through this information with woman. Discuss the causes of preterm labor. Inform gravida of warning signs and symptoms. Reassure woman. Supervise practice timing frequency of contractions.	Woman verbalizes understanding of signs and symptoms of preterm labor. Woman verbalizes understanding and asks appropriate questions. Woman gives return demonstration.
Premature rupture of membranes (PROM).	ND: Potential for injury to fetus, related to PROM. P/G: Injury to fetus from prolapsed cord or sepsis will be prevented or decreased.	*Woman needs to know how to recognize PROM:* Describe rupture of membranes: a gush or trickle of clear watery discharge that seems to come from vagina. Tell woman that a positive diagnosis of PROM must be made at clinic or hospital.	Woman verbalizes understanding of information. Woman knows where to go if symptoms appear.
Absence or change in fetal movements.	ND: Knowledge deficit related to assessment of fetal movement, its change in character, or its absence. P/G: Woman will learn to assess the character and frequency of fetal movement.	*Woman needs to know about fetal movement:* Discuss fetal movements she is experiencing. Provide information on fetal activity. Discuss cessation, diminution, and acceleration of fetal movement.	Woman verbalizes understanding of information. Woman reports any change in fetal activity.
Teaching needs: discomforts. Diminished tolerance to activities of daily living (ADL).	ND: Activity intolerance related to maternal adaptations. P/G: Woman (couple) will learn ways of conserving her energy.	*Woman needs to conserve energy:* Discuss the importance of frequent rest periods during the day. Help the woman form strategies to help her relax while on the job. Discuss ways in which the woman's partner can help her with household duties.	Woman (couple) verbalizes understanding of information. Woman (couple) verbalizes understanding of information.

Continued.

General Nursing Care Plan—cont'd

ASSESSMENT	NURSING DIAGNOSIS (ND), PLAN/GOAL (P/G)	RATIONALE/ IMPLEMENTATION	EVALUATION
Diminished sexual activity.	ND: Altered sexuality patterns related to discomforts of third trimester of pregnancy. P/G: Woman (couple) will learn alternate ways of achieving sexual satisfaction during this time.	*The woman (couple) benefit if they identify and accept changes in sexuality:* Assess couple's sexual relationship. Encourage open discussion. Supply information on alternative methods, positions, etc. Encourage verbalization of fears and anxieties.	Sexual needs are met and are mutually satisfying. Couple verbalizes understanding and accepts changes in sexual patterns.
Problems sleeping.	ND: Sleep pattern disturbance related to late pregnancy. P/G: Woman will learn ways to adjust sleep schedule and positions to aid in sleeping.	*The woman needs to develop strategies to rest and sleep:* Assess woman's level of fatigue and her response to decreased amount of sleep (decreased coping mechanisms, etc.) Suggest strategies such as relaxation techniques, warm bath/shower, reading, warm milk before bed, back rub.	Woman reports increased sleep/rest. Woman's fatigue reduced, coping mechanism increased.
Constipation.	ND: Constipation related to late pregnancy. P/G: Woman will continue to eat fresh fruits, vegetables, and whole-grain products and drink plenty of water to aid in bowel regularity.	*Constipation may be minimized:* Discuss high-fiber diet. Discuss fluid intake. Discourage use of laxatives and cathartics: may cause preterm labor. Discuss exercise.	Woman verbalizes understanding of information.
Urinary frequency.	ND: Altered patterns of urinary elimination related to late pregnancy. P/G: Woman understands information and infection does not occur.	*Urinary frequency and edema can be minimized:* Provide information about third-trimester physiologic changes. Advise woman to lie in left lateral position. Discuss adequate fluid intake. Discourage use of diuretics.	Woman verbalizes understanding of information.
		Discuss ways to prevent UTI, which is one of the leading causes of preterm labor. Discourage long periods of standing or sitting. Suggest use of support hose.	Woman knows signs and symptoms of UTI to report to physician.

General Nursing Care Plan—cont'd

ASSESSMENT	NURSING DIAGNOSIS (ND), PLAN/GOAL (P/G)	RATIONALE/ IMPLEMENTATION	EVALUATION
Expressed emotional anxiety.	ND: Ineffective family/ individual coping, related to adaptations to pregnancy. P/G: Woman (couple) will learn and demonstrate positive coping techniques.	*Intervention can help woman (couple) minimize anxiety and develop coping strategies:* Assess level of anxiety Discuss those areas and situations that cause woman's (couple's) anxiety. Suggest childbirth education classes (prenatal classes). Give reassurance	Resolution of problems occurs through open discussion. Couple attends classes and works through those anxieties related to labor and delivery.
Backache.	ND: Pain: backache related to postural changes and relaxed joints. P/G: Woman reports greater comfort.	*Discomfort of backache can be minimized:* Discuss causes. Teach woman relaxation techniques and exercises. Teach woman about proper body mechanics and good posture. Supply written materials on the above for woman's future reference. Discuss types of shoes and types of heels woman should be wearing.	Woman verbalizes understanding of information. Woman uses proper body mechanics and demonstrates good posture.
Shortness of breath.	ND: Ineffective breathing pattern related to limited diaphragmatic excursion in late pregnancy. P/G: Woman will learn ways to cope with shortness of breath until lightening occurs.	*Measures can help woman cope with shortness of breath:* Discuss posture, exercises, and positioning for sleep using extra pillows. Strongly suggest cessation of smoking.	Woman accepts information and utilizes suggestions given by nurse.
Leg cramps. Varicose veins.	ND: Pain related to maternal adaptations. P/G: Woman will learn self-care strategies to diminish discomfort.	*Discomfort from leg cramps and varicose veins can be minimized:* Discuss diminution of fatigue, amount of milk ingested per day, and adequate calcium intake. Discuss use of maternity support hose. Suggest frequent rest periods and elevation of legs.	Woman verbalizes understanding of information given. Woman asks appropriate questions.

Prenatal Care

Prenatal care will include changes in the pattern of care and modifications in other aspects such as weight gain and diet. Prenatal visits by the mother with multifetal pregnancy are scheduled at least every 2 weeks in the second trimester and weekly thereafter.

Diet and weight control are supervised to allow weight gain of about 50% or more than the average woman with a singleton pregnancy (as much as 18 kg [40 lb] above the woman's ideal nonpregnant weight). Iron and vitamin supplementation is desirable. Attempts are made to prevent preeclampsia—eclampsia and vaginitis; if they do develop, they are treated early and properly.

The considerable uterine distension can cause increase in backache. Elastic stockings or tights may control leg varices.

Abstinence from both coitus and masturbation to the point of orgasm during the last trimester is recommended. This may help prevent preterm labor.

Enforced rest periods, begun as soon as pregnancy is diagnosed, may help avoid untimely early labor. The mother needs to assume the left lateral position.

Untimely early labor should be avoided. Delivery after the thirty-sixth week increases the likelihood of survival of the newborns.

SUMMARY

The prenatal period is one of growth and change in the woman's personal and social context. The schedule of prenatal visits is designed to monitor the individual gravida's pregnancy and responses to care. A heightened readiness for learning is experienced by the gravida and her family. Counseling for self-care, fetal growth and development, and diagnostic tests is offered. Standards for maternity care and employment are shared with expectant parents.

Assessment for maternal and fetal risk factors continues throughout pregnancy and provides the basis for preventive care. The gravida and her family are alerted to danger signs that need immediate medical attention. Prenatal danger signs and recognition of preterm labor are reviewed with each gravida and her family. During the last trimester, discomforts associated with advancing pregnancy and concerns about the approaching labor preoccupy expectant families. The relationship between the health care team and the expectant parents progresses, and the parents-to-be develop in their roles as active participants in their health care.

Women experiencing multifetal pregnancy are at risk and require special nursing care to minimize possible complications for themselves and their fetuses.

LEARNING ACTIVITIES

1. For as many clients as possible, assess their learning needs and note their week of gestation.
2. In a simulated situation, teach self-care measures for the discomforts of pregnancy.
3. In a clinic or physician's office, measure fundal height and auscultate fetal heart rate.
4. Practice taking a sexual history with a classmate. Discuss results in small groups.
5. In small groups discuss cultural influences based on data from interviews with clients or from personal experiences.
6. Observe and record the following in two contrasting settings, for example, a physician's office and a county welfare clinic.
   a. Did the tone and the information provided to the women and their families differ? If so, how?
   b. Did the women have rights, and were they allowed to assert those rights? Did they?
   c. What questions were asked of the clients, and what were the answers? Were those answers adequate?
   d. Compare the visits the student observed with the ideal textbook description of client care.
   e. How did each clinical experience make you feel? Which approach would you use? What are your reasons?
7. Role-play teaching a gravida to recognize preterm labor.

KEY CONCEPTS

- The prenatal period is a preparatory one both physically, in terms of fetal growth and maternal adaptations, and psychologically, in terms of anticipation of parenthood.
- The psychosocial aspects of care are of paramount importance and may well affect the whole course of pregnancy, childbirth, and the adjustment of the new family.
- The gravida's readiness to learn is at a high level, making this an excellent time to help her expand her self-care skills.
- Discomforts and changes of pregnancy can cause anxiety to the gravida and her family and require sensitive attention and a plan for teaching self-care measures.
- Education about healthy ways of using the body (e.g., exercise, body mechanics) is essential given maternal anatomic and physiologic responses to pregnancy.
- Safeguarding the gravida and fetus involves appropriate use of auto seat belts and following standards for maternity care and employment developed by the U.S. Children's Bureau.
- Important components of the initial prenatal visit include detailed and carefully recorded findings from the interview, a comprehensive physical examination, and selected laboratory tests.
- Even in normal pregnancy the nurse must remain alert to hazards such as supine hypotension, danger signs and symptoms, and signs of potential parenting disorders.
- Blood pressure is evaluated on the basis of absolute values and length of gestation and interpreted in the light of modifying factors; normal MAPs during the second trimester are <90 mm Hg.
- In the absence of factors that affect accuracy, measurement of fundal height is one of the indicators of the progress of fetal growth. Auscultation of fetal heart tones is another tool for assessing fetal health status.
- The quiet period of the second trimester gives way to an active period more oriented to the reality of impending childbirth and parenting responsibilities; attention to prebirth preparation is a necessary component of prenatal care.
- Each gravida needs to know how to recognize and report preterm labor.

References

Affonso DD: The Filipino American. In Clark A, editor: Culture/childbearing/health professionals, Philadelphia, 1978, FA Davis Co.

Barry M and Bia F: Pregnancy and travel, JAMA 261(5):728, Feb 3, 1989.

Bernhardt TL et al: Hyperbaric oxygen treatment of cerebral air embolism from orogenital sex during pregnancy, Crit Care Med 16:729, 1988.

Bing E and Colman L: Making love during pregnancy, New York, 1977, Bantam Books, Inc.

Brown MA: Marital support during pregnancy, JOGN Nurs 15(6):475, 1986.

Brown MS: A cross-cultural look at pregnancy, labor, and delivery, Obstet Gynecol Nurs 5:35, 1976.

Bryant, H: Antenatal counseling for women working outside the homes, Birth 12:4, Winter 1985.

Bullard JA: Exercise and pregnancy, Can Fam Physician 27:977, 1981.

Carrington BW: The Afro-American. In Clark AL, editor: Culture/childbearing/health professionals, Philadelphia, 1978, FA Davis Co.

Chang A: Auto safety in pregnancy, a neglected area, Contemp OB/GYN 254:117, 1985.

Clark M: Health in the Mexican-American culture: a community study, Berkeley, 1970, University of California Press.

Cohen, A: Movement as a yardstick for fetal well-being, Contemp OB/GYN 26:61, Aug 1985.

Crosby, WM: Traumatic injuries during pregnancy, Clin Obstet Gynecol 26(4):902, 1983.

Cunningham FG, MacDonald RC, and Gant NF: Williams obstetrics, ed 18, Norwalk Conn, 1989, Appleton & Lange.

Dale E et al: Exercise during pregnancy: effects on the fetus, Can J Appl Sport Sci 7:98, June 1982.

Dawson KP et al: Keeping abreast of the times: the Tauranga infant feeding survey, NZ Med J 89:75, 1979.

Dean J: Pregnancy and exercise: how much and what kind? On this the experts agree: more research is needed, Sportwest 1:30, Dec 1981.

Doucette JS: Is breast-feeding still safe for babies? MCN 3:354, 1978.

Edwards M: Communications: dimensions in childbirth education, Pacific Grove, Calif, 1973, M Edwards.

Fanaroff AA and Martin RJ, editors: Neonatal-perinatal medicine: diseases of the fetus and infant, ed 4, St Louis, 1987, The CV Mosby Co.

Goldsmith MF: Pregnancy Dx? Rx may now include condoms, JAMA 261(5):678, Feb 3, 1989.

Herron MA: One approach to preventing preterm birth, J Perinat Neonat Nurs 2(1):33, 1988.

Hollingsworth AO et al: The refugees and childbearing; what to expect, RN 43:45, 1980.

Horn BM: Northwest coast Indians: the Muckleshoot. In Kay, MA, editor: Anthropology of human birth, Philadelphia, 1982, FA Davis Co.

House JS: Work, stress and social support, Reading, Mass, 1981, Addison-Wesley Publishing Co, Inc.
Howard FM and Hill JM: Drugs in pregnancy, Obstet Gynecol Surv 34:643, 1979.
Hutchinson PL et al: Metabolic and circulatory responses to running during pregnancy, Phys Sportsmed 9:55, Aug 1981.
Iams JD, Johnson FF, and Creasy RK: Prevention of preterm birth, Clin Obstet Gynecol 31(3):599, Sept 1988.
Johnson FF: Assessment and education to prevent preterm labor, MCN 14(3):157, May/June 1989.
Jopke T: Pregnancy: a time to exercise judgment, Phys Sportsmed 11:139, July 1983.
Kay MA, editor: Anthropology of human birth, Philadelphia, 1982, FA Davis Co.
Kendall K: Maternal and child care in an Iranian village. In Leininger M, editor: Transcultural nursing, '79, New York, 1979, Masson Publishing USA.
Krozy RE et al: Auto safety, pregnancy and the newborn, JOGN Nurs 14:1, Jan/Feb 1985.
Leap TL et al: Equal employment opportunity and its implications for personnel practices in the 1980s, Labor Law J 31:669, 1980.
Lee RV: Understanding Southeast Asian mothers-to-be, Childbirth Educ 8(3):32, Spring 1989.
Lee RV et al: Southeast Asian folklore about pregnancy and parturition, Obstet Gynecol 71:243, 1988.
Leviton A: Caffeine consumption and the risk of reproductive hazards, J Reprod Med 33:175, 1988.
Luke B: Does caffeine influence reproduction? MCN 7:240, July/Aug 1982.
Malasanos L et al: Health assessment, ed 4, St Louis, 1990, The CV Mosby Co.
Marbury MC et al: Work and pregnancy, Occup Med vol. 26, 1984.
Martin BJ and Reeb RM: Oral health during pregnancy: a neglected nursing area, MCN 7:350, 1982.
Martin BJ and Reeb RM: The nurse as the first line of defense against periodontal disease, JOGN Nurs 12:333, 1983.
McCary JL: Human sexuality: physiological factors, ed 4, New York, 1982, Van Nostrand Reinhold Co, Inc.
McKay S: Smoking during the childbearing years, MCN 5:46, Jan/Feb 1980.
Meleis AI and Sorrell L: Bridging cultures: Arab American women and their birth experiences, MCN 6:171, 1981.
Mueller L: Pregnancy and sexuality, JOGN Nurs 14:4, July/Aug 1985.
NAACOG: Reproductive health hazards: women in the workplace, vol 11, Feb 1985, NAACOG, 600 Maryland Ave, SW Suite 2000, Washington, DC 20024.
Naeye RL: Coitus and associated amniotic-fluid infections, N Engl J Med 301:1198, 1979.
Naeye RL: Coitus and antepartum hemorrhage, Br J Obstet Gynecol 88:765, 1981.
Increasing culturally relevant practice with Hispanic clients, NPA Bulletin 3(4):23, Nov/Dec 1988.
Nicholson W: Midwives, mothers, and breastfeeding, Nursing Mothers Association of Australia, 5 Glendale St, Nunawading, Victoria 3131, 1985.
Page EW, Villee CA, and Villee DB: Human reproduction: essentials of reproductive and perinatal medicine, ed 3, Philadelphia, 1981, WB Saunders Co.
Riordan JM: A practical guide to breastfeeding, St Louis, 1983, The CV Mosby Co.
Ross MG et al: Breast stimulation contraction test. Presented at the annual meeting of the Society of Perinatal Obstetricians, San Antonio, Feb. 2-4, 1984.
Scott JR et al: Obstetrics and gynecology, ed 6, Philadelphia, 1990, JB Lippincott Co.
Seidel HM et al: Mosby's guide to physical examination, ed 2, St Louis, 1991, The CV Mosby Co.
Snow, L: Folk medical beliefs and their implications for care of patients, Ann Intern Med 81:82, 1974.
Stern, PM: Solving problems of cross-cultural health teaching: the Filipino childbearing family, Image 13:47, 1981.
Stringfellow, L: The Vietnamese. In Clark A, editor: Culture/childbearing/health professionals, Philadelphia, 1978, FA Davis Co.
Wright LM, and Leahey M: Nurses and families: a guide to family assessment and interaction, Philadelphia, 1984, FA Davis Co.
Zalar MK: Sexual counseling for pregnant couples, MCN 1:176, May/June 1976.
Zuspan FP, and Quilligan EJ, editors: Practical manual of obstetric care, St Louis, 1982, The CV Mosby Co.

Bibliography

Alexander LL: The pregnant smoker: nursing implications, JOGN Nurs 16(3):167, 1987.
Arneson S et al: Automobile seat belt practices of pregnant women, JOGN Nurs 15(4):330, 1986.
Bash D: Jewish religious practices related to childbearing, J Nurse Midwife 25(5):39, 1980.
Bentz JM: Missed meanings in nurse/patient communication, MCN 5:55, Jan/Feb 1980.
Bond MB: Reproductive hazards in the workplace, Contemp OB/GYN 28(3):57, 1986.
Brown MA: How fathers and mothers perceive prenatal support, MCN 12(6):414, 1987.
Brown MA: Marital support during pregnancy, JOGN Nurs 15(6):475, 1986.
Brown MA: Social support, stress and health: a comparison of expectant mothers and fathers, Nurs Res 35(2):72, 1986.
Brucker MC and Reedy NJ: Maternity leaves and the Pregnancy Discrimination Act, JOGN Nurs 12:341, 1983.
Bullard JA: Exercise and pregnancy, Can Fam Physician 27:977, 1981.
Carter ER: Quality maternity care for the medically indigent, MCN 11(2):85, 1986.
Chenger P and Kovacik A: Dental hygiene during pregnancy: a review, MCN 12(5):342, 1987.
Clinton JF: Physical and emotional responses of expectant fathers throughout pregnancy and the early postpartum period, Int J Nurs Stud 24(1):59, 1987.
Dameron GW: Helping couples cope with sexual changes pregnancy brings, Contemp Obstet Gynecol 21:23, Feb 1983.
Engstrom, JL: Measurement of fundal height, JOGN Nurs 17(3):172, 1988.
Fast A et al: Low-back pain in pregnancy, Spine 12(4):368, 1987.
Fawcett J and York R: Spouses physical and psychological symptoms during pregnancy and the postpartum, Nurs Res 35(4):144, 1986.

Foster SD: MCN patient teaching, MCN 12(2):131, 1987.
Gill PJ and Katz M: Early detection of preterm labor: ambulatory home monitoring of uterine activity, JOGN Nurs 15(6):439, 1986.
Gross C et al: The Vietnamese American family—and grandma makes three, MCN 6:177, May/June 1981.
Kulin J: Childbearing Cambodian refugee women, Can Nurs p 46, June 1988.
Lee PA: Health beliefs of pregnant and postpartum Hmong women, West J Nurs Res 8(1):83, 1986.
Lewallen LP: Health beliefs and health practices of pregnant women, JOGNN 18(3):245, May/June 1989.
Lindell SG: Education for childbirth: a time for change, JOGNN 17(2):108, March/April 1988.
May KA: Three phases of father involvement in pregnancy, Nurs Res 31:337, 1982.
Mercer RT: She's a multip . . . she knows the ropes, MCN 4:301, Sept/Oct 1979.
Miller SJ: Prenatal nursing assessment of the expectant family, Nurse Pract 11(5):40, 1986.
Moore L et al: Self-assessment: a personalized approach to nursing during pregnancy, JOGN Nurs 15(4):311, 1986.
Poole CJ: Fatigue during the first trimester of pregnancy, JOGN Nurs 15(5):375, 1986.
Queenan JT moderator: Managing pregnancy in patients over 35, Contemp OB/GYN 29(5):180, 1987.
Redman BK: The process of patient education, ed 6, St Louis, 1988, The CV Mosby Co.
Sherwen LN: Psychosocial dimensions of the pregnant family, New York, 1987, Springer Publishing Co, Inc.
Stainton MC: The fetus: a growing member of the family, Fam Relations 34:321, 1985.
Tucker SM et al: Patient care standards, ed 4, St. Louis, 1988, The CV Mosby Co.
Winslow W: First pregnancy after 35: what is the experience? MCN 12(2):92, 1987.

CHAPTER

11 Maternal and Fetal Nutrition

Mary Courtney Moore

Learning Objectives

Correctly define the key terms listed.

Explain optimum maternal weight gain during pregnancy focusing on nutritional values of foods eaten to achieve weight gain.

State recommended daily allowance (RDA) for kcal, protein, vitamins, and minerals during pregnancy.

Give examples of food sources of the nutrients required for optimum maternal nutrition during pregnancy.

Examine the role of nutritional supplements during pregnancy.

List five nutritional risk factors during pregnancy.

Give examples of cultural food patterns and possible dietary problems for two ethnic groups.

Evaluate nutritional status during pregnancy.

Outline and give examples of nursing care related to maternal and fetal nutrition based on the 5-step nursing process.

Key Terms

anemia
anthropometry
blood-forming nutrients
calories
fat-soluble vitamins
food cravings
food taboos
hypervitaminosis
intrauterine growth retardation (IUGR)
iron supplementation
kcal
ketonemia
lactose intolerance
megaloblastic anemia
nutrition risk factors
pattern of weight gain
physiologic anemia of pregnancy
pica
recommended daily allowances (RDAs)
vegetarian diets
water-soluble vitamins

According to the Policy Statement on Nutrition and Pregnancy issued by the American College of Obstetricians and Gynecologists (ACOG):

> A woman's nutritional status before, during and after pregnancy contributes to a significant degree to the well-being of both herself and her infant. Therefore, what a woman consumes before she conceives and while she carries the fetus is of vital importance to the health of succeeding generations.

Considerable resources and information are available to assist a woman in selecting foods and dietary patterns associated with a healthy pregnancy and a healthy outcome. Pregnancy is an especially good time to promote good nutrition since expectant parents may be highly motivated to change poor eating habits.

❑ NUTRITIONAL REQUIREMENTS

Weight Gain During Pregnancy

Optimum weight gain of the mother during pregnancy makes an important contribution to the pregnancy's successful course and outcome. The weight gained during a normal pregnancy will vary among individual women. The average acceptable weight gain for most healthy women of normal weight for height carrying a single fetus is 11 to 12.25 kg (24 to 27 lb). However, fetal outcome is best if women who are underweight before pregnancy gain more than this and women who are obese gain less (Naeye, 1979).

Some of the maternal weight gain is caused by deposition of fat—maternal stores laid down for energy to sustain fetal growth during the latter part of pregnancy and energy for lactation to follow. About 2 to 4 kg (4 to 8 lb) of fat are commonly deposited for these stores, presumably as the result of stimulus by progesterone acting centrally to reset a "lipostat" in the hypothalamus. When the pregnancy is over, the lipostat reverts to its usual nonpregnant level, and the added fat is lost. The average weight of the products of a normal pregnancy are given below.

Products	Weight
Fetus	3400 g (7.5 lb)
Placenta	450 g (1 lb)
Amniotic fluid	900 g (2 lb)
Uterus (weight increase)	1100 g (2.5 lb)
Breast tissue (weight increase)	1400 g (3 lb)
Blood volume (weight increase)	1800 g (4 lb) (1500 ml)
Maternal stores	1800 to 3600 g (4 to 8 lb)
TOTAL	11,000 to 13,000 g (11 to 13 kg; 24 to 28 lb)

Pattern of Weight Gain. The weight gain should be the result of a well-balanced diet in appropriate amounts for age, height, weight, and activity level. Regarding the woman's **pattern of weight gain,** there is general agreement that there should be little weight gain during the first trimester, a rapid increase during the second, and some slowing in the rate of increase during the third. During the first trimester, growth takes place almost entirely in maternal tissue, gain is primarily in maternal tissue during the second trimester and in fetal tissue in the third trimester. About 900 to 1800 g (2 to 4 lb) is an average gain during the first trimester. Thereafter, about 450 g (1 lb) a week during the remainder of the pregnancy is usual.

Deviations in Weight and Weight Gain. Deviations from usual values for either prepregnant weight or weight gain during pregnancy may contribute to adverse perinatal outcome. The following are considered to be deviations from the norm:

1. *Underweight:* prepregnant weight less than 85% of standard weight for age and height. Women who are underweight before pregnancy are more likely than women of normal weight to experience preterm labor and to deliver low-birth-weight (less than 2500 g) infants (Brown et al, 1981; Frentzen, Dimperio, and Cruz, 1988; and Frentzen, Johnson, and Simpson, 1988).
2. *Overweight:* prepregnant weight more than 120% of standard weight for age and height.
3. *Inadequate gain:* gain of 1 kg (2.2 lb) or less per month in the second or third trimester. Weight loss or failure to gain during pregnancy is a sign of nutritional difficulties.
4. *Excessive gain:* gain of 3 kg (6.6 lb) or more per month is likely to be caused by tissue fluid retention rather than by excessive caloric intake. A total weight gain of over 14.5 kg (32 lb) is associated with higher rates of perinatal mortality.

Hazards of Restricting Adequate Weight Gain. Young women in North America enter pregnancy already burdened by cultural obsession with thinness and "dieting." This conscious or unconscious pressure is difficult to dislodge. There are potential hazards, however, for both mother and infant from restricting weight gain during pregnancy. The mother's weight gain and prepregnancy weight are the two strongest influences (except gestational age) on birth weight. Infant birth weights, in turn, have been studied intensively with respect to infant mortality and morbidity, brain development, and learning disabilities in later life. Birth weights serve as practical indicators of the health and nutrition of a population.

The obese woman entering pregnancy faces an increased risk of severe complications, notably hypertensive disorders and diabetes mellitus, which have adverse effects on pregnancy outcome. Obesity should not be equated with overall good nutrition; excessive caloric ingestion may mask other nutritional problems (e.g., anemia, inadequate protein intake). Some persons have advocated restriction of weight gain in such women so that they conclude pregnancy with a net loss. However, the advisability of such a course seems questionable on several grounds. First, dietary restrictions to limit calories may also result in displacement of other nutrients from the diet. Second, optimum protein utilization in pregnancy apparently requires a minimum of approximately 30 kcal/kg/24 hours. This caloric allowance may be excessive, however, if calculated on obese weight. Usually the caloric allowance is based on the desirable weight for height or some intermediate value between the desirable and actual weight. Third, dietary restriction results in catabolism of fat stores, which in turn produces **ketonemia.** Ketonemia might jeopardize the development of the fetus.

Although the importance of adequate weight gain during pregnancy cannot be overemphasized, it is imperative that the pregnant woman not use pregnancy as an excuse for dietary excesses. The woman who gains 18 kg (40 lb) or more is likely to retain much of her weight gain after the birth of her infant (Olsen and Mundt, 1986; Greene et al, 1988). Because obesity and overweight are associated with heart disease, diabetes, and other chronic diseases, dietary counseling during pregnancy should focus on quality, rather than on weight gain alone (Abrams and Laros, 1986; Dohrmann and Lederman, 1986). If the nutritional education focuses positively on the necessity for supplying fetal nutritional needs, the weight gain focus usually becomes secondary.

Nutrient Needs

What nutrients must the mother take to supply the fetus and her own changing body optimumly for this critical gestation period?

During the first trimester (the first 3 months), the fetus is small, so the mother's relative nutrient requirements are increased slowly from normal adult needs. These nutrients are essential during this vital period; only the *quantitative* need for them is not yet greatly increased. The importance of a diet that contains balanced portions of essential nutrients according to individually assessed quantities continues into the second trimester.

The last trimester of pregnancy is the period during which a greater *amount* of key nutrients is required by the fetus, as it lays down stores for growth. This need for increased amounts of certain nutrients is indicated by the **recommended daily allowances (RDAs)** outlined

Table 11-1 **Nutritional Recommendations During Pregnancy**

	Nonpregnant Female RDA (18-24 yr)	RDA for Pregnancy/ Lactation	Reasons for Increased Need During Pregnancy	Food Sources
Calories	2100	2400/2740	Increased BMR,* energy needs; protein sparing†	Carbohydrates; fats; proteins
Protein	46 g	60 g/65 g	Rapid fetal tissue growth; amniotic fluid; placental growth and development; maternal tissue growth: uterus, breasts; increased maternal circulating blood volume: hemoglobin increase, plasma protein increase; maternal storage reserves for labor, delivery, and lactation	Milk; cheese; egg; meat; grains; legumes; nuts
Minerals				
Calcium	800 mg	1200 mg/1200 mg	Fetal skeleton formation; fetal tooth bud formation; increased maternal calcium metabolism	Milk; cheese; yogurt; leafy vegetables
Phosphorus	800 mg	1200 mg/1200 mg	Fetal skeletal formation; fetal tooth bud formation; increased maternal phosphorus metabolism	Milk; cheese; lean meats; yogurt; whole grains
Iron	15 mg	30+ mg (supplement usually required)/‡	Increased maternal circulating blood volume, increased hemoglobin; fetal liver iron storage (primarily in third trimester); high iron cost of pregnancy	Liver; meats; whole or enriched grain; leafy vegetables; nuts; legumes; dried fruits
Zinc	12 mg	15 mg/19 mg	Factor influencing growth	Wheat; bran; milk; liver; shellfish; meat
Iodine	150 μg	175 μg/200 μg	Increased BMR—increased thyroxine production	Iodized salt; sea food
Magnesium	280 mg	320 mg/355 mg	Coenzyme in energy and protein metabolism; enzyme activator; tissue growth, cell metabolism; muscle action	Nuts; soybeans; cocoa; seafood; whole grains; dried beans and peas

Adapted and revised from Williams SR: Nutritional guidance in prenatal care. In Worthington-Roberts BS and Williams SR: Nutrition in pregnancy and lactation, ed 4, St Louis, 1988, The CV Mosby Co. Food and Nutrition Board, RDAs, 10th ed, Research Council, National Academy Press, 1989.

*Basal metabolic rate.

†Provision of adequate nonprotein calories so that protein can be utilized for tissue synthesis and maintenance rather than energy needs.

‡Iron needs during lactation are not substantially different from those of nonpregnant women, but continued supplementation of the mother for 2 to 3 months after parturition is advisable to replenish stores depleted by pregnancy.

by the National Research Council (NRC) (Table 11-1). The recommended allowances provide a margin of safety above minimum requirements to allow for variations of need. For example, the reference woman in the typical RDA table is aged 18 to 24 years, weighs 58 kg (128 lb), is 164 cm (65 in) tall, lives in a temperate climate, and is a normally active, healthy woman. Variations from this state would need to be considered when providing counseling. The increased quantitative need for nourishment by pregnant adolescents should be noted (Chapter 27). The need for individual counseling and for therapeutic use of these recommendations as guidelines is clearly stated by the NRC:

> They are not called 'requirements' because they are not intended to represent merely literal (minimum) requirements of average individuals, but to cover substantially the individual variations in the requirements of normal people.

Table 11-1 Nutritional Recommendations During Pregnancy—cont'd

	Nonpregnant Female RDA (18-24 yr)	RDA for Pregnancy/ Lactation	Reasons for Increased Need During Pregnancy	Food Sources
Fat-soluble Vitamins				
A	800 RE* (4000 IU)	800 RE (4000 IU) 1300 RE (6500 IU)	Essential for cell development, hence tissue growth; tooth bud formation (development of enamel-forming cells in gum tissue); bone growth	Butter; cream; fortified margarine; green and yellow vegetables; liver
D	7.5 μg† (300 IU)	10 μg (400 IU)/ 10 μg (400 IU)	Absorption of calcium and phosphorus, mineralization of bone tissue, tooth buds	Fortified milk; fortified margarine; fish liver oils; egg yolk; butter; liver
E	8 mg alpha-TE‡	10 mg alpha-TE/ 12 mg alpha-TE	Tissue growth, cell wall integrity; red blood cell integrity	Vegetable oils; leafy vegetables; cereals; meat; egg; milk
Water soluble Vitamins				
C	60 mg	70 mg/95 mg	Tissue formation and integrity; cement substance in connective and vascular tissues; increases iron absorption	Citrus fruits; strawberries; melons; tomatoes; chili peppers; green peppers; green leafy vegetables; broccoli; potatoes
Folic acid (folacin)	180 μg	400 μg/280 μg	Increased metabolic demand in pregnancy; prevention of **megaloblastic anemia** in high-risk women; increased heme production for hemoglobin; production of cell nucleus material	Green leafy vegetables; oranges; bananas; liver; potatoes; cantaloupe
B_1 (thiamin)	1.1 mg	1.5 mg/1.6 mg	Coenzyme for energy metabolism	Pork, beef; liver; whole or enriched grains; legumes
B_2 (riboflavin)	1.3 mg	1.6 mg/1.8 mg	Coenzyme in energy metabolism and protein metabolism	Milk; liver; enriched grains; vegetables
B_6 (pyridoxine)	1.6 mg	2.2 mg/2.1 mg	Coenzyme in protein metabolism; increased fetal growth requirement	Wheat; corn; liver; meat
B_{12} (cobalamin)	2 μg	2.2 μg/2.6 μg	Coenzyme in protein metabolism, especially vital cell proteins such as nucleic acid; formation of red blood cells	Milk; egg; meat; liver; cheese
Niacin	15 mg	17 mg/20 mg	Coenzyme in metabolism	Meat; fish; poultry; liver; whole or enriched grains; peanuts

*Retinol equivalents (RE) replace international units (IU).
†400 IU (international units) = 10 μg of pure crystalline vitamin D_3 (cholecalciferol).
‡Total vitamin E activity, estimated to be 80% as alpha-tocopherol and 20% as other tocopherols.

In considering the needs of the normal pregnant woman, therefore, the nutrient elements should be reviewed in terms of the general amount of increased intake indicated, and why this increase is recommended. Factors to be considered include the following:

1. *Uterine-placental-fetal unit.* Placentas of poorly nourished mothers often contain fewer and smaller cells. Poorly developed placentas have a reduced ability to synthesize substances needed by the fetus, to facilitate flow of needed nutrients, and to inhibit passage to potentially harmful substances. Therefore it is understandable that the infant of a poorly nourished mother would be poorly nourished and small-for-gestational-age (SGA) (Chapter 28). Maternal uterine adaptations are discussed in Chapter 8.

2. *Maternal blood volume and constituents.* Total blood volume is known to increase about 33% above normal during pregnancy. Plasma volume increases 50% in nulliparas and more in multiparas. Red blood cell (RBC) production is stimulated during pregnancy. The number of RBCs increases gradually; the expansion of plasma volume proceeds rapidly. This rapid increase in plasma volume results in hemodilution and is referred to as **physiologic anemia of pregnancy.** At the same time, a deficiency of iron or of folic acid may contribute to the development of true **anemia.**

Blood levels of many nutrients, for example, total protein, decrease during pregnancy secondary to hemodilution. Most plasma lipid fractions rise during pregnancy. For example, cholesterol increases from under 200 mg/dl to between 250 and 300 mg/dl.

3. *Maternal mammary changes.* Preparation of mammary glands for lactation is presented in Chapter 18.

4. *Metabolic needs.* Basal metabolic rates (BMRs), when expressed as **kcal** per minute, are about 20% higher in pregnant women than in nonpregnant women. This increase includes the energy cost for tissue synthesis. The increased basal energy need over the entire pregnancy period plus the energy needed for new tissue brings the total energy cost for pregnancy to about 80,000 kcal, or about 300 kcal in 24 hours.

Water. Water as an essential nutrient is commonly overlooked during assessment. Among its many functions, water assists digestion by dissolving food and aiding its transport. Essential during the exchange of nutrients and wastes across cell membranes, water is the main substance of cells, blood, lymph, and other vital body fluids. It also aids in maintaining body temperature.

Drinking 6 to 8 glasses (1500 to 2000 ml) of water and juices every 24 hours is recommended. Other types of fluids may contain ingredients that are best used sparingly or omitted during pregnancy. For instance, caffeine-containing beverages should be discouraged, as should beverages containing the artificial sweetener saccharin. Although aspartame (Nutrasweet), another artificial sweetener, has not been found to have any adverse effects on the normal mother or fetus, its use should be avoided by pregnant women homozygous for phenylketonuria (London, 1988).

Protein. An additional daily allowance of 14 g of protein is recommended throughout pregnancy, raising the 46 g recommended for the normal nonpregnant woman to at least 60 g daily. This represents an increase of about 66%, or two thirds. For a large number of high-risk or active women, however, even more protein is needed—closer to 100 g or about double their previous allowance.

Protein, with its essential constituent, nitrogen, is the nutritional element that is basic to growth. More protein is essential to meet the demands posed by the rapid growth of the fetus; by the enlargement of the uterus, mammary glands, and placenta; by the increase in maternal circulating blood volume and the subsequent demand for increased plasma protein to maintain colloidal osmotic pressure; and by the formation of amniotic fluid and storage reserves for labor, delivery, and lactation.

Milk, meat, eggs, and cheese are complete protein foods of high biologic value. Protein-rich foods also contribute other nutrients such as calcium, iron, and B vitamins. The amounts of these foods that would supply the quantities of protein needed are indicated in the recommended daily food plan (Table 11-2). Additional protein may be obtained from legumes, whole grains, and nuts.

Recommended protein intake is adjusted to the body size of individuals. The following guidelines are suggested:

1. Mature women: 1.3 g protein per kg of pregnant weight
2. Adolescent girls (15 to 18 years of age): 1.5 g protein per kg of pregnant weight
3. Younger girls: 1.7 g protein per kg of pregnant weight

The greater protein intake recommended for adolescents and younger girls is needed to support possible continued maturation. If a multifetal birth (e.g., twins) is expected, additional protein and other nutrients are also needed in the mother's diet.

Calories. Calories should be sufficient to meet energy and nutrient demands and to spare protein for tissue building. Classic studies indicate that a minimum of 36 calories per kg of body weight is required for efficient use of protein during pregnancy. Although only 300 calories additional to the amount ingested by the nonpregnant woman is recommended by the NRC, representing about a 10% to 15% increase over the usual previous intake, this amount is insufficient for

Table 11-2 Daily Food Plan for Pregnancy and Lactation

Food	Nonpregnant Woman	Pregnant Woman	Lactating Woman
Milk, yogurt, cheese, ice cream, skimmed milk or buttermilk (food made with milk can supply part of requirement)	2 C	3-4 C	4-5 C
Meat (lean meat, fish, poultry, cheese, dried beans or peas*)	1 serving (3-4 oz)	2 servings (6-8 oz); include liver frequently	2½ servings (8 oz)
Eggs	1	1-2	1-2
Vegetable† (dark green or deep yellow)	1 serving	1 serving	1-2 servings
Vitamin C–rich food† Good source—citrus fruit, broccoli, strawberries, cantaloupe Fair source—tomatoes, cabbage, greens, potatoes in skin	1 good source or 2 fair sources	1 good source and 1 fair source or 2 good sources	1 good source and 1 fair source or 2 good sources
Other vegetables and fruits	2 servings	4-6 servings	4-6 servings
Bread‡ and cereals (enriched or whole grain)	4-6 servings	6-10 servings	6-10 servings
Butter or fortified margarine	Moderate amount	Moderate amount	Moderate amount

Adapted from Williams SR: Nutrition and diet therapy, ed 6, St Louis, 1989, The CV Mosby Co.
*¾-1 C equals 1 serving.
†Use some raw daily.
‡One slice of bread or ½ cup grain equals 1 serving.

many active or nutritionally deficient women, who may easily need as much as 2500 to 3000 calories a day. The emphasis should be a positive one on ample calories to ensure nutrient and energy needs, not a negative idea of restricting calories.

Minerals

Iron. The changes in maternal red blood volume and cell mass accompanying pregnancy represent a fundamental physiologic adjustment. Since full-term average-for-gestational-age (AGA) infants are born with high hemoglobin levels of 18 to 22 g/dl and with a supply of iron stored in the liver to last 3 to 6 months, the maternal organism must transfer about 300 mg of iron to the fetus during gestation.

If dietary iron is not available to meet the needs of the maternal-placental-fetal unit, fetal iron reserves will not be impaired but maternal iron stores will be depleted and maternal red cell mass will be reduced. If the mother has no iron reserves, which occurs commonly in young women, especially teenagers, maternal hemoglobin levels will drop more than usual and iron-deficiency anemia may be superimposed on the physiologic anemia of pregnancy. **Iron supplementation** is usually started at the first prenatal visit to maintain maternal reserves and to meet fetal requirements during pregnancy (see guidelines for client teaching, p. 310).

Calcium. Almost all the additional calcium required during pregnancy is utilized by the fetus. Because it is virtually impossible to meet these requirements with foods other than dairy products, milk is considered by many to be particularly essential during pregnancy. One liter of milk contains 1200 mg of calcium, precisely the amount suggested in the RDAs. Individuals who do not consume milk or milk products—for example, persons with **lactose** (milk sugar) **intolerance** or dislike of dairy foods—will require calcium supplementation.

Calcium and phosphorus are found in the same foods. If calcium needs are met, adequate phosphorus will be assured.

Sodium. During pregnancy there is a slight increase in the need for most nutrients, including sodium. Routine restriction of sodium is unphysiologic and unfounded. Diets low in calories and sodium place the normal mother and her fetus at unnecessary risk. When sodium is restricted, the maternal organism undergoes a series of hormonal and biochemical changes in an effort to conserve sodium.

Sources of excessive sodium are discouraged, however, since excess sodium may contribute to fluid retention and edema. Excessive sodium is found in many canned and processed foods. Products devoid of nutritive value and excessively high in sodium include pretzels, potato chips, soft drinks, and bouillon cubes. Hidden sources of sodium are present in medications such as bicarbonate of soda. Some people are unaware that table salt contains sodium.

Zinc. The metal zinc is a constituent of numerous enzymes involved in major metabolic pathways. It may be noteworthy that maternal zinc deficiency is highly teratogenic in rats. The incidence of malformations of the central nervous system (CNS) in humans appears to be increased in geographic areas where zinc deficiency is prevalent.

Large intakes of iron and folic acid interfere with absorption of zinc and decrease serum zinc levels (Hambidge et al, 1988). Since iron and folic acid supplements are commonly prescribed during pregnancy, pregnant women should be encouraged to consume good sources of zinc daily (see Table 11-1).

Fat-soluble Vitamins. *Because of the high potential for toxicity, gravidas are advised to take fat-soluble vitamin supplements only as prescribed.*

Vitamin A. The added allowance of vitamin A for pregnancy relates to fetal storage of the vitamin. The RDA can readily be provided by dietary sources. There appears to be no need for routine supplementation. Certain food faddists advocate massive amounts of vitamin A. Pregnant women should be cautioned against this practice. Toxicity related to **hypervitaminosis** A represents a potential danger to both the pregnant woman (liver damage) and to her unborn child (congenital malformations).

Vitamin D. Vitamin D plays an important role in promoting positive calcium balance in pregnancy. It is present naturally in only a few animal foods such as fish liver oils, eggs, butter, and liver. The main food sources are enriched or fortified foods. It is also produced in the skin by the action of ultraviolet light (irradiation) on dehydrocholesterol. Excessive amounts in the mother may cause hypervitaminosis D expressed as hypercalcemia in infants. Since most milk in the United States is fortified with vitamin D at a level of 10 μg per quart, the daily consumption of a quart of milk provides the full allowance of vitamin D and of calcium as well for most gravidas.

Water-soluble Vitamins. The **water-soluble vitamins,** in contrast to those soluble in fat, are readily excreted in urine. The daily diet must supply the RDA because storage is limited. Toxicity with overdosage is less likely than with fat-soluble vitamins.

Folic Acid. The augmented maternal erythropoiesis of pregnancy requires substantially increased amounts of folic acid (folacin). Moreover, because folic acid is intimately involved in DNA synthesis, requirements are particularly high in rapidly growing cells such as fetal and placental tissues. In view of the evidence indicating increased folic acid needs during pregnancy and dietary survey data suggesting that the usual American diet is marginal in folic acid content, authorities have advised routine folic acid supplementation for pregnant women. Evidence suggests that neural tube defects may be more common in infants of women deficient in folic acid.

Other B Vitamins. An important function of thiamin (vitamin B_1), riboflavin (B_2), pyridoxine (B_6), and cobalamin (vitamin B_{12}) is that of coenzyme in metabolism. Suggested increased RDAs during pregnancy can usually be provided by the diet. Low maternal levels of vitamin B_{12} are associated with prematurity and occur more often in smokers than in nonsmokers.

Ascorbic Acid (Vitamin C). The entire requirement of vitamin C may be readily provided by dietary sources. Pregnant women should be cautioned against unprescribed use of any vitamin preparation, including vitamin C. The possibility of beneficial effects of extremely large ascorbic acid supplements for prevention of the common cold has created considerable interest. Aside from the controversial aspect of this type of pharmacologic treatment, its use in pregnancy is open to serious question.

Vitamin and Mineral Supplements. Nutrition counselors (nurses, nutritionists) must assess whether the woman has sufficient knowledge, motivation, and income to follow the nutrition guidance given. If needs can be met through diet, vitamin and mineral supplementation may not be necessary. For some gravidas a careful selection of vitamin and mineral supplements is of some value if problems are anticipated. It must be noted that supplementation cannot compensate for poor food habits. In some instances the prescriptions of supplements may give both the woman and the health care professional a false sense of security.

NUTRITION RISK FACTORS IN PREGNANCY

To assess effectively the nutritional status of the pregnant or lactating woman, the nutrition counselor needs to understand the major **nutrition risk factors.** Nutrition risk factors include those present at the onset of pregnancy and those that may occur during the course of pregnancy.

Risk Factors at the Onset of Pregnancy

See Chapter 27 for a discussion of the nutrition risk factors for pregnant adolescents.

The woman who has had three or more pregnancies within 2 years, as well as the multiparous woman who has progressed from one pregnancy directly to another, is considered to be at increased risk. These women are prone to depleted nutrient stores. This situation can potentially compromise maternal and fetal health and well-being.

Special attention should be paid to the woman's obstetric history. Poor weight gain in pregnancy, pregnancy-induced hypertension (PIH), a previous stillbirth or delivery of a low-birth-weight infant, premature delivery, and perinatal infection are all common in women who are or have been poorly nourished in the past. As a result the woman with a poor reproductive history may need more than usual nutrition guidance.

For economically deprived women there are several programs that help with the purchase of food or that offer supplements, for example, the federal food stamp program and the supplemental food program for women, infants, and children, sometimes known as the WIC program.

A woman may enter pregnancy either having been or continuing to be on a faddish or otherwise nutritionally inadequate diet. Although carefully planned **vegetarian diets** may be completely adequate, the pregnant vegetarian requires careful assessment.

There is also always the possibility that women who indulge excessively in the use of cigarettes, drugs, or alcohol may not consume sufficient quantities of nutritious food. (For detailed discussion, see Chapter 25 and Appendix F).

Medical problems such as anemia, thyroid dysfunction, and chronic medical or surgical gastrointestinal disorders may be associated with interference of ingestion, absorption, or utilization of nutrients. Drugs utilized in treatment of these conditions may also affect nutrition by similar interference. Nutrition counseling should combine general nutrition guidelines for prenatal care *and* diet therapy recommended for a particular woman's medical condition.

Risk Factors During Pregnancy

The iron needed during pregnancy is obtained from maternal iron stores, diet, and supplementation. True anemia occurring during pregnancy is often caused by iron deficiency. Many healthy American women do not have iron stores large enough to meet the demands of pregnancy. Iron supplementation will aid greatly in maintaining the hemoglobin at normal levels.

The cause of PIH is not known. It is characterized by an elevation in blood pressure, proteinuria, and rapid weight gain caused by edema. There is considerable controversy over the influence of nutrition (particularly sodium and protein) on the development of PIH (Zlatnik, 1983; Worthington-Roberts, 1985).

Normal pregnancy is a time of progressive maternal weight gain. The following are presumptive signs of maternal and fetal malnutrition: (1) failure to gain weight (less than 0.9 kg [2 lb] per month during the second and third trimesters), (2) actual weight loss, (3) significant nausea and vomiting during early pregnancy, and (4) poor or delayed uterine-fetal growth.

Inadequate maternal weight gain has been associated with lowered birth weight and evidence of **intrauterine growth retardation (IUGR).** It is therefore important to document the pattern of weight gain in pregnancy, as well as the total amount gained.

Total maternal weight gain during the 40 weeks of pregnancy averages 11.5 kg (25 lb). This amounts to about 1.4 to 1.8 kg (3 to 4 lb) per month. Rapid accumulation of weight in a singleton pregnancy—that is, 0.9 to 2.3 kg (2 to 5 lb) per week results usually from tissue fluid retention and may be associated with PIH. The woman must be assessed carefully for development of this condition.

Excessive weight gain associated with accumulation of fat is less dramatic and is best assessed by evaluating the woman's eating habits and by measuring subcutaneous fat stores by means of skinfold calipers. Sources of energy-rich but nutritionally poor food should be identified and eliminated and moderate exercise should be encouraged if there is no contraindication. Weight reduction in pregnancy or lactation by dietary manipulation or drug administration or both is contraindicated because of potentially adverse and possibly toxic effects on fetal nutrition, growth, and development.

Demands of Lactation

Increased nutritional demands of lactation can also be a risk factor. Storage of 2 or 3 kg of fat during pregnancy provides the gravida with a reservoir of some 14,000 to 24,000 kcal for lactation needs. Ordinarily, fat stores will be gradually utilized for the first 4 to 6 months of lactation.

Without the demands of nursing, fat stores may remain a permanent addition to the maternal frame and increase the potential for obesity with advancing age and parity. A modest reduction in caloric intake after delivery is appropriate for the woman who does not breastfeed her infant. This is particularly true if she uses an oral contraceptive agent. For discussion of nutrition and oral hormone contraception refer to Chapter 6.

❑ NURSING PROCESS IN NUTRITIONAL CARE

Adequate nutrition is vital throughout the life span. During pregnancy, nutrition plays a key role in achieving an optimum outcome for the mother and her unborn baby. Motivation to learn about nutrition is usually higher during pregnancy, as parents strive to "do what's right for the baby." Optimum nutrition cannot eliminate all problems that may arise in pregnancy, but it establishes a good foundation for supporting the needs of the mother and her unborn child.

Assessment

An individual assessment and evaluation of nutritional status must be made at the beginning of prenatal care and continued throughout the pregnancy. The following methods of assessment provide the data necessary to determine need:

1. Interview (individual and family history, dietary assessment)
2. Physical examination, including assessment for skinfold thickness
3. Laboratory tests

Interview

Health History. Data from the pregnant woman's history are among the most important elements in nutrition assessment. These data must include basic information carefully taken from the prenatal record; data that have a bearing on nutritional status. From the obstetric history it is important to note the woman's age, number of pregnancies and their outcomes, and the interval between pregnancies. Several medical problems have nutritional implications. These problems include diabetes mellitus, cystic fibrosis, phenylketonuria (PKU), anemia, and lactose intolerance (White and Owsley, 1983).

Social and Experiential History. Food habits and attitudes cannot be viewed in isolation: life situations and values, as well as physical and emotional factors, must also be considered. Thus if nutrition counseling is to be valid, it must be based on an individual plan of care.

A woman's living situation will have an influence on her eating behavior. Therefore the data on the home setting, housing, life-style, family members, occupation, socioeconomic status, food assistance needs, and family roles and attitudes concerning foods are important.

Nutrition-related folklore and myths need to be identified. Some beliefs may prevent the gravida from complying with sound nutritional guidelines. Cultural-ethnic food and religious practices need to be explored.

It is important to determine special diet practices such as faddish or unusual patterns. Strict vegetarian diets or various forms of pica may be nutritionally unsound. **Pica** refers to the regular and excessive ingestion of nonfood items (e.g., laundry starch or red clay) or of foods with limited nutritional value (e.g., cornstarch) (p. 303).

The use of *all* medications and vitamin and mineral supplements should be discussed with the woman.

Food allergies and milk or lactose intolerance need to be explored (White and Owsley, 1983). Lactose intolerance is a problem for certain individuals and ethnic groups, including blacks, Orientals, and Eskimos. The nurse's help is often needed for the family to plan for protein and calcium intake from sources other than milk. Tofu (soybean curd) and dark molasses contain considerable calcium but no lactose. Of the cheeses, Swiss contains the least lactose. Commercial enzyme preparations are available to hydrolyze (digest) the lactose in milk.

Dietary Assessment. A *nutrition questionnaire* covering the background information is a useful tool in dietary assessment. The California Department of Health Services (1975) developed an excellent instrument to be used specifically by the physician, nurse, or registered dietitian. The nutrition questionnaire groups questions into 11 sections that identify factors that may influence prenatal nutrition (see box, p. 299).

Additional information is gathered with the following questions. How many meals and snacks are served per day and how are these spaced? What is a typical menu? What quantities are served? How are foods selected and cooked? What is the woman's level of understanding of good nutrition? What does she consider to be "good nutrition"? What does she perceive as nutritional problems and solutions?

Several functional gastrointestinal problems are common during pregnancy. Nausea and vomiting, constipation and hemorrhoids, heartburn, or a full feeling may interfere with optimum nutrition. These complaints are highly individual in character. Their existence is usually uncovered during the review of the physical systems.

NUTRITION QUESTIONNAIRE

Name: ______________________________ Date: __________

Please answer the following by checking the appropriate box or filling in the blank. Answer only those questions that apply to you. All information is confidential.

1. a. Before this pregnancy, what was your usual weight? ________ kg (________ lb)
   ☐ Don't know
   b. During your last pregnancy, how much weight did you gain? ________ kg (________ lb)
   ☐ Don't know
   c. How much weight do you expect to gain during this pregnancy? ________ kg (________ lb)
   ☐ Don't know
   d. Have you ever had any problems with your weight?
   ☐ Yes ☐ No If yes, what? ☐ Underweight
   ☐ Overweight ☐ Other ________
2. a. How would you describe your appetite?
   ☐ Hearty ☐ Moderate ☐ Poor
   b. With this pregnancy, have you experienced either of the following? ☐ Nausea ☐ Vomiting
3. How would you describe your regular eating habits?
   ☐ Regular ☐ Irregular
4. a. Indicate the person who does the following in your household:
   Plans the meals ________
   Buys the food ________
   Prepares the food ________
   b. How much is spent on food each week for your household? ________ ☐ Don't know
   How many people does this feed? ________
   c. Indicate the type of kitchen equipment you have in your home:
   ☐ Refrigerator ☐ Hot plate ☐ Stove
5. a. Are you *now* taking any vitamin or mineral supplement?
   ☐ Yes ☐ No
   b. Do you take any pills to control your weight?
   ☐ Yes ☐ No
   c. Do you take diuretic (water) pills?
   ☐ Yes ☐ No
6. a. Are you now on a diet to lose weight?
   ☐ Yes ☐ No
   b. Are you *now* on a special diet (low salt, diabetic, gallbladder, etc.)?
   ☐ Yes ☐ No
   If yes, what kind of diet? ________
   c. If you have been on a special diet in the past, indicate what kind and when. ________
7. a. Is there any food you *cannot* eat?
   ☐ Yes ☐ No
   If yes, what food(s)? ________
   What happens when you eat this food? ________
   b. Do you have any cravings for things such as
   ☐ Cornstarch ☐ Plaster ☐ Dirt or clay
   ☐ Other ________
8. Do you have either of the following problems?
   ☐ Constipation ☐ Diarrhea
9. a. Do you smoke? ☐ Yes ☐ No
   b. Do you drink any alcoholic beverages (liquor, wine, beer)? ☐ Yes ☐ No
10. Are you receiving either of the following?
   ☐ Food stamps ☐ WIC vouchers
11. How do you want to feed your baby?
   ☐ Breast milk ☐ Evaporated milk formula
   ☐ Commercial formula ☐ Undecided

Adapted from Nutrition during pregnancy and lactation, Sacramento, Calif, 1975, Maternal and Child Health Branch, California Department of Health Services.

Physical Examination

Two problems bear on the validity of the physical examination. First, the lack of standard definitions and the nonspecificity of most clinical manifestations of malnutrition result in considerable variation in interpretation of physical signs. Second, pregnancy may complicate specific interpretation of physical signs. Despite these shortcomings the physical assessment of nutritional status can be useful if it is utilized in conjunction with the biochemical analyses and dietary assessment (Table 11-3).

General screening for *dental health status* provides helpful information on nutritional status. The most common clinical nutrition-related disorders that are likely to be encountered during the reproductive years are caries and periodontitis. These conditions cause mechanical and mastication difficulties that interfere with the ingestion of certain types of food.

Anthropometry, the study of human body measurements, provides both short- and long-term indications of the level of nutrition and is therefore a valuable component of the nutrition assessment profile. Assessment of height, weight, and skinfold thickness is performed. Care must be taken to ensure that proper equipment and techniques are used for anthropometric assessment; for example, the scale is calibrated to zero

Table 11-3 Physical Assessment of Nutritional Status

Signs of Good Nutrition	Signs of Poor Nutrition
General appearance	
Alert, responsive	Listless, apathetic, cachectic
Weight	
Normal for height, age, body build	Overweight or underweight
Posture	
Erect, arms and legs straight	Sagging shoulders, sunken chest, humped back
Muscles	
Well developed, firm, good tone, some fat under skin	Flaccid, poor tone, undeveloped, tender, "wasted" appearance, cannot walk properly
Nervous control	
Good attention span, not irritable or restless, normal reflexes, psychologic stability	Inattentive, irritable, confused, burning and tingling of hands and feet, loss of position and vibratory sense, weakness and tenderness of muscles, decrease or loss of ankle and knee reflexes
Gastrointestinal function	
Good appetite and digestion, normal regular elimination, no palpable organs or masses	Anorexia, indigestion, constipation or diarrhea, liver or spleen enlargement
Cardiovascular function	
Normal heart rate and rhythm, no murmurs, normal blood pressure for age	Rapid heart rate, enlarged heart, abnormal rhythm, elevated blood pressure
General vitality	
Endurance, energetic, sleeps well, vigorous	Easily fatigued, no energy, looks tired, apathetic
Hair	
Shiny, lustrous, firm, not easily plucked, healthy scalp	Stringy, dull, brittle, dry, thin and sparse, depigmented, can be easily plucked
Skin (general)	
Smooth, slightly moist, good color	Rough, dry, scaly, pale, pigmented, irritated, easily bruised, petechiae

Adapted from Williams SR: Nutritional guidance in prenatal care. In Worthington-Roberts BS and Williams SR: Nutrition in pregnancy and lactation, ed 4, St Louis, 1988, The CV Mosby Co.

before a weight is taken. Skinfolds are measured with calipers and are best obtained by specially trained nurses or registered dietitians.

Measurements of weight-for-age and weight-for-height are used in assessing obesity, but they do fail to distinguish muscular and skeletal tissue mass from fat. On the other hand, serial weight measurements give a reasonable indication of excessive weight gain and likely obesity.

Lean body mass can be estimated from the triceps skinfold thickness and upper arm circumference. Measurement of skinfold thickness is the most convenient method of objectively assessing relative fatness. In general, two skinfold measurements, one on a limb (left triceps) and one on the trunk (left subscapular), are advised to account for differing distributions of fat.

Erroneous information regarding specific indices such as height and weight measurements can lead to inappropriate conclusions. An incomplete or inaccurate data base can result in poor decisions and client care management.

Laboratory Tests

Laboratory data provide vital baseline information for nutrition assessment at the beginning of pregnancy as well as a means of monitoring nutritional status throughout gestation.

Blood-forming Nutrients. Measures of the **blood-forming nutrients**—iron, folacin, and vitamin B_{12}—are important guides for use in preventing and treating anemias often associated with pregnancy (Chapter 23). The following can be measured in routine tests:

1. Hemoglobin levels
2. Hematocrit levels
3. Mean corpuscular volume (MCV)
4. Mean corpuscular hemoglobin concentration (MCHC)

Table 11-3 Physical Assessment of Nutritional Status—cont'd

Signs of Good Nutrition	Signs of Poor Nutrition
Face and neck	
Skin color uniform, smooth, pink, healthy appearance, not swollen	Greasy, discolored, scaly, swollen, skin dark over cheeks and under eyes, lumpiness or flakiness of skin around nose and mouth
Lips	
Smooth, good color, moist, not chapped or swollen	Dry, scaly, swollen, redness, angular lesions at corners of mouth, fissured, scarred
Mouth, oral membranes	
Reddish pink mucous membranes in oral cavity	Swollen, boggy oral mucous membranes
Gums	
Reddish pink, healthy, no swelling or bleeding	Spongy, bleed easily, marginal redness, inflamed, gums receding
Tongue	
Healthy pink or deep reddish in appearance, not swollen or smooth, surface papillae present, no lesions	Swollen, scarlet and raw, magenta color, beefy, hyperemic and hypertrophic papillae, atrophic papillae
Teeth	
No cavities, no pain, bright, straight, no crowding, well-shaped jaw, clean, no discoloration	Unfilled caries, absent teeth, worn surfaces, mottled, malpositioned
Eyes	
Bright, clear, shiny, no sores at corners of eyelids, membranes moist and healthy pink color, no prominent blood vessels or mound of tissue on sclera, no fatigue circles beneath	Eye membranes pale, redness of membrane, dryness, signs of infection, Bitot's spots, redness and fissuring of eyelid corners, dryness of eye membrane, dull appearance of cornea, soft cornea, blue sclerae
Neck (glands)	
No enlargement	Thyroid enlarged
Nails	
Firm, pink	Spoon shaped, brittle, ridged
Legs, Feet	
No tenderness, weakness, or swelling; good color	Edema, tender calf, tingling, weakness
Skeleton	
No malformations	Bowlegs, knock-knees, chest deformity at diaphragm, beaded ribs, prominent scapulas

5. Serum iron levels and percentage of concentration in saturation
6. Transferrin levels

Other tests include those for vitamin deficiency:

1. MCV
2. Hypersegmented polymorphonuclear leukocytes
3. Serum folic acid
4. RBC folic acid
5. Serum vitamin B_{12}

Serum Albumin. An adequate level of serum albumin is important during pregnancy. Serum albumin helps maintain normal flow of tissue fluids from the circulating blood through the tissue for nourishment of cells and back into circulation by means of capillary fluid shift mechanisms. A protein deficit would contribute to a lowered plasma albumin level and in turn to an imbalance in the fluid shift mechanism, resulting in edema. Hemodilution usually lowers albumin levels during pregnancy. An acceptable level of serum albumin during pregnancy is 3.2 g/dl or above.

Minerals and Vitamins. Depending on individual situations, tests for other vitamin and mineral levels may be performed, including determinations of the water-soluble vitamins (thiamin, riboflavin, niacin, and vitamin C), the fat-soluble vitamins (A, D, E, and K), and trace minerals.

Blood Lipids, Glucose, and Enzymes. Routine testing for urine sugar and ketone bodies is often done to screen for latent diabetes mellitus or gestational glycosuria. However, more definitive tests are necessary for accurate assessment for endocrine disturbances such as diabetes mellitus (Chapter 24). Other tests may be performed, if there is a complicating chronic disease, particularly cardiovascular or renal disease.

Nursing Diagnoses

Each gravida and her family will present the nurse with a unique set of nutritional needs. The nurse formulates appropriate nursing diagnoses based on the identified needs from the assessment data. Following are examples of nutrition-related nursing diagnoses arising from the course of prenatal period:

Altered nutrition, less than body requirements, related to
- Imbalance of intake versus activity expenditures
- Inability to procure food (related to finances or cultural proscription)
- Chewing difficulties secondary to poor dental hygiene

Knowledge deficit related to
- Adequate nutrition or reliance on vitamin-mineral supplementation
- Pica
- Nutrition-related discomforts of pregnancy
- Cultural "superstition"
- Iron supplementation

Potential for injury: fetus, related to
- Overdoses of vitamins

See guidelines for client teaching and nursing care plan in this chapter.

Planning

The information in this chapter is general in nature. A plan is developed for each gravida utilizing content that relates specifically to her and her family's nutritional needs. Collaboration among the nurse, the registered dietitian, and the client is basic to the following step in the nursing process: setting the goals in client-centered terms, prioritizing the goals, and selecting nursing actions that will help the client meet the goals.

The Health Team Approach

The health team approach has been devised as an attempt to meet some of the problems brought about by the rapid increase in population and the equally rapid expansion of scientific knowledge, which has brought an increasing complexity to health care. The rapid advance of science requires the cooperation of a team of specialists who share their special knowledge and learn from each other for the welfare of the client.

Whether functioning in the hospital, the clinic, or the community, the registered dietitian (RD) and the nurse hold positions on the health team in a unique relation to the client. In certain respects they are closest to the client and the family and have the opportunity to help determine many of the client's needs, which include basic nutritional requirements. They must coordinate services and often are the only ones who can help the client understand and participate in her care. They have unparalleled opportunity to practice continuous client-centered care that treats the whole person.

Such practitioners are concerned not merely with the *how* but also with the *why*. More pointedly still, they are concerned with the *who* and realize that their most therapeutic contribution is their genuine involvement and concern. The nurse plays a critical role in providing individualized care by assessing the client, consulting with other members of the health care team and sharing information with them, and referring the client as appropriate.

General ***goals*** directed to the maternity population as a whole include the following:

1. To provide nutrition-related services for all pregnant women and their fetuses or newborns and families
2. To ensure optimum nutrition for women of childbearing age
3. To ensure optimum nutrition for the gravida and her fetus
4. To involve the woman as a participant in her own care

Implementation

Nurses assume many caregiving roles during the prenatal period including supportive and teacher/counselor/advocate.

Supportive Activities

The nurse-client relationship is important in setting the tone for further interactions (Chapter 2). The techniques of listening with an attentive expression, touching, and using eye contact have their place, as does recognition of the client's feelings and her right to express them. One common complaint of gravidas is the weighing-in at the start of a prenatal visit. Weighing-in should be ego-building and psychologically unthreatening. Many women state that they "shake in their boots" while waiting to hear remarks of disgust and condemnation for gaining too much. To avoid this disapproval, some starve themselves the evening before the visit or take diuretics ("water pills"). Both alternatives are detrimental to the health of the mother and her unborn child (Dohrmann and Lederman, 1986).

Nutrition counseling provides the nurse the opportunity to commend the gravida for her knowledge and use of good nutrition practices. The nurse can help the woman set her own goals and make her own decisions.

Teacher/Counselor/Advocate

There are several tools that are useful in providing nutrition information and guidance to the pregnant woman. The tools include a daily food guide, a sample meal pattern and sample menus, and information on ethnic preferences and vegetarian diets.

Daily Food Guide. A diet consisting of a variety of foods from all the basic food groups can supply needed nutrients (see Table 11-2). The increased quantities of essential nutrients needed during pregnancy may be met by skillful planning around a daily food guide based on the RDAs.

It is necessary to show the woman how the daily food guide can be used. Sample daily meal patterns and sample menus are very helpful. A mutually developed plan is more likely to be followed by the client. Gravidas find a collaboratively written shopping list helpful in implementing the planned menus.

Ethnic and Cultural Influences. Consideration of a woman's cultural food preferences enhances the communication between her and her counselor, thus providing a greater opportunity to obtain compliance with a prescribed diet. However, within one cultural group there may occur several variations. Women in most cultures are encouraged to eat a normal diet. The nurse needs to know what constitutes a normal diet for each ethnic group. Thus careful exploration of individual preferences is needed (Table 11-4). The emphasis of counseling is to build an adequate diet utilizing the woman's usual foods and food preferences. To do otherwise is to waste time and energy for both the woman and the nurse.

Although ethnic and cultural food beliefs may conflict with the dietary instruction provided by physicians, nurses, and dietitians, it is often possible for the empathic health care provider to identify cultural beliefs that are congruent with the modern understanding of pregnancy and fetal development. For instance, Southeast Asian folklore discourages alcohol consumption during pregnancy (Lee et al, 1988). Dietary instruction can reinforce and build on this prohibition.

Food taboos are more common than food prescriptions. Vietnamese women are to avoid "unclean" foods such as beef, dog, rat, and snake meat (Hollingsworth et al, 1980). Japanese women are cautioned against hot, spicy, and salty food, as are Filipino and Southeast Asian women. Blacks in the southern United States, Guatemalans, Mexicans, and Mexican-Americans may not eat acid foods or fresh fruits and vegetables (Kay, 1982).

Food taboos often follow the principles of imitative magic, in which physical characteristics of food eaten by the mother may be transmitted to the child. Filipinos avoid eating prunes (Affonso, 1978) and Chinese avoid eating soy sauce (Campbell and Chang, 1973), in both instances to prevent a dark-skinned infant. Campbell and Chang (1973) report that some Chinese mothers shun shellfish during the first trimester, believing it is responsible for allergies in the latter life of the child.

Food cravings during pregnancy are considered normal by many cultures, but the kinds of cravings may be culturally specific (Obeyesekere, 1963; Carrington, 1978). In most cultures women crave acceptable foods, such as chicken, fish, and greens among blacks (Carrington, 1978). Affonso (1978) notes that the Filipinos believe cravings should be satisfied to prevent the premature arrival of the infant.

Women in some cultures desire nonnutritive substances such as laundry starch, clay, and dirt. Desiring or eating of these substances is called **pica**. Causes of pica have been attributed to a variety of reasons and may be engaged in by children, as well as pregnant women. Pica may be a psychologic response of someone needing attention, a truly cultural phenomenon, a response to hunger, or the body's response to needed nutrients. Scientific controversy exists about whether the iron deficiency observed in persons with pica is the cause or the effect of the anemia. Whatever the reason, according to Leiderman et al (1977), a documented sequela is increased iron deficiency anemia because of interference with absorption of necessary nutrients when clay is eaten.

Vegetarian Diet Practices. Vegetarianism has gained popularity in recent years. Foods basic to almost all vegetarian diets are vegetables, fruits, legumes, nuts, and grains.

Vegetarian diets may not satisfy all nutrient requirements for the pregnant or lactating woman. There are several types of vegetarian diets:

1. *Lactoovovegetarian.* The vegetable diet is supplemented with milk, eggs, and cheese. There is no problem in securing adequate protein with this diet.
2. *Lactovegetarian.* The vegetable diet is supplemented with milk and cheese. Milk products add complete protein to this diet.
3. *Strict vegetarian, or vegan.* The all-vegetable diet includes vegetables, fruits, legumes, nuts, and grains but is not supplemented with any animal foods, dairy products, or eggs. More careful planning is required to achieve combinations providing the necessary amounts of the essential amino acids. Vitamin B_{12} deficiency is a potential problem.
4. *Fruitarian.* The fruitarian diet consists of raw or dried fruits, nuts, honey, and olive oil. Potential inadequacy is greater in this diet than in other diets.

Of particular concern is the strict vegetarian (vegan)

Text continues on page 307.

Table 11-4 Characteristic Food Patterns of Some Cultures

Ethnic Group	Milk Group	Meat Group	Fruits and Vegetables	Breads and Cereals	Possible Dietary Problems
American Indian (many tribal variations; many "Americanized")	Fresh milk Evaporated milk for cooking Ice cream Cream pies	Pork, beef, lamb, rabbit Fowl, fish, eggs Legumes Sunflower seeds Nuts: walnut, acorn, pine, peanut butter Game meat	Green peas, beans Beets, turnips Leafy green and other vegetables Grapes, bananas, peaches, other fresh fruits Roots	Refined bread Whole wheat Cornmeal Rice Dry cereals "Fry" bread Tortillas	Obesity, diabetes, alcoholism, nutritional deficiencies expressed in dental problems and iron deficiency anemia Inadequate amounts of all nutrients Excessive use of sugar
Middle Eastern (Armenian, Greek, Syrian, Turkish)	Yogurt Little butter	Lamb Nuts Dried peas, beans, lentils	Peppers Tomatoes Cabbage Grape leaves Cucumbers Squash Dried apricots, raisins	Cracked wheat and dark bread	Fry many meats and vegetables Lack of fresh fruits Insufficient foods from milk group Like sweetenings, lamb fat, and olive oil
Black	Milk Ice Cream Puddings	Pork: all cuts, plus organs, chitterlings	Leafy vegetables Green and yellow vegetables	Cornmeal and hominy grits Rice	Extensive use of frying, "smothering" in gravy, or simmering
	Cheese: longhorn, American	Beef, lamb Chicken, giblets Eggs Nuts Legumes Fish, game	Potato: white, sweet Stewed fruit Bananas, and other fresh fruit	Biscuits, pancakes, white breads Puddings: bread rice Molasses*	Fats: salt pork, bacon drippings, lard, and gravies Enjoy sweets Insufficient citrus and enriched breads Vegetables often boiled for long periods Limited amounts from milk group
Chinese (Cantonese most prevalent)	Milk: water buffalo	Pork sausage† Eggs and pigeon eggs Fish Lamb, beef, goat Fowl: chicken, duck Nuts Legumes Soybean curd (tofu)‡	Many vegetables Radish leaves Bean, bamboo sprouts	Rice/rice flour products Cereals, noodles Wheat, corn, millet seed	Tendency of some immigrants to use more grease in cooking Limited use of milk and milk products Often low in protein, calories, or both May wash rice before cooking, removing vitamins added in fortification Soy sauce (high sodium)

*Light molasses (first extraction): 1 tbsp = 50 calories, 33 mg of calcium, 0.9 mg of iron, 0.01 mg each of vitamins B_1 and B_2; dark molasses (third extraction): 1 tbsp = 45 calories, 137 mg of calcium, 3.2 mg of iron, 0.02 mg of vitamin B_1, 0.04 mg of vitamin B_2, 0.4 mg of niacin.
†Lower in fat content than Western sausage.
‡Good source of protein.

Table 11-4 Characteristic Food Patterns of Some Cultures—cont'd

Ethnic Group	Milk Group	Meat Group	Fruits and Vegetables	Breads and Cereals	Possible Dietary Problems
Filipino (Spanish-Chinese influence)	Flavored milk Milk in coffee Cheese: gouda, cheddar	Pork, beef, goat, deer, rabbit Chicken Fish Eggs Nuts Legumes	Many vegetables and fruits	Rice, cooked cereals Noodles: rice, wheat	Limited use of milk and milk products Tend to prewash rice May have only small portions of protein foods
Italian	Cheese Some ice cream	Meat Eggs Dried beans	Leafy vegetables Potatoes Eggplant Spinach Fruits	Pasta White breads, some whole wheat Farina Cereals	Prefer expensive imported cheeses; reluctant to substitute less expensive domestic varieties Tendency to overcook vegetables Limited use of whole grains Enjoy sweets Extensive use of olive oil Insufficient servings from milk group
Japanese (Isei, more Japanese influence; Nisei, more westernized)	Increasing amounts being used by younger generations	Pork, beef, chicken Fish Eggs Legumes: soya, red, lima beans Tofu Nuts	Many vegetables and fruits Seaweed	Rice, rice cakes Wheat noodles Refined bread, noodles	Excessive salt: pickles, salty crisp seaweed High intake of monosodium L-glutamate (MSG) and soy sauce Insufficient servings from milk group May use refined or prewashed rice
Mexican-Spanish, Mexican-American	Milk Cheese Flan Ice Cream	Beef, pork, lamb, chicken, tripe, hot sausage, beef intestines Fish Eggs Nuts Dry beans: pinto, chick-peas (often eaten more than once daily)	Spinach, wild greens, tomatoes, chilies, corn, cactus leaves, cabbage, avocado, potatoes Pumpkin, zapote, peaches, guava, papaya, citrus	Rice, oats, cornmeal Sweet bread Tortilla: corn, flour Biscuits Vermicelli *(fideo)*	Limited meats primarily due to economics Limited use of milk and milk products Increasing use of flour tortillas over more nutritious corn tortillas Large amounts of lard Abundant use of sugar Tendency to boil vegetables for long periods

Continued.

Table 11-4 Characteristic Food Patterns of Some Cultures—cont'd

Ethnic Group	Milk Group	Meat Group	Fruits and Vegetables	Breads and Cereals	Possible Dietary Problems
Polish	Milk Sour cream Cheese Butter	Pork (preferred) Chicken	Vegetables Cabbage Roots Fruits	Dark rye	Enjoy sweets Tendency to overcook vegetables Limited fruits (especially citrus), raw vegetables, and meats
Puerto Rican	Limited use of milk products Coffee with milk (*café con leche*)	Pork Poultry Eggs (Fridays) Dried codfish Beans (*habichuelas*)	Avacado, okra Eggplant Sweet yams Starchy vegetables and fruits (*viandas*)	Rice Cornmeal	Small amounts of pork and poultry Use fat, lard, salt pork, and olive oil extensively Lack of milk products
Scandinavian: Danish, Finnish, Norwegian, Swedish	Cream Butter	Wild game Reindeer Fish Eggs	Berries Dried fruit Vegetables: cole slaw, roots, avocado	Whole wheat, rye, barley, sweets (molasses for flavoring)	Insufficient fresh fruits and vegetables Enjoy sweets, pickled salted meats, and fish Liberal use of fat
Southeast Asian: Vietnamese, Cambodian	Generally not taken Coffee with condensed cow's milk Plain yogurt Ice cream (rare) Soybean milk	Fish (daily): fresh, dried, salted Poultry/eggs: duck, chicken Pork Beef (seldom) Dry beans Tofu	Seasonal variety: fresh or preserved Green, leafy Yams Corn	Rice: grains, flour, noodles, "cellophane" French bread	Fresh milk products generally not consumed Poultry/eggs may be limited Meat considered "unclean" is avoided Pregnant women prefer a diet high in salt and pepper as well as rice and pork High intake of MSG and soy sauce
Jewish: orthodox	Milk* Cheese*	Meat (bloodless; Kosher prepared): beef, lamb, goat, deer, poultry (all types) Fish with fins and scales only No crustaceans	Wide variety	Wide variety	High intake of sodium

*Milk and milk products not eaten with meat; milk may be taken before the meal or 6 hours following meal; different sets of dishes and silverware are used to serve milk and meat products.

who eliminates all products of animal origin, including meat, poultry, fish, cheese, eggs, and milk. The pregnant woman who practices strict vegetarianism may require assistance in combining plant protein sources to consume adequate amounts of complete protein. Plant proteins are incomplete, which means they are lacking in one or more of the essential amino acids required for optimum growth and maintenance of body tissues. Skillful combination of complementary incomplete proteins, where one protein source will be rich in an amino acid the other protein source lacks, and vice versa, can provide sufficient amounts of complete protein in the diet. Since vitamin B_{12} is found only in animal products and a few fortified foods, the strict vegetarian may need a supplement. Complementary proteins include legumes plus grains (e.g., beans and rice or beans and tortillas) and nuts and seeds plus legumes (e.g., sesame-soybean snack mix). Milk products can be used to complement any incomplete protein. Examples include macaroni and cheese, cereal with milk, bean soup topped with yogurt, and an ice cream sundae with walnuts. A modified food guide for vegetarians is presented in Table 11-5.

Iron Supplementation and Nutrition Counseling. An important responsibility of the nurse is to teach women about meeting nutritional needs for themselves and their unborn babies. Guidelines for client teaching about iron supplementation are given on p. 310. Table 11-6 is another format that can be used for nutrition counseling during pregnancy.

Referral for Additional Services. Individuals with insufficient income to purchase foods may have a nutritionally inadequate diet. Nutrients such as protein and iron are among those more likely to be deficient in diets of low-income groups. To help improve the nutritional quality of the diet, the person with a limited income should be encouraged to participate in federal food programs such as WIC and the food stamp program. Nutrition education and counseling are important to ensure the benefits of such programs.

The referral system has two functions. First, a comprehensive network of services can offer solutions to problems that a particular program may not have the resources to solve. Second, the referral system informs women about a program by making them aware of their needs for benefits from that service. Food assistance programs, such as the WIC program, are a particularly good example of resources that can be tapped for pregnant women.

A sample nursing care plan designed to meet the specific needs of a client is on p. 309.

Evaluation

Evaluation is a continuous process that begins during assessment. To be effective, evaluation is based on measurable outcome criteria. Nurses are accountable for measuring and documenting client outcomes. The criteria reflect the parameters used to measure the goals for care. The maternal and fetal areas consistently assessed as indicators of maternal and fetal well-being and the clinical findings that represent normal response are presented as outcome criteria in Table 11-6. These criteria are used as a basis for selecting appropriate nursing actions and evaluating their effectiveness.

Table 11-5 Modified Food Guide for Vegetarian Diets During Pregnancy

	Recommended Number of Servings	
Food Group	Lactovegetarian	Lactoovovegetarian
Milk	5	5
Protein		
Eggs (2 = 1 serving)	0	1
Legumes	3	3
Nuts	1	1
Fruits and vegetables		
Vitamin C	3	3
Vitamin A	2	2
Other	4	3
Whole grain products	7	6
Others (e.g., butter or margarine)	1	1

Table 11-6 Examples of Nutrition Counseling During Pregnancy

Goals	Nursing Actions	Outcome Criteria
Woman will know reason for increased nutrient and energy needs during pregnancy.	Explain that pregnancy is like building a house (the baby). You need materials (nutrients) and labor (energy). If you do not have enough materials or labor, the house will not be big or strong. This is also true for the baby.	Woman will explain why she needs more nutrients and energy while she is pregnant.
Woman will know additional nutrients needed during pregnancy and how to fulfill this need. Woman will meet her nutrient needs.	Explain that although all nutrient needs are increased during pregnancy, seven nutrients are particularly essential: calories, protein, calcium, iron supplements, vitamin A, vitamin C, and folic acid. Use 24-hr recall to point out areas of concern. Discuss daily food guide (see Table 11-2).	Woman will identify which nutrients should be increased, including calories, protein, calcium, iron, vitamin A, vitamin C, and folic acid. Woman will suggest how she might fulfill these needs.
Woman will know suggested weight gain pattern and components of total weight gain during pregnancy.	Explain that suggested weight gain pattern is about 1.4 kg (3 lb) in first trimester, 4.5 kg (10 lb) in second, and 4.5 kg (10 lb) in third. Discuss components of total weight gain as follows: 27%, fetus 12%, placenta and fluid in uterus 50%, increased maternal organs (uterus, fat, breasts) 10%, increased blood volume	Woman will explain what suggested weight gain pattern is and will list following components that make up total weight gain: 27%, fetus 12%, placenta and fluid in uterus 50%, increase in maternal organs 10%, increased blood volume
Woman will know that good nutrition leads to suggested weight gain in pregnancy.	Explain that monitoring weight is a way to measure whether fetus is receiving adequate supply of nutrients.	Woman will state that adequate supply of nutrients promotes optimum development of infant and suggested weight gain.
Woman will achieve steady weight gain.	Explain that steady weight gain indicates that fetus is receiving adequate nutrients.	Woman will state how much she has gained.
Woman will know how her weight gain compares with average weight gain.	Record weight gain at each visit. Discuss weight gain pattern.	Completed each time throughout second and third trimesters. Woman will state how her weight gain compares to average.
Woman will know that poor nutrition can lead to anemia, preeclampsia-eclampsia, obesity, or preterm labor.	Explain that poor nutrition during pregnancy may lead to several problem conditions. Poor supply of iron, folic acid, protein, or vitamin C may lead to anemia. Generally poor nutrition may lead to preterm labor. Poor selection of food may lead to obesity.	Woman will identify following problems that may result from poor nutrition in pregnancy: anemia, preeclampsia-eclampsia, obesity, and preterm labor.

Adapted from Pregnancy protocol for nutrition counseling, Phoenix, 1978, Nutrition Services, Arizona Department of Health; and Detroit, 1979, Nutrition Division, City of Detroit Department of Health.

Specific Nursing Care Plan

MATERNAL/FETAL NUTRITION

Laura is a 22-year-old married woman who is 10 weeks pregnant with her second child. John, her first child, now a healthy 18 months of age, was born at term weighing 3500 g (7 lb 12 oz). Laura expressed concern that she would not have enough calcium because she "just had a baby 18 months ago and never could stand drinking milk." During the dietary assessment she reveals that she cannot drink orange juice. During her last pregnancy she drank caster oil in orange juice for "chronic constipation." History, physical examination, and laboratory results are not remarkable.

ASSESSMENT	NURSING DIAGNOSIS (ND), PLAN/GOAL (P/G)	RATIONALE/ IMPLEMENTATION	EVALUATION
Laura is 10 weeks pregnant; first baby 18 months old. Laura does not drink milk. Laura cannot drink orange juice.	ND: Altered nutrition potential: less than body requirements related to inability to drink milk or orange juice. P/G: Laura will consume adequate intake of nutrients present in milk and orange juice.	*Adequate intake of nutrients present in milk and orange juice must be assured:* Encourage her to choose sources she likes and can afford. Compose a list of foods specifying serving sizes.	Laura is able to choose alternate sources of nutrients. Laura ingests sufficient quantities of nutrients to meet RDA requirements and her own needs.
Laura is concerned because she is unable to use the usual food sources of nutrients.	ND: Self-esteem disturbance related to perceived lack of self-control in meeting nutritional needs. P/G: Laura will increase her perceived control of what happens to her and will enhance her self-concept.	*Perceived control of events and enhanced self-concept increase ability to cope:* Compliment her on her expressed concern and her knowledge of needed nutrients and on choosing equivalent alternatives. Discuss with her the four food groups and distribution of nutrients. Help her write out shopping list and sample menus including serving size.	Laura participates in her own care. Laura practices problem solving by exploring alternatives and making choices to meet changing needs. Laura indicates satisfaction in her new skills.
Laura states she had chronic constipation during her first pregnancy. Assess her understanding of constipation, and her usual methods of prevention and treatment. Assess usual bowel habits, daily fluid intake, dietary intake of roughage, exercise regimen, if any.	ND: Knowledge deficit related to constipation during pregnancy, its prevention and treatment with nonpharmaceutical means. P/G: Knowledge deficit is removed. ND: Constipation related to knowledge deficit of self-help methods of prevention and treatment. P/G: Laura will augment coping skills using self-help measures without pharmaceuticals.	*Knowledge of nonpharmaceutic means of prevention or treatment of constipation increases self-care ability:* Review maternal adaptations to pregnancy that alter alimentary function. Teach methods of prevention and treatment. Help her incorporate knowledge into menu plan as necessary and set schedule for water intake, bowel elimination, exercise. Commend her on her participation in problem solving.	Laura is able to state physiologic basis of constipation. Laura learns methods of preventing/relieving constipation with nonpharmaceutical means. Laura does not experience constipation. Laura utilizes methods of preventing constipation.

Guidelines for Client Teaching
IRON SUPPLEMENTATION

ASSESSMENT

1. Gravida is in her second trimester. She mentions that she has been ingesting dry laundry starch because "all pregnant women crave it."
2. Woman is chewing ice from a paper cup while waiting to be seen by the physician.
3. Laboratory values: hemoglobin 10.2 g/dl; hematocrit, 34%.

NURSING DIAGNOSES

Altered nutrition: less than body requirements related to pica and the ingestion of nonnutritive substances.

Knowledge deficit related to pica and its possible significance.

Knowledge deficit related to proper nutrition, iron deficiency, and its effect on woman and her fetus.

GOALS

Short-term

Gravida starts taking iron supplement, as prescribed, immediately.

Gravida's laboratory data for hemoglobin and hematocrit indicate beginning improvement with the next test.

Gravida stops ingesting dry laundry starch.

Intermediate

Gravida continues to take iron supplements as long as prescribed.

Gravida understands anemia and its potential effects on her and her baby.

Gravida eats foods that are nutritionally sound.

Long-term

Woman and her baby do not suffer any adverse effects of anemia.

REFERENCES AND TEACHING AIDS

Printed instructions for using iron supplements.

Hospital-supplied pamphlets on nutrition, including information on food groups and supplements.

Laboratory slips showing woman's blood values.

RATIONALE/CONTENT	TEACHING ACTION
Knowledge provides a basis for decision-making re nutrition. Gravida may not know about pica, therefore the nurse will share the following:	
Pica is a learned behavior. Cravings are not uncommon; if diet is well-balanced, occasional indulgence is probably not harmful. Many cultures have specific beliefs about cravings and "making the baby" or ease of delivery. Nonnutritive foods may provide unwanted calories, interfere with the absorption of iron, and contribute to iron-deficiency anemia.	Few women are willing to volunteer information on pica, so sensitive questioning is necessary to uncover the practice. Discuss the reasons for woman's cravings. Provide information on this practice without demeaning the woman's underlying cultural beliefs. Encourage discussion and questions.
Information facilitates understanding of the condition: Discuss woman's laboratory report. Define hemoglobin, hematocrit, red blood cells, anemia; explain values and normal parameters.	Review, assess woman's level of understanding. Discuss clinical significance of the differences.
Knowledge provides the foundation for improving nutrition: Discuss building blood through diet. Explain types and amounts of bloodforming nutrients. Explain that food sources of nutrients, such as liver and other red meats, dried beans, dried fruit, deep green vegetables, eggs, and enriched cereals, provide sources of iron.	Review; help woman identify food sources of nutrients in her current diet; praise her. Assist with menu selection to meet woman's preferences and her cultural prescriptions and proscriptions. Involve family members in planning dietary intake if possible.

Guidelines for Client Teaching—cont'd

RATIONALE/CONTENT	TEACHING ACTION
Knowledge of medical therapy for iron deficiency anemia supports client compliance:	Review this information
Discuss building blood through iron supplementation (30 to 60 mg of elemental iron [150 to 300 mg of ferrous sulfate]). Explain that iron is absorbed most readily in the ferrous form in the presence of acid, before meals, but iron tablets on an empty stomach are highly irritating. Explain that enteric forms of iron supplementation are less effective because of poor absorption beyond the duodenum. Identify foods that decrease iron absorption: milk, cereal, and eggs. Discuss side effects of iron supplementation: stools become dark-green to black in appearance; they may become more formed, contributing to constipation, or become loose; and gastric irritation and bad taste may occur.	Discuss and plan proper administration: Divide daily dose into 3 equal doses. Take tablets with a citrus fruit juice, which is a good source of vitamin C, or with vitamin C, 500 mg orally, once daily. Take tablets after eating food that does not include cereal, eggs, or milk. Time medication to fit woman's (family's) mealtime and her convenience. After the first trimester and nausea has subsided, woman may be able to take the tablet with orange juice between meals. Review side effects sensitively.
Monitor woman's progress—within 1 week there is an increase in the number of reticulocytes (immature red blood cells) and in the rate of hemoglobin synthesis.	Review woman's laboratory findings that confirm her improvement and provide her with tangible proof of her success; give appropriate praise.
Children need to be protected from accidental poisoning: Review need to secure medications from children.	Review safety precautions against accidental ingestion of chemicals.

EVALUATION The nurse can be assured that teaching was effective when her laboratory report shows improvement in anemia (e.g., increase in reticulocyte count, mean corpuscular hemoglobin, hemoglobin, and hematocrit). The woman will indicate she has dark stools, can and does choose appropriate foods, and reduces or eliminates pica. The woman verbalizes her understanding of pica and anemia, and their potential effects on her and her fetus.

SUMMARY

Nutrition is an important component of care during the prenatal period. Scientific research has identified the nutrient needs for optimum body function, growth, development, maintenance and repair of body tissues, and prevention of disease. The nurse is in a strategic position to assist clients directly or through collaboration with a registered dietitian to meet their nutrition needs. Among the nurse's tools are a sound knowledge of maternal physiologic adjustments to pregnancy and nutritional needs and the nursing process.

LEARNING ACTIVITIES

1. At the prenatal clinic, assess the nutritional status of a selected client utilizing your observational skills for physical signs and symptoms either during a physical examination or as the client is involved in other clinic routines.
2. Interview a client at the prenatal clinic utilizing the nutrition questionnaire and develop a daily food plan for her based on this formation.
3. Describe your own nutritional status and dietary strengths and weaknesses; your positive and negative eating habits; the influence of your culture, religion, and ethnic group on your dietary practices; your attitudes toward overweight and underweight persons; and how your views and beliefs about nutrition may influence women when providing care for prenatal clients.
4. Use the material compiled in activity 3 for discussion with peers about their views and beliefs. People of varying backgrounds may be able to offer additional insights into each others' problems with acceptance of clients' varying attitudes and practices.
5. Use the cultural preferences listed in Table 11-4 to develop sample menus for 1 day for clients coming from three of the backgrounds listed, taking into account the availability of ethnic and specialty foods and the constraints of an average income. (You may also want to take a research trip to several stores in the area to check for availability of special foods.)

KEY CONCEPTS

- A woman's nutritional status before, during, and after pregnancy contributes to a significant degree to the well-being of both herself and her infant, and is of vital importance to the health of succeeding generations.
- Many physiologic changes occurring during pregnancy influence the need for nutrients and the efficiency with which the body uses them.
- There are potential hazards for both mother and infant from restricting weight gain and salt during pregnancy.
- Water is an essential nutrient.
- Iron and folic acid supplementation are recommended during pregnancy.
- The nurse and the client are influenced by cultural and personal values and beliefs during nutrition counseling.
- Factors such as frequent pregnancies and insufficient income put the gravida at nutritional risk before and during pregnancy.

References

Abrams BF and Laros RK, Jr: Prepregnancy weight, weight gain, and birth weight. Am J Obstet Gynecol 154:503, 1986.
Affonso DD: The Filipino American. In Clark AL, editors: Culture/childbearing/health professionals, Philadelphia, 1978, FA Davis Co.
Brown JW et al: Influence of pregnancy weight gain on the size of infants born to underweight women, Obstet Gynecol 57:13, 1981.
California Department of Health Services: Nutrition during pregnancy and lactation, Sacramento, Calif, 1975, Maternal and Child Health Branch, CDHS.
Campbell T and Chang B: Health care of the Chinese in America, Nurs Outlook 21:245, 1973.
Carrington BW: The Afro-American. In Clark AL, editor: Culture/childbearing/health professionals, Philadelphia, 1978, FA Davis Co.
Dohrmann KR and Lederman SA: Weight gain in pregnancy, JOGN Nurs 15(6):446, 1986.
Frentzen BH, Dimperio DL, and Cruz AC: Maternal weight gain: effect on infant birth weight among overweight and average-weight low-income women, Am J Obstet Gynecol 159:1114, 1988.
Frentzen BH, Johnson JWC, and Simpson S: Nutrition and hydration: relationship to preterm myometrial contractility, Obstet Gynecol 70:887, 1988.
Greene GW et al: Postpartum weight change: how much of the weight gained in pregnancy will be lost after delivery? Obstet Gynecol 71:701, May, 1988.
Hambidge KM et al: Acute effects of iron therapy on zinc status during pregnancy, Obstet Gynecol 70:593, 1988.
Hollingsworth AO et al: The refugees and childbearing: what to expect, RN 43:45, 1980.
Kay MA, editor: Anthropology of human birth, Philadelphia, 1982, FA Davis Co.
Lee RV et al: Southeast Asian folklore about pregnancy and parturition, Obstet Gynecol 77:643, 1988.
Leiderman PH et al: Culture and infancy, New York, 1977, Academic Press, Inc.
London RS: Saccharin and aspartame: are they safe to consume during pregnancy? J Reprod Med 33:17, Jan, 1988.
Naeye RL: Weight gain and the outcome of pregnancy, Am J Obstet Gynecol 135:3, 1979.
Obeyesekere G: Pregnancy cravings (dola-duka) in relation to social structure and personality in a Sinhalese village, Am Anthropol 65:323, 1963.
Olsen LC and Mundt MH: Postpartum weight loss in a nurse-midwifery practice, J Nurse Midwife 31:177, Jul/Aug, 1986.
White JE and Owsley VB: Helping families cope with milk, wheat, and soy allergies, MCN 8:423, Nov/Dec, 1983.
Worthington-Roberts B: Nutrition deficiencies and excesses: impact on pregnancy, part 1, J Perinat 5:9, Summer, 1985.
Zlatnik FJ and Burmeister LF: Dietary protein and preeclampsia, Am J Obstet Gynecol 147:345, 1983.

Bibliography

Alexander LL: The pregnant smoker: nursing implications, JOGN Nurs 16(3):167, 1987.
Barnico LM and Cullinane MM: Maternal phenylketonuria: an unexpected challenge, MCN 10:108, March/April, 1985.
Cagle CS: Professionally speaking: access to care and prevention of low birth weight, MCN 12(4):235, 1987.
Choi EC: Unique aspects of Korean-American mothers, JOGN Nurs 15(5):394, 1986.
Cunningham FG, MacDonald PC, and Gant NR: Williams obstetrics, ed 18, Norwalk, Conn, 1989, Appleton & Lange.
Food and Nutrition Board: Recommended dietary allowances, rev ed, Washington, DC, 1980, National Academy of Sciences—National Research Council.
Frank DW et al: Nutrition in adolescent pregnancy, J Calif Perinatal Assoc 1:21, 1983.
Grosso C et al: The Vietnamese American family . . . and grandma makes three, MCN 6:177, 1981.
Gulick EE, Franklin CM, and Elinson M: Food beliefs and food behaviors among minority pregnant women, J Perinat 6(3):197, 1986.
Haworth JC et al: Fetal growth retardation in cigarette-smoking mothers is not due to decreased maternal food intake, Am J Obstet Gynecol 137:719, 1980.
Jacobson HN: Diet therapy and the improvement of pregnancy outcome, Birth 10:29, Spring, 1983.
Laboratory indices of nutritional status in pregnancy, pub no F-427, Washington, DC, Sept 1977, National Academy of Sciences—National Research Council.

Lenke RR and Levy HL: Maternal phenylketonuria and hyperphenylalaninemia, N Engl J Med 303:1202, 1980.
Lipson A et al: Maternal hyperphenylalaninemia and fetal effects, J Pediatr 104:216, 1984.
Leonard LG: Pregnancy and the underweight woman, MCN 9(5):331, Sept/Oct, 1984.
Luke B: Megavitamins and pregnancy: a dangerous combination, MCN 10:18, Jan/Feb, 1985.
Moore L et al: Self-assessment: a personalized approach to nursing during pregnancy, JOGN Nurs 15(4):311, 1986.
Naeye RL: Teenaged and pre-teenaged pregnancies: consequences of the fetal-maternal competition for nutrients, Pediatrics 67:146, 1981.
Naeye RL: Effects of maternal nutrition on fetal and neonatal survival, Birth 10:109, Summer, 1983.
Orque MS, Bloch B, and Ahumada-Monrroy LS: Ethnic nursing care: a multicultural approach, St Louis, 1983, The CV Mosby Co.
Queenan JT, moderator: Managing pregnancy in patients over 35, Contemp OB/GYN 29(5):180, 1987.
Seidel HM et al: Mosby's guide to physical examination, St Louis, 1987, The CV Mosby Co.
Williams SR: Nutrition and diet therapy, ed 6, St Louis, 1989, The CV Mosby Co.
Willson JR and Carrington ER: Obstetrics and gynecology, ed 8, St Louis, 1987, The CV Mosby Co.
Winslow W: First pregnancy after 35: what is the experience? MCN 12(2):92, 1987.
Worthington-Roberts B: Nutrition deficiencies and excesses: impact on pregnancy, part 2, J Perinat 5:12, Fall, 1985.

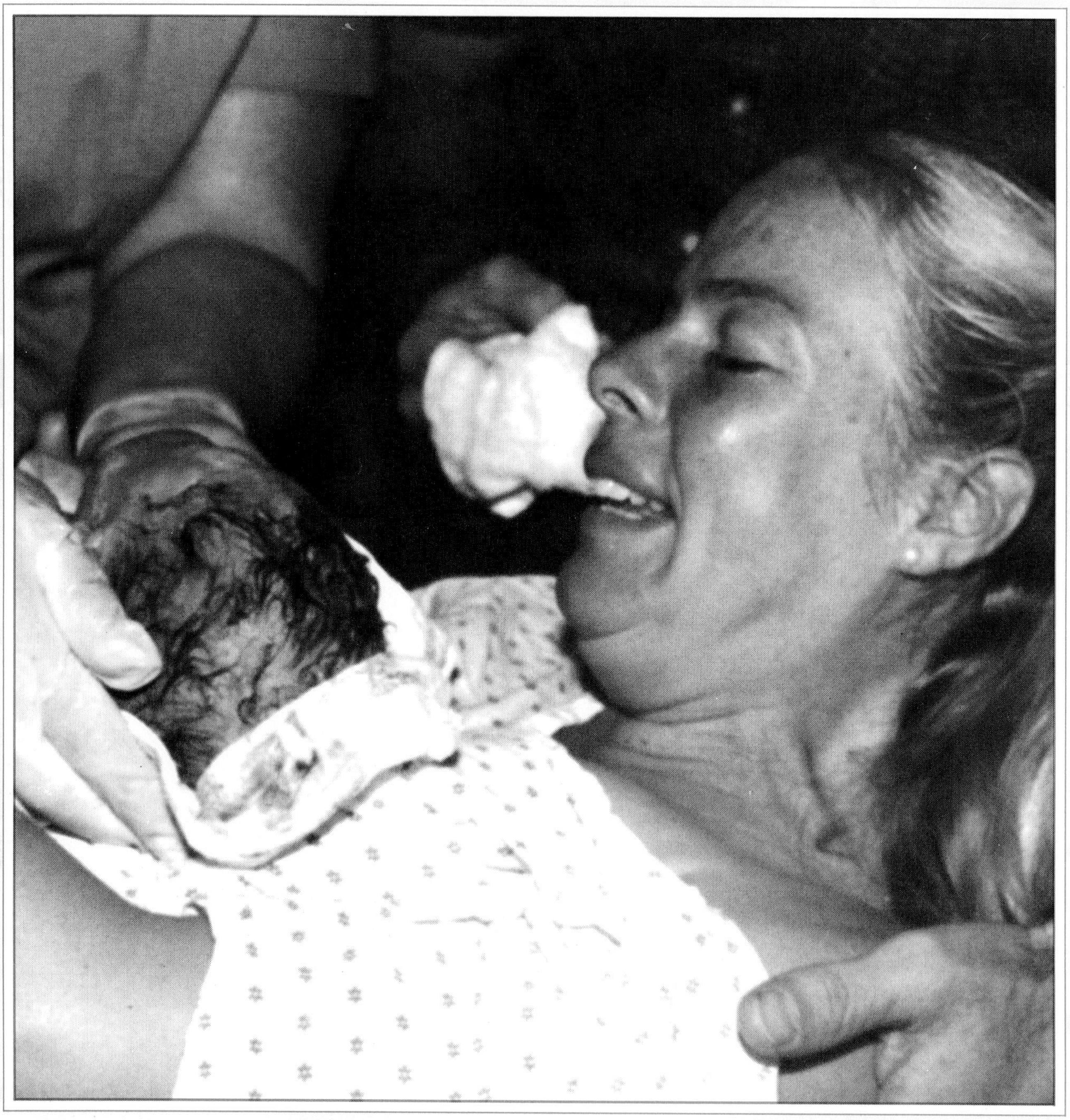

UNIT

III

NORMAL CHILDBIRTH

CHAPTER

12 Essential Factors and Processes of Labor

Vicki Akin

Learning Objectives

Correctly define the key terms listed.

Explain the five essential factors that affect the labor process.

Describe the anatomic structure of the bony pelvis.

Differentiate the four types of pelves.

Delineate the diameters of the pelvic inlet, cavity, and outlet and state the normal measurements.

Review the anatomy of the fetal skull and state the normal measurements.

Summarize the process of molding of the fetal head during labor.

Describe the mechanism of labor.

Assess the maternal anatomic and physiologic adaptations to labor.

Explain the fetal adaptations to labor.

Key Terms

attitude
biparietal diameter
bloody show
breech presentation
bregma
cephalic presentation
denominator
descent
diagonal conjugate
engagement
expulsion
Ferguson's reflex
fontanel
four stages of labor
gate-control theory
gynecoid pelvis
lie
lightening
mechanism of labor
molding
partograms
position
powers
presentation
presenting part
restitution
station
suboccipitobregmatic diameter
vertex

During pregnancy, the mother and the fetus prepare to accommodate themselves to each other during the labor process. The fetal-placental unit has grown and developed in preparation for extrauterine life. The mother has undergone various physiologic adaptations during the period of gestation that prepare her for the birth process and role of mother. Labor and delivery is the culmination of the childbearing cycle and is an intense period during which the products of conception are expelled from the uterus. To implement nursing care in labor the nurse must use the nursing process. The essential factors and processes of labor must be understood along with the maternal and fetal adaptations to labor. The family's adaptations to childbirth are discussed in Chapter 9. In this chapter, essential terms are in **bold print.** Some of the important terms are defined below:

parturition Childbirth, birthing, the birth process
parturient A woman in labor
labor A coordinated sequence of involuntary uterine contractions that result in effacement and dilatation of the cervix and voluntary bearing-down efforts that result in delivery; the actual expulsion of the products of conception—the fetus and placenta
toko- and **toco-** (Greek) Combining forms meaning childbirth or labor
eutocia Normal labor
prodromal labor Early or premonitory manifestations of impending labor; events before the onset of true labor

❑ ESSENTIAL FACTORS IN LABOR

Five essential factors affect the process of labor and delivery. These are easily remembered as the five P's:

1. Passenger
   a. Fetus: gestational age, size, lie, presentation, position and attitude of the fetus; number of fetuses
   b. Placenta: type, sufficiency of, and site of insertion

2. Passageway
   a. Configuration and diameters of the maternal pelvis
   b. Distensibility of the lower uterine segment, cervical dilatation, and capacity for distension of pelvic floor, vaginal canal, and introitus
3. Powers
   a. Primary powers: intensity, duration, and frequency of uterine contractions
   b. Secondary powers: bearing-down efforts
4. Position of the mother: standing, walking, side-lying, squatting, hands and knees
5. Psychologic response: previous experiences, emotional readiness, preparation, cultural-ethnic heritage, support systems, and environment

Four of the five factors will be discussed in this chapter; the fifth factor, psychologic response, will be covered in Chapter 15.

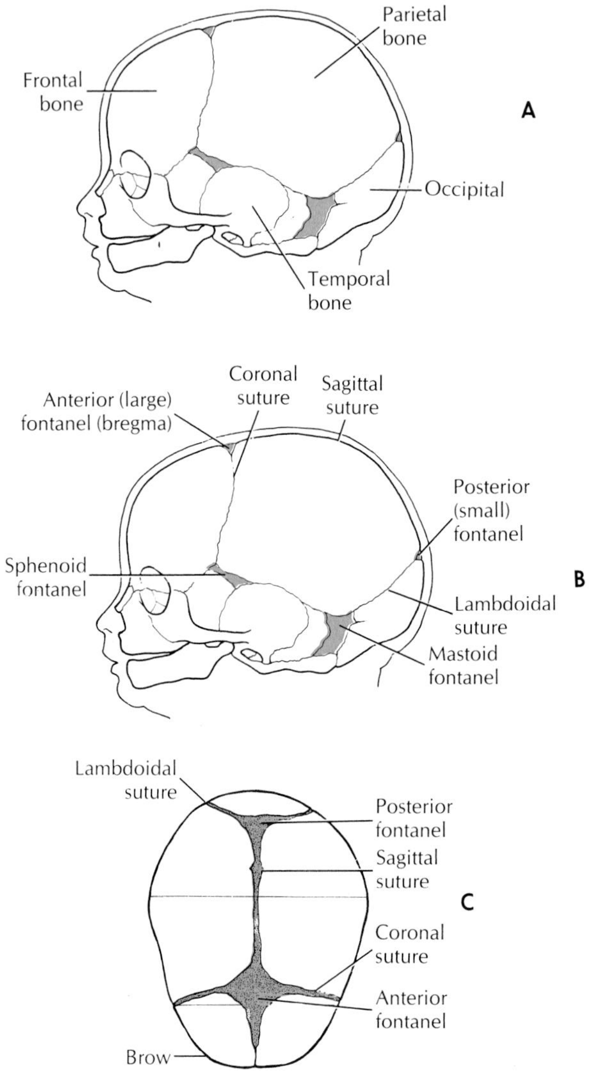

Fig. 12-1 Fetal head at term. **A**, Bones. **B** and **C**, Sutures and fontanels.

Passenger

The passage of the fetus through the birth canal is a result of several interacting factors. It is influenced by the size of the fetal head and shoulders, the dimensions of the bony pelvis, and fetal presentation, position, and attitude.

Fetus

Because of its size and relative rigidity, the **fetal head** has a major effect on the birth process. The external cranial vault is composed of two parietal bones, two temporal bones, the frontal bone, and the occipital bone (Fig. 12-1, *A*). These bones are united by membranous **sutures:** the **sagittal,** lambdoidal, coronal, and frontal. The membrane-filled spaces called *fontanels* (Fig. 12-1, *B* and *C*) are located where the sutures intersect. The two most important fontanels are the anterior and posterior fontanels. During labor, vaginal palpation of fontanels and sutures identifies fetal presentation and position. Assessment of their size reveals information about the age and well-being of the newborn.

The larger of the two fontanels, the **anterior fontanel,** or **bregma,** is diamond-shaped and is at the junction of the sagittal, coronal, and frontal sutures. It ossifies by 18 months of age. The **posterior fontanel** is at the junction of the sutures of the two parietal bones and the one occipital bone and is therefore triangular in shape. It is smaller than the anterior fontanel and closes 6 to 8 weeks after birth. The sutures and fontanels allow the brain to continue growing.

The bones of the cranial vault are not firmly united, and slight overlapping of the bones, or **molding** of the shape of the head, occurs during labor. This capacity of the bones to slide over one another permits adaptation to the various diameters of the maternal pelvis. Molding can be extensive, but with most newborns the head assumes its normal shape within 3 days of birth.

Principal measurements of the fetal skull are in centimeters (Fig. 12-2). The **biparietal diameter** is the largest transverse diameter. Of the anteroposterior diameters shown in Fig. 12-2, it can be seen that the attitudes of flexion or extension allow diameters of different sizes to enter the maternal pelvis. With the head in complete flexion, **suboccipitobregmatic diameter,** the smallest diameter, presents and enters the true pelvis easily (Fig. 12-3).

Because of their mobility, the position of the **shoulders** (the shoulder girdle) can be altered during labor, so that one shoulder may occupy a lower level than the other. This permits a small shoulder diameter to nego-

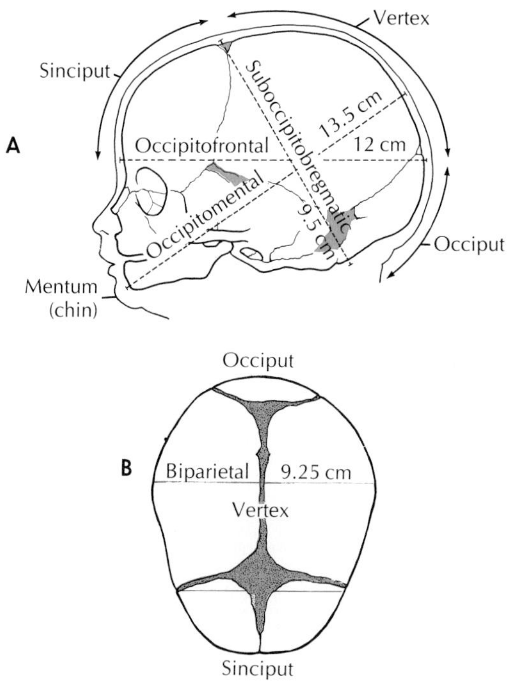

Fig. 12-2 Cephalic landmarks. **A,** Cephalic presentations: occiput, vertex, and sinciput; and cephalic diameters: suboccipitobregmatic, occipitofrontal, and occipitomental. **B,** Cephalic presentations and biparietal diameter.

tiate the passageway. The circumference of the hips, or pelvic girdle, is usually small enough not to create problems.

Lie is the relationship of the long axis (spine) of the fetus to the long axis (spine) of the mother. There are two lies: *longitudinal,* or vertical, in which the long axis of the fetus is parallel with the long axis of the mother, and *transverse,* or horizontal, in which the long axis of the fetus is at a right angle to that of the mother (Figs. 12-4 and 12-5). Longitudinal lies are either cephalic (head) or sacral (breech) presentations, depending on the fetal structure that first enters the mother's pelvis.

Presentation refers to the part of the fetus that enters the pelvic inlet first and leads through the birth canal during labor at term. The three main presentations are cephalic (head first), 96%; breech (buttocks first), 3%; and shoulders, 1%.

Presenting part refers to the leading, or most dependent portion of the fetus, lying over the internal os of the cervix. It is the part on which the caput succedaneum, a localized, easily identifiable edematous area of the scalp, forms and is the part first felt by the examining finger during a vaginal examination.

Attitude is the relationship of the fetal body parts to each other. The fetus assumes a characteristic posture (attitude) in utero partly because of the mode of fetal growth and partly because of accommodation to the shape of the uterine cavity. The shape of the fetus is roughly ovoid, the back is markedly flexed, the head is flexed on the chest, the thighs are flexed at the knee joints, and the arches of the feet rest on the anterior surface of the legs. This attitude is called *general flexion.* The arms are crossed over the thorax, and the umbilical cord lies between the arms and the legs.

Denominator refers to that part of the presentation that indicates or determines the position of the fetus in utero. In a **cephalic presentation,** the denominator is the occiput; in a **breech presentation,** it is the sacrum; in a face presentation, the mentum; and in a brow presentation, the denominator is the sinciput.

Position is the relationship of the denominator (occiput, sacrum, mentum [chin], or sinciput) to the front, back, or sides of the mother's pelvis. The maternal pelvis has a 360-degree circumference. Eight points that are 45-degrees apart are the pelvic landmarks, and the position of the fetus is determined by the relationship

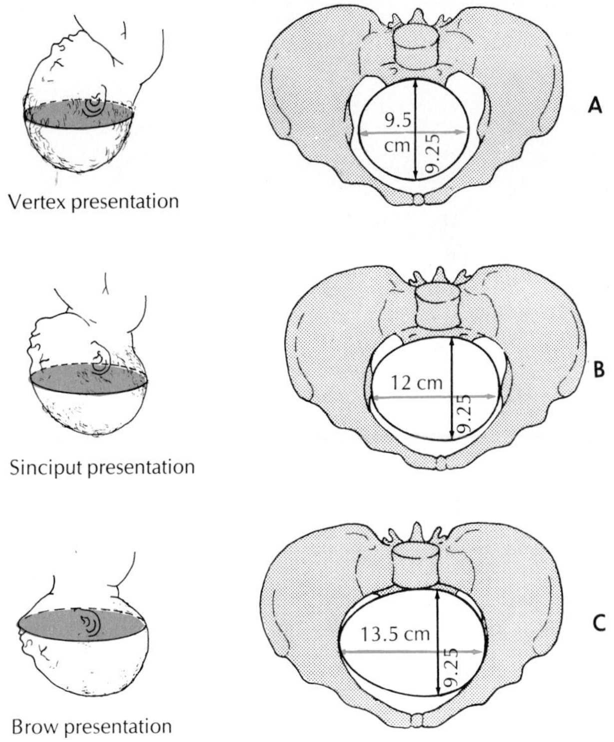

Fig. 12-3 Head entering pelvis. Biparietal diameter is indicated in black. **A,** Suboccipitobregmatic diameter: complete flexion of head on chest so that smallest diameter enters. **B,** Occipitofrontal diameter: moderate extension (military attitude) so that large diameter enters. **C,** Occipitomental diameter: marked extension (deflection) so that largest diameter, which is too large to permit head to enter pelvis, is presenting.

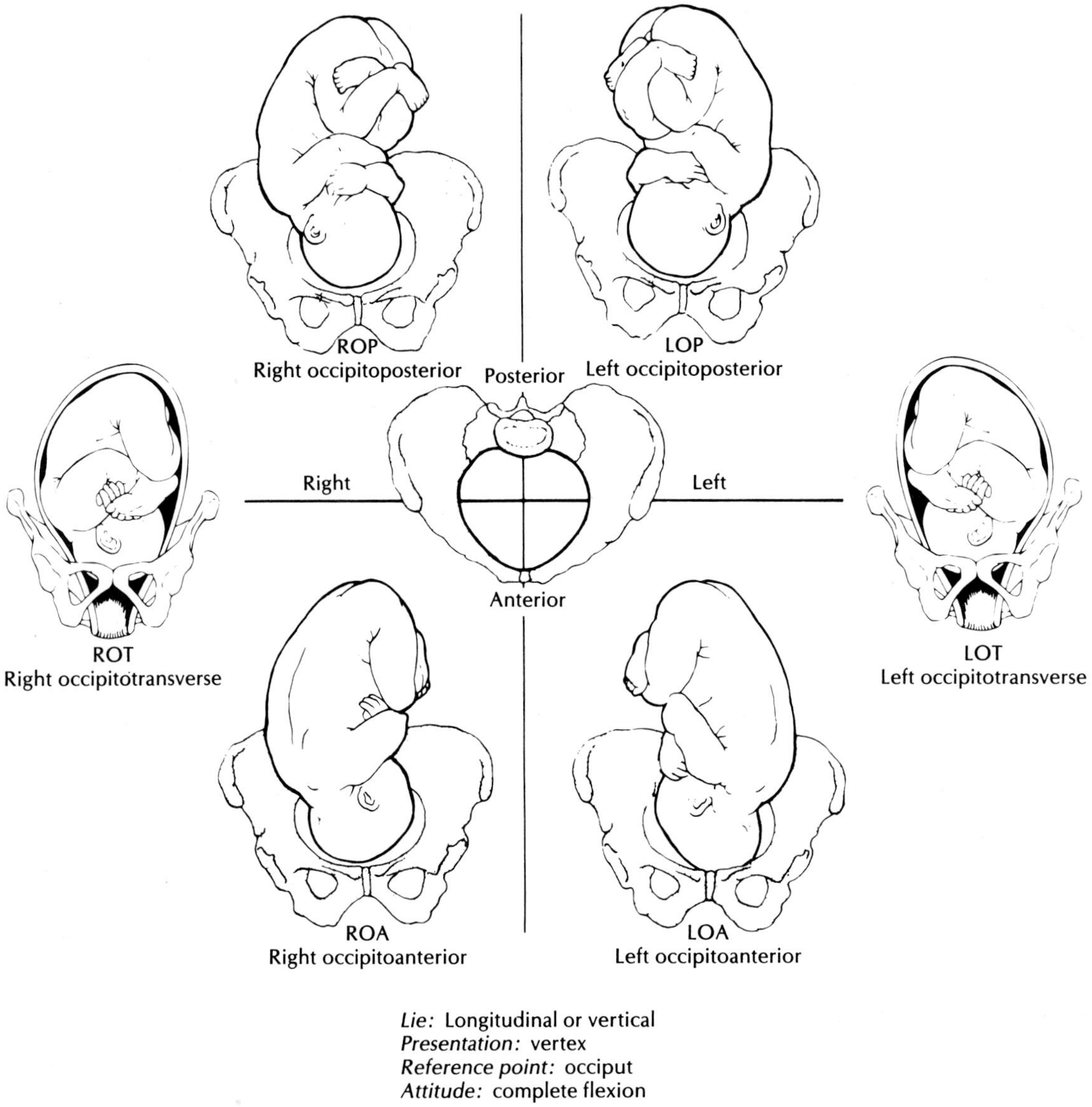

Fig. 12-4 Examples of fetal vertex (occiput) presentations in relation to front, back, or side of maternal pelvis.

of the denominator to one of these landmarks. Position is described in abbreviated form determined by the first letter of each key word. For example, right occipitoanterior position is written as ROA; right occipitotransverse is abbreviated as ROT. There are eight positions for each denominator (Table 12-1; see Fig. 12-4).

Engagement indicates that the largest transverse diameter of the presentation has passed through the maternal pelvic inlet or brim. In a well-flexed cephalic presentation, the biparietal diameter (9.25 cm) is the widest (see Fig. 12-3, *A*). Engagement can be determined by abdominal or vaginal examination.

Station is the relationship of the presenting part of the fetus to an imaginary line drawn between the maternal ischial spines. Station is expressed in terms of centimeters above or below the spines. For example, when the presenting part is 1 cm above the spines, it is noted as being minus one (see Fig. 12-19).

When the presenting part is 1 cm below the spines, however, the station is said to be plus one. At the level of the spines, the station is referred to as zero. The station of the presenting part should be determined when labor begins to keep accurate documentation of the rate of descent of the fetus during labor.

Placenta

Since the most common site for implantation of the fertilized ovum is the fundal part of the uterus, the de-

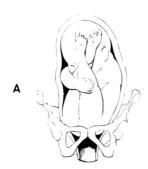

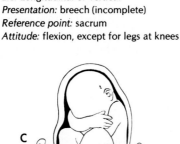

Frank breech

Lie: Longitudinal or vertical
Presentation: breech (incomplete)
Reference point: sacrum
Attitude: flexion, except for legs at knees

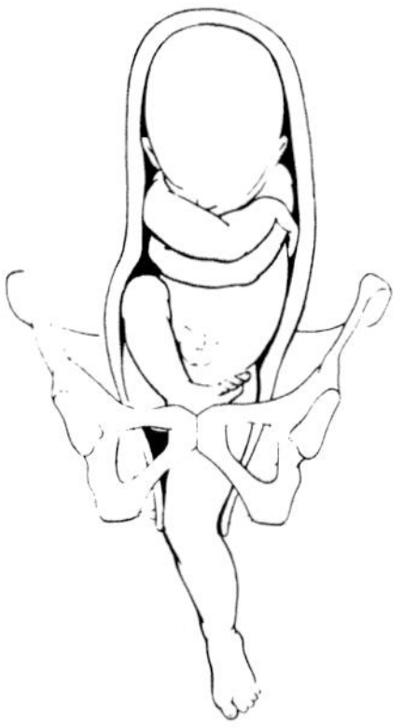

Single footling breech

Lie: Longitudinal or vertical
Presentation: breech (incomplete)
Reference point: sacrum
Attitude: flexion, except for one leg extended at hip and knee

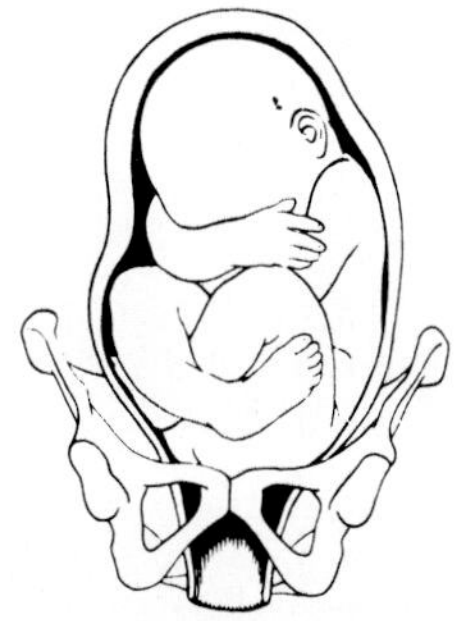

Complete breech

Lie: Longitudinal or vertical
Presentation: breech (sacrum and feet presenting)
Reference point: sacrum (with feet)
Attitude: general flexion

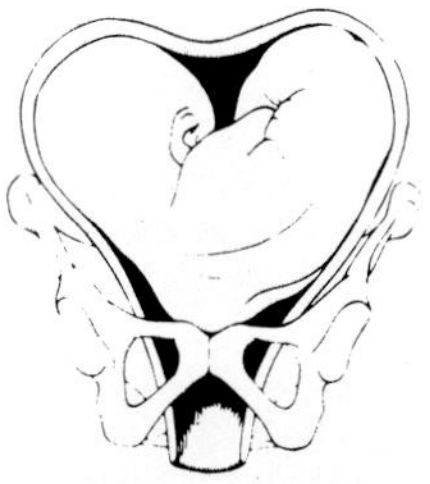

Shoulder presentation.

Lie: Transverse or horizontal
Presentation: shoulder
Reference point: scapula (Sc)
Attitude: flexion

Fig. 12-5 Fetal presentations. **A** to **C**, Breech (sacral) presentation. **D**, Shoulder presentation.

veloped placenta rarely impedes the process of labor. Placenta-related problems are included with content on hemorrhage in Chapter 23.

Passageway

The passageway, or birth canal, is composed of the rigid bony pelvis and the soft tissues of the cervix, pelvic floor, vagina, and introitus.

Bony Pelvis

The anatomy of the bony pelvis was reviewed in Chapter 8. A further discussion of the importance of pelvic configurations as they relate to the labor process is necessary at this point.

Assessment of the bony pelvis may be performed during the first prenatal evaluation and need not be repeated if the pelvis is of adequate size and suitable

Table 12-1 **Fetal Lie, Presentation, and Position**

	Presenting Part	Example of Position
LONGITUDINAL LIE		
Cephalic		
Vertex	Occiput	Left occipitotransverse (LOT)
Brow	Brow	Left brow anterior (LBA)
Face (chin) (rare)	Mentum	Right mentoposterior (RMP)
Pelvic		
Breech	Sacrum	Right sacroanterior (RSA)
TRANSVERSE LIE		
Shoulder	Scapula	Right scapuloanterior (RScA)

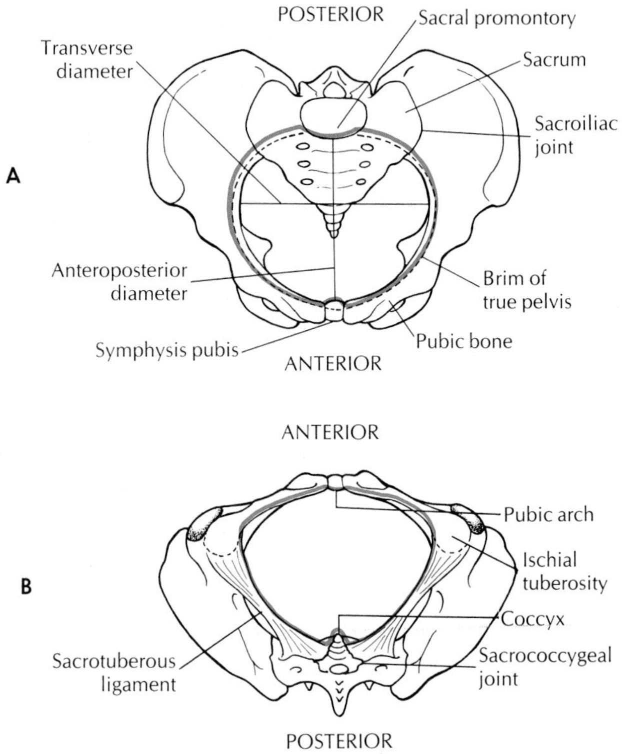

Fig. 12-6 Female pelvis. **A,** Pelvic brim from above. **B,** Pelvic outlet from below.

shape. In the third trimester of pregnancy, the examination of the bony pelvis may be more thorough and the results more accurate because there is relaxation of pelvic joints and ligaments. The four pelvic joints are the symphysis pubis, the right and left sacroiliac joints, and the sacrococcygeal joint (Fig. 12-6). The hormones of pregnancy, especially the ovarian hormone progesterone, cause the development of considerable mobil ity. Widening of the symphyseal joint and instability may cause pain in any or all of the joints.

Because the examiner does not have direct access to the bony structures and because the bones are covered with varying amounts of soft tissue, estimates of size and shape are approximate. Precise bony pelvis measurements can be determined using computed tomography and ultrasound, or x-ray films. However, x-ray examination is rarely done.

The bony pelvis is separated by the brim, or inlet, into two parts: the **false pelvis** and the **true pelvis** (see Fig. 4-17). The false pelvis is that part above the brim and is of no obstetric interest.

The true pelvis is divided into three planes: the inlet, or brim; the midpelvis, or cavity; and the outlet.

The **pelvic inlet,** or brim, of the pelvis, is formed anteriorly by the upper margins of the pubic bone, laterally by the iliopectineal lines along the innominate bones, and posteriorly by the anterior, upper margin of the sacrum, and the sacral promontory (see Figs. 4-17 and 12-6, *A*).

The **pelvic cavity,** or midpelvis, is a curved passage having a short anterior wall and a much deeper concave posterior wall. It is bounded by the posterior aspect of the symphysis pubis, the ischium, a portion of the ilium, the sacrum, and coccyx (see Fig. 4-17).

The **pelvic outlet** when viewed from below is ovoid, somewhat diamond-shaped, bounded by the pubic arch anteriorly, the ischial tuberosities laterally, and the tip of the coccyx posteriorly (Fig. 4-17). In the latter part

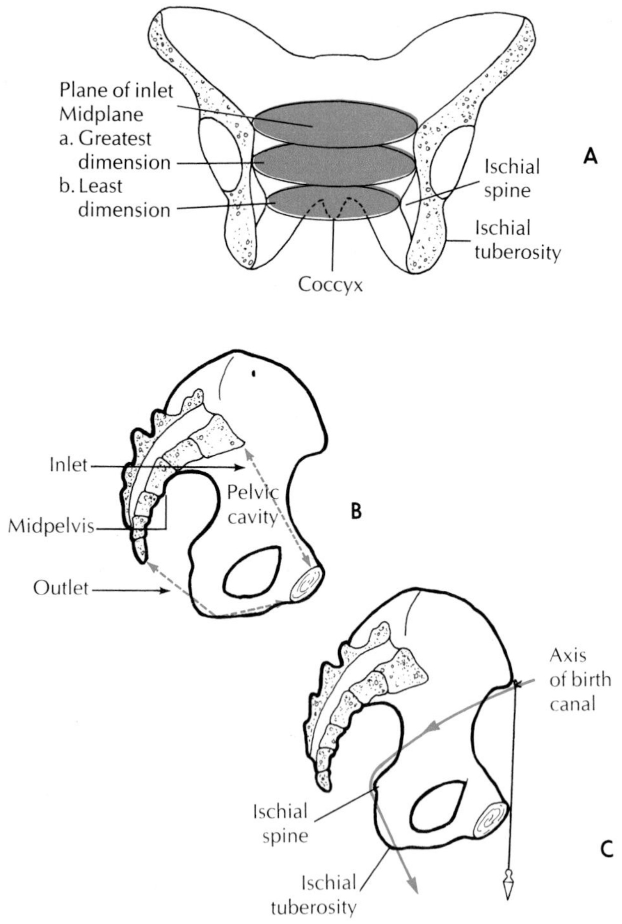

Fig. 12-7 Pelvic cavity. **A,** Inlet and midplane. Outlet not shown. **B,** Cavity of true pelvis. **C,** Note curve of sacrum and axis of birth canal.

of pregnancy the coccyx is movable (unless it has been broken in a fall while skiing or skating, for example, and has fused to the sacrum during healing).

The pelvic canal varies in size and shape at various levels. The diameters at the plane of the pelvic inlet, midpelvis, and outlet, plus the axis of the birth canal (Fig. 12-7), determine whether vaginal delivery is possible and the manner by which the fetus may pass down the birth canal (mechanism of labor).

The **subpubic angle,** which indicates the type of pubic arch, together with the length of the pubic rami and the intertuberous diameter, is of great importance. Because the presenting part must pass beneath the pubic arch, a narrow subpubic angle will be less favorable than a rounded, wide arch. Measurement of the subpubic arch is shown in Fig. 12-8. A summary of obstetric measurements is given in Table 12-2. The most important measurements are depicted in Figs. 12-8 through 12-11.

The four basic types of pelves are classified as follows:

1. Gynecoid (the classic female type)
2. Android (resembling the male pelvis)
3. Anthropoid (resembling the pelvis of anthropoid apes)
4. Platypelloid (the flat pelvis)

The **gynecoid pelvis** is the most common, with major gynecoid pelvic features present in 50% of all women. Significant anthropoid features are present in 24% of women; android configuration occurs in 23%; and the remaining 3% of women have platypelloid pelvic features. Examples of pelvic variations are given in Table 12-3 and Fig. 12-12. Female and male pelves are compared in Fig. 12-13.

Table 12-2 Obstetric Measurements

Plane of inlet (superior strait). The principal pelvic diameters of the plane of the inlet are as follows:		
Conjugates		
Diagonal	12.5-13 cm	From *inferior border* of symphysis pubis to sacral promontory
Obstetric: measurement that determines whether presenting part can engage or enter superior strait	1.5-2 cm less than diagonal (radiographic)	From *posterior surface* of symphysis pubis to sacral promontory (normally ≥10 cm)
True (vera) (anteroposterior)	≥11 cm (12.5) (radiographic)	From *upper margin* of symphysis pubis to sacral promontory
Transverse diameter	≥13 cm	Usually colon obscures this by filling left pelvis
Oblique diameter (R or L)	≥12.75 cm	From sacroiliac joint on one side to opposite iliopectineal prominence
Midplane of pelvis. The midplane of the pelvis normally is its largest plane and the one of greatest diameter.		
Anteroposterior diameter	≥11.5 cm	From midsymphysis to sacrum (at fused second and third sacral vertebras)
Transverse diameter (interspinous diameter)	10.5 cm	Narrowest transverse diameter in the midplane
Posterior sagittal diameter	4.5 cm	Segment of anteroposterior diameter dorsal to line between ischial spines; although midplane is comparatively large, critical shortening of interspinous or posterior sagittal diameter of midplane may cause pelvic dystocia
Plane of pelvic outlet. The outlet presents the smallest plane of the pelvic canal. It encompasses an area including the lower portion of the symphysis pubis, the ischial tuberosities, and the tip of the sacrum. The significant diameters are as follows:		
Anteroposterior diameter	11.9 cm	From lower border of symphysis pubis to tip of sacrum; coccyx may be displaced posteriorly during labor and is not considered to be a fixed bone
Transverse diameter (intertuberous diameter)	≥8 cm	From inner border of one ischial tuberosity to other
Posterior sagittal diameter	9 cm	Projected from tip of sacrum to a point in space where intertuberous diameter transects anteroposterior projection

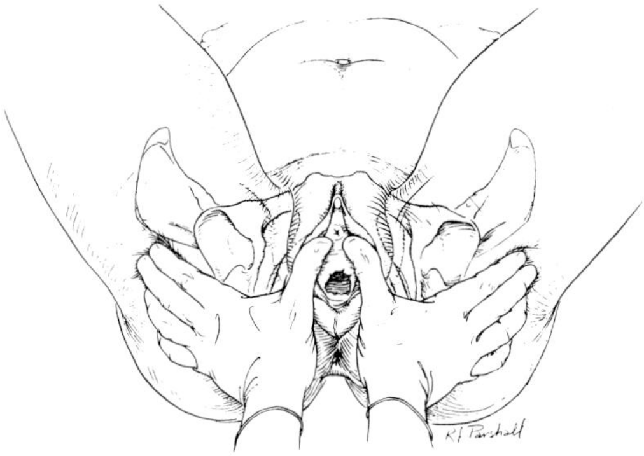

Fig. 12-8 Estimation of angle of subpubic arch. Using both thumbs, examiner externally traces descending rami down to tuberosities. (From Malasanos L et al: Health assessment, ed 3, St Louis, 1990, The CV Mosby Co.)

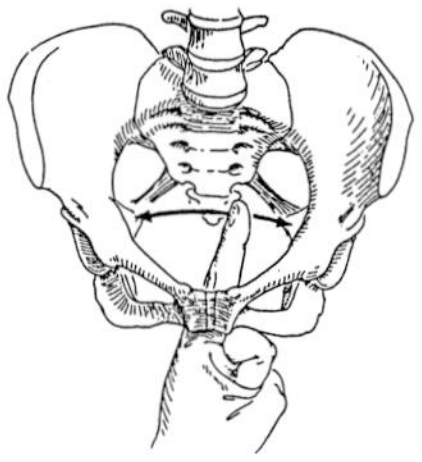

Fig. 12-10 Measurement of interspinous diameter. (From Malasanos L et al: Health assessment, ed 4, St Louis, 1990, The CV Mosby Co.)

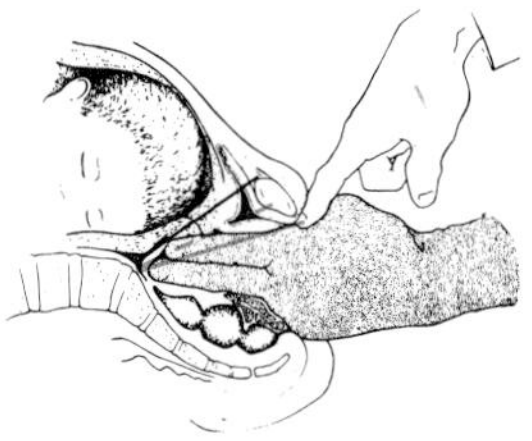

Fig. 12-9 Length of **diagonal conjugate** (solid colored line), obstetric conjugate (broken colored line), true conjugate (black line).

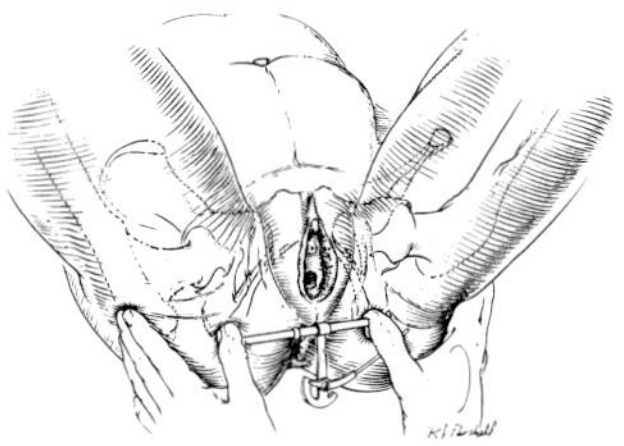

Fig. 12-11 Use of Thom's pelvimeter to measure intertuberous diameter. (From Malasanos L et al: Health assessment, ed 4, St Louis, 1990, The CV Mosby Co.)

Table 12-3 Comparison of Pelvic Types

	Gynecoid (50% of Women)	Android (23% of Women)	Anthropoid (24% of Women)	Platypelloid (3% of Women)
Brim	Slightly ovoid or transversely rounded Round	Heart shaped, angulated Heart	Oval, wider anteroposteriorly Oval	Flattened anteroposteriorly, wide transversely Flat
Depth	Moderate	Deep	Deep	Shallow
Side walls	Straight	Convergent	Straight	Straight
Ischial spines	Blunt, somewhat widely separated	Prominent, narrow interspinous diameter	Prominent, often with narrow interspinous diameter	Blunted, widely separated
Sacrum	Deep, curved	Slightly curved, terminal portion often beaked	Slightly curved	Slightly curved
Subpubic arch	Wide	Narrow	Narrow	Wide
Usual mode of delivery	Vaginal Spontaneous Occipitoanterior position	Cesarean Vaginal Difficult with forceps	Forceps/spontaneous occipitoposterior or occipitoanterior position	Spontaneous

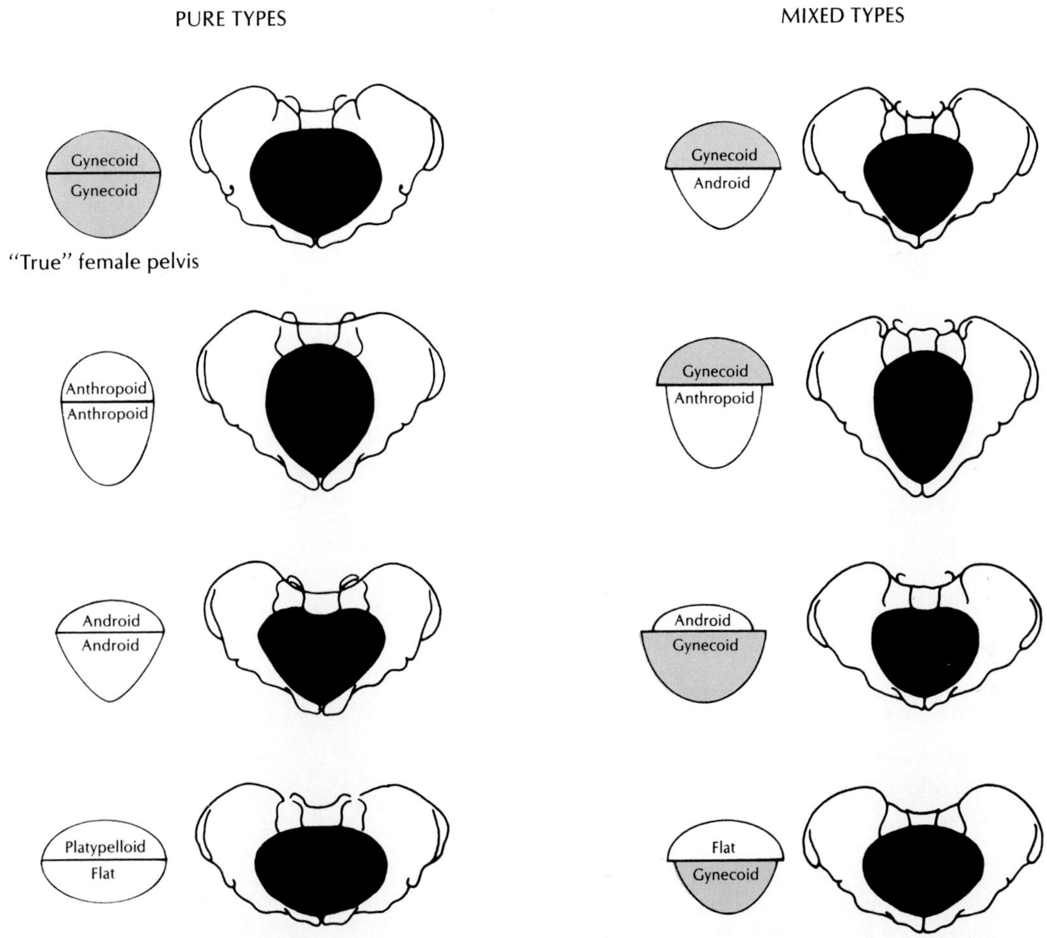

Fig. 12-12 Female pelves; pure and mixed types. Note the differences in shapes of inlets.

Soft Tissues

The soft tissues of the passageway include the distensible lower uterine segment, cervix, pelvic floor muscles, vagina, and introitus.

Before labor begins, the uterus is composed of the uterine body (corpus) and cervix (neck). After labor has begun, the uterine contractions cause the uterine body to differentiate into a thick and muscular upper segment and a thin-walled passive muscular lower segment tube. A physiologic retraction ring separates the two segments (Fig. 12-14). The lower uterine segment gradually distends to accommodate the intrauterine contents as the wall of the upper segment becomes thicker and its capacity is reduced.

The downward pressure caused by contraction of the fundus is transmitted to the cervix. The cervix then

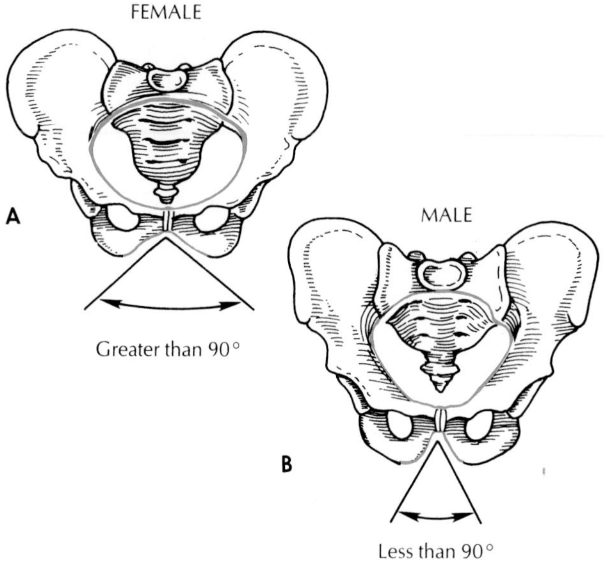

Fig. 12-13 Pelves. **A**, Gynecoid, female. **B**, Android, male. Compare shape of brim and angle of subpubic arch.

effaces (thins) (Fig. 12-14, *B* and *C*) and dilates (opens) (Fig. 12-14, *C* and *D*) sufficiently to allow **descent** of the presenting part into the vagina. Actually, the cervix is drawn upward and over the presenting part as the **vertex** or breech descends.

The pelvic floor is a muscular diaphragm that separates the pelvic cavity above from the perineal space below. This structure helps the presenting part of the fetus rotate anteriorly during the second stage of labor and directs it downward and forward along the lower straits of the birth canal. The vagina in turn distends to permit passage of the fetus into the external world. As noted earlier, the soft tissues of the vagina develop throughout pregnancy until at term the vagina can dilate to accommodate the fetus.

Powers

The forces acting to expel the fetus and placenta are derived from the **primary powers,** the involuntary uterine contractions. After the first stage of labor, **secondary powers,** voluntary bearing-down efforts, augment the force of the involuntary contractions.

Primary Powers

Contractions originate at pacemaker points in the myometrium near the uterotubal junction. From the pacemaker points, contractions move over the uterus like a wave. Successive downward waves of contractions are separated by short rest periods. The following is a description of the primary forces from Willson and Carrington (1987).

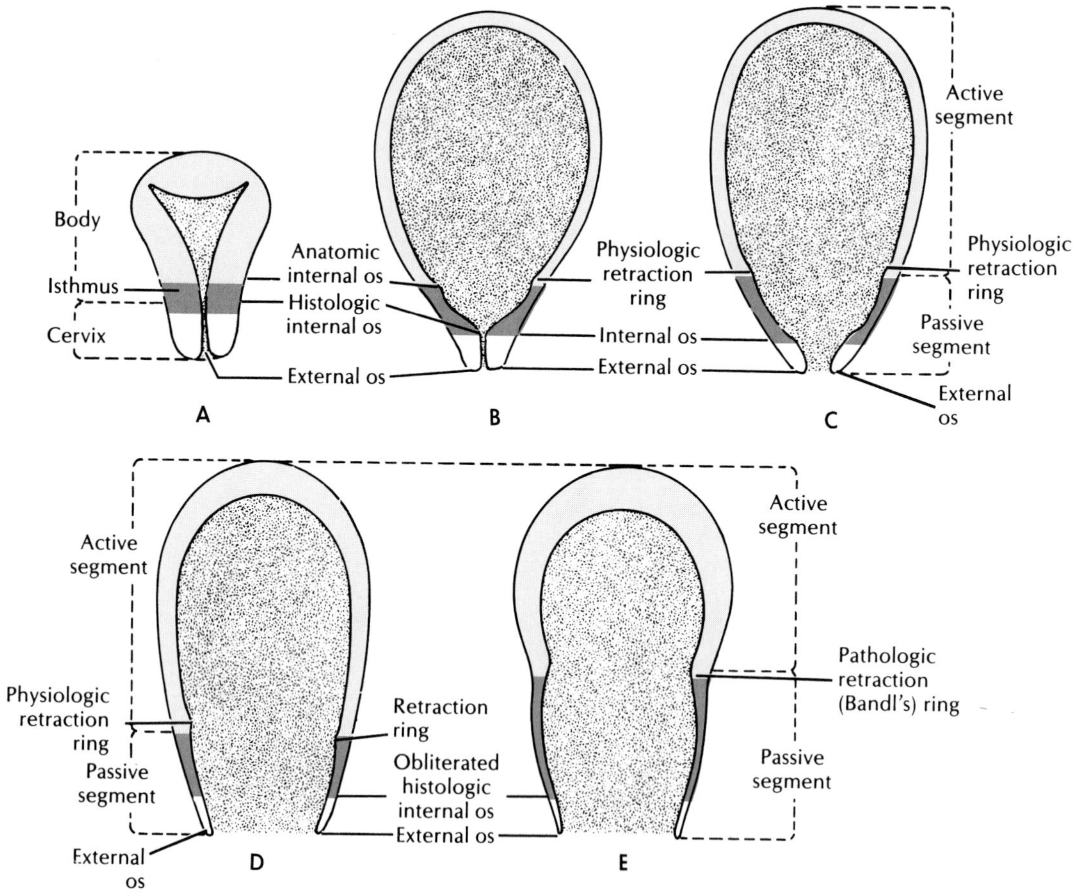

Fig. 12-14 Progressive development of segments and rings of uterus at term. Note comparison between **A,** nonpregnant uterus, **B,** uterus at term, and **C,** uterus in normal labor in early first stage, and **D,** second stage. Passive segment is derived from lower uterine segment (isthmus) and cervix, and physiologic retraction ring is derived from anatomic internal os. **E,** Uterus in abnormal labor in second-stage dystocia. Pathologic retraction (Bandl's) ring that forms under abnormal conditions develops from physiologic ring. (Modified from Willson JR and Carrington, ER: Obstetrics and gynecology, ed 8, St Louis, 1987, The CV Mosby Co.)

The ultimate effect . . . of a normal labor contraction . . . is a gradient of force directed from the fundus to the least active and weakest area of the uterus, the cervix. This is called *fundal dominance.* The force generated by each contraction is applied to the amniotic fluid and directly against the pole of the infant that occupies the upper segment. Therefore each time the muscle contracts, the uterine cavity becomes smaller, and the presenting part of the infant or the forebag of waters lying ahead of it is pushed downward into the cervix. This tends to force it open, or *dilate* it.

A more potent factor in cervical dilatation, however, is the *retraction of the upper segment.* As this area of the uterus becomes shorter and thicker, it pulls the lower segment and the dilating cervix upward around the presenting part at the same time the uterus contracting directly against the fetus tends to push it through the cervical opening (Fig. 12-15). The cervix opens or is dilated by a combination of these two factors but retraction is probably more important than the pressure of the presenting part, since dilatation will occur even though the presenting part does not descend into it. A *completely dilated cervix* that will permit a term infant to pass through it has a diameter of about 10 cm.

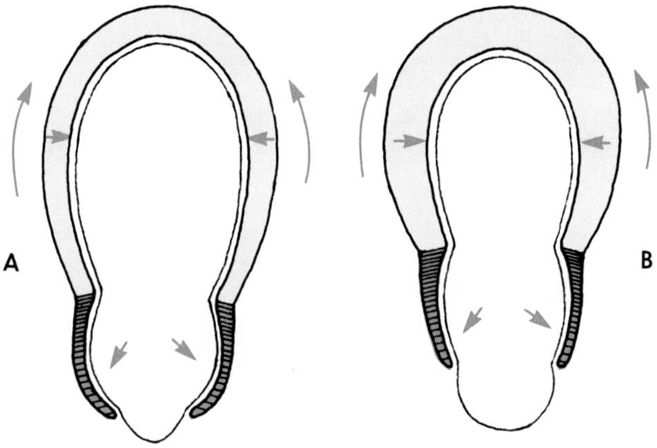

Fig. 12-15 Lower uterine segment and cervix are pulled up (retracted) as the fetus and amniotic sac are pushed downward. **A,** Cervix is effaced and partially dilated. **B,** Cervical dilatation is complete. Cervix is being pulled upward as presenting part descends. Intrauterine space is decreasing. (From Willson JR and Carrington ER: Obstetrics and gynecology, ed 8, St Louis, 1987, The CV Mosby Co.)

The primary powers are responsible for the effacement and dilatation of the cervix and descent of the fetus. **Effacement** of the cervix means the shortening and thinning of the cervix during the first stage of labor. The cervix, normally 2 to 3 cm in length and about 1 cm thick, is obliterated or "taken up" by a shortening of the uterine muscle bundles during the thinning of the lower uterine segment in advancing labor. Eventually only a thin edge of the cervix can be palpated when effacement is complete. Effacement generally is advanced in nulliparas at term before more than slight dilatation occurs. In multiparas, effacement and dilatation of the cervix tend to progress together. Degree of effacement is expressed in percentages (e.g., a cervix is 50% effaced) (Fig. 12-16).

Dilatation of the cervix is the enlargement or widening of the cervical os and the cervical canal during the first stage of labor. The diameter increases from perhaps less than 1 cm to approximately 10 cm to allow delivery of a term fetus. When the cervix is fully dilated (and completely retracted), it can no longer be palpated (Fig. 12-16).

Dilatation of the cervix occurs by the drawing upward of the musculofibrous components of the cervix with strong uterine contractions. Pressure exerted by the amniotic fluid while the membranes are intact or force applied by the presenting part also encourages cervical dilatation. Scarring of the cervix as a result of infection or surgery may retard cervical dilatation.

Secondary Powers

As soon as the presenting part reaches the pelvic floor, the woman experiences an urge to push, a voluntary bearing-down effort (secondary power). The bearing-down effort is similar to that used in the process of defecation. However, a different set of muscles is used; the parturient contracts her diaphragm and abdominal muscles and pushes out the contents of the birth canal. Bearing-down results in increased intraabdominal pressure. The pressure compresses the uterus on all sides and adds to the power of the expulsive forces. The secondary forces have no effect on cervical dilatation; they are of considerable importance in aiding the expulsion of the infant from the uterus and vagina after the cervix is fully dilated.

Any voluntary bearing-down efforts by the woman earlier in labor are counterproductive to cervical dilatation. Straining will exhaust the woman and cause cervical trauma (p. 393).

Position of The Mother

The mother's position affects her anatomic and physiologic adaptations to labor. Her cardiac output normally increases during labor as uterine contractions return blood into the maternal vascular bed (see Table 12-4). The increase in cardiac output is possible if the maternal position prevents compression of the descending aorta and ascending vena cava. Increased cardiac output improves blood flow to the uterofetoplacental unit and the maternal kidneys.

Gravity is added to the psychologic benefits of various positions. In general, if the woman is in the upright position, uterine contractions are stronger and more ef-

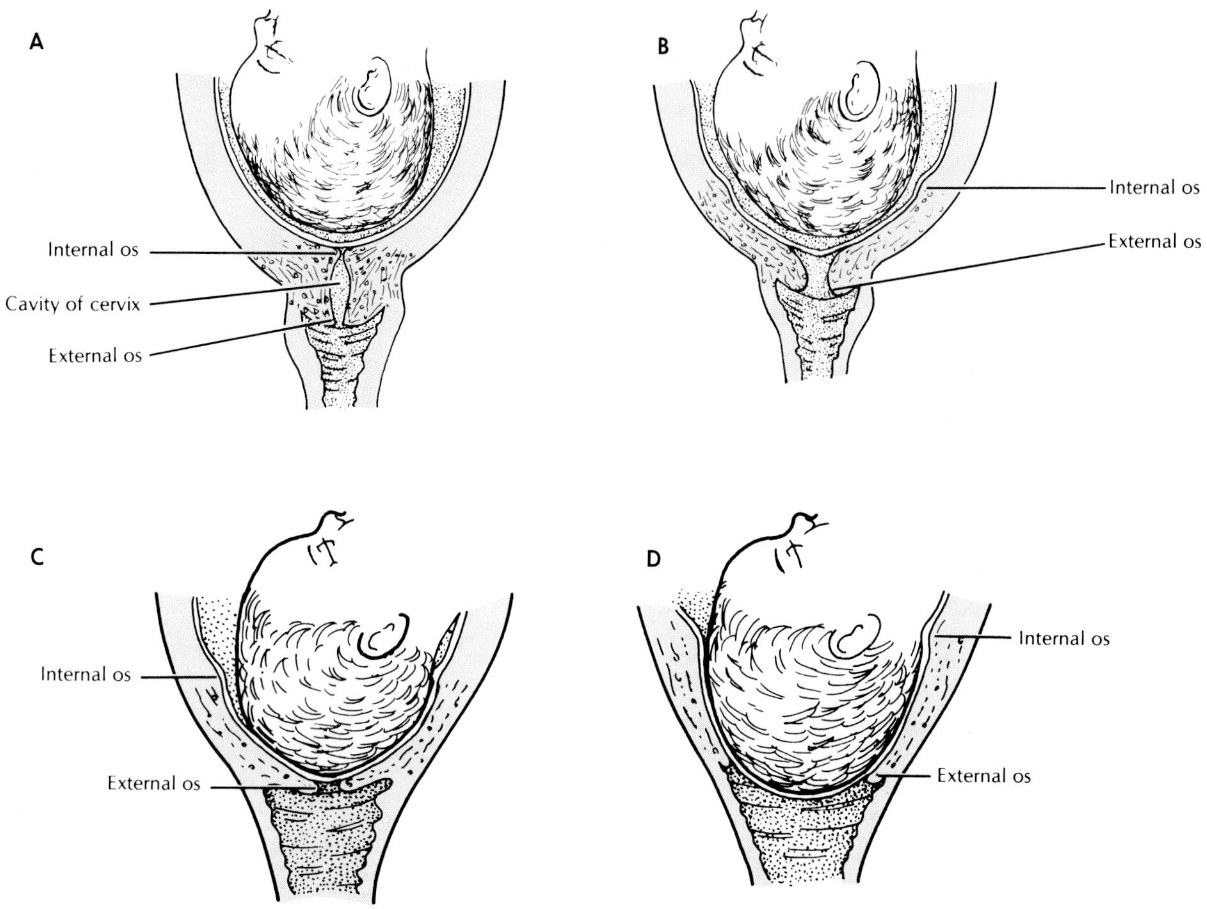

Fig. 12-16 Cervical effacement and dilatation. Note how cervix is drawn up around presenting part (internal os). Membranes are intact, and head is not well applied to cervix. **A,** Before labor. **B,** Early effacement. **C,** Complete effacement (100%). Head is well applied to cervix. **D,** Complete dilatation (10 cm). Some overlapping of cranial bones. Membranes still intact.

ficient, and the duration of labor is shorter. The upright position includes standing, walking, and squatting. Frequent changes in position relieve fatigue and improve circulation to body parts. Maternal position changes enlist gravity to aid fetal descent through the birth canal.

Squatting during the second stage moves the uterus forward, thereby straightening the long axis of the birth canal (McKay, 1984). As the fetus descends in the birth canal, the pressure of the presenting part on stretch receptors of the pelvic floor stimulates the woman's bearing-down reflex. Stimulation of the stretch receptors in turn stimulates the release of oxytocin from the posterior pituitary (**Ferguson's reflex**). Oxytocin increases the intensity of the uterine contractions. In a sitting position, such as squatting, abdominal muscles work in greater synchrony with uterine contractions during bearing-down efforts.

❑ PROCESS OF LABOR

Prodromal signs and symptoms are among the first indicators that the reproductive system is preparing for the childbirth.

Reproductive System Changes

In nulliparas the uterus gradually sinks downward and forward about 2 weeks before term, when the fetus's presenting part (usually the fetal head) descends into the true pelvis. This settling is called **lightening** or "dropping" and usually happens gradually (Fig. 12-17). After lightening, women feel less congested and breathe more easily. However, there is usually more bladder pressure as a result of this shift and consequently a return of urinary frequency. In multiparas, lightening may not take place until after uterine contractions are established and true labor is in progress.

Persistent low backache and sacroiliac distress as a result of relaxation of the pelvic joints may be described. Occasionally strong, frequent, but irregular uterine (Braxton Hicks') contractions may be identified by the gravida.

Prodromal labor events are experienced before the onset of true labor. The vaginal mucus becomes more profuse in response to the extreme congestion of the vaginal mucus membranes. Brownish or blood-tinged cervical mucus may be passed (**bloody show**). The cervix becomes soft (ripens) and partially effaced and may begin to dilate. The membranes may rupture spontaneously.

Two other phenomena are common in the days preceding labor: (1) loss of 0.5 to 1.5 kg (1 to 3 lb) in weight, caused by water loss resulting from electrolyte shifts that in turn are produced by changes in estrogen and progesterone levels, and (2) a burst of energy. Women speak of a burst of energy that they often use to clean the house and put everything in order. This activity has been described as the "nesting instinct."

The onset of true labor cannot be ascribed to a single cause. Many factors, including changes in the maternal uterus, cervix, and pituitary gland are involved. Hormones produced by the normal fetal hypothalamus, pituitary, and adrenal cortex probably contribute to the **initiation of labor.** Progressive uterine distension, increasing intrauterine pressure, and aging of the placenta seem to be associated with increasing myometrial irritability. This is a result of increased concentrations of estrogen and prostaglandins, and decreasing progesterone levels. In actuality, many factors may be responsible for initiating labor. The mutually coordinated effects of these factors result in strong, regular, rhythmic uterine contractions. Normally, these factors working in concert terminate in the birth of the fetus and the delivery of the placenta. It is still not completely understood how certain alterations trigger others and how proper checks and balances are maintained.

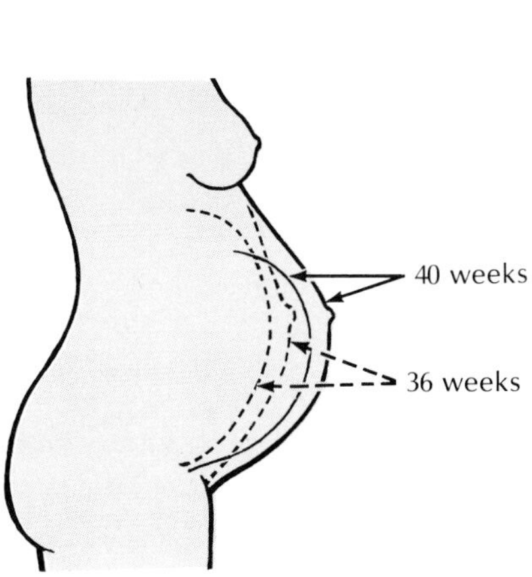

Fig. 12-17 Lightening.

Afferent and efferent nerve impulses to and from the uterus alter its contractility. Although nerve impulses to the uterus will stimulate contractions, the denervated uterus still contracts well during labor because oxytocin in the circulating blood is a regulator of labor. Therefore some women who are paralyzed can still give birth vaginally.

Mechanism of Labor

The female pelvis has varied contours and diameters at different levels, and the presenting part of the passenger is large in proportion to the passage. For delivery to occur, the fetus must adapt to the birth canal during the descent. The turns and other adjustments necessary in the human birth process are termed the **mechanism of labor** (Fig. 12-18). The cardinal movements of the mechanisms of labor that occur in a vertex presentation are **engagement, descent, flexion, internal rotation, extension,** and **external rotation.** The fetus is born by **expulsion.** Although these phases will be discussed separately, a combination of movements is occurring simultaneously; for example, engagement involves both descent and flexion.

Engagement. When the biparietal diameter of the head passes the pelvic inlet, the head is said to be engaged in the pelvic inlet. In most nulliparous women this occurs before the onset of active labor because the firmer abdominal muscles direct the presenting part into the pelvis. In multiparous women with more relaxed abdominal musculature, the head often remains freely movable above the pelvic brim until labor is established. In the majority of cases the head of a normal-sized fetus enters the pelvis with the sagittal suture transverse to the pelvic inlet (Fig. 12-4, ROT or LOT).

Descent. Descent refers to the progress of the presenting part through the pelvis. As **partograms** (labor curves) (Figs. 15-7 and 15-8) indicate, there is little progress in descent during the latent phase of the first stage of labor. Descent becomes more rapid in the latter part of the active phase when the cervix has dilated to 5 to 7 cm. It is apparent especially when the membranes have ruptured.

Descent depends on three forces: (1) pressure of the amniotic fluid, (2) direct pressure of the contracting fundus on the fetus, and (3) contraction of the maternal diaphragm and abdominal muscles in the second stage. The effects of these forces are modified by the size and shape of the maternal pelvic planes and the size and capacity of the fetal head to mold.

The degree of descent is gauged by the station of the presenting part (Fig. 12-19). The speed of the descent increases in the second stage of labor. In nulliparas this descent is slow but steady; in multiparas the descent may be rapid. Progress in the descent of the presenting part is determined by abdominal palpation (Leopold's maneuvers) (Chapter 15) and vaginal examination until the presenting part can be seen at the introitus.

Flexion. As soon as the descending head meets resistance from the cervix, pelvic wall, or pelvic floor, flexion normally occurs, and the chin is brought into more intimate contact with the fetal chest (see Fig. 12-18, *B*). Flexion permits the smaller suboccipitobregmatic diameter (9.5 cm) rather than the larger diameters to present to the outlet.

Internal Rotation. The maternal pelvic inlet is widest in the transverse diameter. Therefore the fetal head passes the inlet into the true pelvis in the occipitotransverse position (see Fig. 12-4). The outlet is widest in the anteroposterior diameter, however. To exit, the fetal head must rotate. Internal rotation begins at the level of the ischial spines but is not completed until the presenting part reaches the lower pelvis. As the occiput rotates anteriorly, the face rotates posteriorly. With each contraction the fetal head is guided by the bony pelvis and the muscles of the pelvic floor. Eventually the occiput will be in the midline beneath the pubic arch. The head is almost always rotated by the time it reaches the pelvic floor (see Fig. 12-18, C). Both the levator ani muscles and the bony pelvis are important for anterior rotation. Previous childbirth injury or regional anesthesia compromises the function of the levator sling.

Extension. When the fetal head reaches the perineum to be born, it is deflected anteriorly by the per-

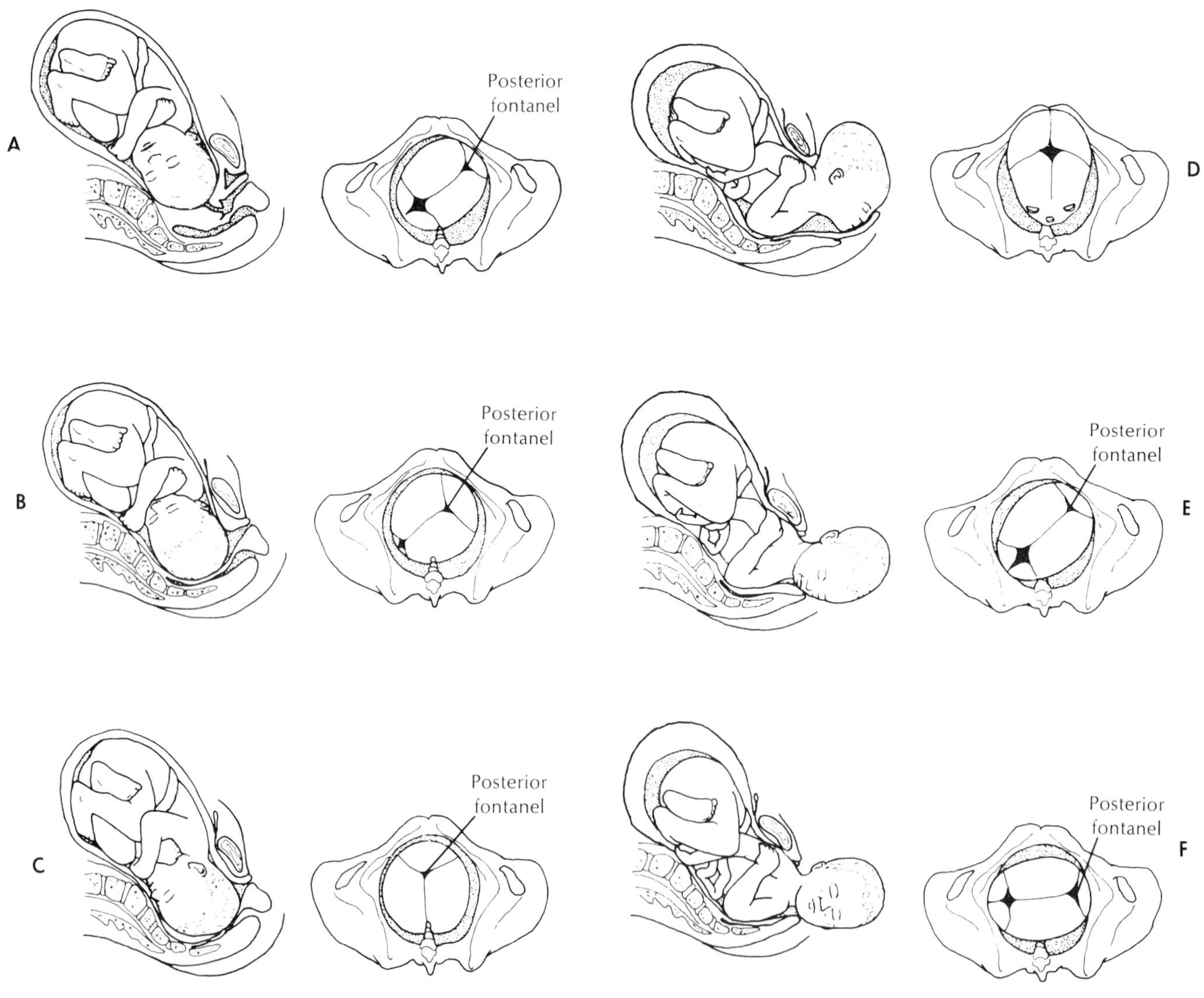

Fig. 12-18 Mechanism of labor in left occipitoanterior (LOA) presentation. **A,** Engagement and descent. **B,** Flexion. **C,** Internal rotation to OA. **D,** Extension. **E,** Restitution. **F,** External rotation.

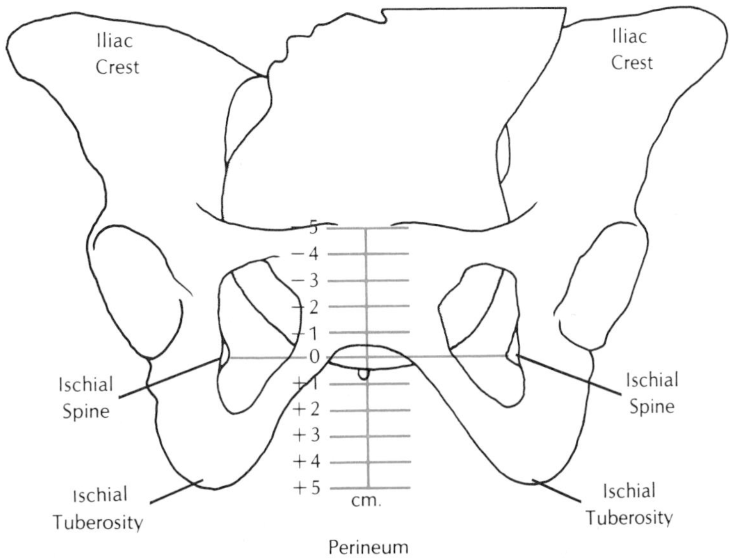

Fig. 12-19 Stations of presenting part or degree of descent. Silhouette shows head of infant approaching station +1. (Courtesy Ross Laboratories, Columbus, Ohio.)

ineum. The occiput acts as the fulcrum as it passes under the lower border of the symphysis pubis. As a result the head is born by extension: first the occiput, then the face, and finally the chin (see Fig. 12-18, *D*).

Restitution and External Rotation. After delivery of the head, it rotates briefly to the position it occupied when it was engaged in the inlet. This movement is referred to as **restitution** (see Fig. 12-18, *E-F*). The 45-degree turn realigns the infant's head with her or his back and shoulders. The head can then be seen to rotate further. External rotation occurs as the shoulders engage and descend in maneuvers similar to those of the head. As noted earlier, the anterior shoulder descends first. When it reaches the outlet, it rotates to the midline and is delivered from under the pubic arch. The posterior shoulder is guided over the perineum until it is free of the introitus.

Expulsion. After delivery of the shoulders, the head and shoulders are lifted up toward the mother's pubic bone and the trunk of the baby is delivered by a movement of lateral flexion in the direction of the symphysis pubis. When the baby is completely born, birth is complete. *This* is the end of the second stage of labor and *the time* is recorded on the records.

Stages of Labor

Normal labor (eutocia) is recorded when the woman is at or near term, without complications, when a single fetus presents by vertex, and when labor is complete within 24 hours.

The course of normal labor is remarkably constant and consists of three concomitant subprocesses: (1) regular progression of uterine contractions, (2) effacement and progressive dilatation of the cervix, and (3) progress in descent of the presenting part. **Four stages of labor** are recognized.

The **first stage of labor** is considered to last from the onset of regular uterine contractions to full dilatation of the cervix. Commonly the onset of labor is difficult to establish; the woman may be admitted to the labor floor just before delivery so that the beginning of labor may be only an estimate. The first stage is much longer than the second and third combined. Great variability is the rule, however, depending on the essential factors discussed earlier. Some multiparas may reach full dilatation in less than 1 hour, or, uncommonly, a nullipara may reach complete dilatation of the cervix in 24 hours.

The first stage of labor has been divided into two phases: a *latent phase* and an *active phase.* Transition is a part of the active phase of the first stage of labor. During the latent phase there is more progress in effacement of the cervix and little increase in descent. During the active phase there is more rapid dilatation of the cervix and descent of the presenting part. If the degree of dilatation and descent is plotted in a graph, it forms an S curve. This curve can be used as a basis for assessment of progress in labor (Figs. 15-7 and 15-8).

The **second stage of labor** lasts from full dilatation of the cervix to delivery of the fetus. Labor of up to 2 hours is considered within the normal range for the second stage.

The **third stage of labor** lasts from delivery of the fetus to delivery of the placenta. The placenta normally separates with the third or fourth strong uterine contraction after the infant has been delivered. Then it should be delivered with the next uterine contraction after placental separation. Placental separation usually begins with the contraction that delivers the baby's trunk and is normally completed with the first contraction after the birth of the baby. However, delivery of the placenta within 45 to 60 minutes is generally considered within normal limits.

The **fourth stage of labor** arbitrarily lasts about 2 hours after delivery of the placenta. It is the period of immediate recovery, when homeostasis is reestablished. It serves as an important period of observation for complications, such as abnormal bleeding.

There are no absolute values for the normal length of the first stage of labor (Willson and Carrington, 1987). Variations may reflect differences in the client population or in clinical practice. Friedman (1978) provides statistical upper limits for the first and second stages of labor:

	Nulliparous	**Multiparous**
First stage		
Latent phase	20 hours	14 hours
Active phase	1.2 cm per hour	1.5 cm per hour
Second stage	2 hours	1.5 hours

The duration of the third stage will be 15 to 30 minutes or even longer if the physician waits for the mother to expel the placenta herself. When the placental stage is managed actively, its duration can be less than 5 minutes (Willson and Carrington, 1987).

A description of the labor experience of a significant number of parturients is given in Figs. 15-7 and 15-8. Friedman and Sachtleben (1965) used this information to predict the duration of normal labor for the first and second stages.

The mother and fetus must adapt anatomically and physiologically during the birth process. Accurate assessment of the parturient and fetus requires a knowledge of expected adaptations.

❑ MATERNAL ADAPTATIONS

A thorough understanding of maternal adaptations to pregnancy (Chapter 8) is fundamental to anticipating and meeting the parturient's needs. Table 12-4 summarizes normal adaptations by body systems, including objective and subjective symptomatology.

Discomfort During Labor

The discomfort experienced during labor has two origins. During the *first stage* of labor, uterine contractions cause (1) cervical dilatation and effacement and (2) uterine ischemia (decreased blood flow and therefore local oxygen deficit) from contraction of the arteries to the myometrium.

The discomfort from cervical changes and uterine ischemia is *visceral.* The discomfort is located over the lower abdomen and radiates to the lumbar area of the back and down the thighs. Usually the woman experiences discomfort only during contractions and is free of pain between contractions.

During the *second stage* of labor, the stage of expulsion of the baby, the woman experiences perineal or *somatic* pain. Perineal discomfort results from traction on the peritoneum and uterocervical supports during contractions. It can also be produced by expulsive forces or from pressure by the presenting part on the bladder, bowel, or other sensitive pelvic structures.

Pain may be *local,* with cramplike pain and a tearing or bursting sensation because of distension and laceration of the cervix, vagina, or perineal tissues. It may also be *referred,* with the discomfort felt in the back, flanks, or thighs. Emotional tension from anxiety and fear may increase pain and perception of pain during labor (see Dick-Read method, p. 220).

Pain impulses during the first stage of labor are transmitted through the spinal nerve segment of T11-12 and accessory lower thoracic and upper lumbar sympathetic nerves. Pain impulses during the second stage of labor are carried through S1-4 and the parasympathetic system. Pain experienced during the third stage, as well as so-called afterpains, is uterine, similar to that experienced early in the first stage of labor. Areas of discomfort are illustrated in Fig. 12-20.

Pain results in both psychic responses and reflex physical actions. The quality of physical pain has been described as pricking, burning, aching, throbbing, sharp, nauseating, or cramping. Pain in childbirth gives rise to symptoms that are identifiable. It may cause increased activity of the sympathetic nervous system. As a result there are changes in blood pressure, pulse, respirations, and skin color. Bouts of nausea and vomiting and excessive perspiration are also commonplace. Certain affective expressions of suffering are familiar to all. Affective changes include increasing anxiety with lessened perceptual field, writhing, crying, groaning, gesturing (hand clenching and wringing), and excessive muscular excitability throughout the body. Childbirth pain is of a limited duration (at most 2 to 3 days).

Perception of Pain. Although the pain threshold is remarkably similar in all people regardless of sexual, social, ethnic, or cultural differences, these differences play a definite role in the individual's perception of the pain experience. The reasons for the effects of such factors as culture, use of counterstimuli, or distraction in coping with pain are not fully understood. The mean-

Table 12-4 Maternal Anatomic and Physiologic Adaptation to Labor

Body System	Normal Adaptation to Labor	Observable Findings
Cardiovascular		
Cardiac output	Increases; during each contraction 400 ml blood is emptied from uterus into maternal vascular system	Pulse slows; BP increases; no alteration in FHR
WBC	Mechanism unknown; possible WBC level changes secondary to physical/emotional stress	$\geq 25{,}000/mm^3$
Peripheral vascular system	Response to cervical dilatation; compression of vessels by fetus passing through birth canal	Malar flush; hot or cold feet; hemorrhoids
Respiratory		
Rate	Increased physical activity with increased oxygen consumption	Rate increases
Acid/base balance	Hyperventilation may be cause of increased pH early in labor; pH returns to normal by end of first stage	No change if hyperventilation is controlled
Renal		
Fluids/electrolytes	Diaphoresis	Possible temperature elevation
	Increased insensible water loss through respirations	Thirst
	Occasionally NPO	
Bladder	Becomes an abdominal organ starting with the second trimester	When filling, palpable above symphysis pubis
	Deterrents to spontaneous voiding: tissue edema secondary to pressure from presenting part, discomfort, sedation, embarrassment	Possible inability to void spontaneously
Urine constituents	Breakdown of muscle tissue from the physical work of labor	1 + proteinuria
Integument	Great distensibility in area of vaginal introitus; degree of distensibility varies with the individual	Minute tears in skin around vagina
Musculoskeletal	Marked increase in muscle activity (in addition to uterine activity)	Diaphoresis; fatigue; 1 + proteinuria; ? increased temperature
	Backache and joint ache (unrelated to fetal position) secondary to increased joint laxity at term	Verbal/nonverbal cues indicating back discomfort
	Leg cramps secondary to labor process and pointing of toes	Verbal/nonverbal cues
Neurologic	Sensorium alterations change as woman moves through phases of first stage of labor and as she moves from one stage to the next	Euphoria to increased seriousness to amnesia between contractions to elation or fatigue after delivery
	Discomfort (see discussion on pain during childbirth)	Verbal/nonverbal cues absent or minimal
	Endogenous endorphins and encephalins and physiologic anesthesia of perineal tissues with decreased perception of discomfort	
Gastrointestinal	Mouth breathing, dehydration, emotional response to labor	Verbal/nonverbal cues indicating dry mouth
	Decreased motility and absorption; delayed stomach emptying time	Nausea/vomiting of undigested foods eaten after onset of labor
	Nausea as a reflex response to full cervical dilatation	Nausea/vomiting; belching
	History of diarrhea concurrent with onset of labor or	Verbal cue
	Presence of hard or impacted stool in rectum	Palpable on vaginal examination; fecal material extruded during delivery
Endocrine	Level of estrogen increases; levels of progesterone, prostaglandins, and oxytocin decrease	Labor is initiated and maintained
	Metabolism increases	Blood glucose may decrease

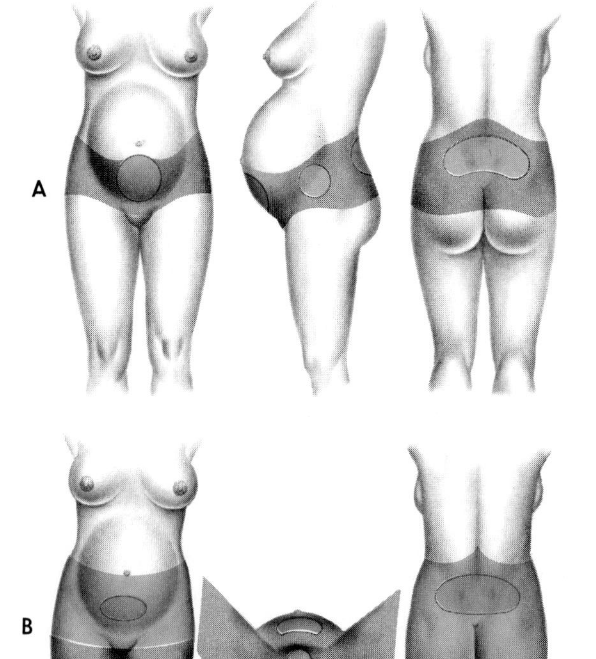

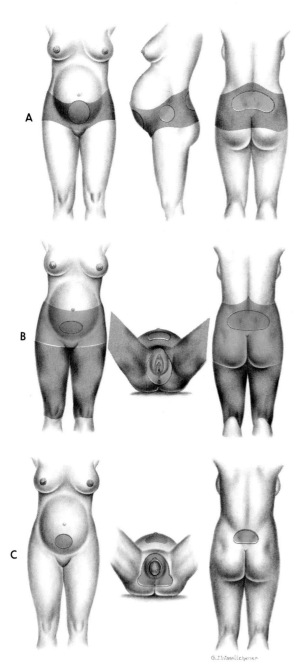

Fig. 12-20 Discomfort during labor. **A**, Distribution of labor pain during first stage. **B**, Distribution of labor pain during later phase of first stage and early phase of second stage. **C**, Distribution of labor pain during later phase of second stage and actual birth. (Gray shading indicates areas of mild discomfort; light colored shading indicates areas of moderate discomfort; dark colored areas indicate intense discomfort.)

ing of pain and the verbal and nonverbal expressions given to pain are apparently learned from interactions within the primary social group. It is personalized for each individual. As pain is experienced, people develop various coping mechanisms to deal with it. Pain or the possibility of pain that has unknown qualities can induce fear in which anxiety borders on panic. Fatigue and sleep deprivation magnify pain. Parity may affect perception of labor pain (Gaston-Johansson, Fridh, and Turner-Norveli, 1988).

At times, pain stimuli that are particularly intense can be ignored. It may be that certain nerve cell groupings within the spinal cord, brain stem, and cerebral cortex have the ability to modulate the pain impulse through a blocking mechanism. This **gate-control theory** is helpful in understanding the approaches used in education-for-childbirth programs or the use of hypnosis in labor. According to this theory, local physical stimulation such as massage or stroking of the woman in labor can balance the pain stimuli. It is thought to work by closing down a hypothetical "gate" in the spinal cord, thus blocking pain signals from reaching the brain. Also, when the laboring woman performs neuromuscular and motor skills, activity within the spinal cord itself further modifies the transmission of pain. Cognitive activities of concentration on breathing and relaxation skills require selective and directed cortical activity, which activates and closes the gating mechanism as well. The gate-control theory emphasizes the need for a supportive setting for birth. In such an environment the laboring woman can relax and allow the various higher mental activities to be implemented.

❑ FETAL ADAPTATIONS

Fetal heart rate (FHR) monitoring provides reliable and predictive information about the condition of the fetus as it relates to oxygenation (Chapter 14). Stresses to the uterofetoplacental unit result in characteristic FHR patterns. It is important for the nurse to have a basic understanding of the factors involved in fetal oxygenation and of the fetal responses that reflect adequate fetal oxygenation.

The placenta serves as a link between the fetal and maternal circulations. Uterine spiral arterioles must pass through the full thickness of the myometrium to reach the intervillous space. The maternal blood spurts through these arterioles into the intervillous space. Oxygen, nutrients, and inherent warmth are absorbed by the thin-walled fetal capillaries contained within the chorionic villi of the placenta. These are eventually carried to the fetus by the umbilical vein. Carbon dioxide and fetal waste products circulate back to the placenta through the umbilical arteries and fetal capillaries in the chorionic villi. Here they cross back through the intervillous space to the maternal circulation.

The average FHR at term is 140 beats per minute (bpm); the normal range is 120 to 160 bpm. Earlier in gestation the FHR is higher, with an average of approximately 160 bpm at 20 weeks' gestation. The rate decreases progressively as the maturing fetus reaches term. The normal range of pH in an adult is 7.35 to 7.45. The average fetal range is 7.30 to 7.35.

Uterofetoplacental circulation can be affected by many factors. These factors include maternal position, uterine contractions, blood pressure, and umbilical cord blood flow. Maternal position is discussed earlier in this chapter and in Chapter 15. Uterine contractions during labor tend to increase circulation through the spiral arteries and subsequent perfusion through the intervillous space. This stress seems to be well within the ability of the fetus to compensate for in most gestations. The fetus is exposed to increased pressure as she or he is moved passively through the birth canal during the mechanism of labor. Usually umbilical cord blood flow is undisturbed by uterine contractions or fetal position.

Normal Adaptations to Stress of Labor

A healthy fetus with an adequate uterofetoplacental circulation will respond in fairly predictable ways to stresses. Transitory accelerations and slight decelerations can be expected in response to spontaneous fetal movement, vaginal examination, fundal pressure, uterine contractions, and abdominal palpation. These changes prepare the fetus for initiating respirations after birth. During vaginal delivery, 7 to 42 ml of amniotic fluid is squeezed out of the fetal lungs. Normally, fetal Po_2 falls from 80 to 15 mm Hg, arterial Pco_2 rises from 40 to 70 mm Hg, and arterial pH falls below 7.35. These changes stimulate chemoreceptors in the aorta and carotid bodies to initiate respirations immediately after birth.

SUMMARY

A firm grasp of the theory of essential factors and processes in labor and maternal and fetal adaptations is only half of the preparation a nurse needs to implement the nursing process with parturients. Although anatomic and physiologic considerations are important, it is equally important to understand the family's adaptation to childbirth. Family responses and adaptation are discussed in Chapter 15.

LEARNING ACTIVITIES

1. Use an anatomic model of the bony pelvis (if possible a cloth model) with a fetal doll to demonstrate the following: (1) maternal pelvic measurements; (2) lie, presentation, and position; (3) the cardinal movements of a mechanism of labor; and (4) the different pelvic types.
2. In the nursery palpate the sutures and the anterior and posterior fontanels of a newborn. Close your eyes and imagine performing a vaginal examination to determine the position of a fetus in utero.
3. Attend a series of childbirth classes to learn what is taught about childbirth to the public. Share your different experiences with the other students in your group.
4. Role play instruction of a multipara who is 38 weeks pregnant and has had precipitous deliveries. She wants to know more about the signs and symptoms of labor and is very anxious about the delivery. Explain to her about the birth process and provide emotional support.
5. Provide nursing care in labor and delivery to as many different families as possible to observe and assess for the differences and similarities in the following situations:
   A. False vs. true labor.
   B. Intensity of uterine contractions in an obese vs. small client. (Palpate the abdomen through a few contractions and observe the fetal monitor for the recording of these contractions.)
   C. Primigravida vs. multiparous labor. (Observe for the intensity, duration, and different perceptions of their labor.)
6. Identify an ethnic population in your area and research their different childbearing customs. Observe families in the clinical setting for their responses to labor, including how the mother expresses pain, who supports the mother during labor, and how the family participates in the childbirth process.

References

Friedman EA: Labor: clinical evaluation and management, ed 2, New York, 1978, Appleton-Century-Crofts.

Friedman EA and Sachtleben MR: Station of the fetal presenting part, Am J Obstet Gynecol 93:522, 1965.

Gaston-Johansson F, Fridh G, and Turner-Norvell K: Progression of labor pain in primiparas and multiparas, Nurs Res 37(2):87, 1988.

McKay S: Squatting: an alternate position for the second stage of labor, MCN 9:181, May/June, 1984.

Willson JR and Carrington ER: Obstetrics and gynecology, ed 8, St Louis, 1987, The CV Mosby Co.

KEY CONCEPTS

- Five essential factors affect the process of labor and delivery.
- Because of its size and relative rigidity, the fetal head has a major effect on the birth process.
- The diameters at the plane of the pelvic inlet, midpelvis, and outlet, plus the axis of the birth canal, determine whether vaginal delivery is possible and the manner by which the fetus may pass down the birth canal (mechanism of labor).
- The forces acting to expel the fetus and placenta are derived from involuntary uterine contractions during the first stage of labor, which are augmented by voluntary bearing-down efforts during the second stage.
- The mother's position affects her anatomic and physiologic adaptations to labor.
- The cardinal movements of the mechanism of labor are descent, flexion, internal rotation, extension, external rotation, and expulsion of the baby.
- Many factors, including changes in the maternal uterus, cervix, and pituitary gland, are involved in the initiation of labor.
- An understanding of maternal adaptations to pregnancy is fundamental to anticipating and meeting the parturient's needs.
- Discomfort during labor has two origins: visceral pain during the first stage and somatic pain during the second stage.
- A healthy fetus with an adequate uterofetoplacental circulation will respond in fairly predictable ways to stresses.

Bibliography

Carlson J et al: Maternal position during parturition in normal labor, Obstet Gynecol 68:433, 1986.

Cunningham FG, MacDonald PC, and Gant NR: Williams obstetrics, ed 18, Norwalk, Conn, 1989, Appleton & Lange.

Curry J: Pregnancy health fair, Can Nurse, p. 26, June 1988.

Dundes L: The evolution of maternal birthing position, Am Public Health 77:5, 636, 1987.

Feetham SL: Acute and chronic pain in maternal-child health, MCN 9:249, July/Aug, 1984.

Liggins GC: New concepts of what triggers labor, Contemp OB/GYN 19(5):131, 1982.

Malasanos L et al: Health assessment, ed 4, St Louis, 1990, The CV Mosby Co.

McKay S and Roberts J: Second stage labor: what is normal? JOGN Nurs 14:101, March/April, 1985.

Miller J and Pelham D: The facts of life, New York, 1984, Viking Penguin, Inc.

Okita JR et al: Initiation of human parturition, Am J Obstet Gynecol 142:432, 1982.

Roberts J and Kriz D: Delivery positions and perineal outcome, Nurse Midwife 29(3):186, 1984.

Romond JL and Baker IT: Squatting in childbirth: a new look at an old tradition, JOGN Nurs 14:406, Sept/Oct, 1985.

Scott JR et al: Danforth's obstetrics and gynecology, ed 6, Philadelphia, 1990, JB Lippincott Co.

CHAPTER

13 Pharmacologic Control of Discomfort

Irene M. Bobak

Learning Objectives

Correctly define the key terms listed.

Discuss the types of analgesia and anesthesia used during labor.

Compare the types of pharmacologic control of discomfort by stage of labor and method of delivery.

Discuss the use of naloxone (Narcan).

Relate each stage of the nursing process in the management of labor discomfort.

Key Terms

agonist-antagonist compounds
analgesia
anesthesia
ataractics
epidural blood patch
cricoid pressure
local infiltration anesthesia
lumbar epidural anesthesia
meninges
narcotic analgesics
narcotic antagonist
paracervical block
pudendal block
regional analgesia
spinal (subarachnoid) anesthesia
systemic analgesia

Nursing care of the woman in labor may include pharmacologic control of discomfort. Medications for discomfort can be used throughout all stages of labor. The nurse must be knowledgeable to provide competent, comprehensive nursing care during labor.

❑ ANALGESIA AND ANESTHESIA

The use of analgesia and anesthesia was not generally accepted as part of obstetric management until Queen Victoria used chloroform during the birth of her son in 1853. Much study has gone into the development of pharmacologic control of discomfort during the birth period. The goal of researchers is to develop methods that will provide adequate pain relief to women without adding to maternal or fetal risk.

Nursing management of obstetric analgesia and anesthesia combines the nurse's expertise in maternity care with a knowledge and understanding of anatomy and physiology, and of medications and their desired and undesired side effects and methods of administration.

Some terms used in this chapter are defined to assist the reader:

anesthesia The loss of all sensation

analgesia The loss of pain sensation or the raising of one's threshold for pain perception

analgesic Relieving pain; an agent that relieves pain without causing unconsciousness

agonist An agent that "activates or excites"

antagonist An agent or substance that tends to nullify the action or effect of another

Analgesia can be induced by positive conditioning and analgesic drugs. A basic understanding of the normal course of labor and delivery and proper physical and psychologic preparation by the gravid woman will reduce perception of pain during childbirth. Especially important is good antenatal care in its broadest sense; reassurance and suggestion are beneficial. Participation in childbirth preparation classes such as those proposed by Grantly Dick-Read or psychoprophylaxis by Lamaze (1972) or Bradley (1974) should do much to alleviate distress (Chapter 9).

The type of analgesic or anesthetic to be used is chosen in part by the stage of labor and by the method of delivery (see box, p. 338).

Sedatives such as barbiturates relieve anxiety, promote relaxation, and induce sleep only in prodromal or

PHARMACOLOGIC CONTROL OF DISCOMFORT BY STAGE OF LABOR AND METHOD OF DELIVERY

FIRST STAGE	SECOND STAGE

Systemic analgesia*
  Narcotics
  Analgesic potentiators
Paracervical block
Peridural block (continuous)
  Lumbar epidural
  Caudal
Subarachnoid spinal (continuous)
  Local
  Morphine
	Local infiltration of perineum
	Pudendal nerve block
	Peridural block ("one shot")
	  Lumbar epidural
	  Caudal
	Subarachnoid spinal ("one shot," "saddle block")
	Inhalation
	  Analgesia
	  Anesthesia

VAGINAL BIRTH	**ABDOMINAL BIRTH**
Local infiltration Pudendal block Peridural block Subarachnoid spinal Inhalation analgesia	Subarachnoid spinal Peridural block Inhalation—general anesthesia

*Administered by labor nurse.

early latent labor and in the absence of pain. If the woman has pain, sedatives given without an analgesic may increase apprehension and cause the mother to become hyperactive and disoriented (Scott et al, 1990). Undesirable side effects include respiratory and vasomotor depression of both the mother and newborn. Because of these disadvantages, barbiturates are seldom used (Scott et al, 1990).

Systemic Analgesia

When personnel trained in **regional analgesia** are not available, **systemic analgesia** remains the major method of analgesia for the woman in labor (Scott et al, 1990). Systemic analgesics cross the blood-brain barrier to provide central analgesic effects. They also cross the placental barrier. Effects on the fetus depend on the maternal dosage, the pharmacokinetics of the specific drug, and the route and timing of administration. Intravenous (IV) administration is often preferred over intramuscular (IM) administration because the onset of the drug effect is faster and more reliable. Classes of analgesic drugs used include narcotic drugs, narcotic agonist-antagonist compounds, and tranquilizers. Tranquilizers used are analgesic-potentiating drugs (**ataractics**).

Narcotic Analgesic Compounds. Opium-related **narcotic analgesics,** for example, morphine and meperidine (Demerol), are especially effective for the relief of severe, persistent, or recurrent pain. They have no amnesic effect. Meperidine overcomes inhibitory factors in labor and may even relax the cervix (see medication cards at back of book).

Meperidine is the most commonly used narcotic for women in labor (Scott et al, 1990). After IV injection, onset is rapid (30 seconds), and maximum effect is reached in 5 to 10 minutes. Peak effect after IM injection is reached in 40 to 50 minutes, with a duration of about 3 hours. To minimize neonatal depression, birth should ideally occur before 1 hour or after 4 hours after IM injection. Since tachycardia is a possible side effect, meperidine is used cautiously for parturients with cardiac disease. For other nursing considerations, see medication card at back of text.

Morphine is an effective analgesic. However, peak analgesic effect is delayed for about 20 minutes after IV injection and for 1 to 2 hours after IM administration. Analgesia may persist for up to 6 hours. Neonatal depression is greater than with meperidine since the neonatal blood-brain barrier is more permeable to morphine. During labor, morphine should be given in 1 to 2 mg increments to a total dose limited to 10 mg.

Naloxone (Narcan) should be available in case the mother or neonate exhibit excessive central nervous system (CNS) depression (see below). Narcosis of the neonate may be exhibited by respiratory depression, hypotonia, lethargy, and a delay in temperature regulation. Alterations of neurologic and behavioral responses may be evident for 72 hours after birth. Meperidine may be present in the neonate's urine for up to 3 weeks. Some depression of attention and social responsiveness may be evident for up to 6 weeks (Briggs, Freeman, and Yaffe, 1986).

Mixed Narcotic Agonist-Antagonist Compounds. In the doses used during labor, mixed narcotic **agonist-antagonist compounds** such as butorphanol (Stadol) and nalbuphine (Nubain) provide analgesia without causing respiratory depression of the mother or neonate. Both IM and IV routes are used for administration. Butorphanol (1 to 3 mg IM; 0.5 to 2 mg IV) or nalbuphine (0.2 mg/kg SC/IM; 0.1 to 0.2 mg/kg IV) may be given during the first stage of labor. If the woman has a preexisting narcotic dependency, the antagonist effect of these compounds will cause her to immediately exhibit symptoms of narcotic withdrawal.

Narcotic Antagonists. If a narcotic, such as morphine or meperidine, has been administered to a parturient, naloxone, or the new **narcotic antagonist** naltrexone, promptly reverses the narcotic effects, including respiratory depression of the newborn. Therefore a narcotic antagonist is especially valuable if labor is more rapid than expected. If given to the mother approximately 10 to 15 minutes before delivery, the narcotic antagonist will counteract maternal and neonatal narcotic effects. Naloxone can be given to the newborn (see medication cards at back of book). Some physicians prefer postdelivery administration, because an exact dose for the neonate can be determined.

With the administration of naloxone, pain also returns. Naloxone also counters the effect or stress-induced elevated levels of endorphins.

Analgesic-potentiators (Ataractics). Phenothiazines, so-called tranquilizer drugs, have the property of augmenting most of the desirable but few of the undesirable effects of analgesics or general anesthetics. These drugs do not relieve pain but decrease anxiety and apprehension, as well as potentiate narcotic effects. This category includes compounds such as promethazine (Phenergan), propiomazine (Largon), hydroxyzine (Vistaril), and promazine (Sparine).

As little as 50 mg of meperidine can be effective for the relief of pain during labor when given with, for example, 25 mg of hydroxyzine. Besides potentiating the effects of the analgesic, the **ataractic** (tranquilizer) also acts as an antinauseant and antiemetic. Fetal or neonatal problems rarely develop with these doses. The combination can be administered safely until the end of the first stage of labor. Usual dosages include the following: Promethazine 25 to 50 mg IM or 15 to 25 mg IV; Promazine 50 mg IM or 5 to 10 mg IV; hydroxyzine 25 to 50 mg IM. Since hydroxyzine is only given by IM injection, onset of effect is slower and less predictable.

Nerve Block Analgesia and Anesthesia. A variety of compounds are used in obstetrics to produce peripheral and regional analgesia and anesthesia. Most of these drugs are related chemically to cocaine and carry the suffix *-caine.* This helps identify a local anesthetic.

The principal pharmacologic effect of local anesthetics is the temporary interruption of the conduction of nerve impulses, notably pain. Examples of common agents given in 0.5% to 1% solutions include lidocaine (Xylocaine), bupivacaine (Marcaine), chloroprocaine (Nesacaine), tetracaine (Pontocaine), and mepivacaine (Carbocaine).

Rarely, individuals are sensitive (allergic) to one or more local anesthetics. Testing with minute amounts of the drug to be used may determine such sensitivity. When excessive amounts of a regional anesthetic are injected, initially the CNS is stimulated. Stimulation may be followed by depression, hypotension, and other serious adverse effects. Atropine, antihistaminic drugs, oxygen, and supportive measures should bring relief. Therefore *adequate hydration is a prerequisite.* An IV line is placed before initiation of this type of anesthesia. Should maternal and fetal resuscitation be needed, left uterine displacement *must* be maintained.

Local Infiltration Anesthesia. Local infiltration anesthesia is commonly used when an episiotomy is to be done and when time or the fetal head position does not permit a pudendal block to be administered (Scott et al, 1990). Anesthesia is produced by injecting an average of 10 to 20 ml of local anesthetic with 1% lidocaine or 2% chloroprocaine into the skin and then subcutaneously into the region to be anesthetized. Epinephrine often is added to the solution to intensify the anesthesia in a limited region and to prevent excessive bleeding and systemic effects by constricting local blood vessels (Hahn, Oestreich, and Barkin, 1986). Repeated injection will prolong the anesthesia as long as needed.

Pudendal Block. Pudendal block is useful for the second stage of labor, episiotomy, and delivery. It does not relieve pain from uterine contractions. Pudendal nerve block is administered 10 to 20 minutes before perineal anesthesia is needed. Once the presenting part descends through the cervix, vaginal and soon pudendal distension occur. Under these circumstances, vaginal and perineal pain can be eliminated by a pudendal anesthetic block (Fig. 13-1, *A*). The pudendal nerve traverses the sacrosciatic notch just medial to the tip of the ischial spine on each side. Injection of an anesthetic solution at or near these points will anesthetize the pudendal nerves peripherally (Fig. 13-2). The transvaginal approach is usually used since it is less painful for the woman, has a higher success rate, and has less chance of fetal complications (Scott et al, 1990). Pudendal block does not change maternal hemodynamic or respiratory functions, vital signs, or fetal heart rate (FHR). The bearing-down reflex is lessened or lost completely. Anesthetic effect is insufficient to permit instrumental vaginal delivery except for low forceps; and it does not allow uterine exploration or manual removal of the placenta (Scott et al, 1990).

Spinal (Subarachnoid) Anesthesia. In **spinal (subarachnoid) anesthesia,** local anesthetic is injected through the third, fourth, or fifth lumbar interspace into the subarachnoid space (Figs. 13-3 and 13-4), where the medication mixes with cerebrospinal fluid (see Fig. 13-1, C). This single-injection technique is useful for delivery, but not for labor. For vaginal delivery, the anesthetic solution is administered during the second stage of labor when delivery is imminent (e.g., fetal head is on the perineum.)

The low spinal ("saddle") injection is made with the woman in a sitting position, her legs over the side of the delivery table, and her feet supported on a stool. The nurse stands in front of her. The woman rests her chin on her chest, arches her back "like a rainbow," and leans on the nurse for support. The nurse comforts and coaches her. This posture is assumed to widen the intervertebral space for ease in inserting the spinal nee-

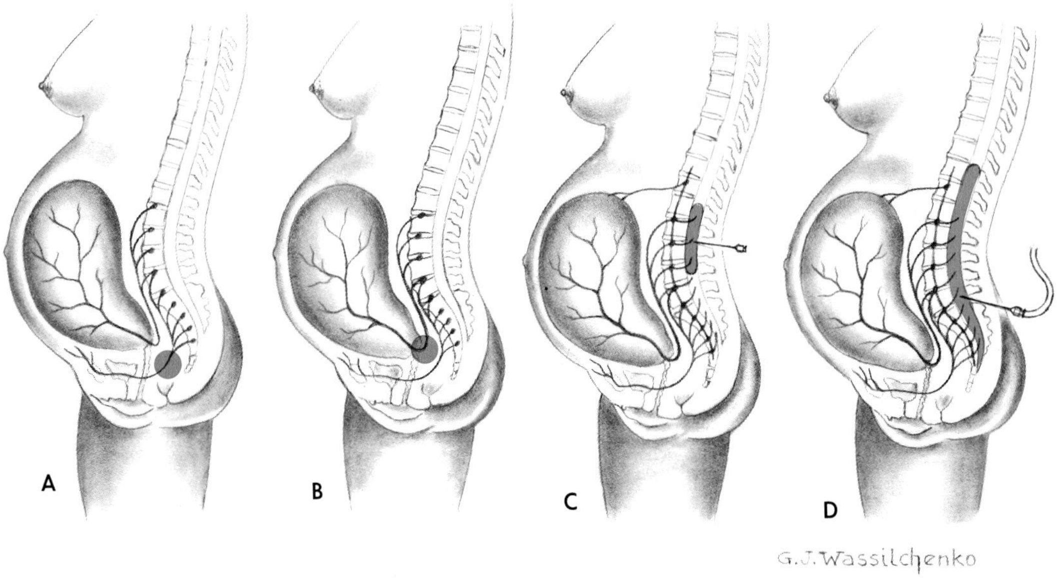

Fig. 13-1 Pain pathways and sites of pharmacologic nerve blocks. **A,** Pudendal block; suitable during second and third stages of labor and for repair of episiotomy. **B,** Paracervical (uterosacral) block: suitable during first stage of labor. **C,** Lumbar sympathetic block (one type of subarachnoid block): given as shown, suitable during first stage of labor. **D,** Epidural block: suitable during all stages of labor and for repair of episiotomy.

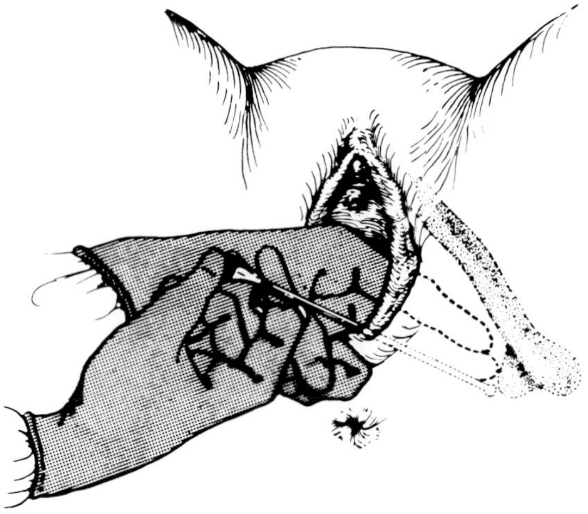

Fig. 13-2 Pudendal block. Use of needle guide ("Iowa trumpet") to locate correct position. (Modified from Benson RC: Handbook of obstetrics and gynecology, ed 5, Los Altos, Calif, 1974, Lange Medical Publications.)

dle and to allow the heavy anesthetic solution to gravitate downward. The injection is made between contractions to avoid an unexpectedly high block. Once the anesthetic has been injected, the woman remains upright for a period of 30 seconds to 2 minutes (as directed by the anesthesiologist) to permit downward diffusion. Then the woman is assisted to a supine position. She must remain supine with the head elevated slightly. Onset of anesthesia usually occurs within 1 to 2 minutes after injection. Duration of anesthesia is 1 to 3 hours, depending on the anesthetic used.

Marked hypotension, decreased cardiac output, and respiratory inadequacy tend to occur during any spinal anesthesia. Therefore the woman is hydrated with IV fluids before injection of anesthetic to decrease the potential for sympathetic blockade hypotension. After injection, maternal blood pressure, pulse, respirations, and FHR must be checked and recorded every 5 to 10 minutes. If signs of serious hypotension or fetal distress develop, oxygen should be given by mask. The physician may administer vasopressors such as ephedrine. The rate of IV fluid infusion may be increased if marked hypotension develops. Since the mother is not able to sense her contractions, she must be instructed when to bear down. After delivery of the placenta the mother will need assistance to move back to her recovery bed. She must remain flat in bed for a minimum of 8 hours to prevent postlumbar (intrathecal) puncture (spinal) headache. A small, flat pillow may be used for her head.

Advantages of spinal anesthesia include ease of administration and absence of fetal hypoxia with maintenance of normotension. Maternal consciousness is maintained, excellent muscular relaxation is achieved, and blood loss is not excessive. Usually, no other anesthetic agents (e.g., inhalation drugs) are required. If stirrups are used for delivery, care must be taken to position them properly (Chapter 15). Spinal anesthesia may be the method of choice for women with severe respiratory problems or with liver, kidney, or metabolic disease.

Disadvantages of spinal anesthesia include drug reactions (e.g., allergy), rare chemical myelitis or infection, hypotension, and high spinal anesthesia with respiratory paralysis. There is an increased need for operative delivery (episiotomy, low forceps extraction) because of elimination of voluntary expulsive efforts. After delivery, there is an increased tendency for bladder and uterine atony, and spinal headache (see discussion below).

Spinal (Postpuncture) Headache. Leakage of cerebrospinal fluid from the site of puncture of the **meninges** (membranous coverings of the spinal cord) is thought to be the major factor in the beginning of spinal headache. Headache may be postural and occur only in the head-up or sitting or standing position. Presumably, with postural changes, the diminished volume of cerebrospinal fluid allows traction on pain-sensitive CNS structures. Headache and auditory and visual problems may persist for days or weeks.

The likelihood of this unpleasant complication, however, can be reduced if the anesthesiologist uses a small-gauge spinal needle and avoids multiple punctures of the meninges. Positioning the woman absolutely flat in bed (with only a small, flat pillow for her head) for at least 8 hours has been recommended to prevent postspinal headache, but there is no definitive evidence that this procedure is effective. Positioning the woman on her abdomen is thought to decrease the loss of fluid through the puncture site. Hyperhydration has been claimed to be of value, but there is no compelling evidence to support its use (Cunningham, MacDonald, and Gant, 1989).

Creation of an **epidural blood patch** (a patch repairing a tear or a hole in the dura mater around the spinal cord) has proven efficacious. To form a patch, a few milliliters of the woman's blood without anticoagulant is injected epidurally at the site of the spinal tap (Fig. 13-5), forming a clot that covers the hole and prevents further fluid loss. Saline similarly injected in larger vol-

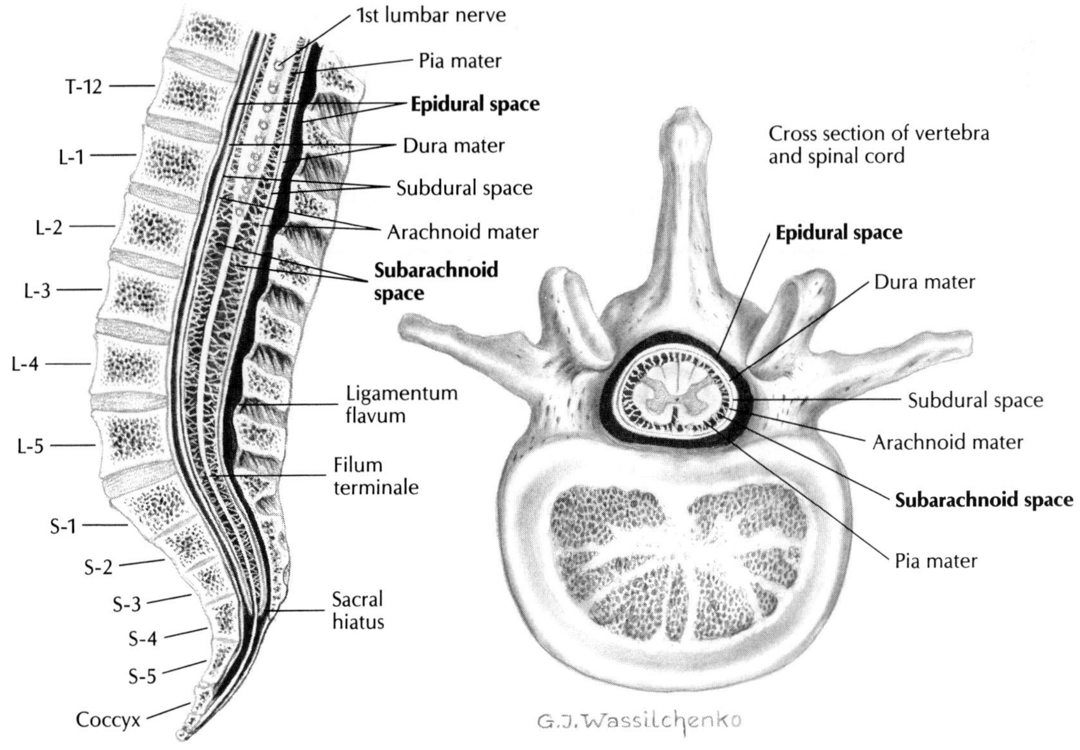

Fig. 13-3 Membranes and spaces of spinal cord.

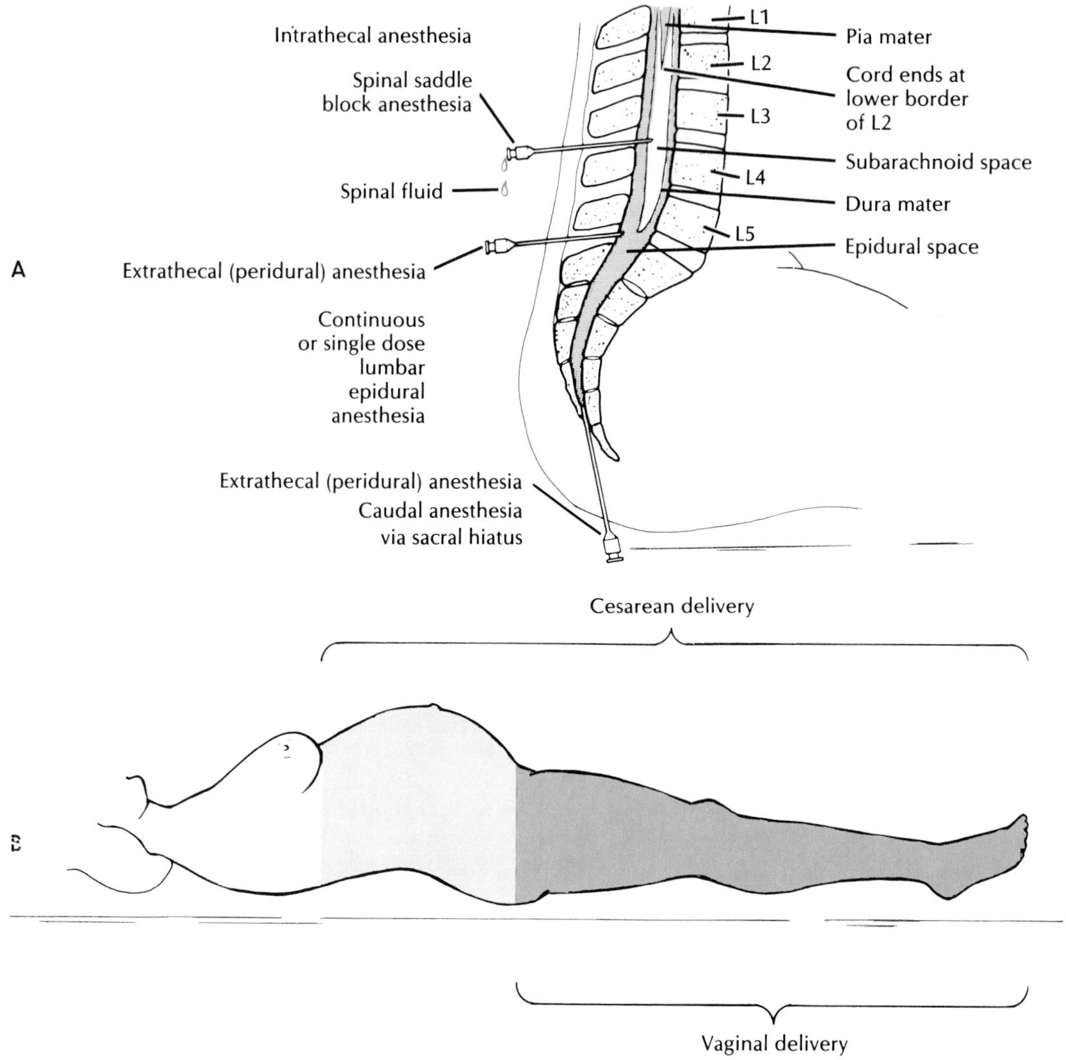

Fig. 13-4 **A,** Regional block anesthesia in obstetrics. **B,** Level of anesthesia necessary for cesarean delivery and for vaginal delivery. (Courtesy Ross Laboratories, Columbus, Ohio.)

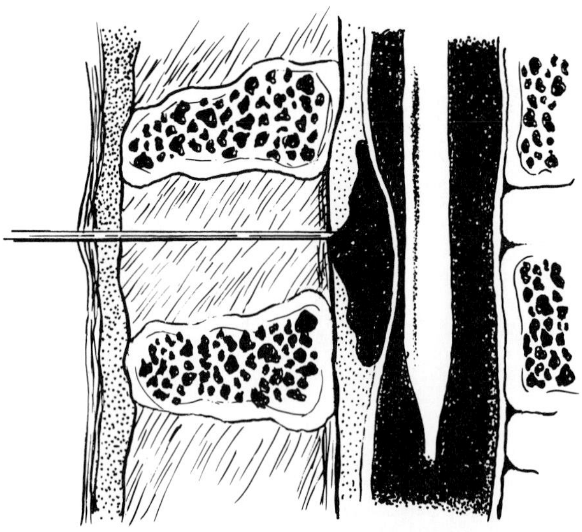

Fig. 13-5 Blood patch therapy for spinal headache.

umes has also been claimed to provide relief. Abdominal support with a girdle or abdominal binder seems to afford relief and is worth trying. The headache may be remarkably improved by the third day and absent by the fifth day for some women.

Epidural Block. Relief from the pain of uterine contractions and delivery, both vaginal and abdominal, can be accomplished by injecting a suitable local anesthetic into the epidural (peridural) space (see Figs. 13-3 and 13-4). The portal of entry into this space for obstetric analgesia and anesthesia is through either a lumbar intervertebral space or caudally through the sacral hiatus and sacral canal. A single injection or repeated doses through an indwelling plastic catheter results in excellent analgesia-anesthesia (Fig. 13-1, *D*).

Complete **lumbar epidural anesthesia** for the discomfort of labor and vaginal delivery requires a block from T-10 to S-5. For abdominal delivery, a block is essential from at least T-8 to S-1. The diffusion of epidural anesthesia depends on the location of the catheter tip, the dose and volume of anesthetic agent used, and the woman's position (e.g., horizontal, or head-up position) (Cunningham, MacDonald, and Gant, 1989).

The caudal space is the lowest extent of the epidural, or peridural, space (see Figs. 13-3 and 13-4). Emerging from the dural sac a few inches higher, a rich network of sacral nerves passes downward through the caudal space. A suitable anesthetic solution filling the caudal canal may eliminate the sensation of pain carried via the sacral nerves to produce anesthesia suitable for vaginal delivery. Higher levels with continuous caudal technique provide both analgesia in the first and second stages of labor and anesthesia for delivery.

The mother is hydrated with 500 to 1000 ml lactated Ringer's solution intravenously within 20 minutes before the block. Facilities for cardiopulmonary resuscitation, including oxygen and suction, must be immediately available.

For introduction of epidural anesthesia, the woman is positioned as for a spinal injection or in a modified Sims' position (Fig. 13-6). For modified lateral Sims' position, the woman is placed on her left side, shoulders parallel, legs slightly flexed, and back arched.

For introduction of caudal anesthesia, the woman is placed in a modified knee-chest or Sims' position, with the upper leg well flexed at the hip and knee, and the lower leg extended. The injection site is cleansed and draped. Once the needle and fine plastic catheter have been inserted into the caudal canal (see Figs. 13-3 and 13-4), a test dose is given. After 5 minutes the anesthesiologist checks the anal sphincter for relaxation and the temperature of the lower extremities. Relaxation of the anal sphincter and increased warmth of the feet indicate proper placement of the catheter in the caudal canal. The remainder of the dose is then given. Relief is experienced in a few minutes, and repeated doses may be administered as the effect wears off. The catheter and syringe are taped securely in position so that the

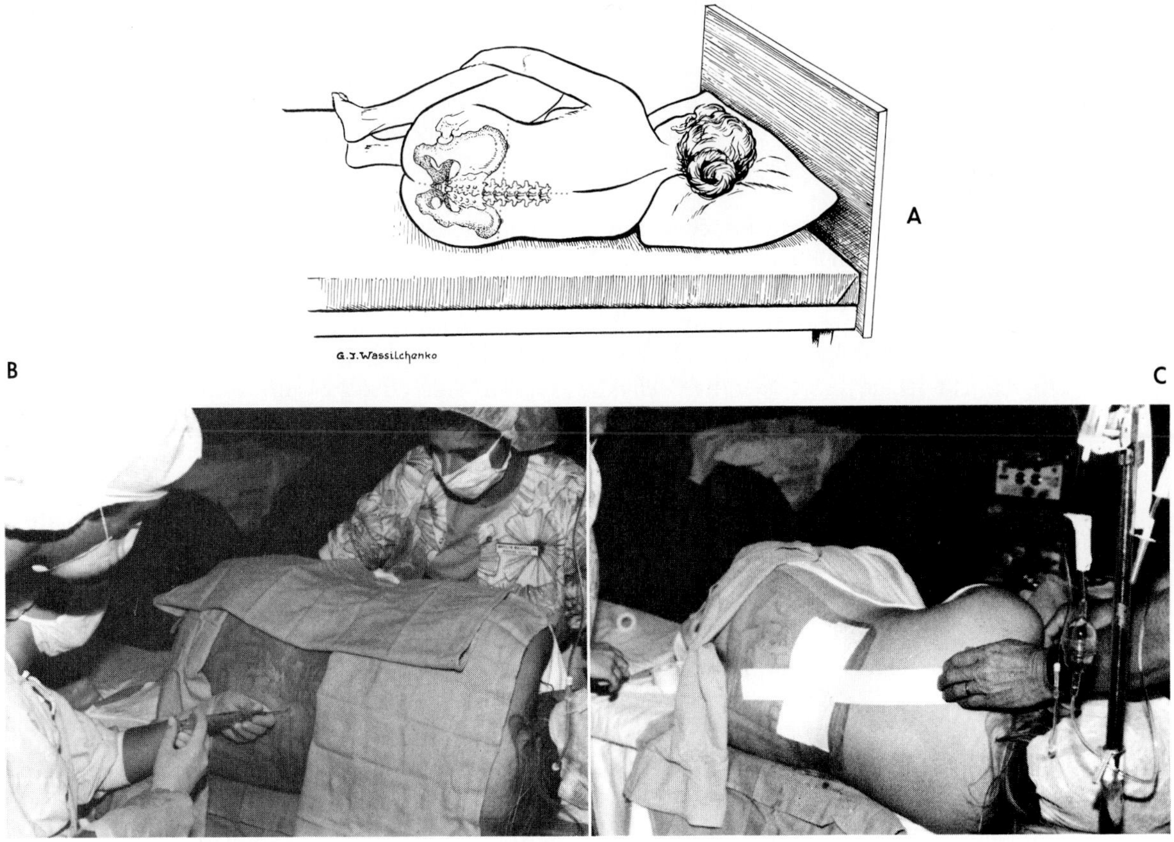

Fig. 13-6 **A,** Lateral decubitus position for epidural and subarachnoid block and anatomic landmarks to locate needle insertion site. **B,** Epidural anesthesia. Skin has been prepared with antiseptic solution (povidone-iodine) (Betadine). Area is draped with sterile towels. Nurse continues to support woman. **C,** Catheter is taped to woman's back; port segment is taped near her shoulder. (**B** and **C** courtesy Stanford University Hospital, Stanford, Calif.)

woman is free to move about in bed. The blood pressure, pulse, respirations, and FHR must be measured and recorded every 15 minutes.

The woman is positioned preferrably on her left side to avoid weight of the uterus on the ascending vena cava and descending aorta. Oxygen is available should hypotension occur despite maintenance of IV fluid and displacement of maternal uterus to the left. The anesthesiologist may need to inject ephedrine and accelerate IV fluid infusion.

The FHR and progress in labor must be monitored carefully. The parturient will not be aware of changes in strength of uterine contractions or descent of the presenting part. Occasionally depression of contractions may result, necessitating augmentation of labor with oxytocin. She will need coaching to push, and low forceps will be required to complete delivery. After the third stage, she will need assistance to move to the recovery bed.

The *advantages* of a continuous block are numerous: fetal distress is rare, but it may occur with rapid absorption or marked hypotension; the mother remains alert and cooperative, airway reflexes remain intact, and only partial motor paralysis develops; and good relaxation is achieved and blood loss is not excessive. Dose, volume, and type of anesthetic can be modified to allow the mother to push, to produce perineal anesthesia, and to permit forceps or even abdominal delivery if required (Cunningham, MacDonald, and Gant, 1989).

The *disadvantages* of a continuous block include the following: special training and experience are required by the anesthesiologist. Since a considerable amount of the drug must be used, reactions or rapid absorption of the anesthetic agent may result in hypotension, convulsions, or paresthesia. The incidence of operative delivery is increased because the woman cannot bear down effectively. Occasionally accidental high spinal anesthesia (and later, spinal headache) may follow inadvertent perforation of the dural (thecal) membrane when administering lumbar epidural anesthesia.

For some women, the anesthetic selected is not effective, and a second form of anesthesia is required. Establishment of effective pain relief with maximum safety takes time. Consequently, in case of rapid labor, the potential for pain relief during labor and for delivery is not realized. Therefore peridural anesthesia for women of higher parity in active labor is likely to prove not worth the bother, risk, and expense (Cunningham, MacDonald, and Gant, 1989).

Intraspinal Narcotics. There is a high concentration of narcotic receptors along the pain pathway in the spinal cord, in the brain stem, and in the thalamus. Since these receptors are specific for narcotics, a small quantity produces marked analgesia lasting for several hours. These receptors are reached by injecting medication through a catheter placed in the epidural or subarachnoid space. Pain transmission is blocked. Since there is no associated sympathetic blockade, resultant maternal hypotension is not a problem. If given during labor, the woman feels contractions, but no pain is noted by her or her observers. Since the pushing reflex is not lost and motor power remains intact, the woman's ability to bear down during the second stage of labor is preserved. Maternal vital signs are normal during labor.

Fentanyl may be used alone. Its effects last up to 90 minutes. When added to the local anesthetic at the time of epidural administration, it extends the duration of anesthesia. There are no cardiovascular effects. However, fentanyl does not provide adequate analgesia for second-stage labor pain, episiotomy, or delivery (Cunningham, MacDonald, and Gant, 1989).

The most common indication for intraspinal narcotics is for the relief of postoperative pain. Women who deliver by the abdominal route are given intraspinal morphine 1 hour after surgery through the catheter. The catheter is then removed, and the women are pain-free for 24 hours. Ability to be up with ease and to care for the baby are two of the advantages to epidural morphine. The women usually cannot believe the effects of the morphine on pain. Early ambulation and freedom from pain facilitate bladder emptying. To women who have had a previous cesarean delivery with the usual postoperative pain, the effects of the intraspinal morphine seem miraculous. The nurse caring for the woman who has been given intraspinal morphine generally is amazed at the mother's ease in ambulation and relative freedom from pain.

The side effects of intraspinal morphine are nausea, vomiting, pruritus (itching), urinary retention, and delayed respiratory depression. The serious concern is for delayed respiratory depression. The woman is observed frequently and is placed on an apnea monitor for 24 hours (Fig. 13-7). Antiemetics, antipruritics, and naloxone are used to relieve the nausea, vomiting, pruritus, and respiratory depression. These symptoms may be treated with promethazine or metoclopramide (Reglan). Hospital protocols provide specific directives for treatment of postintraspinal narcotic side effects. Many obstetricians feel that the benefits of intraspinal injection are not sufficient to warrant its routine use.

Contraindications to Subarachnoid and Peridural Blocks. Some contraindications to epidural analgesia apply equally to caudal and subarachnoid blocks (Scott et al, 1990):

1. *Client refusal.*
2. *Antepartum hemorrhage.* Acute hypovolemia

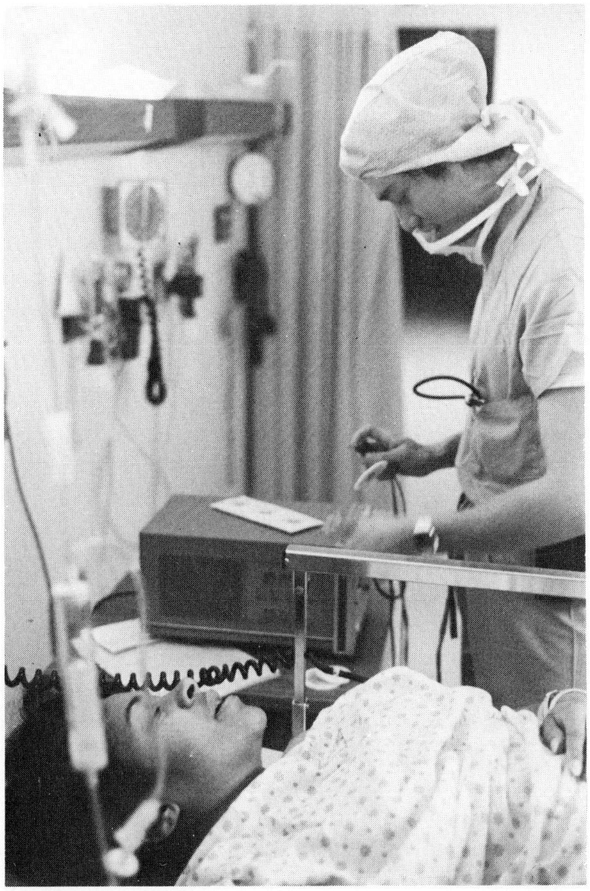

Fig. 13-7 After epidural anesthesia for cesarean delivery, anesthetist applies apnea monitor on woman.

leads to increased sympathetic tone to maintain the blood pressure. Any anesthetic technique that blocks the sympathetic fibers can lead to significant hypotension that can endanger the mother and baby.

3. *Anticoagulant therapy or bleeding disorder.* If a woman is receiving anticoagulant therapy or has a bleeding disorder, injury to a blood vessel may result in a hematoma. The hematoma may compress the cauda equina or the spinal cord and lead to serious CNS sequelae.
4. *Infection at the injection site.* Infection can be spread through the peridural or subarachnoid spaces if the needle traverses an infected area.
5. *Tumor at the injection site.* A tumor at the injection site is an unusual but definite contraindication.
6. *Allergy to anesthetic drug.*

Relative contraindications to intraspinal blocks include CNS disorders, extensive back surgery, morbid obesity or anatomic abnormality in which landmarks cannot be identified, and current or prior disease of the CNS (Scott et al, 1990).

Paracervical (Uterosacral) Block. **Paracervical block** is given during the acceleration phase (Friedman curve, Fig. 15-7 and p. 380) of the first stage of labor to relieve pain from cervical dilatation and distension of the lower uterine segment. For paracervical anesthesia, a dilute local anesthetic drug (e.g., 5 ml of 1% procaine) is injected just beneath the mucosa adjacent to the outer rim of the cervix (9 and 3 o'clock positions) after the cervix is more than 5 cm dilated. A needle guide (e.g., the "Iowa trumpet") is useful but not indispensable for transvaginal administration (Fig. 13-8). Relief from discomfort is noticed within approximately 5 minutes. Excellent pain relief lasts for at least 1 hour.

Anesthesia extends from the lower uterine segment and cervix to the upper one third of the vagina (see Fig. 13-1, *B*); there is no perineal anesthesia. Although there may be a transient depression of contractions,

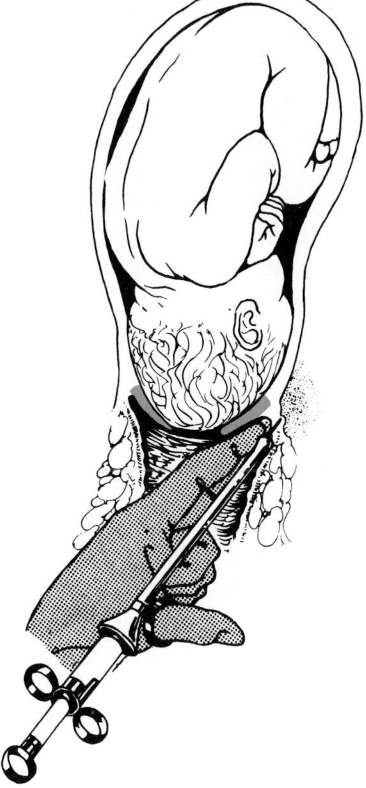

Fig. 13-8 Paracervical block. Note the position of the hand and fingers in relation to the cervix and fetal head and the shallow depth of the needle insertion. Note also that no undue pressure is applied at the vaginal fornix by the fingers or needle guide. (From Benson RC: Handbook of obstetrics and gynecology, ed 7, Los Altos, Calif, 1980, Lange Medical Publications.)

there is little or no effect on the labor. Repeat injections may be given until the cervix is dilated to 8 cm, whereupon another method, such as pudendal block, may be necessary.

Paracervical block anesthesia may cause fetal intoxication because of rapid absorption of the drug. When the anesthetic is injected into the tissues lateral to the cervix, it is picked up by the circulation, which quickly involves the uterus and placenta. When overdosage occurs, the fetus may exhibit bradycardia because of the quinidine-like effect of the anesthetic on the myocardium or, as recent research indicates, because of a reduction in uterine blood flow. In addition, CNS medullary depression may develop, and the neonate may show vascular collapse and apnea at delivery. Hematomas can develop at the site of injection if a uterine vessel is damaged.

Because of these potential complications, paracervical block may not be the method of choice for labor but remains an option for anesthesia during abortion or other gynecologic procedures.

Inhalation Analgesia

Self-administration of inhalation gases may be helpful, especially during the second stage of labor. The mother breathes subanesthetic concentrations of inhalation anesthetic; if given properly, the woman remains conscious but has profound pain relief. An example of this type of anesthetic is methoxyflurane (Penthrane). The route is usually self-administered from a capsule and mask strapped to the wrist. The physician sets the desired concentration and the woman inhales the drug during contractions. The goal of this method is for the woman to remain conscious while profound analgesia, as well as some amnesia for painful events, is achieved.

The nurse must stay with the woman and never administer the drug for her because overdose is a risk. The nurse must also monitor vital signs closely (be alert for cardiac arrhythmias) every 30 minutes and FHR every 15 minutes. The woman should remain conscious and not become delirious or excited. The nurse alerts the physician and removes the analgesic from the woman's hand if the mother has cardiac arrhythmia or loses consciousness or if FHR abnormalities occur. Today these inhalation analgesics are rarely used.

Inhalation analgesics such as nitrous oxide (50%) are nontoxic when administered with ample air or oxygen (50%). Nitrous oxide is administered by trained personnel during contractions or continuously. The goal is analgesia. If the woman has used lysergic acid diethylamide (LSD) at some time in the past, she is not a candidate for this type of analgesia, since she will usually experience a "flashback" or "trip."

General Anesthesia

General anesthesia is rarely indicated for uncomplicated vaginal delivery. It may be necessary if the woman refuses or there is a contraindication to regional anesthesia, or if fetal indications necessitate rapid delivery. The woman is not awake with this method, and there is danger of vomiting followed by aspiration and respiratory depression. It is safer than regional anesthesia for hypovolemic clients, however, and does not depress the newborn unless the mother is anesthetized deeply. A commonly used anesthetic is thiopental (Pentothal). Administered IV, thiopental produces rapid induction of anesthesia but depresses the newborn. It is useful in controlling maternal convulsions. Halothane (fluothane) inhalation relaxes the uterus quickly and facilitates intrauterine manipulation, version, and extraction. The desired effect is general loss of sensitivity to touch, pain, and other stimulation.

If general anesthesia is being considered, the nurse gives the woman nothing by mouth and sees that an IV infusion is established. The nurse premedicates the woman with a nonparticulate oral antacid such as sodium citrate (30 ml) to increase gastric pH to neutralize acid contents of the stomach. If there is sufficient time, some physicians also order a histamine (H_2) blocker such as cimetidine to decrease production of gastric acid and metoclopramide to increase gastric emptying (Scott et al, 1990). Sometimes the nurse is asked to assist with **cricoid pressure** before intubation. Priorities for recovery room care are to maintain open airway, maintain cardiopulmonary functions, and prevent postpartum hemorrhage. Routine postpartum care is organized to facilitate parent-child attachment as soon as possible and to answer the mother's questions. When appropriate, the nurse assesses the mother's readiness to see the baby and her response to the anesthesia and to the event that necessitated general anesthesia delivery (e.g., giving birth by cesarean delivery when vaginal delivery was anticipated).

Combination Anesthesia for Cesarean Birth. Light general anesthesia, considered by many to be ideal for cesarean delivery, is achieved with a combination of thiopental, nitrous oxide–oxygen, and succinylcholine. The woman is given 100% oxygen for 3 minutes, followed by almost simultaneous rapid administration of thiopental and succinylcholine. During intubation, cricoid pressure is maintained to prevent aspiration of vomitus (Fig. 13-9). Cricoid pressure is often maintained by the nurse. When the woman is somnolent, a nitrous oxide–oxygen mixture is given. Excellent tolerance of the anesthetic is widely reported. Rapid resuscitation of the mother and even small-for-gestational-age (SGA) and growth-retarded infants can be achieved.

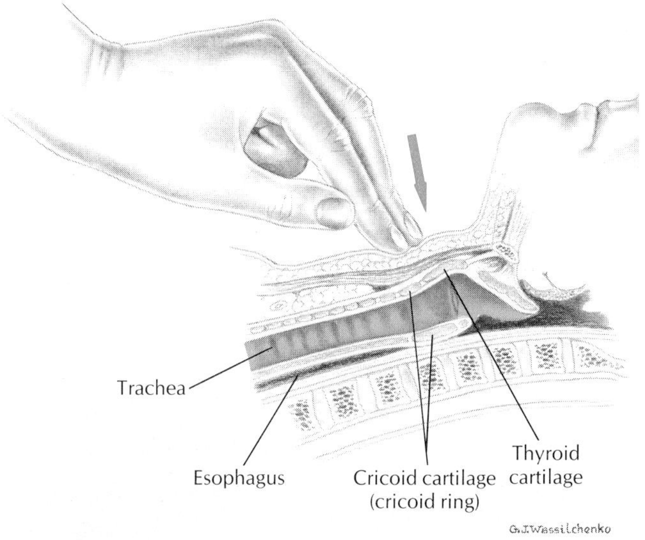

Fig. 13-9 Technique of applying pressure on cricoid cartilage to occlude esophagus prevents pulmonary aspiration of gastric contents during anesthesia induction.

Drug Effects on Neonate

There is an ongoing debate concerning the effects of epidural anesthesia on the neonate's neurobehavioral responses. Studies of associations between neurobehavioral outcome and epidural anesthesia are far from consistent (Avard and Nimrod, 1985). One author found a beneficial effect (Hodgkinson et al, 1977). Some authors found that neonates did not score as well on neurobehavioral tests (Rosenblatt et al, 1981). Others found no difference (Abboud et al, 1982; Marx, 1984). However, the findings suggest a mild transient effect on newborn behavior.

Assessment

Before Administration of Medication

The assessment of the parturient, her fetus, and her labor is a joint effort of the nurse and the physicians (obstetrician and anesthesiologist), who then consult with the woman. The needs of each woman are different. Many factors enter into the nursing assessment to determine choice of analgesia and anesthesia.

History. The woman's prenatal chart is read for relevant information. In addition to identifying data, the woman's parity, estimated date of delivery, and complications and medications during pregnancy are noted. History of allergies are noted carefully and displayed prominently. History of smoking and neurologic and spinal disorders are noted.

Interview. Interview data establishes time and type of food taken at last meal; existing respiratory condition (cold, allergy); and unusual reactions to medications, cleansing agents, or tape. The woman is asked about childbirth preparation classes. Her preparation and preferences for management of discomfort are noted. Her knowledge of choices for management of discomfort is assessed.

The woman is asked about the onset of labor and status of membranes; or, the reason for this admission is determined—induction of labor, cesarean delivery. The events since the woman's last contact with the physician are reviewed (e.g., infections, diarrhea, change in fetal behavior). If verbal and physical signs are suggestive, the nurse inquires about substance abuse: type of drug used, time of last use, method of administration.

Physical Examination. The character and status of this labor and fetal response are assessed (Chapters 12 and 15). The nurse notes the degree of hydration by assessing intake and output, moisture of mucous membranes, and skin turgor. Evidence of skin infection near sites of possible needle insertion are recorded and reported. Signs of apprehension such as fist clenching and restlessness are noted.

If the woman is in labor, maternal and fetal vital signs; uterine contractions; and cervical effacement and dilatation, station, and anticipated time until delivery are all considered. The gravida's perception of discomfort and her expressed need for medication add to the data base. Bladder distension is noted. Length of labor and degree of fatigue are important considerations.

Laboratory Tests. Laboratory tests are reviewed for anemia (hemoglobin and hematocrit), coagulopathy (bleeding disorder), and infection (white cell count and differential). The prenatal record is reviewed for a history of infection (blood test, urinalysis, culture and sensitivity) and other concurrent disorders (tests for substance abuse).

The types of antenatal diagnostic studies (contraction stress test [CST], amniocentesis [Chapter 22]) and findings are noted.

The choice of analgesia and anesthesia varies by phase and stage (see box, p. 338).

After Administration of Medication

The nurse monitors and records the woman's response to medication: level of pain relief, level of apprehension, return of sensations and perception of pain, and allergic or untoward reactions (e.g., hypotension, respiratory depression). The nurse continues to monitor maternal vital signs, blood pressure, strength and frequency of uterine contractions, changes in the cervix and station of the presenting part, presence of the bearing-down reflex, bladder filling, and state of hydration. Fetal response following administration of analgesia or anesthesia is vital. The woman is asked if she (or the family) has any questions. The nurse assesses the woman's and her family's understanding of the need for ensuring her safety (e.g., keeping side rails up, calling for assistance as needed).

The time between the administration of a narcotic and the time of the baby's birth are noted.

Nursing Diagnoses

Following are some examples of nursing diagnoses relevant to pharmacologic control of discomfort during the birth period:

Pain related to
- The processes of labor

Situational low self-esteem related to
- Negative perception of behavior

Knowledge deficit related to
- Procedure for nerve block analgesia
- Expected sensation during nerve block analgesia
- Mother's role during nerve block analgesia
- Options for analgesia and anesthesia

Potential for dystocia or injury to bladder related to
- Loss of sensation after regional anesthesia

Inability to bear down during second stage related to
- Loss of sensation after regional anesthesia

Family processes, altered, related to
- Unmet expectations of labor and delivery

Planning

For each woman a plan is developed that relates specifically to her clinical and nursing problems. The plan involves the mother and family and incorporates their priorities and preferences. The nurse, in collaboration with the physician and parturient, selects those aspects of care relevant to the individual client. The ***goals*** for nursing care related to pharmacologic control of discomfort include the following:

1. The mother will achieve adequate pain relief without adding to maternal risk (e.g., through appropriate medication, dosage, and timing and route of administration)
2. The unborn and newborn will maintain well-being and adjustment to extrauterine life
3. The family will know their needs and rights in relation to use of analgesia or anesthesia

Implementation

Nurses assume many caregiving roles during the childbirth period. The nurse-clinician's roles can be categorized as supportive and teacher/counselor/advocate. A specific nursing care plan is given on p. 349.

Supportive Activities

This brief discussion is probably one of the most significant in this text. The woman's *perception* of her behavior during labor is of utmost importance. If she had planned a nonmedicated birth, then needs and accepts medication, her self-esteem will falter. Verbal and nonverbal acceptance of her behavior is given as necessary and reinforced by visiting her the day after delivery if possible. Explanations about fetal response to maternal discomfort, the effects of maternal fatigue, and the medication itself are supportive measures. In some instances the husband needs support if he was planning on a nonmedicated delivery.

Parents may feel reassured somewhat by hearing that medication is sometimes indicated for the baby's benefit. A reasonable amount of stress is harmless to the mother and to labor progress, and actually benefits the fetus by promoting adaptation to labor and birth. Excessive stress (as yet undefined in perinatal medicine), however, causes increased maternal catecholamine production, which may be related to dysfunctional labor and fetal and neonatal distress and illness (Simkin, 1986a,b).

Teacher/Counselor/Advocate

Informed Consent. The anesthesiologist and obstetrician are responsible for informing gravidas of the alternative methods of pharmacologic pain relief available in the hospital setting. The description of the anesthetic techniques is essential to informed consent, even if the woman has received information about analgesia and anesthesia earlier in her pregnancy. This interview should take place just before or early in labor so the woman has time to consider the alternatives. The obstetric nurse plays a part in the informed consent by clarifying or describing the procedures or by acting as a client's advocate and asking the anesthesiologist for further explanations. The explanation of the procedure to be used for anesthesia must include maternal position for administering the anesthetic, skin preparation, degree of discomfort, time requirement, and interval before the anesthetic is effective. The woman must be informed that the anesthetic is not always effective and that there are potential side effects for both mother and fetus.

Specific Nursing Care Plan

ANALGESIA FOR PAIN DURING LABOR

Rose N. is a 31-year-old woman in active labor. At her last vaginal examination the physician found her to be 7 cm/90%/+2. Her contractions are coming every 2½ to 3 minutes and lasting 30 to 45 seconds. Rose and her husband attended childbirth education classes and are doing well with the breathing techniques. However, the pain of the contractions is getting too intense for Rose. The physician has ordered meperidine 50 mg and promethazine 25 mg to help her stay in control and decrease her anxiety.

ASSESSMENT	NURSING DIAGNOSIS (ND), PLAN/GOAL (P/G)	RATIONALE/ IMPLEMENTATION	EVALUATION
Rose is in active labor experiencing acute pain. Rose communicates verbally and nonverbally her anxiety and decreased coping mechanisms.	ND: Pain, related to increasing frequency and intensity of uterine contractions. P/G: Rose will state she has the relief she wants and she and fetus remain well. ND: Ineffective individual coping related to increased intensity and frequency of labor contractions. P/G: Rose experiences minimum anxiety and remains in control.	*Pain of contractions and other labor-related effects can be diminished:* Provide comfort measures. Provide information about analgesics. Assist Rose and husband with relaxation techniques, breathing exercises, abdominal effleurage, and back rubs. Provide emotional support.	Rose is more calm and verbalizes less discomfort. Rose is lucid and in control.
Assess vital signs, blood pressure, labor pattern, and FHR immediately after analgesia is given and at intervals indicated by hospital protocol.	ND: Potential for fetal and maternal compromise related to medication. P/G: Rose indicates she is more comfortable and she, her labor, and the fetus suffer no adverse sequelae.	*Prompt intervention is vital:* Observe Rose for comfort level. Observe Rose for side effects such as: hives, shortness of breath, and altered sensorium. Monitor for change in labor pattern. Monitor FHR for distress.	Rose's vital signs, blood pressure, and FHR remain within normal limits. Normal labor pattern continues. Rose experiences no adverse side effects.
Rose is apologetic for taking analgesic medication.	ND: Situational low self-esteem related to inability to cope with labor without medication. P/G: Rose and her husband do not feel as though they have failed because medication was needed.	*Participation in decision-making supports self-esteem:* Assess Rose's (couple's) behavior. Support Rose's decision. Assist Rose through relaxation and breathing techniques to regain and maintain control. Provide verbal and nonverbal acceptance of her choice. Praise her (their) efforts.	Rose feels good about decision and maintains control during her labor.

Timing of Administration. Many medication orders are written to be given on the nurse's judgment. These orders require clinical knowledge and expertise.

Other types of analgesia and anesthetics are the responsibility of the anesthesiologist. It is often the nurse who alerts the physician that a parturient is in need of pharmacologic relief of discomfort. The box on p. 338 lists pharmacologic control by stage of labor and method of delivery. A review of the origins of discomfort in Chapter 12 provides the basis for understanding the parturient's changing needs during labor.

Preparation for Procedures. The nurse reviews or validates the woman's choices for relief from discomfort and clarifies the mother's information, as necessary. The woman needs an explanation of the procedure and what will be asked of her (e.g., to maintain flexed position during insertion of epidural). The woman benefits from knowing how the medication is to be given, the degree of discomfort to expect from administration of the medication, sensations she can expect, skin preparation, time requirement for administration, and interval before medication "takes hold." The nurse explains the need for keeping the bladder empty. If an indwelling epidural catheter is threaded and the woman feels a momentary twinge down her leg, hip, or back, she is assured that it is not a sign of injury.

For paracervical and pudendal blocks a long needle is used (see Fig. 13-8). The sight of this needle may be frightening. The woman can be reassured that only the tip of the needle will be inserted.

Instrumental Activities

Accuracy in monitoring the progress of labor is the basis for clinical judgment in the need for pharmacologic control of discomfort. Knowledge of medications used during childbirth is essential. The most effective route of administration for each woman is selected. The medication is prepared and administered correctly.

The preferred route of administration is through IV tubing. The medication is given slowly in small doses at the *beginning* of three to five consecutive contractions (Petree, 1983). Since uterine blood vessels are constricted during contractions, the medication stays within the maternal vascular system for several seconds before the uterine blood vessels reopen. Through this method of injection, the amount of drug crossing the placenta to the fetus is minimized. With decreased placental transfer, the mother's degree of pain relief is maximized. The IV route has the following results:

Pain relief is obtained with small doses of the drug.
Onset of pain relief is more predictable.
Duration of effect is more predictable.

IM injections of analgesics, although still used, are no longer the preferred route of administration to the laboring woman. Identified disadvantages of the IM route include the following:

Onset of pain relief is delayed for several minutes.
Higher doses of medication are required.
Medication is released from the muscle tissue at an unpredictable rate and is available for transfer across the placenta to the fetus.

IM injections are given in the upper arm if regional anesthesia is planned later in the labor. This is because the autonomic blockage from the regional (e.g., epidural) anesthesia increases blood flow to the gluteal region and accelerates absorption of the drug. The maternal plasma level of the drug necessary to bring pain relief usually is reached 45 minutes after IM injection, followed by a decline in plasma levels. The maternal drug levels (after IM injections) are unequal because of uneven distribution (maternal uptake) and metabolism. The advantage of using the IM route is quick administration.

An IV line is established before nerve blocks such as paracervical, peridural, and subarachnoid spinal and general anesthesia are introduced. Lactated Ringer's solution is often the infusate of choice. Infusion solutions without dextrose are preferred, especially when the solution needs to be infused rapidly (e.g., in the presence of severe dehydration or to maintain blood pressure). Solutions containing dextrose raise maternal blood glucose levels rapidly, necessitating the release of insulin; fetal or neonatal hypoglycemia may result. In addition, dextrose changes osmotic pressure so that fluid is excreted from the kidneys more rapidly. Therefore lactated Ringer's and normal saline solutions are the preferred infusates.

The woman needs assistance in assuming and maintaining the correct position for peridural and spinal anesthesia (see pp. 339 and 343).

Following a nerve block the woman is protected by raised side rails, constant attendance, and a call bell within easy reach. She must be protected from prolonged pressure on an anesthetized part (e.g., lying on one side with weight on one leg; tight bedclothes on feet). If stirrups are used, the nurse pads them, adjusts both stirrups at the same level and angle, places both of the woman's legs into them simultaneously avoiding pressure to the popliteal angle, and applies restraints without restricting circulation.

The woman's record during childbirth serves as a documented means of communication among all members of the health care team. Documentation of the events is mandatory to meet legal requirements. Precise records also serve as a reservoir for research study.

Evaluation

Evaluation is a continuous process. The nurse can be relatively assured that care was effective if the goals for care (p. 348) are met: the mother has adequate pain relief without risk; the unborn and newborn maintain well-being; and the family knows their needs and rights in relation to analgesia and anesthesia.

SUMMARY

Nursing management of obstetric analgesia and anesthesia combines the nurse's expertise in obstetrics with knowledge and understanding of techniques, drugs, and their potential complications. The physiologic requirements of the woman (e.g., adequate hydration, preventing hypotension) receiving pharmacologic control of discomfort have been presented. Effects on the unborn and newborn baby (e.g., uterine blood flow, oygenation, and glucose) have been discussed. The key is to provide the childbearing family with a choice in pain relief. It is then the duty of caring professionals to provide the safety in that choice by using their knowledge of drugs and techniques (Petree, 1983).

LEARNING ACTIVITIES

1. Develop a nursing care plan for a client who is to receive regional nerve block analgesia/anesthesia for labor and delivery.
2. Attend a prenatal education class during which pharmacologic relief of discomfort is discussed. Compare and contrast the information presented with that which is presented in a nursing class.
3. In the clinical setting, interview a client who received no analgesia/anesthesia and one who did. Compare and contrast their feelings about their birth experience.
4. Discuss the concept of informed consent in relation to obstetric analgesia/anesthesia.
5. Interview several obstetricians and several obstetric nurses regarding their preferences for analgesia/anesthesia for labor clients. Compare and contrast the preferences of these professionals.
6. In the clinical setting assess the emotional status of a client who planned to have an unmedicated birth experience, but instead opted for narcotic analgesia (meperidine) as a result of her inability to cope with the discomfort of her labor.

KEY CONCEPTS

- The type of analgesic or anesthetic to be used is chosen in part by the stage of labor and the method of delivery.
- Narcotic effects can be potentiated with ataractics and reversed with an antagonist.
- Pharmacologic control of discomfort during labor requires collaboration among the nurse, obstetrician, anesthesiologist, and parturient.
- The nurse must understand medications, their expected effect, potential side effects, and methods of administration.
- Placement of an IV line and maternal hydration are essential during regional nerve blocks.
- Maternal analgesia/anesthesia potentially affect neonatal neurobehavioral response.

References

Abboud TK et al: Maternal, fetal and neonatal responses after epidural anesthesia with bupivacaine, 2-chloroprocaine or lidocaine, Anesth Analg 61:638, 1982.

Avard DM and Nimrod CM: Risks and benefits of obstetric epidural analgesia: a review, Birth 12:215, Winter, 1985.

Bradley RA: Husband-coached childbirth, New York, 1974, Harper & Row Publishers, Inc.

Briggs GC, Freeman RK, and Yaffe SJ: Drugs in pregnancy and lactation, ed 2, Baltimore, 1986, Williams & Wilkins.

Cunningham FG, MacDonald PC, and Gant NF: Williams obstetrics, ed 18, Norwalk, Conn, 1989, Appleton & Lange.

Dick-Read G: Childbirth without fear, ed 2, New York, 1959, Harper & Row, Publishers, Inc.

Hahn AB, Oestreich DJ, and Barkin RL: Mosby's pharmacology in nursing, ed 16, St Louis, 1986, The CV Mosby Co.

Hodgkinson R et al: Neonatal neurobehavioral tests following vaginal delivery under ketamine, thiopental, and extradural anesthesia, Anesth Analg 56:548, 1977.

Lamaze F: Painless childbirth, New York, 1972, Pocket Books.

Marx GF: Pain relief during labor—more than comfort, J Calif Perinat Assn 4:36, Winter, 1984.

Petree B: A nursing perspective of obstetrical analgesia/anesthesia, NAACOG update series, 1:lesson 12, 1983.

Rosenblatt DB et al: The influence of maternal analgesia on neonatal behavior. II. Epidural bupivacaine, Br J Obstet Gynaecol 88:407, 1981.

Scott JR et al: Danforth's obstetrics and gynecology, ed 6, Philadelphia, 1990, JB Lippincott Co.
Simkin P: Stress, pain, and catecholamines in labor. I. A review, Birth 13(4):227, 1986a.
Simkin P: Stress, pain, and catecholamines in labor. II. A pilot survey of new mothers, Birth 13(4):234, 1986b.

Bibliography

Booth T: Relaxation for childbirth, Int Childbirth Educ, 2(2):43, 1987.
Cheek TG and Gutsche BB: Epidural analgesia for labor and vaginal delivery, Clin Obstet Gynecol 30(3):515, 1987.
Chestnut DH: Regional anesthesia, other than epidural, for labor and vaginal delivery, Clin Obstet Gynecol 30(3):530, 1987.
Collins BA: The role of the nurse in labor and delivery as perceived by nurses and patients, JOGN Nurs 15(5):412, 1986.
Donovan M, editor: Pain control, Nurs Clin North Am, Sept, 1987.
Garite TJ and Ray D: Intrauterine resuscitation with tocolysis, Contemp OB/GYN 31(3):24, 1988.
Haight K: What you should know about epidural analgesia, Nurs '87 17(9):58, 1987.
Henrikson ML and Wild LK: A nursing process approach to epidural anesthesia, JOGN Nurs 17(5):316, 1988.
Inturrisi M, Camenga CF, and Rosen M: Epidural morphine for relief of postpartum, postsurgical pain, JOGN Nurs 17(4):238, 1988.
Jankowski H and Wells S: Self-administered medications for obstetric patients, MCN 12(3):199, 1987.
Lowe NK: Parity and pain during parturition, JOGN Nurs 16(5):340, 1987.
Lynn N: ICEA review: pain theory and childbirth, Int Childbirth Educ 2(2):21, 1987.
McCaffery M: Patient-controlled analgesia: more than a machine, Nurs '87 17(11):62, 1987.
McGilvray R: Over the counter drugs in pregnancy, Int Childbirth Educ 2(2):37, 1987.
Pearson J: Some women's experiences of epidurals, Int Childbirth Educ 2(2):19, 1987.
Pedersen H and Finster M: Selection and use of local anesthetics, Clin Obstet Gynecol 30(3):505, 1987.
Rimar JM: Epidural morphine for analgesia following a cesarean, MCN 11(5):345, 1986.
Sarno AP and Phelan JP: Intrauterine resuscitation of the fetus, Contemp OB/GYN 32(1):143, 1988.
Simkin P: Comfort measures for labor, Int Childbirth Educ 2(2):5, 1987.

CHAPTER 14 Fetal Monitoring

Susan M. Tucker

Learning Objectives

Correctly define the key terms listed.

Explain baseline fetal heart rate and evaluate periodic changes.

Discuss fetal heart rate monitoring by periodic auscultation and electronic methods.

Identify typical signs of fetal distress and appropriate nursing interventions.

Review nursing standards for electronic fetal monitoring.

Key Terms

accelerations
amnioinfusion
antepartum monitoring
baseline fetal heart rate (FHR)
bradycardia
decelerations
electronic fetal monitoring (EFM)
fetal distress
intrauterine catheter
meconium-stained amniotic fluid
prolonged decelerations
smooth (flat) baseline
spiral electrode
supine hypotensive syndrome
tachycardia
tocotransducer
ultrasound transducer
uterine activity
uteroplacental insufficiency
variability

❑ HISTORY

It was not until the seventeenth century that the first fetal heart tones were heard or described. Periodically during the next 200 years, physicians would describe fetal heart tones and uterine souffle in medical journals. Then in 1917 David Hillis, an obstetrician at Chicago Lying-In-Hospital, reported on a head stethoscope, or fetoscope, as it is used today. In 1922 J.B. DeLee, the chief of staff at the same institution, published a report regarding a similar instrument. A controversy developed because DeLee claimed to have had the idea before Hillis' report. The instrument eventually became known as the DeLee-Hillis stethoscope and has remained essentially unchanged in design and use.

In 1958 Edward Hon of the Yale University School of Medicine published a report on continuous fetal electrocardiographic (ECG) monitoring from the maternal abdomen. Obstetricians Caldeyro-Barcia of Uruguay in 1966 and Hammacher in Germany in 1967 reported their observations of fetal heart rate (FHR) patterns associated with fetal distress. Based on their work the first generation of commercially available fetal monitors was produced in the late 1960s. Technologic advances continue to improve the quality and accuracy of the tracings.

❑ FETAL STRESS

Since labor represents a period of stress for the fetus, continuous monitoring of fetal health is instituted as part of the nursing care during labor. The fetal oxygen supply must be maintained during labor to prevent severe debilitating conditions after birth. Fetal stress can result in death in utero or shortly after birth. The fetal oxygen supply can be reduced in a number of ways:

1. Reduction of blood flow through the maternal vessels as a result of maternal hypertension or hypotension (systolic blood pressure of 100 mm Hg in brachial artery is necessary for placental perfusion).
2. Reduction of the oxygen content of the maternal blood as a result of hemorrhage or severe anemia.
3. Alterations in fetal circulation, occurring with compression of the cord, placental separation, or head compression (head compression causes increased intracranial pressure and vagal nerve stimulation with slowing of the heart rate).

Fetal well-being during labor can be measured by the *response of the FHR to uterine contractions.* In general, a reassuring FHR pattern is characterized by: a FHR between 120 and 160 beats per minute (bpm) with normal baseline variability, no ominous periodic changes, and accelerations of FHR with fetal movement.

A normal uterine activity pattern in labor is characterized by: contractions every 2 to 5 minutes, duration of contractions less than 90 seconds, intensity of contractions less than 100 mm Hg pressure, 30 seconds or more from the end of one contraction to the beginning of the next contraction, and an average intrauterine pressure of 15 mm Hg or less between contractions.

Baseline Fetal Heart Rate

The intrinsic rhythmicity of the fetal heart and the fetal autonomic nervous system control the FHR. An increase in sympathetic response results in acceleration of the FHR. An augmentation in parasympathetic response produces a slowing of the FHR. Usually there is a balanced increase of sympathetic and parasympathetic response during contractions, with no observable change in the FHR.

Baseline fetal heart rate (FHR) is the average rate when the woman is not in labor or is between contractions. At term this average is about 135 bpm, a decrease from 155 bpm early in pregnancy. The normal range at term is 120 to 160 bpm.

Tachycardia is a baseline FHR above 160 bpm. It can be considered an early sign of fetal hypoxia and can result from maternal or fetal infection, such as with prolonged rupture of membranes with amnionitis; maternal hyperthyroidism, or fetal anemia; as well as in response to drugs such as atropine, hydroxyzine (Vistaril), or ritodrine.

Bradycardia is a baseline FHR below 120 bpm. (Bradycardia should be distinguished from prolonged deceleration patterns, which are *periodic changes* that are described later in this chapter.) It can be considered a later sign of fetal hypoxia and is known to occur before fetal demise. Bradycardia can result from placental transfer of drugs such as anesthetics, prolonged compression of the umbilical cord, maternal hypothermia, and maternal hypotension. Maternal **supine hypotensive syndrome,** caused by uterine pressure (the weight of the gravid uterus) on the vena cava, decreases the return of blood flow to the maternal heart, which then reduces maternal cardiac output and blood pressure. These responses in the mother subsequently result in a decrease in the FHR and fetal bradycardia. Table 14-1 contrasts tachycardia with bradycardia.

Variability of the FHR can be described as the normal irregularity of the cardiac rhythm. Variability is described as being short-term or long-term. Short-term

Table 14-1 Tachycardia and Bradycardia

	Tachycardia	Bradycardia
Definition	FHR above 160 bpm lasting longer than 10 min	FHR below 120 bpm lasting longer than 10 min
Cause	Early fetal hypoxia Maternal fever Parasympatholytic drugs (atropine, hydroxyzine) Beta-sympathomimetic drugs (ritodrine, isoxsuprine) Amnionitis Maternal hyperthyroidism Fetal anemia Fetal heart failure Fetal cardiac arrhythmias	Late fetal hypoxia Beta-adrenergic blocking drugs (propranolol; anesthetics for epidural, spinal, caudal, and pudendal blocks) Maternal hypotension Prolonged umbilical cord compression Fetal congenital heart block
Clinical significance	Persistent tachycardia in absence of periodic changes does not appear serious in terms of neonatal outcome (especially true if tachycardia is associated with maternal fever); tachycardia is an ominous sign when associated with late decelerations, severe variable decelerations, or absence of variability	Bradycardia with good variability and absence of periodic changes is not a sign of fetal distress if FHR remains above 80 bpm; bradycardia caused by hypoxia is an ominous sign when associated with loss of variability and late decelerations
Nursing intervention	Dependent on cause; reduce maternal fever with antipyretics as ordered and cooling measures; oxygen* at 10-12 L/min may be of some value; carry out physician's orders based on alleviating cause	Dependent on cause; intervention not warranted in fetus with heart block diagnosed by ECG; oxygen at 10-12 L/min may be of some value; carry out physician's orders based on alleviating cause

*Some hospital protocols specify oxygen rates of 7-8 L/min.

variability is the change in FHR from one beat to the next. This is because even though a fetal heart may beat 140 times over the course of a minute, there are moments in that minute when the heart rate is 134 or 146. This normal irregularity or unevenness from one heart beat to the next is termed *short-term variability*. *Long-term variability* appears as rhythmic cycles (or waves) from the baseline, and there are generally 3 to 5 cycles per minute. All monitors can present evidence of long-term variability whether the woman is monitored internally or externally. Only the internal signal source from a **spiral electrode** can accurately assess short-term variability (Fig. 14-1). However, monitors with autocorrelation can closely approximate short-term variability when the external signal source, the **ultrasound transducer**, is used.

Absence of variability or a **smooth (flat) baseline** is considered an ominous sign of fetal distress. Decreased variability can result from fetal hypoxia and acidosis, as well as from certain drugs that depress the central nervous system (CNS), including analgesics, narcotics (meperidine [Demerol]), barbiturates (secobarbital [Seconal] and pentobarbital [Nembutal]), tranquilizers (diazepam [Valium]), ataractics (promethazine [Phenergan]), and general anesthetics. In addition a temporary decrease in variability can occur when the fetus is in a sleep state. These sleep states do not usually last longer than 30 minutes before average variability resumes. Table 14-2 contrasts key differences between increased and decreased variability.

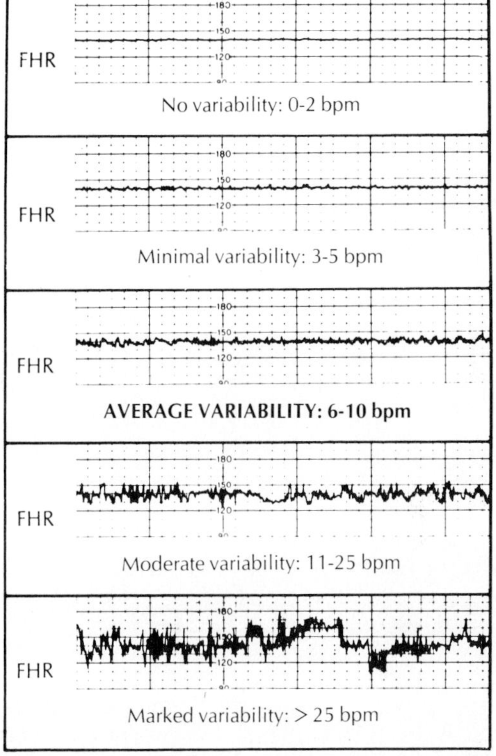

Fig. 14-1 Fetal heart rate variability. Short- and long-term variability tend to increase and decrease together. (From Tucker SM: Pocket guide to fetal monitoring, St Louis, 1988, The CV Mosby Co.)

Periodic Changes in FHR

Periodic changes in the FHR are referred to as accelerations or decelerations, and the latter are described

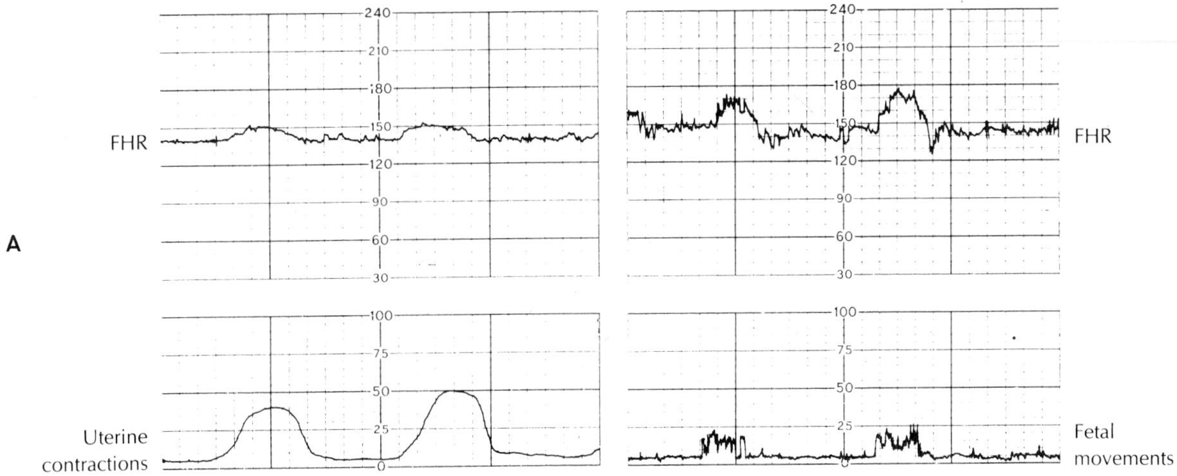

Fig. 14-2 **A**, Acceleration of FHR with uterine contractions. **B**, Acceleration of FHR with fetal movement. (From Tucker SM: Pocket guide to fetal monitoring, St Louis, 1988, The CV Mosby Co.)

Table 14-2 Increased and Decreased Variability

	Increased Variability	Decreased Variability
Cause	Early mild hypoxia Fetal stimulation by the following: Uterine palpation Uterine contractions Fetal activity Maternal activity	Hypoxia/acidosis CNS depressants Analgesics/narcotics Meperidine Alphaprodine (Nisentil) Morphine Pentazocine (Talwin) Barbiturates Secobarbital Pentobarbital Amobarbital (Amytal) Tanquilizers (diazepam) Ataractics Promethazine (Phenergan) Propiomazine (Largon) Hydroxyzine (Vistaril) Promazine (Sparine) Parasympatholytics (Atropine) General anesthetics Prematurity Fetal sleep cycles Congenital abnormalities Fetal cardiac arrhythmias
Clinical significance	Significance of marked variability not known; increased variability from a previous average variability, earliest FHR sign of mild hypoxia	Benign when associated with periodic fetal sleep states, which last 20 to 30 min; if caused by drugs, variability usually increases as drugs are excreted Decreased variability considered ominous if caused by hypoxia/asphyxia; occurring with late decelerations, decreased variability associated with fetal acidosis and low Apgar scores
Nursing intervention	Observe FHR tracing carefully for any sign of fetal distress including decreasing variability and late decelerations; if using external mode of monitoring, consider using internal mode (spiral electrode)	Dependent on cause; intervention not warranted if associated with fetal sleep states or temporarily associated with CNS depressants; consider application of internal mode (spiral electrode) with physician; assist physician with fetal blood sampling for pH if ordered; prepare for delivery if so indicated by physician

as early, late, or variable depending on their characteristics of timing, shape, and repetitiveness in relation to uterine contractions. **Accelerations** (caused by dominance of the *sympathetic* response) are usually encountered with breech presentations (Fig. 14-2, *A*). Pressure applied to the infant's buttocks results in accelerations, whereas pressure applied to the head results in decelerations. Accelerations may occur, however, during the second stage of labor in cephalic presentations. Accelerations (Fig. 14-2, *B*) of the FHR occurring during fetal movement are indications of fetal well-being (nonstress test, Chapter 22).

Decelerations (caused by dominance of *parasympathetic* response) may be benign or ominous. The three types of decelerations that are encountered during labor are early, late, and variable. FHR decelerations are described by their relation to the onset and end of a contraction and by their shape.

Early deceleration (slowing of heart rate) in response to compression of the fetal head is normal and usually does not indicate fetal distress (Fig. 14-3, *A*). The deceleration is characterized by a uniform shape and an early onset corresponding to the rise in intrauterine pressure as the uterus contracts. It is not a common oc-

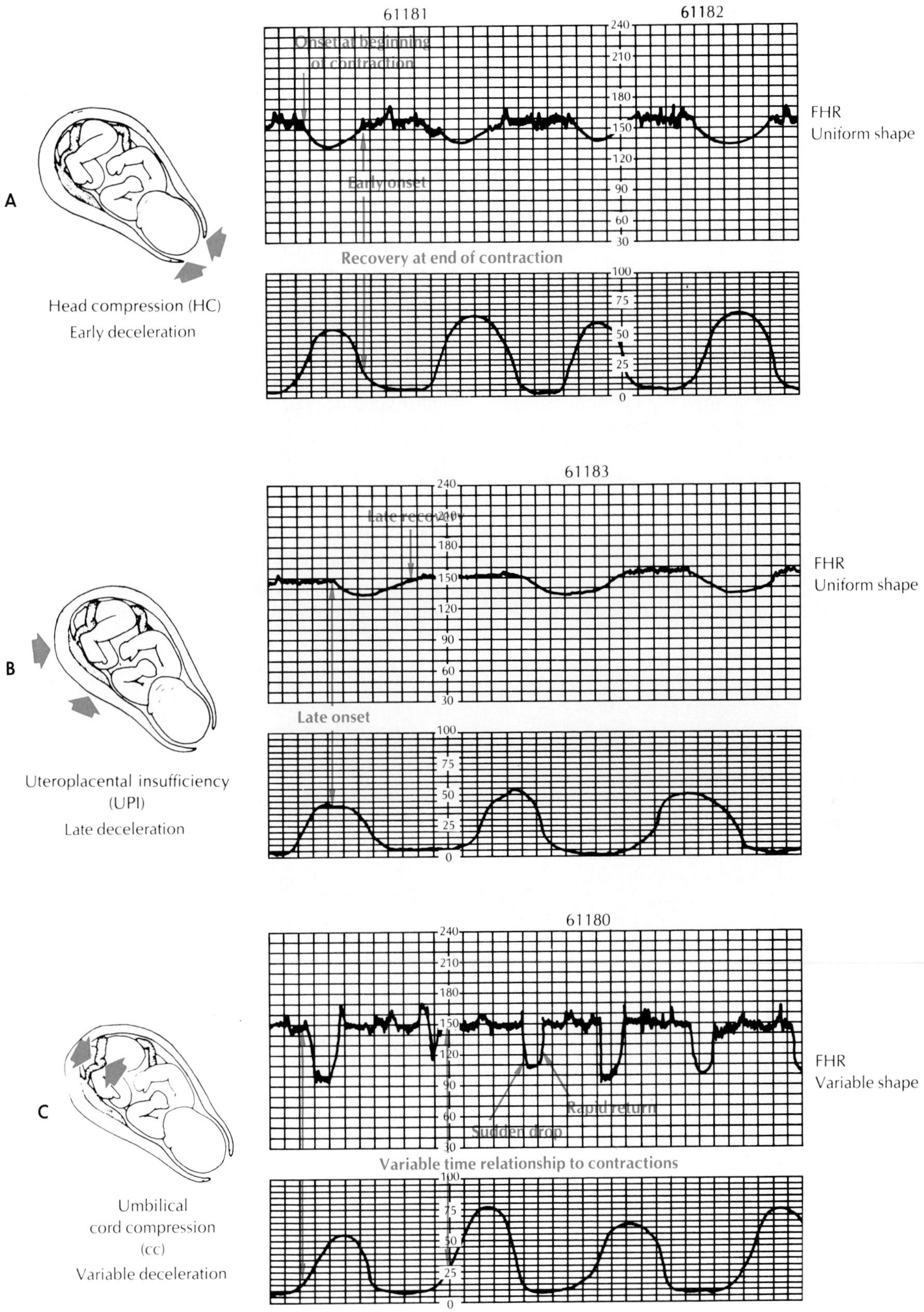

Fig. 14-3 **A,** Early decelerations caused by head compression. **B,** Late deceleration caused by utero-placental insufficiency. **C,** Variable deceleration caused by cord compression.

currence. When present it usually occurs during the first stage of labor when the cervix is dilated 4 to 8 cm. Early deceleration is sometimes seen during the second stage when the parturient is pushing. Early decelerations as a response to fetal head compression can occur during vaginal examinations, as a result of fundal pressure, during placement of the internal mode for fetal monitoring, and during uterine contractions.

Early decelerations are considered to be a benign pattern, therefore interventions are not necessary. The value of identifying early decelerations is to be able to distinguish them from late or variable decelerations, which can be nonreassuring, and for which interventions are appropriate. Table 14-3 contrasts accelerations of FHR with early decelerations.

Late decelerations are caused by **uteroplacental insufficiency** and appear as a smooth, curvilinear, uniform heart rate pattern that mirrors the pattern of intrauterine pressure during a contraction. However, the deceleration necessarily begins *after* the contraction has been established and consistently *persists into the interval after the contraction* (Fig. 14-3, *B*). Late deceleration patterns when persistent or recurrent usually indicate fetal hypoxia because of deficient placental perfusion. Persistent and repetitive late decelerations are associated with fetal hypoxia and acidosis. They should be considered an ominous sign when they are uncorrectable, especially if they are associated with decreased variability and tachycardia. Late decelerations caused by maternal supine hypotensive syndrome are usually correctable when the woman turns to her side to displace the weight of the gravid uterus off the vena cava. This allows a better return of maternal blood flow to the heart, which increases cardiac output and blood pressure.

Late decelerations caused by uteroplacental insufficiency can result from uterine hyperstimulation with oxytocin, pregnancy-induced hypertension (PIH), postmature syndrome, amnionitis, small-for-gestational-age (SGA) fetus, maternal diabetes, placenta previa, abruptio placentae, conduction anesthetics (producing maternal hypotension), maternal cardiac disease, and maternal anemia.

Variable decelerations are those occurring anytime during the uterine contracting phase and are caused by compression of the umbilical cord. Table 14-4 contrasts late deceleration with variable deceleration. The appearance of variable deceleration patterns is different than the early and late decelerations, which mirror the uterine contraction. In contrast, variable decelerations

Table 14-3 Acceleration and Early Deceleration

	Acceleration	Early Deceleration
Description	Transitory increase of FHR above baseline (see Fig. 14-2)	Transitory decrease of FHR below baseline concurrent with uterine contractions (see Fig. 14-3, *A*)
Shape	May resemble shape of uterine contraction	Uniform shape; mirror image of uterine contraction
Onset	Variable; often precedes or occurs simultaneously with uterine contraction	Early in contraction phase before peak of contraction
Recovery	Variable	By end of contraction as uterine pressure returns to its resting tone
Amplitude	Usually 15 bpm above baseline	Usually proportional to amplitude of contraction; rarely decelerates below 100 bpm
Baseline	Usually associated with average baseline variability	Usually associated with average baseline variability
Occurrence	Variable; may be repetitive with each contraction	Repetitious (occurs with each contraction); usually between 4 and 7 cm dilatation and in second stage of labor
Cause	Spontaneous fetal movement Vaginal examination Breech presentation Occiput posterior position Uterine contractions Fundal pressure Abdominal palpation	Head compression resulting from following: Uterine contractions Vaginal examination Fundal pressure Placement of internal mode of monitoring
Clinical significance	Acceleration with fetal movement signifies fetal well-being representing fetal alertness or arousal states	Reassuring pattern not associated with fetal hypoxia, acidosis, or low Apgar scores
Nursing intervention	None required	None required

Table 14-4 Late Deceleration versus Variable Deceleration

	Late Deceleration	Variable Deceleration
Description	Transitory decrease in FHR below baseline rate in contracting phase (see Fig. 14-3, *B*)	Abrupt transitory decrease in FHR that is variable in duration, intensity, and timing related to onset of contractions (Fig. 14-3, C)
Shape	Uniform; mirror image of uterine contraction	Variable; characterized by sudden drop in FHR in V or U shape
Onset	Late in contraction phase; after peak of contraction; low point of deceleration occurs well after peak of contraction	Variable times in contracting phase; often preceded by transitory acceleration
Recovery	Well after end of contraction	Return to baseline is rapid, sometimes with transitory acceleration or acceleration immediately preceding and following deceleration; slow return to baseline with severe variable decelerations
Deceleration	Usually proportional to amplitude of contraction; rarely decelerates below 100 bpm	*Mild:* decelerates to any level, less than 30 sec with abrupt return to baseline *Moderate:* decelerates above 80 bpm, any duration with abrupt return to baseline *Severe:* decelerates below 70 bpm for greater than 30 sec with slow return to baseline
Baseline	Often associated with loss of variability and increasing baseline rate	Mild variables usually associated with average baseline variability; moderate and severe variables often associated with decreasing variability and increasing baseline rate
Occurrence	Occurs with each contraction; proportional to strength and duration of contractions	Variable; commonly observed late in labor with fetal descent and pushing
Cause	Uteroplacental insufficiency caused by the following: Uterine hyperactivity or hypertonicity Maternal supine hypotension Epidural or spinal anesthesia Placenta previa Abruptio placentae Hypertensive disorders Postmaturity Intrauterine growth retardation (IUGR) Diabetes mellitus Amnionitis	Umbilical cord compression caused by the following: Maternal position with cord between fetus and maternal pelvis Cord around fetal neck, arm, leg, or other body part Short cord Knot in cord Prolapsed cord
Clinical significance	Nonreassuring, worrisome pattern associated with fetal hypoxia, acidosis, and low Apgar scores; considered ominous if persistent and uncorrected, especially when associated with fetal tachycardia and loss of variability	Variable decelerations occur in about 50% of all labors and are usually transient, correctable, and not associated with low Apgar scores; mild variable decelerations reassuring; decelerations progressing from moderate to severe are associated with fetal acidosis, hypoxia, and low Apgar scores; severe variable decelerations with good baseline variability just before delivery usually well tolerated
Nursing intervention	Change maternal position Correct maternal hypotension Elevate legs Increase rate of maintenance IV Discontinue oxytocin if infusing Administer oxygen* at 10 to 12 L/min with tight face mask Assist with fetal blood sampling if ordered Assist physician with termination of labor if pattern cannot be corrected	Change maternal position; if decelerations do not yet meet criteria for mild variable deceleration, proceed with measures below. Discontinue oxytocin if infusing Administer oxygen* at 10-12 L/min with tight face mask Assist with vaginal or speculum examination, fetal blood sampling If cord is prolapsed, examiner will elevate fetal presenting part with cord between gloved fingers until cesarean delivery is accomplished Assist with amnioinfusion if ordered Assist with delivery

*Some hospital protocols specify 7-8 L/min.

are often a U shape or V shape characterized by a rapid descent and ascent to and from the nadir (or depth) of the deceleration (Fig. 14-3, C).

Variable decelerations may be related to partial, brief compression of the cord. If encountered in the first stage of labor, they can usually be eliminated by changing the mother's position, such as from one side to the other. Administration of oxygen by face mask to the mother is sometimes of value. They are most commonly encountered during the second stage of labor as a result of cord compression during fetal descent. Variable decelerations are associated with neonatal depression only when cord compression is severe or prolonged (e.g., tight nuchal cord, short cord, knot in cord, prolapsed cord). Variable decelerations occur in about half of all labors and are usually a temporary and correctable phenomenon with maternal position change. A nonreassuring sign is variable deceleration with a very slow return to baseline and decreasing variability or deceleration below 70 bpm for longer than 30 to 45 seconds. **Amnioinfusion** may be considered by some physicians in parturients who have oligohydramnios (insufficient amniotic fluid). In this procedure normal saline is infused via the intrauterine catheter into the uterine cavity in an attempt to add fluid around the umbilical cord and thus prevent its compression during contractions.

Prolonged Decelerations

Prolonged decelerations are difficult to classify, since they can occur in many situations.

Generally the benign causes are pelvic examination, application of spiral electrode, rapid fetal descent, and sustained maternal Valsalva maneuver.

Other prolonged decelerations are caused by progressive severe variable decelerations, sudden umbilical cord prolapse, and hypotension produced by spinal or epidural anesthesia. Paracervical anesthesia, a tetanic contraction, and maternal hypoxia, which may occur during a seizure, often produce prolonged decelerations. When the duration of the deceleration is longer than 2 to 3 minutes, a loss of variability with rebound tachycardia usually occurs. Occasionally, a period of late decelerations follows. These responses normally clear spontaneously. However, when a prolonged deceleration is seen late in the course of severe variable decelerations or during a prolonged series of late decelerations, the prolonged deceleration may occur just before fetal death.

The nurse's responsibility on seeing a prolonged deceleration is to notify the physician immediately and initiate treatment of fetal distress (see Nursing Intervention, Table 14-4).

❑ MONITORING TECHNIQUES

Periodic Auscultation: FHR

Periodic auscultation of the fetal heart may reveal tachycardia, bradycardia, or arrhythmia that may occur during the brief examination (Fig. 14-4).

In the low-risk woman auscultation of the FHR may be done every 15 minutes in the first stage of labor and every 5 minutes during the second stage of labor. In both instances, auscultation is done for a period of 30 (preferably 60) seconds immediately after a uterine contraction. However, nonreassuring and potentially ominous FHR patterns may not occur during the periods of auscultation and may pass unrecognized by the examiner.

An improved method that is more likely to aid in diagnosing fetal compromise in the high-risk pregnancy is the counting of FHR during sequential contractions

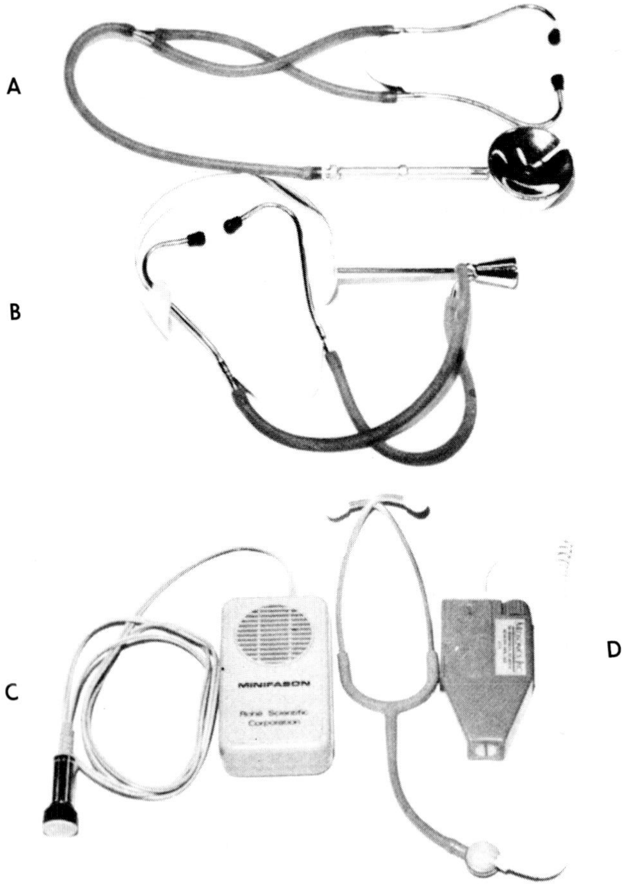

Fig. 14-4 **A,** Leffscope. **B,** DeLee-Hillis scope. **C,** Ultrasound fetoscope; amplifies sound to those in immediate area. **D,** Ultrasound stethoscope; amplifies mechanical movement of fetal heart to listener by means of ear pieces. (From Ingalls AJ and Salerno MC: Maternal and child health nursing, ed 5, St Louis, 1983, The CV Mosby Co.)

and for a full 3 minutes thereafter. Persistent, postcontraction bradycardia (e.g., FHR of 100 bpm, or a persistent drop of 30 bpm or more below baseline) or gross irregularity indicates fetal distress.

The woman becomes anxious if the examiner cannot count the FHR. For the inexperienced listener it often takes time to locate the heartbeat and find the area of maximum intensity. The mother can be told that the nurse is "finding the spot where the sounds are loudest." If it has taken considerable time to locate them, offer the mother an opportunity to hear them too, to reassure her. If the examiner cannot locate the FHR, an experienced nurse should be asked for assistance.

There are two modes of electronic monitoring. The external mode employs the use of external transducers placed on the maternal abdomen to assess heart rate and uterine activity. The internal mode uses a spiral electrode applied to the fetal presenting part to assess the fetal ECG and the **intrauterine catheter** to assess uterine activity and pressure. A brief description contrasting the external and internal modes of **electronic fetal monitoring (EFM)** is provided in Table 14-5.

External EFM-FHR

Continuous EFM has a lower false-normal rate than intermittent auscultation of the FHR (Quirk and Miller, 1986). Separate transducers monitor the FHR and uterine contractions (Fig. 14-5). The *ultrasound transducer* acts through the reflection of high-frequency sound waves from a moving interface, in this case the fetal heart and valves. Therefore short-term variability and beat-to-beat changes in the FHR cannot be assessed by this method. It is also difficult to reproduce a continuous and precise record of the FHR because of artifacts introduced by fetal and maternal movement. The FHR tracing is printed on a strip chart. Once the *area of maximum intensity of FHR* has been located, conductive gel is applied to the surface of the ultrasound transducer, and the transducer is then positioned over this area.

The **tocotransducer** (tocodynamometer) measures **uterine activity** transabdominally. A pressure-sensitive surface on the side next to the abdomen is depressed by uterine contractions or fetal movement. The device is placed over the fundus above the umbilicus. The tocotransducer can measure and record the frequency, regularity, and duration of uterine contractions but not their intensity. This method is especially valuable during the first stage of labor in women with intact membranes or for use in the nonstress test (NST) or oxytocin challenge test (OCT).

The equipment is easily applied by the nurse but must be repositioned as the mother or fetus changes

Table 14-5 External and Internal Modes of Monitoring

External Mode	Internal Mode
FETAL HEART RATE (FHR)	
Ultrasound transducer: High-frequency sound waves reflect mechanical action of the fetal heart. Used during the antepartum and intrapartum period. *Phonotransducer:* Microphone amplifies sound, reflects excessive noise when woman is in labor. Used infrequently for **antepartum monitoring.** *Abdominal electrodes:* Fetal ECG is obtained when electrodes are properly positioned. Used infrequently for antepartum monitoring because of ease and reliability of ultrasound transducer.	*Spiral electrode:* Electrode converts fetal ECG as obtained from the presenting part to FHR via a cardiotachometer. This method can only be used when membranes are ruptured and cervix sufficiently dilated during the intrapartum period. Electrode penetrates fetal presenting part 1.5 mm and must be on securely to ensure a good signal.
UTERINE ACTIVITY	
Tocotransducer: This instrument monitors frequency and duration of contractions by means of pressure-sensing device applied to the maternal abdomen. Used during both the antepartum and intrapartum periods.	*Intrauterine catheter:* This instrument monitors frequency, duration, and *intensity of contractions.* Catheter filled with sterile water is compressed during contractions, placing pressure on a strain gauge converting the pressure into millimeters of mercury on the uterine activity panel of the strip chart. It can be used when membranes are ruptured and cervix sufficiently dilated during the intrapartum period.

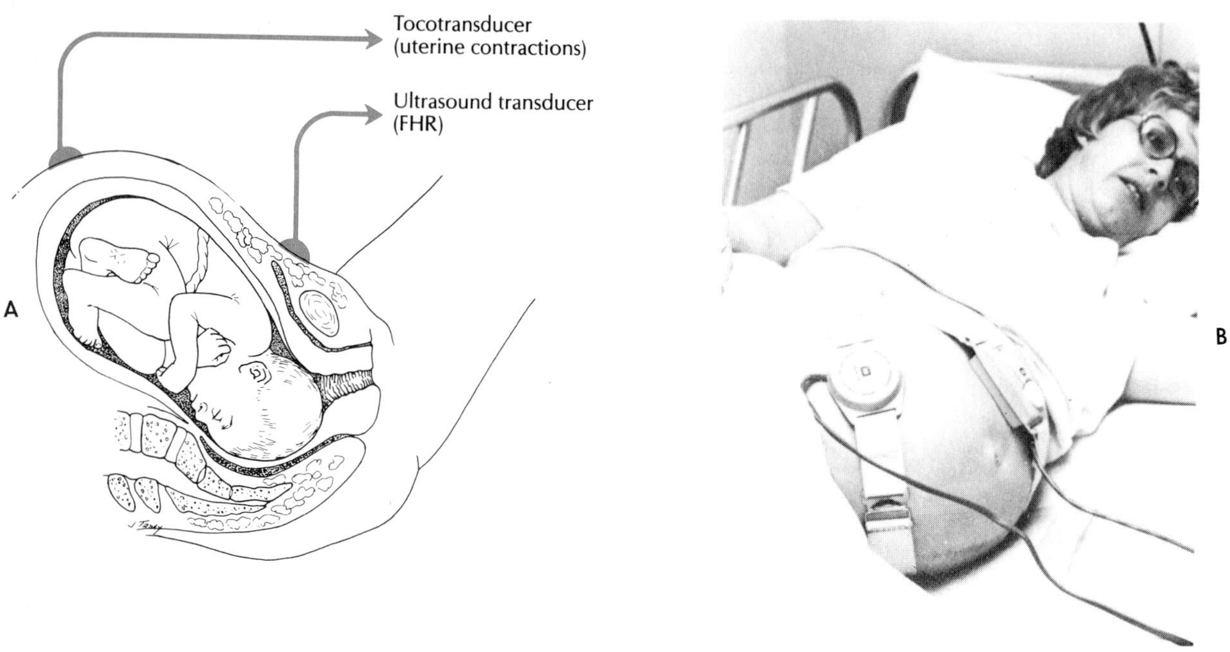

Fig. 14-5 Diagrammatic representation of external noninvasive fetal monitoring with tocotransducer and ultrasound transducer, **A**, with ultrasound transducer placed below umbilicus and tocotransducer placed on uterine fundus. **B**, Note that client is lying in left lateral position. (**B** from Tucker SM: Fetal monitoring and fetal assessment in high-risk pregnancy, St Louis, 1978, The CV Mosby Co.)

position. The woman is asked to assume a semi-sitting position or left-lateral position (see Fig. 14-5, *B*). The equipment is removed periodically to permit washing of the applicator sites and giving of back rubs. This type of monitoring confines the woman to bed. Portable telemetry monitors allow observation of the FHR and uterine contraction patterns by means of centrally located electronic display stations. These portable units permit ambulation during electronic monitoring.

Internal EFM-FHR

The technique of continuous internal monitoring provides an accurate appraisal of fetal well-being during labor (Fig. 14-6). For this type of monitoring the membranes must be ruptured, the cervix sufficiently dilated, and the presenting part low enough for placement of the electrode. A small electrode attached to the presenting part yields a continuous FHR on the fetal monitor strip. A catheter filled with sterile water is introduced into the uterine cavity. The fluid acts as a transmitter of changes in uterine pressure because, as the uterus contracts, it compresses the fluid-filled catheter, placing pressure on the monitor strain gauge or pressure transducer, which is then converted into a pressure reading in millimeters of mercury. The normal range during a contraction is 50 to 75 mm Hg. The

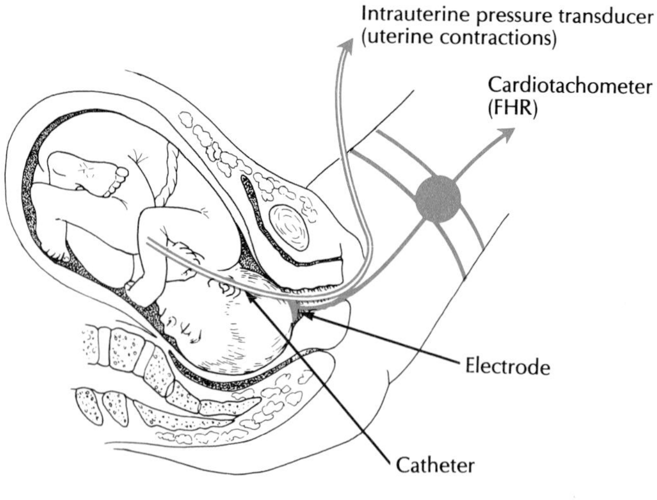

Fig. 14-6 Diagrammatic representation of internal invasive fetal monitoring with intrauterine catheter and spiral electrode in place (membranes ruptured and cervix dilated).

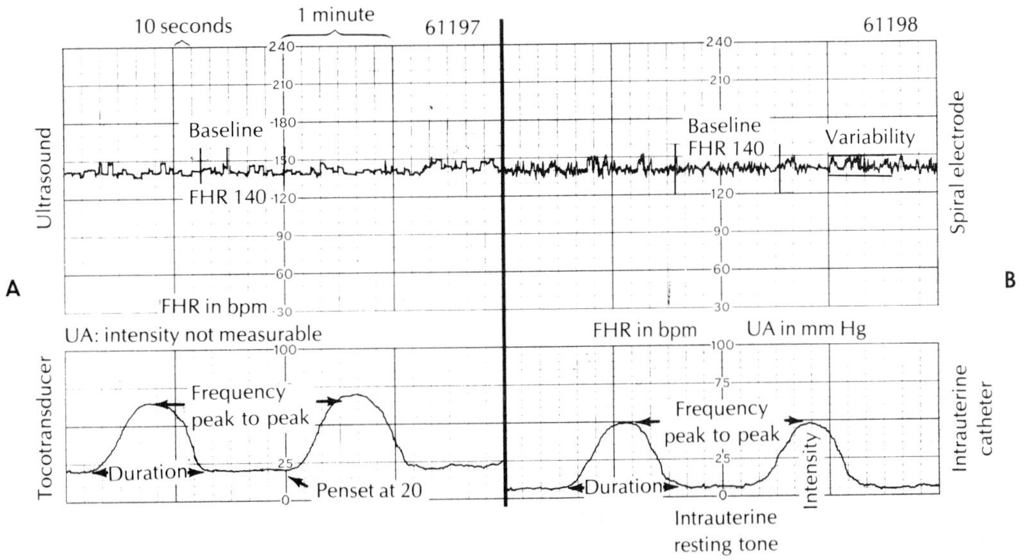

Fig. 14-7 Display of FHR and uterine activity on chart paper. **A,** External mode with ultrasound and tocotransducer as signal source. **B,** Internal mode with spiral electrode and intrauterine catheter as signal source. (From Tucker SM: Pocket guide to fetal monitoring, St Louis, 1988, The CV Mosby Co.)

display of FHR and uterine activity on the chart paper differs for the two modes of electronic monitoring (Fig. 14-7). *Note that each small square represents 10 seconds; each larger box of 6 squares equals 1 minute.*

Fetal Blood Sampling

It is thought that fetal acidosis occurs as a result of hypoxia. As a part of the intrapartum fetal monitoring process, it may be useful to determine the fetal capillary pH, although the exact role of this procedure remains controversial (ACOG, 1989). Because blood gas values can vary so rapidly with transient circulatory changes, the use of fetal blood sampling during the intrapartum period is not routinely warranted. Some of the factors causing this variability include maternal acidosis or alkalosis, caput succedaneum, stage of labor, and time relationship of scalp sampling to uterine contraction (Tucker, 1988).

The procedure is performed by a physician who obtains the sample from the fetal scalp transcervically after rupture of membranes. The scalp is swabbed with a disinfecting solution before the puncture is made. The sample is collected and sent to the laboratory for analysis.

Meconium-stained Amniotic Fluid. The passage of meconium from the fetal bowel before birth may indicate fetal distress. Peristalsis of the bowel increases during hypoxia, and the contents are likely to be expelled. Although the presence of **meconium-stained amniotic fluid** is not always an indication of fetal difficulty, its presence requires immediate notification of the physician (Chapter 22).

Pattern Recognition and Nursing Standards: EFM

Many factors must be evaluated to determine if an FHR pattern is reassuring or nonreassuring. This includes an assessment and evaluation of baseline rate, variability, accelerations, and decelerations, as well as consideration of the frequency and strength of uterine contractions. These factors must be evaluated based on other obstetric information, including parity, maternal and obstetric complications, progress in labor, and analgesia or anesthesia. The estimated time interval until delivery must also be considered. Intervention and interruption of labor are therefore based on clinical judgment of a complex, integrated process.

It is the responsibility of the labor and delivery room nurse to assess FHR patterns, perform independent nursing interventions, and report nonreassuring patterns to the physician.

Nurses planning to work with electronic monitors require additional education and training in their use. In addition to knowing how to apply the monitor and interpret tracings, the nurse needs to know how to trouble-shoot the monitor. A checklist for fetal monitoring equipment is presented in the box on p. 364.

CHECKLIST FOR FETAL MONITORING EQUIPMENT

Name: ______________________ Evaluator: ______________________
Date: ______________________

Items to be Checked | Items to be Checked

PREPARATION OF MONITOR
1. Is the paper inserted correctly?
2. Are transducer cables plugged into the appropriate outlet of the monitor?

ULTRASOUND TRANSDUCER
1. Has ultrasound transmission gel been applied to the crystals?
2. Was the FHR tested and noted on the chart paper?
3. Does a signal light flash with each heart beat?
4. Is the strap secure and snug?

TOCOTRANSDUCER
1. Is the tocotransducer firmly strapped where the least maternal tissue is in evidence?
2. Has it been applied without gel or paste?
3. Was the pen-set knob adjusted between 20 and 25 mm marks and noted on chart paper?
4. Was this setting done between contractions?
5. Is the strap secure and snug?

SPIRAL ELECTRODE
1. Are the wires attached firmly to the posts on the leg plate?
2. Is the spiral electrode attached to the presenting part of the fetus?
3. Is the inner surface of the leg plate covered with electrode paste?
4. Is the leg plate properly secured to the woman's thigh?

INTERNAL CATHETER/STRAIN GAUGE*
1. Is the strain gauge located about half the height of the uterus (approximately at maternal xiphoid)?
2. Is the catheter filled with sterile water?
3. Is the black line on the catheter visible at the introitus?
4. Is it noted on the chart paper that the stopcock was opened to room air (reading 0 on paper)?
5. Was the uterine activity (UA) tested for 10 seconds?
6. Is the stopcock turned off to the syringe during monitoring?

CHARTING
1. Are testings of FHR and UA written on chart paper at least every 4 hours?
2. Is the chart paper properly labeled with the following:
   a. Woman's name
   b. Identification number
   c. Date
   d. Time monitor attached and mode
   e. High-risk conditions (pregnancy-induced hypertension, diabetes, etc.)
   f. Membranes intact or ruptured
   g. Gestational age
   h. Dilatation and station
3. Are the following noted?
   a. Maternal position and repositioning in bed
   b. Vaginal examinations
   c. Epidural anesthesia
   d. Medication given
   e. BP and temperature, pulse, respiration (TPR)
   f. Voidings
   g. O_2 given
   h. Emesis
   i. Pushing
   j. Fetal movement
   k. Notations of baseline or periodic changes
   l. Any change in mode of monitoring
   m. Adjustments of equipment, i.e.
      (1) Relocation of transducers
      (2) Flushing catheter
      (3) Replacement of electrode
      (4) Replacement of catheter
      (5) Time lapse when changing recording paper

From Tucker SM: Pocket guide to fetal monitoring, St Louis, 1988, The CV Mosby Co.
*New internal catheters are solid, without syringes or stopcocks.

❑ FETAL DISTRESS

Fetal distress is a compromise in fetal well-being. It can be an acute or chronic condition, depending on antepartum and intrapartum events, with the possibility of an acute insult superimposed on a condition of chronic fetal distress.

The goal of intrapartum FHR monitoring is the early detection of mild fetal hypoxia and the prevention of severe fetal hypoxia. The nurse must be thinking continually in terms of whether FHR pattern is reassuring and whether one can consider that fetal oxygenation is good. A differentiation can be made of reassuring patterns, nonreassuring or warning FHR patterns generally indicative of mild fetal hypoxia, and worrisome or ominous patterns where there is evidence of severe fetal hypoxia. Reassuring FHR patterns are given in the following list:

1. Baseline FHR in the normal range of 120 to 160 bpm with no periodic changes and average baseline variability
2. Early decelerations
3. Mild variable decelerations

4. Accelerations

Nonreassuring (warning) FHR patterns are given in the following list:

1. Progressive increase or decrease in baseline heart rate
2. Tachycardia of 160 bpm or above
3. Progressive decrease in baseline variability

Administration of oxygen to the mother may be of some value with the preceding patterns.

Ominous FHR patterns and the appropriate nursing intervention are given in Table 14-6.

Potentially ominous FHR patterns are given in the following list:

1. Severe variable decelerations (FHR less than 70 bpm lasting longer than 30 to 60 seconds with rising baseline, decreasing variability, and/or slow return to baseline)
2. Late decelerations of any magnitude—especially those that are repetitive and uncorrectable with a decreasing variability or rising baseline
3. Absence of variability
4. Prolonged deceleration
5. Severe bradycardia

Nursing interventions for fetal distress can include changing the maternal position; discontinuing oxytocin; increasing parenteral fluid infusion rate; and administering oxygen according to physician's order. The nursing intervention should be based on the presenting FHR pattern as described previously in the discussion of various patterns and the summary provided in Table 14-6 on nursing interventions for potentially ominous FHR patterns. The decision for medical intervention or termination of labor achieved by expeditious vaginal or cesarean delivery is made by the physician.

SUMMARY

Nursing care of the woman in labor may include fetal and maternal monitoring. The nurse's knowledge and competence in this area can have a significant impact on the woman's labor experience.

Normal FHR patterns correlate with high Apgar scores and lower neonatal morbidity. An abnormal pattern is equated with fetal hypoxia, low Apgar scores, and high neonatal morbidity in many but by no means all cases. Because FHR patterns suggesting hypoxia may occur in the absence of fetal distress, intermittent and continuous FHR assessments are screening rather than diagnostic devices. Nursing responsibilities in implementing intrapartum FHR monitoring have been developed by the Nurses' Association of the American College of Obstetrics and Gynecology (NAACOG) (now called the Organization for Obstrical, Gynecologic, and Neonatal Nurses (Appendix B).

Table 14-6 Ominous FHR Patterns and Nursing Interventions

Ominous FHR Patterns	Nursing Intervention
Severe variable deceleration; definition: FHR below 70 bpm lasting longer than 30-60 sec with any of following: Rising baseline FHR Decreasing variability Slow return to baseline; may be with "overshoot" (FHR goes above baseline then returns immediately to baseline)	With severe variable deceleration: Change maternal position Perform vaginal or speculum examination or both Discontinue oxytocin if infusing Administer oxygen at 10-12 L/min by tight face mask Delivery considered by physician if pattern cannot be corrected to meet criteria of mild variable deceleration
Late decelerations of any magnitude—more serious if associated with decreasing variability or rising baseline	Intervene in step-by-step approach, proceeding to next step *only* if pattern is uncorrected Keep woman on side Correct maternal hypotension; elevate legs or change bed position, increase rate of maintenance IV infusion Discontinue oxytocin if infusing Administer oxygen at 10-12 L/min by tight face mask Assist physician with fetal pH if done; pH if done; pH >7.2: repeat pH in 10 to 15 min; pH <7.2: prepare for immediate delivery Expeditious delivery considered by physician if pattern cannot be corrected
Absence of variability	Correct identifiable cause; if uncorrectable, assist physician with delivery
Prolonged deceleration	As above
Severe bradycardia	As above

KEY CONCEPTS

- Fetal well-being during labor is measured by the response of the FHR to uterine contractions.
- FHR characteristics include the baseline FHR and periodic changes in FHR.
- Monitoring techniques of fetal well-being include FHR assessment and watching for presence of meconium-stained amniotic fluid.
- It is the responsibility of the labor and delivery room nurse to assess FHR patterns, perform independent nursing interventions, and report nonreassuring patterns to the physician.
- The NAACOG has established nursing standards for EFM.

LEARNING ACTIVITIES

1. Study at least 10 actual or sample fetal monitor strips and determine:
   a. FHR baseline
   b. Variability
   c. Contraction interval, duration, intensity, and resting tone
   d. Periodic changes, if any
2. For activity 1., describe the appropriate nursing actions for each sample in writing; exchange and compare their descriptions with those developed by other students.
3. Role-play a mother in the first stage of labor who is upset and unknowledgeable of the uses of the fetal monitor and a nurse who is using the equipment in an actual case for the first time. Make suggestions concerning actions that would be supportive and reassuring.

References

American Academy of Pediatrics/American College of Obstetricians and Gynecologists: Guidelines for perinatal care, Elk Grove Village, Ill, 1988, AAP/ACOG.

Fields LM: Electronic fetal monitoring: practices and protocols for the intrapatum patient, J Perinat Neonat Nurs 1(1):5, 1987.

Quirk JG and Miller FC: FHR tracing characteristics that jeopardize the diagnosis of fetal well-being, Clin Obstet Gynecol 29(1):12, 1986.

Tucker SM: Pocket guide to fetal monitoring, St Louis, 1988, The CV Mosby Co.

Bibliography

American College of Obstetricians and Gynecologists: Standard for obstetric-gynecologic services, ed 7, Washington, DC, 1989, ACOG.

Collins BA: The role of the nurse in labor and delivery as perceived by nurses and patients, JOGN Nurs 15(5):412, 1986.

Cunningham FG, MacDonald PC, and Gant NF: Williams' obstetrics, ed 18, Norwalk, Conn, 1989, Appleton & Lange.

Funk M and Buerkle L: Intrauterine treatment of fetal tachycardia, JOGN Nurs 15(4):298, 1986.

Galvan B, Van Mullem C, and Brockhuizen F: Using amnioinfusion for the relief of repetitive variable decelerations during labor, JOGN Nurs 19(3):222, 1989.

Garite TJ and Ray D: Intrauterine resuscitation with tocolysis, Contemp OB/GYN 31(3):24, 1988.

Garite TJ and Towers C: Seeking the cause of transient bradycardia, Contemp OB/GYN 28(3):36, 1986.

Sarno AP and Phelan JP: Intrauterine resuscitation of the fetus, Contemp OB/GYN 32(1):143, 1988.

Schifrin BS: Polemics in perinatology: the future of fetal monitoring, J Perinatol 6(4):331, 1986.

Scott JR et al: Danforth's obstetrics and gynecology, ed 6, Philadelphia, 1990, JB Lippincott Co.

Triolo PK: Prepared childbirth, Clin Obstet Gynecol 30(3):487, 1987.

CHAPTER 15 Nursing Care During Labor and Delivery

Vicki Akin

Learning Objectives

Correctly define the key terms listed.

Review the factors involved in the initial assessment of the woman in labor.

Summarize the subsequent assessment of progress during the four stages of labor.

Identify nursing diagnoses and develop an appropriate plan of care throughout the four stages of labor.

Evaluate the role of supportive persons in relation to the four stages of labor.

Explain the ways in which the nurse can assist support persons.

Outline the preparation for birth in the delivery room.

Summarize the nurse's role with the parturient and her family during the second stage of labor.

Discuss assessment of the neonate during the third stage of labor.

Describe in detail the logical order of emergency childbirth.

Outline the nurse's role in the care of the new mother with an episiotomy or a laceration.

Identify priorities of maternal care immediately after delivery.

Prioritize measures to prevent hemorrhage.

Formulate measures to prevent bladder distension.

Explain measures to facilitate parent-infant interaction.

Summarize measures to promote comfort and support emotional needs.

Review transfer of mother and newborn to postdelivery area.

Key Terms

active phase
afterpains
Apgar score
area of maximum impulse
atony
bearing down
bonding
caul
cervical dilatation
crowning
descent
descent phase
duration (of contractions)
effacement
effleurage
episiotomy
eye prophylaxis
Ferguson's reflex
frequency (of contractions)
Hawthorn effect
hemorrhage
hemorrhoids
hyperventilation
hypovolemic shock
intensity (of contractions)
involution
lacerations
latent phase
lithotomy position
living ligature
lochia
mini-prep
nuchal cord
ophthalmia neonatorum
orthostatic hypotension
partogram
placental separation
regularity (of contractions)
retained placental fragments
ring of fire
Ritgen's maneuver
show
Sims' position
slow breathing
splanchnic engorgement
transcutaneous electrical nerve stimulation (TENS)
transitional phase
uterine hypotonia
Valsalva maneuver
vocalization
Wharton's jelly

The labor process is an exciting and anxious time for the woman and her family. Labor for most women begins with the first uterine contraction, continues with hours of the hard work of dilatation and delivery, and ends as the woman begins the attachment process with her infant.

This chapter presents the four stages of labor. Each stage is described in detail, including nursing assessments, therapeutic nursing interventions, and possible complications of labor. There are many cultural practices that surround the birthing process and these will be discussed throughout the stages of labor. The labor and delivery nurse can assist the family both physically and psychosocially to a safe and satisfying delivery.

❑ FIRST STAGE OF LABOR

Nursing care of the woman during the first stage of labor is directed toward safe delivery of a live, healthy baby to a couple who have had a happy and fulfilling childbirth experience. If a hospital delivery has been elected, the woman is admitted to the labor unit (Fig. 15-1). An alternative birth setting, such as home or birthing center, may have been chosen. The first stage of labor is characterized by the onset of symptoms the expectant mother has been prepared to recognize during the prenatal period. The time has arrived for the birth of the baby.

The first stage of labor begins with the onset of regular uterine contractions and culminates when the cervix has reached full dilatation. Care of the woman in labor begins with the woman's report of the following:

1. Onset of progressive, regular uterine contractions that increase in strength, frequency, and duration
2. Rupture of the membranes
3. Bloody vaginal discharge (bloody show)

When the woman and her partner arrive at the labor unit, the nurse should greet them warmly, call them by name, and extend a welcome to them. On admission to the unit, assessment of the woman is the most important priority.

Assessment

Initial Assessment

The admission form can be used to guide the nurse's assessment of the woman in labor. The data for the admission record is obtained from several sources and includes review of the prenatal record; interview information; obtaining baseline physiologic parameters; laboratory results; psychological, social, and cultural factors; and assessment of the woman's current clinical status.

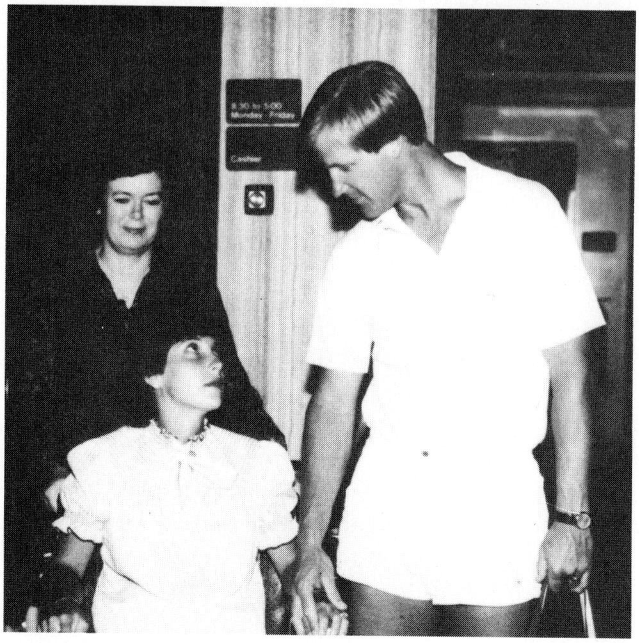

Fig. 15-1 Couple arrives on labor/birth unit accompanied by maternal grandmother. (Courtesy Marjorie Pyle, RNC, Lifecircle, Costa Mesa, Calif.)

Prenatal Record. Before the nurse's first meeting with the woman who is in labor, a review of the woman's prenatal record is made. Significant items are noted. If the woman has not had any prenatal care, the needed information must be obtained on admission. It is best to complete her data base before active labor begins.

Age is important. The needs of a 12-year-old girl and those of a 42-year-old woman vary in some respects. **Height and weight** are also significant. A woman who stands 145 cm (4 ft 10 in) and weighs 77 kg (170 lb) may require interventions different from those needed by the woman who also weighs 77 kg but is 177.5 cm (5 ft 11 in) tall. **General health,** any **medical conditions,** and history of **surgical interventions** are carefully noted.

Parity and gravidity are recorded (Chapter 8). Previous obstetric experience is reviewed for the following:

1. Problems: spontaneous abortions, preterm labors, stillbirths, premature rupture of membranes, bleeding, hypertension, anemia, gestational diabetes, infections (especially sexually transmitted diseases)
2. Type of labors: duration of labors, anesthesia used
3. Type of deliveries: normal spontaneous vaginal delivery (NSVD), forceps assisted, cesarean
4. Condition of babies at birth: weight, **Apgar**

scores, singleton (one baby) or multifetal (twins, triplets) births

Pertinent information on the present pregnancy includes the date of the last normal menstrual period (LNMP), date of quickening, growth of height of the fundus, and estimated weight of the fetus. These data are used to confirm the expected date of delivery (EDD). The woman's vital signs, blood pressure, weight and pattern of weight gain, and results of urinalysis help confirm the normalcy of this pregnancy. The fetal heart rate (FHR) and its location provide a baseline against which the nurse can compare findings of initial assessment.

Data noted include the gestational week of initial visit, diagnostic studies done, and problems encountered. The medications used during this pregnancy are carefully documented.

Laboratory tests performed during this pregnancy and the findings are recorded. These tests include the initial blood test for blood group and Rh factor, hemoglobin and hematocrit, hepatitis B surface antigen (HB_sAG), antibodies, and sickle cell trait, if indicated.

To complete the admission form, the nurse uses the assessment techniques of interviewing, physical examination, and laboratory tests. Each of these techniques will be discussed.

Interview. Any information not found in the prenatal record is requested on admission. Pertinent data include birth plan, choice of infant feeding method, anesthesia, and pediatrician. A client profile is obtained; this profile indicates the woman's preparation for childbirth, supportive persons desired and available, and ethnic or cultural expectations or needs.

The woman's chief complaint or reason for coming to the hospital is determined. The chief complaint may be that her "bag of waters has broken," with or without contractions. In this case she is in for an **obstetric check.** The obstetric check is reserved for women who are unsure about onset of labor. This designation allows time on the unit for diagnosis of labor without official admission, and minimizes or avoids cost to the client.

The woman may have been scheduled for induction of labor (Chapter 26). Induction of labor and other complications of labor, such as premature rupture of membranes, require special alterations in the nursing care plan. However, even in those instances much of the nursing care remains the same.

The onset of labor may be difficult to determine even for the experienced gravida. The woman is asked to recall the events of the previous days. She is assessed for the prodromal signs of labor (Chapter 12) and for the onset of regular contractions. She is asked to describe the following:

1. Frequency and duration of contractions.
2. Location and character of discomfort from contractions (i.e., back pain, suprapubic discomfort).
3. Persistence of contractions despite changes in maternal position, when walking or lying down.
4. Presence and character of vaginal discharge or show.
5. Status of amniotic membranes, such as gush or seepage of fluid. If there is a discharge that may be amniotic fluid, she is asked the date and time the fluid was first noted. In many instances a sterile speculum examination is utilized to confirm that the membranes are ruptured.

These questions also help the nurse determine the degree of progress by determining the character of the contractions and the nature of the vaginal discharge. Bloody show must be distinguished from bleeding. **Show** is pink in color and feels sticky from the mucus it contains. It is scant to begin with and increases with effacement and dilatation of the cervix. A woman may report a scant brownish discharge that may be attributed to cervical trauma as a result of vaginal examination or coitus within the last 48 hours.

In case general anesthesia may be required at a moment's notice, it is important to know about the woman's respiratory status. The nurse asks if the woman has a "cold" or related symptoms, "stuffy nose," sore throat, or cough. Allergies are rechecked, including allergies to drugs routinely used, such as meperidine (Demerol) or mepivacaine (Carbocaine). Some allergic responses cause swelling of mucous membranes of the respiratory system. Because vomiting and subsequent aspiration into the respiratory tract can complicate an otherwise normal labor, the nurse records the type and time of the woman's last meal.

This initial interview helps confirm the onset of true labor and provides information on the woman's current clinical condition.

False labor may be experienced from the thirty-eighth week of pregnancy onward. It can be disheartening for the woman and her partner to find that the contractions she is having are not true labor contractions and that she must return home to await the onset of true labor. (For a comparison of true and false labor, see guidelines for client teaching, p. 370).

The nullipara, because of eagerness to complete labor, may come to the hospital early in the first stage. If she lives near the hospital, she may be asked to return home to wait for further progress either in frequency and strength of contractions or in amount of show. She is encouraged to walk about but is asked to restrict ingestion to clear fluids. If the woman lives a considerable distance from the hospital, she may be admitted and the same care given.

Guidelines for Client Teaching

DISTINGUISHING TRUE LABOR FROM FALSE LABOR

ASSESSMENT

1. Woman pregnant for first time.
2. Woman expresses a desire to learn the difference between true and false labor.

NURSING DIAGNOSES

Knowledge deficit related to the difference between true and false labor.
Anxiety related to lack of knowledge.

GOALS

Short-term

Woman will verbalize understanding of true vs. false labor.

Intermediate

Woman can palpate contractions for practice.

Long-term

Woman verbalizes confidence and can apply knowledge of breathing with onset of true labor.

REFERENCES AND TEACHING AIDS

Printed materials containing comparison between true and false labor and the doctor/clinic/hospital's number.

RATIONALE/CONTENT	TEACHING ACTIONS
Knowledge of false or prodromal labor patterns provides a basis for decision making: Define false contractions as mild, intermittent, painless contractions that occur during pregnancy and aid in keeping uterine tone and facilitate placental perfusion. As pregnancy progresses these contractions become more frequent and are felt as a tightening of the abdomen. Woman may obtain relief with walking or lying down. These contractions do not increase in intensity over time, nor is there a change in interval time between each contraction.	Discuss this with the woman/couple. Encourage questions. Have woman/couple place hands on her abdomen to try and feel for this tightening.
Describe contractions of true labor as contractions that occur regularly, with intensity increasing and intervals between them shortening. May be located in lower back or feel like gastrointestinal (GI) upset, may be accompanied by diarrhea.	Explain how true labor works to dilate and efface the cervix. Use available illustrations or audiovisual materials.
Knowledge of signs and symptoms of labor provides a basis for individual coping: Discuss show—in true labor this is usually present as a pinkish mucus that may contain mucous plug from cervix. There is no show in false labor unless woman has had a vaginal examination within last 48 hours; mucus may be brownish stained.	Discuss the mucous plug and its purpose. Show the woman a picture or illustration of what a bloody show would look like.
Discuss rupture of membranes as true sign of labor and need to report this to physician or nurse-midwife immediately.	Describe slow leak or sudden gush of fluid.
Discuss cervix—becomes effaced and dilated as time progresses. No change with false labor.	
Discuss **descent** of fetus—progressive as labor continues. No descent of fetus in false labor.	Explain how fetus moves down into the true pelvis.
Discuss fetal movement—no significant change in true labor. May intensify for a short time or remain the same with false labor.	Encourage discussion and questions.

EVALUATION Teaching has been effective when all goals have been obtained. Woman is able to feel, time, and describe false vs. true labor contractions. Woman is able to verbalize the difference between false and true labor. Woman recognizes when true labor begins.

Psychologic Responses. The woman's general appearance and behavior (and that of her partner) provide valuable clues as to the type of supportive care she will need. The nurse notes the following:

1. *Verbal interaction.* Is the woman talkative or mute? Does she talk to staff members freely or only in response to questions? How does she talk to her support person? Does that person do all the talking?
2. *Body posture and set.* Is the woman relaxed or tense? What is her anxiety level? Does she lie rigidly on her back or sit up tailor fashion (see Fig. 10-11, B)? Where does her partner sit?
3. *Perceptual acuity.* Does the woman report horror stories of labor she has heard of or does she have unrealistic expectations of labor? Does her anxiety level require repeated explanations? Does she understand what the nurse says? Can she repeat what has been said or demonstrate that she understands (e.g., use the call bell correctly)?
4. *Energy level.* Does the woman look tired? How much rest has she had in the previous few days? Does excitement mask a depleted energy reserve?
5. *Discomfort or pain.* How much does the woman relate what she is experiencing? How does she react to a contraction?
6. *Cultural background.* Does the woman's ethnic/cultural heritage define any prescriptions or proscriptions for her behavior or the care she receives during labor? What are her expectations of the hospial, the staff, and her family members?

Physical Examination

The initial examination confirms the onset of true labor. The findings serve as a baseline for assessing the woman's progress from that point in time. Although some complications of labor are anticipated, others appear only in the clinical course of labor. Knowledge of pregnancy, careful initial assessment, and follow-up of progress are necessary during normal labor, as well as during an abnormal labor (see danger signs box, above).

DANGER SIGNS

During Labor

1. Intrauterine pressure above 75 mm Hg
2. Contractions lasting longer than 60 seconds
3. Contractions occuring more than every 2 minutes
4. Fetal bradycardia, tachycardia
5. Irregular FHR
6. Absence of fetal heart beat
7. Thick meconium staining or bloody amniotic fluid
8. Umbilical cord as presenting part
9. Declining or arrested progress in dilatation/effacement of cervix and descent of fetal part

Vaginal Examination. The vaginal examination reveals whether the woman is in true labor and enables the examiner to determine if the membranes have ruptured (Fig. 15-2). Labor is initiated by spontaneous rupture of the membranes (SROM) in almost 25% of gravidas. The lag period, rarely exceeding 24 hours, precedes the onset of labor. The length of uterine inactivity is directly related to the duration of pregnancy. If the woman is only 32 weeks pregnant, for example, several days may pass before labor begins. If she is at term, labor usually ensues within 12 hours of rupture of the membranes. After a delay of 24 hours, the woman is said to have premature or prolonged rupture

A

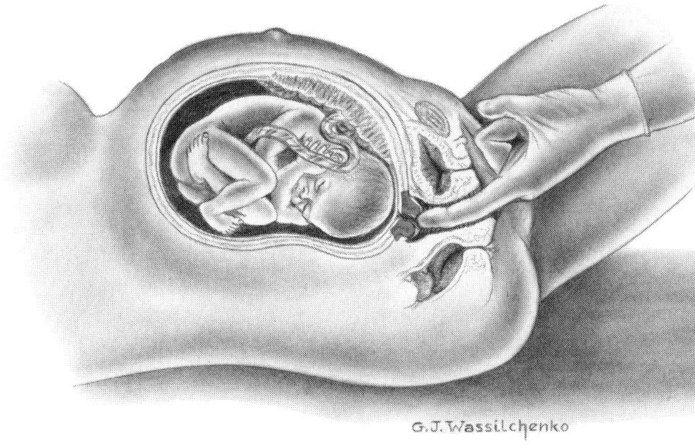

B

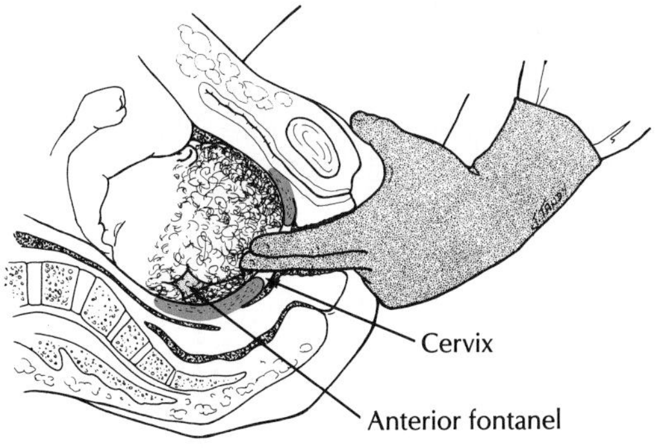

Fig. 15-2 Vaginal examination. **A,** Undilated, uneffaced cervix. Membranes intact. **B,** Palpation of sagittal suture line. Cervix effaced and partially dilated.

PROCEDURE 15-1
TESTS FOR RUPTURE OF MEMBRANES

DEFINITION

Affirmation of rupture of membranes or leakage of amniotic fluid by using definitive diagnostic measures.

PURPOSE

To determine if membranes have ruptured.
To determine if fluid leakage is urine or amniotic fluid.

EQUIPMENT

Nitrazine paper; sterile glove, water, swab; microscope, clean glass slide; Nile blue stain.

NURSING ACTIONS	RATIONALE
Nitrazine Test for pH	
Explain procedure to woman (couple).	Diminishes anxiety and assists her (them) to maintain sense of control.
Procedure	
Use Nitrazine paper, a dye 1-1 impregnated test paper for pH.	Differentiates amniotic fluid, which is slightly alkaline, from urine and purulent material (pus), which are acidic.
Wearing a sterile glove lubricated with water, place a piece of test paper at the cervical os.	Maintains asepsis. Avoids affecting pH. Ensures testing for amniotic fluid.
OR	
Use a sterile, cotton-tipped applicator to dip deep into vagina to pick up fluid; touch applicator to test paper.	Maintains asepsis. Ensures testing for amniotic fluid.
Read results:	Completes the test.
Membranes probably intact: Yellow pH 5.0 Olive yellow pH 5.5 Olive green pH 6.0	Identifies vaginal and most body fluids that are acidic.
Membranes probably ruptured: Blue-green pH 6.5 Blue-gray pH 7.0 Deep blue pH 7.5	Identifies amniotic fluid that is alkaline.
Realize that false tests are possible because of presence of bloody show, insufficient amniotic fluid, or semen.	Minimizes misdiagnosis.
Remove gloves and wash hands.	Implements universal precautions while handling body fluids (Chapter 23).
Chart results: positive or negative.	Provides data base.
Test for Ferning or Fern Pattern (usually performed by physician)	
Explain procedure to client/couple.	Reduces anxiety.
Wash hands, apply gloves, obtain specimen of fluid (usually with sterile speculum examination).	Minimizes nosocomial infection.
Spread a drop of fluid from vagina on a clean glass slide with a sterile, cotton-tipped applicator.	Prepares specimen for assessment. Maintains asepsis.
Allow fluid to dry.	Prepares specimen.
Assess slide under microscope: observe for appearance of ferning (a frondlike crystalline pattern) (do not confuse with cervical mucus test, when high levels of estrogen are responsible for the ferning).	Supports finding of ruptured membranes.
Observe for absence of ferning.	Alerts staff to possibility that specimen was inadequate or that specimen was urine, vaginal discharge, or blood.
Remove gloves and wash hands.	Implements universal precautions when handling body fluids (Chapter 23).
Chart results: either a positive or negative fern test.	Provides a data base.

PROCEDURE 15-1—cont'd

NURSING ACTIONS	RATIONALE
Test for Lanugo Hairs or Fetal Squamous Cells (usually performed by physician)	
Explain procedure to client/couple.	Reduces anxiety.
Wash hands and apply gloves.	Prevents nosocomial infection.
Aspirate fluid from posterior vaginal vault with sterile aspiration syringe.	Obtains specimen.
	Maintains asepsis.
Place on clean glass slide.	Prepares specimen for assessment.
Observe under microscope for presence of fetal lanugo hairs or fetal squamous cells.	Supports finding of ruptured membranes.
Stain with Nile blue stain to identify fetal cells because some squamous cells that contain lipids stain yellow; other squamous cells and hairs stain blue.	Supports finding of ruptured membranes.
Assess findings.	Provides data for analysis.
Remove gloves and wash hands.	Implements universal precautions when handling body fluids (Chapter 23).
Chart results: Nile blue stain shows some squamous cells and some blue squamous cells and hair.	Provides data base.

of the membranes (PROM). If they are ruptured, the nurse notes the color and character of the amniotic fluid, asks for the time of rupture, and checks the vaginal discharge with phenaphthazine (Nitrazine paper) for pH (positive = dark blue) because pH is weakly basic at 7.2 (see Procedure 15-1).

The following steps should be included in the vaginal examination:

1. The nurse assembles all the equipment needed, including single sterile glove, antiseptic solution or soluble gel, and a light source.
2. The woman is prepared through explanation of procedure and draping her to prevent chill and protect privacy.
3. The nurse washes her hands and applies sterile gloves using aseptic technique. The nurse explains to the woman as she gently inserts first and middle fingers into the vagina.
4. The woman is assessed for the following:
   a. Dilatation and effacement of cervix.
   b. Presenting part, position, station, and if vertex, any molding of the head.
   c. Intact membranes.
   d. Presence of stool in rectum.
5. The woman is helped to a comfortable position and the nurse reports and records all of the above data.

Assessment Procedures. Complete and accurate assessment on admission provides the basis for ongoing care. Minimum assessment guidelines and normal limits of maternal progress during the first stage of labor are presented in Tables 15-1 and 15-2 (pp. 378 and 379). Physical examinations include the following:

1. Vital signs and blood pressure
2. Urine specimen
3. Brief physical assessment: heart, lungs; presence of edema of the legs, face, hands, or sacrum; deep tendon reflexes and clonus (Chapters 10 and 23)
4. Abdominal palpation: Leopold's maneuvers
5. Auscultation of the FHR
6. Uterine contractions

The assessment procedures that follow can be used as a basis for teaching women and their families. The purpose, equipment needed, and nursing actions and rationale of each procedure can be shared with the woman. All procedures are preceded by thorough handwashing. The procedures and findings are explained to the woman whenever possible. Universal precautions and precautions for invasive procedures are taken as needed (Chapter 23). Findings and the time the procedure is performed are carefully noted and initialed on the chart. Handwashing is also important *after* the examinations. Accurate charting is done as soon after interaction with a client is possible.

Vital Signs and Blood Pressure. Vital signs and blood pressure (BP) are assessed on admission of the client to the hospital. Findings are assessed for normalcy and are used for comparison with future values. If the BP is elevated, it should first be determined whether the correct size of BP cuff has been used, and BP should then be reassessed 30 minutes later to obtain a true reading after the woman has relaxed. The woman should also be encouraged to lie on her left side and not in a supine position to avoid supine hypotension and fetal distress (see Fig 15-9). The temperature is assessed to monitor for signs of infection.

Urine Specimen. A urine specimen is obtained to gather data about the pregnant woman's health. It is a convenient and simple procedure that can provide information about her hydration status (specific gravity, color, amount), nutritional status (ketones), or possible complications, for example, pregnancy-induced hypertension (PIH) (protein). The results can be obtained quickly and will help the nurse determine appropriate interventions.

Leopold's Maneuvers. Leopold's maneuvers are abdominal palpations performed to determine fetal presentation, lie, position, and engagement. These maneuvers are utilized with every woman to determine where to place the ultrasonic transducer. The maneuvers also provide information regarding the size of the fetus and the amount of amniotic fluid within the uterus. The four maneuvers provide a systematic examination. Proficiency in determining presentation and position by abdominal palpation requires considerable practice, so every opportunity to learn must be used to perform the technique. Gross maternal obesity, excessive amniotic fluid (hydramnios), or tumors may make it difficult to feel the fetal contours (see Procedure 15-2 and Fig. 15-3).

Auscultation of FHR. The area of maximum impulse (MI) of the FHR is the location of the maternal abdomen where the FHR is heard the loudest. The MI is

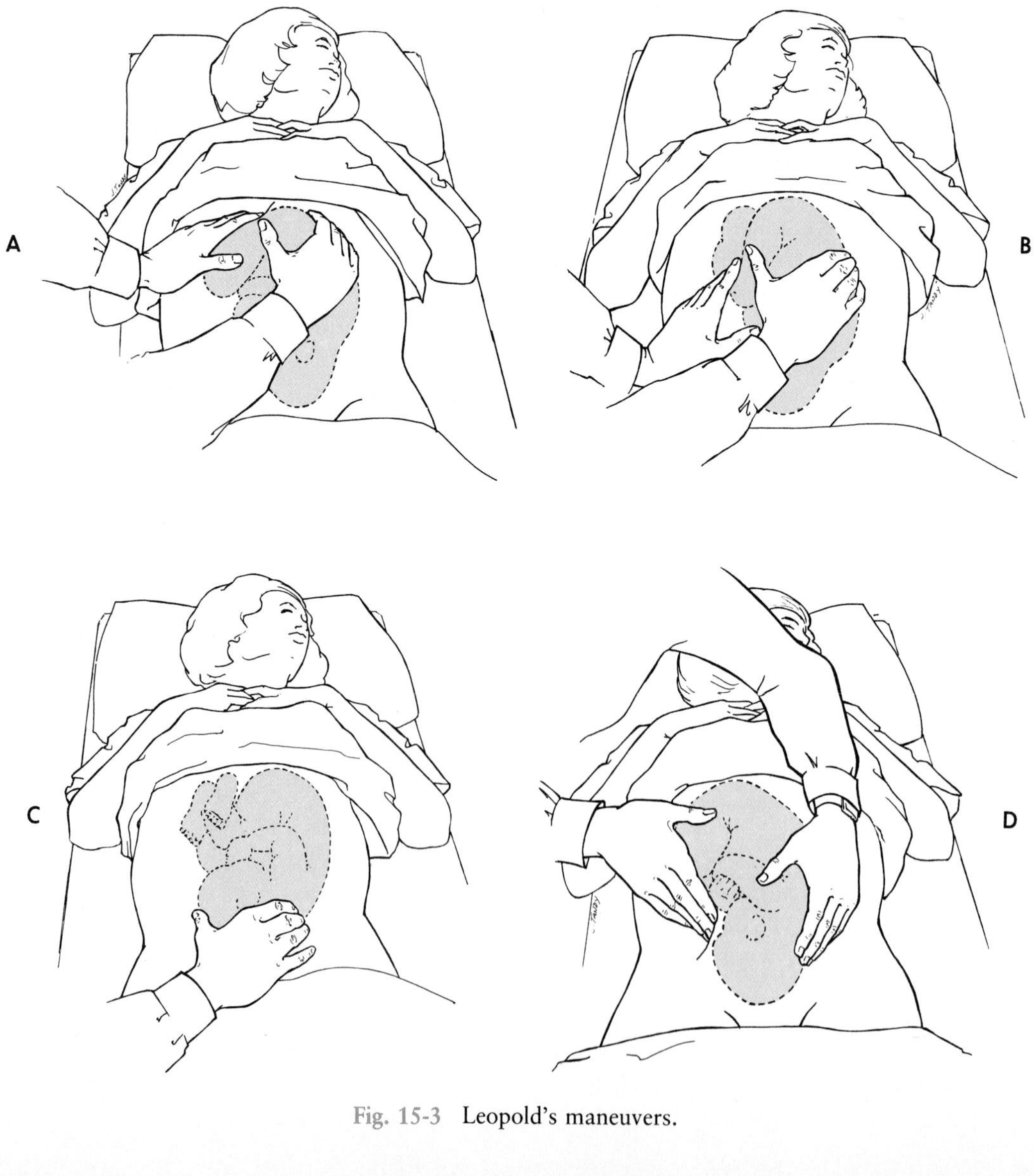

Fig. 15-3 Leopold's maneuvers.

PROCEDURE 15-2
LEOPOLD'S MANEUVERS

DEFINITION

Four maneuvers for assessing fetal position by external palpation of the mother's abdomen.

PURPOSE

To identify number of fetuses.
To identify fetal presentation, lie, presenting part, degree of descent, and fetal attitude.
To identify point of maximum intensity (PMI) of FHR in relation to the woman's abdomen.
To monitor the descent and internal rotation of the fetus.

EQUIPMENT

Fetal monitoring device.

NURSING ACTIONS	RATIONALE
Wash hands.	Prevents nosocomial infection.
Ask woman to empty bladder.	Increases maternal comfort during examination. Facilitates accurate assessment.
Position woman supine with one pillow under her head and with her knees slightly flexed.	Ensures comfort. Relieves tension of abdominal musculature.
Place small rolled towel under woman's right hip.	Displaces uterus to left off of major blood vessels. (Avoids supine hypotensive syndrome, Fig. 15-9).
If right-handed, stand on woman's right, facing her:	Facilitates examination by using dominant hand.
1. Identify fetal part that occupies the fundus. The head feels round, firm, freely movable, and palpable by ballottement; the breech feels less regular and softer (Fig. 15-3, *A*).	Identifies fetal lie (vertical or horizontal) and presentation (vertex or breech).
2. Using palmar surface of one hand, locate and palpate the smooth convex contour of the fetal back and the irregularities that identify the small parts (feet, hands, elbows) (Fig. 15-3, *B*).	Assists in identifying fetal presentation.
3. With the right hand, determine which fetal part is presenting over the inlet to the true pelvis. Gently grasp the lower pole of the uterus between the thumb and fingers, pressing in slightly (Fig. 15-3, C). If the head is presenting and not engaged, determine the attitude of the head.	Confirms presenting part. Helps identify degree of descent. If the presenting part is not engaged, it can be rocked from side to side; if engaged, it cannot be rocked.
4. Turn to face gravida's feet. Using two hands, outline the fetal head (Fig. 15-3, *D*) with palmar surface of fingertips.	When presenting part has descended deeply, only a small portion of it may be outlined. Palpation of cephalic prominence assists in identifying attitude of head. If the cephalic prominence is found on the same side as the small parts, the head must be flexed, and the vertex is presenting (Fig. 15-3, *D*). If the cephalic prominence is on the same side as the back, the presenting head is extended (Fig. 15-3, C).
Determination of PMI of FHR:	
Wash hands.	Prevents nosocomial infection.
Perform Leopold's maneuvers.	Locates fetal back, presentation, and position.
Auscultate FHR (Figs. 15-4, 15-5 and 10-8).	Assists in estimating PMI.
Apply monitor prn (Chapter 14).	Assists in assessing fetal well-being.
Wash hands.	Implements universal precautions (Chapter 23) when handling body fluids.
Chart fetal presentation, position, and lie; whether presenting part is flexed or extended, engaged or free floating.	Provides data base for future findings. Provides data base for next steps in the nursing process.
Use hospital's protocol for charting (e.g., "Vtx, LOA, floating")	Promotes collaboration with other members of the health care team.

Continued.

PROCEDURE 15-2—cont'd

NURSING ACTIONS	RATIONALE
Chart PMI of FHR using a two-line figure to indicate the four quadrants of the maternal abdomen, right upper quadrant (RUQ), left upper quadrant (LUQ), left lower quadrant (LLQ), and right lower quadrant (RLQ):	Provides data base for future comparison. Provides data base for nursing process.
The umbilicus is the point where the lines cross. The PMI for the fetus in vertex presentation, in general flexion with the back on the mother's right side, is commonly found in the mother's right lower quadrant, and is recorded with an "x" or with the FHR as follows:	Assists other examiners.

RUQ	LUQ
RLQ	LLQ

x	

or

140	

also an aid in determining the fetal position (Figs. 15-4 and 15-5). In vertex and breech presentations, with the head well flexed on the fetal chest, the FHR is heard loudest through the fetal back. In vertex presentations the FHRs commonly are heard below the mother's umbilicus in a lower quadrant of the abdomen (Fig. 15-4, *A* and *B*). In breech presentations the FHRs are usually heard loudest above the level of the umbilicus (Fig 15-4, *C* and 15-5, A). As the fetus undergoes descent and internal rotation, the MI changes and is found to move downward and to the midline. In Fig. 15-4, *B*, the MI of the fetus in the right occipitoanterior (ROA) position is seen to move to the midline just over the symphysis pubis. Just before delivery the fetal position is occipitoanterior (OA) and the fetal back is directly above the symphysis pubis. (See also Chapter 14 for fetal monitoring).

Uterine Contractions. The primary powers, the uterine contractions, and their functions are described in detail in Chapter 12. There are three methods of assessing contractions: by the subjective description given by the woman, by palpation and timing by a nurse or physician, and by electronic monitoring devices (Chapter 14).

Each contraction exhibits a wavelike pattern; it begins with a slow increment, gradually reaches an acme, and then diminishes rather rapidly (decrement). This is followed by an interval of rest (intrauterine pressure is 8 to 15 mm Hg), which is broken when the next contraction begins (Fig. 15-6).

In describing a uterine contraction, reference is made to the following characteristics:

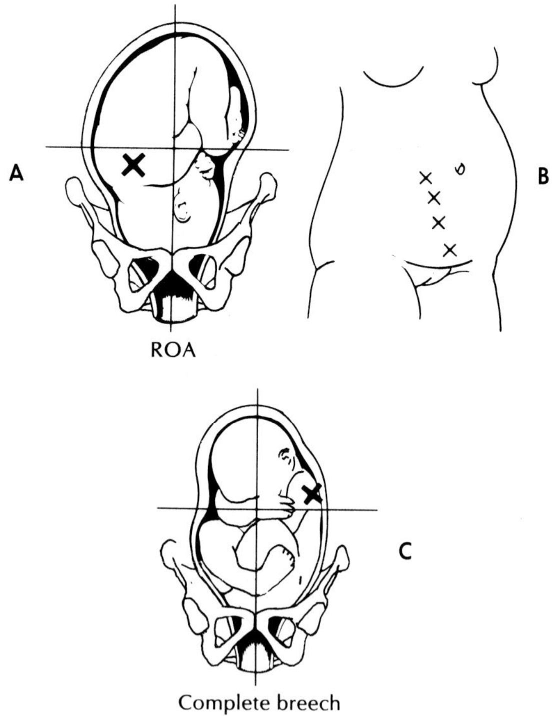

Lie: vertical
Presentation: breech (sacrum and feet presenting)
Reference point: sacrum (with feet)
Attitude: general flexion

Fig. 15-4 The area of the FHR. **A**, With fetus in ROA position. **B**, Change in area of MI as fetus undergoes internal rotation from ROA to OA for delivery. **C**, With fetus in LSP (left sacrum posterior) position. (**A** and **C** courtesy Ross Laboratories, Columbus, Ohio.)

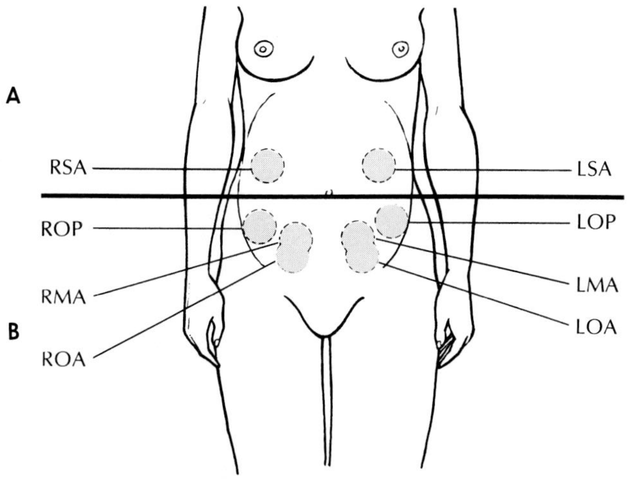

Fig. 15-5 Areas of maximum intensity of FHR for differing positions: *RSA*, right sacrum anterior; *ROP*, right occipitoposterior; *RMA*, right mentum anterior; *ROA*, right occipitoanterior; *LSA*, left sacrum anterior; *LOP*, left occipitoposterior; *LMA*, left mentum anterior; and *LOA*, left occipitoanterior. **A**, Presentation is *breech* if FHR is heard *above* umbilicus. **B**, Presentation is *vertex* if FHR is heard *below* umbilicus.

1. **Frequency.** Contractions occur intermittently throughout labor. They may begin at about 20 to 30 minutes apart and become closer together until, at the height of the expulsive efforts, they are as frequent as every 2 to 3 minutes.
2. **Regularity.** Contractions occur with increasing regularity as labor becomes established. There is more consistency in the intervals between contractions.
3. **Duration.** The length of time a contraction lasts increases from 30 seconds to between 60 and 90 seconds near full dilatation of the cervix. Then the duration of the contraction becomes about 60 seconds during the second stage until delivery of the fetus is accomplished.
4. **Intensity.** The strength of the contraction also increases as labor progresses; from weak contractions noted early in labor to strong expulsive contractions (intrauterine pressure measured at 50 to 75 mm Hg measured with an intrauterine pressure catheter [IUPC]) near the time of delivery.

Palpation of uterine contractions is less precise than electronic monitoring devices for determining the intensity of uterine contractions. Practice is required to discern between mild, moderate, and strong contractions. The definitions of these descriptive terms are as follows:

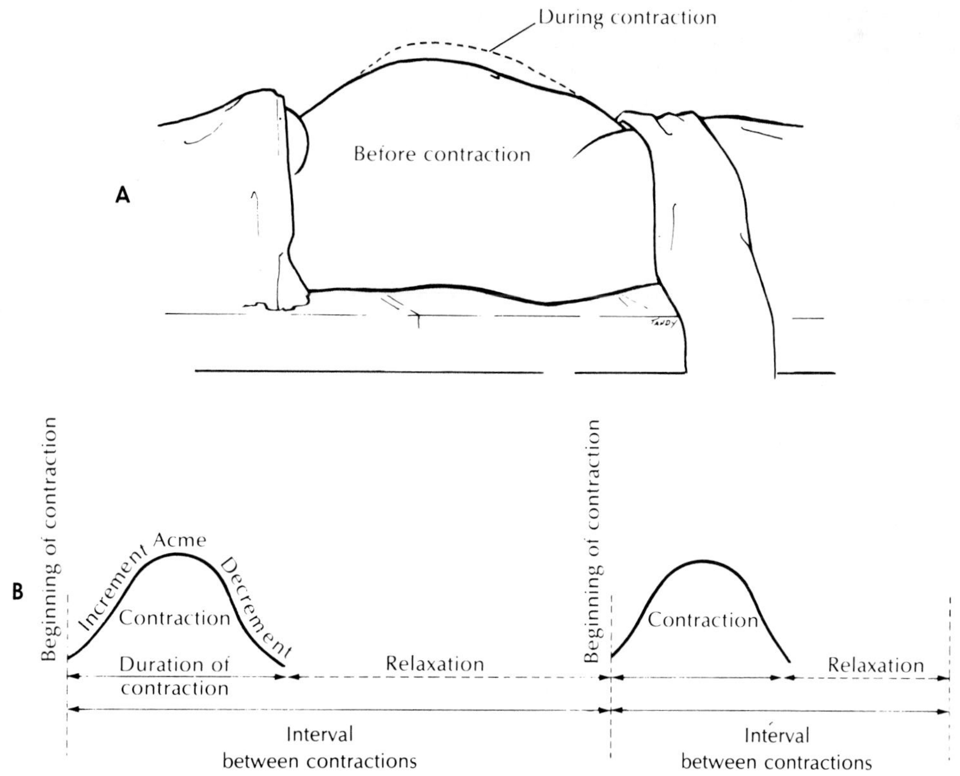

Fig. 15-6 Assessment of uterine contractions. **A**, Abdominal contour before and during uterine contraction. **B**, Wavelike pattern of contractile activity.

mild contractions Slightly tense fundus that is easy to indent with fingertips
moderate contractions Firm fundus that is difficult to indent with fingertips
strong contractions Rigid, boardlike fundus that is almost impossible to indent

In most cases the woman is not aware of the sensation of the contracting of the uterus until each contraction is fairly well established. Commonly, her description of the end of a contraction is related to the end of pain sensation (felt in the lower part of the uterus, not in the fundus). This sensation may persist after the cessation of the actual contraction. Therefore the woman's description of each contraction may not be as accurate as that obtained by the nurse by abdominal assessment.

Subsequent Assessment During Labor

Findings from initial assessments serve as a basis for comparison with expected symptomatology of labor (Table 15-1; guidelines for client teaching, p. 370). As-

Table 15-1 Maternal Progress in First Stage of Labor Within Normal Limits

	Phases Marked by Cervical Dilatation*		
Criterion	0-3 cm	4-7 cm	8-10 cm Transition
DURATION	About 8-10 hr	About 3 hr	About 1-2 hr
CONTRACTIONS			
Magnitude (strength)	Mild	Moderate	Strong to expulsive
Rhythm	Irregular	More regular	Regular
Frequency	5-30 min apart	3-5 min apart	2-3 min apart
Duration	10-30 sec	30-45 sec	45-60 (few to 90) sec
DESCENT			
Station of presenting part	Nulliparous: 0	About +1 to +2 cm	+2 to +3 cm
	Multiparous: 0 to −2 cm	About +1 to +2 cm	+2 to +3 cm
SHOW			
Color	Brownish discharge, mucous plug or pale, pink mucus	Pink to bloody mucus	Bloody mucus
Amount	Scant	Scant to moderate	Copious
BEHAVIOR AND APPEARANCE	Excited; thoughts center on self, labor, and baby; may be talkative or mute, calm or tense; some apprehension; pain controlled fairly well; alert, follows directions readily; open to instructions	Becoming more serious, doubtful of control of pain, more apprehensive; desires companionship and encouragement; attention more inner directed; fatigue evidenced; malar flush; has some difficulty following directions	Pain described as severe; backache common; feelings of frustration, fear of loss of control, and irritability surface; vague in communications; amnesia between contractions; writhing with contractions; nausea and vomiting, especially if hyperventilating; hyperesthesia; circumoral pallor, perspiration on forehead and upper lips; shaking tremor of thighs; feeling of need to defecate, pressure on anus

*The pace of progress in cervical dilatation (according to Friedman and Sachtleben, 1965) varies as follows: from 0 to 2 cm (latent phase), progress is slow; from 2 to 4 cm (phase of acceleration), pace quickens; from 4 to 9 cm (phase of maximum acceleration), pace is most rapid; and from 9 to 10 cm (phase of deceleration), pace slows again (see Figs. 15-7 and 15-8).
In the nullipara, effacement is often complete before dilatation begins; in the multipara, it occurs simultaneously with dilatation.

Table 15-2 Minimum Assessment of Progress of First Stage of Labor

	Cervical Dilatation		
	0-5 cm	6-7 cm	8-10 cm
Vital signs*	Every 4 hr	Every 4 hr	Every 4 hr
Blood pressure (BP)	Every 60 min	Every 30 min	Every 30 min
Contractions	Every 30 min to 1 hr	Every 15 min	Every 5-10 min
Fetal heart rate (FHR)	Every 15 min†	Every 15 min†	Every 5 min†
Show	Every 60 min	Every 30 min	Every 10-15 min
Behavior, appearance, energy level	Every 30 min	Every 15 min	Every 5 min
Vaginal examination‡	To be done only for following reasons: 1. To confirm diagnosis when symptoms indicate change (e.g., strength, duration, or frequency of contractions; increase in amount of bloody show; membranes rupture; or woman feels pressure on her rectum) 2. To determine whether dilatation and descent are sufficient for administration of analgesic or anesthetic 3. To reassess progress if labor takes longer than expected 4. To determine station of presenting part		

*If membranes have ruptured, check temperature every 2 hours.
†For a period of 30 seconds immediately after a uterine contraction (Zuspan and Quilligan, 1982).
‡In presence of vaginal bleeding, physician performs vaginal examination, usually under double setup, or ultrasonography.

sessment is continuous throughout labor. The routine for assessment of progress and of the continued well-being of the mother and fetus is usually set on a minimum level by hospital policy (Table 15-2). Any unusual findings would prompt more frequent performance of assessment procedures.

The symptomatology of progress in labor is well defined (Table 15-1). The character of the woman's uterine contractions, her behavior, and her appearance correlate with the phase of labor she is experiencing. The woman's culture, fatigue, and other factors may affect how she deals with labor.

The woman's response to labor may also be reflected in vital signs and BP. Fear, anxiety, and fatigue can cause alterations in the baseline findings. Continued fetal well-being is monitored through assessment of the FHR and of the character of the amniotic fluid discharge.

Careful assessment provides the cues for selection and implementation of nursing actions. *The nurse assumes much of the responsibility for making the assessment of progress. It is the nurse's responsibility to keep the physician or midwife informed about progress and any deviations from normal findings.*

Uterine Contractions, Cervical Dilatation, and Descent. A general characteristic of effective labor is regular uterine activity. Uterine activity is not directly related to labor progress. Minimum activity may cause rapid progress in some women. For other women a large amount of uterine activity may produce slow progress or no progress.

Several methods are available for evaluation of uterine contractions. To assess uterine contractions, explain to woman the purpose of palpating her abdomen, and then palpate using the sensitive fingertips, not the palmar surface of the hand. The fingers are kept moving over the uterus as the contraction proceeds from increment, to acme, through decrement to relaxation (Fig. 15-6, *B*).

When uterine activity is discussed it must be related to (1) its effect on progress in cervical effacement and dilatation and descent of the presenting part and (2) its effect on the fetus (see fetal monitoring). Graphing labor progress with both cervical dilatation and station (descent) of the presenting part validates the normal progress of labor. It also facilitates early identification of deviations from normal patterns. The normal pattern of cervical dilatation and descent in a nulliparous labor is shown in Fig. 15-7, *A*. The pattern in a parous labor is shown in Fig. 15-7, *B*.

Each time an assessment is made, the findings are plotted on a **partogram** (a graphic chart) and a pattern emerges (Fig 15-8). In addition to recording the findings on the partogram, the nurse is responsible for notifying the physician should an abnormal pattern emerge. Therefore an understanding of the partogram is necessary.

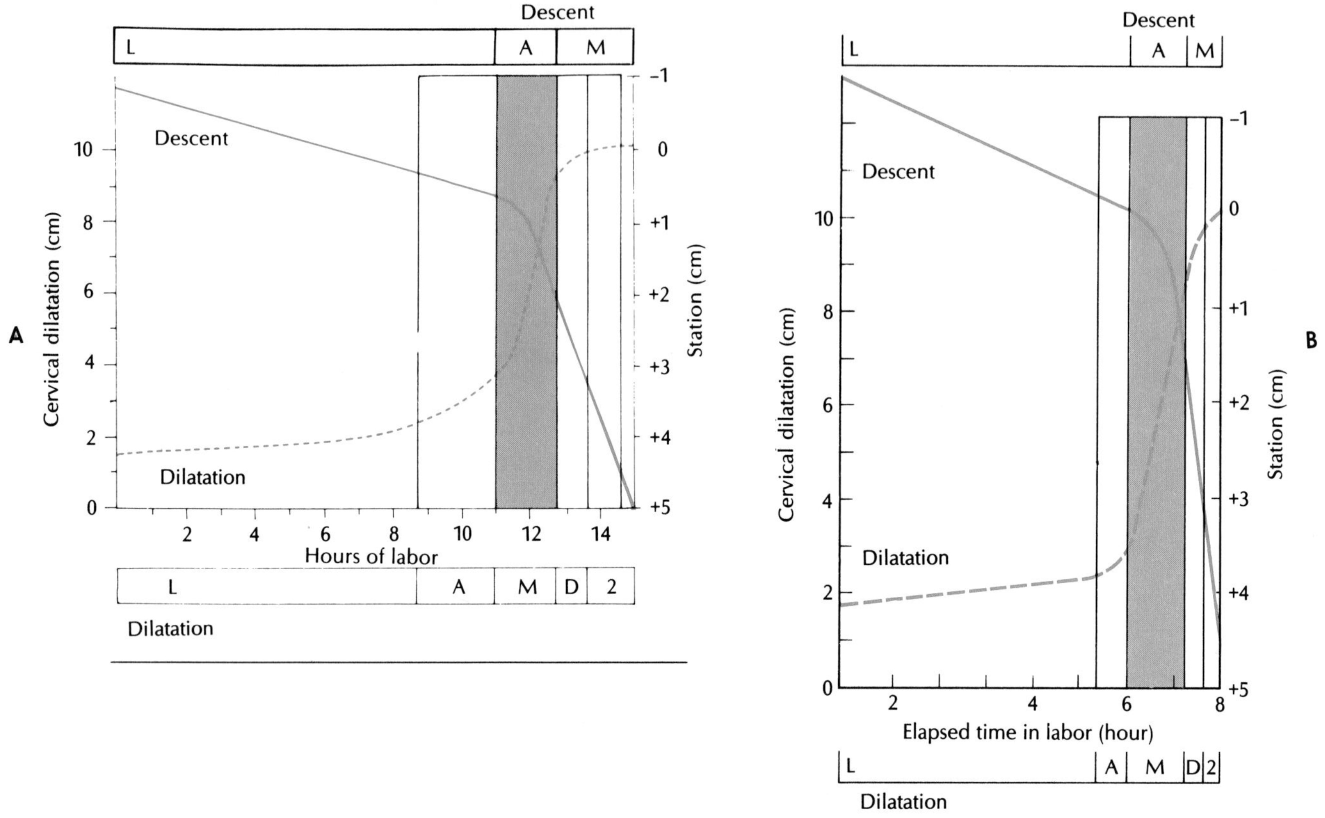

Fig. 15-7 Partogram showing relationship between cervical dilatation and descent of presenting part. **A,** Nulliparous labor. **B,** Multiparous labor. (**B** adapted from Friedman EA and Sachteben MR: Am J Obstet Gynecol 93:522, 1965.)

Cervical Effacement. Effacement precedes cervical dilatation in the nullipara and it often accompanies dilatation in the multipara. The process of effacement plays a role in dilatation. As the cervix is retracted upward, it becomes a part of the lower uterine segment. The "taking up" of the cervix reduces the length of the cervix from about 2 cm to a few millimeters when it is 100% effaced. This upward pull on fibers of the lower uterus and downward push on the fetus presses the presenting part onto the cervix. As uterine contraction and retraction continue, the cervical os dilates (opens) progressively. Effacement does not appear on the partogram.

Cervical Dilatation. On the partogram the phases of cervical dilatation are identified by the letters L, A, M, and D. A number, for example, "2," refers to the stage of labor. The **latent phase** (L) of the first stage of labor is that time between the onset of labor and onset of acceleration. The **active phase** begins with the **acceleration phase** (A) and spans the time between the onset of the upward curve of cervical dilatation and full dilatation of the cervix. Friedman (1978) divides the active phase into three parts: (1) *acceleration phase* (A), (2) *phase of maximum slope* (M), and (3) *deceleration phase* (D). The dotted line in Fig. 15-7 denotes cervical dilatation. The rate of cervical dilatation is indicated by the symbol "O" in Fig. 15-8. A line drawn through the symbols depicts the slope of the curve.

Descent. Located over the graph are the letters L, A, and M. The L refers to the latent phase of minimum descent. Active descent (A) generally begins when the cervical dilatation curve reaches its phase of maximum slope. The rate of descent reaches its maximum at the beginning of the deceleration phase of cervical dilatation. Maximum descent (M) continues in a linear manner until the perineum is reached (Zuspan and Quilligan, 1982). In Fig. 15-7 the solid line shows the rate of descent. In Fig. 15-8, station is indicated with an "X." A line drawn through the Xs reveals the pattern of descent.

Rupture of Membranes and Amniotic Fluid. SROM may occur at any time during labor. Rupture of membranes must be noted and confirmed, and amniotic fluid assessed. Tests for assessing rupture of membranes are discussed in Procedure 15-1. (See nursing care plan, pp. 390-391). The routine for assessment of

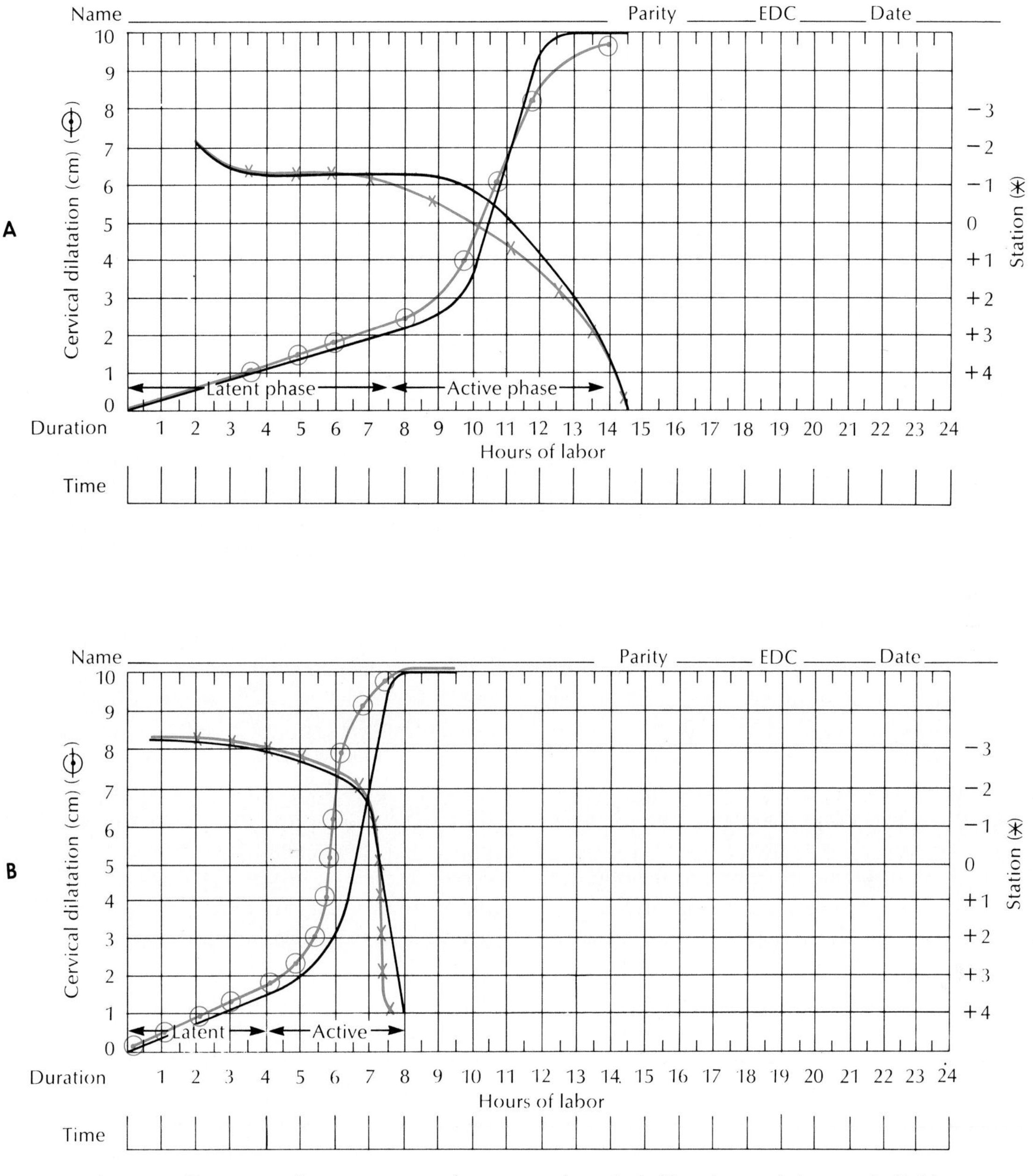

Fig. 15-8 Partogram for assessment of patterns of cervical dilatation and descent. Individual woman's labor patterns *(colored)* superimposed on prepared labor graph *(black)* for comparison. **A**, Nulliparous labor. **B**, Multiparous labor.

amniotic fluid includes the following (see danger signs box, right).

Amniotic fluid is normally pale straw colored. If it is greenish brown, the fetus has probably undergone a hypoxic episode resulting in relaxation of the anal sphincter. Passage of meconium from the bowel is a sequel to hypoxia.* Yellow-stained fluid may indicate fe-

*May also be seen in response to maternal marijuana use (Chapter 25).

DANGER SIGNS

Rupture of Membranes

1. Premature rupture of membranes (PROM)
2. Bloody, foul-smelling, or meconium-stained fluid
3. Change in FHR pattern
4. Signs of fetal distress
5. Preterm labor contractions

tal hypoxia that occurred 36 hours or more before rupture of the membranes or fetal hemolytic disease (Rh or ABO incompatibility, intrauterine infection).

Meconium-stained amniotic fluid may be a normal finding in breech presentation. Frank meconium may often be seen exuding into the birth canal. However, even in the case of a breech presentation the passage of meconium may indicate fetal distress and not just pressure on the fetal rectum. Although meconium-stained fluid may be noted with fetal asphyxia, *its presence is not always diagnostic of prospective fetal distress.* However, it should be promptly reported and recorded, and the FHR monitored closely. Port wine-colored amniotic fluid is one indicator of premature separation of the placenta (abruptio placentae) (Chapter 23).

Amniotic fluid normally looks like water and has a characteristic odor. Thick consistency and unpleasant odor are associated with infection.

A normal range for the amount of amniotic fluid is 500 to 1200 ml. *Hydramnios,* an excessive amount of amniotic fluid (more than 2000 ml), is commonly associated with congenital anomalies in the neonate (Chapter 28).

Oligohydramnios, an abnormally small amount or virtual absence of amniotic fluid (less than 500 ml) may be accompanied by such abnormalities as agenesis or malformation of the ears. In the presence of oligohydramnios, genitourinary tract anomalies, particularly renal agenesis may be seen (Chapter 28).

Complications associated with ruptured membranes may include infection, prolapsed cord, and preterm labor. Once the membranes have ruptured, the "clock of infection" begins to tick.* Prophylactic antibiotic therapy rarely will protect against chorioamnionitis. In most cases such treatment results in the development of antibiotic-resistant strains of many pathogenic organisms. The maternal temperature and vaginal discharge are assessed frequently for early identification of developing infection. For a discussion of herpetic vaginal or perineal lesions and mode of delivery, see Chapter 23.

Stress in Labor. Since labor represents a period of stress for the fetus, continuous monitoring of fetal health is instituted as part of the nursing care during labor (Chapter 14).

Women and their families approach labor with a feeling of satisfaction that the preparatory phase of pregnancy is now at an end; within a relatively short time their child will be born. However, most women have two major concerns. The first concerns the child; the woman may ask, "Will my child be all right?" Second, she may ask, "Will my labor be as expected? How will I act? Will I be okay?

*Ascending infection may involve intact membranes and may be the direct cause of PROM (Chapter 23).

"Will I be Able to Cope?" Exploring the woman's first question regarding the health of her child is probably not appropriate at this time. The prenatal record may provide information indicating cause for legitimate concern. Her other concerns need to be assessed further at this time. The plan for this labor may be noted in her prenatal record. Preferences may be recorded for the following:

1. Medicated or unmedicated labor
2. Support person she wants with her—husband, mother, coach, other
3. Electronic monitor or not
4. Episiotomy or not

Some women and couples want an active role in decision making: others want to leave it all in the hands of the physicians and nurses. Each individual has self-expectations as well as expectations of others. Regardless of the actual labor and delivery experience, the woman's or couple's *perception of the experience* is most positive when events and performance meet expectations. It is particularly important for the nurse to meet their expectations of the nursing role.

Women from various cultures are taught from childhood the "right" way to behave during labor. They are taught that they should moan, scream, remain silent, or be totally anesthetized, depending on the culture. If a woman can follow through with the social expectations of her culture, she perceives herself as having mastery, as having had control over her labor. Her self-esteem receives a boost. The nurse should explore with the woman what she expects from herself as well as from the nurse and other staff members. The nurse can then help the woman in achieving her goals or provide support and understanding if the goals cannot be met.

The woman's level of anxiety may rise when she does not understand what is being said. Observe the facial expression and body language of the woman who has just been examined vaginally when the physician, within the parturient's hearing, tells the nurse, "She's a primigravida, EDD 2 weeks from now. She's 50% effaced but I can barely get a fingertip in there. She had bloody show but she'll have to drop the head some yet. If her membranes don't rupture by themselves, I'll pop them myself. The contractions are weak now; they'll have to get a lot harder to get the job done. Do a miniprep on her." The woman who is unfamiliar with these terms could understandedly panic. Many of the terms—bloody show, drop the head, membranes rupture—sound violent and could conjure up thoughts of injury or pain. If the woman perceives her "weak" contractions as painful, she may become tense anticipating the more intense uterine contractions that are needed "to get the job done."

By explaining unfamiliar terms to the woman and preparing her for sensations and procedures that will follow, the nurse can alleviate anxiety. By encouraging the woman or couple to ask questions and providing honest, understandable answers, the nurse can play a significant role in achieving a satisfying birth experience.

The father, coach, or significant other also experiences stress during labor. The nurse can assist and support by identifying needs and expectations and helping that person meet them. What role does this person expect to play? Is he or she nervous or anxious? Have the couple attended childbirth classes? The nurse should ascertain what role the support person intends to fulfill and whether he or she is prepared. The nurse must be sensitive to needs and provide teaching support as appropriate.

Nursing Diagnoses

Nursing diagnoses lend direction to types of nursing actions needed to implement a plan of care. When establishing nursing diagnoses, the nurse analyzes the significance of findings collected during assessment.

Initial assessment

Impaired verbal communication related to
- Foreign language barrier

Knowledge deficit related to
- Lack of previous experiences or preparation-for-parenthood classes

Anxiety related to
- Knowledge deficit regarding physical examination procedures

Potential for injury related to
- Lack of prenatal testing of blood and urine

Subsequent assessments

Pain related to
- Intense contractions

Fluid volume deficit related to
- Decreased fluid intake

Impaired gas exchange related to
- Hyperventilation

Impaired physical mobility related to
- Station of fetal presenting part
- Status of fetal membranes
- Fetal monitoring

Altered patterns of urinary elimination related to
- Reduced fluid intake
- IV fluids
- Bed rest
- Lack of privacy
- Analgesia
- Anesthesia

Assessment of stress during labor

Impaired gas exchange, fetal, related to
- Maternal position

Spiritual distress, maternal, related to
- Inability to meet expectations of self

Ineffective family coping: compromised, related to
- Knowledge deficit of comfort measures that can be used for parturient

Planning

During this important step, ***goals*** are set in client-centered terms, and the goals are prioritized. Nursing actions are selected, with the client where appropriate, to meet the goals. Planning with the client is essential for the implementation of goals. Throughout the first stage of labor the woman will:

1. Demonstrate normal progression of labor as exhibited by the Friedman curve
2. Express satisfaction with the assistance of her support person and nursing staff
3. Verbalize her desires for participation in labor and participate as tolerated throughout labor
4. Continue normal progression of labor while the FHR remains within normal range without signs of distress
5. Maintain adequate hydration status through oral or intravenous intake
6. Void every 2 hours to prevent bladder distension
7. Encourage participation of support person by verbalizing discomfort and indicating measures that help reduce discomfort and promote relaxation

Implementation

Standards of Care

Standards of care guide the nurse in preparing for and implementing procedures with the expectant mother (Chapter 3). Protocols for care include the following:

1. Check the physician's orders
2. Assess the physician's orders for appropriateness and correctness; for example, perineal shave, enema (when not to carry out these procedures)
3. Check labels on intravenous (IV) solutions, drugs, and other materials used for nursing care
4. Check expiration date on any packs of supplies used for ordered procedures
5. Ensure that information on the woman's identification band is correct (also check that identification band is accurate, for example, if she has allergies, the band is the appropriate color)
6. Employ an empathic approach when giving care:
   a. Use words the woman can understand when explaining procedures

   b. Establish a rapport with the woman and her support person(s)
   c. Be kind, caring, and competent when performing necessary procedures
   d. Be aware that pain and discomfort is as the woman describes
   e. Repeat instructions as necessary and ensure that they are understood by the woman
   f. Carry out appropriate comfort measures, for example, mouth care and back care, and ensure support person is coping
   g. Always wash hands before beginning and after completion of nursing care
7. Complete procedures, for example, label specimens, record procedures on chart regarding maternal and fetal well-being
8. Facilitate uterine perfusion by preventing supine hypotension (Fig. 15-9, *D*).

Emergency Interventions

Prolapsed Umbilical Cord. Prolapse of the umbilical cord occurs when the cord lies below the presenting part of the fetus when the membranes are ruptured. Prolapse of the cord means that a loop of cord is displaced below the presenting part with the membranes intact. Prolapsed cord occurs in about one in 400 deliveries (Fig. 15-10). Two factors contribute to this situation: a long cord and an unengaged presentation or malpresentation, for example, a breech presentation or shoulder presentation. When the presenting part does not fit into the lower uterine segment, as in polyhy-

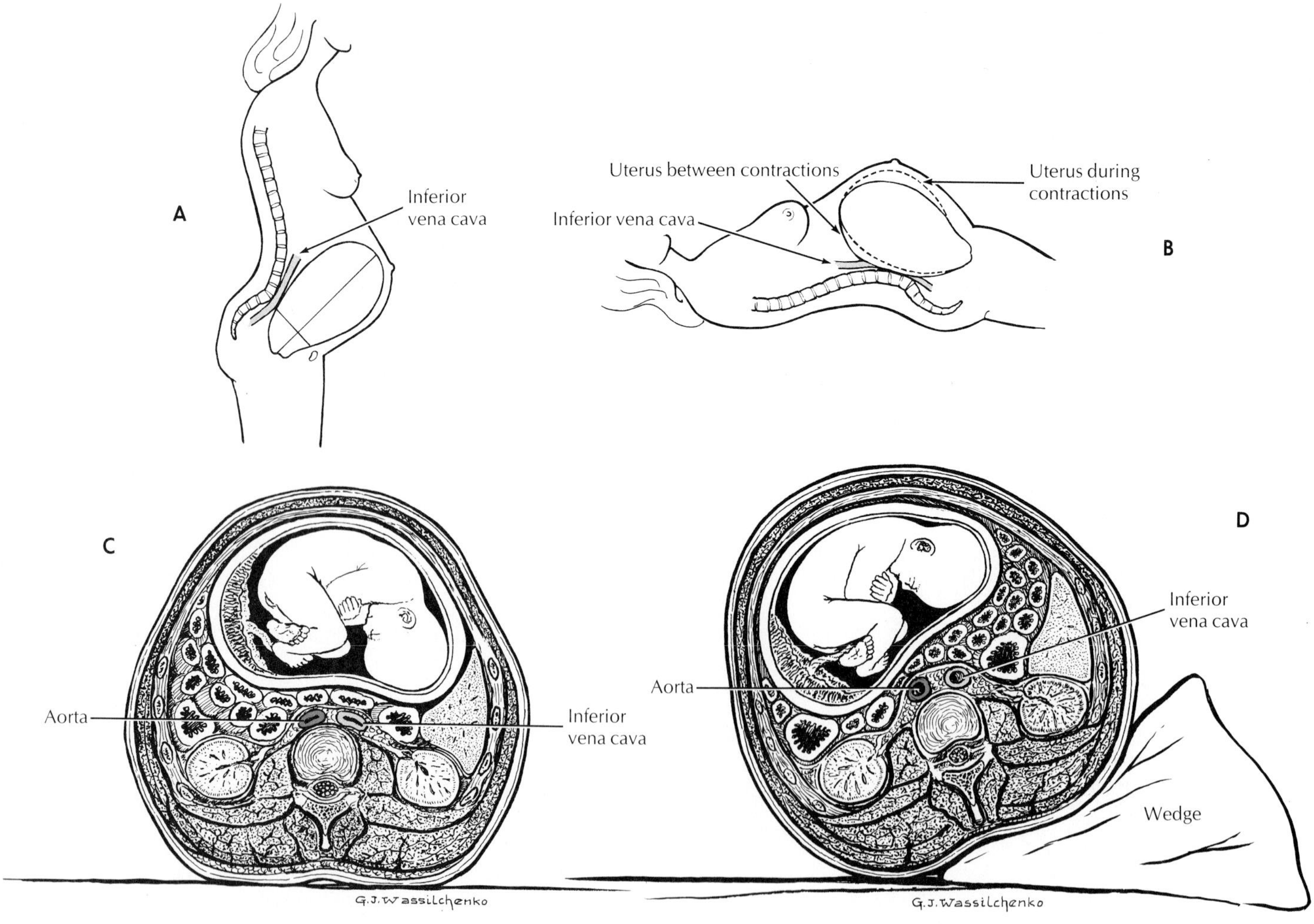

Fig. 15-9 Supine hypotension. Note relationship of gravid uterus to ascending vena cava in standing posture, **A**, and in supine posture, **B**. **C**, Compression of aorta and inferior vena cava with woman in supine position. **D**, Relieved by use of a wedge pillow placed under woman's right side.

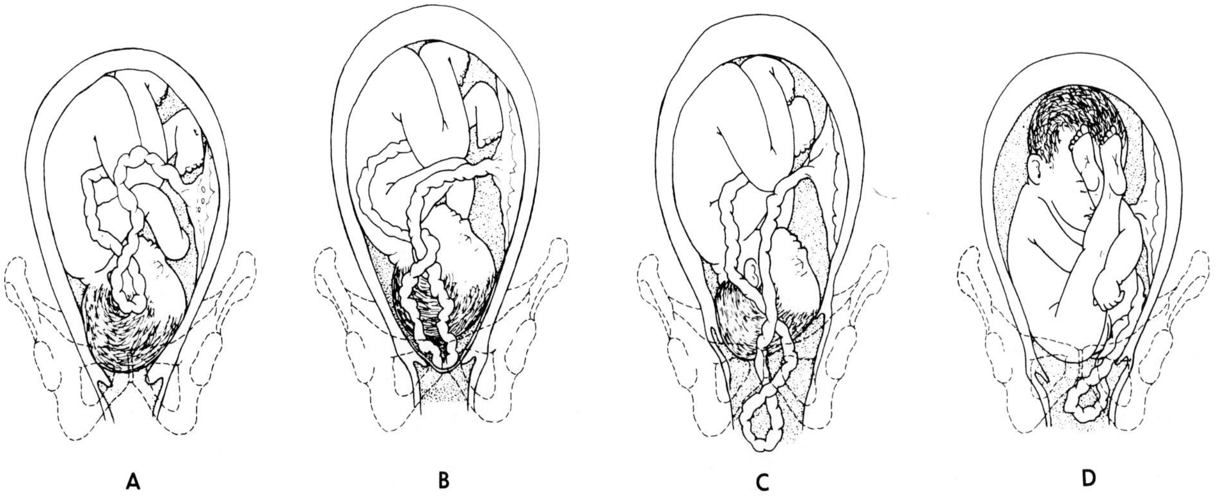

Fig. 15-10 Prolapse of umbilical cord. Note pressure of presenting part on umbilical cord, which endangers fetal circulation. **A,** Occult (hidden) prolapse of cord. **B,** Complete prolapse of cord. Note membranes are intact. **C,** Cord presenting in front of fetal head and may be seen within vagina. **D,** Frank breech presentation with prolapsed cord.

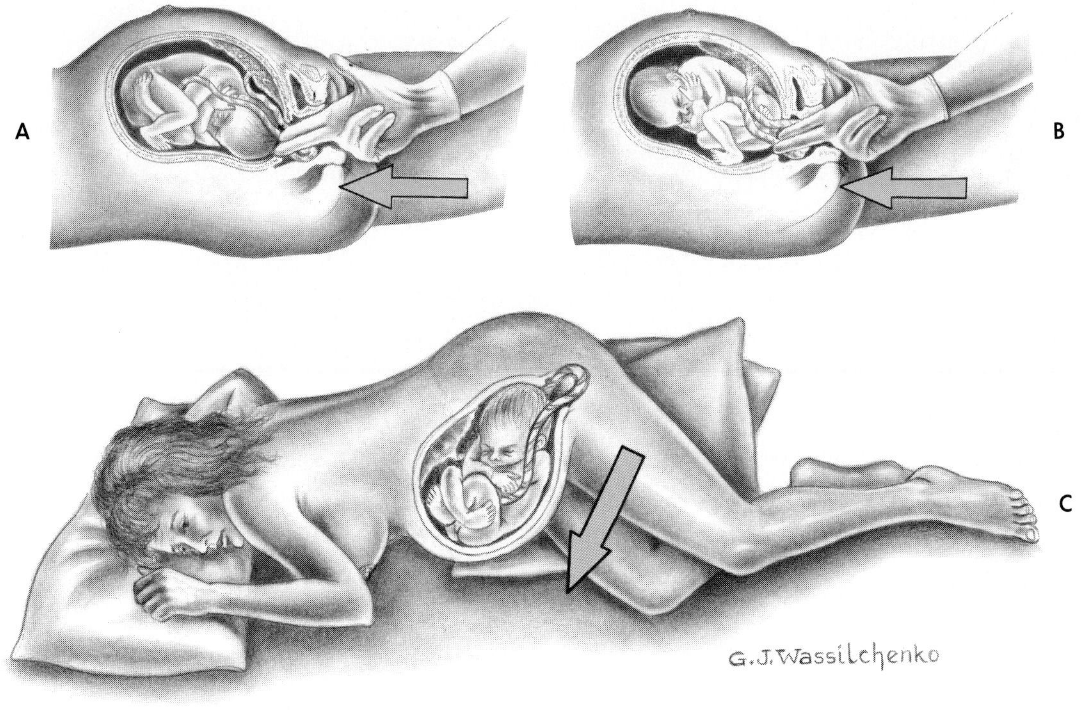

Fig. 15-11 Arrows indicate direction of pressure against presenting part to relieve compression of prolapsed umbilical cord. Pressure exerted by examiner's fingers in **A,** vertex presentation, and **B,** in breech position. **C,** Gravity relieves pressure with woman in modified Sims' position with hips elevated as high as possible with pillows.

dramnios or when the membranes rupture, a sudden gush of amniotic fluid may cause the cord to be displaced downward. Similarly the cord may prolapse during artificial rupture of the membranes (AROM) if the presenting part is high. A small fetus also may not fit snugly into the lower uterine segment and as a result, cord prolapse is more likely to occur. Other factors predisposing to cord prolapse and associated with a high presenting part are multiparity, cephalopelvic disproportion, and placenta previa. Prolapse of the cord is difficult to diagnose; however, an alert nurse or physician may make the diagnosis on vaginal examina-

EMERGENCY PROCEDURE

PROLAPSE OF CORD

DEFINITION

Protrusion of the umbilical cord in advance of the presenting part.

PURPOSE

To stop compression of the umbilical cord.
To stop umbilical cord from drying out.
To facilitate a delivery that will be the least harmful to mother and fetus.

EQUIPMENT

Fetoscope or doppler; sterile gloves; towels; oxygen equipment; IV fluid and equipment; sterile, normal saline.

NURSING ACTIONS	RATIONALE
Preprocedure	
Explain what is happening to woman (couple). Explain procedure.	Reduces anxiety and elicits cooperation of a woman (couple).
Call for assistance.	Need for additional personnel to prepare for delivery
Procedure	
Glove the examining hand quickly and insert two fingers into the vagina to the cervix. With one finger on either side of the cord or both fingers to one side, exert upward pressure against the presenting part to relieve compression of the cord (Fig. 15-11, *A* and *B*). Apply a rolled towel under the woman's right hip.	Maintains asepsis. Relieves compression from the presenting part. Prevents supine hypotensive syndrome.
Place woman into extreme Trendelenburg's or modified Sims' position (Fig. 15-11, C).	Allows gravity to pull presenting part down and relieve compression of the cord.
Notify physician immediately.	Physician assistance is urgent.
If cord is protruding from vagina wrap loosely in a sterile towel wet with warm sterile normal saline.	Stops cord from drying out and becoming nonfunctioning.
Administer oxygen by mask 10 to 12 L/min to the woman until delivery is accomplished.	Increases oxygen to fetus.
Start IV fluids or increase existing drip rate.	Increases circulating fluid volume to uterus. Maintains maternal blood pressure and hydration.
Deliver fetus immediately. If cervix completely dilated, vaginal delivery is possible.	Allows for a favorable outcome and good prognosis for mother and baby.
If cervical dilatation incomplete, cesarean delivery is the method of choice.	Decreases trauma to mother and baby.
Postprocedure	
Vaginal delivery: assess mother and baby for trauma or untoward effects. Pediatrician should examine infant in nursery. Assess mother for emotional stress and trauma.	Stressful situation may be followed by physical or emotional sequela. Be alert for any problems. Any high-risk delivery should have a pediatrician or neonatalogist in attendance to care for the infant.
Cesarean delivery: same as above, add postoperative assessment and observation of postanesthesia problems.	
Chart incident and results of treatment.	Provides data base for future comparison. Provides information for implementation of nursing process. Promotes collaboration between members of health care team.

DANGER SIGNS

Prolapsed Cord

1. Premature rupture of membranes
2. Presenting part not engaged
3. Fetal distress or abnormal FHR pattern
4. Protruding cord from vagina

tion after a sudden gush of fluid (see danger signs box, above). Prompt recognition is important, since fetal hypoxia from prolonged cord compression (more than 5 minutes) usually results in central nervous system (CNS) damage or demise of the fetus (see danger signs box, above).

Pressure on the cord is relieved by applying direct pressure on the presenting part by the examiner's fingers and by having the woman assume Trendelenburg's position until delivery is accomplished (see emergency procedure, p. 386, and Fig. 15-11). Cesarean birth is essential unless the cervix is fully dilated. If the cervix is completely dilated, rapid forceps delivery or vacuum extraction of the head or extraction of a breech presentation may be possible (Chapter 26). Prompt delivery in the most appropriate manner is imperative for the safety of the mother and fetus.

Fetal Distress or Abnormal FHR Patterns. Fetal distress may occur at any time during the labor process. The physician must be informed immediately. The nurse reports the nursing measures implemented, and the fetal response to the interventions instituted. For further discussion, see Chapter 14.

Inadequate Uterine Relaxation. Uterine contractions can be stressful to both the mother and the fetus. To prevent possible damage to the fetus and unnecessary stress to the mother, the nurse assesses the strength, duration, and frequency of contractions to

EMERGENCY PROCEDURE
INADEQUATE UTERINE RELAXATION

DEFINITION

Inadequate resting tone between uterine contractions. May cause fetal distress caused by poor delivery of oxygen to the placenta and fetus.

PURPOSE

To increase uterine muscle relaxation. To increase placental perfusion.

EQUIPMENT

Oxygen mask or cannula; mechanical oxygen source; IV fluid without oxytocin added; terbutaline 1 ml ampule.

NURSING ACTIONS	RATIONALE
Preparation	
Assess problem by monitoring labor and its effects on the fetus.	Uterine contractions are monitored continuously during labor. FHR observed for unusual patterns.
Explain procedure to woman.	Elicits cooperation through understanding.
Procedure	
Change maternal position. Turn woman to her left side, if that is ineffectual, put woman in modified Sims' position (Fig. 15-11, C).	Increases placental perfusion and increases oxygen delivered to the fetus.
Stop oxytocin infusion (if there is one running) and replace it with a maintenance IV.	Stop stimulation of the uterine muscle. Allows uterine muscle to relax.
Notify physician.	Allows collaboration in decision-making and informs him/her of possible problems.
If ordered, administer terbutaline 0.25 mg IVP	Decreases or stops uterine contractions, to decrease stress on fetus.
Administer oxygen by face mask or nasal cannula at 10 to 12 L/min until physician arrives and decides course of action.	Increases amount of oxygen available to the uterus and the fetus.
Record problems observed and actions taken by medical/nursing personnel.	Provides information for future care and collaboration.

identify abnormal contraction patterns. If the nurse identifies inadequate relaxation of the uterus, (e.g., contractions lasting longer than 90 seconds, relaxation between contractions inadequate or less than 30 seconds), the nursing actions in the emergency procedure on p. 387 must be implemented without delay.

Admission to the Labor Unit

First impressions are vivid. The woman and her partner are welcomed by name and introduced to staff members who will be involved in the woman's care. The nurse then determines whether the woman wishes her partner to stay throughout assessment and other admission procedures. The partner is incorporated into the assessment and admission process through orientation and explanation. Family members not participating in this process are directed to the appropriate waiting area. The woman is asked to undress and get into bed. Her personal belongings are put away safely. For legal reasons, most hospitals have a checklist or other method of recording the woman's belongings that becomes part of her permanent record. If the woman prefers to wear some items of her own (such as knee socks), these are noted on her chart.

The woman's understanding of the use of the call bell (or light) is checked. She is told the reasons that bathroom privileges are permitted or not. If the membranes have ruptured, she is told to remain in bed until assessment for potential prolapse of the umbilical cord is completed. The routine of care is reviewed, that is, which techniques will be used to assess progress, the reasons for using them, and how the woman or couple may assist in reporting her progress. For the minimum schedule for assessment of progress during the first stage of labor, see Table 15-1.

If the woman has not already done so, she signs the necessary papers giving permission for care for herself and her newborn. Her identification bracelet is secured. Legally a permit for care must be signed before the woman receives any medication or any procedures are instituted.

The nurse inquires if the woman came by car and ensures that the vehicle is properly parked. Some women, especially those who arrive in labor unexpectedly, welcome the offer of a telephone to notify their families. In some instances the nurse may have to make the calls for the woman.

The nurse should minimize the woman's anxiety by explaining terms commonly used during labor. While reviewing the prenatal record, the nurse can add short definitions for technical terms and abbreviations. The woman's interest and response guide the nurse in choosing the depth and breadth of the explanations. The nurse's openness and willingness to explain can be reassurance in itself—it indicates to the woman that there need be no "secrets." A general nursing care plan for admission of a woman in labor follows on p. 390.

Fluid Intake, Voiding, Bowel Elimination, and General Hygiene. Intake, elimination, and general hygiene are basic human needs. The parturient also has these same needs. However, nursing care of the parturient is modified somewhat. A summary of nursing actions and rationales is presented in Table 15-3.

Maternal Position During Labor. A great deal of discussion both within the nursing profession and among consumers of maternity care revolves around the way a woman should be positioned during labor. Should she be kept in bed, or should she be allowed to walk about, stand, sit, squat, or kneel? There is no "right" position. Should she deliver in the dorsal or semirecumbent position where most medical techniques and procedures can be best applied, or should she be allowed to adopt the position that she finds most comfortable without regard for the convenience of conventional obstetric practices (Romney and White, 1984)? Research has shown that women in the upright position during labor and birth have stronger and more effective uterine contractions. This results in shorter labor duration and increased comfort. Variation in the positions that women assume during the birth process has not been dictated as much by physiology as by culturally oriented patterned behavior.

Much research is being directed toward a better understanding of the physiologic and psychic effects of maternal position in labor. It is important to appreicate that clinical entities such as fetal presentations or mechanisms of labor may be helped or hindered by maternal posture.

Support Measures

Important components of the nursing care of the woman in labor relate to helping the parturient participate to the extent she wishes in the delivery of her infant, meeting the woman's goals for herself, helping the parturient conserve her energy, and helping control the woman's discomfort.

The nurse acts as an advocate for the woman and her family. Couples who have attended childbirth education programs will know something about the labor process, coaching techniques, and comfort measures (Chapter 9). The staff's role is to be supportive and keep them informed of progress. Even if the couple has not attended such classes, the various techniques may be taught to a degree during the early phase of labor. The nurse will be expected to do more of the coaching and give supportive care. If the woman is alone, the nursing staff acts as the substitute family, coaching and supporting.

Table 15-3 Fluid Intake, Voiding, Bowel Elimination, and General Hygiene

Need	Nursing Actions	Rationale
Fluid Intake		
Oral	Per physician's orders, offer clear fluids, small amounts of ice chips, hard candy, or lollipops.	Meets standard of care; provides hydration; provides calories; absorbs quickly and is less likely to be vomited; provides positive emotional experience.
IV	Establish and maintain IV.	Maintain hydration.
Nothing by mouth (NPO)	Inform family of NPO and rationale.	A precautionary measure if anesthesia is a possibility; deters vomiting and its possible sequelae.
	Provide mouth care.	Promotes comfort.
Voiding	Encourage voiding at least every 2 hours.	A full bladder may impede descent of presenting part; overdistention may cause bladder atony and injury and difficulty in voiding postnatally.
Ambulatory	Ambulate to bathroom per physician's orders, *if:*	Reinforces normal process of urination.
	The presenting part is engaged, or The membranes are not ruptured, and	Precautionary measure against prolapse of umbilical cord.
	The woman is not medicated.	Precautionary measure against injury.
Bedrest	Offer bedpan.	Prevents hazards of bladder distension and ambulation.
	Turn on the tap water to run; pour warm water over the vulva; and give positive suggestion.	Encourages voiding.
	Provide privacy.	Shows respect for gravida.
	Put up side rails on bed. Place call bell within reach.	Prevents injury from fall.
	Offer washcloth for hands.	Maintains cleanliness and comfort.
	Wash vulvar area.	Maintains standard of care.
Catheterization	Catheterize per physician's order per hospital protocols.	Prevents hazards of bladder distension.
	Insert catheter between contractions.	Minimizes discomfort.
	Avoid force if obstacle to insertion is noted.	"Obstacle" may be caused by compression of urethra by presenting part.
	If presenting part is low, introduce 2 fingers of free hand into introitus to apply upward pressure on presenting part while other hand inserts the catheter.	Minimizes potential for injury and subsequent infection to urethra.
Bowel Elimination	After careful assessment *experienced* nurse ambulates woman to bathroom or offers bedpan.	Women often misinterpret rectal pressure from the presenting part as the need to defecate.
General Hygiene		
Showers/bed baths	Assess for progress in labor.	Determines appropriateness for the activity.
	Supervise showers closely if gravida is in true labor.	Prevents injury from fall; labor may accelerate.
	Suggest allowing warm water to strike lower back.	Aids relaxation; increases comfort.
Vulva	Mini-prep if ordered.	Facilitates cutting and repair of episiotomy.
Oral hygiene	Offer toothbrush, mouthwash, or wash the teeth with an ice-cold wet washcloth every hour.	Refreshes mouth; improves morale; helps counteract dry, thirsty feeling.
Hair	Brush, braid per gravida's wishes	Improves morale.
Hand-washing	Offer washcloths before and after voiding and prn.	Maintains cleanliness; improves morale and comfort.
Face	Offer cool washcloth	Improves morale; relief from diaphoresis.
Gowns/linens	Change prn; fluff pillows.	Improves morale and comfort, probably through the Hawthorn effect.

General Nursing Care Plan

FIRST STAGE OF LABOR

ASSESSMENT	NURSING DIAGNOSIS (ND), PLAN/GOAL (P/G)	RATIONALE/ IMPLEMENTATION	EVALUATION
Term pregnancy. Admission to labor unit in labor. Latent phase of labor. Assess level of knowledge.	ND: Anxiety, mild, related to excitement of onset of labor and fear of unknown. ND: Knowledge deficit related to latent phase of first stage of labor. P/G: Woman (and her support person) verbally and nonverbally communicates less anxiety, more comfort, and ability to collaborate with her care.	*Relaxation and reduction of stress increase woman's ability to cope with labor:* Support woman's knowledge of labor. Explain all procedures in simple language. Orient woman and support person to environment. Support woman's preference for breathing and relaxation techniques to be used at this time. Provide comfort measures. Monitor vital signs, FHR, and progress of labor. Provide privacy.	Woman remains calm and retains psychologic and physiologic control.
Diminished oral intake: monitor intake and output; vital signs, FHR, blood pressure, respirations, amount of diaphoresis, and urine specific gravity	ND: Fluid volume deficit related to decreased intake and increased loss of fluid with the work of labor. P/G: Woman remains appropriately hydrated.	*Hydration is essential for adequate blood supply to mother and fetus:* Explain to woman and support person why oral fluids are decreased or restricted at this time. Start and maintain an IV infusion. Provide ice chips or sips of clear fluids if allowed. Provide mouth care as needed.	Woman's temperature, skin turgor, and moisture of mucous membranes remain normal. Specific gravity of urine remains within normal limits. Woman verbalizes understanding of procedures and information given. Woman does not suffer the fatigue associated with dehydration.
Rupture of membranes: baseline data of maternal vital signs and FHR; fetal lie, station, presentation, and position; status of membranes (bulging?); character of vaginal discharge.	ND: Potential for injury, maternal and fetal, related to contamination, infection, prolapsed cord, abnormal fetal position. P/G: Woman and fetus are not compromised as a result of rupture of membranes.	*Rupture of membranes increases potential for maternal infection and fetal hypoxia:* Maintain asepsis during vaginal examinations. Change soiled linen and underpads frequently. Continue to monitor: maternal vital signs (especially temperature and pulse); FHR for tachycardia; vaginal secretions; fetal lie and position, using Leopold's maneuvers. Observe for physical signs and umbilical cord prolapse, and implement emergency procedure, prn (p. 386):	Woman verbalizes understanding of procedures and information. Woman reports subjective symptoms as necessary. Woman and infant are not compromised as a result of rupture of membranes. FHR indicates continued fetal well-being. Fetal scalp pH indicates continued fetal well-being. Cesarean delivery is accomplished in a timely fashion; mother and infant are in good condition.

General Nursing Care Plan—cont'd

ASSESSMENT	NURSING DIAGNOSIS (ND), PLAN/GOAL (P/G)	RATIONALE/ IMPLEMENTATION	EVALUATION
		Reposition woman to left lateral position or other positions as necessary. Provide oxygen by nasal cannula or face mask as necessary. Increase rate of infusion of maintenance IV fluid. Assist with fetal scalp blood sampling as necessary. Assist with preparation for surgery as necessary.	
First stage of labor. Woman in active phase. Baseline data: maternal vital signs; FHR; labor pattern. Degree of perceived discomfort.	ND: Pain related to increasing frequency and intensity of uterine contractions. P/G: Mother reports decreased discomfort; FHR remains within normal limits.	*Reduction of pain increases woman's ability to cope with labor:* Assess woman's verbal and nonverbal communication. Promote the use of psychoprophylactic breathing techniques. Provide comfort measures. Assess vital signs, including blood pressure, FHR, frequency, and intensity of uterine contractions. Administer analgesics as ordered.	Woman verbalizes understanding of information presented. Woman utilizes breathing method of choice. Baseline data remains within normal limits.
Bladder fullness. Epidural anesthesia. Decreased oral intake. Unable to ambulate to bathroom.	ND: Altered patterns of urinary elimination related to discomfort, effects of analgesia, anesthesia, or fetal position. P/G: Bladder will be emptied periodically.	*Empty bladder promotes comfort:* Offer bedpan or help to bathroom frequently; catheterize prn. Assess for side effects from analgesics or anesthetics. Monitor IV or oral fluids.	Bladder fullness is prevented.
Woman in stressful and threatening situation.	ND: Ineffective individual coping related to anxiety, fear, and decreased problem-solving capability. P/G: Woman utilizes coping strategies appropriate to each stage of labor with assistance of coach.	*Reduction of stress enables woman to cope with progression of labor:* Assess anxiety level. Assess behavior of support person and its effect on the woman. Provide information. Provide comfort measures. Assist woman and support person in focusing on breathing and relaxation techniques to maintain control. Give quiet reassurance. Support woman's decision for pain medications.	Woman remains calm and in control. Support person provides necessary help and reassurance to woman. Woman and support person express satisfaction with their behavior during labor and with the management of their labor.

Comfort measures vary with the situation. The nurse can draw on the couple's repertoire of comfort measures learned during the pregnancy.

The **Hawthorn effect** is the "phenomenon that occurs when a person in pain begins to feel more comfortable as the nurse talks soothingly, fluffs a pillow, and promises to stay nearby. Positive support, especially by one in authority, enhances the ability to cope with stress" (Jimenez, 1983 a, b).

The comfort measures to be discussed below include maintaining a comfortable, supportive atmosphere in the labor and delivery area; using touch therapeutically; providing nonpharmacologic management of discomfort; and administering analgesics when necessary; but, most of all, just *being there.*

Labor and Delivery Area. Labor rooms need to be light and airy. However, the bright overhead lights are turned off when not needed. In some hospitals, couples are urged to bring pillows or pictures to help make the hospital surrounding more homelike.

The room temperature is kept at a comfortable level—between 20° and 22.2° C (68° and 72° F). Although most women feel warm during labor, a number complain of feeling cold. A warm blanket placed over the woman and one wrapped around her feet are comforting. Many woman wish to wear socks. For those who feel too warm, a cool moist cloth placed on the forehead can be soothing, as can ice chips given for sucking (where permissible).

Touch. Most women respond positively to touch in labor. They appreicate gentle handling by the staff. **Effleurage** (a light rhythmic stroking over the woman's abdomen in rhythm with breathing during contractions [see Fig. 10-16]) may be effective in helping them relax between contractions. Counterpressure against the sacrum during a contraction results in relief from discomfort (Fig. 15-12). Back rubs, including over the sacral area and the buttocks (especially for women who have been in labor a long time), every hour or two and as necessary between contractions help ease tension. If possible, warm foot baths followed by foot massage can result in general body relaxation. Accupressure has also been found to assist women in the labor process.

The woman's awareness of the soothing qualities of touch changes as labor progresses. Many women develop hyperesthesia (increased sensitivity, especially in the skin) as labor progresses. They may tell their coach to "leave me alone," or they may say, "Don't touch me." The partner who is unprepared for this normal response may feel rejected and may react by withdrawing active support. The nurse can point out that this response on the part of the woman is a positive indication that the first stage is ending and that the transition stage is approaching. The woman's aggressive behavior

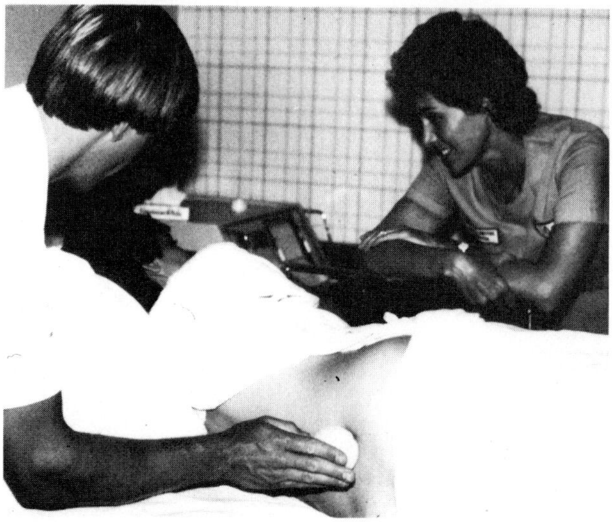

Fig. 15-12 Father applies sacral pressure with a tennis ball while nurse provides verbal encouragement. (Courtesy Marjorie Pyle, RNC, Lifecircle, Costa Mesa, Calif.)

is accepted; negative comments toward the woman are unwarranted and inappropriate.

Nonpharmacologic Management of Discomfort. The alleviation of pain is important. Commonly it is not the amount of pain the woman experiences, but *whether she meets her goals for herself in coping with the pain* that influences her perception of the birth experience as "good" or "bad." The observant nurse looks for cues to identify the woman's desired level of control in the management of pain and its relief.

The origins of discomfort during labor, the symptomatology of pain, pain threshold, and gate-control theory of pain and pharmacologic control of discomfort are discussed in Chapter 13. The pain associated with parturition was accepted as a necessary part of childbirth until the discovery of the first anesthetics, nitrous oxide and ethyl ether. Since then much research has gone into the development of methods of pain control that bring effective relief for the mother without harm to the child. The perfect solution is yet to be found; therefore at times the safety of the child must take precedence over the comfort of the mother.

Nonmedicated methods of relief of discomfort are taught in many different types of prenatal preparation classes. Whether or not a woman or couple has attended these classes or read from the various books and magazines on the subject, the nurse can teach techniques to relieve discomfort during labor. Following are some nonmedicated methods of managing discomfort during labor.

Focusing and Feedback Relaxation. Some women bring a favorite device for use in focusing attention.

Others choose some fixed object in the labor room. As the contraction begins, they may focus on this object to reduce their perception of pain. This technique, coupled with feedback relaxation, helps the woman work with her contractions rather than against them. The coach monitors this process, giving the woman cues as to when to begin the breathing techniques. After the degree of relaxation has been assessed, relaxation techniques practiced in the prenatal period can be reviewed. The coach also keeps her from being disturbed by routine examinations for progress and checking of FHR. These procedures are postponed until the contraction is completed.

Breathing Techniques. Different approaches to childbirth preparation stress varying techniques for using breathing as a "tool" to help the woman maintain control through contractions. In the first stage, breathing techniques can promote relaxation of abdominal muscles and thereby increase the size of the abdominal cavity. This lessens friction and discomfort between the uterus and the abdominal wall. Since the muscles of the genital area also become more relaxed, they do not interfere with descent. In the second stage, breathing is used to increase abdominal pressure and thereby assist in expelling the fetus. It is also used to relax the pudendal muscles to prevent precipitate expulsion of the head.

For those couples who have prepared for labor by practicing such techniques, occasional reminders to the couple may be all that is necessary. For those who have had no preparation, instruction in simple breathing and relaxation can be given early in labor and is often surprisingly successful. Motivation is high, and learning readiness is enhanced by the reality of labor.

1. *Cervical dilatation to 3 cm.* As the woman feels the onset of a contraction, she takes a deep, cleansing breath in through the nose and out through pursed lips. Then she is encouraged to concentrate on slow, rhythmic chest breathing (6 to 9 breaths per minute) through the contraction (Fig. 15-13). When the contraction is over, she takes a final deep breath in and then "blows the contraction away" through pursed lips. She may focus on a chosen fixed point or simply close her eyes.

2. *Cervical dilatation of 4 to 7 cm.* Breathing during this phase is similar to that advocated in the early phase. When cervical dilatation reaches 5 cm, some women begin to concentrate seriously on the strength of the contractions and the discomfort accompanying them. At this time a change to a shallower, lighter breathing can be suggested (no more than 16 breaths per minute to prevent hyperventilation). Other women can be helped by changing to slow abdominal breathing. Another technique that is often successful is to have the woman slowly raise her abdomen as she breathes in, following the support person's hand "up to the ceiling" or "out to the side of the bed" (if she is in side-lying position). This focusing mechanism results in the lifting of the abdominal wall away from the contracting uterus.

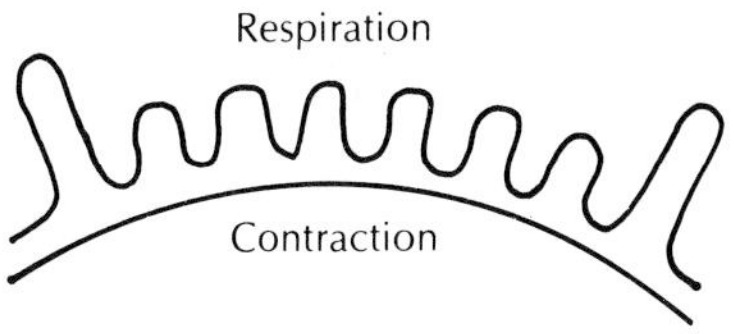

Fig. 15-13 Slow chest breathing. (From Phillips CR: Family-centered maternity/newborn care, ed 2, St Louis, 1987, The CV Mosby Co.)

3. *Cervical dilatation of 8 to 10 cm: transition.* The most difficult time to maintain control during contractions comes when the cervical dilatation reaches 8 to 10 cm. This period is also called the **transitional phase.** Even for the woman who has prepared for labor, concentration on breathing techniques is difficult to maintain. The type used may be the 4:1 pattern: breath, breath, breath, puff (as though blowing out a candle). This ratio may increase to 6:1 or 8:1. These patterns begin with the routine cleansing breath and end with a deep breath exhaled to "blow the contraction away."

An undesirable side effect of this type of breathing may be **hyperventilation.** The woman must be aware of the accompanying symptoms of the resultant *respiratory alkalosis*: lightheadedness, dizziness, tingling of fingers, or circumoral numbness. Alkalosis may be overcome by having the woman breathe into a paper bag or mask that is tightly held around the mouth and nose. This enables her to rebreathe carbon dioxide and replace the bicarbonate ion. She can breathe into her cupped hands if no bag is available.

As the fetal head reaches the pelvic floor, the woman will experience the urge to push and will automatically begin to exert downward pressure by contracting her abdominal muscles. Descent cannot continue until the cervix is fully dilated and the presenting part is free to move down the birth canal. Pushing before full dilatation is reached compresses the cervix between the fetal head and the pubic bone. This compression *may result in fetal distress or in cervical edema.* It may even slow the dilatation process. The woman can control the urge to push by taking panting breaths or by slowly exhaling through pursed lips. This is good practice for the type of breathing to be used as the fetal head is slowly delivered (see p. 407).

Transcutaneous Electrical Nerve Stimulation. The application of pressure to or rubbing of a part of the body that is sore is an age-old remedy to relieve discomfort. Effleurage and sacral pressure or massage are two methods that have brought relief to many women during the first stage of labor. The gate-control theory may supply the reason for the effectiveness of these measures (Chapter 12). **Transcutaneous electrical nerve stimulation (TENS)** may operate on the same principle. TENS may also be effective because of the "placebo effect;" that is, confidence in TENS may stimulate the release of endogenous opiates (enkephalins) in the woman's body and thus alleviate the discomfort.

Two pairs of electrodes are taped on either side of the thoracic and sacral spine. Continuous mild electrical currents are applied from a battery-operated device. During a contraction the woman increases the stimulation by turning control knobs on the device. Women describe the sensation as a tingling or buzzing and pain relief as good or very good. The use of TENS poses no risk to the mother or fetus. TENS is credited with reducing or eliminating the need for analgesia and with increasing the woman's perception of control over the experience.

The nurse assists the mother who is using TENS by explaining the device and its use, by carefully placing and securing the electrodes, and by closely evaluating its effectiveness.

Sociocultural Aspects of Pain Management. The quality of the nurse-client relationship is a factor in the woman's ability to cope with the discomfort of the labor process. The nurse who is aware of sociocultural aspects of helping and coping acts as a protective agent for the woman. The responsibility for initiating and maintaining such a therapeutic relationship rests with the nurse. An area in which the nurse and the pregnant woman from different cultures could misunderstand each other is pain.

A study of nurses from the United States, Japan, Puerto Rico, Korea, Thailand, and Taiwan revealed that nurses from diverse cultures make different inferences about physical pain and psychologic distress (Davitz, Davitz, and Higuchi, 1977). Nurses sampled from the United States were midway between the other national groups and showed the smallest variability. An important implication of these findings is that Oriental national groups differ among themselves in terms of response to pain, just as one would expect groups from various Western societies to differ.

Indochinese women walk around during labor and do not ask for medication. These women and others exert great self-control, to the point that the nurse may not recognize an impending delivery (Hollingsworth, 1980). Black women commonly find comfort in having another woman such as a mother or sister pray with them during the discomfort of labor. Based on these data, the nurse need not label clients from the same cultural group as alike in their responses to pain. Not all Orientals are stoic, nor do all Western people respond to pain in the same manner. Zborowski (1952) found that people of Irish, Jewish, Italian, and "old American" descent respond to pain differently.

General Nursing Actions. Even if the laboring woman and her partner (or family or support persons) are well prepared, the nurse remains an important member of the childbirth team. Labor is a crisis time, and all people, no matter how well prepared, enter labor with some level of anxiety. The following are some helpful actions that the nurse as a support person can use to offer both verbal and practical support during labor:

1. Remember that labor is stressful, even if the couple is prepared. Continually encourage relaxation. Do not leave them totally alone. Provide company when they need it—and privacy when they need it.
2. Minimize adverse environmental stimuli. Control glaring lights. Decrease traffic flow and noise in the birth setting.
3. Remind the mother that she is to select the *position* in which she feels most comfortable during labor and to change her position whenever she wishes. Encourage walking in early labor.
4. Provide privacy and a space with adequate room temperature and ventilation.
5. Talk of contractions, not pains.
6. Relax and get as near to the woman's level as possible. Sit by the bedside. Do not tower over her. Use touch as appropriate.
7. Adjust the labor bed to provide a comfortable position (usually elevating the top of the bed to 45 degrees). The woman should never be flat on her back because the weight of the uterine contents puts too much pressure on major blood vessels, thus reducing the blood flow back to the brain. Use pillows to support all dependent body parts.
8. Use comfort measures such as cold cloths, backrubs, and ice chips. Showers or tub baths may be taken depending on the progress of labor.
9. Try effleurage. It is best done by the woman herself, although it may be done for her.
10. Carry on a conversation if necessary only between contractions.
11. Talk with the father or other support person. Give reassurance and remember that the coach also has needs for nourishment, rest, and elimination. Let him know where the bathroom is and where food may be purchased. Also, reassure him that you will stay with the laboring woman if he needs to leave for a while to tend to his own needs.
12. Do not ask irrelevant questions. Keep talk to a

minimum. It uses energy needed to cope. Be aware of attitudinal changes as labor progresses.
13. Keep your voice well modulated at all times.
14. Remind the mother to urinate frequently. A full bladder can slow down the descent of the baby.
15. Encourage rest between contractions.
16. Keep the couple informed of what is happening: how many centimeters dilated, station, effacement, and fetal position.
17. Assure the mother she is doing well, offer encouragement, agree with her if she says it hurts but offer positive comments, too.
18. Do not distract the woman during contractions. Wait until a contraction is over to perform a nursing procedure.
19. Remember that transition (8 to 10 cm) may be the most intense time during labor. Because the woman may fall asleep between contractions, they may get ahead of her, so assist with identification of onset of contractions.
20. During the actual birth stage, trust the woman and work with her body. This is not an athletic contest; the goal is pelvic floor release and relaxation. Encourage a series of quick breaths, holding one for 5 seconds while pushing with grunting sounds or expiratory vocalizations (Table 15-5), and then taking another breath. Give verbal support such as, "Beautiful! Go with it!" You might even give the woman a mirror so that she can watch her own progress as she pushes the baby out.
21. If the couple is giving birth in the delivery room, give the father or other support person the clothes to wear in the delivery room well in advance so that there is no last-minute rush.
22. As you encourage relaxation, encourage *release* toward your touching hand on her body. This will help the woman increase her body awareness.
23. Always encourage the breathing that *feels* right for each woman. She may have practiced one type of breathing before labor only to find that it is not helpful during a certain part of labor. If this happens, be flexible. Encourage her to find what is working for her and stick with it.
24. There is no failure! Some people who have prepared faithfully for a "natural" childbirth will not be able to achieve that goal because of circumstances beyond their control. They may need analgesia, anesthesia, or a cesarean birth. If they are disappointed, encourage them to talk about their disappointment and then help them work through it by emphasizing that there is no failure. When they have achieved a meaningful and safe birth experience, they have achieved their goal.
25. Throughout the entire labor process be constantly and consistently aware of the needs of the fetus. When the couple has prepared diligently for labor and are extremely intent on what they are doing, it is often easy for the support person to get caught up in that intensity and feel reluctant to do any procedure that might "spoil" their experience, Continually think of yourself as a fetal advocate and use your knowledge and skills to make sound judgments that will lead to a meaningful and safe birth experience for all family members.
26. Share in the couple's joy if their expectations have been met, or their grief if they have not.

The helpful actions for labor support given in this unit are useful for all laboring women (Table 15-4). However, if there is no family or friend to support the laboring woman, then the nurse's role becomes even more crucial. A woman should never have to labor alone! If the realities of staffing shortages prevent constant attendance to women laboring alone, seek labor support persons from community volunteer groups. Until labor support groups can be formed, you can communicate openly and honestly with women laboring alone. Inform them of the constraints on your time. Let them know where you will be when you leave their side, how they can communicate with you, and when you will be back.

Father During Labor

Involving the father in the birth of his child dispels feelings of alienation, isolation, impotence, helpless inaction, and insignificance. *Ethnic definition and role expectations govern the type and degree of the individual's involvement.*

Individual preference for a kind of involvement spans a full spectrum of possibilities. Different men seek different types of involvement. What are their hopes and expectations for this experience for themselves and their partners? What is the nurse's role in relation to their decisions? These questions will be discussed in the following sections.

Nurses should recall their feelings the first time they witnessed a woman in active labor. The father's experience can be no less intense. In addition, the woman in labor is not a client to him; she is birthing their baby.

During the delivery the father may see facial and physical expressions of pain, drainage from the mother's vagina, fecal discharge, episiotomy, and forceps delivery. He may hear the mother moaning and grunting, heaving or vomiting; he may hear routine hospital noises (such as page systems, sterilizer buzzers, and fe-

Table 15-4 Woman's Expected Responses and Support Person's Actions During Labor

Woman	Support Person
DILATATION OF CERVIX 0-3 CM (contractions 10-30 sec long, 5-30 min apart, mild to moderate)	

Mood: alert, happy, excited, mild anxiety
Settles into labor room; selects focal point
Rests or sleeps if possible
Uses breathing techniques
Uses effleurage; focusing and relaxation techniques
	Provides encouragement, feedback for relaxation, companionship
	Assists with contractions
	  Uses focusing techniques
	  Concentration on breathing technique
	Uses comfort measures
	  Position most comfortable for woman
	  Keeps woman aware of progress, explains procedures and routines
	  Gives praise
	  Offers ataractics as ordered (Chapter 13).

DILATATION OF CERVIX 4-7 CM (contractions 30-40 sec long, 3-5 min apart, moderate to strong)	

Mood: seriously labor oriented, concentration and energy needed for contractions, alert, more demanding
Continuous relaxation, focusing techniques
Uses breathing techniques
	Acts as buffer, limits assessment techniques to between contractions
	Assists with contractions
	  May need to encourage woman to help her maintain breathing techniques
	Uses comfort measures
	  Positions woman on side
	  Encourages voluntary relaxation of muscles of back, buttocks, thighs, and perineum; effleurage
	  Uses counterpressure to sacrococcygeal area
	  Encourages and praises
	  Keeps woman aware of progress
	  Offers analgesics and anesthetics as ordered
	  Checks bladder, encourages to void
	  Gives mouth care, ice chips

DILATATION OF CERVIX 8-10 CM (transition) (contractions 45-60-90 sec long, 2-3 min apart, strong)	

Mood: irritable, intense concentration, symptoms of transition
Continues relaxation, needs greater concentration to do this
Breathing techniques
Uses 4:1 breathing pattern if possible
Uses panting to overcome response to urge to push
	Stays with woman, provides constant support
	Assists with contractions
	  Probably will need to remind, reassure, and encourage to reestablish breathing pattern and concentration
	  If sedated or drowsy, woman needs warning to begin breathing pattern before contraction becomes too intense
	  If woman begins to push, institutes panting respirations
	Uses comfort measures
	  Accepts woman's inability to comply with instructions
	  Accepts irritable response to helping, such as counterpressure
	  Supports woman who has nausea and vomiting, gives mouth care as needed, gives reassurance regarding symtomatology of end point of first stage
	Uses countertension techniques (effleurage and voluntary relaxation)
	  Keeps woman aware of progress, tells woman when time to push

tal monitoring devices) and protests about fathers who "don't belong in the delivery room." He may smell vaginal drainage, fecal drainage, vomitus, and cleaning solutions. The emergence of the baby can be both frightening and exciting. The nurse can assist the father by offering explanations and assurance during this often overwhelming experience.

Father in Labor Suite. "He'll just be underfoot." "He'll add confusion and increase the chance of infections and the number of lawsuits." These typical statements for years kept the father apart from his wife and child. These fears proved largely unfounded when fathers were reunited with their laboring wives. Fathers proved helpful, comforting, and reassuring to their wives. There was no change in the incidence of infection or lawsuits. Furthermore, it was found that it was easier for the physician and parents to cope with the birth of a child with a defect when both parents were active participants on an adult-to-adult level with the physician.

The father may be an adjunct to the nurse-physician team in several ways. For example, he may assist with comfort measures such as pillows, ice chips, washcloths to forehead, and back rubs. He may provide almost constant companionship to offset the aloneness of labor and the anxiety it can foster. Should something occur when the nurse or physician is out of the room, the father can call for help. In addition, he is usually better equipped to interpret the mother's wishes and needs to the staff.

Participation in the birth is ego building. The father *can* be of assistance; his presence *is* important. When the father is active and supportive, the mother turns to him. The physician remains the medical-surgical expert, without taking on the father or husband-surrogate role as well. The couple's future relationship and their relationship with their child may be positively influenced. Mutuality is fostered when the mother can turn to the father and say, "I could never have done it without you. You were my pillar of strength."

Supporting Father During Labor. Supporting the father, as well as the mother, in labor elevates the nurse's role. It is another step forward from merely providing custodial care to enacting a therapeutic role. Supporting the father reflects the nurse's orientation and commitment to the person, the family, and the community. Therapeutic nursing actions convey to the father several important concepts.

First, he is of value as a person. He is not a comic strip character, inept and bungling or idle, nervous, and inconsequential. Second, he can learn to be a partner in the mother's care. Finally, childbearing is a partnership.

Even if the father enters the labor unit without any parent education classes, he can be taught "on the job," and his choices can be supported. The nurse can support the father in the following ways:

1. Regardless of the degree of involvement desired, orient him to the maternity unit, including wife's labor room and what he can do there (sleep, telephone), restroom, cafeteria, waiting room, nursery, visiting hours, and names and functions of personnel present.
2. Respect his or their decisions as to his degree of involvement, whether the decision is active participation in the delivery room or just being kept informed. When appropriate, provide data on which he or they can base decisions; offer freedom of choice as opposed to coercion one way or another. This is *their* experience and *their* baby.
3. Indicate to him when his presence has been helpful and continue to reinforce this throughout labor.
4. Offer to teach him comfort measures to the degree he wants to know them. Reassure him that he is not assuming the responsibility for observation and management of his wife's labor, but supporting her as she progresses.
5. Communicate with him frequently regarding her progress and his needs. Keep father informed of procedures to be performed, what to expect from procedures, and what is expected of him.
6. Prepare him for changes in her behavior and physical appearance.
7. Remind him to eat; offer snacks and fluids if possible.
8. Relieve him as necessary; offer blankets if he is to sleep in a chair by the bedside. Acknowledge the stress of the situation on each partner and identify normal responses. The nonjudgmental attitude of staff helps the father and mother accept their own and the other parent's behavior.
9. Attempt to modify or eliminate unsettling stimuli (such as extra noise, extra light, chatter)

A well-informed father can make a significant contribution to the health and well-being of the mother and child, their family interrelationship, and his self-esteem. It has been found that a significantly lower percentage of women suffered postdelivery emotional upsets when their partners received support and assistance from prenatal classes, physicians, and nurses throughout the childbearing cycle.

Culture and Father Participation. Many hospitals encourage the father's presence during labor and delivery. If he is not able to be there, another significant person may be present. In several cultures the father may be available, but his presence with the mother may not be appropriate and he may resist involvement at this time. His behavior could be misconstrued by the nursing staff as lack of concern, caring, or interest.

Griffith (1982) identifies the importance of the affectional bond between a Mexican woman and her mother and sisters or other female relatives in regard to home-related activities such as childbearing. This is also true for many other groups, and the presence of another woman or women is highly desired. If childbearing occurs in the hospital, at least one woman must be present for assistance, Southeast Asians (Hollingsworth et al, 1980), blacks (Carrington, 1978; Johnson and Snow, 1978), and American Indians (Farris, 1978; Horn, 1982) and some of the major cultural groups indicating a preference for a woman's assistance during childbearing.

According to Pillsbury (1978), the Chinese husband is not allowed in the delivery room, lest he become polluted by the woman's blood. A nurse from a different culture might think it odd that a Chinese husband did not seem to have given any emotional support to his wife during labor and delivery. However, Chinese women have significant others who can provide emotional support—mothers, inlaws, cousins, other members of the extended family, or close friends.

In India all attendants at birth are women; men are totally excluded (Flint, 1982). On the other hand, in Guatemala, a husband may assist his wife and the midwife during delivery (Cosminsky, 1982). During the labor process of the Navajo in the Southwestern United States, people passing by the hogan (home) are encouraged to enter and provide support for the mother (Newton, 1972). Because of the wide variation in who comprises the preferred person or persons, it is critical for the nurse to determine from the woman and her family what persons are wanted during labor and delivery.

Grandparents During Labor

Support of grandparents is similar to that provided the father as discussed in the preceding pages. The nurse acts as a role model for parents by treating grandparents with dignity and respect, by acknowledging the value of their contributions to parental support, and by recognizing the difficulty parents have in witnessing their child's discomfort or crisis, regardless of the child's age.

Of particular value is the availability of another person or persons to relieve the father or coach. This may be necessary to assist the parturient with walking, especially if IV poles are to be pushed; and to help the parturient when she needs two tasks performed simultaneously.

Whenever possible the nurse offers the grandparent emotional support. This can be done by providing liquid refreshment even if unsolicited and by initiating discussion with open-ended questions or statements, such as "It is sometimes hard to watch a daughter in labor. . . ."

These nursing actions are therapeutic for the entire family unit. According to Barnard (1978), "Rather than compete with family members, we can use them, provide support to them, and teach them. The family's influence will far outlast our contact with the client. If we can improve this social unit's ability to care, we will have a powerful health care system indeed." Support for the mother of a laboring woman—mothering *her* mother—is an important place to begin (Stephany, 1983).

Siblings During Labor

Preparation for acceptance of the new child helps with the attachment process. Parents, brothers and sisters, and other extended family members benefit from *cognitive rehearsal* for the new addition to the family. Preparation for and participation during pregnancy and labor may help the older children accept this change. The older child or children become *active* participants who are important to the family (Bliss, 1980). Rehearsal for the event before labor is essential. Preparation for the entire family includes the additional support person who is to be responsible for the older children during the entire childbirth process.

The age and developmental level of the children influence their responses. The child under 2 years of age shows little interest in pregnancy and labor; for the older child the experience may reduce fears and misconceptions. Preparation is adjusted to the age and developmental level of the child. Most parents have a "feel" for the maturational level and ability to cope of their children. Preparation includes description of anticipated sights and sounds. The children must learn that their mother will be working hard. She will not be able to talk to them during contractions. She may groan and pant at times. Labor is uncomfortable, but their mother's body is made for the job. The sights, sounds, smells, and behavior of participants will be similar to those for which fathers are prepared. Films are available for preparing older preschool and school-age children for participating in the birth experience.

Leonard et al (1979) observed the behavior of children present during labor, delivery, and the postpartum period. In general the preschool-age children tended to interact eagerly with their parents during early labor. They were seen to withdraw from the happenings as labor progressed. None of the children seemed to become acutely distressed during the experience. However, children need to feel free to ask questions and express personal feelings (Daniels, 1983).

Preparation for Giving Birth in the Delivery Room

If any woman in labor, be she a nullipara or multipara, states: "The baby is coming!" it is too late for transfer to the delivery room (or if in a birthing room, it may be too late to have the physician present). The birth is imminent. Prepare to assist with the delivery until the physician arrives. (See Emergency Childbirth, p. 416).

The delivery room nurse is responsible for ensuring that the facility is properly prepared and that all supplies and equipment are in working order at all times. This should be routinely checked at the beginning of the nurse's shift. The role of the woman's partner is reviewed and suitable delivery area clothing may be provided. It is essential that the woman's record be up-to-date, because her condition can change quickly.

All nursing care and the woman's or couple's responses must be recorded to ensure continuity of care, ensure appropriate assessment of the woman's progress, and document the nursing and other care given. Courts of law insist that the nursing and medical care that is not documented on the client's record may not have been given.

The following are suggestions for preparation for delivery. These items may vary among different facilities so that the protocols from each facility's procedure manual should be consulted.

1. Scrubbing facilities, scrub brushes, cuticle sticks, cleaning agent, and masks are available.
2. The following have been done:
   a. Sterile gowns and gloves for physician or nurse-midwife, sterile drapes and towels for draping the woman, and sterile instruments and other supplies (such as bulb syringes, sutures, and anesthetic solutions) are arranged for convenience in use on sterile table.
   b. Sterile basin and water for hand washing during delivery process are readied for use.
   c. Supplies for cleansing vulva are available (sterile basin, sterile water, and cleaning solution).
   d. Delivery area is warmed and free of drafts.
   e. Infant receiving blankets and heated crib are readied. Material for prophylactic care of infant's eyes is available (see p. 415).
3. Equipment is in working order: delivery table (bed or chair), overhead lights, and mirror.
4. Emergency equipment, anesthesia, laryngoscope, and supplies are available and in working order if needed for emergency situations such as control of maternal hemorrhage or fetal respiratory distress.
5. Additional supplies (anesthetics, oxytocics for injection, and obstetric forceps) are available.
6. Woman's record is up-to-date and ready for use in delivery area. In areas such as the labor unit, recordings are made concomitantly as symptoms are noted, assessments are made, and care is given. It is imperative to have recordings complete at all times.

Transfer to the Delivery Room*

Nullipara:	when the presenting part begins to distend the perineum
Multipara:	when the cervix is 8 to 9 cm dilated

Evaluation

Evaluation of progress and outcomes is a continuous activity during the first stage of labor. Each interaction with the mother-to-be and her family must be carefully evaluated by the nurse; the degree to which formulated goals for care are being met must be critically appraised. If the evaluation process identifies that results fall short of achieving any goal, further assessment, planning, and implementation are imperative to attain the correct nursing care for the woman and her family.

❑ SECOND STAGE OF LABOR

The second stage of labor is the stage of expulsion of the fetus. It extends from full cervical dilatation (10 cm) through the birth of the baby. The three phases of the second stage are **latency/resting, descent,** and **final transition.** There is a rhythmic nature to the second stage of labor (Carr, 1983). The rhythm and movement emerge for the woman encouraged to listen to her body as she progresses through this stage. A woman will normally respond by changing body positions, pushing when she has an urge to push, vocalizing as she bears down. If a woman is confined to bed in a recumbent position this rhythmic urge to push is lost. The rhythm is also lost if she is moved to another room and placed on a delivery table in the lithotomy position, as has been the custom in North America for the past 30 years. Fortunately this is changing, with LDR (labor, delivery, and recovery) rooms becoming more and more common. In most societies labor and delivery occur in the same room.

*In many facilities, it is now common practice to have the woman labor, deliver, and recover in the LDR (Labor, Delivery, and Recovery) room, thus alleviating the added stress of transfer to a new and often strange environment at a critical time in the childbirth process.

"In the majority of cases, labor and delivery are physiologic processes, and do not, in the true sense, require 'management' " (Scott et al, 1990). In response to the question of whether the obstetrician should interfere with the process of labor during the second stage, Warrington (1842) replied, "He should let it alone if he has ascertained the position is correct."

Assessment

The only positive objective sign that the second stage of labor has begun is when no cervix can be felt on vaginal examination (Myles, 1985). Other signs that suggest the onset of the second stage include the following:

1. Sudden appearance of sweat on upper lip
2. An episode of vomiting
3. An increased bloody show
4. Shaking of extremities
5. Increased restlessness; verbalization that "I can't go on"
6. Involuntary bearing-down efforts

These signs commonly appear at the time the cervix reaches full dilatation (Myles, 1985; Scott et al, 1990). Other indicators for assessing progress during each phase of the second stage can be found in Table 15-5.

Assessment is continuous during the second stage of labor. The specific type and timing of assessments are determined by hospital protocol.

In the second stage *each* contraction is monitored for frequency, strength, duration, intensity, and fetal response. Descent of the presenting part is confirmed by vaginal examination until the presenting part can be seen at the introitus. The degree of bladder filling is as-

Table 15-5 Maternal Progress in Second Stage of Labor

Criterion	Latent-Resting (10-20 min)	Descent	Final/Transition
Contractions	Period of physiologic lull for all criteria		
Magnitude (intensity)		Significant increase	Overwhelmingly strong Expulsive
Frequency	Period of peace and rest (Carr, 1983; Mahan and McKay, 1984)	2½ min	2½ min
Duration		90 sec	90 sec
Descent		Increases and **Ferguson's reflex*** activated	Rapid
Show: color and amount		Significant increase in dark red bloody show	Fetal head visible at introitus; bloody show accompanies birth of head
Spontaneous bearing-down efforts	Slight to absent except with peaks of strongest contractions (Carr, 1983)	Increased urgency to bear down	Greatly increased
Vocalization		Grunting sounds or expiratory vocalization (Carr, 1983; Mahan and McKay, 1984)	Grunting sounds and expiratory vocalizations continue
Maternal behavior (Carr, 1983)	Experiences sense of relief that transition to second stage is finished Feels fatigued and sleepy Feels a sense of accomplishment and optimism, since the "worst is over" Feels in control	Senses increased urgency Alters respiratory pattern: has short 4 to 5 sec breath-holds with regular breaths in between, 5-7 times per contraction Makes grunting sounds or expiratory vocalizations	Expresses sense of extreme pain Expresses feelings of powerlessness Shows decreased ability to listen or concentrate on anything but giving birth Describes the **"ring of fire"**† Often shows excitement immediately following delivery of head

*Ferguson's reflex. Pressure of presenting part on stretch receptors of pelvic floor stimulates release of oxytocin from posterior pituitary, resulting in more intense uterine contractions.
†Ring of fire. Burning sensation of acute pain as vagina stretches and fetal head crowns.

sessed, since a full bladder can impede descent of the head and affect uterine contractions.

Maternal pulse and BP are checked every 30 minutes. The BP is obtained between contractions. The presence of amnesia between contractions is noted. The partner's or father's response is assessed.

If the FHR is monitored intermittently with a fetoscope, it is checked after every contraction or every 5 minutes. If continuous FHR monitoring is used (Chapter 14), the nurse checks the tracings on the monitor with each contraction. Mild, brief bradycardia and decelerations can occur in 90% or more of women during the second stage of labor (Mahan and McKay, 1984). If recovery of the FHR from the deceleration is prompt after the contraction and expulsive forces cease, these episodes are not of major concern. (Cunningham, MacDonald, and Gant, 1989).

All protocols include assessment of show and amniotic fluid. Show is checked for evidence of excessive bleeding. Amniotic fluid is checked for meconium staining, odor, and amount (see Procedure 15-1, p. 372). Amniotic fluid is normally odorless but an odor can be detected when intrauterine infection (amnionitis) is present. Vaginal examinations are avoided or the number restricted whenever possible.

Duration of Second Stage

There is considerable controversy over the precise duration of the second stage and the time limits that should be regarded as normal. Friedman's curves for nulliparous and multiparous women are commonly used to assess the progress of the second stage. A second stage of more than 2 hours for a nullipara and 1 hour for a multipara is considered abnormal and must be reported to a physician. Other factors that must be considered are the FHR pattern, the descent of the presenting part, the quality of the uterine contractions, and the fetal scalp blood pH (Mahan and McKay, 1984). The range and average duration of the second stage of labor based on Friedman's data vary with parity:

Parity	Range (min)	Average (min)
Nulliparas	25 to 75	57
Multiparas	13 to 17	14.4

The nurse should be aware of the danger signs during labor (p. 371).

Yeates and Roberts (1984) compared the duration of the second stage when women engage in coached pushing or are allowed to push spontaneously when they feel the urge. Their findings are based on a small sample but suggest that spontaneous pushing may be the most effective in aiding in the descent and rotation of the newborn.

Nursing Diagnoses

Nursing diagnoses lend direction to the nursing action needed to implement care. Before establishing diagnoses the nurse analyzes the significance of the findings collected during assessment. Following are some nursing diagnoses indicating potential areas for concern during the second stage.

Potential for injury to mother and fetus related to
- Persistent use of Valsalva maneuver

Situational low self-esteem related to
- Knowledge deficit of normal, beneficial effects of vocalizations during bearing-down efforts
- Inability to carry out plan for unmedicated birth

Ineffective individual coping related to
- Coaching that contradicts woman's physiologic urge to push

Pain related to
- Bearing down efforts and distension of the perineum

Anxiety related to
- Inability to control defecation with bearing down efforts

Knowledge deficit related to
- Inexperience with reasons for perineal sensation

Potential for injury to mother related to
- Inappropriate positioning of mother's legs in stirrups

Situational low-self-esteem of father related to
- Inability to support mother during final stage of labor

Planning

In both the second and third stages of labor planning must be completed with speed and accuracy. Goals must be set and prioritized and may change as the second stage progresses. Nurses' ability and adaptability in relation to planning care will depend on their experience, which will influence their competence. A specific nursing care plan for a woman in the second stage of labor is provided on p. 402.

Goals for the second stage of labor may include that the woman will:
1. Actively participate in the labor process
2. Sustain no injury during the labor process (nor will the fetus)
3. Obtain comfort and support from family members of choice

Specific Nursing Care Plan

HYPERVENTILATION AND SPONTANEOUS RUPTURE OF MEMBRANES

Judy S. is a 30-year-old multipara in labor. She is assessed as being 8 cm dilated, station +2, membranes intact when her husband brings her to the labor and delivery area. Judy and her husband have been through prepared childbirth classes and she is doing her breathing exercises with each contraction. As the nurse is helping Judy into the bed, her membranes rupture with a gush of clear fluid. The nurse immediately assesses the FHR and the fluid that was lost.

The contractions are now coming faster and harder and Judy is starting to hyperventilate. She starts complaining of numbness of her fingers and around her mouth and lightheadedness. The nurse tries to calm her breathing pattern down and gives her a bag to breathe into.

ASSESSMENT	NURSING DIAGNOSIS (ND), PLAN/GOAL (P/G)	RATIONALE/ IMPLEMENTATION	EVALUATION
Spontaneous rupture of membranes (SROM) Station +2 8 cm dilated Multipara	ND: Potential for injury to mother or newborn related to rapid delivery. ND: Potential for infection related to delayed delivery after SROM. P/G: Fetal status, amniotic fluid, and progress of labor are within normal limits: infection does not occur; physician or midwife is present for birth.	*Rupture of membranes increases potential for fetal hypoxia:* Assess FHR and progress of labor. Assess the color of the fluid—normally straw-colored. Assess character of the fluid—normally looks like water and has a characteristic odor. Assess amount of fluid lost—an excessive amount, polyhydramnios, or an abnormally small amount, oligohydramnios, signals congenital anomalies. Record findings and notify physician or midwife.	Fetal status remains within normal limits. Progress of labor continues within normal limits. Woman understands reasons for procedures.
Numbness in fingers and around mouth Lightheadedness Rapid respiratory rate	ND: Impaired gas exchange related to respiratory alkalosis. ND: Altered cardiopulmonary tissue perfusion related to hyperventilation and respiratory alkalosis. P/G: Mother resumes normal breathing pattern with no signs or symptoms of alkalosis; FHR stays within normal limits.	*Hyperventilation interferes with adequate gas exchange:* Provide a paper bag for the woman to breathe into. She may also breathe into cupped hands, if no bag is available. Explain to woman what is happening and how rebreathing her own air is therapeutic. Coach woman to breathe without hyperventilation. Identify stress (e.g., anxiety, knowledge deficit, or discomfort) that may underlie woman's hyperventilation; relieve the identified stress.	Woman ceases to hyperventilate and signs and symptoms are relieved. FHR remains within normal limits. Concurrent stress is relieved.

Implementation

The nurse implements plans to monitor constantly the events of the second stage and mechanism of delivery, maternal physiologic and emotional responses to the second stage, paternal response to the second stage, and fetal response to the stress of the second stage.

The nurse continues to provide comfort measures for the mother such as positioning, mouth care, maintaining clean, dry bedding, and avoiding extraneous noise, conversation, or other distractions (e.g., laughing, talking of attending personnel in or outside the labor area). The woman is encouraged to indicate other support measures she would like.

If the mother is to be transferred to another area for delivery, the nurse makes the transfer early enough to avoid rushing the client. The delivery area is also readied for the birth.

Maternal Position. The woman may want to assume various positions such as squatting. For this position a firm surface is required, and the woman will need side support. In a birthing bed a squat bar is available to assist (Fig. 15-14). Another position is the side-lying position with the upper leg held by the nurse or coach or placed on a pillow. Some women prefer Fowler's position (can be attained with the support of a wedged pillow or with the father supporting the woman). Others prefer the hands and knees or standing position when bearing down. When a woman is in the standing position, with weight being borne on both femoral heads, the pressure in the acetabulum will increase the transverse diameter of the pelvic outlet by up to 1 cm. This can be helpful if descent of the head is delayed as a result of failure of the occiput to rotate from the lateral (transverse diameter of pelvis) to the anterior position. The woman may also want to sit on the toilet to push, since many women are concerned about stool incontinence during this stage. These women must be closely monitored and removed from the toilet before delivery becomes imminent.

Bearing-down Efforts. As the fetal head reaches the pelvic floor most women experience the urge to push. Automatically the woman will begin to exert downward pressure by contracting her abdominal muscles while relaxing her pelvic floor. This **bearing down** is an involuntary reflex response to the pressure of the presenting part on stretch receptors of pelvic musculature. A strong expiratory grunt may accompany the push. When coaching women to push, the nurse encourages them to push as *they* feel like pushing rather than giving a prolonged push on command. The nurse monitors the woman's breathing so that the woman does not hold her breath more than 5 seconds at a time. Prolonged breath-holding may trigger the **Valsalva maneuver,** which results from the woman's closing the glottis, thereby increasing intrathoracic and cardiovascular pressure. In addition, holding the breath for more than 5 seconds diminishes the perfusion of oxygen across the placenta and results in fetal hypoxia. The nurse reminds the woman to take deep breaths to refill her lungs following each contraction.

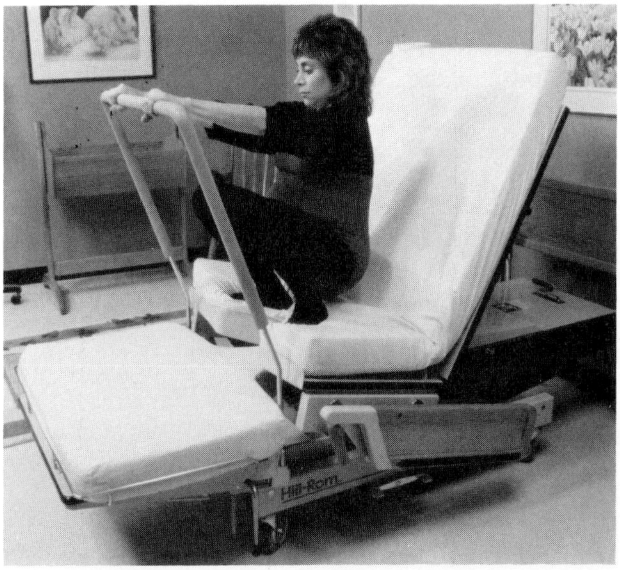

Fig. 15-14 Birth bed for a single-room maternity care—labor, delivery, recovery, and postpartum care (LDRP). (Courtesy The Borning Corp, Spokane, Wash.)

To ensure slow delivery of the fetal head, the nurse encourages the woman to control the urge to push. The urge to push is controlled by coaching the woman to take panting breaths or to exhale slowly through pursed lips as the baby's head crowns. The woman needs simple, clear directions from *one* coach.

Amnesia between contractions is often pronounced in the second stage, and the woman may have to be roused to cooperate in the bearing-down process. Parents who have attended childbirth classes may have devised a set of verbal cues for the parturient to follow. It is helpful if they print these on a card that may be attached to the head of the bed so that the nurse can better substitute as coach if the partner has to leave.

Fetal Heart Rate. FHR must be checked as noted previously. If the rate begins to drop or if there is a loss of variability, prompt treatment must be initiated. The woman can be turned on her left side to reduce the pressure of the uterus against the ascending vena cava and descending aorta (Fig. 15-9), and oxygen can be administered by mask at 10 to 12 L/min. This is often all that is required to restore the normal rate. If the FHR does not return to normal immediately, quickly notify the physician, since medical intervention to hasten the birth may be indicated.

Support of the Father/Coach. During the second stage the woman needs continuous support and coaching. The coaching process can be physically and emotionally tiring for the father/coach. The nurse can offer him nourishment, fluids, and short breaks. If the father is to attend the delivery, he is given instructions as to donning cover gown, mask, hat, and shoes and he is advised as to areas in which he has freedom to move and what support he can give to his wife (some are prepared to do coaching for pushing and panting) (Table 15-6).

Birth Beds and Chairs. There is no single position for childbirth. Labor is a dynamic, interactive process between the mother's uterus, pelvis, and voluntary muscles. Angles between the baby and mother's pelvis constantly change as the infant turns and flexes down the birth canal. If able to, a mother will constantly change position in labor. The birth bed (Fig. 15-15) changes shape according to the mother's needs. She can squat, kneel, recline, or sit, choosing the position most comfortable for her. At the same time, there is excellent exposure for examination, electrode placement, fetal scalp sampling, and delivery. With the birth bed the mother has full control of both seat and back functions and can adjust her position for maximum comfort. The mother and fetus can maintain a close personal contact and a new degree of involvement in the birth process if they desire. The bed can be positioned for administer-

Table 15-6 Expected Responses and Support Person's Actions During Second Stage of Labor

Woman's Responses	Nurse/Support Person's Actions
LATENT/RESTING PHASE	
Experiences a short period (10-20 min) of peace and rest	Encourages woman to listen to her body (Carr, 1983) Continues support measures If descent phase does not begin after 20 min, suggests upright position to encourage progression of descent
DESCENT PHASE	
Senses increased urgency to bear down as Ferguson's reflex is elicited Notes increase in intensity of uterine contractions Demonstrates change in respiratory pattern (e.g., 5-second breath-holds, 5-7 per contraction) Makes grunting sounds or expiratory vocalizations	Endorses respiratory pattern (short breath-holds with glottis closed) Stresses normalcy and benefits of grunting sounds and expiratory vocalizations Encourages pushing *with* urge to push Encourages/suggests maternal movement and position changes (upright, if descent is not occurring) If descent is occurring, encourages woman to listen to her body regarding movement and position change Discourages long breath-holding If transfer to a delivery room cannot be avoided, nurse transfers her early to avoid rushing or offers her option of walking to DR if permitted If descent is too fast, places woman in lateral recumbent position to slow descent (Carr, 1983)
FINAL/TRANSITIONAL PHASE	
Behaves in manner similar to transition during first stage (8-10 cm) Experiences a sense of severe pain and powerlessness (Carr, 1983) Shows decreased ability to listen Concentrates on delivery of baby until head is born Experiences contractions as overwhelming in intensity Reports "ring of fire" as head crowns Maintains respiratory pattern of 3 to 5, 5-second breath-holds per contraction followed by forced expiration Eases head out with short expirations Responds with excitement and relief after head is born	Encourages slow, gentle pushing (Carr, 1983) Explains that "blowing away the contraction" facilitates a slower birth of the head Provides mirror or guides woman to see/touch emerging fetal head (best to extend over 2 to 3 contractions) to help her understand the perineal sensations Coaches relaxation of mouth, throat, and neck to relax pelvic floor Applies warm compresses to perineum to aid relaxation

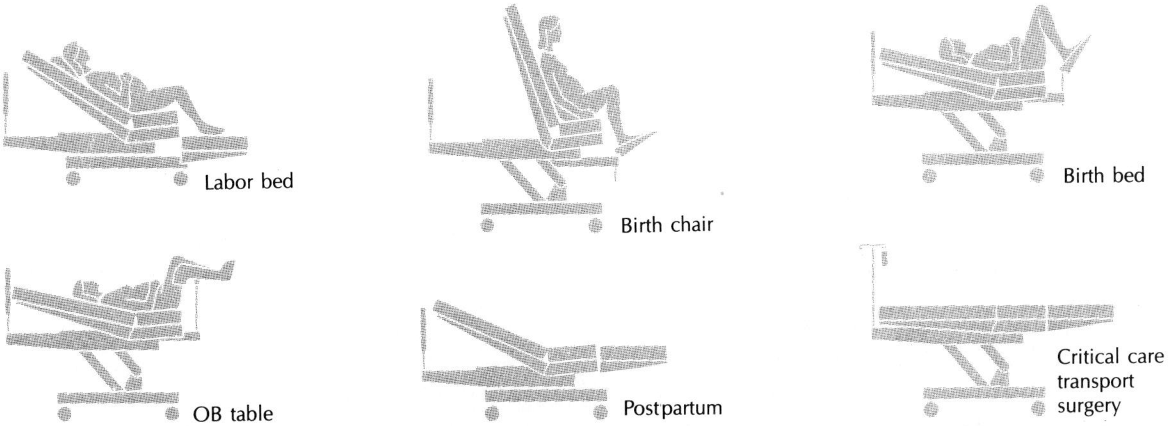

Fig. 15-15 The versatility of today's birth bed makes it practical in a variety of settings. (Courtesy Hill-Rom.)

ing anesthesia, the V-shaped perineal cut-out is adaptable to both spontaneous birth and forceps and the bed can be used to transport to surgery in the event of a cesarean birth.

Birth chairs may also be used and may provide women with a better physiologic position during childbirth, although some women feel restricted by a chair. Potentially there is both a physiologic and psychologic advantage to the upright position. The mother can see the birth as it occurs and also maintain *en face* contact with the attendant (Balaskis, 1983). Most chairs are designed so if an emergency occurs the chair can be adjusted to the horizontal or Trendelenberg position. However, some evidence is offered for a higher incidence of postpartum hemorrhage when a chair is used. Coltrell and Shannahan (1986) found that there is also an increased risk of perineal edema caused by the pressure of the rim of the chair, which may obstruct venous return from the perineal region.

In some hospitals oversize beanbag chairs are being used for both labor and delivery. These chairs mold around and support the mother in whatever position she selects. These chairs are of paticular value for mothers who seek active involvement in the birth process.

Preparation for Birth in a Delivery Room

If the woman is to be transferred to a delivery area for completion of the birth process, the nurse uses the guidelines for transfer to the delivery room given on p. 399.

Delivery Room Birth Table. Delivery rooms are specifically designed to facilitate care during delivery (Fig. 15-16). The delivery table is designed with many features: the entire table can be raised or lowered, and the head or foot may be raised or lowered. A wedge pillow or bolster can be inserted under the top of the mattress to raise it slightly, or the head of the table can be raised to prevent supine hypotension and to facilitate pushing. The table is equipped with stirrups for supporting the legs and handle grips to aid in bearing down. If stirrups are used, the bed can be "broken"; that is, the lower half of the bed can be lowered and rolled back to fit under the top half.

Supplies, Instruments and Equipment. The delivery table is prepared and instruments are arranged on the instrument table (Fig. 15-17). Standard procedures are followed for gloving, identifying and opening sterile packages, adding sterile supplies to the instrument table, and unwrapping and handing sterile instruments to the physician or nurse-midwife. Fig. 15-18 illustrates the proper sequence for perineal cleansing. The crib and equipment are readied for the support and stabilization of the infant (Fig. 15-16, C).

Birth in a Delivery Room. The woman will need assistance to move from the labor bed to the delivery table. If this is done between contractions, the mother can help, but because of her awkwardness, she cannot be rushed.

The position assumed for delivery may be **Sims' position** (if this is the case, the attendant will need to support the upper leg), dorsal position, or lithotomy position.

The **lithotomy position** has been the position most commonly used for delivery in Western cultures although this is changing slowly. The lithotomy position makes it more convenient for the physician to deal

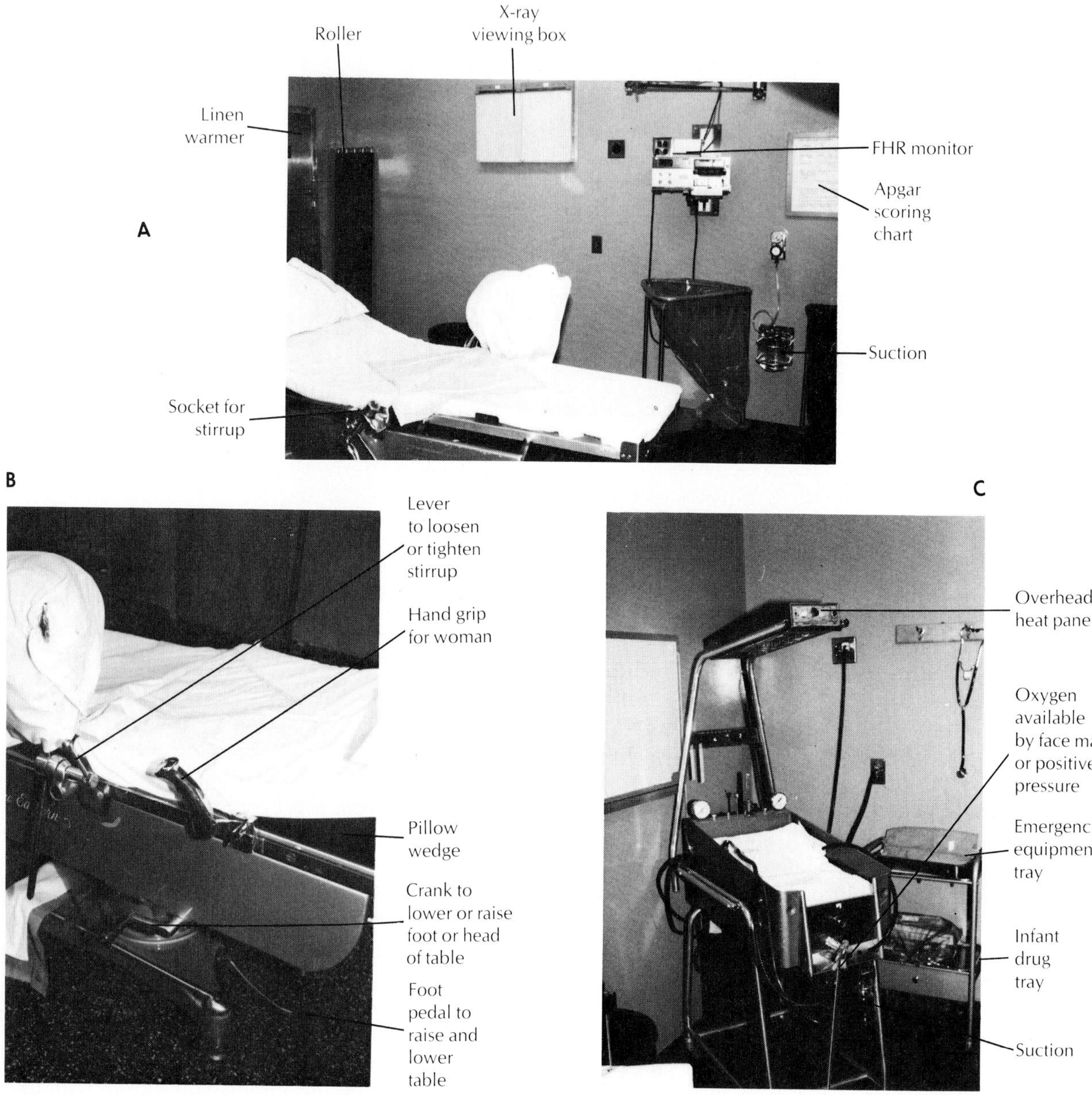

Fig. 15-16 Delivery room.

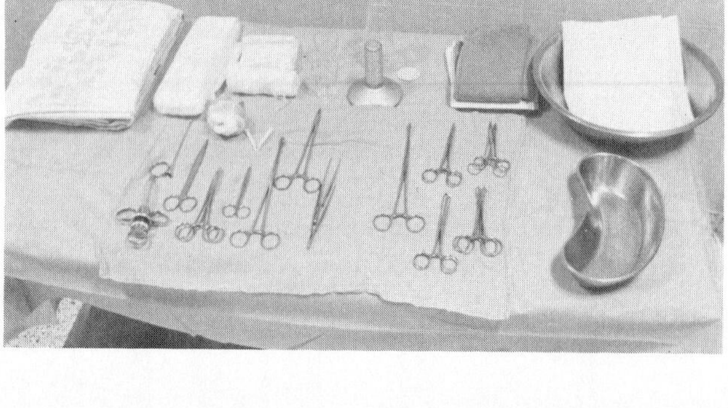

Fig. 15-17 Instrument table (all equipment sterile). *Top, left to right:* receiving blanket, perineal pad, vaginal roll, medicine glasses (for anesthetic agent), hand cover for spotlight, urine specimen bottle, towels, and placenta bowl and paper towel for covering scales. *Bottom, left to right:* syringe (anesthetic) needle guard, episiotomy scissors, bulb syringe (covered with gauze for aspirating newborn), two artery forceps, scissors, cord clamp, ring forceps, needle holder, thumb forceps (for repair of episiotomy), extra instruments (ring forceps, small artery forceps, toothed forceps, Allis clamps and sharp hook forceps for holding drapes in place), and kidney basin.

with any complications that arise. The buttocks are brought to the edge of the table, and the legs are placed in stirrups. Care must be taken to pad the stirrups, raise and place both legs simultaneously, and adjust the shanks of the stirrups so that the calfs of the legs are supported. There should be no pressure on the popliteal space. If the stirrups are uneven in height, the woman can develop strained ligaments in her back as she bears down. This strain causes considerable discomfort in the postdelivery period. The lower portion of the table may be dropped down and rolled back under the table.

Once the woman is positioned for delivery, the vulva is washed thoroughly with soap and water or a surgical disinfectant (Fig. 15-18). A **mini-prep** may be performed at this time, shaving the area between the vagina and anus. The physician or midwife dons cap and mask, scrubs hands, and puts on the sterile gown and gloves. The woman may then be draped with sterile towels and sheets. The husband or coach helps the mother remember not to touch the sterile drapes.

The circulating nurse will continue to coach and encourage the parturient. Once the woman's legs are in the stirrups, the handle grips can be used to exert counter pressure. The nurse will check FHR after every contraction or with continual electronic monitoring and notify the physician as to the rate and regularity. The equipment for taking the BP should be readied for instant use if signs of shock develop. However, the readings are distorted (increased) by the increase in thoracic and abdominal pressures as the woman pushes. A reading will be taken after delivery before transferring the woman to the recovery room. An oxytocic medication such as Syntocinon may be prepared for administration after delivery. Observations and procedures are recorded on the chart.

Fathers are encouraged to be present at the birth of their infants if this is in keeping with their cultural expectations. The psychologic closeness of the family unit is maintained, and the father can continue the supportive care given in labor. The father needs as much opportunity as does the mother to initiate the attachment process with the baby. Studies indicate, however, that it is the continuous long-term contact between father and child that acts to cement the bonds and that there is no immediate "magic moment" of bonding.

The father is usually gowned in a clean scrub outfit and wears a cap and a mask. These supplies need to be provided in ample time for him to don them before the delivery. If the couple has decided that the father is not to be present, their decision should be respected.

Contact with parents is maintained by touch, verbal comforting instructions as to reasons for care, and sharing in parents' joy at birth of their child. The nurse notes and records the time of birth (i.e., when infant is born completely).

Mechanism of Delivery: Vertex Presentation

The nurse who is knowledgeable about the mechanism of delivery has increased skills as support person and teacher/counselor/advocate. While most of the time the delivery remains in the hands of the obstetrician or nurse-midwife, there may be a time when the nurse must assist the woman to give birth (p. 416). The nurse's knowledge of the birth process provides a basis for client preparation before and during delivery.

The nurse reviews with the woman or couple the mechanics of labor (Chapter 12). Once the cervix is fully dilated, descent occurs. The vertex advances with each contraction and recedes slightly as the contraction wanes; descent is constant, and late in the second stage the head reaches the pelvic floor. *Bulging of the perineum* occurs during the **descent phase** when the fetal presenting part is distending the perineum but is not

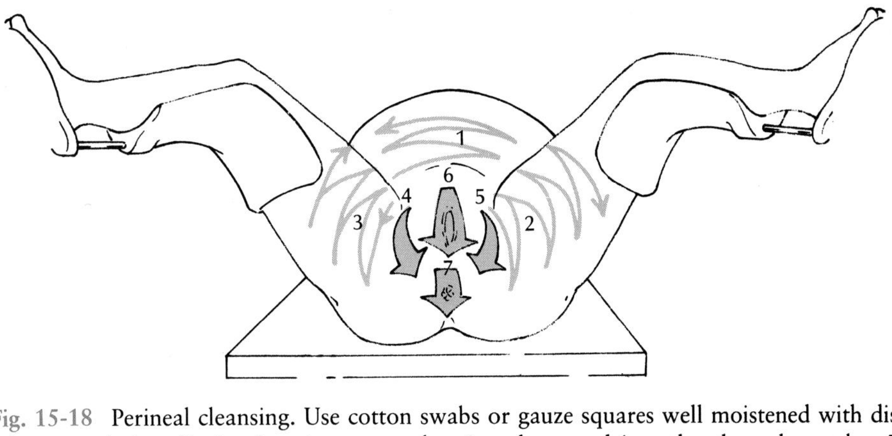

Fig. 15-18 Perineal cleansing. Use cotton swabs or gauze squares well moistened with disinfectant solution. Begin cleansing at number 1 and proceed in order through number 7. Discard swab after each step. Finish cleansing with wash of sterile water.

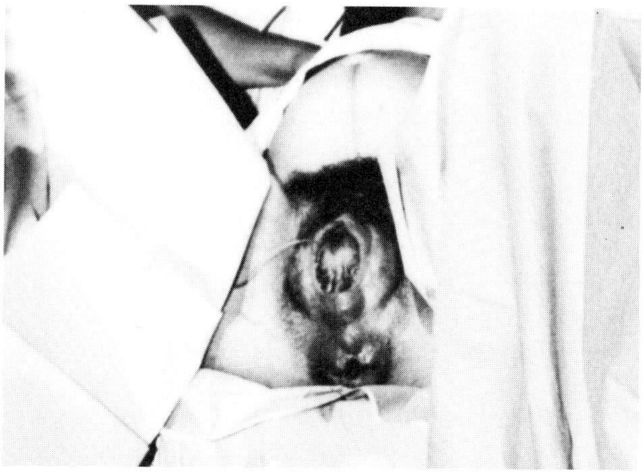

Fig. 15-19 Oval-shaped appearance of introitus. Note prominent anal hemorrhoids as head distends perineum. (Courtesy Marjorie Pyle, RNC, Lifecircle, Costa Mesa, Calif.)

yet visible at the introitus. The occiput generally rotates anteriorly, and with voluntary bearing down efforts, the head appears to the introitus (Fig. 15-19). Although more and more head may be seen with each push, **crowning** occurs when the head's widest part (the biparietal diameter) distends the vulva just before birth. Immediately before delivery, the perineal musculature becomes greatly distended. If an **episiotomy** is necessary, it is done at this time to minimize soft tissue damage (p. 419). The head delivers by extension and following delivery restitutes in line with the shoulders. Interiorly the shoulders rotate into the anteroposterior diameter of the pelvis; external rotation of the head is observed. The body is born by lateral flexion.

The three phases of a spontaneous delivery of the fetus in a vertex presentation are (1) delivery of the head, (2) delivery of the shoulders, and (3) delivery of the body and extremities.

Delivery of Head. The vertex first appears, followed by the forehead, face, chin, and neck. The speed of delivery of the head must be controlled, or sudden birth of the head may cause severe **lacerations** through the anal sphincter or even into the rectum (p. 419). The physician or nurse-midwife controls the birth of the head by (1) applying pressure against the rectum, drawing it downward to aid in flexing the head as the back of the neck catches under the symphysis pubis; (2) then applying upward pressure from the coccygeal region (modified **Ritgen's maneuver**) (Fig. 15-20), to extend the head during the actual delivery, thereby protecting the musculature of the perineum; and (3) assisting the mother with voluntary control of the bearing down efforts by coaching her to pant. In addition to protecting the maternal tissues, gradual delivery is imperative to prevent fetal intracranial injury.

The membranes may not be ruptured before delivery. During birth of the head these membranes look like a hood covering the head. This hood of intact amniotic membranes covering the head during birth is known as a **caul.** In Scotland a child born with a caul is thought to be gifted with "second sight."

The umbilical cord often encircles the neck (**nuchal cord**) but rarely so tightly as to cause hypoxia. The cord should be slipped gently over the head (Fig. 15-21, *A*). If the loop is tight or if there is a second loop, the cord is clamped twice, severed between the clamps, and unwound from around the neck before the delivery is continued. Mucus, blood, or meconium in the nasal or oral passages may prevent the newborn from breathing. Moist gauze sponges are used to wipe the nose and mouth. A bulb syringe is inserted into the mouth and oropharynx first to aspirate contents. Next, the nares are cleared while the head is being supported (see discussion of suctioning the neonate, Chapter 17).

Delivery of Shoulders. Before the shoulders can deliver they must engage in the pelvic inlet. Internal rotation of the shoulders, accompanied by restitution (Fig. 15-22, *A*) and external rotation of the head, oc-

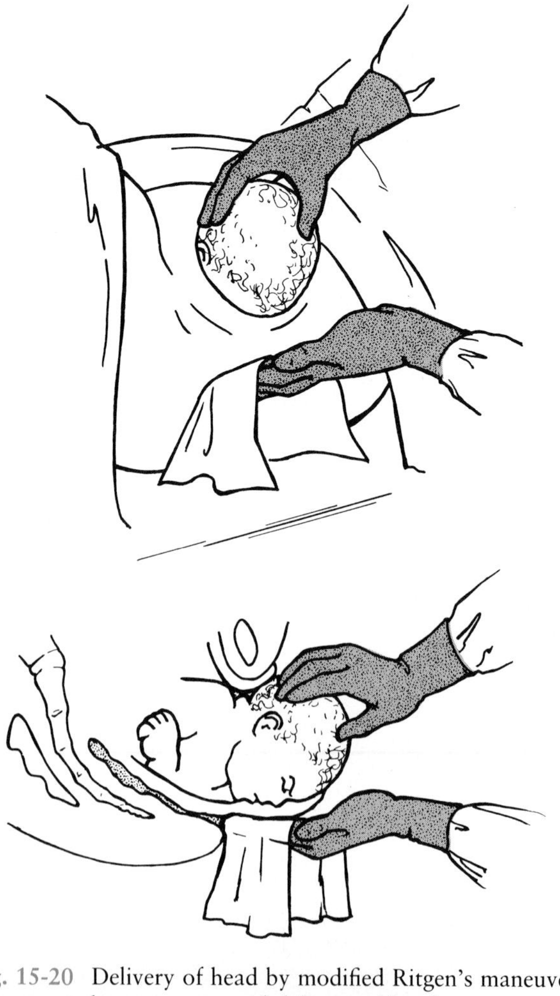

Fig. 15-20 Delivery of head by modified Ritgen's maneuver. Note control to prevent rapid delivery of head.

A

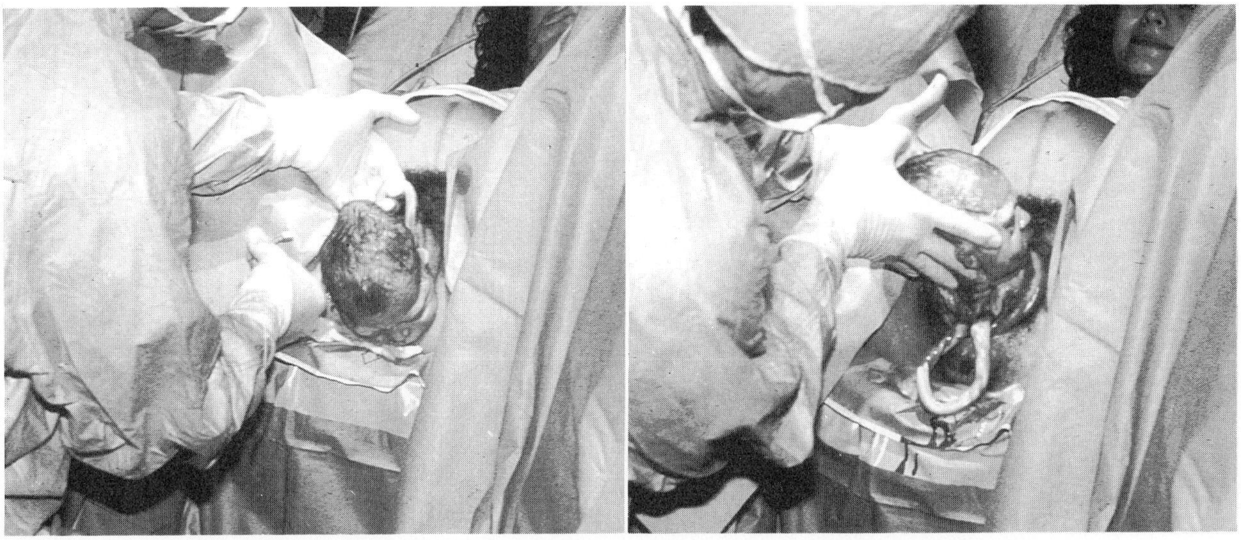

B

Fig. 15-21 **A,** Loosening nuchal cord. **B,** Birth of posterior shoulder. (Courtesy Marjorie Pyle, RNC, Lifecircle, Costa, Mesa, Calif.)

A

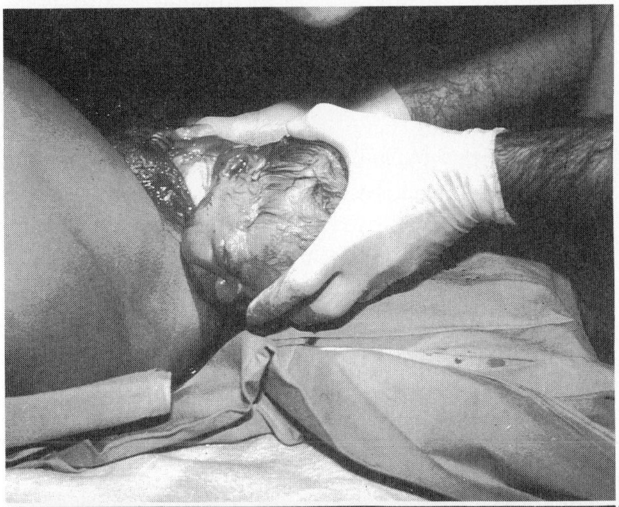

Fig. 15-22 Mechanism of labor. **A,** Restitution. **B,** External rotation. **C,** Slow expulsion of fetus/newborn. Note bulb syringe in hand in **B.** (Courtesy Marjorie Pyle, RNC, Lifecircle, Costa Mesa, Calif.)

B

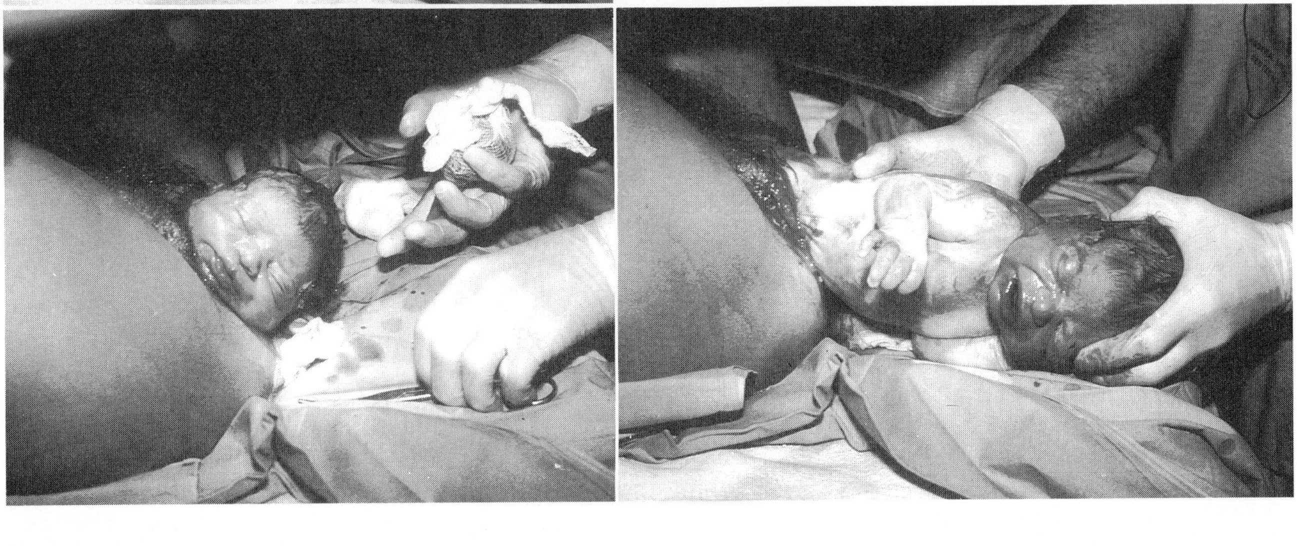

C

curs (Fig. 15-22, *B*), and the shoulders now lie in the anteroposterior diameter of the inlet (see also Fig. 12-18, *E, F*). The shoulders can now pass through the pelvic cavity. While awaiting rotation, the physician wipes the baby's face with sterile gauze squares and uses the bulb syringe to clear the nose of mucus, ready for the baby's first breath.

The head is drawn downward and backward by the obstetrician or midwife to help the anterior shoulder impinge beneath the arch of the symphysis and slide beneath the pubic arch. Normally the anterior shoulder is delivered with this slight downward traction toward the perineum. The posterior shoulder distends the perineum, and to prevent perineal trauma, the head is lifted toward the symphysis pubis, the shoulder being delivered over the perineum (see Fig. 15-21, *B*) (Myles, 1985).

Delivery of Body and Extremities. Expulsion (Fig. 15-22, C) is controlled so that it occurs slowly. Lateral flexion is continued, the weight of the baby is supported by the doctor's or midwife's lower hand (Fig. 15-22, C), again to prevent perineal trauma. Slight rotation of the body to the right or left may be used to facilitate the birth. The time of birth is considered the precise time when the entire body is out of the mother. This must be recorded on the record.

Siblings During The Second Stage. A young child may become frightened by the intensity of the second stage. Sights such as rupture of the membranes and sounds such as their mother's moans, screams, and grunts can be unsettling (Quinlan, 1983). The child present during delivery needs someone to be close and to give explanations simply and calmly. The child may want to be held. Long-term effects on young children witnessing birth are not yet known.

Evaluation

Evaluation of outcomes is an ongoing activity. During each encounter with the woman and her family during the second stage of labor the nurse evaluates the degree to which goals for care are being met. If the evaluation shows that results fall short of achieving any goal, further assessment, planning, and implementation are warranted.

THIRD STAGE OF LABOR

The third stage of labor extends from the birth of the baby until the delivery of the placenta. The goal in the management of the third stage of labor is the prompt separation and expulsion of the placenta, achieved in the easiest, safest manner.

The placenta is attached to the decidual layer of the thin endometrium of the basal plate by numerous, randomized, fibrous anchor villi—much like a postage stamp is attached to a sheet of postage stamps. After the fetus is delivered, in the presence of strong uterine contractions, the placental site is markedly reduced in size. This reduced size causes the anchor villi to break and the placenta to separate from its attachments. Normally the first few strong contractions 5 to 7 minutes after the birth of the baby shear the placenta from the basal plate. A placenta will not be easily freed from a flaccid (relaxed) uterus because the placental site is not reduced in size.

Assessment

Placental separation is indicated by the following (Fig. 15-23):

1. A firmly contracting fundus
2. A change in the uterus from a discoid to a globular ovoid shape, as the placenta moves to the lower segment
3. A sudden gush of dark blood from the introitus
4. Apparent lengthening of the umbilical cord as the placenta gets closer to the introitus
5. A vaginal fullness (the placenta) noted on vaginal or rectal examination, or fetal membranes seen at the introitus

Whether the placenta presents by the shiny fetal surface (Schultze mechanism) or whether it turns to show first its dark roughened maternal surface (Duncan's mechanism) is of no clinical importance. After the placenta with its membranes is born, it is examined for intactness to be certain that no portion of it remains in the uterine cavity (that is, no retained fragments of the placenta or membranes) (Fig. 15-24).

Maternal Physical Status

Physiologic changes after delivery are profound. The cardiac output is increased rapidly as maternal circulation to the placenta ceases and the pooled blood from the lower extremities is mobilized. The pulse rate slows in response to the change in cardiac output. Pulse rates tend to remain slightly slower than before pregnancy during the first 7 to 10 days after delivery.

The BP usually returns to the woman's usual nonpregnant levels shortly after delivery. Several factors contribute to an elevated blood pressure: the excitement of the second stage, certain medications, and the time of day (blood pressure is highest during the late afternoon). Analgesics and anesthetics may lead to hypotension in the hour following birth.

Even as the physician or nurse-midwife is completing the third stage of labor, the nurse observes the

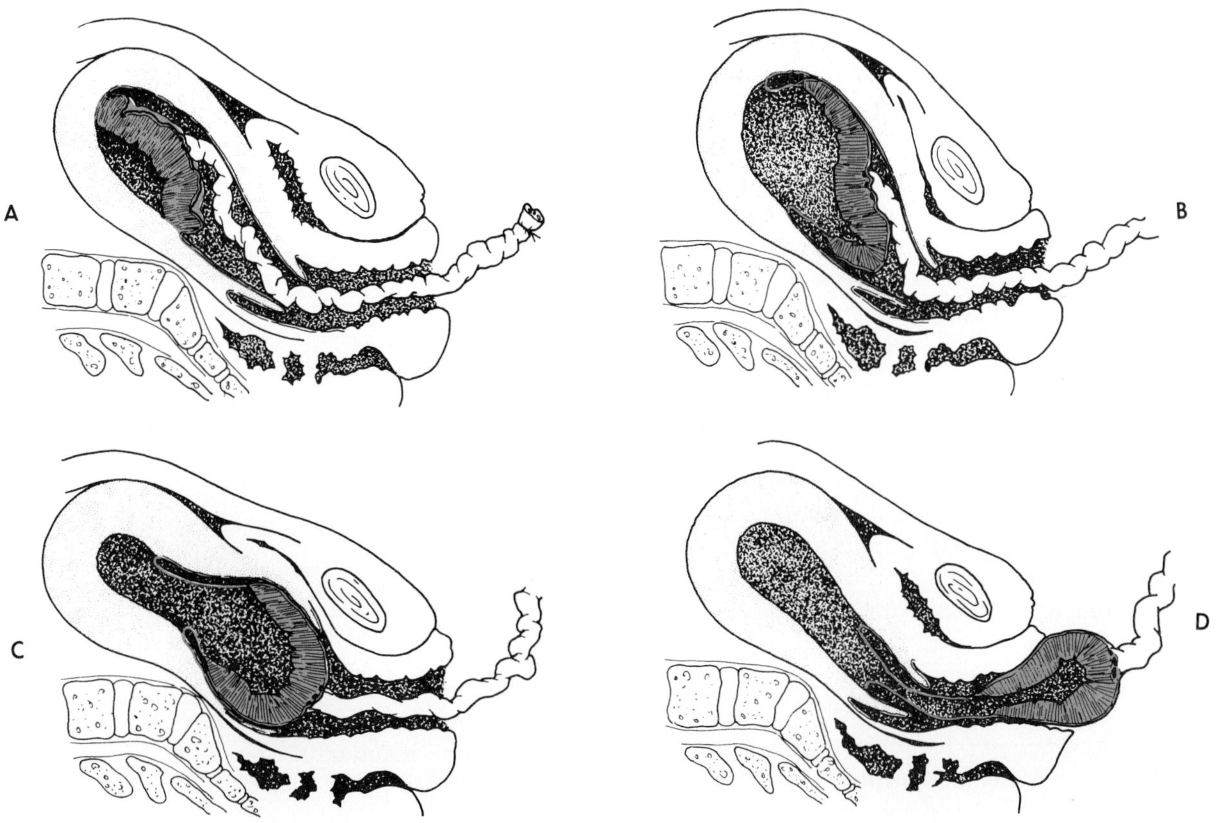

Fig. 15-23 Third stage of labor. **A,** Placenta begins by separating in central portion with retroplacental bleeding. Uterus changes from discoid to globular shape. **B,** Placenta completes separation and enters lower uterine segment. Uterus is globular in shape. **C,** Placenta enters vagina, cord is seen to lengthen, and there may be increase in bleeding. **D,** Expression (birth) of placenta and completion of third stage.

mother for signs of an altered level of consciousness (LOC) or alteration in respirations. Because of the rapid cardiovascular changes (e.g., the increased intracranial pressure during pushing and the rapid increase in cardiac output), this period represents the risk of *rupture of a preexisting cerebral aneurysm* and of pulmonary emboli. The risk of *pulmonary amniotic fluid emboli* arises from another source as well. As the placenta separates, there is a possibility of amniotic fluid entering the maternal circulation if the uterine musculature does not contract rapidly and well. The incidence of these possible complications is small; however, the alert nurse can contribute to their immediate recognition and the prompt initiation of therapy.

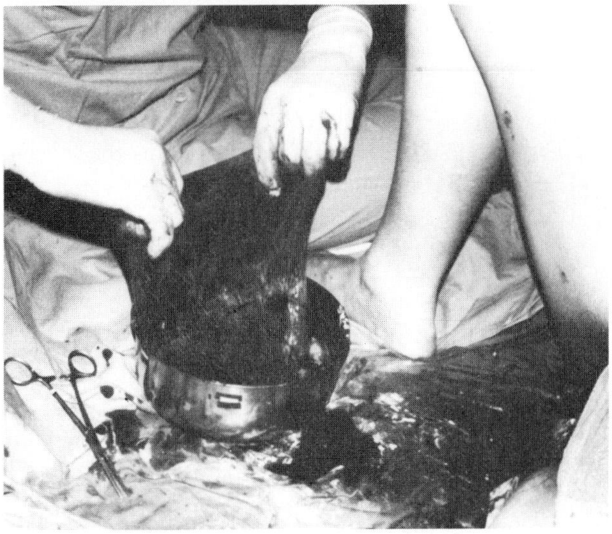

Fig. 15-24 Examination of the placenta. (Courtesy Marjorie Pyle, RNC, Lifecircle, Costa Mesa, Calif.)

Nursing Diagnoses

Before establishing nursing diagnoses, the nurse correlates the events of the third stage and the mother's physical and emotional responses to the third stage of labor. The following are examples of nursing diagnoses:

Ineffective individual (mother) coping related to

- Lack of preparation for sensations that occur during third stage of labor

Knowledge deficit related to

- Procedure for delivery of placenta

Planning

Planning for this stage focuses on the woman's rapid physiologic changes and timely intact delivery of the placenta. Concomitantly, the emotional environment of the family is maintained.

Goals for the third stage of labor may include:

1. The placenta is expelled and blood loss is less than 500 ml
2. The mother is prepared for the sensations she will experience
3. Mother and family initiate the **bonding** process

Implementation

To assist the mother in delivery of placenta, the nurse or physician instructs the woman to push when signs of separation have occurred. If an oxytocin medication is ordered, the nurse administers the medication in the dosage and by the route indicated by the physician or nurse-midwife. If possible, the placenta should be expelled by maternal effort during a uterine contraction but assistance such as *alternate compression* and *elevation of the fundus,* plus *minimum,* controlled traction on the umbilical cord may be employed to facilitate delivery of the placenta and membranes. When the third stage is complete and tears or episiotomy are sutured (p. 419), the vulva area is gently cleansed with sterile water by the physician or nurse-midwife. The circulating nurse or the physician performs the following:

1. Applies a sterile perineal pad
2. Removes the drapes if used, or places dry linen under the buttocks
3. Repositions the delivery table or bed
4. Lowers the mother's legs simultaneously from the stirrups if she is in lithotomy position
5. Assists the woman onto her bed if she is to be transferred from the delivery area to the recovery area; the nurse should request assistance to move the woman from a delivery table onto a bed if the woman has had anesthesia and does not have full use of her lower extremities
6. Dresses the woman in a clean gown and covers her with a warmed blanket
7. Raises the side rails of the bed during the transfer (in some hospitals, the mother is given the baby to hold during the transfer; in some hospitals, the father carries the baby; in other hospitals, the nurse carries the baby either to the nursery or to the recovery area for the duration of the mother's recovery period)

If the woman labors, gives birth, and recovers in the same bed and room, she is refreshed as described above. After the woman is discharged, the delivery area is cleaned as necessary.

The Family During the Third Stage. Most parents enjoy being able to handle, hold, explore, and examine the baby immediately after birth. Both parents can assist with the thorough drying of the infant. The infant may be wrapped in a receiving blanket and placed on the mother's abdomen. If skin-to-skin contact is desired, the unwrapped infant may be placed on the mother's abdomen and then covered with a warm blanket.

The mother may cut the cord or the cord may be left long enough so that the father can clamp it and cut off the extra portion. The mother can hold the infant next to her skin to maintain the baby's body heat and provide skin contact; care must be taken to keep the head warm as well. It is the nurse's responsibility to make sure the baby is kept warm and is in no danger of slipping from the parent's grasp.

Many women wish to begin to breastfeed their infants at this time to take advantage of the infant's alert state and to stimulate the production of oxytocin that promotes contraction of the uterus. Others wish to wait until the infant, mother, father, and older siblings are together in the recovery room.

While the physician carries out the postdelivery vaginal examination and, if necessary, repairs the episiotomy, the mother usually feels discomfort. Therefore while the process is being completed, the infant can be weighed and measured, wrapped in warm blankets, and given to the father to hold.

Parent-Newborn Relationships. The mother's reaction to the sight of her newborn may range from excited outbursts of laughing, talking, and even crying to apparent apathy. A polite smile and nod may acknowledge the comments of nurses and physicians. Occasionally the reaction is one of anger or indifference; the mother turns away from the baby, concentrates on her own pain, and sometimes makes hostile comments. These varying reactions can arise from pleasure, exhaustion, or deep disappointment. Whatever the reaction and cause may be, the mother needs continuing acceptance and support from all the staff. A written form accompanying the baby's chart should record the parent's reaction at birth. How do parents *look?* What do they *say?* What do they *do?*

Some warning signs in parent-child relationships ap-

WARNING SIGNS: PARENT-NEWBORN RELATIONSHIPS IMMEDIATELY AFTER DELIVERY

1. Passive reaction, either verbal or nonverbal (parents do not touch, hold, or examine baby or talk in affectionate terms or tones about baby)
2. Hostile reaction, either verbal or nonverbal (parents make inappropriate verbalization, glances, or disparaging remarks about physical characteristics of child)
3. Disappointment over sex of baby
4. No eye contact
5. Nonsupportive interaction between parents (if interaction seems dubious, talk to nurse and physician involved with delivery for further information)

Reproduced by permission from Gray JD et al: Semin Perinatal 3:95, Jan, 1979.

parent immediately following delivery are listed in the box, above).

Siblings, who may have appeared only remotely interested in the final phases of the second stage, experience renewed interest and excitement and should be encouraged to hold the new family member (Fig. 15-25).

Parents are responsive to praise of their newborn. Many require reassurance that the blue appearance of the baby after delivery is normal until respirations are well established. The reason for the molding of the baby's head must be reviewed with parents. Information about hospital routine as to future parent-child contacts can be repeated. The hospital staff, by their interest and concern, can do much to make this a satisfying experience for parents, family, and significant others.

Evaluation

Evaluation of outcomes is an ongoing activity. During each encounter with the new mother during the third stage of labor, the nurse evaluates the degree to which goals for care are being met. If the evaluation shows that results fall short of achieving any goal, further assessment, planning, and implementation are warranted.

Care of the Newborn

Care immediately following delivery focuses on assessing and stabilizing the newborn. The nurse has primary responsibility for the infant during this period, because the physician will be involved with delivery of the placenta and care of the mother. The nurse must be alert for any signs of distress and initiate appropriate interventions.

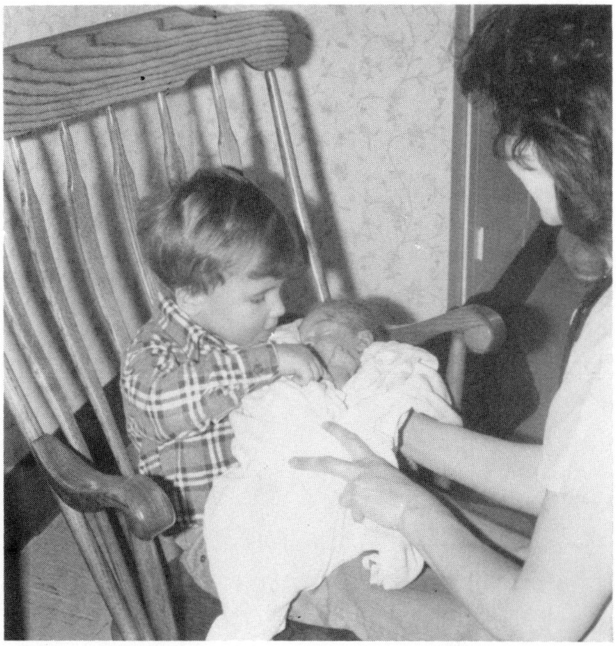

Fig. 15-25 Nurse helps big brother become acquainted with new baby sister.

Assessment

Before birth, the nurse evaluates the maternal history, including labor, to identify potential problems for the neonate and alerts the nursery to any potential problems. Although an extensive examination will be performed later, a minimum examination of the newborn is completed immediately after birth.

The **Apgar Score** permits a rapid and semiquantitative assessment based on five signs indicative of the physiologic state of the neonate (Fig 17-1): ***heart rate,*** based on auscultation with stethoscope; ***respiration,*** based on observed movement of chest wall, ***muscle tone,*** based on degree of flexion and movement of the extremities; ***reflex ability,*** based on response to gentle slaps on the soles of the feet; and ***color*** (pallid, cyanotic, or pink). The 5-minute score correlates with neonatal mortality and morbidity. In addition, the nurse makes the following assessments and records findings:

1. Assesses respirations and neonate's ability to keep airway clear
2. Estimates infant's health status using Apgar rating at 1 and 5 minutes of age
3. Examines the cord for anomalies and verifies the presence of two arteries and one vein (Fig. 15-26), checks cord clamp is in place (Figs. 15-27 and 15-28)
4. Collects cord blood from placenta for analysis (Rh factor, blood grouping, and hematocrit)
5. Assesses weight, length, head circumference, and gestational age

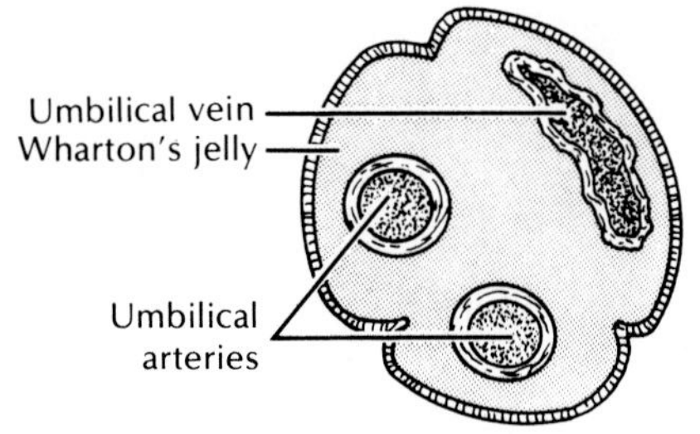

Fig. 15-26 Cross section of umbilical cord. Note collapsed appearance of thin-walled umbilical vein and contour of thicker, muscular-walled arteries.

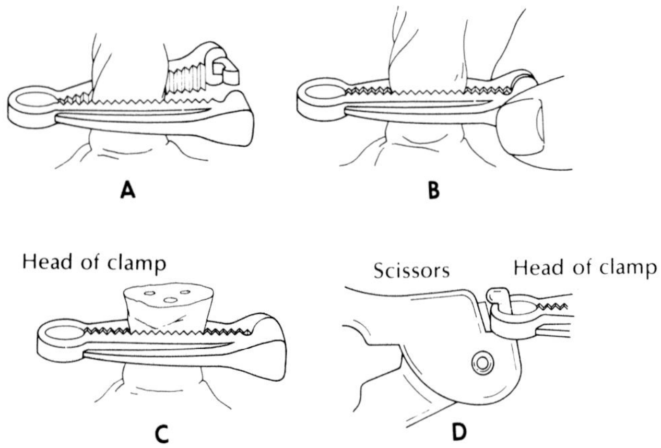

Fig. 15-27 Hollister cord clamp. **A**, Position clamp close to umbilicus. **B**, Secure cord. **C**, Cut cord. **D**, Remove clamp, using scissors, after cord dries (about 24 hours).

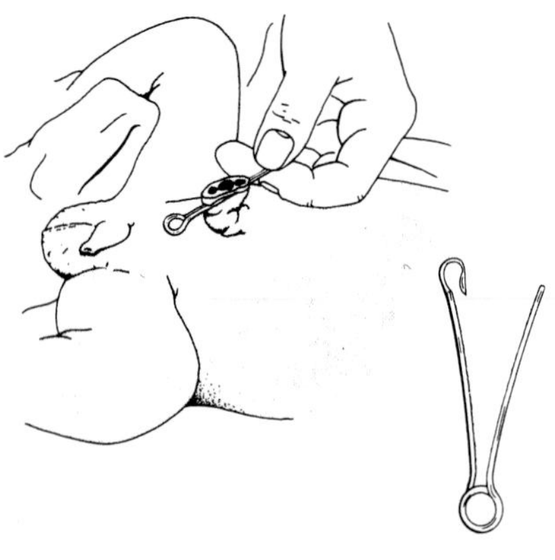

Fig. 15-28 Hesseltine cord clamp.

6. Notes passage of meconium or urine
7. Performs minimum physical examination and assessment of neonate such as the following (see Chapter 16 for more in-depth discussion and techniques):
   a. *External:* notes skin color, staining, peeling, or wasting (dysmaturity); considers length of nails and development of creases on soles of feet; checks for presence or absence of breast tissue; assesses nasal patency by closing one nostril at a time while observing the infant's respirations and color; notes meconium staining of cord, skin, fingernails, or amniotic fluid (may indicate fetal hypoxia; offensive odor may indicate intrauterine infection)
   b. *Chest:* palpates for site of maximum cardiac impulse and auscultates for rate and quality of heart tones and murmurs, compares and notes character of respirations and presence of rales or rhonchi by holding stethoscope in each axilla
   c. *Abdomen:* verifies presence of a domed abdomen and absence of anomalies; assesses umbilical cord (Chapter 16)
   d. *Neurologic:* checks muscle tone and reflex reaction and appraises Moro's reflex; palpates large fontanel for fullness or bulge; notes by palpation the presence and sizes of the sutures and fontanels
   e. *Other observations:* notes gross structure malformations obvious at birth (described in general terms and recorded on delivery record)
8. Assesses parents' response to newborn and to each other; assessment of the parent-child relationship is discussed under the nursing care of the mother during the fourth stage of labor (see p. 424)

Nursing Diagnoses

Nursing diagnoses lend direction to the type of nursing actions needed to implement a plan of care. Before establishing nursing diagnoses, the nurse analyzes the significance of findings collected during assessment. Following are some examples of nursing diagnoses:

Ineffective airway clearance related to
- Airway obstruction with mucus and amniotic fluid

Ineffective thermoregulation related to
- Environmental factors
- Amniotic fluid moisture

Altered health maintenance related to
- Congenital disorders

Table 15-7 Nursing Care of the Neonate

Intervention	Rationale
AIRWAY	
Hold baby with head lowered (10 to 15 degrees)	Uses gravity to help remove fluids
Suction oral pharynx with small bulb syringe as soon as head is born	Expedites drainage and prevents aspiration of amniotic fluid, mucus, and blood (maternal)
Suction nares next	Prevents inspiration following stimulation of nares before mouth is clear
Avoid deep suctioning with catheter, if possible	May cause bradycardia or laryngospasm or both
Avoid suspending neonate by ankles	Results in hyperextension of baby whose entire development occurred in flexed position
CORD CLAMPING	
Immediately following birth, neonate is kept at about the same level as uterus, until cord clamp is applied or until cord has stopped pulsating	If neonate is held above level of uterus, gravity drains blood to placenta
Without "stripping" it, cord is clamped close to umbilicus approximately 30 seconds after birth if neonate appears normal and mature	Ordinarily it is unwise to strip cord before clamping and cutting because postdelivery red blood cell destruction will be increased and hyperbilirubinemia may ensue; in addition, polycythemia (increased number of red blood cells) increases blood viscosity, leading to cardiopulmonary problems
Cord is clamped 8 to 10 cm from umbilicus if there is a possibility for exchange transfusion	Permits access to umbilical vessels
Assess cord for two arteries and one vein (see Fig. 15-26)	Absence indicates need for further assessment
ATTACHMENT AND WARMTH	
Unless immediate intervention is required, dry infant and place on mother's abdomen, covering both; or wrap infant in warm blanket first	Facilitates attachment Assures and relaxes mother
Caution parents to keep neonate's head covered	Prevents cold stress
Permit mother to breastfeed as desired	Facilitates uterine contractions and expulsion of placenta
APGAR SCORE	
Appraise neonate at 1 minute and again at 5 minutes, using Apgar scoring method (see p. 413 and Fig. 17-1)	Permits rapid and semiquantitative assessment based on signs indicative of physiologic state; 5-minute score correlates with neonatal mortality and morbidity
EYE PROPHYLAXIS	
Instill medication per agency policy (Fig. 15-29)	Meets legal requirements
NEWBORN WEIGHT AND LENGTH	
Weigh and measure the neonate; this may be delayed until the fourth stage	Parents are usually anxious to know and want to share data with relatives and friends.
IDENTIFICATION	
Identify the neonate by one of a number of techniques *before mother or baby leaves the delivery area.*	Although rare, an occasional mix-up in the identity of newborns occurs; identification and care to check both mother's and baby's ID numbers prevent unnecessary anxiety and legal complications

Planning

During this important step, goals are set in client-centered terms. The goals are prioritized. Nursing actions are selected, with the client where appropriate, to meet the goals. ***Goals*** for the infant during the recovery period include:

1. Airway remains clear
2. Temperature remains within normal limits
3. Potential injury is avoided
4. The bonding process is facilitated

Implementation

Events move rapidly during this time period. Assessment must be followed quickly by appropriate implementation. The physician/midwife may be concentrating on the progress of the third stage for the mother. The nurse assumes responsibility and accountability for accurate assessment of and timely intervention for the newborn.

Initiation and maintenance of respiration is the top priority. Abnormal breathing must be recognized and treated (see danger signs box, p. 491, and emergency procedure, p. 495, Chapter 17).

Nursing actions that usually apply to this period include a variety of activities. Among them are actions relevant to the care of the airway, cord clamping, attachment and warmth, Apgar score, eye prophylaxis, measurement of weight and length, and identification. A summary of these nursing actions and the rationale for each are given in Table 15-7.

Eye Prophylaxis. Instillation of a prophylactic agent in the eyes of all newborns is mandatory in the United States. In some Canadian institutions the parents may sign a form refusing **eye prophylaxis.** In the United States, if the family objects to this treatment, the physician must request the parents to sign an informed consent and note their refusal in the neonate's record. The agent used for prophylaxis varies according to hospital protocols. Canadian hospitals have not recommended the use of silver nitrate since 1986. In some institutions instillation of eye prophylaxis is delayed until an hour or so after birth. This facilitates eye contact and enhances attachment. The Centers for Disease Control specify that a delay of up to 2 hours is safe.

Evaluation

Evaluation of nursing care and outcomes is an ongoing activity in the care of both mother and baby. During the third stage of labor, the nurse evaluates the degree to which goals for care are being met. If the evaluation shows that results fall short of achieving any goal, further assessment, planning, and implementation are warranted.

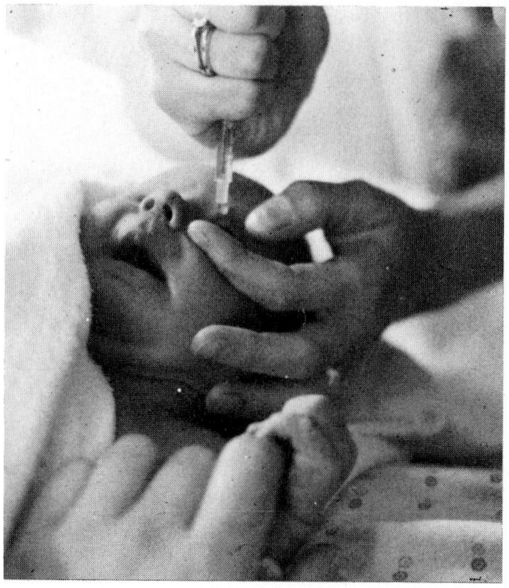

Fig. 15-29 Instillation of ophthalmic erythromycin drops using needleless syringe. Drops are instilled into conjunctival sac.

❑ EMERGENCY CHILDBIRTH

Even under the best of circumstances there will probably come a time when the maternity nurse will be required to deliver an infant without medical assistance. Consider the precipitous multipara who arrives at the community hospital fully dilated in the middle of the night. As it is impossible to prevent an impending delivery, the maternity nurse needs to be able to function independently and to be skilled in safely delivering a vertex fetus.

The following measures are necessary for the emergency birth of a fetus in the vertex position:

1. The woman will usually assume the position most suitable for her. If she is in a bed and there is time, elevate the head of the bed about 45 degrees. This position, in addition to facilitating perfusion of the uterus, allows you to maintain eye-to-eye contact with the woman. Occasionally the woman will assume the crawling position, on hands and knees. Some women will stand and lean over a bed or their support person's shoulder. Others will assume a side-lying position.
2. Reassure the woman verbally with eye-to-eye contact and a calm, relaxed manner. If there is someone else available (e.g., the father), that

person could help support her in position, assist with coaching, and compliment her on her efforts.

3. Wash your hands with soap and water or wash-and-dry pledgets if possible.
4. Place under woman's buttocks whatever clean material is available. *Do not* break the table if no physician is available.
5. Avoid touching the vaginal area to decrease the possibility of infection. (If there is time, scrub your hands and fingernails for 5 minutes before touching the parturient.) If hands are clean or sterile gloves are available, massage or support perineum as needed. Use Universal Precautions for body fluids at all times (Chapter 23).
6. The perineum thins and distends. As the head begins to crown, the birth attendant should do the following:
   a. Tear the amniotic membrane (caul) if it is still intact.
   b. Instruct the woman to pant or pant-blow, thus avoiding the urge to push.
   c. Place the flat side of the hand on the exposed fetal head and apply *gentle* pressure toward the vagina to prevent the head from "popping out." The mother may participate by placing her hand under yours on the emerging head.

      NOTE: Rapid delivery of the fetal head must be prevented because it is followed by a rapid change of pressure within the molded fetal skull, which may result in dural or subdural tears, and it may cause vaginal or perineal lacerations.
7. Instruct the mother to pant or pant-blow as you check for an umbilical cord. If the cord is around the neck, try to slip it up over the baby's head or pull *gently* to get some slack so that it can slip down over the shoulders.
8. Support the fetal head as restitution (external rotation) occurs. After restitution, with one hand on each side of the baby's head, exert *gentle* pressure downward so that the anterior shoulder emerges under the symphysis pubis and acts as a fulcrum; then as *gentle* pressure is exerted in the opposite direction, the posterior shoulder, which has passed over the sacrum and coccyx, is delivered.
9. Be alert! Hold the baby securely because the rest of the body may deliver quickly. The baby will be slippery!
10. Cradle the baby's head and back in one hand and the buttocks in the other, keeping the head down to drain away the mucus. Use a bulb syringe to remove mucus if one is available.

    NOTE: Do not hold the baby upside down by the ankles because to do so (1) hyperextends the spine, which has been flexed since conception; (2) increases intracranial pressure and the danger of capillary rupture; (3) may cause direct tissue trauma to the ankles; and (4) increases the possibility of dropping a wet, slippery baby.
11. Dry the baby rapidly (to prevent rapid heat loss), keeping the baby at the same level as the mother's uterus.

    NOTE: Keep the baby at the same level to prevent gravity flow of baby's blood to or from the placenta and the resultant hypovolemia or hypervolemia. Also, do not "milk" the cord: hypervolemia can cause respiratory distress initially or hyperbilirubinemia subsequently (Chapter 28); and if isoimmunization has occurred, the baby may receive an additional inoculation of harmful antibodies (e.g., anti-Rh positive or anti-A or anti-B antibodies).
12. As soon as the infant is crying, place the baby on mother's abdomen, cover baby (remember to keep head warm too) with her clothing, and have her cuddle baby. Compliment her (them) on a job well done and on the baby if appropriate. (If something appears to be the matter with the baby, do not lie!) She may wish to expose the part of the baby that will be touching her skin for skin-to-skin contact.

    NOTE: Soon after the **Wharton's jelly** in the cord is exposed to cool air and shrinks and the infant cries, the umbilical vessels stop pulsating and the blood flow ceases. The baby's presence on the mother's abdomen stimulates the release of oxytocin from the posterior pituitary and thus stimulates uterine contractions, which aid in placental separation.
13. *Wait* for the placenta to separate; *do not* tug on the cord.

    NOTE: Injudicious traction may tear the cord, separate the placenta, or invert the uterus. Signs of placental separation include a slight gush of dark blood from the introitus, lengthening of the cord, and change in uterine contour from discoid to globular shape.
14. Instruct the mother to push to deliver the separated placenta. Gently ease out the placental membranes, using an up-and-down motion until membranes are removed. If delivery is occurring outside of the hospital setting, to minimize complications do not cut the cord without proper clamps or ties and a sterile cutting tool and inspect the placenta for intactness. Place the baby on the placenta and wrap the two together for additional warmth.

NOTE: There is no hurry to cut the cord. The infant will not lose blood through the placenta because the cord circulation ceases (clots) within minutes of birth. If a cord tie is needed, use technique in Fig. 15-30.

15. Check the firmness of the uterus. Gently massage the uterus and demonstrate to the mother how she can massage her own uterus properly.
16. Clean the area under the mother's buttocks.
17. Prevent or minimize hemorrhage.
    a. Hemorrhage from uterine atony.
        (1) *Gently* massage fundus to stimulate uterine musculature to contract.
        NOTE: Overstimulation may fatigue the myometrium and cause atony.
        (2) Put the baby to the breast as soon as possible. Sucking or nuzzling and licking the breast stimulate the release of oxytocin from the posterior pituitary.
        NOTE: If the baby does not nurse, manually stimulate the mother's breasts.
        (3) If medical assistance is delayed, do not allow the mother's bladder to become distended.
        (4) Expel any clots from her uterus.
        NOTE: The fundus should be firm to prevent accidental inversion during this procedure. While holding the bottom of the uterus just above the symphysis pubis, apply gentle pressure on the firm fundus downward toward the vagina.
    b. Hemorrhage from perineal lacerations.
        (1) Apply a clean pad to the perineum.
        (2) Instruct the mother to press her thighs together.
18. Comfort or reassure the mother and her family or friends. Keep her and the baby warm. Give her fluids if available and tolerated.

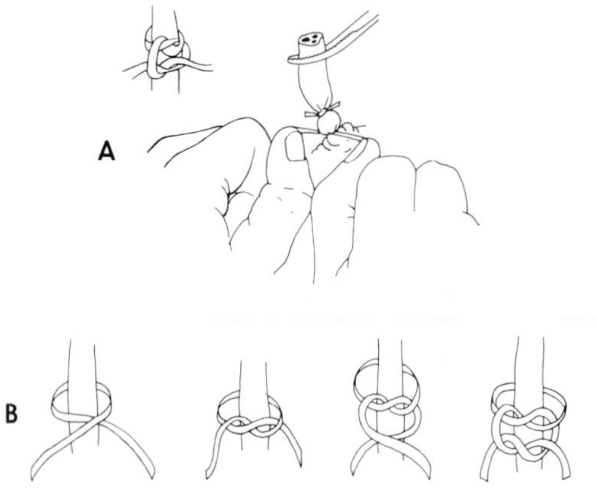

Fig. 15-30 Technique of tying off umbilical cord using **A**, soft flat tape to prevent cutting through cord as it is drawn tight and **B**, square knot to prevent slippage.

19. If this is a multifetal birth, identify the infants in order of birth.
20. Make notations on the birth.
    a. Fetal presentation and position.
    b. Presence of cord around neck or other parts and number of times cord encircles part.
    c. Color, character, and amount of amniotic fluid.
    d. Time of delivery.
    e. Estimated time of Apgar score, resuscitation, and ultimate condition of baby.
    f. Sex of baby.
    g. Approximate time of placental expulsion, its appearance, and completeness.
    h. Maternal condition: affect, amount of bleeding, and status of uterine contractions.
    i. Any unusual occurrences during the delivery (i.e., maternal or paternal response, verbalizations, or gestures to birth or newborn).

Lateral Sims' Position for Emergency Delivery

A lateral Sims' posture may be the position of choice for delivery when (1) the delivery is progressing rapidly and there is insufficient time for slow distension of the perineum; (2) the fetal head seems too large to pass through the introitus without laceration, and episiotomy is not possible; or (3) the apparent size of the fetus is consistent with possible shoulder dystocia.

In the lateral Sims' position, less stress is placed on the perineum and better visualization of the perineum is possible. In the event of shoulder dystocia, lateral Sims' posture increases the space needed for delivery.

Emergency Delivery of Preterm Infant

The actual process of birthing the preterm infant does not vary from that of the term infant. However, the care of the infant after birth requires some modification as follows:

1. Warmth is essential.
2. Minimize handling, maintain a clear airway, and feed and change the infant.
3. Nutrition may be a problem if a medical facility is not available. Although the infant may be unable to nurse at the breast, slow feeding is important, using a medicine dropper, for example.
4. Gently stimulate the preterm infant to breathe. When the infant "forgets" to breathe, rubbing the back or the soles of the feet is usually effective.
5. Transport the infant to a medical facility equipped to handle preterm infants as early as possible (Chapter 28).

❑ CHILDBIRTH TRAUMA

Episiotomy

An episiotomy is an incision made in the perineum to enlarge the vaginal outlet. Episiotomies are performed more commonly in the United States and Canada than in Europe. The use of the side-lying position for delivery is routinely used in Europe while the position with legs in stirrups is more commonly used in the United States and Canada. With the side-lying position there is less tension on the perineum and a gradual stretching of the perineum is possible. As a result the indications for use of episiotomies are less.

The proponents of use of the episiotomy maintain it serves the following purposes:

1. Prevents tearing of the perineum. The clean and properly placed incision heals more properly than does a ragged tear. Some conditions that predispose a woman to perineal tearing and are therefore indications for episiotomy are a large infant, rapid labor in which there is not sufficient time for stretching of the perineum to take place, a narrow subpubic arch with a constricted outlet, and malpresentations of the fetus (e.g., face).
2. May minimize prolonged and severe stretching of the muscles supporting the bladder or rectum, which may later lead to stress incontinence or to vaginal prolapse.
3. Reduces duration of the second stage, which may be important for maternal reasons (e.g., a hypertensive state) or fetal reasons (e.g., persistent bradycardia).
4. Enlarges the vagina in case manipulation is needed to deliver an infant, for example, in a breech presentation or for application of forceps.

Those who are opposed to the *routine* use of episiotomies maintain that:

1. The perineum can be prepared for delivery through use of the Kegel's exercises and massage in the prenatal period. Use of Kegel's exercises in the postpartum period improves and restores the tone of the perineal muscles.
2. Lacerations may occur even with the use of an episiotomy.
3. Pain and discomfort from episiotomies can interfere with mother-infant interactions and the reestablishment of parental sexual intercourse.
4. Episiotomies *are indicated* (a) if the well-being of the mother or fetus is in jeopardy, to shorten the second stage of labor, (b) if the infant is preterm and cerebral hemorrhage is a possibility because of capillary fragility, (c) if the infant is large (greater than 4000 g [9 lb]), or (d) in most forceps and breech deliveries (Pernoll and Benson, 1987).

The type of episiotomy is designated by site and direction of the incision (Fig. 15-31).

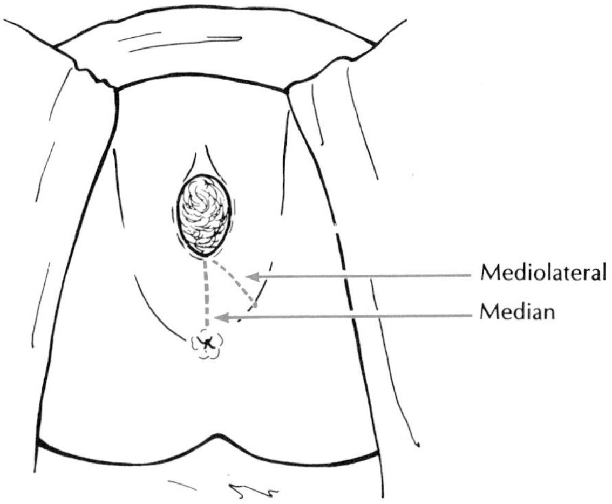

Fig. 15-31 Types of episiotomies.

Median episiotomy is the one most commonly employed. It is effective, easily repaired, and generally the least painful. Occasionally there may be an extension through the rectal sphincter (third-degree laceration) or even into the anal canal (fourth-degree laceration). Fortunately primary healing and a good repair usually will be followed by good sphincter tone.

Mediolateral episiotomy commonly is employed in operative delivery when posterior extension is likely. Although a fourth-degree laceration may thus be avoided, a third-degree laceration may occur. Moreover, as compared with a median episiotomy, blood loss is greater and the repair more difficult and painful. Repair of left mediolateral episotomy is shown in Fig. 15-32.

Lacerations

Most acute injuries and lacerations of the perineum, vagina, uterus, and their support tissues occur at parturition, and their management is an obstetric problem. Some childbirth injuries to the supporting tissues, whether they were acute or nonacute and whether they were repaired or not, may become gynecologic problems later in life.

The soft tissues of the birth canal and adjacent structures suffer some damage during every delivery. Damage is usually more pronounced in nulliparas because the tissues are firmer and more resistant than in multiparas. Perineal skin and vaginal mucosa may appear intact, obscuring numerous small lacerations in underlying muscle and its fascia. Damage to pelvic supports is usually easily apparent and thus is repaired after delivery.

The individual woman's tendency to sustain lacerations varies; for example, the soft tissue in some

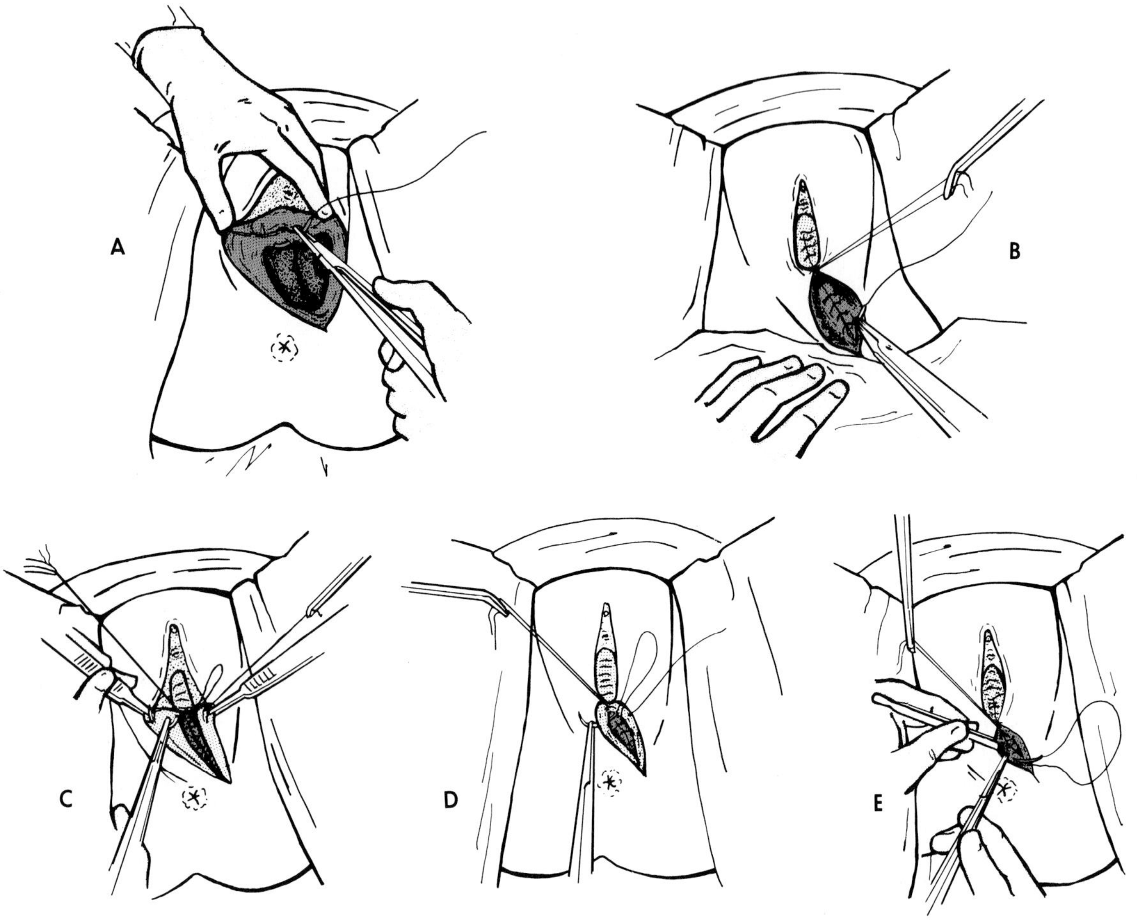

Fig. 15-32 Repair of left mediolateral episiotomy. **A** and **B**, Repair of levator muscle and its severed fascia. Attendant approximates cut edge of vaginal orifice, using forceps to exert traction on suture of bulbocavernous muscles. **C**, Repair of cut ends. **D**, Repair of muscle and fascial components of urogenital diaphragm. **E**, Closure of skin edges. Sutures are placed just under dermis so that no sutures are visible when skin edges are approximated.

women may be less capable of distension. Heredity may be a factor. For example, the tissue of very light-skinned women, especially those with reddish hair, is not as readily distensible as that of a darker-skinned woman. Women whose tissues show a tendency to lacerate may also exhibit varicose veins and diastasis recti abdominis. These women may also heal less efficiently.

Immediate repair promotes healing and limits residual damage, as well as decreases the possibility of infection. After every delivery the cervix, vagina, and perineum are inspected immediately. During the early days postdelivery, the nurse and physician carefully inspect the perineum and evaluate lochia and symptoms to identify any previously missed damage (Chapters 19 and 21).

Perineal Lacerations. Perineal lacerations usually occur as the fetal head is being born. The extent of the laceration is defined on the basis of depth.

1. *First degree.* Laceration extends through the skin and structures superficial to muscles.
2. *Second degree.* Laceration extends through muscles of perineal body.
3. *Third degree.* Laceration continues through anal sphincter muscle.
4. *Fourth degree.* Laceration also involves the anterior rectal wall.

Lacerations in the lower vagina occur along one or both lateral walls (sulci), rather than up the midline. At least the fascia of the elevator ani muscle is injured in all but the most superficial perineal tears. Perineal injury is often accompanied by small lacerations in the medial surfaces of the labia minora below the pubic rami and to the sides of the urethra and clitoris. Lacerations in this greatly vascular area result in profuse bleeding.

Immediate repair with absorbable suture (Fig. 15-33) is indicated. Third- and fourth-degree lacerations

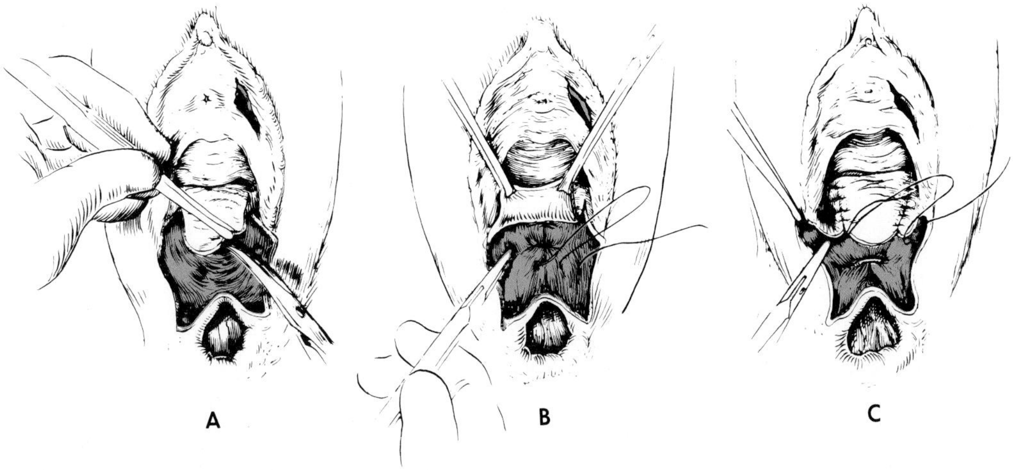

Fig. 15-33 Perineal lacerations. **A,** Bilateral sulcus tears, periurethral tear, and separation of anal sphincter. **B,** Exposure and approximation of levator ani structures. **C,** Approximation of torn bulbocavernosus muscle. (From Wellson JR: Atlas of obstetric technic, ed 2, St Louis, 1969, The CV Mosby Co.)

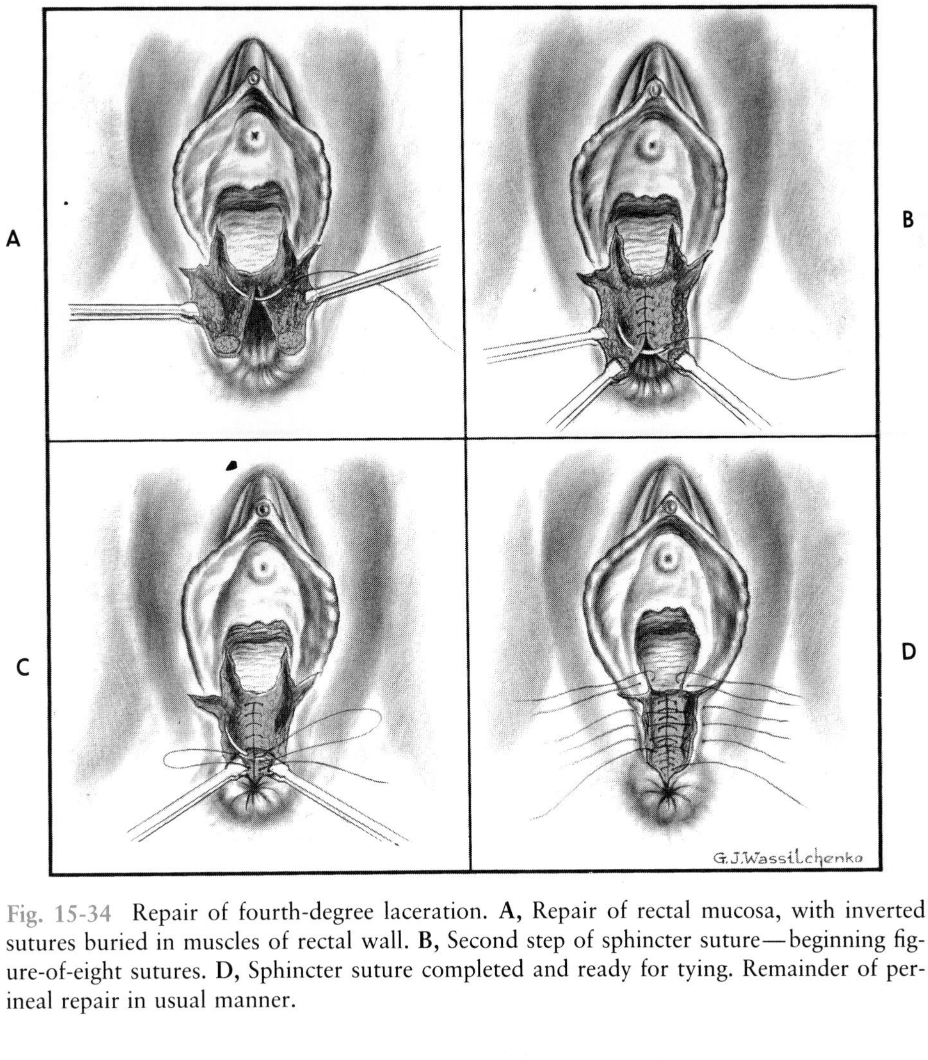

Fig. 15-34 Repair of fourth-degree laceration. **A,** Repair of rectal mucosa, with inverted sutures buried in muscles of rectal wall. **B,** Second step of sphincter suture—beginning figure-of-eight sutures. **D,** Sphincter suture completed and ready for tying. Remainder of perineal repair in usual manner.

require special attention so that the woman retains fecal continence. Postdelivery nursing care is discussed in Chapters 19 and 21. The woman's comfort is increased and healing is promoted by measures taken to ensure soft stools for a few days. Antimicrobial therapy is not deemed necessary.

When the levator ani (including the iliococcygeus and pubococcygeus muscles, which form the slinglike support of pelvic viscera) is not involved, simple perineal injuries usually heal without permanent disability regardless of whether they were repaired. However, the *vaginal introitus may gape* if torn or severed (episiotomy) ends of superficial perineal muscles (e.g., bulbocavernosus) are not well approximated during repair.

The ends of the torn or severed anal sphincter muscles must be repaired adequately to avoid *fecal incontinence* (Fig. 15-34). It is easier to repair a new perineal injury to prevent sequelae than it is to correct long-term damage.

Vaginal Lacerations. Vaginal lacerations often accompany perineal lacerations. Vaginal lacerations tend to extend up the lateral walls (sulci) and, if deep enough, to involve the levator ani. Additional injury may occur high in the vaginal vault near the level of the ischial spines. Vaginal vault lacerations may be circular and may result from forceps rotation, especially in the presence of cephalopelvic disproportion (CPD) (Chapter 26).

A cervical or vaginal laceration extending into the broad ligament should *not* be repaired vaginally. Laparotomy with evacuation of the resultant hematoma and hemostatic repair or hysterectomy will be required (Pernoll and Benson, 1987).

The location of the lacerations and the rapid and profuse bleeding make it difficult to expose and repair these tears. Late sequelae and management depend on the injury and the results of subsequent repair of injuries to the levator ani (Chapter 24).

Cervical Injuries. The greatest percentage of cervical injuries are obstetric in origin and occur when the cervix is being retracted over the advancing fetal head. Obstetrically acquired *cervical lacerations* usually occur at the lateral angles of the external os; most are shallow and bleeding is minimal (Fig. 15-35). More extensive lacerations may extend to the vaginal vault or beyond the vault into the lower uterine segment; serious bleeding may occur. Extensive lacerations may follow injudicious attempts to enlarge the cervical opening artificially or to deliver the fetus before full cervical dilatation is achieved.

Anterior lip incarceration can occur. Occasionally the cervix is injured if the anterior lip is trapped between the fetal head and the pubic bone, an event that occurs most often when there is some degree of cephalopelvic disproportion (Chapter 26). Since the trapped (incarcerated) cervix cannot be retracted upward

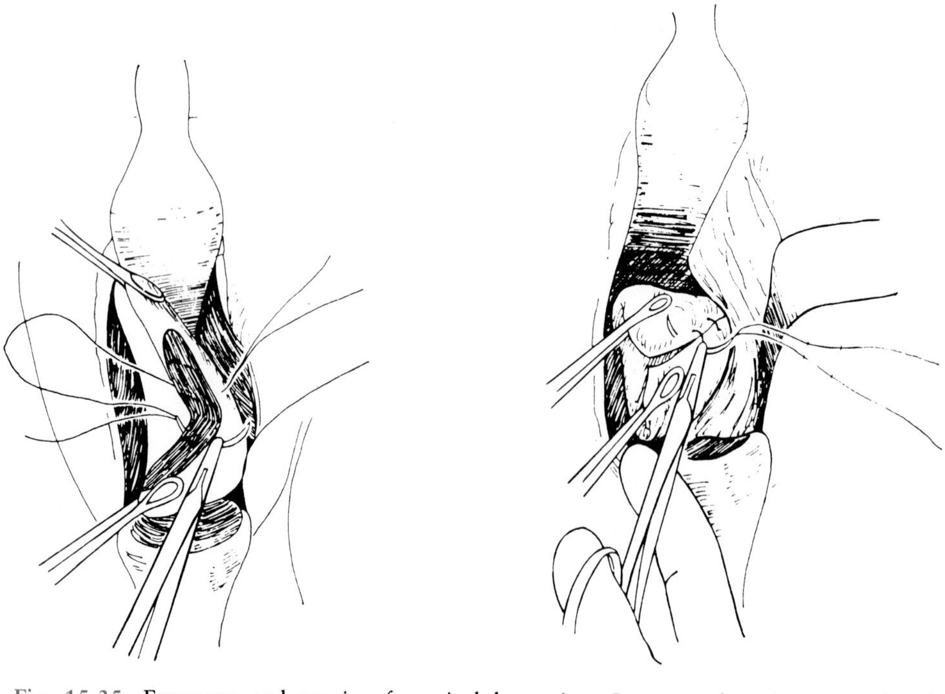

Fig. 15-35 Exposure and repair of cervical laceration. Interrupted sutures are placed through entire thickness of cervix. (From Willson JR et al: Obstetrics and gynecology, ed 7, St Louis, 1983, The CV Mosby Co.)

around the descending head, the lower uterine segment above it thins excessively and may rupture. The anterior lip becomes edematous, bruised and almost black in color, and diffused with blood. The condition is exacerbated by women pushing before full dilatation of the cervix (p. 393). Unless the anterior lip is freed by pushing the head upward and easing the cervix over the head, the entire cervix may be torn loose; this condition is called *annular amputation*.

Uterine Rupture. The most serious of childbirth injuries, rupture of the uterus, occurs approximately once in 1500 to 2000 deliveries. Although the uterus may rupture during pregnancy, the uterine wall usually gives way during the stresses of labor. Hysterectomy may be indicated if the uterus is severely damaged. Uterine rupture is discussed in Chapter 26.

❑ FOURTH STAGE OF LABOR

The fourth stage of labor, the stage of recovery, is a critical period for the mother and newborn, who are not only recovering from the physical process of birth, but are also initiating new relationships.

During the first 2 hours after the birth, the maternal organism makes its initial readjustment to the nonpregnant state, and body systems begin to stabilize. The newborn continues with the transition from intrauterine to extrauterine existence. Since many parents are opting for early discharge from the hospital, and others must leave because of diagnosis related group (DRG) and insurance requirements, the health care team must be reasonably assured that there is no potential for disruption in these normal processes for the mother or newborn. The nurse's skills as a technician, teacher/counselor/advocate, and support person can make a critical difference during the fourth stage. Some important terms are defined below:

puerperium Variable period, usually 6 to 8 weeks, that begins with the delivery of the placenta and ends either with the resumption of ovulatory menstrual periods or when involuntary changes that result in the nonparous state are complete (e.g., after postdelivery hysterectomy); the postpartum period; the postnatal period; the postdelivery period.

p. immediate The first 24 hours after delivery.

involution Process that results in the healing of the birth canal and the return of the uterus and all systems to or almost to the prepregnant state. Generally, changes reflect reversals of the anatomic and physiologic adaptations to pregnancy.

lochia Uterine discharge after delivery.

atonic uterus A lack of tone in the uterine muscle caused by interference with the ability of the muscle to contract and retract.

Assessment

If the nurse has not previously cared for the new mother, assessment begins with review of the prenatal and labor record. In many institutions the labor nurse now follows the woman through the initial 2 hours after delivery. Of primary importance are conditions that could predispose the mother to hemorrhage (such as precipitous labor, large baby, grand miltiparity, or induced labor), which is a potential danger during the fourth stage of labor.

To help the nurse provide comprehensive care, a worksheet is suggested. On a busy unit even experienced nurses appreciate a checklist. During the first hour in the recovery room, physical assessment of the mother is frequent. All factors except temperature are assessed every 15 minutes for 1 hour. After the fourth 15-minute assessment, if all parameters have stabilized within the normal range, assessment is repeated twice more at 30-minute intervals. The physical assessment of the mother during the fourth stage of labor is given in Procedure 15-3). The area of examination and purpose, the method of assessment, and findings within normal limits are discussed briefly.

Nursing Diagnoses

Nursing diagnoses lend direction to the type of nursing action needed to implement a plan of care. Before establishing nursing diagnoses, the nurse analyzes the significance of findings collected during assessment. Examples of nursing diagnoses include the following:

Potential for hemorrhage,* related to
- Uterine atony

Urinary retention related to
- Effects of labor and delivery on urinary tract sensation

Pain related to
- Childbirth trauma

Potential for injury related to
- Early ambulation

Potential altered parenting related to
- Postpartum pain or fatigue

Altered family processes related to
- Addition of new member

Ineffective breastfeeding related to
- Lack of experience

*Not approved by the North American Nursing Diagnosis Association (NANDA) at this time.

PROCEDURE 15-3

ASSESSMENT DURING FOURTH STAGE OF LABOR

DEFINITION

Physical assessment of woman in the immediate postpartum period.

PURPOSE

To monitor the new mother's physical recovery from childbirth through accurate assessment of vital signs and blood pressure, uterine involution and lochial discharge, bladder function, and condition of perineum.

EQUIPMENT

Blood pressure cuff and sphygmomanometer; thermometer; light source; prn supplies: gloves, perineal pads, wash cloth, soap, warm water, towels, ice bags.

NURSING ACTIONS	RATIONALE
Assemble equipment.	Saves time and avoids leaving woman until after assessment is completed.
Explain procedure.	Reduces anxiety and elicits cooperation.
Wash hands.	Prevents nosocomial infection.
Blood pressure	
Measure per assessment schedule	Provides data base for diagnosis of complications (e.g., hemorrhage), usually stabilizes at prelabor values during first hour.
Pulse:	
Count pulse, assess rate, amplitude (indicating volume), rhythm and symmetry, regularity.	Provides data base for diagnosis of complications; usually stabilizes at prelabor levels during first hour.
Temperature	
Determine temperature.	Provide data base for diagnosis of complications; usually stabilizes within normal range during first hour, or slight elevation to 38° C (100.4° F) related to dehydration.
Fundus	
Apply gloves, prn.	Implements universal precautions.
Position woman with knees flexed.	Relieves tension on abdomen and facilitates palpation.
Just below umbilicus, cup hand, press firmly into abdomen.	Locates fundus.
If fundus is firm (and bladder is empty), with uterus in midline, measure its position relative to woman's umbilicus. Lay fingers flat on abdomen under umbilicus; measure how many fingerbreadths fit between umbilicus and top of fundus.	Monitors uterine involution. Provides data base for possible deviations from normal (e.g., atonic uterus, **retained placental fragments**).
If fundus is *not* firm, stimulate "living ligature" to regain tone and expel any clots before measuring distance from umbilicus.	Facilitates more accuracy in assessment and assists in prevention of hemorrhage.
Place hands appropriately, massage gently only until firm.	Avoids overstimulation, which causes muscle fatigue and relaxation.
Expel clots while keeping hands placed as in Fig. 15-36. With upper hand, firmly apply pressure downward toward vagina; observe perineum for amount/size of expelled clots. Measure height of firm fundus.	Removes clots, which prevent uterus from retaining tone. Support of uterus during expulsion of clots prevents its inversion. Allows nurse to assess expelled clots.
Bladder	
Assess distension by noting location and firmness of uterine fundus and by observation and palpation of bladder. Distended bladder is seen as a suprapubic rounded bulge that is dull to percussion and fluctuates like a water-filled balloon. When bladder is distended, uterus may be boggy, well above umbilicus, and usually to woman's right side.	Identifies bladder fullness. Overdistension displaces uterus upward and usually to the right of the midline and prevents efficient uterine contractions, which may lead to hemorrhage.

PROCEDURE 15-3—cont'd

NURSING ACTIONS	RATIONALE
Bladder—cont'd	
Assess bladder function. Ask woman to void; measure amount of urine voided.	Identifies degree of return of normal bladder function.
Catheterize prn. Reassess and compare findings with signs of an empty bladder: fundus firm, in midline; bladder nonpalpable.	Identifies possible need for intervention (e.g., catheterization). Overdistension causes maternal discomfort, is a significant factor in uterine hemorrhage and can result in bladder atony.
Lochia	
Observe lochia on perineal pads and on linen under mother's buttocks. Determine amount and color; note size and number of clots; note odor.	Provides data base to differentiate between lochia of normal involution and discharge signaling complication such as infection or hemorrhage.
Observe perineum for source of bleeding (e.g., episiotomy, lacerations).	Allows for comparison with normal findings: Lochia rubra is moderate and may contain some small clots. Odor of normal menstrual flow. Lochia does not come out in a continuous trickle or in spurts.
Perineum	
Ask or assist woman to turn on her side and flex upper leg on hip. Lift upper buttock. Observe perineum in good lighting.	Provides data base to differentiate between birth trauma within normal limits and possible complications. Allows comparison with normal findings: vaginal birth: mild edema or labial swelling: slight bruising. Episiotomy or laceration repair is intact, dry, mildly edematous but not inflamed.

Planning

During the planning step, ***goals*** are set in client-centered terms. The goals are prioritized. Nursing actions are selected, with the client where appropriate, to meet the goals. Goals for the fourth stage of labor may include that the woman will:

1. Saturate no more than one pad per hour
2. Void within 6 to 8 hours after delivery
3. Verbalize acceptance of labor process after expressing concerns
4. Begin the bonding process with infant and family
5. Verbalize increased comfort following initiation of comfort measures

Implementation

During the fourth stage of labor, the nurse must organize care to include observation of vital signs, provision of comfort measures, education of the mother, and care of the infant. Nursing concerns include prevention of hemorrhage, prevention of urinary bladder distension, maintenance of comfort, maintenance of cleanliness, maintenance of fluid balance and nutrition, support of parental emotional needs, and promotion of maternal and infant care education. The guidelines for client teaching that follow include assessment findings, nursing actions, teaching, and evaluation for emotional and physical factors during the fourth stage of labor.

Prevent Hemorrhage

Assessments are designed for early identification of events that may lead to **hemorrhage.** The mother's temperature, pulse, and BP are assessed and recorded and should be within normal limits. The pulse rate will generally be between 60 and 70 bpm. If the pulse rate is over 90 bpm, investigation and continued supervision are necessary. The temperature may be below normal because of loss of body heat. On occasion it may be over 37.2° C (99° F.) because of dehydration, long labor, or lack of fluids. After a difficult labor, systolic BP less than 110 mm Hg and accompanied by a pulse over 100 bpm, is usually the result of hemorrhage or shock.

The uterus must be palpated at frequent intervals to

Text continued on p. 429.

Guidelines for Client Teaching
PHYSICAL FACTORS DURING THE FOURTH STAGE OF LABOR

ASSESSMENT

1. Woman has given birth within the last 2 hours.
2. Physical parameters must be observed to avoid harm to postpartum woman.
3. Uterus must remain firm to prevent hemorrhage.
4. Urinary bladder must be emptied periodically to prevent distension and boggy, or atonic uterus.
5. Watch for verbal and nonverbal cues of pain and discomfort.
6. Woman complains of fatigue.
7. Woman has elevated temperature.
8. Woman's fluid intake (oral and intravenous) limited.
9. Woman states she is hungry.
10. Effects of analgesia or anesthesia wearing off.

NURSING DIAGNOSES

Pain related to episiotomy, **hemorrhoids,** involution of the uterus, full bladder.
Knowledge deficit related to the fourth stage of labor.
Potential fluid volume deficit related to decreased oral fluid intake and IV administration.
Altered nutrition: potential for less than body requirements, related to having nothing by mouth during labor and delivery.
Impaired skin integrity related to lacerations of the perineum or episiotomy.
Sleep pattern disturbance related to labor and delivery.
Activity intolerance related to fatigue.
Potential for infection related to alteration in skin integrity.

GOALS

Short-term

Woman will get rest and sleep.
Woman's hunger and thirst will be satisfied.
Woman's bladder will be emptied periodically.
Woman's pain and discomfort will be diminished.
Anesthesia from delivery will wear off.

Intermediate

Woman's perineal swelling will start to subside and healing will begin.
Woman's fundus will remain firm and lochia rubra will remain within normal limits.
Woman will ambulate with assistance to the bathroom to void.

Long-term

Woman will ambulate to bathroom by herself to void.
Woman will begin self-care activities.
Uterus will begin to involute.

REFERENCES AND TEACHING AIDS

Prelabor and delivery counseling using pamphlets and booklets explaining the physiologic changes that take place during the fourth stage of labor.

RATIONALE/CONTENT	TEACHING ACTIONS
Direct care and education of the woman will decrease incidence of postpartum hemorrhage, therefore the nurse shares the following: Uterus must remain firm to become the **living ligature.** When uterus becomes boggy, or atonic, living ligature is no longer working to stop excessive bleeding. If gentle massage does not work, further assessment must be performed. When lochia is heavy, reassessment of source of bleeding, uterine tone, and bladder distension must be made. Clots should be expelled. Note size and amount.	Identify for woman the location and size of the uterus. Show mother how to massage uterus gently to firm up uterine fundus. Explain what the term *involution* means. Discuss lochia and clot formation. Give rationale for assessing, discuss meaning of terms. Teach woman about expected regression (color and amount) during involution. Explain that atony and subsequent hemorrhage can be the result of a distended bladder. Bleeding may be from another source. Intrauterine clots prevent the living ligature from working.
Bladder distension can lead to postpartum hemorrhage, therefore the nurse will: Assess woman's intake of fluids, oral and intravenous.	Discuss rationale for keeping bladder empty; prevent uterine atony and trauma to bladder.
Assess rate of diuresis as evidenced by bladder filling. Assess woman's ability to void. Share information related to diuresis and postdelivery bladder function	Provide privacy, sound of running water, fluids to drink. If available, expose urinary meatus to vapors from spirits of peppermint. Offer analgesia to assist woman to relax urinary meatus. Suggest she void while in sitz bath or while using surgigator. Discuss possible catheterization if trauma and edema to tissues or anesthesia impairs normal urination pattern.

Guidelines for Client Teaching—cont'd

RATIONALE/CONTENT	TEACHING ACTIONS
The possibility of hemorrhage can be reduced through stimulation of endogenous oxytocin and the woman can be assisted to meet her goal to breastfeed:	
Review the benefits to the newborn (who is healthy and ready to nurse) and to her. See guidelines for client teaching: breastfeeding, Chapter 18.	Show woman how to put the infant to breast and explain that nipple stimulation results in the release of oxytocin, which causes the uterus to contract and assists involution.
Comfort can be increased by a variety of methods, therefore the nurse will teach:	
Discomfort is normal and measures can reduce discomfort of:	Validate that woman's discomfort is expected and interventions are available to help.
Episiotomy: positioning, icepacks, medication (local or systemic). **Afterpains:** warm blanket, empty bladder, medication.	Implement care (icepacks, medications); share rationale and expected outcomes.
Hydration is essential for health maintenance, therefore the nurse will teach that: Drinking small amounts of fluids slowly prevents nausea and vomiting. There is a relationship between fluid deficit and temperature rise and fatigue.	Provide explanations. Maintain IV fluids or provide oral fluids, as ordered. Caution against drinking large amounts at one time or rapidly.
Nutrition is essential for health maintenance, therefore the nurse will teach that: Giving birth consumes considerable energy. There is a relationship between food deficit and fatigue and rate of recovery.	Provide rationale. Provide foods as ordered. Begin postpartum nutrition counseling.
Bladder elimination is essential for health maintenance, therefore the nurse is aware that: Overdistension can lead to bladder atony and delayed recovery. Urine retention can predispose to bladder infection.	Provide rationale for need to prevent bladder distension. Encourage woman to void. Catheterize as needed, per physician's order.
Safety is essential to health maintenance, therefore the nurse will teach that: Postdelivery splanchnic engorgement predisposes the woman to **orthostatic hypotension.**	Request that woman ask for assistance to ambulate. Put side rails up and call bell within reach, and provide rationale.
Recovery from effects of analgesia/anesthesia varies: Some analgesics affect the woman's balance. Spinal anesthesia requires a period of bed rest with only a small flat pillow under the woman's head	Help woman maintain flat position for specified time after spinal anesthesia, and provide rationale.
Childbirth increases the woman's vulnerability to infection because of a variety of reasons, including fluid and calorie deficit and tissue trauma.	Explain rationale to promote comfort and healing and to prevent infection. Demonstrate perineal care. Teach woman signs and symptoms to report after discharge home.

EVALUATION The nurse can be reasonably assured that teaching and care were effective when all goals for care have been achieved. The uterus retains tone. Mother locates and massages uterus. The lochia is moderate or less with no clots or just a few small clots. The mother voids completely so that uterus is firm, in midline, and below umbilicus; her bladder is emptied without additional trauma and by using strict aseptic technique. Mother understands cause of possible sensation of afterpains during breastfeeding. Woman's nonverbal and verbal responses validate that she is comfortable, and she is able to rest comfortably. Woman is well hydrated (elevated temperature and fatigue take time to resolve). Her hunger is satisfied. She takes oral fluids and foods without difficulty. Before ambulating, woman requests assistance, ambulates without difficulty, and incurs no injury. Woman understands rationale for all care provided her.

Guidelines for Client Teaching
EMOTIONAL FACTORS DURING THE FOURTH STAGE OF LABOR

ASSESSMENT

1. Woman has completed labor and given birth within previous 2 hours.
2. Woman gives verbal cues that suggest failure, loss of self-esteem (e.g., "I was such a baby").
3. Woman embarrassed about behavior during labor and delivery (e.g., "I'm sorry for screaming").
4. Woman and other family members express desire to hold newborn.
5. Woman indicates desire to breastfeed.
6. Woman (couple) talks about met and unmet expectations.
7. Woman (couple) reacts to newborn.

NURSING DIAGNOSES

Situational low self-esteem related to labor and delivery experience.
Potential altered parenting related to care of newborn.
Knowledge deficit related to care of newborn, breastfeeding, and process of integration of the birth experience.

GOALS

Short-term

Woman (couple) will relive and replay birth experience.
Woman will begin to feel comfortable with her behavior.
Woman will begin to breastfeed, if desired.
Woman (couple) will begin to bond with newborn.

Intermediate

Woman (couple) will resolve feelings of birth experience and begin to feel satisfaction from the process.
Woman will gain satisfaction from breastfeeding.
Woman (couple) and family will become attached to newborn.

Long-term

Woman (couple) will have positive memories of the birth experience.
Woman will continue to derive satisfaction from breastfeeding.
Woman (couple) will provide love and care for the new infant.

REFERENCES AND TEACHING AIDS

Printed material explaining normal reactions to labor and delivery processes.
Breastfeeding information (see client teaching: breastfeeding, Chapter 18).
Pamphlets and booklets describing newborn care.

CONTENT/RATIONALE	TEACHING ACTIONS
Integration of the birth experience is essential to foster maternal self-esteem, therefore the nurse is aware that: Women approach labor with certain self-expectations. "Normal" behavior during labor includes behaviors that are unacceptable to many people, such as loss of control, moaning, belching, grunting. Normal amnesia, medications, and labor preclude a clear recall of events; gaps in recall or misinterpretations prevent positive coping and self-esteem.	Implement communication techniques (Chapter 1). Encourage and listen to mother's replay of her experience. Phrase questions and answers in manner that indicates that her responses during all stages of labor were within expected range.
Parent-child attachment is dependent on many variables, therefore the nurse is aware that: Attachment to newborn is a continuous process. Fatigue of either mother or baby may delay but will not adversely influence attachment response.	Assess woman's readiness (absence of sedation or fatigue) and newborn's condition. Wrap baby warmly. Position baby in woman's arms for maximum safety. Ensure woman's comfort. Point out newborn's individual characteristics. Help the mother put baby to breast if she wishes to.
Cultural variations may affect interactions between family members, therefore the nurse is aware that: Each ethnic and cultural group and individual couple have developed workable ways for family interactions. There is no one "right" way.	Meet family's ethnic and cultural expectations for care by: Accepting degree of involvement of individuals regarding overt expression of joy or love. Accepting family's desires regarding newborn (e.g., some may want newborn to be cared for in nursery).

EVALUATION Woman gives nonverbal cues that she is beginning to accept her behavior and the experience. Woman (couple) begins attachment process. Family indicates satisfaction with the experience.

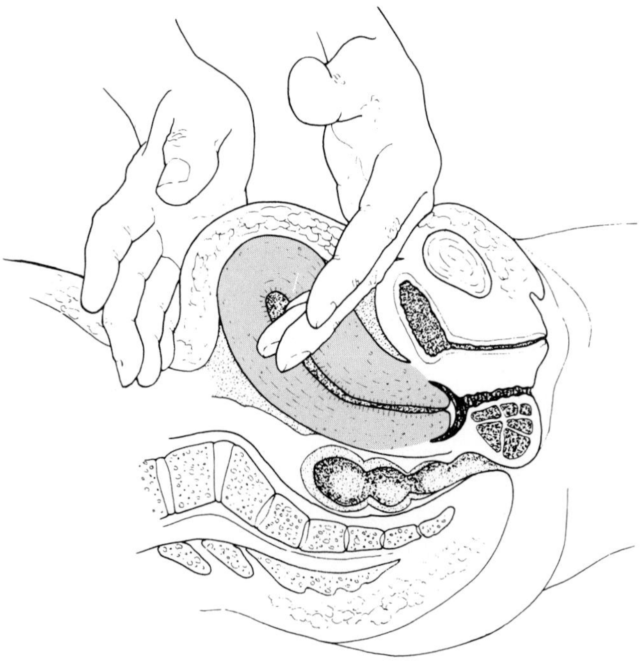

Fig. 15-36 Palpating fundus of uterus during first hour after delivery. Note that upper hand is cupped over fundus; lower hand dips in above symphysis pubis and supports uterus while it is massaged gently.

ascertain that it is not filling with blood (Fig. 15-36). The pad must be checked frequently to ensure that blood is not excessive (Fig. 15-37). Lochia may be described as scant, light, moderate, or heavy (profuse). Normally, the fundus is firm or may be returned to a state of firmness with intermittent gentle massage. As noted earlier, *atony (relaxation) of the uterine musculature* may occur. As the relaxed uterus distends with blood and clots, blood vessels in the placental site are not clamped off by the "living ligature," and bleeding results.

NOTE: To express clots it is necessary to express gently the acccumulated blood and clots before the uterus will contract again. First, make certain the fundus is firm, then support the base of the uterus with one hand while pressing gently on the uterus in the direction of the vagina with the other hand. If atony is not controlled by this treatment, medical intervention must be instituted (Chapter 23).

As the effect of the oxytocic medication administered after delivery wears off, the amount of lochia will increase because the myometrium relaxes somewhat. The nurse *always checks* under the mother's buttocks, as well as on the perineal pad. Bleeding may flow between the buttocks onto the linens under the mother while the amount on the perineal pad is slight. A perineal pad that is soaked through from tail to tail contains approximately 100 ml of blood. Higgins (1982) found that most nurses overestimate blood loss, but were consistent in their observations. When hemorrhage is suspected, the nurse should save all peripads and underpads for the physician or midwife to assess. If a pad is found to be soaked through in 15 minutes, or if blood is seen pooled under the buttocks, continuous observation of blood loss, vital signs, and maternal color and behavior is essential.

Another potential source of hemorrhage is the development of a hematoma under the vaginal mucosa or in the connective tissue of the vulva. This may occur as a result of injury to a blood vessel during the delivery or in repairing the laceration/episiotomy. The bleeding may be slow but continuous as the blood oozes from the vessel and distends the surrounding tissue. In many cases this distension of the tissue may not be visualized by the nurse. The initial complaint by the woman is that of severe and intense pressure and/or pain in the perineal or rectal area. The nurse should carefully inspect the perineum, monitor vital signs, and report all findings to the physician immediately, with emphasis placed on the woman's complaint of pain.

A vulvar hematoma may be visualized as the swelling increases. It is usually unilateral and becomes purplish. A vaginal hematoma is usually only found through manual examination. A soft mass may be palpated through a vaginal or rectal examination. The blood loss with this type of hematoma may be excessive. It is not unusual to have a loss of 500 ml or more.

The hematoma continues to be evaluated, and if it remains small there will be no treatment necessary, since the hematoma will reabsorb. However, many times it is necessary for the nurse to prepare the woman for surgical incision and evacuation of the hematoma. The procedure is performed with general anesthesia or regional anesthesia where the clots are removed and there is ligation of the blood vessel. Nursing care after the procedure includes careful monitor-

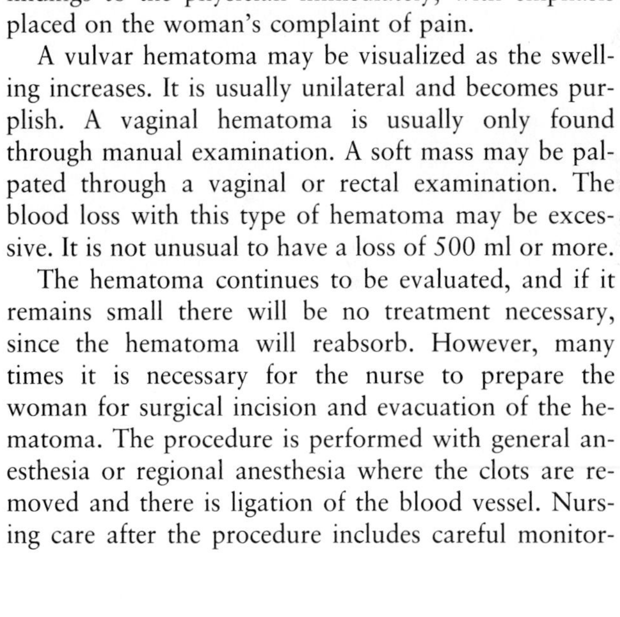

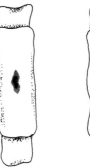

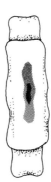

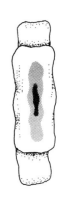

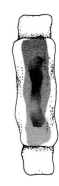

Fig. 15-37 Peripad-saturation volumes.

ing of the perineum and blood loss, maintenance of IV fluids, monitoring of vital signs and lab work, preparing for a possible blood transfusion, and administering prescribed antibiotics as prophylaxis against infection (see Chapter 23 for additional information).

If bleeding is in the form of a continuous trickle or is seen to come in spurts, lacerations of the vagina or cervix or the presence of an unligated vessel in the episiotomy are suspected. The woman will most likely be returned to the delivery area to permit visualization of the site and surgical correction.

Hypovolemic Shock. Hemorrhage and early hemorrhagic shock may occur in an otherwise normal fourth stage of labor. Prompt identification and intervention usually result in rapid stabilization of the woman's pulse, BP, and other signs. The danger signs box below is a quick reference for signs and symptoms of **hypovolemic shock.** Interventions are presented in the emergency procedure for hypovolemic shock below.

Bladder Distension

Palpation to determine the amount of *bladder distension* should accompany palpation of the fundus. The full bladder forces the uterus upward and to the

EMERGENCY PROCEDURE
HYPOVOLEMIC SHOCK

DEFINITION

State of physical collapse and prostration caused by massive blood loss, circulatory malfunction, and inadequate tissue perfusion.

PURPOSE

To identify and control bleeding.
Prompt replacement of blood and fluid volumes.
Prevention of total collapse and death.

EQUIPMENT

IV fluid; IV tubing, needles, angiocaths; aromatic spirits of ammonia; oxytocic medication; oxygen with nasal prongs or mask.

NURSING ACTIONS	RATIONALE
Preprocedure	
Observe mother for persistent heavy bleeding: the soaking of a second perineal pad in 15 minutes, may or may not be accompanied by a change in vital signs, skin color, or behavior.	Fast diagnosis leads to quick action and a favorable prognosis. Blood volume still sufficient for body to compensate for loss.
Assess mother for signs of shock (i.e., feels light-headed, sick feeling in stomach, sees "stars," starts to act anxious, ashen or grayish color appears, skin feels cool and clammy, exhibits air hunger). Pulse rate increases as blood pressure falls.	Compensatory mechanisms becoming ineffective. Sympathetic nervous system stimulated. Hypoxia of brain cells. Hypoxia of tissue cells. β-adrenergic receptor stimulation. Attempt made to compensate for tissue hypoxia and metabolic acidosis.
Procedure	
Call for help immediately—summon help *to you.*	*Do not leave* the woman.
Tilt woman onto her side and raise her legs *high.* Increase flow of IV drip.	Increases circulating blood volume; prevents supine hypotension.
If uterus is atonic, massage gently and expel clots to allow uterus to contract; compress uterus manually, as needed, using two hands. Add oxytocic to IV drip, as ordered.	Prevents further loss of blood by stimulating uterine contractions. Stimulates uterine contractions.
Break ampule of aromatic amonia, a respiratory stimulant; give oxygen by face mask or nasal prongs at 8 to 10 L/min.	Facilitates oxygen by stimulating respirations and increasing available oxygen.
Reassure woman (couple).	Decreases anxiety.
Postprocedure	
Chart incident and medical and nursing interventions employed. Chart results of treatments.	Provides data base for future comparison. Provides information for implementation of nursing process.

DANGER SIGNS

Hypovolemic Shock

1. Persistent significant bleeding—perineal pad soaked within 15 minutes; *may not be accompanied by a change in vital signs or maternal color or behavior.*
2. Mother states she feels light-headed, "funny," "sick to my stomach," or sees "stars"
3. Mother begins to act anxious, or exhibits air hunger
4. Woman's color turns ashen or grayish
5. Temperature of skin feels cool and clammy
6. Increasing pulse rate
7. Falling BP
8. Intense perineal pain

right of the midline. Such a position interferes with the contractility of the uterine muscles, and hemorrhage results. In addition to the possibility of causing uterine relaxation, distension of the urinary bladder can result in atony of the bladder wall. Atony leads to urinary retention, which provides a favorable environment for infection. A specific nursing care plan for a client with bladder distension is on p. 432.

A nurse encourages the woman to void naturally, employing one or more of the following: placing a bedpan under the mother, giving her water to drink if the physician has ordered oral fluids, turning on the water faucet, pouring warm water over the perineum, helping her walk to the bathroom (if ordered), and providing privacy. If after these meaures the woman cannot void, most physicians write an order for catheterization.

Spirits of peppermint are sometimes used to aid the woman to void naturally. "Spirits" are concentrated alcohol solutions of volatile substances; they are also known as essences. Spirits of peppermint give off vapors. These vapors have an external, local relaxing effect on the sphincter muscle of the urinary meatus. Use of peppermint spirits may make it unnecessary to catheterize. The nurse places a bedpan under the woman and pours a few drops of peppermint spirits *into the bedpan.* The vapors rise to flow over the vulvar area, the urinary meatus relaxes, and urine is released. Nothing touches the woman except the vapors; the woman feels no sensation, only notices the aroma of peppermint. Most hospitals do not require a physician's order for the technique.

Maintain Comfort

The mother is settled comfortably in bed. A new mother needs to remain in bed for at least 2 hours even if she has an unmedicated delivery. The rapid decrease in intraabdominal pressure after birth results in dilatation of blood vessels supplying the intestines (known as splanchnic engorgement). **Splanchnic engorgement** pools blood in the viscera. Therefore when the woman stands up, she may feel faint (orthostatic hypotension). Women and their families need to be forewarned so that they know to call for assistance, especially the first time or two that the woman ambulates.

The woman who has received analgesics needs to be watched until she is fully recovered from the medication (i.e., vital signs are stable within her normal range, and she is fully awake). A woman who has had saddle block anesthesia will need to remain flat in bed. She must remain on her side, abdomen, or back with her head raised not more than 15 to 20 cm (6 to 8 in) for 6 to 12 hours to prevent development of a spinal headache (Chapter 13). An increase in oral fluids and extraabdominal pressure applied over the uterus also helps prevent "spinal headache."

Maintain Cleanliness. Cleanliness is another measure that increases the mother's comfort. The vulva is cleansed and a sterile pad placed in position, buttocks dried, and any wet linen removed so that the woman will be a warm and comfortable. While demonstrating good handwashing technique and gloving before touching the woman's perineal area, the nurse explains the actions to the woman. The nurse reminds the mother to cleanse the vulval area using a separate tissue for one wipe from front to back, to repeat until clean, and then to wash her hands.

A peribottle of warm water is also used for comfort and cleanliness. Some hospitals routinely offer a bed bath during this period. If the woman is ambulatory she may wish to shower. A shower chair and call light within reach provide for the woman's safety if she should become faint.

The nurse's attention to the mother's needs demonstrates a sense of caring. The woman feels more comfortable even if the same amount of discomfort is still present (Hawthorn effect).

Prevent Discomfort

Uterine contractions may result in discomfort known as *afterpains.* The volume within the uterus is decreased after delivery. The force of the myometrial contractions is considerable; the intrauterine pressure is much greater than that during labor, reaching 150 mm Hg or more.

During the first 2 hours after delivery, uterine contractions are regular and strong, especially in multiparas. The nurse adds to the woman's comfort by performing the following measures:

1. Explaining the normal physiology of afterpains
2. Helping the mother keep her urinary bladder empty

Specific Nursing Care Plan

NEW MOTHER WITH BLADDER DISTENSION

Stacey Lewis, a 25-year-old first-time mother is 2 hours postdelivery with epidural anesthesia. She is complaining of pain in her abdomen and inability to void. On examination you find her fundus firm 3 cm above the umbilicus and off to the right. Lochia is moderate and rubra. Perineum is edematous. Urinary bladder is full and palpable at the symphysis pubis. Stacey has asked that her baby be taken to the nursery because she "can't deal with her right now" because the labor was so long and painful.

ASSESSMENT	NURSING DIAGNOSIS (ND), PLAN/GOAL (P/G)	RATIONALE/ IMPLEMENTATION	EVALUATION
New mother—2 hours postpartum. Pain in abdomen Bladder distension. Adequate intake and output. Fundus firm, above umbilicus, and not in midline. Lochia not excessive. Episiotomy.	ND: Pain, related to distended bladder. ND: Altered patterns of urinary elimination: distension, related to increased bladder filling and retention of urine from birth trauma, edema, or regional anesthesia. P/G: Stacey empties bladder without assistance and relieves pain of distension.	*Pain and swelling from birth trauma may prevent emptying of bladder leading to hemorrhage:* Assist Stacey to bathroom, or assist her on bedpan; run water from faucet; pour warm water over perineum; use sitz bath; use spirits of peppermint. Administer analgesic if inability to void is caused by perineal discomfort. If all nursing measures fail, obtain doctor's order to catheterize.	Stacey voids and empties bladder unassisted. Stacey verbalizes discomfort and pain are relieved. If catheterization is necessary, Stacey suffers no adverse sequelae, (e.g., infection).
Stacey not interested in interaction with newborn. Lack of appropriate parental behaviors. Stacey states had a long labor Assess maternal physical discomfort.	ND: Altered parenting related to mother's physical condition and emotional lability. P/G: Stacey's physical problems will be resolved and maternal-infant attachment will be initiated.	*Relaxation and elimination of physical discomfort increases woman's ability to bond with infant:* Increase Stacey's comfort through rest, relaxation techniques, local medication to perineum, analgesia, and food; acknowledge that she has just accomplished a significant event. When Stacey indicates readiness: introduce her to newborn, pointing out special qualities; undress infant and encourage Stacey to touch her and observe newborn characteristics; demonstrate care of newborn; and assist her in newborn care. Provide information on the process and time that can be involved in the development of attachment.	Stacey's comfort will improve and mother-infant attachment is observed by health care providers before discharge.

3. Providing a warmed blanket to the mother's abdomen
4. Administering analgesics ordered by the physician
5. Encouraging relaxation and breathing exercises

As the bladder fills it presses against the uterus causing it to relax. The uterus attempts to stay firm by increasing the force of contractions, thereby increasing the discomfort of afterpains. Gentle massage of the fundus increases uterine contractions, thereby intensifying afterpains. To help the new mother cope with the discomforts of assessment measures, the nurse explains what is being done and why, and then encourages the woman to perform the procedure.

The *episiotomy* area or *hemorrhoids* may contribute to the new mother's discomfort. Ice packs wrapped in gauze or a chemical ice pack may be placed over the episiotomy. Cold therapy is used to numb the area and to minimize the amount of edema that occurs, thus reducing discomfort. The ice pack is most effective in minimizing edema if it is used for the first hour or two after delivery. The physician may order any one of several antiseptic or anesthetic ointments or sprays to ease discomfort in the perineal area. A side-lying position relieves direct pressure on the area.

If the woman has had a saddle block or other regional anesthetic, the nurse's description of sensations to expect as the anesthetic wears off can be reassuring. Women describe the sensation as tingling or prickly, much like that experienced by people after they have been sitting crosslegged for a long time and the legs have "gone to sleep."

Some women experience intense *tremors* after delivery that resemble the shivering of a chill. The chilling may be related to the sudden release of pressure on pelvic nerves. According to another theory, chilling may be symptomatic of a fetus-to-mother transfusion that sometimes occurs during placental separation. The feeling of a chill may be a reaction to epinephrine (adrenaline) production during delivery. The nurse can help the woman relax or feel comforted by providing her with warm blankets and an explanation that the tremors are commonly seen after delivery and are not related to infection. The warm blanket also provides a means of "mothering the mother." This helps restore her energy so she can move from a focus on herself to a focus on her baby.

If the nurse administers analgesics, the sedating effect of these analgesics necessitates such protective care as raising side rails, placing call bell within reach, and cautioning about remaining in bed. The woman must be warned about any expected dizziness or drowsiness resulting from the medications.

Maintain Fluid Balance (Hydration) and Meet Nutritional Needs

Because of the restrictions on fluid intake and the loss of fluids (blood, perspiration, or emesis) during labor, many women are thirsty and request fluids soon after giving birth. Clear fluids, such as apple juice or tea, and toast can be given unless contraindicated. The nurse records the type of fluids and foods ingested; the time, the amount, and the mother's tolerance. Many parents wish to have a champagne toast at this time. The nurse needs to caution the mother if analgesia has been given and provide safety measures. The physician may order continued parenteral fluids at a "keep open" rate in the event of hemorrhage or need for IV medications.

Support Parental Emotional Needs

It is acceptable for the nurse to share openly in the excitement and emotion of birth. The nurse assists the parents by accepting any expressions of disappointment about the child's sex or appearance and reassures them that these feelings are normal. The nurse may reassure the mother that her behavior during labor was acceptable if the mother appears worried about this. The new mother may need to talk about her labor and may endeavor to fill in gaps that she cannot remember, particularly if the delivery was hurried (Affonso, 1977).

Psychic states of new mothers range from euphoria, a feeling of well-being, to a sleepy state marked by an unawareness of surroundings. As noted earlier, first reactions of new mothers and fathers to their newborns vary widely. These reactions give the obstetric team cues to use in individualizing plans of care. Women who have experienced long, difficult labors or who are in pain are commonly too exhausted to extend interest to the child. The nurse can offer to take the baby to the nursery until the mother is rested. The father can be invited to accompany the nurse to the nursery at this stage (Fig. 15-38). After sufficient rest a mother's attitude can be surprisingly different. The child unwanted for diverse reasons may continue to be rejected or given only mild interest. The attitude of the father is often reflected in the mother. His pleasure arouses a responsive pleasure, or his disappointment arouses corresponding disappointment.

Ethnic or cultural origins dictate behaviors that are deemed appropriate for special occasions. Some parents may not be able to express their delight openly; others wish to welcome the newcomer noisily.

The single or teenage mother may express mixed emotions at the birth of the baby. The nurse can help her express her emotions, involve any significant other, family, or friends', or refer her to a social worker.

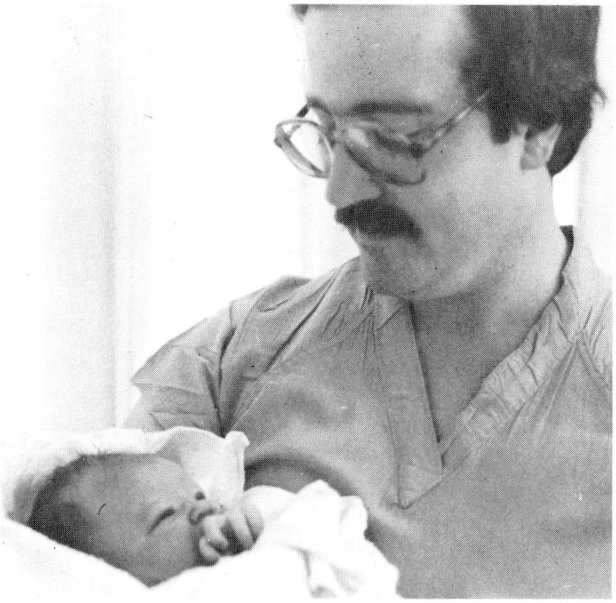

Fig. 15-38 A proud father's pensive moment with his son. (Courtesy Stanford University Medical Center, Stanford, Calif.)

Some mothers, particularly with their firstborn, are surprised and disturbed by the passivity or disinterest they experience on seeing their long-awaited infant. The nurse can reassure the mother of the normalcy of these feelings. The idealized "mother love" does not necessarily appear right after delivery. The gradual growth of such love comes to some as they assume the care and responsibility for their child.

The nurse can facilitate parent-child attachment or acquaintance by providing a warm, quiet, dimly lighted environment. An infant responds by opening the eyes. Parents are encouraged to hold the infant ***en face.*** In the *en face* position, parents and newborns gaze into each others eyes. Newborns focus best at about 20.3 cm (8 in) distance. Body odor can be noticed (mothers have remarked that each child smells different). Skin contact between mother and baby should be encouraged during this time. Newborn temperatures remain stable if mother and newborn are placed chest-to-chest and covered by a blanket. The mother is encouraged to explore her baby and put her baby to the breast, if she plans to breastfeed. Immediately after birth the baby has a strong desire to suck, so this early feed is most encouraging for the mother and bonding is promoted.

Transfer from Recovery Area

When the new mother's condition has stabilized and interventions after delivery have been completed, she is ready to be transferred to the postpartum unit. To ensure continuity of care the recovery nurse must document the type of labor and delivery, any unusual observations, anesthesia or analgesia administered, condition of perineum, and any notable events since delivery. Assessment data, including gravidity, parity, and age of mother should be noted. The condition and sex of the newborn, relevant social factors (i.e., baby to be given up for adoption), and any medication to be continued should also be recorded.

This information must also be documented for the nursing staff in the newborn nursery. Additionally, specific information should be provided regarding the infant's Apgar scores, weight, voiding, and feeding since delivery. Nursing interventions that have been completed (i.e., eye prophylaxis, vitamin K injection) should also be recorded.

Evaluation

Evaluation of progress and outcomes is a continuous activity through the fourth stage of labor. Physiologic recovery from pregnancy and labor, and development of parent-infant attachment and new family interrelationships are evaluated by the nurse. The degree to which formulated goals of care are being met must be critically appraised. If the evaluation process identifies that results fall short of achieving any goal, further assessment, planning, and implementation are imperative to attain the correct nursing care for the woman and her family.

SUMMARY

The childbearing family has many special needs and concerns throughout the labor process. Parents arrive during the first stage of labor with a perception of how they want to labor and deliver their child. Hospitals have become consumer oriented and offer alternatives to the traditional birth setting. The family is encouraged to actively participate in the birth options of their choice.

Nursing care begins with the initial assessment during the admission procedure and a plan of care is begun that can be modified and updated throughout the labor process. Nurses must utilize their expertise in caring for the physical needs of the woman and family in providing for a safe delivery of the infant and recognize and appropriately intervene for complications.

The nurse is also sensitive to the cultural orientation of the woman and family and modifies the plan of care to reflect these preferences. All family members (grandparents, siblings, father of baby) are integral parts of the birthing team are supported in their support of the laboring woman.

Throughout the fourth stage of labor, the nurse continues to modify the plan of care and prepare the woman for the tasks of the postpartum period as well as for care of the infant. This is accomplished through education and physical and emotional support of both the woman and her family. The plan of care continues during the postpartum period and beyond if continued support is required.

LEARNING ACTIVITIES

1. Role-play the following situations:
   a. The nurse interacting with mother and father who are expressing disappointment over the sex of the child; with the husband hinting that this is his wife's fault.
   b. The mother who does not want fundal massage.
   c. The nurse interacting with parents of a different culture, who express avoidance behaviors toward the child.
   d. A teenage mother who is indifferent to the labor and delivery process.
   In each situation the group should evaluate the responses of all participants and suggest alternative actions, responses and reasons for responses.
2. Rehearse appropriate nursing actions for a client who may be experiencing hemorrhage.
3. Evaluate the birth settings available, the procedures, and the nursing personnel, physicians, or midwives at your institution. Assess their potential effect on parent-newborn bonding.
4. In a group, discuss responses to the first delivery you have observed. Express both negative and positive feelings and explore their causes.
5. Observe several clients in different stages of labor. Begin to develop some generalizations about each stage and share these observations in a group setting.
6. Admit clients to the labor suite, collect data for assessment, and prepare a plan of care based on the nursing diagnoses you have developed. Include in your plan potential problems and nursing interventions.
7. Diagram on partograms the cervical dilatations and stations of the fetal presenting part of both nulliparous and multiparous women during labor and compare findings. Discuss how results differ, whether they follow the normal labor curve, how you account for any deviations from normal, and how to alter your plan of care for the client.
8. Research various cultures' attitudes, perceptions, and beliefs in relation to childbirth and compare with your own. Explain to group how these factors might affect the behavior of parents and grandparents and nurses during the labor process.

References

Affonso D: Missing pieces: a study of postpartum feelings, Birth Fam J 4:159, Winter, 1977.
Balaskis J: Active birth, London, 1983, Unicorn.
Barnard R: The family and you, MCN 3:83, 1978.
Bliss J: New baby in the family, Can Nurs 76:42, 1980.
Carr KG: Management of the second stage of labor, NAACOG Update series, lesson 9, vol 1, 1983.
Carrington BW: The Afro-American. In Clark AL, editor: Culture/childbearing/health professionals, Philadelphia, 1978, FA Davis Co.
Cosminsky S: Knowledge and body concepts of Guatemalan midwives. In Kay MA, editor: Anthropology of human birth, Philadelphia, 1982, FA Davis Co.
Cunningham FG, MacDonald PC, and Gant NF: Williams obstetrics, ed 18, Norwalk, Conn, 1989, Appleton & Lange.
Daniels MB: The birth experience for a sibling: Description and evaluation of a program, J Nurs Midwife 28(5):15, 1983.
Davitz LL, Davitz JR, and Higuchi Y: Cross-cultural inferences of physical pain and psychological distress, Nurs Times 73:556, 1977.
Farris L: The American Indian. In Clark AL, editor: Culture/childbearing/health professionals, Philadelphia, 1978, FA Davis Co.
Flint M: Lockmi: an Indian midwife. In Kay MA, editor: Anthropology of human birth, Philadelphia, 1982, FA Davis Co.
Friedman FA: Labor: clinical evaluation and management, ed 2, New York, 1978, Appleton-Century-Crofts.
Friedman EA and Sachtleben MR: Station of the presenting part, Am J Obstet Gynecol 93:522, 1965.
Griffith S: Childbearing and the concept of children, JOGN Nurs 11:181, 1982.
Higgins PG: Measuring nurses' accuracy of estimating blood loss, J Adv Nurs 7:175, 1982.
Hollingsworth AO et al: The refugees and childbearing: what to expect, RN 43:45, 1980.
Horn BM: Northwest coast Indians: the Muckleshoot. In Kay MA, editor: Anthropology of human birth, Philadelphia, 1982, FA Davis Co.
Jimenez SL: Application of the body's natural pain relief mechanisms to reduce discomfort in labor and delivery, NAACOG Update Series, lesson 1, vol 1, 1983a.
Jimenez SL: The pregnant woman's comfort guide, Englewood Cliffs, NJ, 1983b, Prentice-Hall, Inc.
Johnsen NM and Gaspard ME: Theoretical foundations for a prepared sibling class, JOGN Nurs 14:237, May/June, 1985.
Johnson SM and Snow LF: The profile of some unplanned pregnancies. In Bauwens EE, editor: The anthropology of health, St Louis, 1978, The CV Mosby Co.
Leonard CH et al: Preliminary observations on the behavior of children present at the birth of a sibling, Pediatrics 64:949, 1979.
Mahan CS and McKay S: Are we overmanaging second stage labor? Contemp OB/GYN 24:37, Dec, 1984.
Myles M: Textbook for midwives, ed 10, Edinburgh, 1985, Churchill Livingstone, Inc.
Newton N: Childbearing in broad perspective: pregnancy, birth and the newborn baby, Boston, 1972, Delacorte Press.
Orque MS et al: Ethnic nursing care: a multicultural approach, St Louis, 1983, The CV Mosby Co.

KEY CONCEPTS

- The onset of labor may be difficult to determine even for the experienced gravida.
- Although some complications of labor are anticipated, others appear only in the clinical course of labor.
- The nurse assumes much of the responsibility for making the assessment of progress and keeping the physician informed about that progress and any deviations from normal findings.
- Although meconium-stained fluid may be noted with fetal asphyxia, its presence is not always diagnostic of prospective fetal distress.
- The woman's level of anxiety may rise when she does not understand what is being said to her about her labor because of the medical terminology used or because of a language barrier.
- Prolapsed umbilical cord requires prompt recognition and therapy to prevent fetal hypoxia.
- Coaching, support, and comfort measures help the woman use her energy constructively in relaxing and working with the contractions.
- The nurse can be a positive influence in promotion of family integration of the birth process.
- The nurse who is aware of the sociocultural aspects of childbirth is able to incorporate those expectations into the plan of care.
- The woman needs continuous monitoring, support, and coaching during the second stage of labor.
- If the woman states that "the baby is coming," immediate delivery should be anticipated.
- There are five signs that placental separation has occurred and the placenta is ready to be expelled; before placental separation, excessive traction can result in immediate or delayed injury to the mother.
- Most parents (families) enjoy being able to handle, hold, explore, and examine the baby immediately after birth. The nurse should assist in this process and be alert for warning signs of an impaired relationship.
- As the neonate makes the transition from intrauterine to extrauterine life, initiation and maintenance of respiration and prevention of cold stress are crucial priorities.
- The fourth stage of labor, the stage of recovery, is a critical period for the mother and newborn.
- Primary nursing concern during this period is the prevention of hemorrhage. Other concerns include bladder distension, safety, comfort, and nutrition.
- The nurse can facilitate mother-infant attachment by meeting the new mother's physical, support, and teaching needs.
- Regardless of parity, marital status, or age, new mothers can benefit from explanations for the various nursing actions during the immediate puerperium.

Pernoll ML and Benson RC: Current obstetric and gynecologic diagnosis and treatment, ed 6, Los Altos, Calif, 1987, Appleton & Lange.

Quinlan P: Genevieve's birth at Pithiviers, Birth 10:187, Fall, 1983.

Pillsbury BLK: "Doing the month": confinement and convalescence of Chinese women after birth, Soc Sci Med 12:11, 1978.

Romney ML and White VGL: Current practices in labor. In Field PA, editor: Perinatal nursing, Edinburgh, 1984, Churchill Livingstone, Inc.

Scott JR et al: Danforth's obstetrics and gynecology, ed 6, Philadelphia, 1990, JB Lippincott Co.

Stephany T: Supporting the mother of a patient in labor, JOGN Nurs 12(5):345, 1983.

Warrington J: The obstetric catechism, Philadelphia, 1842, Crolius and Clading.

Yeates J and Robers J: A comparison of 2 bearing down techniques during the second stage of labor, J Nurs 29:3, 1984.

Zborowski M: Cultural components in responses to pain, J Soc Issues 3:16, 1952.

Zepeda M: Selected maternal infant care practices of Spanish-speaking people, JOGN Nurs 11:371, 1982.

Zuspan FF and Quilligan EJ, editors: Practice manual of obstetric care, St. Louis, 1982, The CV Mosby Co.

Bibliography

Amderberg GJ: Initial acquaintance and attachment behavior of siblings with the newborn, JOGN Nurs 17(1):49, 1988.

Bates B and Turner AN: Imagery and symbolism in the birth practices of traditional cultures, Birth 12:29, Spring, 1985.

Bjorkman LA Du E: Childbirth care for Hmong families, MCN 10(6):382, 1985.

Bloom KC: Assisting the unprepared woman during labor, JOGN Nurs 13:303, Sept/Oct, 1984.

Brucker MC: Pain control of the fourth stage, NAACOG Newsletter 14(8):1, 1987.

Carlson J et al: Maternal position during parturition in normal labor, Obstet Gynecol 68:443, 1986.

Collins BA: The role of the nurse in labor and delivery as perceived by nurses and patients, JOGN Nurs 15(5):412, 1986.

Coltrell BH and Shannahan MD: Effect of the birth chair duration of second stage labor and maternal outcome, Nurs Res 35:364, 1986.
Dundes L: The evolution of maternal birthing positions, Am J Public Health 77:636, Sept/Oct, 1987.
Field PA: Maternity nurses: how parents see us, Int J Nurs Stud 24(3):1981, 1987.
Gorrie TM: Postpartal nursing diagnosis, JOGN Nurs 15(1):52, 1986.
Griffith R and Hare M: Do women really want natural childbirth, Midwives Chronicle 98(1167):92, 1985.
Grosso C et al: The Vietnamese American family . . . and grandma makes three, MCN 6:177, 1981.
Hageman JR et al: Delivery room management of meconium staining of the amniotic fluid and the development of meconium aspiration syndrome, J Perinatal 8(2):127, 1988.
Hans A: Postpartum assessment: the psychological component, JOGN Nurs 15(1):49, 1986.
Haun N: Nursing care during labor, Can Nurs 80:26, Oct, 1984.
Honig JC: Preparing school-age children to be siblings, MCN 11(1):37, 1986.
Horn M and Manion J: Creative grandparenting: bonding the generations, JOGN Nurs 14(3):233, 1985.
Howe CL: Physiologic and psychosocial assessment in labor, Nurs Clin North Am 17(1):49, 1982.
Kintz DL: Nursing support in labor, JOGN Nurs 16:126, March/April, 1987.
Konrad CJ: Helping mothers integrate the birth experience, MCN 12(4):268, 1987.
Kowba MD and Schwirian PM: Direct sibling contact and bacterial colonization in newborns, JOGN Nurs 14:412, Sept/Oct, 1985.
Leboyer F: Birth without violence, New York, 1976, Alfred A Knopf, Inc.
Leininger M: Transcultural nursing: an essential knowledge and practice field for today, Can Nurs 80:41, Dec, 1984.
Lehrman E: Birth in the left lateral position: an alternative to the traditional delivery position, J Nurs Midwife 30:193, July/Aug, 1985.
MacDonald J: Birth attendants: another choice, Can Nurse 80:22, Oct, 1984.
Maloney R: Childbirth education classes: expectant parent's expectations, JOGN Nurs 14:245, May/June, 1985.
Marecki M et al: Early sibling attachment, JOGN Nurs 14:418, Sept/Oct, 1985.
McKay S: Squatting: an alternative position for the second stage of labor, MCN 9:181, May/June, 1984.
McKay S and Mahan CS: Ways to upgrade postpartal care, Contemp OB/GYN 27:63, Nov, 1985.
McKay S and Roberts J: Second stage labor: what is normal, JOGN Nurs 14:101, March/April, 1985.
Mercer R and Stainton MC: Perceptions of the birth experience: a cross-cultural comparison, Health Care for Women International 5:29, 1984.
Poole C: Educating new labor and delivery room nurses, JOGN Nurs 14:459, Nov/Dec, 1985.
Ramona J and Baker I: Squatting in childbirth: a new look at an old tradition, JOGN Nurs 14:406, Sept/Oct, 1985.
Roberts JE et al: A descriptive analysis of involuntary bearing-down efforts during the expulsive phase of labor, JOGN Nurs 16:48, Jan/Feb, 1987.
Romond JL and Baker IT: Squatting in childbirth: a new look at an old tradition, JOGN Nurs 14:406, Sept/Oct, 1985.
Rosse MA and Lindell SG: Maternal positions and pushing techniques in a nonprescriptive environment, JOGN Nurs 15:203, May/June, 1986.
Shannahan M and Cottrell B: The effects of birth chair delivery on maternal perceptions, JOGN Nurs 18(4):323, 1988.
Stote KM: Nursing diagnosis and the childbearing woman, MCN 11:13, Jan/Feb, 1986.
Turner M et al: The birth chair: an obstetric hazard, J Obstet Gynecol 6:232, April, 1986.
Whaley LF and Wong DL: Nursing care of infants and children, ed 4, St Louis, 1991, The CV Mosby Co.
Willson JR and Carrington ER: Obstetrics and gynecology, ed 8, St Louis, 1988, The CV Mosby Co.
Winslow W: Perinatal nursing education, Can Nurs, p 31, June, 1988.

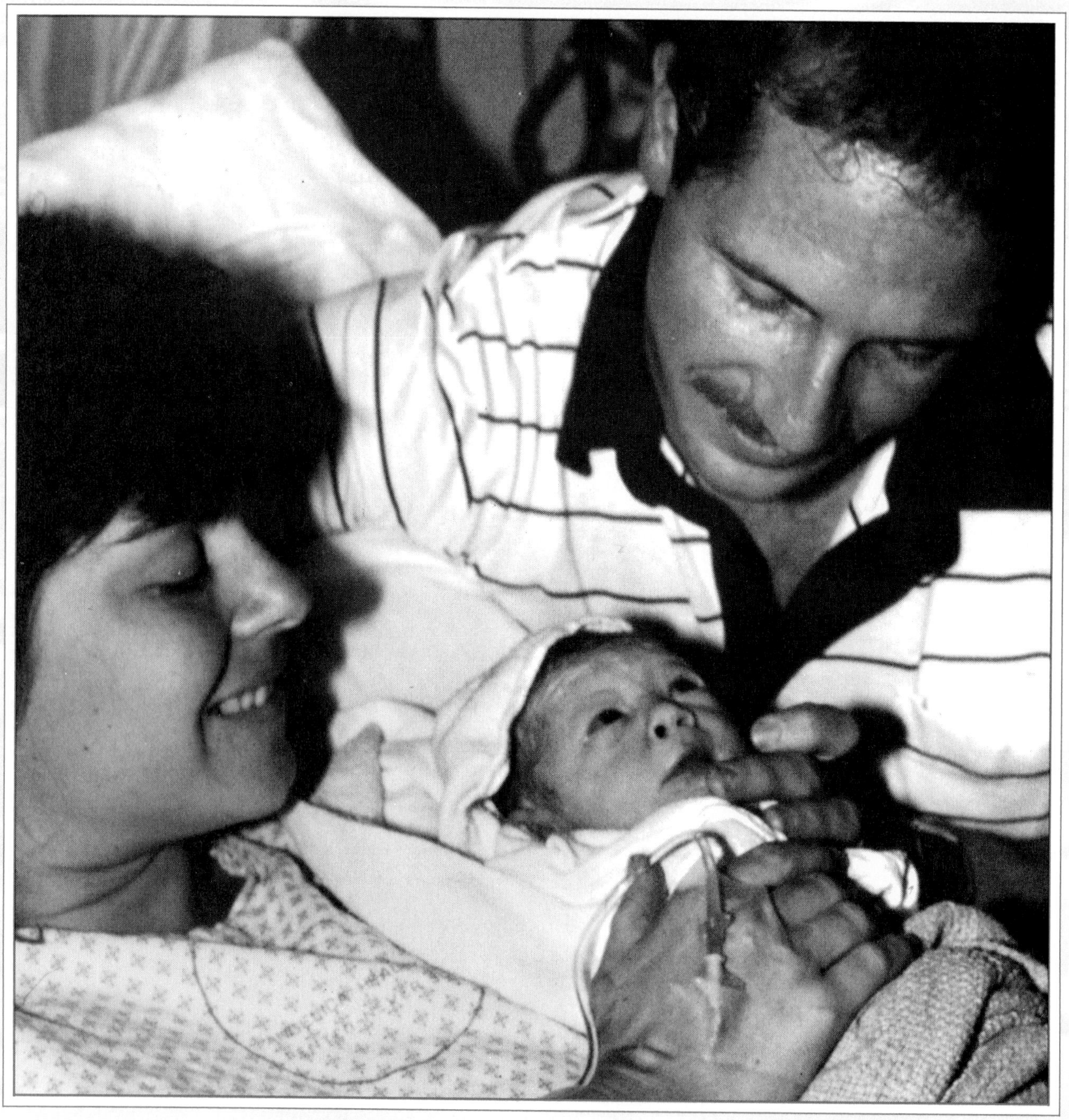

UNIT

IV

NORMAL NEWBORN

CHAPTER

16 Normal Newborn

Shannon E. Perry

Learning Objectives

Correctly define the key terms listed.

List biologic characteristics for the following systems of the newborn: cardiovascular, hematopoietic, respiratory, renal, gastrointestinal, hepatic, immune, integumentary, reproductive, skeletal, neuromuscular, thermogenetic.

Compare and contrast these systems with those of the adult.

Describe the behavioral characteristics of the newborn.

Summarize the newborn's biologic and behavioral characteristics in a manner easily understood by parents.

Key Terms

Brazelton neonatal behavioral assessment scale
cardiovascular system changes
cold stress
fluid and electrolyte balance
hematopoietic characteristics
hyperbilirubinemia
immune system status
integumentary characteristics
newborn stools
neuromuscular system
newborn reflexes
periods of reactivity
reproductive system characteristics
respiratory patterns
responses to environmental stimuli
sensory behaviors
skeletal system
sleep-wake cycles
state-related behaviors
thermogenesis
transition period

The newly born infant must accomplish a number of developmental tasks to establish and maintain a physical existence apart from the mother. By term gestation, the fetus's various anatomic and physiologic systems have reached a level of development and functioning that permits a separate existence from the mother. At birth, the newborn infant manifests behavioral competencies and a readiness for social interaction.

Newborn infants pass through phases of instability in the first 6 to 8 hours after birth. These phases are termed the **transition period** between intrauterine and extrauterine existence. The first phase lasts up to 30 minutes after birth and is called the ***first period of reactivity.*** The ***second period of reactivity*** occurs at about the fourth to eighth hour after birth (see p. 933). This sequence occurs in all newborns, regardless of gestational age or type of delivery (vaginal or cesarean). There will be variations, however, in the length of time the periods last, depending on amount and kind of stress experienced by the fetus.

❑ BIOLOGIC CHARACTERISTICS

The profound biologic adaptations that occur at birth make possible the newborn infant's transition from intrauterine to extrauterine life. These adaptations set the stage for future growth and development. The neonatal period, from birth through day 28, represents a time of dramatic physical change for the newborn.

Cardiovascular System

The **cardiovascular system changes** markedly after birth. There is closure of the foramen ovale, ductus arteriosus, and ductus venosus. The umbilical arteries and vein and the hepatic arteries become ligaments (Fig. 16-1).

The infant's first breath inflates the lungs and thereby reduces pulmonary vascular resistance to the pulmonary blood flow. As a result there is a drop in pulmonary artery pressure. This sequence is the major mechanism by which pressure in the *right atrium declines.* The increased pulmonary blood flow returned to the left side of the heart *increases* the pressure in the *left atrium.* This change in pressures causes a functional closure of the foramen ovale. Temporary reversal of flow through the foramen ovale may occur with crying and lead to mild cyanosis during the first few days of life.

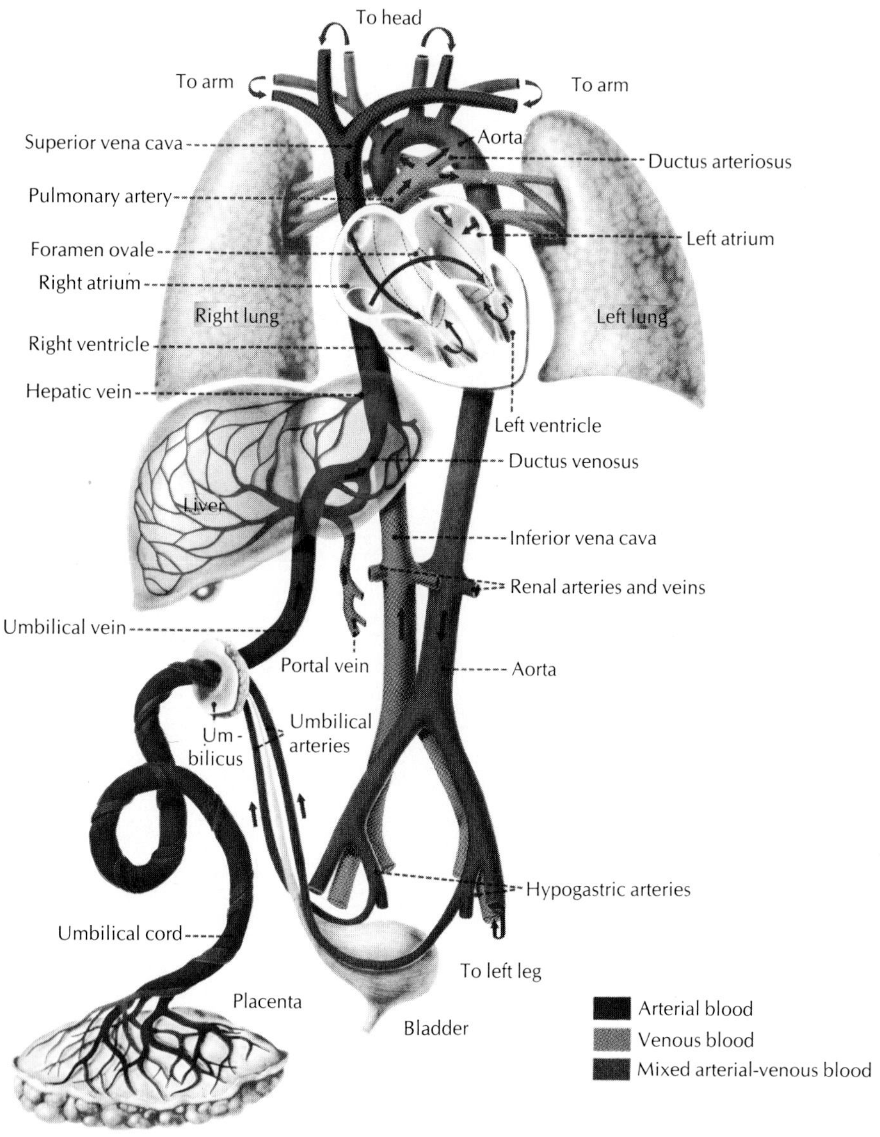

Fig. 16-1 Fetal circulation. *Before birth.* Arterialized blood from the placenta flows into the fetus through the umbilical vein and passes rapidly through the liver into the inferior vena cava; it flows through the foramen ovale into the left atrium, soon to appear in the aorta and arteries of the head. A portion bypasses the liver through the ductus venosus. Venous blood from the lower extremities and head passes predominantly into the right atrium, the right ventricle, and then into the descending pulmonary artery and ductus arteriosus. Thus the **foramen ovale and the ductus arteriosus act as bypass channels,** allowing a large part of the combined cardiac output to return to the placenta without flowing through the lungs. Approximately 55% of the combined ventricular output flows to the placenta; 35% perfuses body tissues; and the remaining 10% flows through the lungs (Behrman and Vaughan, 1987). *After birth.* The foramen ovale closes; the ductus arteriosus closes and becomes a ligament; the ductus venosus closes and becomes a ligament; and the umbilical vein and arteries close and become ligaments. (Courtesy Ross Laboratories, Columbus, Ohio.)

The ductus arteriosus constricts in response to the establishment of a Po_2 level of about 50 mm Hg in the arterial blood. Eventually it occludes and becomes a ligament. With the clamping and severing of the cord, the umbilical arteries and vein and the ductus venosus close immediately and are converted into ligaments. The hypogastric arteries also occlude and become ligaments. The changes in blood flow with birth of the infant have the effect of transforming the circulatory system. Before birth the two ventricles act in parallel, with shunts adjusting possible unequal outputs, while after birth the two pumps act in series (Behrman and Vaughan, 1987).

Heart Rate and Sound. The heart rate averages 140 beats per minute (bpm) at birth with variations noted during sleeping and waking states. At 1 week of age the mean heart rate is 128 bpm asleep and 163 bpm awake; at 1 month of age it is 138 bpm asleep and 167 bpm awake. Sinus arrhythmia (irregular heart rate) may be considered a physiologic phenomenon in infancy and an indication of good heart function (Lowrey, 1986).

Heart sounds after birth reflect the series action of the heart pump. They are described as the familiar "lub, dub, lub, dub" sound. The "lub" is associated with closure of the mitral and tricuspid valves at the beginning of systole and the "dub" with closure of the aortic and pulmonic valves at the end of systole. The "lub" is the first heart sound and the "dub" the second heart sound. The normal cycle of the heart starts with the beginning of systole (Guyton, 1986). Heart sounds during the neonatal period are higher pitched, shorter in duration, and of greater intensity than those of adults. The first sound is typically louder and duller than the second sound, which is sharp in quality. Most heart murmurs heard during the neonatal period have no pathologic significance, and more than half disappear by 6 months.

By term gestation, the infant's heart lies midway between the crown of the head and the buttocks, and the axis is more transverse than that of the adult. The point of maximum impulse (PMI) in the newborn infant is at the fourth intercostal space and to the left of the midclavicular line. The PMI is often visible.

Blood Pressure and Volume. Blood pressure in infants varies from day to day during the first month of life. A drop in systolic blood pressure (about 15 mm Hg) the first hour after birth is common. Values from several hours after delivery through the neonatal period average a systolic pressure of 78 and a diastolic pressure of 42 (see discussion of Doppler technique, Chapter 22). Crying and moving result in changes in blood pressure, especially systolic.

Blood volume in the newborn ranges from 80 to 110 ml/kg during the first several days and doubles by the end of the first year. Proportionately, the newborn has approximately 10% greater blood volume and nearly 20% greater red blood cell mass than the adult. However, the newborn's blood is about 20% less plasma volume when compared by kilogram of body weight with the adult. The infant born prematurely will have a relatively greater blood volume than the term newborn. This is because the preterm infant has a proportionately greater plasma volume, not a greater red blood cell mass.

A number of differences in the circulatory dynamics of the newborn result from early or late clamping of the cord. Late clamping results in an expansion of blood volume from the so-called placental transfusion, an increase of close to 60%. This in turn causes an increase in the size of the heart, increased systolic blood pressure, and a higher respiratory rate.

Hematopoietic System

Hematopoietic characteristics of the newborn include certain variations from the hematopoietic system of the adult. There are differences in red blood cells and leukocytes and relatively few differences in platelets.

At birth the average values of hemoglobin and red blood cells are higher than those values in the adult. These fall and reach the average levels of 11 to 17 g/dl and 4.2 to $5.2/mm^3$, respectively, by the end of the first month. The blood values may be affected by delayed clamping of the cord, which results in a rise in hemoglobin, red blood cells, and hematocrit. The source of the sample is another significant factor, since capillary blood will give higher values than venous blood. Also, the time after birth when the blood sample was obtained is significant, since the slight rise in red blood cells after birth is followed by a substantial drop. At birth the infant's blood contains about 80% fetal hemoglobin, but because of the shorter life span of the cells containing fetal hemoglobin, the percentage falls to 55% by 5 weeks and 5% by 20 weeks. Fortunately iron stores generally are sufficient to sustain normal red blood cell production for 6 months, and thus the slight brief anemia is not serious. Delayed clamping of the cord increases available iron, as 80 ml of placental blood yields 50 mg of iron (Cunningham, MacDonald, and Gant, 1989).

Leukocytosis, with the white blood cell count approximately $18,000/mm^3$, is normal at birth. The number, largely polymorphs, increases to about 23,000 to $24,000/mm^3$ during the first day after birth. A resting level of $11,500/mm^3$ normally is maintained during the neonatal period. Serious infection is not well tolerated by the newborn, and a marked increase in the white blood cell count is unlikely even in critical sepsis. In most instances sepsis is accompanied by a decline in white cells, particularly in neutrophils. The activity of the marrow is accurately reflected by the number of circulating cells—both erythrocytes and leukocytes. The early high white blood cell count of the newborn decreases rapidly (see Appendix G).

Platelet count and aggregation are essentially the same in newborn infants as in adults. One exception is the infant of a mother who has taken aspirin or chlorpromazine, both of which interfere with the release of adenosine diphosphate (ADP). Otherwise bleeding tendencies in the newborn are rare, and unless there is a marked vitamin K deficiency, clotting is sufficient to prevent hemorrhage.

The infant's blood group is established early in fetal life. However, during the neonatal period there is a gradual increase in the strength of the agglutinogens present in the red blood cell membrane.

Respiratory System

At birth, air must be substituted for fluid that has filled the respiratory tract to the alveoli. During the course of normal vaginal delivery, amniotic fluid is squeezed or drained from the newborn's lungs. After delivery the major portion of the fetal lung fluid is absorbed across the alveolar membrane into the blood capillaries. This is largely a result of the pressure gradient from alveoli to interstitial tissue to blood capillary. Reduced vascular resistance also accommodates this flow of lung fluid; however, it is the diminished intravascular pressure that is ultimately responsible.

Initial breathing is probably the result of a reflex triggered by pressure changes, chilling, noise, light, and other sensations related to the birth process. In addition the chemoreceptors in the aorta and carotid bodies initiate neurologic reflexes when the arterial Po_2 falls from 80 to 15 mm Hg, arterial Pco_2 rises from 40 to 70 mm Hg, and arterial pH falls below 7.35. (When these changes are extreme, however, depression ensues.) In most cases an exaggerated respiratory reaction follows within 1 minute of birth, and the infant takes a first gasping breath and cries.

With the first breath the infant develops a considerable negative intrathoracic pressure. Air is drawn in, and about half of this remains as residual pulmonary volume. Normally only a few breaths are required to expand the lungs well; subsequently the pressure will be lower than at the onset of respiration.

Abnormal respiration and failure to completely expand the lungs retard the egress of fetal lung fluid from alveoli and interstices into the pulmonary circulation. Retention of fluid in turn alters pulmonary function.

Certain **respiratory patterns** are characteristic of the normal term newborn. After respirations are established, they are shallow and irregular, ranging from 30 to 60 breaths per minute, with short periods of apnea (less than 15 seconds). These short periods of apnea occur most often during the active (rapid eye movement [REM]) sleep cycle and decrease in frequency and duration with age. Apneic periods over 15 seconds in duration should be evaluated.

Newborn infants are obligatory nose breathers. The reflex response to nasal obstruction is opening the mouth to maintain an airway. This response is not present in most infants until 3 weeks after birth. Therefore cyanosis or asphyxia may occur with nasal blockage.

The chest circumference is approximately 30 to 33 cm (12 to 13 in) at birth. The ribs of the infant articulate with the spine at a horizontal rather than a downward slope; consequently the rib cage cannot expand with inspiration as readily as does the adult's. Neonatal respiratory function is largely a matter of diaphragmatic contraction. The negative intrathoracic pressure is created by the descent of the diaphragm, much like negative pressure is created in the barrel of a syringe when medication is drawn up by retracting the plunger. The newborn infant's chest and abdomen rise simultaneously with inspiration. *Seesaw respirations are not normal* (Fig. 16-2).

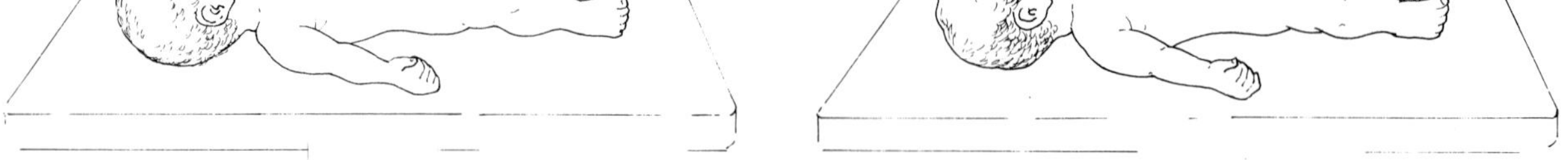

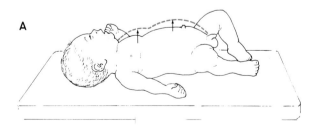

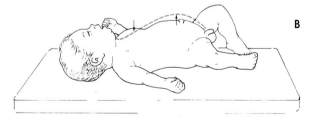

Fig. 16-2 **A,** Normal respiration. Chest and abdomen rise with inspiration. **B,** Seesaw respiration. Chest wall retracts and abdomen rises with inspiration. (Courtesy Mead Johnson & Co., Evansville, Indiana.)

Auscultation of the chest of a newborn infant reveals loud, clear breath sounds that seem very near, because little chest tissue intervenes. Several significant differences exist between the respiratory system of the newborn infant and the adult:

1. Newborn infants are obligate nose breathers.
2. The newborn infant's tongue is relatively large (macroglossia), whereas the glottis and trachea are small.
3. All lumens of the newborn infant are narrower and more easily collapsed.
4. Respiratory tract secretions of the newborn infant are more abundant than those of the adult.
5. The mucous membranes of the newborn infant are more delicate and therefore more susceptible to trauma. The ciliated columnar epithelium just below the vocal cords is especially prone to edema.
6. The alveoli of the newborn infant are more sensitive to changes in pressures.
7. The capillary network of the newborn infant is less well developed. Capillaries are more friable (more easily damaged) and have less well developed vasoconstrictive and dilatative ability.
8. The newborn infant's bony rib cage and respiratory muscles are not as well developed.

Renal System

At term gestation the kidneys occupy a large portion of the posterior abdominal wall. The bladder lies close to the anterior abdominal wall and is partially an abdominal, as well as a pelvic, organ. In the newborn almost all palpable masses in the abdomen are renal in origin.

Kidney function comparable to that of the adult is not approached until the second year of life. The newborn has a narrow range of chemical balance and safety. Diarrhea, infection, or improper feeding can lead rapidly to acidosis and fluid imbalances—dehydration or edema. Renal immaturity also limits the newborn infant's ability to excrete drugs.

Small amounts of urine are usually present in the bladder at birth; however, the newborn may not void for 12 to 24 hours. Voiding after this period is frequent. Six to ten voidings a day of pale, straw-colored urine are indicative of adequate fluid intake. The usual urinary output by 10 days is 50 to 300 ml/24 hours.

Differences in **fluid and electrolyte balance** from adult physiologic response include the following:

1. The distribution of extracellular and intracellular fluid differs from that of the adult. About 40% of the body weight of the newborn is extracellular fluid, whereas in the adult it is 20%.

2. The rate of exchange of extracellular fluid is different. The newborn daily takes in and excretes 600 to 700 ml of water, which is 20% of the total body fluid, or 50% of the extracellular fluid. In contrast, the adult exchanges 2000 ml of water, which is 5% of the total body fluid and 14% of the extracellular fluid.

3. The composition of body fluids shows variations. There is a higher concentration of sodium, phosphates, chloride, and organic acids and a lower concentration of bicarbonate ions. These findings mean that the newborn is in a compensated acidotic state and in a state of potential manifest edema.

4. The glomerular filtration rate is about 30% to 50% of that of the adult. This results in a decreased ability to remove nitrogenous and other waste products from the blood. However, the newborn's ingested protein is almost totally metabolized for growth.

5. The decreased ability to excrete excessive sodium results in hypotonic urine compared to plasma.

6. The sodium reabsorption is decreased as a result of lowered sodium-potassium-activated adenosine triphosphatase (ATPase) activity.

7. The newborn can dilute urine down to 50 milliosmols (mOsm). The capacity to dilute urine exceeds the capacity to concentrate it. There is some limitation in the ability to increase urinary volume.

8. The newborn can concentrate urine to 600 to 700 mOsm compared with the adult's capacity of 1400 mOsm. The inability to concentrate urine is not absolute, but in terms of adult function, it is somewhat limited.

9. The newborn has a higher renal threshold for glucose.

Gastrointestinal System

In the adequately hydrated newborn infant the mucous membrane of the mouth is moist and pink. Pallor and cyanosis of the mucous membrane are normally not present. Drooling of mucus is common in the first few hours after birth. There are no clefts in the palate. Retention cysts, small whitish areas (Epstein's pearls), may be found on the gum margins and at the juncture of the hard and soft palate. The cheeks are full because of well-developed sucking pads. These, like the labial tubercles (sucking calluses) on the upper lip, disappear when the sucking period is over.

A special mechanism present in normal newborns weighing more than 1500 g coordinates the breathing, sucking, and swallowing reflexes necessary for oral feeding. Sucking in the newborn takes place in small bursts of three or four sucks at a time. In the term newborn, longer and more efficient sucking attempts occur in only a few hours. The newborn infant is unable to move food from the lips to the pharynx; therefore it is necessary to place the nipple (breast or bottle) well inside the baby's mouth. Peristaltic activity in the esophagus is uncoordinated in the first few days of life. It quickly becomes a coordinated pattern in normal infants, and they swallow easily.

Bacteria are not present in the infant's gastrointestinal tract at birth. Soon after birth, oral and anal orifices permit entrance of bacteria and air. Bowel sounds can be heard 1 hour after birth. Generally the highest bacterial concentration is found in the lower portion of the intestine, particularly in the large intestine. The normal intestinal flora help synthesize vitamin K, folic acid, and biotin.

The capacity of the stomach varies from 30 to 90 ml depending on the size of the infant. Emptying time for the stomach is highly variable. Several factors, such as time and volume of feedings, type and temperature of food, and psychic stress, may affect the emptying time. This can range from 1 to 24 hours. Regurgitation may be noted in the neonatal period. The cardiac sphincter and nervous control of the stomach are still immature.

Digestion. Two principal types of cells make up the lining of the stomach. The first type, chief cells, synthesizes and secretes pepsinogen, which aids protein digestion. The second type, parietal cells, secrete hydrochloric acid, which forms the gastric acidity. The enzyme pepsin and gastric acidity are necessary for preliminary digestion of milk before its entrance into the small intestine. The infant's gastric acidity at birth normally equals the adult level but is reduced within a week and may remain reduced for 2 to 3 months. The reduction in gastric acidity may lead to "colic." Infants with colic usually remain awake, crying in apparent distress between 2 feedings, often the same ones every day. Nothing seems to appease them. They appear to "grow out" of this behavior by age 3 months.

Further digestion and absorption of nutrients occur in the small intestine. This complex process is made possible by pancreatic secretions, secretions from the liver through the common bile duct, and secretions from the duodenal portion of the small intestine.

The newborn infant's ability to digest carbohydrates, fats, and proteins is regulated by the presence of certain enzymes. Most of these are functional at birth. One exception is *amylase,* produced by the salivary glands after about 3 months and by the pancreas at about 6 months of age. This enzyme is necessary to convert starch into maltose. The other exception is *lipase,* also secreted by the pancreas; it is necessary for the digestion of fat. Thus the normal newborn is capable of digesting simple carbohydrates and proteins but has a limited ability to digest fats (see Chapter 18 for more detail).

Stools. At birth the lower intestine is filled with meconium. Meconium is formed during fetal life from the amniotic fluid and its constituents, intestinal secretions, and shed mucosal cells. Meconium is greenish black and viscous and contains occult blood. The first meconium passed is sterile, but within hours all meconium passed contains bacteria. The first passage of meconium occurs within 24 hours in 90% of normal infants. Most of the rest do so within 36 hours (Cunningham, MacDonald, and Gant, 1989).

The number of **newborn stools** varies considerably during the first week and are most numerous between the third and sixth days. Transitional stools (thin, slimy, and brown to green because of the continued presence of meconium) are passed from the third to sixth day. Newborns fed early pass stool sooner than those fed later (Boyer and Vidyasagar, 1987). The stools of breastfed babies and bottle-fed babies differ. The stools of the breastfed baby are loose, golden yellow in color, and nonirritating to the infant's skin. It is normal for the baby to have a bowel movement with each feeding or a bowel movement every 3 to 4 days. Even if the latter is the case, the stools remain loose and unformed. The stools of the bottle-fed baby are formed but soft, are pale yellow, and have a typical stool odor. They tend to be irritating to the baby's skin. The number of stools decreases in the first 2 weeks from five or six each day (after every feeding) to one to two per day.

Distension of the stomach muscles causes a corresponding relaxation and contraction of the muscles of the colon. As a result, infants often have bowel movements during or just after a feeding. (Breastfed babies are more likely to stool during a feeding than bottle-fed babies.) Stooling at these times has been attributed to the gastrocolic reflex.

The infant develops an elimination pattern by the second week of life. With the addition of solid food the infant's stool gradually assumes the characteristics of an adult's stool.

Feeding Behaviors. Variations occur among infants regarding interest in food, symptoms of hunger, and amount ingested at any one time. The amount that the infant takes at any one feeding depends, of course, on the size of the infant; but other factors seem to play a part: if put to breast, some infants nurse immediately, whereas others require a learning period of up to 48 hours before nursing can be said to be effective. Random hand-to-mouth movement and sucking of fingers have been seen in utero. These actions are well developed at birth and are intensified with hunger.

Hepatic System

The liver performs a number of functions, one of which is to control the amount of circulating unbound bilirubin. The pigment bilirubin is derived from the hemoglobin released with the breakdown of red blood cells (90% to 95%). The remaining pigment is derived from the myoglobin in muscle cells. The hemoglobin is phagocytized by the reticuloendothelial cells, converted to bilirubin, and released in an unconjugated form. Unconjugated bilirubin, termed *indirect bilirubin,* is relatively insoluble and is almost entirely bound to circulating albumin, a plasma protein. The unbound bilirubin can leave the vascular system and permeate other extravascular tissues (e.g., the skin, sclera, and oral mucous membranes). The resultant yellow coloring is termed *jaundice.*

In the liver the unbound bilirubin is conjugated with glucuronide in the presence of the enzyme glucuronyl transferase. The conjugated form of bilirubin is excreted from liver cells as a constituent of bile. It is termed *direct bilirubin* and is soluble. Along with other components of bile, direct bilirubin is excreted into the biliary tract system that carries the bile into the duodenum. Bilirubin is converted to urobilinogen and stercobilin within the duodenum through the action of the bacterial flora. Urobilinogen is excreted in urine and feces; stercobilin is excreted in the feces (Fig. 16-3). Total serum bilirubin is the sum of conjugated (direct) and unconjugated (indirect) bilirubin.

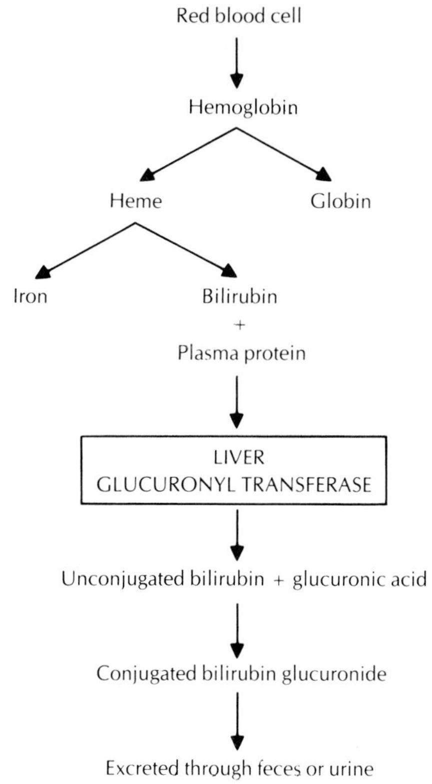

Fig. 16-3 Formation and excretion of bilirubin. (From Whaley L and Wong D: Essentials of pediatric nursing, ed 3, St Louis, 1989, The CV Mosby Co.)

The full-term newborn's liver is usually sufficiently mature and the production of glucuronyl transferase great enough to conjugate the circulating unconjugated bilirubin. Adequate serum albumin–binding sites are also available unless the infant experiences asphyxia neonatorum, cold stress, or hypoglycemia. Maternal prebirth ingestion of drugs such as sulfa drugs and aspirin can reduce the amount of serum albumin–binding sites in the newly born. Although the newborn has the functional capacity to convert bilirubin, physiologic hyperbilirubinemia occurs in most infants.

Physiologic Hyperbilirubinemia. Physiologic **hyperbilirubinemia,** or neonatal jaundice, is a normal occurrence in 50% of full-term and 80% of preterm newborns. Asian and American-Indian newborns appear to have increased physiologic jaundice regardless of feeding method (Auerbach and Gartner, 1987). Korones (1986, p. 321) noted that neonatal jaundice occurs because:

1. The newborn has a higher rate of bilirubin production. The number of fetal red blood cells per kilogram of weight is greater than the adult. The fetal red blood cells have a shorter survival time, 40 to 90 days compared to 120 days in the adult.
2. There is considerable reabsorption of bilirubin from the neonatal small intestine.

Although neonatal jaundice is considered benign, bilirubin may accumulate to hazardous levels and become pathologic (Chapter 28). Linn and associates (1985) reported ethnic differences in the rate of hyperbilirubinemia. They reported that 49.2% of Oriental, 20% of white, and 12.1% of black newborns had bilirubin levels of 10 mg/dl or higher. The risk of hyperbilirubinemia is increased with delayed clamping of the cord. Physiologic jaundice fulfills the following specific criteria (Korones, 1986, p. 321):

> (1) The infant is otherwise well; (2) in term infants, jaundice first appears after 24 hours and disappears by the end of the seventh day; (3) in premature infants, jaundice is first evident after 48 hours and disappears by the ninth or tenth day; (4) serum unconjugated bilirubin concentration does not exceed 12 mg/100 ml, either in term or preterm infants; (5) hyperbilirubinemia is almost exclusively of the unconjugated variety, and conjugated (direct) bilirubin should not exceed 1 to 1.5 mg/100 ml; (6) daily increments of bilirubin concentration should not surpass 5 mg/100 ml. Bilirubin levels in excess of 12 mg/100 ml may indicate either an exaggeration of the physiologic handicap or the presence of disease. *At any serum bilirubin level, the appearance of jaundice during the first day of life or persistence beyond the ages previously delineated usually indicates a pathologic process.*

Jaundice is noticeable first in the head and then progresses gradually toward the abdomen and extremities because of the newborn infant's circulatory pattern (cephalocaudal developmental progression). The appearance of jaundice in the various body locations gives a rough estimate of the circulating levels of unbound bilirubin. For example, when jaundice appears over the nose, the circulating level of unbound bilirubin is approximately 3 mg; levels at which other body areas appear jaundiced are as follows:

Approximate Level of Hyperbilirubinemia by Cephalocaudal Distribution

Nose: 3 mg/dl	Abdomen: 10 mg/dl
Face: 5 mg/dl	Legs: 12 mg/dl
Chest: 7 mg/dl	Palms: 20 mg/dl

Several nursery practices may influence the appearance and degree of physiologic hyperbilirubinemia. *Early feeding* tends to keep the serum bilirubin level low by stimulating intestinal activity and the passage of meconium and stool. Removal of intestinal contents prevents the reabsorption (and recycling) of bilirubin from the gut.

Chilling of the newborn may result in acidosis and raise the level of free fatty acids. In the presence of acidosis, albumin binding of bilirubin is *weakened* and bilirubin is freed. Bilirubin is *displaced* from its serum albumin–binding sites by the free fatty acids and as unbound bilirubin can be deposited in body tissues. ***Kernicterus***, the most serious complication of neonatal hyperbilirubinemia, is caused by the precipitation of bilirubin in neuronal cells, resulting in their destruction (see Chapter 28). Cerebral palsy, epilepsy, and mental retardation are expected in survivors.

There is an increase in the number of mothers and infants being discharged from the hospital between 2 and 48 hours after birth and others who have elected birth at home. As a result the professional attendant may not be available to assess pathologic rises in circulating unbound bilirubin. *Therefore all parents need instruction in how to assess jaundice and to whom to report the findings* (see Chapter 18).

Jaundice Associated with Breastfeeding. Two types of jaundice are associated with breastfeeding: breast*feeding* jaundice and breast *milk* jaundice. Breastfeeding jaundice occurs earlier than breast milk jaundice and is associated with the breastfeeding pattern. Breast milk jaundice is thought to be caused by the presence of an enzyme in the milk and lasts longer than breastfeeding jaundice.

Breastfeeding jaundice usually becomes apparent about the third day of life. There is no other apparent clinical cause. Dehydration, lack of fluid, and weight loss are not causes (DeCarvalho et al, 1981). Recent research has documented that the number of breastfeedings during the first 3 days of life are related to bilirubin levels and display a significant relationship (Lascari, 1986). The greater the number of feedings, the lower the bilirubin level (DeCarvalho et al, 1982; Lascari, 1986). The number of feedings per day should be eight or more. The mother is encouraged to feed around the clock. Early breastmilk colostrum is a natural laxative that helps promote passage of meconium. Consequently early, frequent nursings will enhance meconium excretion and decrease bilirubin levels.

Breastfed babies may have higher bilirubin levels than bottlefed babies (Kivlahan and James, 1984; DeCarvalho et al, 1985; Lascari, 1986). ***Breast milk jaundice*** is defined as increasing indirect hyperbilirubinemia after the first week of life. Jaundice from ingestion of breast milk occurs in 0.5% to 2% of fullterm newborns (Saul and Warburton, 1984). It is thought that an enzyme present in the milk of some women inhibits the enzyme glucuronyl transferase, which is necessary for the conjugation of bilirubin. Although breast milk jaundice is a form of physiologic jaundice, it occurs after the mature milk has come in, usually about the fifth or sixth day of life in a thriving infant whose mother is lactating well. This type of jaundice usually persists longer—up to 6 weeks—than breastfeeding jaundice. Unconjugated bilirubin rises beyond physiologic limits (15 to 20 mg/dl) by the seventh day. The levels subside by 5 to 10 mg if breastfeeding is discontinued for 12 to 24 hours; then usually 3 to 5 days pass before the previous high level is again reached. Mothers are encouraged to maintain their milk supply during this test period by pumping or manually expressing the milk. Mothers need reassurance that nothing is wrong with their milk (Lascari, 1986).

Although the indirect bilirubin level may range from 10 to 30 mg/dl during this time, no cases of bilirubin encephalopathy related to breast milk jaundice have been reported (Brovten et al, 1985).

Immune System

All newborns, especially preterm newborns, are at risk for infection, one of the major causes of newborn illness and death during the first few months of life. This is because the newborn cannot limit pathogens to the portal of entry because of hypofunction of the inflammatory and immune responses (Medici, 1983).

Medici (1983, p. 25) summarizes the newborn's **immune system status** as follows:

> The term and preterm neonate has an increased incidence of infection for the first four to six weeks of life. This reflects the immaturity of a number of protective systems which significantly increases the risk of infection in this patient population. Natural barriers such as the acidity of the stomach or the production of pepsin and trypsin which maintain sterility of the small intestine are not fully developed until three to four weeks. The membrane protective IgA is missing from the respiratory and urinary tracts, and unless the newborn is

breast fed, it is absent from the gastrointestinal tract as well. The immune system is in great part suppressed; possibly this is a mechanism for preventing maternal recognition of paternal antigens with subsequent rejection of the fetus. Finally, the qualitative and quantitative response of the inflammatory response is depressed because of decreased initiation factors and sluggish responses of the phagocytic cells.

Integumentary System

Knowledge of **integumentary characteristics** is basic to providing nursing care to newborns and their families. Several characteristics are discussed here. The epidermis (skin) of the term newborn possesses the characteristic five layers (strata) of the adult: germinativum, spinosum, granulosum, corneum, and on the palmar and plantar surfaces, stratum lucidum underneath the stratum corneum. In the newborn the stratum corneum is thin and fused with the vernix caseosa (a reason for not removing the vernix at birth). The stratum corneum later becomes the effective skin barrier.

The intact skin of the newborn acts as an effective barrier to infection; however, the fragility of the skin makes it more vulnerable to disruption of the surface when traumatized by too vigorous handling, rubbing, or excoriation.

The term infant has an erythematous skin (beefy red) for a few hours after birth, after which it fades to its normal color. It often appears blotchy, especially over the extremities. The hands and feet appear slightly cyanotic. This bluish discoloration, *acrocyanosis,* is caused by vasomotor instability, capillary stasis, and a high hemoglobin level; it is normal, transient in occurrence, and persists over the first 7 to 10 days, especially with exposure to cold.

The healthy term newborn is plump, and the skin may be slightly tight, suggesting fluid retention. Fine *lanugo hair* may be noted over the face, shoulders, and back. Actual edema of the face and *ecchymosis* (bruising) may be noted as a result of face presentation or forceps delivery.

Caput Succedaneum. Caput succedaneum is a localized, easily identifiable edematous area of the scalp (Fig. 16-4, *A*). The sustained pressure of the presenting vertex against the cervix results in compression of local vessels, thus slowing venous return. The slower venous return causes an increase in tissue fluids within the skin of the scalp, and an edematous swelling develops. This boggy edematous swelling present at birth extends across suture lines of the fetal skull and disappears spontaneously within 3 to 4 days.

Cephalhematoma. Cephalhematoma is a collection of blood between a skull bone and its periosteum. Therefore a cephalhematoma never crosses a cranial suture line (Fig. 16-4, *B*). Cephalhematoma is caused by pressure during delivery. Bleeding may occur with spontaneous delivery from pressure against the maternal bony pelvis. Low forceps delivery, as well as difficult forceps rotation and extraction, may also cause bleeding. This soft, fluctuating, irreducible fullness does not pulsate or bulge when the infant cries. It appears several hours after birth or the day after delivery or becomes apparent following absorption of a caput succedaneum (Fig. 16-4, *A*). It is usually largest on the

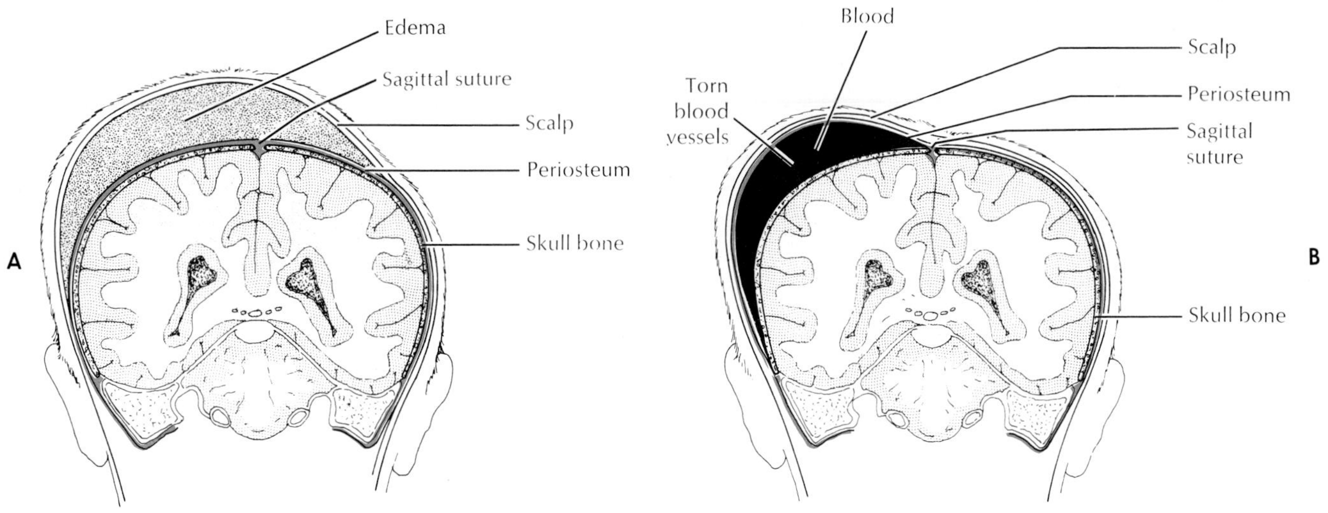

Fig. 16-4 Differences between caput succedaneum and cephalhematoma. **A,** Caput succedaneum: edema of scalp noted at birth; crosses suture line. **B,** Cephalhematoma: bleeding between periosteum and skull bone appearing within first 2 days; does not cross suture lines.

second or third day, by which time the bleeding stops. The fullness of cephalhematoma spontaneously resolves in 3 to 6 weeks. It is not aspirated because infection may develop if the skin is punctured.

As the hematoma resolves, the hemolysis of red blood cells occurs. Hyperbilirubinemia may result after the newborn is home. Therefore the parents are instructed to observe the newborn for jaundice and may be asked to bring the infant in to be rechecked before the usual 4-week visit.

Desquamation. Desquamation of the skin of the term infant does not occur until a few days after birth. Its presence at birth is an indication of postmaturity.

Sweat and Oil Glands. Sweat glands are present at birth but do not function effectively (i.e., do not respond to increases in ambient or body temperature), perhaps because the neurogenic stimuli are still immature. There is some fetal *sebaceous* (oil) *gland* hyperplasia and secretion of sebum as a result of the hormonal influences of pregnancy. Vernix caseosa, a cheeselike substance, is a product of the sebaceous glands. Distended sebaceous glands, noticeable in the newborn, particularly on the cheeks and nose, are known as *milia.* Although sebaceous glands are well developed at birth, they are only minimally active during childhood. They become more active as androgen production increases before puberty.

Mongolian Spots. Mongolian spots, bluish-black areas of pigmentation, may appear over any part of the extensor surface of the body, including the extremities. They are more commonly noted on the back and buttocks. These pigmented areas are noted in babies whose origins are from the shores of the Mediterranean, Latin America, Asia, Africa, or a number of other areas in the world. They are more common in dark-skinned individuals regardless of race. They fade gradually over a period of months or years.

Telangiectatic Nevi. Known as "stork bites," telangiectatic nevi are pink and easily blanched (Fig. 16-5, *A*). They appear on the upper eyelids, nose, upper lip, lower occiput bone, and nape of the neck. They have no clinical significance and fade between the first and second years.

Nevus Vasculosus. The strawberry mark, or nevus vasculosus, is the second most common type of capillary hemangioma (Fig. 16-5, *B*). It consists of dilated, newly formed capillaries occupying the entire dermal and subdermal layers with associated connective tissue hypertrophy. The typical lesion is a raised, sharply demarcated, and bright or dark red, rough-surfaced swelling that resembles a strawberry. Lesions are usually single but may be multiple; 75% occur in the head region. These lesions can remain until the child is of school age or sometimes even longer.

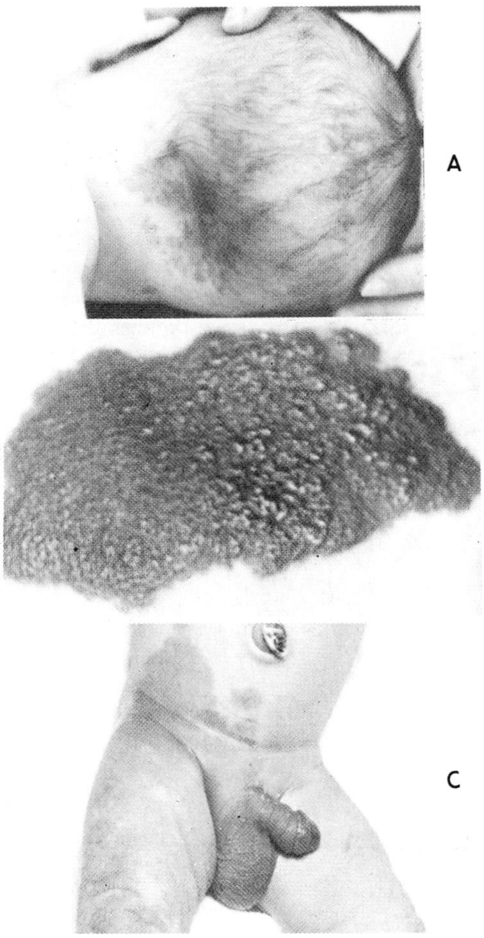

Fig. 16-5 **A,** Telangiectatic nevi (stork bite). **B,** Strawberry mark, or nevus vasculosus. **C,** Port-wine stain, or nevus flammeus. (Courtesy Mead Johnson & Co., Evansville, Indiana.)

Nevus Flammeus. A port-wine stain, or nevus flammeus, is usually observed at birth and is composed of a plexus of newly formed capillaries in the papillary layer of the corium. It is red to purple, varies in size, shape, and location, and is not elevated (Fig. 16-5, *C*). True port-wine stains do not blanch on pressure and do not disappear spontaneously.

Erythema Toxicum. A transient rash, erythema toxicum is also called *erythema neonatorum,* or "fleabite" dermatitis. It has lesions in different stages, erythematous macules, papules, or small vesicles, and may appear suddenly anywhere on the body. The rash is thought to be an inflammatory response. Eosinophils, which help decrease inflammation, are found in the vesicles. The rash is found only in term neonates (36 or more weeks gestational age) during the first 3 weeks after birth (Medici, 1983). Although the appearance is alarming, it has no clinical significance and requires no treatment.

Reproductive System

The newborn differs from the adult in several **reproductive system characteristics.** Knowledge of these characteristics is important to nurses who plan nursing care of newborns and their families.

Female. At birth the ovaries contain thousands of primitive germ cells. These represent the full complement of potential ova, since no oogonia form after delivery in term infants. The ovarian cortex, which is made up primarily of primordial follicles, forms a thicker portion of the ovary in the newborn than in the adult. The number of ova decreases from birth to maturity by approximately 90%.

Hyperestrogenism of pregnancy followed by a drop after delivery results in a mucoid vaginal discharge and even some slight blood spotting ("withdrawal bleeding"). The infant's uterus also responds by undergoing involution in the first weeks of life and decreasing in size and weight. External genitals are usually edematous with increased pigmentation. In term newborn infants, labia majora and minora obscure the vestibule (Fig. 16-6, *A*). Vaginal or hymenal tags are common findings and have no clinical significance.

Male. The testes descend into the scrotum in 90% of newborn boys. Although this percentage drops with preterm birth, by 1 year of age the incidence of undescended testes in all boys is less than 1%. Spermatogenesis does not occur until puberty (see Chapter 7).

A tight prepuce (foreskin) is a common finding in newborns. The urethral opening may be completely covered by the prepuce, which may not be retractable for 3 to 4 years.

External genitals in the term newborn are increased in size and pigmentation in response to maternal estrogen. The scrotal sac is covered with rugae (Fig. 16-6, *B*).

Swelling of Breast Tissue. Swelling of the breast tissue in newborn infants of both sexes is caused by the hyperestrogenism of pregnancy. In a few newborns a thin discharge (witch's milk) can be seen. The finding has no clinical significance, requires no treatment, and will subside as the maternal hormones are eliminated from the newborn infant's body.

Skeletal System

The cephalocaudal direction of development is evident in total body growth. The head at term is one fourth of the body length. The arms are slightly longer than the legs.

The face is small in relation to the skull, which is large and heavy in comparison. Cranial size and shape can be distorted by molding.

There are two curvatures in the vertebral column: thoracic and sacral. When the infant gains head control, another curvature occurs in the cervical region.

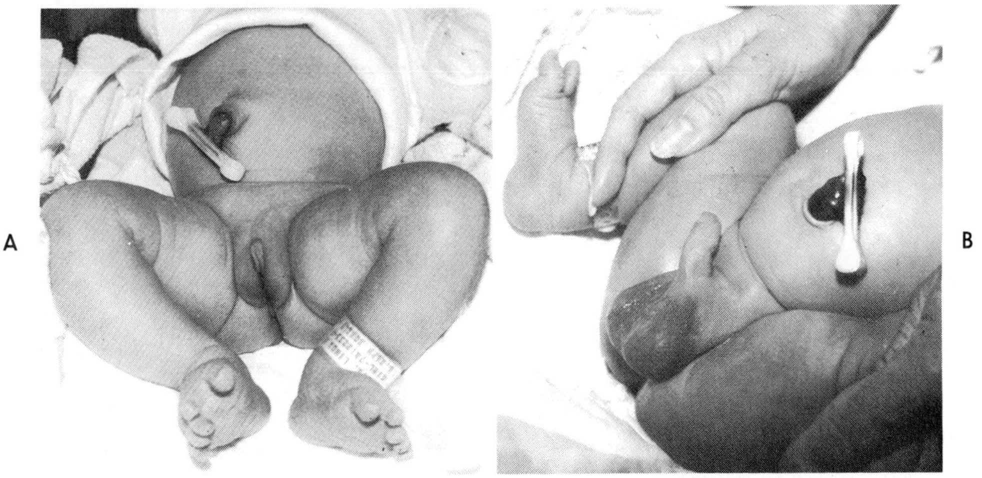

Fig. 16-6 **A,** Genitals in female term infant. Note mucoid vaginal discharge. **B,** Genitals in male infant. Uncircumcised penis. Rugae cover scrotum, indicating term gestation. Cord has been swabbed with ethylene blue to prevent infection.

In newborn infants there is a significant separation of the knees when the ankles are held together, which results in an appearance of bowlegs. At birth, there is no apparent arch to the foot.

Neuromuscular System

Before the late 1950s, the human newborn was thought to be immature and disorganized, functioning at the brainstem level. Neurobehavioral assessment of the newborn was primarily an evaluation of primitive reflexes and muscle tone. Today, the term newborn is recognized as a vital, responsive, and reactive being. The newborn's sensory development and capacity for social interaction and self-organization are remarkable (Fanaroff and Martin, 1987).

Postdelivery growth of the brain follows a predictable pattern of rapid growth during infancy and early childhood (more gradual during the remainder of the first decade and minimal during adolescence). The cerebellum ends its growth spurt, which began at about 30 gestational weeks, by the end of the first year. This is perhaps why it is vulnerable to nutritional or other trauma in early infancy (see discussion of newborn nutrition, Chapter 18, and kernicterus, Chapter 28).

The brain requires glucose as a source of energy and a relatively large supply of oxygen for adequate metabolism. Such requirements signal a need for careful assessment of the newborn infant's ability to maintain an open airway and of respiratory conditions requiring oxygen therapy. The necessity for glucose requires careful monitoring of those newborn infants who may have hypoglycemic episodes.

Spontaneous motor activity may be seen in transient tremors of mouth and chin, especially when crying, and of extremities, notably the arms and hands; these tremors are normal. Persistent tremors or tremors involving the total body may be indicative of pathologic conditions. Marked tonicity, clonicity, and twitching of facial muscles are signs of convulsions. There is a need to differentiate among normal tremors (as described above), tremors of hypoglycemia (Chapter 24), and pathologic conditions (Chapter 28) so that corrective care can be instituted, as necessary.

Neuromuscular control in the newborn, although still very limited, can be noted. If newborns are placed facedown on a firm surface, they will turn their heads to the side to maintain an airway. They attempt to hold their heads in line with their bodies if they are raised by their arms.

There are differences among ethnic groups in neuromuscular development (Freedman, 1979). Various **newborn reflexes** promote their safety and an adequate food intake. This is described further in this chapter under behavioral characteristics of the newborn.

Thermogenetic System

Thermogenesis means the production of heat (thermo = heat, genesis = origin). Effective neonatal care is based on the maintenance of an optimum thermal environment. In homoiothermic individuals the narrow limits of normal body temperature are maintained by producing heat in response to its dissipation. Hypothermia from excessive heat loss is a prevalent and dangerous problem in newborn infants. The newborn's ability to produce heat often approaches the capacity of the adult. However, the tendency toward rapid heat loss in a suboptimum thermal environment is increased in the newborn and is often hazardous.

Heat Production. The shivering mechanism of heat production is rarely operable in the newborn. Nonshivering thermogenesis is accomplished primarily by ***brown fat*** and secondarily by increased metabolic activity in the brain, heart, and liver. Brown fat is located in superficial deposits in the interscapular region and axillas, as well as in deep deposits at the thoracic inlet, along the vertebral column, and around the kidneys. Brown fat has a richer vascular and nerve supply than does ordinary fat. Heat produced by intense lipid metabolic activity in brown fat can warm the newborn by increasing heat production as much as 100%. Reserves of brown fat, usually present for several weeks after birth, are rapidly depleted with cold stress. The less mature the infant, the less reserve of this essential fat is available at birth.

Heat Loss. Heat loss occurs in four ways:

1. *Convection:* the flow of heat from the body surface to cooler ambient air. For this reason nursery ambient temperatures are kept at 24° C (75° F), and newborns are wrapped to protect them from the cold.
2. *Radiation:* the loss of heat from the body surface to cooler solid surfaces not in direct contact but in relative proximity to each other. Nursery cribs and examining tables are placed away from outside windows.
3. *Evaporation:* the loss of heat that occurs when a liquid is converted to a vapor. In the newborn, heat loss by evaporation occurs as a result of vaporization of moisture from the skin. This process is invisible and is known as insensible water loss (IWL). This heat loss can be intensified by not drying the newborn directly after birth or by bathing and drying the infant too slowly.
4. *Conduction:* the loss of heat from the body surface to cooler surfaces in direct contact. The newborn when admitted to the nursery is placed in a warmed bed to minimize heat loss. Loss of heat must be controlled to protect the newborn. As noted above, control of the modes of heat loss is the basis for caregiving policies and techniques.

Temperature Regulation. Anatomic and physiologic differences among the newborn, child, and adult are notable:

1. The newborn's thermal insulation is less than an adult's. Blood vessels are closer to the surface of the skin. Changes in environmental temperature alter that of blood, thereby influencing temperature-regulating centers in the hypothalamus.
2. The newborn has a larger body surface to body weight (mass) ratio. The flexed position that the newborn assumes is a safeguard against heat loss because it substantially diminishes the amount of body surface exposed to the hostile thermal environment.
3. The newborn's vasomotor control is less well developed. However, the ability to constrict subcutaneous and skin vessels is as efficient in preterm infants as it is in adults.
4. The newborn produces heat primarily by nonshivering thermogenesis.
5. The newborn's sweat glands have little homoiothermic function until the fourth week or later of extrauterine life.

In response to the discomfort of lower environmental temperature, the normal term infant may try to increase body temperature by crying or by increased motor activity. Crying increases the work load, and the cost of energy (calories) may be expensive, particularly in a compromised infant.

Cold Stress. Cold stress imposes metabolic and physiologic problems on all newborn infants, regardless of gestational age and condition. The respiratory rate is increased as a response to the increased need for oxygen when the oxygen consumption increases significantly in cold stress. Oxygen consumption and energy in the cold-stressed newborn are diverted from maintaining normal brain cell and cardiac function and growth to thermogenesis for survival.

If the newborn infant cannot maintain an adequate oxygen tension, vasoconstriction follows and jeopardizes pulmonary perfusion. As a consequence, arterial blood gas levels of Po_2 are decreased, and the blood pH drops. These changes aggravate existing respiratory distress syndrome (RDS), also known as hyaline membrane disease (HMD) (see Chapter 28 for a discussion of RDS and HMD). Moreover, decreased pulmonary perfusion and oxygen tension may maintain or reopen the right-to-left shunt across the patent ductus arteriosus (fetal circulation).

The basal metabolic rate is increased with cold stress. If cold stress is protracted, anaerobic glycolysis occurs, resulting in increased production of acids. Metabolic acidosis develops, and if there is a defect in respiratory function, respiratory acidosis also develops. Excessive fatty acids displace the bilirubin from the albumin-binding sites. The increased level of circulating unbound bilirubin that results increases the risk of kernicterus even at serum bilirubin levels of 10 mg/dl or less (see Chapter 28 for a discussion of kernicterus).

❑ BEHAVIORAL CHARACTERISTICS

The healthy newborn infant must achieve both biologic and behavioral tasks to develop normally. Behavioral characteristics form the basis of the social capabilities of the newborn. Through the first half of this century the focus of developmental research was on **newborn responses to environmental stimuli.** Newborn infants were considered to have been born with neither personality nor ability to interact.

Today it is recognized that newborns are well equipped to begin social interactions with their parents. The behavioral characteristics of the newborn represent a second phase in human development. The first phase, fetal phase, of development was discussed in Chapter 7. Research now indicates that the individual personalities and behavioral characteristics of newborn infants play a major role in the ultimate relationship between infants and their parents.

Brazelton (1973) and others have noted the importance of the behavioral states of the newborn. It is their contention that the behavioral responses of newborn infants are indicative of cortical control, responsiveness, and eventual management of the infant's environment. They emphasize the importance of newborn infant-parent interaction. By their responses infants act to either consolidate relationships or alienate the persons in their immediate environment. By their actions they encourage or discourage attachment and caregiving activities. The development of parent-child love does not occur without feedback. The absence of feedback because of separation or incorrectly interpreted feedback can impair the growth of parental love.

One of the first tasks parents must accomplish is to become aware of the unique behavioral responses of their newborn infant. Brazelton (1969) demonstrated that normal newborns differ in such things as activity (active, average, quiet), feeding patterns, sleeping patterns, and responsiveness from the moment of birth. The **Brazelton neonatal behavioral assessment scale** is used to rate the newborn's unique characteristics, dependent (in part) on the newborn's sleep-wake state. Brazelton suggested that the parents' reaction to their newborn infants is determined in part by these differences.

Sleep-Wake Cycles

Variations in *state of consciousness* of newborn infants are called the **sleep-wake cycles** (Brazelton,

1973). They form a continuum with deep sleep, narcosis, or lethargy at one end and extreme irritability at the other end. There are two sleep states—deep sleep and light sleep—and four wake states—drowsiness, quiet alert, active alert, and crying. Brazelton (1973) has noted that the newborn's state of consciousness is the most important element in assessing the newborn's reactions to stimulation. This state is affected by a number of variables: hunger, dehydration, exhaustion.

As shown in Table 16-1 and Fig. 16-7, each state

Table 16-1 Behavioral States and State Behavior

	Characteristics of State				
State	Body Activity	Eye Movements	Facial Movements	Respiratory Pattern	Level of Response
SLEEP STATES					
Deep sleep	Nearly still, except for occasional startle or twitch	None	Without facial movements, except for occasional sucking movement at regular intervals	Smooth and regular	Threshold to stimuli is very high so that only very intense and disturbing stimuli will arouse infants.
Light sleep	Some body movements	Rapid eye movements (REM), fluttering of eyes beneath closed eyelids	May smile and make brief fussy or crying sounds	Irregular	More responsive to internal and external stimuli. When these stimuli occur, infants may remain in light sleep, return to deep sleep, or arouse to drowsy.
AWAKE STATES					
Drowsy	Activity level variable, with mild startles interspersed from time to time. Movements usually smooth	Eyes open and close occasionally, are heavy-lidded with dull, glazed appearance	May have some facial movements; often there are none, and face appears still	Irregular	Infants react to sensory stimuli although responses are delayed. State change after stimulation frequently noted.
Quiet alert	Minimal	Brightening and widening of eyes	Faces have bright, shining, sparkling looks	Regular	Infants attend most to environment, focusing attention on any stimuli that are present. Optimum state of arousal.
Active alert	Much body activity; may have periods of fussiness	Eyes open with less brightening	Much facial movement; faces not as bright as quiet alert state	Irregular	Increasingly sensitive to disturbing stimuli (hunger, fatigue, noise, excessive handling).
Crying	Increased motor activity, with color changes	Eyes may be tightly closed or open	Grimaces	More irregular	Extreme response to unpleasant external or internal stimuli.

From Barnard KE et al: Behavioral states and state behaviors. In Early parent-infant relationships, copyright 1978 by the March of Dimes Birth Defects Foundation, White Plains, NY. Reprinted by permission.

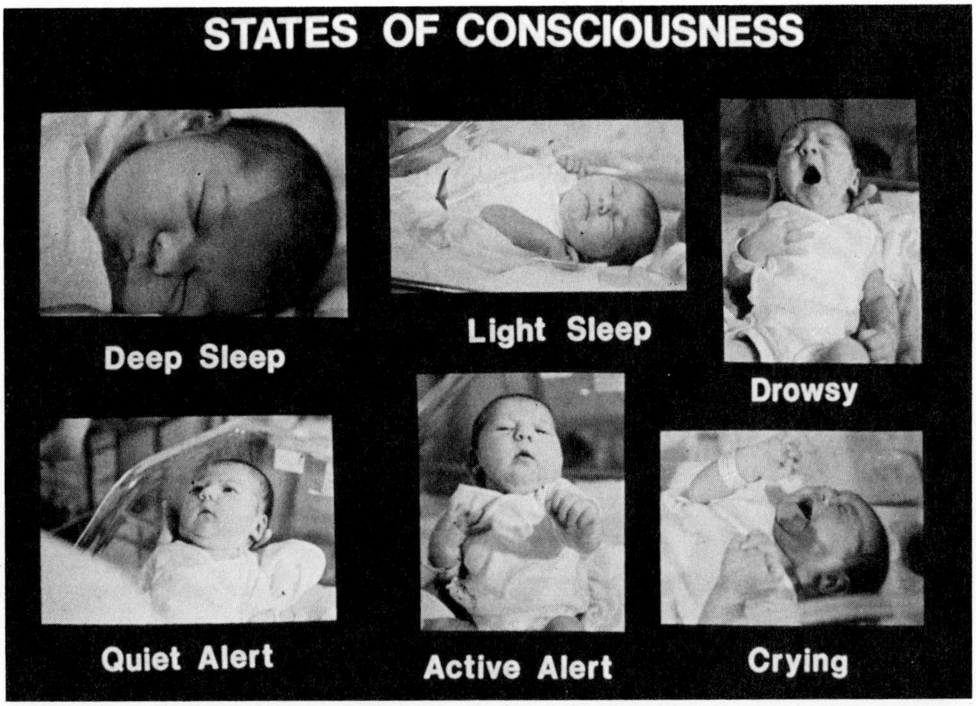

Fig. 16-7 Summary of sleep-wake states of newborn. States of consciousness: deep sleep, light sleep, drowsy, quiet alert, active alert, crying. (Courtesy March of Dimes.)

has its distinguishing characteristics and **state-related behaviors.** The quiet alert state is also termed the optimum state of arousal. During this state newborn infants may be observed smiling, vocalizing, or moving in synchrony. Even during the first day of life, smiling is evident in a surprising number of infants (Wolff, 1969). Newborn infants seem to watch their parents' faces carefully and respond to other persons talking to them. They move their bodies in coordination with the parent's voice and the simultaneous movement of the parent's body (Condon and Sander, 1974). Brazelton (1969) noted that this synchronous movement gives feedback to the speaker and encourages more interaction. Infants have been shown to imitate facial gestures (tongue protrusion, opening the mouth) by 2 weeks of age (Meltzoff and Moore, 1977). Many infants begin a type of vocalizing by the time they are 2 weeks of age, making cooing, small, throaty noises while feeding.

The infant employs purposeful behavior to maintain the optimum state of arousal: (1) active withdrawal by increasing physical distance, (2) a rejecting motion of pushing away with hands and feet, (3) decreasing sensitivity by falling asleep or breaking eye contact by turning the head, or (4) use of signaling behavior, fussing, or crying (Brazelton, 1973). Use of such behaviors permits infants to quiet themselves and reinstate readiness to interact again.

The newborn sleeps a total of about 17 hours a day, with the periods of wakefulness gradually increasing. By the fourth week of life, some infants are staying awake from one feeding session to the next.

Other Factors Influencing Newborn's Behavior

Several other variables, in addition to sleep-wake state, affect the newborn's responses. These are discussed below.

The *gestational age* of the infant and level of central nervous system (CNS) maturity will affect observed behavior. An infant with an immature CNS will have an entire body response to a pinprick of the foot. The mature infant will withdraw the foot. CNS immaturity will also be reflected in reflex development and sleep-wake cycles.

Length of *time* to recuperate from labor and birth will affect the behavior of newborn infants as they attempt to become initially organized. Time since the last feeding and time of day may influence newborns' responses.

Environmental events and *stimuli* will have an effect on the behavioral responses of newborn infants. Nurses in intensive care nurseries observe that infants respond to loud noises, bright lights, monitor alarms, and tension in the unit. It has been well documented that newborn infants are affected by nonverbal behavior in the environment. Newborn infants of mothers who are tense have more muscle activity and their heart rates change parallel to their mothers during feeding. In addition, the newborn responds differently to animate and inanimate stimulation.

There is controversy concerning the effects on newborn infant behavior of *maternal medication* (analgesia, anesthesia) during labor. Some researchers have noted that infants of mothers who were given medications may continue to demonstrate poor state organization beyond the fifth day (Murray et al, 1981). Others maintain that the effect can be beneficial or that there is no effect (Chapter 13).

Some of the most interesting research findings have been the differences in infant behavior across *cultures* (Freedman, 1979). Chinese-American infants were found to have more self-quieting activities, fewer state changes, and more rapid responses to consoling activities than white American infants. The Zinacanteco Indians in southern Mexico demonstrated greater motor maturity and increased ability to maintain quiet alert states for longer times than American infants (Brazelton, 1969).

Sensory Behaviors

From birth, infants possess **sensory behaviors** that indicate a state of readiness for social interaction. Newborn infants are able to use behavioral responses effectively in establishing their first dialogues. These responses, coupled with the newborns' "baby appearance" (the face is proportioned so that the forehead and eyes are larger than the lower portion of the face) and their smallness and helplessness, rouse feelings of wanting to hold, protect, and interact with them.

Vision. The newborn infant's eyes drift off target because muscle control and coordination are immature. This glancing away permits the image being viewed to fall on the fovea (retinal area of clearest vision) more directly. The clearest visual distance is 17 to 20 cm (7 to 8 in), which is about the distance the newborn infant's face is from the mother's face as she breastfeeds or cuddles. Newborn infants are sensitive to light. They will frown if a bright light is flashed in their eyes and will turn toward a soft red light. If the room is darkened, they will open their eyes widely and look about. This is noticeable when the delivery area is darkened after birth.

Response to movement is noticeable. If a bright object is shown to newborns (even at 15 minutes of age), they will follow it with their eyes, and some will even turn their heads to do so. Because human eyes are bright shiny objects, newborns will track them.

Visual acuity is surprising; even at 2 weeks of age infants can distinguish patterns with stripes 3 mm (1/8 in) apart. They prefer to look at black and white patterns rather than plain surfaces, even if the latter are brightly colored (Fantz, 1963). They also prefer more complex patterns to simple ones. They prefer novelty (changes in pattern) by 2 months of age. This is significant knowledge, since it means the infant of a few weeks of age is capable of responding actively to an enriched environment.

From birth onward, infants are able to fix their eyes and gaze intently at objects. They gaze at their parents' faces and respond to changes in them with apparent imitative effect. This ability permits parents and children to gaze into each other's eyes, and a subtle communication pattern is thereby set up. Some researchers have indicated that there may be an ethnic component to this pattern. Freedman (1979) reported a study comparing Navaho and Anglo mothers in their efforts to get their babies' attention. The Anglo mothers became animated, smiled, and used gestures and high-pitched vocal sounds. The Navaho mothers gazed quietly at their babies until their eyes met and the infant gazed quietly back. It is conjectured that such responses may persist over time and influence behavior. Whether such conjectures are true or not, the need to have eye contact is a compelling one (Robson, 1967). Children of blind parents and parents who have blind children must circumvent this obstacle for the formation of a relationship.

Hearing. It has been demonstrated that newborns correctly looked toward sound presented alternately to them on the right and the left side. Newborns can discriminate frequencies of sound in the range of the human voice (Clifton et al, 1981).

Even more discrete differentiation of sound can be demonstrated by a newborn's consistent, preferential turning toward the sound of his mother's voice immediately after birth (Brazelton, 1977; De Casper and Fifer, 1980). This occurs even when another female voice has previously captured the newborn's attention. The phenomenon can be demonstrated to mothers with consistent success.

Truby and Lind (1965) recorded and analyzed the cry of newborns. They discovered that cry imprints produced for each newborn had, like footprints and fingerprints, an individual uniqueness. When a newborn's cry print was compared with the mother's speech patterns, unmistakable similarities were present. Infants of mute mothers did not cry or cried strangely. It was hypothesized that the fetus receives and stores speech features from the mother through hearing and listening while in utero (Truby, 1971).

All these studies indicate a selective listening to the maternal voice sounds and rhythms during intrauterine life that prepare newborns for recognition and interaction with their primary caregivers.

Newborns are accustomed in the uterus to hearing the regular rhythm of the mother's heartbeat. As a result they respond by relaxing and ceasing to fuss and cry if a regular heartbeat simulator is placed in their cribs.

Touch. Sensory pathways for kinesthetic (movement) and tactile (touch) activities are the first to complete myelinization in the newborn infant. The newborn's responses to touch suggest this sensory system is well prepared to receive and process tactile messages. Many of the reflexes of the newborn are elicited in response to tactile stimulation (see Table 16-3).

The new mother uses touch as one of the first interaction behaviors: fingertip touch, soft stroking of the face, and gentle massage of the back. Since touch between strangers is avoided in some cultures, it would seem that this automatic maternal touching behavior evidences an already intimate relationship. Birth trauma or stress and depressant drugs taken by the mother decrease the newborn infant's sensitivity to touch or painful stimuli.

Taste. Newborns have repeatedly demonstrated a preference for sweet fluids over sour or bitter ones. Facial expressions indicating newborn response to taste have been recorded in a series of studies. The facial expressions of a selected variety of people were photographed as various tastes were presented (Steiner, 1979). Preterm and normal newborns; anencephalic newborns; mentally retarded, facially deformed, or congenitally blind adolescents; and normal adults showed the same responses. Sour fluids precipitated puckering of the lips; bitter fluids caused retching or spitting, and sweet tastes resulted in relaxed expressions interpreted as enjoyment and satisfaction. These studies demonstrate not only the newborn's response to various tastes but also the strength of the taste response and its independence from cortical levels of the nervous system.

It is generally accepted that young infants are particularly oriented toward the use of their mouths both for meeting their nutritional needs for rapid growth and for releasing tension through sucking. The early development of circumoral sensation and muscle activity as well as taste would seem to be preparation for survival in the extrauterine environment.

Smell. Several researchers have tested newborn response to odors. The findings demonstrate not only a preference for smells deemed pleasant by adults but also that newborns have the ability to learn and remember.

The significance of smell in maternal identification of offspring and vice versa in the animal world is well documented. Maternal identification of the human newborn by smell has not been studied as extensively. Stainton (1985) noted that mothers reported their infants smell different from birth onward.

Response to Environmental Stimuli

Each newborn has a predisposed capacity to handle the multitudinous stimuli in the external world (Brazelton, 1961). Individual variations in the primary reaction pattern of newborns have been described and termed *temperament* (Thomas et al, 1961, 1970). The style of behavioral response to stimuli is guided by the temperament that affects the newborn's sensory threshold, ability to habituate, and response to maternal behaviors.

Habituation. The newborn is able to control the type and amount of incoming stimuli processed with the ability to *habituate.* Habituation is a phenomenon in which the response to stimuli is decreased after repeated presentation of the stimuli. In the term newborn this can be demonstrated in several ways. Shining a bright light into a newborn's eyes will cause a startle or squinting the first two to three times and possibly a hand or arm will be brought up over the eyes. The third or fourth flash will elicit a diminished response and by the fifth or sixth flash, the infant ceases to respond (Brazelton, 1973, 1977). The same response pattern holds true for the sounds of a rattle, a bell, or a pinprick to a heel. A newborn presented with new stimuli will become wide-eyed and alert, gaze for a time, but eventually show a diminished interest.

As well as shutting out repetitive stimuli, the ability to habituate enables the newborn to select stimuli that potentiate continued learning about the social world and to avoid overload. The intrauterine experiences seem to have programmed the newborn to be especially responsive to human voices, soft lights, soft sounds, sweet tastes, and perhaps patting and rubbing.

Habituation is an early form of learning. The newborn quickly learns the constant sounds in a newborn nursery and in the home environment and is able to sleep in their midst. The selective responses of the newborn indicate cerebral organization capable of remembering and making choices. The ability to habituate is dependent on state of consciousness, hunger, fatigue, and temperament. These factors also affect consolability, cuddliness, irritability, and crying.

Consolability. Korner (1971) reported on studies conducted over several years that describe variations in the ability of newborns to console themselves or to be consoled. In the crying state, most newborns will initiate one of several ways to reduce their distress and move to a lower state. Hand-to-mouth movements are common with or without sucking, as well as alerting to voices, noises, or visual stimuli in the environment.

Cuddliness. The degree to which newborns will mold into the contours of the person holding them varies. Korner and Thoman (1970) tested the effect of body contact and vestibular stimulation in both soothing babies and creating alertness. The vestibular stimulation of being picked up and moved had the greater effect. Schaffer and Emerson (1964) classified newborns into "cuddlers," "noncuddlers," and an "intermediate group."

Irritability. Some newborns cry longer and harder than others. For some the sensory threshold seems low. They are readily upset by unusual noises, hunger, wetness, or new experiences and respond intensely. Others with a high sensory threshold require a great deal more stimulation and variation to reach the active, alert state (Korner, 1971).

Crying. Crying in an infant may signal hunger, pain, desire for attention, or fussiness. As mother and infant become more adept at interpreting each other's behavior, some mothers state that they are able to distinguish the reasons for crying.

■ I can tell when she's hungry. Crying starts in a plaintive way and then becomes more and more demanding. When she is hurt, she lets out a startled yell as though she couldn't believe it was happening to her. Sometimes when she is put down to sleep, she starts a kind of talking cry, jerky and demanding; it gets louder, and if nothing happens, fades away in little spurts. The fussy cry is the hardest to take—nothing seems to work; like a complaining sound it goes on and on.

A report such as this means that the mother and baby are communicating effectively.

Infants use crying as signaling behavior to attract the attention of a caregiver and to communicate. As depicted in the scenario above, newborn infants have distinguishable cries. A hunger cry is often loud and prolonged, not ceasing until the infant is fed. A pain cry is higher pitched and piercing. A fussy cry may be lower pitched and varying in intensity. Infants have individual patterns of communication and the parents must learn to distinguish their own infant's cries.

Temperament. The behavioral styles of infants and children "show distinct individuality in temperament in the first weeks of life, independently of their parents' handling or personality style"; "the original characteristics of temperament tend to persist in most children over the years" (Chess, 1969; Chess and Thomas, 1977).

Chess (1969, p. 749) developed nine categories of primary reactivity to evaluate behavioral style:

1. Activity level: motor functions and the diurnal proportion of active to inactive periods.
2. Rhythmicity: the regularity and predictability of bodily functions and sleep-wake cycle.
3. Approach or withdrawal: the response to a new stimulus.
4. Adaptability: the speed and ease with which current behavior is modified in response to environmental changes.
5. Intensity of reaction: the energy in a response regardless of its quality or direction.
6. Threshold of responsiveness: the intensity of stimuli required to evoke a response.
7. Quality of mood: the proportion of happy behavior to unhappy behavior.
8. Distractibility: the efficacy of external stimuli in changing the direction of ongoing behavior.
9. Attention span and persistence: the length of time one activity is pursued and the effect of distraction.

These nine categories were then grouped into three major patterns of behavioral style or temperament:

1. The easy child who demonstrates regularity in bodily functions, readily adapts to change, has a predominantly positive mood, a moderate sensory threshold, and approaches new situations or objects with a response of moderate intensity.
2. The slow-to-warm-up child who has a low activity level, withdraws on first exposure to new stimuli, is slow to adapt, low in intensity of response, and is somewhat negative in mood.
3. The difficult child who is irregular in bodily functions, intense in reactions, generally negative in mood, resistant to change or new stimuli, and often cries loudly for long periods.

The human newborn possesses sensory receptors capable of responding selectively to various stimuli present in the internal and external environment. The infant also possesses individual characteristics that define him or her as a unique personality.

❑ PHYSICAL ASSESSMENT

The nurse uses knowledge of the biologic and behavioral characteristics of the newborn as a basis for the care of the infant and the teaching and counseling of the parents.

Biologic characteristics are demonstrated through physical assessment. Average findings, normal variations, and deviations from normal range are displayed in Table 16-2. These findings provide a data base for implementing the nursing process with newborns (and their families) discussed in Chapter 17.

The physical assessment includes a neurologic assessment of the newborn's reflexes. This provides useful information about the infant's nervous system and state of neurologic maturation. Many of the reflex behaviors are important for survival, for example, sucking and rooting. Others act as safety mechanisms, for instance, gagging, coughing, and sneezing. The assessment needs to be carried out as early as possible because abnormal signs present in the early neonatal period may disappear. They may reappear months or years later as abnormal functions. Table 16-3 gives the techniques for eliciting significant reflexes and characteristic responses.

Table 16-2 **Physical Assessment of Newborn**

Area Assessed and Appraisal Procedure	Normal Findings		Deviations from Normal Range: Possible Problems (Etiology)
	Average Findings	Normal Variations	
POSTURE			
Inspect newborn before disturbing for assessment Refer to maternal chart for fetal presentation, position, and type of birth (vaginal, surgical), since newborn readily assumes prenatal position	Vertex: arms, legs in moderate flexion; fists are clenched Newborn resists having extremities extended for examination or measurement and may cry when this is attempted Crying ceases when allowed to reassume curled-up fetal position Normal spontaneous movement is bilaterally asynchronous (legs move in bicycle fashion) but equally extensive in all extremities	Frank breech: legs are more straight and stiff; newborn will assume intrauterine position in repose for a few days Prenatal pressure of limb or shoulder may cause temporary facial asymmetry (Fig. 16-8) or resistance to extension of extremities	Hypotonia, relaxed posture while awake (prematurity or hypoxia in utero, maternal medications) Hypertonia (drug dependence, CNS disorder) Opisthotonos (CNS disturbance) Limitation of motion in any of extremities (see Extremities, below)
VITAL SIGNS			
Heart rate and pulses Thorax (chest) Inspection Palpation Auscultation Apex: mitral valve Second interspace, left of sternum: pulmonic valve	Pulsations visible in left midclavicular line; fifth intercostal space Apical pulse; fourth intercostal space 120-140 bpm Quality: *first sound* (closure of mitral and tricuspid valves) and *second sound* (closure of aortic and pulmonic valves) should be sharp and clear	100 (sleeping) to 160 (crying); may be irregular for brief periods, especially after crying Murmurs, especially over base or at left sternal border in interspace 3 or 4 (foramen ovale anatomically closes at about 1 year)	Tachycardia: persistent; ≥170 (RDS) Bradycardia: persistent; ≤120 (congenital heart block) Murmurs (may be functional) Arrhythmias: irregular rate

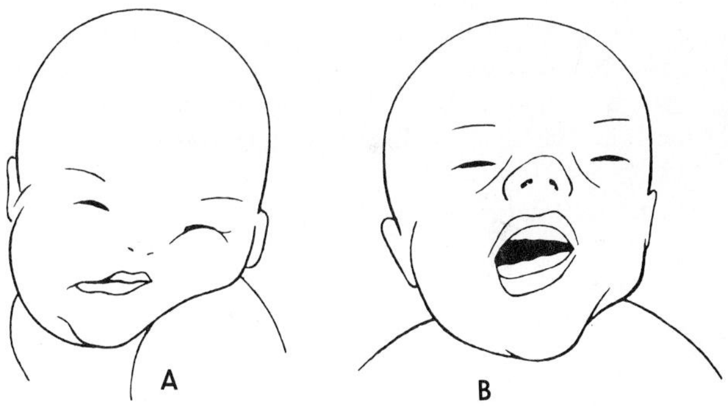

Fig. 16-8 **A,** Facial asymmetry from prenatal pressure. **B,** Lopsided appearance disappears spontaneously in time. (Courtesy Mead Johnson & Co., Evansville, Indiana.)

Continued.

Table 16-2 Physical Assessment of Newborn—cont'd

Area Assessed and Appraisal Procedure	Normal Findings: Average Findings	Normal Findings: Normal Variations	Deviations from Normal Range: Possible Problems (Etiology)
VITAL SIGNS—cont'd			
Heart rate and pulses—cont'd Second interspace, right of sternum: aortic valve Junction of xiphoid process and sternum: tricuspid valve			Sounds Distant (pneumomediastinum) Poor quality Extra Heard on right side of chest: dextrocardia; often accompanied by reversal of intestines
Femoral pulse palpation: flex thighs on hips; place fingers along inguinal ligament about midway between symphysis pubis and iliac crest; feel bilaterally simultaneously	Femoral pulses should be equal and strong		Weak or absent femoral pulses (hip dysplasia, coarctation of aorta, thrombophlebitis)
Temperature Axillary: method of choice until 6 years of age Rectal: before passage of meconium, check for patent anus; insert thermometer with great caution, gently; hold in place for 90 sec, keeping legs immobilized Electronic: thermistor probe (avoid taping over bony area)	Axillary: 37° C (98.6° F) Rectal: may be misleading—even in cold stress may remain unchanged until metabolic activity can no longer maintain core temperature Temperature stabilization by 8-10 hours of age Shivering mechanism undeveloped	36.5°-37.2° C (97.6°-99° F) Heat loss: 200 kcal/kg/min from evaporation, conduction, convection, radiation	Subnormal (prematurity, infection, low environmental temperature, inadequate clothing, dehydration) Increased (infection, high environmental temperature, excessive clothing, proximity to heating unit or in direct sunshine, drug addiction, diarrhea and dehydration) Temperature not stabilized by 10 hours after birth (if mother received magnesium sulfate, newborn is less able to conserve heat by vasoconstriction; maternal analgesics may reduce thermal stability in newborn)
Respiratory rate and effort Observe respirations when infant is at rest Count respirations for full minute Apnea monitor Listen for sounds audible without stethoscope Observe respiratory effort	40/min Tend to be shallow, and when infant is awake, irregular in rate, rhythm, and depth No sounds should be audible on inspiration or expiration Breath sounds: bronchial; loud, clear, near	30-60/min May appear to be Cheyne-Stokes with short periods of apnea and with no evidence of respiratory distress First period (reactivity): 50-60/min Second period: 50-70/min Stabilization (1-2 days): 30-40/min	Apneic episodes: ≥15 sec (preterm or premature infant: "periodic breathing," rapid warming or cooling of infant) Bradypnea: ≤25/min (maternal narcosis from analgesics or anesthetics, birth trauma) Tachypnea: ≥60/min (RDS, aspiration syndrome, diaphragmatic hernia)

Table 16-2 Physical Assessment of Newborn—cont'd

Area Assessed and Appraisal Procedure	Normal Findings: Average Findings	Normal Findings: Normal Variations	Deviations from Normal Range: Possible Problems (Etiology)
VITAL SIGNS—cont'd Respiratory rate and effort—cont'd			Sounds Rales, rhonchi, wheezes (fluid in lungs) Expiratory grunt (narrowing of bronchi) Distress evidenced by nasal flaring, retractions, chin tug, labored breathing (RDS, fluid in lungs)
Blood pressure (BP) (usually assessed only if a problem is suspected) Electronic monitor BP cuff: BP cuff width affects readings; use cuff 2.5 cm (1 in) wide and palpate radial pulse	75/42 (approximately) At birth Systolic: 60-80 mm Hg Diastolic: 40-50 mm Hg At 10 days Systolic: 95-100 mm Hg Diastolic: slight increase	Varies with change in activity level: awake, crying, sleeping	Difference between upper and lower extremity pressures (coarctation of aorta) Hypotension (sepsis, hypovolemia) Hypertension (coarctation of aorta)
WEIGHT* Put protective liner cloth or paper in place and adjust scale to 0 (Fig. 16-9) Weigh at same time each day Protect newborn from heat loss	Female 3400 g (7 lb 8 oz) Male 3500 g (7 lb 11 oz) Regain birth weight within first 2 weeks	2500-4000 g (5 lb 8 oz to 8 lb 13 oz) Acceptable weight loss: 10% or less Caucasian baby generally weighs ½ lb more than infants of other races Second baby weighs more than first	Weight ≤2500 g (prematurity, small for gestational age, rubella syndrome) Weight ≥4000 g (large for gestational age, maternal diabetes, heredity: normal for these parents) Weight loss over 10% (dehydration)

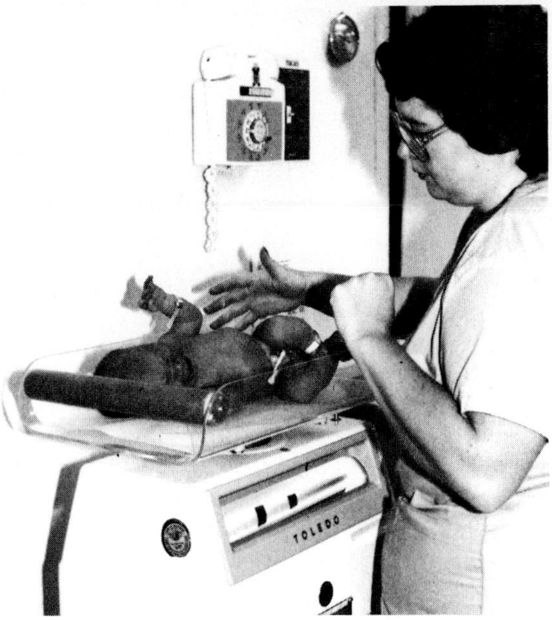

Fig. 16-9 Weighing infant. Note hand is held over infant as safety measure. Scale is covered to provide warmth and protection against cross infection.

*NOTE: Weight, length, and head circumference should all be close to same percentile for any child.

Continued.

Table 16-2 **Physical Assessment of Newborn—cont'd**

Area Assessed and Appraisal Procedure	Normal Findings: Average Findings	Normal Findings: Normal Variations	Deviations from Normal Range: Possible Problems (Etiology)
LENGTH			
Measure recumbent length from top of head to heel; difficult to measure in full-term infant because of presence of molding, incomplete extension of knees (Fig. 6-10, *C*)	50 cm (20 in)	45-55 cm (18-22 in)	<45 or >55 cm (chromosomal aberration, heredity: normal for these parents)
HEAD CIRCUMFERENCE			
Measure head at greatest diameter: occipitofrontal circumference (Fig. 16-10, *A*) May need to remeasure on second or third day after resolution of molding and caput succedaneum	33-35.5 cm (13-14 in) Circumferences of head and chest may be about the same for first 1 or 2 days after birth	32-36.8 cm (12½-14½ in)	Small head ≤32 cm: microcephaly (rubella, toxoplasmosis, cytomegalic inclusion disease) Hydrocephaly: sutures widely separated, circumference ≥4 cm more than chest Increased intracranial pressure (hemorrhage, space-occupying lesion)

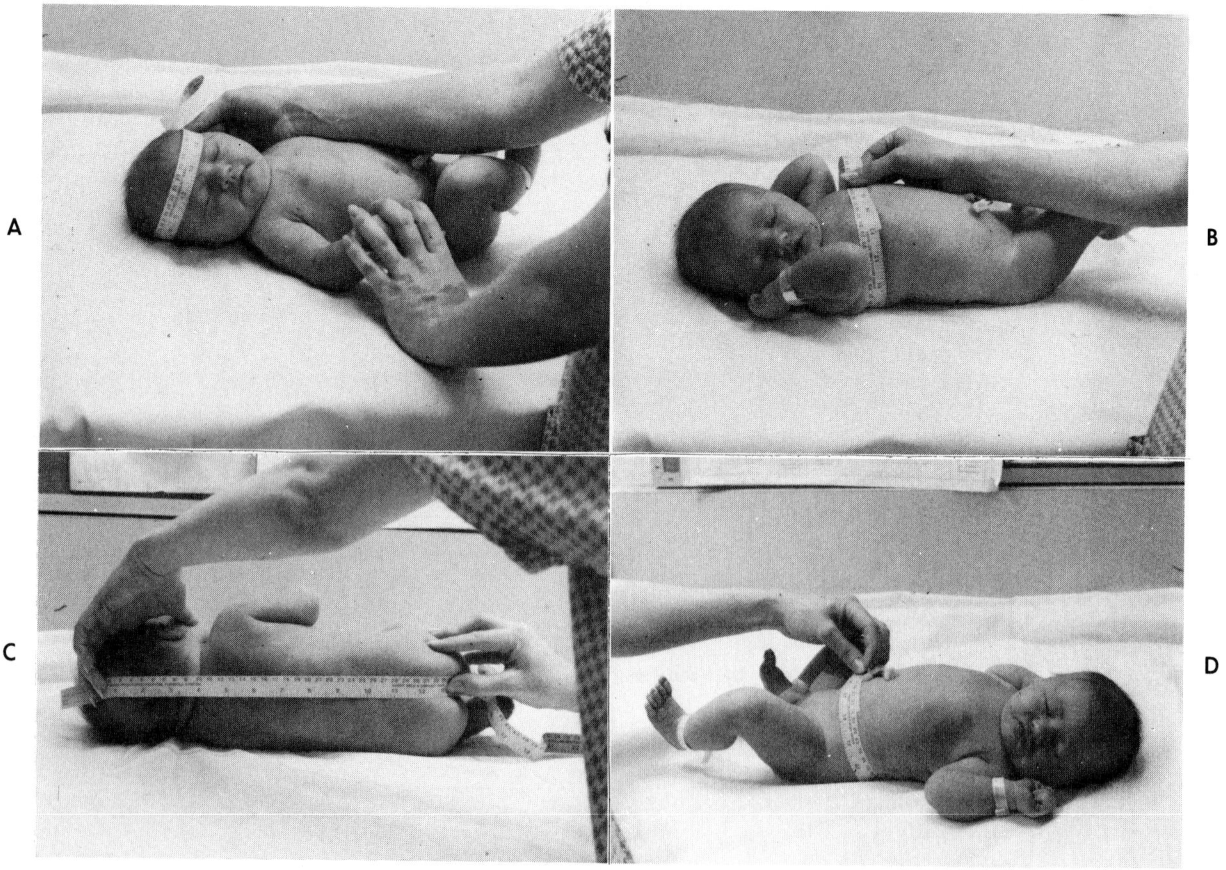

Fig. 16-10 Measurements. **A,** Circumference of head. **B,** Circumference of chest. **C,** Length, crown to rump. To determine total length, length of legs is included. **D,** Abdominal circumference.

Table 16-2 Physical Assessment of Newborn—cont'd

Area Assessed and Appraisal Procedure	Normal Findings: Average Findings	Normal Findings: Normal Variations	Deviations from Normal Range: Possible Problems (Etiology)
CHEST CIRCUMFERENCE			
Measure at nipple line (Fig. 16-10, *B*)	2 cm (3/4 in) less than head circumference; averages between 30-33 cm (12-13 in)		≤30 cm (prematurity) Postmaturity (some small-for-gestational age [SGA] and some large-for-gestational age [LGA])
ABDOMINAL CIRCUMFERENCE			
Measure below umbilicus (Fig. 16-10, *C*) (not usually measured unless specific indication)	Abdomen enlarges after feeding because of lax abdominal muscles Same size as chest		Enlarging abdomen between feedings (Abdominal mass or blockage in intestinal tract)
INTEGUMENT			
Color			
Inspection and palpation Inspect naked newborn in well-lit, warm area without drafts; natural daylight provides best lighting Inspect newborn when quiet and when active	Varies with ethnic origin; skin pigmentation begins to deepen right after birth in basal layer of epidermis Generally pink Acrocyanosis, especially if chilled	Mottling Harlequin sign Plethora Telangiectases ("stork bites" or capillary hemangiomas) Erythema toxicum neonatorum ("newborn rash") Milia	Dark red (prematurity) Pallor (cardiovascular problem, CNS damage, blood dyscrasia, blood loss, twin transfusion, nosocomial infection) Cyanosis (hypothermia, infection, hypoglycemia, cardiopulmonary diseases, cardiac, neurologic, or respiratory malformations)
		Petechiae over presenting part	Petechiae over any other area (clotting factor deficiency, infection)
		Ecchymoses from forceps in vertex births or over buttocks and legs in breech births	Ecchymoses in any other area (hemorrhagic disease, traumatic birth)
Check for jaundice	None at birth	Physiologic jaundice occurs in 50% of term infants	Jaundice within first 24 hr (Rh isoimmunization) Gray (hypotension, poor perfusion)
Birthmarks			
Inspect and palpate for location, size, distribution, characteristics, color	Transient hyperpigmentation Areolae Genitals Linea nigra	Mongolian spotting Infants of black, Oriental, and American Indian origin; 70% Infants of white origin: 9%	Hemangiomas Nevus flammeus: port-wine stain Nevus vasculosus: strawberry mark Cavernous hemangiomas
Condition			
Inspect and palpate for intactness, smoothness, texture, edema	No skin edema Opacity: few large blood vessels seen indistinctly over abdomen	Slightly thick; superficial cracking, peeling, especially of hands, feet No blood vessels seen; a few large vessels clearly seen over abdomen Some fingernail scratches	Edema on hands, feet; pitting over tibia Texture thin, smooth, or of medium thickness; rash or superficial peeling seen Numerous vessels easily seen over abdomen (prematurity)

Continued.

Table 16-2 Physical Assessment of Newborn—cont'd

Area Assessed and Appraisal Procedure	Normal Findings: Average Findings	Normal Findings: Normal Variations	Deviations from Normal Range: Possible Problems (Etiology)
INTEGUMENT—cont'd			
Condition—cont'd			Texture thick, parchment-like; cracking, peeling (postmaturity) Skin tags; webbing Papules, pustules, vesicles, ulcers, maceration (impetigo, candidiasis, herpes, diaper rash)
Hydration and consistency Weigh infant routinely Inspection and palpation Gently pinch skin between thumb and forefinger over abdomen and inner thigh to check for turgor Check subcutaneous fat deposits (adipose pads) over cheeks, buttocks	Dehydration: best indicator is loss of weight After pinch is released, skin returns to original state immediately	Normal weight loss after birth is up to 10% of birth weight May feel puffy Amount of subcutaneous fat varies	Loose, wrinkled skin (prematurity, postmaturity, dehydration: fold of skin persists after release of pinch) Tense, tight, shiny skin (edema, extreme cold, shock, infection) Lack of subcutaneous fat, clavicle or ribs prominent (prematurity, malnutrition)
Check voiding	Voids within 24 hrs of delivery Voids 6-10 times per day		
Vernix caseosa Observe amount		Amount varies; usually more is found in creases, folds	Absent or minimal (postmaturity) Excessive (prematurity)
Observe its color and odor before bath or wiping If not readily apparent over total body, check in folds of axilla and groin	Whitish, cheesy, odorless		Yellow color (possible fetal anoxia 36 hours or more before birth, Rh or ABO incompatibility) Green color (possible in utero release of meconium or presence of bilirubin) Odor (possible intrauterine infection)
Lanugo Inspect for this fine, downy hair: amount, distribution	Over shoulders, pinnas of ears, forehead	Amount varies	Absent (postmaturity) Excessive (prematurity, especially if lanugo is abundant and long and thick over back)
HEAD			
Palpate skin	See Integument, p. 463	Caput succedaneum; may show some ecchymosis	Cephalhematoma
Inspect shape and size	Makes up one fourth of body length Molding (Fig. 16-11)	Slight asymmetry from intrauterine position	Molding Severe molding (birth trauma) Lack of molding (prematurity, breech presentation, cesarean birth)

Continued.

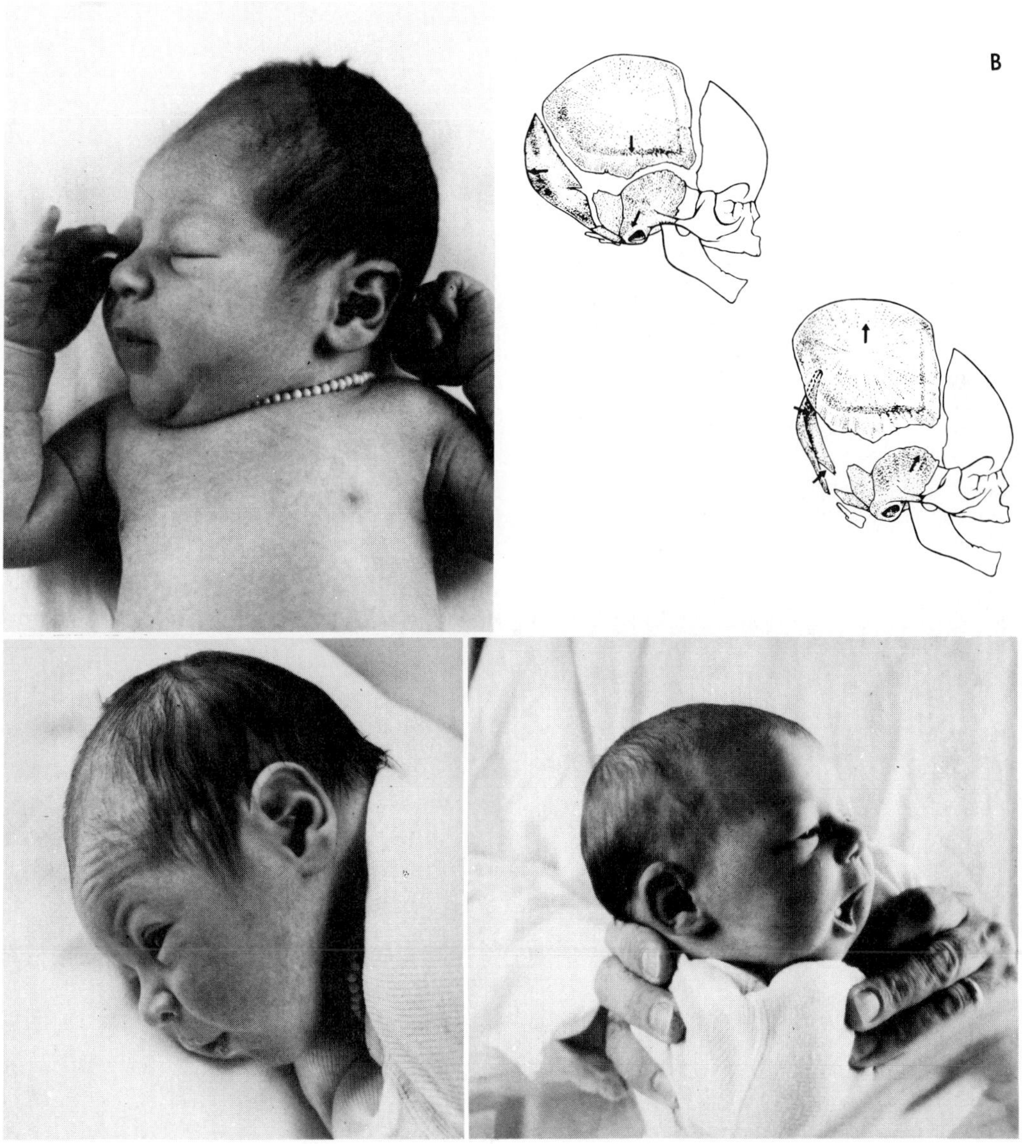

Fig. 16-11 Molding. **A**, Significant molding, soon after birth. **B**, Schematic of bones of skull when molding is present. **C**, Some resolution of molding on second or third day of life. **D**, Molding resolved.

Table 16-2 Physical Assessment of Newborn—cont'd

Area Assessed and Appraisal Procedure	Normal Findings: Average Findings	Normal Findings: Normal Variations	Deviations from Normal Range: Possible Problems (Etiology)
HEAD—cont'd			
Palpate, inspect, measure fontanels	Anterior fontanel 5 cm diamond; increases as molding resolves Posterior fontanel triangle; smaller than anterior	Fontanel size varies with degree of molding Fontanels may be difficult to feel because of molding	Fontanels Full, bulging (tumor, hemorrhage, infection) Large, flat, soft (malnutrition, hydrocephaly, retarded bone age, hypothyroidism) Depressed (dehydration) Large mastoid and sphenoid fontanels (hydrocephaly)
Palpate sutures	Sutures palpable and not joined	Sutures may overlap with molding	Sutures Widely spaced (hydrocephaly) Premature synostosis closure
Inspect pattern, distribution, amount of hair; feel texture	Silky, single strands, lies flat; growth pattern is toward face and neck	Amount varies	Fine, wooly (prematurity) Unusual swirls, patterns, hairline or coarse, brittle (endocrine or genetic disorder)
EYES (Fig. 16-12)			
Placement on face	Eyes and space between eyes each ⅓ the distance from outer-to-outer canthus		
Symmetry in size, shape	Symmetric in size, shape		
Eyelids: size, movement, blink	Blink reflex Epicanthal folds: normal racial characteristic	Edema if silver nitrate instilled	Epicanthal folds when present with other signs (chromosomal disorders such as Down's syndrome, cri du chat syndrome)
Discharge	None	Some discharge if silver nitrate used	

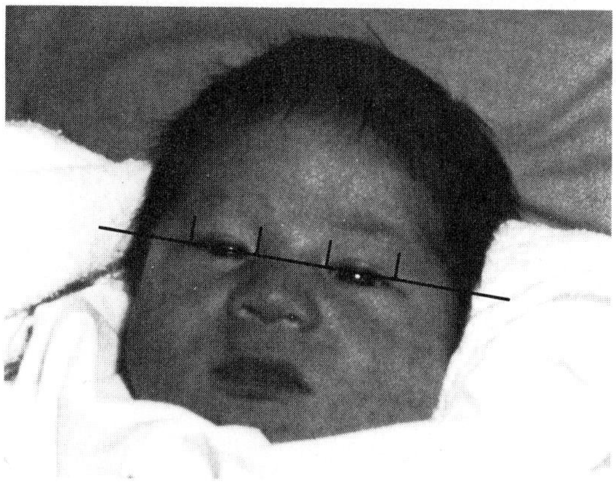

Fig. 16-12 Eyes. Pseudostrabismus. Inner epicanthal folds cause eyes to appear malaligned; however, corneal light reflexes fall perfectly symmetric. Eyes are symmetric in size and shape and well placed.

Table 16-2 **Physical Assessment of Newborn—cont'd**

Area Assessed and Appraisal Procedure	Normal Findings: Average Findings	Normal Findings: Normal Variations	Deviations from Normal Range: Possible Problems (Etiology)
EYES—cont'd			
Eyeballs: presence, size, shape	No tears Both present and of equal size; both round, firm	Occasionally has some tears Subconjunctival hemorrhage	Agenesis or absence of one or both eyeballs Small eyeball size (rubella syndrome) Lens opacity or absence of red reflex (congenital cataracts, possibly from rubella) Lesions: coloboma, absence of part of iris (congenital) Pink color of iris (albinism) Jaundiced sclera (hyperbilirubinemia) Discharge: purulent (infection)
Pupils	Present, equal in size, react to light		Pupils: unequal, constricted, dilated, fixed (intracranial pressure, medications, tumors)
Eyeball movement	Random, jerky, uneven, can focus momentarily, can follow to midline	Transient strabismus or nystagmus until third or fourth month	Persistent strabismus Doll's eyes (increased intracranial pressure) Sunset (increased intracranial pressure)
Eyebrows: amount, pattern	Distinct (not connected in midline)		
NOSE			
Observe shape, placement, patency, configuration of bridge of nose	Midline Apparent lack of bridge, flat, broad Some mucus but no drainage Obligatory nose breathers Sneezes to clear nose	Slight deformity from passage through birth canal	Copious drainage, with or without regular periods of cyanosis at rest and return of pink color with crying (choanal atresia, congenital syphilis) Malformed (congenital syphilis, chromosomal disorder) Flaring of nares (respiratory distress)
EARS			
Observe size, placement on head, amount of cartilage, open auditory canal	Correct placement: line drawn through inner and outer canthi of eye should come to top notch of ear (at junction with scalp) (Fig. 16-13) Well-formed, firm cartilage	Size: small, large, floppy Darwin's tubercle (nodule on posterior helix)	Agenesis Lack of cartilage (prematurity) Low placement (chromosomal disorder, mental retardation, kidney disorder) Preauricular tags Size: may have overly prominent or protruding ears

Continued.

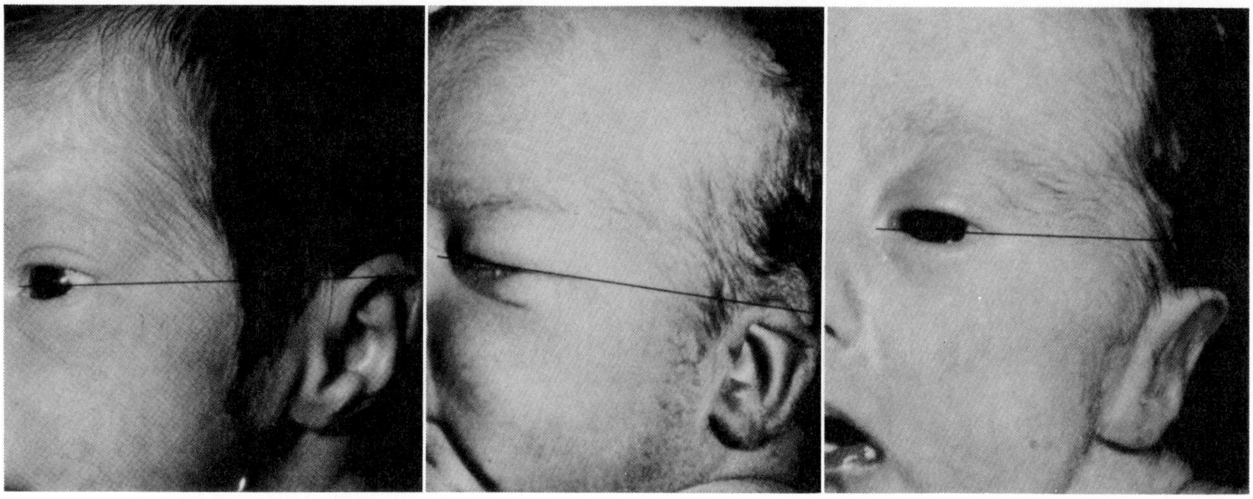

A B C

Fig. 16-13 Placement of ear insertion on head in relation to line drawn from inner to outer canthus of eye. **A,** Normal position. **B,** Abnormally angled ear. **C,** True low-set ear. (Courtesy Mead Johnson & Co., Evansville, Indiana.)

Table 16-2 Physical Assessment of Newborn—cont'd

Area Assessed and Appraisal Procedure	Normal Findings: Average Findings	Normal Findings: Normal Variations	Deviations from Normal Range: Possible Problems (Etiology)
EARS—cont'd			
Hearing	Responds to voice and other sounds	State influences response	Deaf: no response to sound
FACIES			
Observe overall appearance of face	Infant looks "normal"; features are well placed, proportionate to face, symmetric	"Positional" deformities (see Fig. 16-8)	Infant looks "odd" or "funny" Usually accompanied by other features, such as low-set ears and other structural disorders (hereditary, chromosomal aberration)
MOUTH			
Inspection and palpation Placement on face Lips: color, configuration, movement	Symmetry of lip movement	Transient circumoral cyanosis	Gross anomalies in placement, size, shape (cleft lip and/or palate, gums) Cyanosis; circumoral pallor (respiratory distress, hypothermia) Asymmetry in movement of lips (seventh cranial nerve paralysis)
Gums	Pink gums		

Table 16-2 **Physical Assessment of Newborn—cont'd**

Area Assessed and Appraisal Procedure	Normal Findings: Average Findings	Normal Findings: Normal Variations	Deviations from Normal Range: Possible Problems (Etiology)
MOUTH—cont'd			
Tongue: attachment, mobility, movement, size	Tongue does not protrude, is freely movable; symmetric in shape, movement	Short frenulum	Macroglossia (prematurity, chromosomal disorder) Excessive saliva (esophageal atresia, tracheoesophageal fistula) Micrognathia (Pierre Robin or other syndrome) Teeth: predeciduous or deciduous (hereditary) Thrush: white plaques on cheeks or tongue that bleed if touched *(Candida albicans)*
Cheeks	Sucking pads inside cheeks		
Palate (soft, hard) Arch Uvula	Soft and hard palates intact Uvula in midline	Anatomic groove in palate to accommodate nipple; disappears by 3-4 years of age	
Saliva: amount, character		Epstein's pearls (Bohn's nodules): whitish, hard nodules on gums or roof of mouth	
Chin	Distinct chin		
Reflexes Rooting Sucking Extrusion	Reflexes present	Reflex response dependent on state of wakefulness and hunger	
NECK			
Inspection and palpation Length Movement of head Sternocleidomastoid muscles; position of head Trachea: position; thyroid gland Reflex response (Table 16-3)	Short, thick, surrounded by skinfolds; no webbing Head held in midline, i.e., sternocleidomastoid muscles are equal; no masses Freedom of movement from side to side and flexion and extension; cannot move chin past shoulder Thyroid not palpable	Transient positional deformity apparent when newborn is at rest: head can be moved passively	Webbing Restricted movement; head held at angle (torticollis [wryneck], opisthotonos) Masses (enlarged thyroid) Distended veins (cardiopulmonary disorder) Skin tags Absence of head control (prematurity; Down's syndrome)
CHEST			
Inspection and palpation Shape Clavicles Ribs Nipples: size, placement, number Breast tissue Respiratory movements Amount of cartilage in rib cage Auscultation Heart tones and rate and breath sounds (see Vital signs, above)	Almost circular; barrel shaped Symmetric chest movements; chest and abdominal movements synchronized during respirations Breast nodule: approximately 6 mm in term infant Nipples prominent, well formed; symmetrically placed	Occasional retractions, especially when crying Breast nodule: 3-10 mm Secretion of witch's milk Tip of sternum may be prominent	Bulging of chest (pneumothorax, pneumomediastinum) Malformation (funnel chest—pectus excavatum) Fracture of clavicle (trauma) Nipples Supernumerary, along nipple line (congenital) Malpositioned or widely spaced (congenital) Lack of breast tissue (prematurity) Poor development of rib cage and musculature (prematurity) Sounds: bowel sounds (see Abdomen, below) Retractions with or without respiratory distress (prematurity, RDS)

Continued.

Table 16-2 Physical Assessment of Newborn—cont'd

Area Assessed and Appraisal Procedure	Normal Findings: Average Findings	Normal Findings: Normal Variations	Deviations from Normal Range: Possible Problems (Etiology)
ABDOMEN			
Inspect, palpate, and smell umbilical cord	Two arteries, one vein (AVA) Whitish gray Definite demarcation between cord and skin; no intestinal structures within cord Dry around base; drying Odorless Cord clamp in place for 24 hr	Reducible umbilical herniation	One artery (internal anomalies) Bleeding or oozing around cord (hemorrhagic disease) Redness or drainage around cord (infection, possible persistence of urachus) Hernia: herniation of abdominal contents into area of cord (e.g., omphalocele); defect covered with thin, friable membrane, may be extensive (congenital) Gastroschisis: congenital fissure of abdominal cavity (congenital) Meconium stained (intrauterine distress)
Inspect size of abdomen and palpate contour (Fig. 16-10, *D*)	Rounded, prominent, dome shaped because abdominal musculature is not fully developed Liver may be palpable 1-2 cm below right costal margin No other masses palpable No distension	Some diastasis of abdominal musculature	Distension at birth (ruptured viscus, genitourinary masses or malformations: hydronephrosis; teratomas, abdominal tumors) Mild (aerophagia, overfeeding, high gastrointestinal tract obstruction) Marked (lower gastrointestinal tract obstruction, imperforate anus) Intermittent or transient (aerophagia, overfeeding) Partial intestinal obstruction (stenosis of bowel) Annular pancreas (congenital) Malrotation of bowel or adhesions (congenital) Sepsis (infection)
Auscultate bowel sounds and note number, amount, and character of stools, and behavior—crying, fussiness—before or during elimination	Sounds present within 1-2 hours after birth Meconium stool passes within 24-48 hours after birth		Scaphoid, with bowel sounds in chest and respiratory distress (diaphragmatic hernia)
Color		Linea nigra may be apparent; possibly caused by hormone influence during pregnancy	

Table 16-2 **Physical Assessment of Newborn—cont'd**

Area Assessed and Appraisal Procedure	Normal Findings		Deviations from Normal Range: Possible Problems (Etiology)
	Average Findings	Normal Variations	
ABDOMEN—cont'd			
Movement with respiration	Respirations primarily diaphragmatic; abdominal and chest movements synchronous		Decreased abdominal breathing (intrathoracic disease, diaphragmatic hernia)
GENITALS (See Fig. 16-6)			
Girl			
Inspection and palpation			
General appearance	Female genitals	Increased pigmentation caused by pregnancy hormones	Ambiguous genitals—enlarged clitoris with urinary meatus on tip; fused labia (chromosomal disorder; maternal drug ingestion)
Clitoris	Usually edematous		
Labia majora	Usually edematous; cover labia minora in term newborns	Edema and ecchymosis following breech birth	
Labia minora	May protrude over labia majora	Blood-tinged discharge from pseudomenstruation caused by pregnancy hormones	Stenosed meatus (congenital) Labia majora widely separated and labia minora prominent (prematurity)
Discharge	Smegma		
Vagina	Orifice open Mucoid discharge Hymenal/vaginal tag present	Some vernix caseosa may be between labia	Absence of vaginal orifice or imperforate hymen (congenital) Fecal discharge (fistula)
Urinary meatus	Beneath clitoris; hard to see—watch for voiding	Rust-stained urine (uric acid crystals) (to determine whether rust color is caused by uric acid or blood, wash under running warm tap water; uric acid washes out, blood does not)	
Boy			
Inspection and palpation			
General appearance	Male genitals	Increased size and pigmentation caused by pregnancy hormones	Ambiguous genitals (congenital)
Penis	Meatus at tip of penis		
Urinary meatus seen as slit			Urinary meatus not on tip of glans penis (hypospadias, epispadias)
Prepuce	Prepuce (foreskin) covers glans penis and is not retractable	Prepuce removed if circumcised Size of genitals varies widely	
Scrotum	Large, edematous, pendulous in term infant; covered with rugae	Scrotal edema and ecchymosis if breech birth Hydrocele, small, noncommunicating	Scrotum smooth and testes undescended (prematurity, cryptorchidism) Hydrocele Inguinal hernia (congenital) Round meatal opening (congenital)
Rugae (wrinkles)			
Testes	Palpable on each side	Bulge palpable in inguinal canal	
Urination	Voiding within 24-48 hr, stream adequate, amount adequate	Rust-stained urine (uric acid crystals)	Undescended (prematurity)
Reflexes			
Erection	Erection may occur spontaneously and when genitals are touched		
Cremasteric	Testes are retracted, especially when newborn is chilled		

Continued.

Table 16-2 Physical Assessment of Newborn—cont'd

Area Assessed and Appraisal Procedure	Normal Findings: Average Findings	Normal Findings: Normal Variations	Deviations from Normal Range: Possible Problems (Etiology)
EXTREMITIES			
General			
Inspection and palpation Degree of flexion Range of motion Symmetry of motion Muscle tone	Assumes position maintained in utero Attitude of general flexion Full range of motion, spontaneous movements	Transient (positional) deformities	Limited motion (malformations) Poor muscle tone (prematurity, maternal medications, CNS, anomalies) Positive scarf sign
Clavicles	Intact		Crepitus/fracture (trauma)
Arms			
Inspection and palpation Color Intactness Appropriate placement Number of fingers Palpate humerus Joints Shoulder Elbow Wrist Fingers Reflex: grasp	Longer than legs in newborn period Contours and movement are symmetric 5 on each hand Fist often clenched with thumb under fingers Full range of motion; symmetric contour Brachial pulses palpable and equal	Slight tremors may be seen at times Some acrocyanosis, especially when chilled Single palmar crease on one hand common in Asian babies	Assymmetry of movement (fracture/crepitus, brachial nerve trauma, malformations) Asymmetry of contour (malformations, fracture) Amelia or phocomelia (teratogens) Webbing of fingers: syndactyly Absence or excess of fingers Palmar creases Simian line seen with short, incurved little fingers (Down's syndrome) Strong, rigid flexion; persistent fists; fists held in front of mouth constantly (CNS disorder) Increased tonicity, clonicity, prolonged tremors (CNS disorder)
Legs			
Inspection and palpation Color Intactness Length—in relation to arms and body and to each other Major gluteal folds Number of toes Femur Head of femur as legs are flexed on hips and abducted; placement in acetabulum; femoral pulses	Appear bowed since lateral muscles more developed than medial muscles Major gluteal folds even Femur should be intact No click should be heard; femoral head should not override acetabulum Soles well lined (or wrinkled) over two thirds of foot in term infants	Feet appear to turn in but can be easily rotated externally, also positional defects tend to correct while infant is crying Acrocyanosis	Amelia, phocomelia (chromosomal defect, teratogenic effect) Webbing, syndactyly (chromosomal defect) Absence or excess of digits (chromosomal defect, familial trait) Femoral fracture (difficult breech delivery) Congenital hip dysplasia/dislocation Absent femoral pulses Soles of feet Few lines: (prematurity) Covered with lines (postmaturity)

Table 16-2 Physical Assessment of Newborn—cont'd

Area Assessed and Appraisal Procedure	Normal Findings: Average Findings	Normal Findings: Normal Variations	Deviations from Normal Range: Possible Problems (Etiology)
EXTREMITIES—cont'd			
Legs—cont'd			
Inspection and palpation Joints Hip Knee Ankle Toes Reflexes	Plantar fat pad gives flat-footed effect		Congenital clubfoot Hypermobility of joints (Down's syndrome) Yellowed nail beds (meconium staining) Temperature of one leg differs from that of the other (circulatory deficiency, CNS disorder) Asymetric movement (trauma, CNS disorder)
BACK			
Anatomy			
Inspection and palpation Spine Shoulders Scapulae Iliac crests Base of spine—pilonidal area	Spine straight and easily flexed Infant can raise and support head momentarily when prone Shoulders, scapulae, and iliac crests should line up in same plane	Temporary minor positional deformities, which can be corrected with passive manipulation	Limitation of movement (fusion or deformity of vertebra) Pigmented nevus with tuft of hair when located anywhere along the spine is often associated with spina bifida occulta Spina bifida cystica (meningocele, myelomeningocele)
Reflexes (spinal related) Test reflexes			
ANUS			
Inspection and palpation Placement Number Patency Test for sphincter response (active "wink" reflex) Observe for following: Abdominal distension Passage of meconium Passage of fecal drainage from surrounding orifices	One anus with good sphincter tone Passage of meconium within 24 hr after birth Good "wink" reflex of anal sphincter	Passage of meconium within 48 hours after birth	Low obstruction: anal membrane (congenital) High obstruction: anal or rectal atresia (congenital) Drainage of fecal material from vagina in female or urinary meatus in male (rectal fistula)
STOOLS	Meconium followed by transitional and soft yellow stools (see p. 446)		

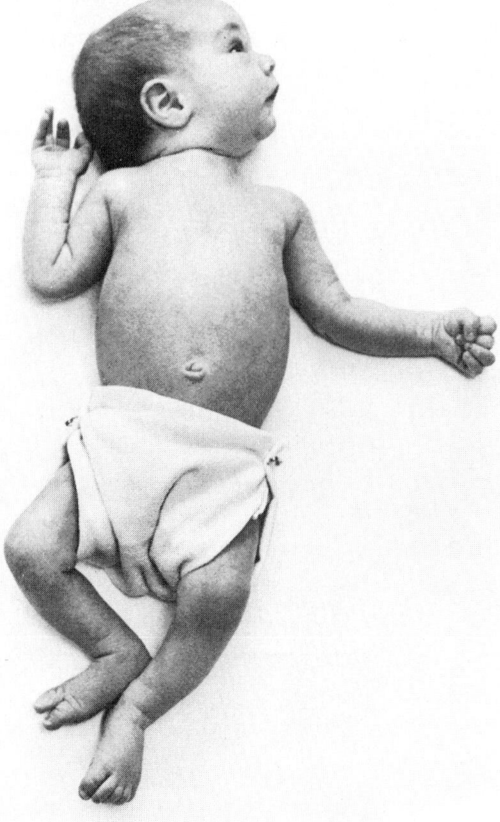

Fig. 16-14 Classic pose in spontaneous tonic neck reflex. (Courtesy Mead Johnson & Co., Evansville, Indiana.)

A

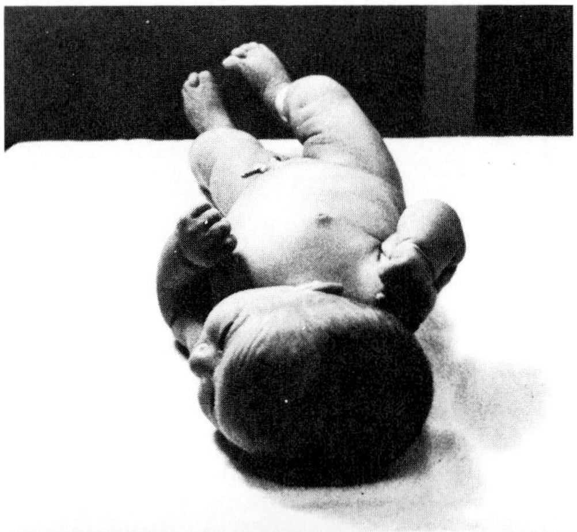

B

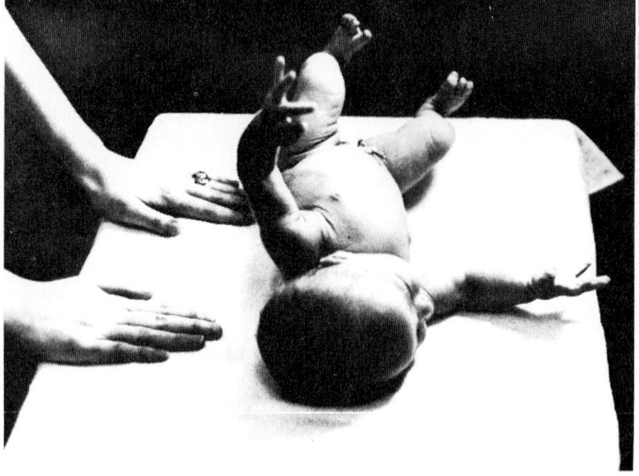

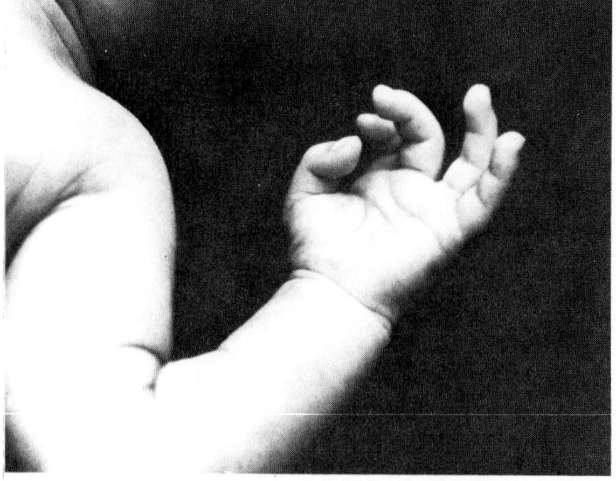

C

Fig. 16-15 **A,** Position of rest. **B,** Moro's reflex consists predominantly of abduction and extension of arms. **C,** Interesting subtlety of Moro's response in newborn infants is C position of fingers: digits extend, except finger and thumb, which are often semiflexed, forming shape of C. (Courtesy Mead Johnson & Co., Evansville, Indiana.)

Table 16-3 Assessment of Newborn's Reflexes

Reflex	Eliciting the Reflex	Characteristic Response	Comments
Sucking and rooting	Touch infant's lip, cheek, or corner of mouth with nipple	Infant turns head toward stimulus, opens mouth, takes hold, and sucks	Difficult if not impossible to elicit after infant has been fed; if weak or absent, consider prematurity or neurologic defect Parental guidance Avoid trying to turn head toward breast or nipple; allow infant to root Disappears after 3-4 months but may persist up to 1 year
Swallowing	Feed infant; swallowing usually follows sucking and obtaining fluids	Swallowing is usually coordinated with sucking and usually occurs without gagging, coughing, or vomiting	If weak or absent, may indicate prematurity or neurologic defect Suck and swallow often uncoordinated in preterm infant
Extrusion	Touch or depress tip of tongue	Newborn forces tongue outward	Disappears at about fourth month
Glabellar (Myerson's)	Tap over forehead, bridge of nose, or maxilla of newborn whose eyes are open	Newborn blinks for first 4 or 5 taps	Continued blinking with repeated taps is consistent with extrapyramidal disorder
Tonic neck or "fencing" (Fig. 16-14)	With infant falling asleep or sleeping, turn head quickly to one side	With infant facing left side, arm and leg on that side extend; opposite arm and leg flex (turn head to right, and extremities assume opposite postures)	Responses in legs are more consistent Complete response disappears by 3-4 months; incomplete response may be seen until third or fourth year After 6 weeks persistent response is sign of possible cerebral palsy
Grasp Palmar Plantar	 Place finger in palm of hand Place finger at base of toes	Infant's fingers curl around examiner's fingers; toes curl downward	Palmar response lessens by 3-4 months; parents enjoy this contact with infant; plantar response lessens by 8 months
Moro (Fig. 16-15)	Hold infant in semisitting position; allow head and trunk to fall backward to an angle of at least 30 degrees Place infant on flat surface; strike surface to startle infant	Symmetric abduction and extension of arms; fingers fan out and form a C with thumb and forefinger; slight tremor may be noted; arms are adducted in embracing motion and return to relaxed flexion and movement Legs may follow similar pattern of response Preterm infant does not complete "embrace," instead, arms fall backward because of weakness	Present at birth; complete response may be seen until 8 weeks* of age; body jerk only, between 8-18 weeks; absent by 6 months if neurologic maturation is not delayed; may be incomplete if infant is deeply asleep; give parental guidance about normal response Asymmetric response; possible injury to brachial plexus, clavicle, or humerus Persistent response after 6 months: possible brain damage

*All durations for persistance of reflexes are based on time elapsed since 40 weeks' gestation, that is, if this newborn was born at 36 weeks' gestation, add 1 month to all time limits given.

Continued.

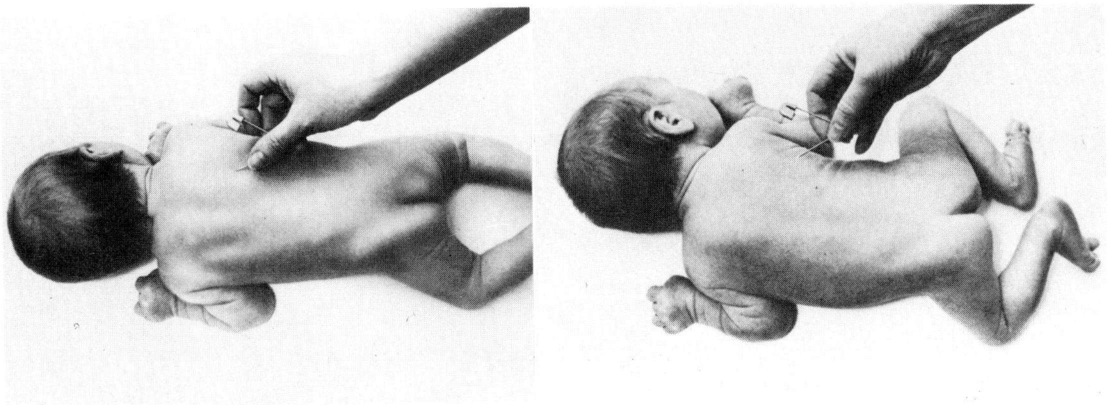

Fig. 16-16 Trunk incurvation reflex. In prone position, infant responds to linear skin stimulus (pin or finger) along paravertebral area by flexing trunk and swinging pelvis toward stimulus. With transverse lesions of cord, there will be no response below that level. Complete absence of response suggests general depression or nervous system abnormality. Response may vary but should be obtainable in all infants, including preterm ones. If not seen in the first few days, it is usually apparent by 5 to 6 days. (Courtesy Mead Johnson & Co., Evansville, Indiana.)

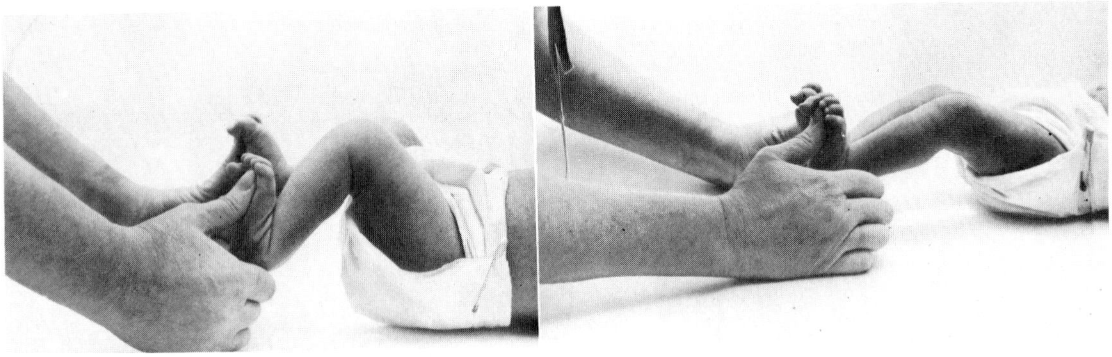

Fig. 16-17 Magnet reflex. With child in supine position and lower limbs semiflexed, light pressure is applied with fingers to both feet. Normally, while examiner's fingers maintain contact with soles of feet, lower limbs extend. Absence of this reflex suggests damage to spinal cord or malformation. Weak reflex may be seen following breech presentation *without* extended legs or may indicate sciatic nerve stretch syndrome. Breech presentation *with* extended legs may evoke an exaggerated response. (Courtesy Mead Johnson & Co., Evansville, Indiana.)

Table 16-3 Assessment of Newborn's Reflexes—cont'd

Reflex	Eliciting the Reflex	Characteristic Response	Comments
Startle	Loud noise of sharp hand clap elicits response; best elicited if newborn is 24-36 hr old or older	Arms abduct with flexion of elbows; hands stay clenched	Should disappear by 4 months Elicited more readily in preterm newborn (inform parents of this characteristic)
Pull-to-sit (traction)	Pull infant up by wrists from supine position with head in midline	Head will lag until infant is in upright position; then head will be held in same plane with chest and shoulder momentarily before falling forward; infant will attempt to right head	Depends on general muscle tone and maturity and condition of infant
Trunk incurvation (Galant) (Fig. 16-16)	Infant should be prone on flat surface; run finger down back about 4-5 cm (1½-2 in) lateral to spine, first on one side, and then down other	Trunk is flexed and pelvis is swung toward stimulated side	Response disappears by fourth week
Magnet (Fig. 16-17)	Infant should be supine; partially flex both lower extremities and apply pressure to soles of feet	Both lower limbs should extend against examiner's pressure	
Crossed extension (Fig. 16-18)	Infant should be supine; extend one leg, press knee downward, stimulate bottom of foot; observe opposite leg	Opposite leg flexes, adducts, and then extends	

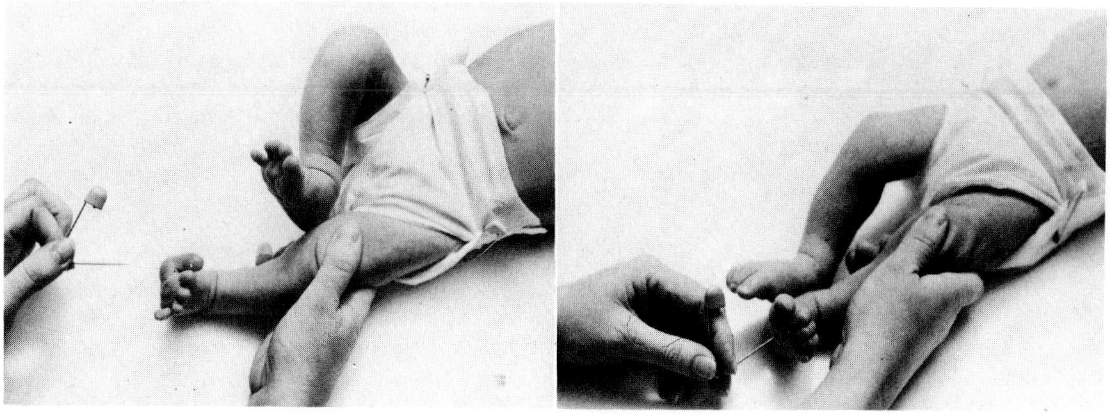

Fig. 16-18 Crossed extension reflex. With child in supine position, examiner extends one of infant's legs and presses knee down. Stimulation of sole of foot of fixated limb should cause *free* leg to flex, adduct, and extend as if attempting to push away stimulating agent. This reflex should be present during newborn period. Absence of response suggests a spinal cord lesion; weak response suggests peripheral nerve damage. (Courtesy Mead Johnson & Co., Evansville, Indiana.)

Continued.

Table 16-3 Assessment of Newborn's Reflexes—cont'd

Reflex	Eliciting the Reflex	Characteristic Response	Comments
Babinski's sign (plantar) (Fig. 16-19)	On sole of foot, beginning at heel, stroke upward along lateral aspect of sole, then move finger across ball of foot	All toes hyperextend, with dorsiflexion of big toe—recorded as a positive sign	Absence requires neurologic evaluation; should disappear after 1 year of age
Placing	Hold infant in vertical position; stroke top of one foot under table edge	Leg flexes and extends	
Stepping or "walking"	Hold infant vertically, allowing one foot to touch table surface	Infant will simulate walking, alternating flexion and extension of feet; term infants walk on soles of their feet, and preterm infants walk on their toes	Normally present for 3-4 weeks
Neck righting	Place newborn in supine position and turn head to one side	Shoulder and trunk and then pelvis will turn to be in alignment with head	Disappears at 10 months of age; absence: implications same as for absent tonic neck reflex
Otolith righting	Hold newborn erect and tilt body	Head returns to erect, upright position	Absence: implications same as for absent tonic neck reflex
Crawling	Place newborn on abdomen	Newborn makes crawling movements with arms and legs	Should disappear about 6 weeks of age
Deep tendon	Use finger instead of percussion hammer to elicit patellar, or knee jerk, reflex; newborn must be relaxed	Reflex jerk is present; even with newborn relaxed, nonselective overall reaction may occur	
Landau	Over a crib or a table, using two hands, suspend infant in prone position	Infant attempts to hold spine in horizontal plane	Absence suggests need for neurologic examination

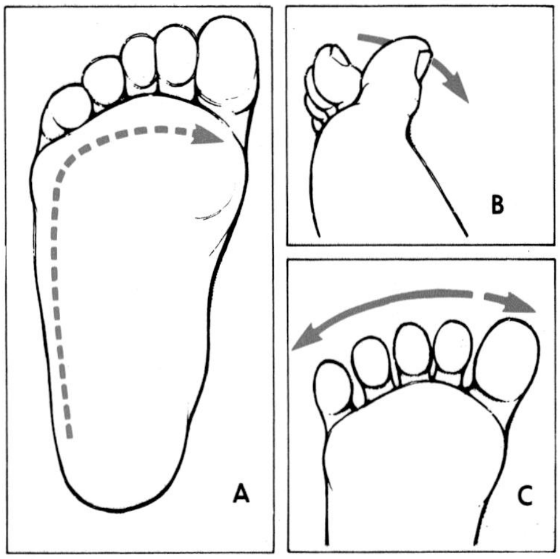

Fig. 16-19 Babinski's reflex. **A,** Direction of stroke. **B,** Dorsiflexion of big toe. **C,** Fanning of toes. (From Whaley LF and Wong DL: Nursing care of infants and children, ed 4, St Louis, 1991, The CV Mosby Co.)

Table 16-3 Assessment of Newborn's Reflexes—cont'd

Reflex	Eliciting the Reflex	Characteristic Response	Comments
Yawn, stretch, burp, hiccup, sneeze	Spontaneous behaviors	May be slightly depressed temporarily because of maternal analgesia or anesthesia, fetal hypoxia, or infection	Parental guidance Most of these behaviors are pleasurable to parents Parents need to be assurred that behaviors are normal Sneeze is usually response to lint, etc., in nose and not an indicator of a cold No treatment is needed for hiccups
Sweat		Sweat response usually not present in term infant; may be seen in infants with cardiac disorder	Parental guidance Amount of clothing for infant: indoors, outside Room temperature
Shiver		Shiver response usually not present in term infant; if seen, check infant for postmaturity	See "Sweat" above
Kernig's sign	Flex thigh on hip and extend leg at knee	Procedure should be accomplished easily and without inflicting pain	Pain and resistance to extension of knee suggest meningeal irritability
Brudzinski's sign	Place infant in supine position; flex neck and observe knees	Infant does not move legs when neck is flexed	Spontaneous flexion of knees suggest meningeal irritability
Paradoxic irritability	Infant cries when touched and held; ascertain that infant is not hungry; hold and cuddle infant	Infant usually responds by quieting down	Continued irritability suggests meningeal irritability

SUMMARY

During the period of infancy the infant within the "protective envelope of nurturing adults" (Brazelton, 1982) can learn complex coping mechanisms and control systems. These in turn help the infant to be alert, to pay attention, and to master rules of communication. The newborn and adult learn about each other and about themselves—a feeling of mutuality, of identification with the "other" is accomplished.

LEARNING ACTIVITIES

1. Observe a normal newborn immediately after birth and in follow-up periods for several days. Write reports on daily observations, including both physiologic and behavioral data; compare and contrast data, and identify questions for further research.
2. Prepare teaching materials on changes and challenges to one of the newborn's body systems that could be used for educating a new-parent class. Present the material prepared to the group for discussion and additional suggestions.
3. For those who have baby books of themselves, share these with the class. In group discussion, discuss what items in the books were considered important when the data were recorded, and what changes you might suggest for a baby book to be kept today.
4. Research theories of newborn behavior and sensory abilities before 20 years ago and over the last 10 years. Discuss changes in attitude and expectations toward the newborn and how these might affect treatment and care of the newborn.

KEY CONCEPTS

- By term the infant's various anatomic and physiologic systems have reached a level of development and functioning that permits a physical existence apart from the mother and sensory capabilities that indicate a state of readiness for social interaction.
- There are several significant differences between the respiratory, renal, and thermogenetic systems in the newborn and those of the adult that have import for nursing care.
- At any serum bilirubin level, the appearance of jaundice during the first day of life or persistence of jaundice usually indicates a pathologic process.
- Chilling of a newborn, even a healthy term newborn, may result in acidosis and raise the level of free fatty acids.
- Many reflex behaviors are important for the newborn's survival.
- The individual personalities and behavioral characteristics of infants play a major role in the ultimate relationship between infants and their parents.
- Behavioral responses of infants are indicative of cortical control, responsiveness, and eventual ability to manage her or his environment.
- The development of parent-child love does not occur without feedback.
- Sleep-wake cycles and other factors influence the newborn's behavior.
- Each newborn has a predisposed capacity to handle the multitude of stimuli in the external world.

References

Auerbach KG and Gartner LM: Breastfeeding and human milk: their association with jaundice in the neonate, Clin Perinatol 14(1):89, 1987.

Behrman RE and Vaughan VC, III: Nelson's textbook of pediatrics, ed 13, Philadelphia, 1987, WB Saunders Co.

Boyer DB and Vidyasagar D: Serum indirect bilirubin levels and meconium passage in early fed normal newborns, Nurs Res 36:174, 1987.

Brazelton TB: Psychophysiologic reactions in the neonate. I. The value of observation of the neonate, J Pediatr 58:508, 1961.

Brazelton TB: Infants and mothers, ed 1, New York, 1969, Dell Publishing Co.

Brazelton TB: Effect of maternal expectations on early infant behavior, Early Child Dev Care 2:259, 1973.

Brazelton TB: The remarkable talents of the newborn, Paper presented at Parent to Infant Attachment Conference, Cleveland, November 6, 1977.

Brazelton TB: Joint regulation of neonate-parent behavior. In Tronick EZ, editor: Social interchange in infancy: affect, cognition, and communication, Baltimore, 1982, University Park Press.

Brovten D et al: Breastmilk jaundice, JOGN Nurs 14(3):220, 1985.

Chess S: Individuality and baby care, Dev Med Child Neurol 11:749, 1969.

Chess S and Thomas A: Temperament and the parent-child interaction, Pediatr Ann 6(9):26, 1977.

Clifton RK et al: Newborns' orientation toward sound: possible implications for cortical development, Child Dev 52:833, 1981.

Condon WS and Sander LW: Neonate movement is synchronized with adult speech: interactional participation and language acquisition, Science 183:99, 1974.

Cunningham FG, MacDonald PC, and Gant NF: Williams obstetrics, ed 18, Norwalk, Conn, 1989, Appleton & Lange.

DeCarvalho M et al: Effects of water supplementation on physiological jaundice in breast-fed babies, Arch Dis Child 56:568, 1981.

De Carvalho M et al: Frequency of breast-feeding and serum bilirubin concentration, Am J Dis Child 136:737, 1982.

DeCarvalho M et al: Fecal bilirubin excretion and serum bilirubin concentrations in breast-fed and bottle-fed infants, J Pediatr 107:786, 1985.

DeCasper AJ and Fifer WP: Of human bonding: newborns prefer their mothers' voices, Science 208:1174, 1980.

Fanaroff AA and Martin RJ: Neonatal-perinatal medicine: diseases of the fetus and infant, ed 4, St Louis, 1987, The CV Mosby Co.

Fantz RL: Pattern vision in newborn infants, Science 140:296, 1963.

Freedman DG: Ethnic differences in babies, Hum Nature 2(1):36, 1979.

Guyton AC: Textbook of medical physiology, ed 7, Philadelphia, 1986, WB Saunders Co.

Kivlahan C and James EJP: The natural history of neonatal jaundice, Pediatrics 74:364, 1984.

Korner AF: Individual differences at birth: implications for early experiences and later development, Am J Orthopsychiatry 41:608, 1971.

Korner AF and Thoman EB: Visual alertness in neonates as evoked by maternal care, J Exp Child Psychol 10:67, 1970.

Korones SB: High-risk newborn infants: the basis for intensive nursing care, ed 4, St Louis, 1986, The CV Mosby Co.

Lascari AD: "Early" breast-feeding jaundice: clinical significance, J Pediatr 108:156, 1986.

Linn S et al: Epidemiology of neonatal hyperbilirubinemia, Pediatrics 75(4):770, 1985.

Lowrey G: Growth and development of children, ed 8, Chicago, 1986, Year Book Medical Publishers.

Martin G: Newborns pacified by tapes of their own crying, Brain/Mind Bull 6(16):2, 1981.

Medici MA: The fight against infection: neonatal defense mechanisms, J Calif Perinat Assoc 3(2):25, 1983.

Meltzoff AN and Moore MK: Imitation of facial and manual gestures by human neonates, Science 198:75, 1977.
Murray AD et al: Effects of epidural anesthesia on newborns and their mothers, Child Dev 52:71, 1981.
Robson KS: The role of eye-to-eye contact in maternal-infant attachment, J Child Psychol Psychiatry 8:13, 1967.
Saul K and Warburton D: Increased incidence of early-onset hyperbilirubinemia in breast-fed versus bottle-fed infants, J Perinatol 4(3):36, 1984.
Schaffer H and Emerson P: Patterns of response to physical contact in early human development, J Child Psychol Psychiatry 5:1, 1964.
Stainton C: Origins of attachment, culture and cue sensitivity. Unpublished doctoral dissertation, University of California, San Francisco, 1985.
Steiner JE: Human facial expressions in response to taste and smell stimulation, Adv Child Dev Behav 13:257, 1979.
Thomas A et al: Individuality in responses of children to similar environmental situations, Am J Psychiatry 117:798, 1961.
Thomas A et al: The origin of personality, Sci Am 223:102, 1970.
Truby HM: Prenatal and neonatal speech, "pre-speech," and an infantile-speech lexicon, Word 27(1-2-3):57, 1971.
Truby H and Lind J: Cry sounds of the newborn infant. In Lind J, editor: Newborn infant cry, Acta Paediatr Scand 163(suppl):7, 1965.
Whaley LF and Wong DL: Nursing care of infants and children, ed 4, St Louis, 1991, The CV Mosby Co.
Wolff PH: Observations on newborn infants, Psychosom Med 21:110, 1969.

Bibliography

Anderson GC et al: Development of sucking in term infants from birth to four hours postbirth, Res Nurs Health 5:21, 1982.
Apostalakis EMB and Cha CC: Visual preferences of preterm and term infants, J Calif Perinat Assoc 2(1):61, 1982.
Cernoch J and Perry SE: The importance of odors in mother-infant interactions, Matern Child Nurs J 12(3):147, 1983.
Clark DA: Times of first void and first stool in 500 newborns, Pediatrics 60:457, 1977.
Collis PM: The testing and comparison of the intra-uterine sound against other methods for calming babies, Midwives Chron 97(1161):336, 1984.
Davis V: The structure and function of brown adipose tissue in the neonate, JOGN Nurs 9:368, 1980.
Dodman N: Newborn temperature control, Neonatal Network 5(6):19, 1987.
Fantz RL and Miranda SB: Newborn infant attention to form of contour, Child Dev 46:224, 1975.
Fleming J: Common dermatologic conditions in children, MCN 6:346, 1981.
Gill NE et al: Transitional newborn infants in a hospital nursery: from first oral cue to first sustained cry, Nurs Res 33:213, 1984.
Keefe MR: Comparison of neonatal nighttime sleep-wake patterns in nursery versus rooming-in environments, Nurs Res 36:140, 1987.
Ludington-Hoe S: What can newborns really see? Am J Nurs 83:1286, 1983.
Schachter J et al: Heart rate and blood pressure in black newborns and white newborns, Pediatrics 58:283, 1976.
Wolff PH: Observations on the early development of smiling. In Stone LJ et al, editors: The competent infant: research and commentary, New York, 1973, Basic Books, Inc, Publishers.

CHAPTER

17 Nursing Care of the Normal Newborn

Shannon E. Perry

Learning Objectives

Correctly define the key terms listed.

Discuss the components of assessment of the newborn from the antenatal, intranatal, and postnatal periods.

Explain what is meant by a safe environment.

Review procedures for heel stick, assisting with venipuncture, collection of urine specimen, and restraining the infant.

Compare methods of maintaining an adequate oxygen supply.

Outline in detail the emergency procedure for cardiopulmonary resuscitation and relieving airway obstruction.

Discuss methods to maintain the infant's temperature.

Describe precautions in administering an intramuscular injection to a newborn.

Discuss phototherapy and guidelines for teaching parents about it.

Explain circumcision: purposes, methods, postoperative care, and parent teaching.

Determine each daily care activity.

Review anticipatory guidance for parents.

Key Terms

acid mantle
anticipatory guidance
apnea
bilirubin
bradypnea
bulb syringe
cardiopulmonary resuscitation (CPR)
clovehitch restraint
common cold
cradle cap
DeLee mucus-trap catheter
excoriation
galactosemia
hyperbilirubinemia
hypothermia
mummy technique
phenylketonuria (PKU)
phimosis
phototherapy
prepuce
respiratory distress
tachypnea
thermistor probe
thyroxine

During the neonatal period the prenatal and postdelivery characteristics of the infant merge. Gradually the former disappear as the infant grows and matures outside the womb. Although most infants make the necessary biopsychosocial adjustment to extrauterine existence without undue difficulty, their well-being depends on the care they receive from others. The nursing care described in this chapter is based on careful assessment of biologic and behavioral responses and formulation of nursing diagnoses. It includes planning and implementing appropriate nursing actions and evaluating their effectiveness.

Assessment

Routine assessment of the infant is a continuous process. Whenever any care is given to a newborn, observations and recordings of the child's progress are made. At the beginning of each 8-hour shift the following assessments are made, compared with the norm, and recorded:

1. Temperature
2. Respiratory rate, rhythm, and effort
3. Breath sounds
4. Heart rate and rhythm
5. Skin color
6. Activity level and muscle tone

Feeding and elimination behavior is recorded as it occurs.

The first *assessment* of the infant is done at birth, using the Apgar scoring technique and a brief *physical assessment* (Chapter 15). An assessment for gestational age may be done within the first 2 hours after birth (Chapter 28).

Admission to the Nursery

Having verified the infant's identification with the transfer nurse from the delivery unit, the nursery nurse places the baby in a warm environment and begins the admission assessment, which includes pertinent information from the mother's prenatal record and the record of events during the mother's labor and the newborn's birth. Often a form such as the one in Fig. 17-1 is used to record findings. This form shows at a glance, significant data from the antenatal period through nursery admission. An example of newborn nursery routine orders is shown in the box below.

Physical Examination

A thorough physical examination is done within 24 hours after delivery, when the newborn's temperature is stabilized. The *goal* of this examination is to compile a complete record of the newborn that will act as a data base for subsequent assessment and care. Having the parents present during this examination permits prompt discussion of parental concerns, and involves the parents actively in the health care of their child from birth. At the same time, *parental interactions with the child* can be observed; this aids in early diagnosis of concerns in parent-child relationships and learning needs.

> **ROUTINE ADMISSION ORDERS**
>
> Vital signs: on admission and q 30 min × 2, q1h × 2, then q8h
> Weight, length, and head and chest circumference on admission; then weigh daily
> Erythromycin ophthalmic ointment 5 mg/g 1 line each eye (ou)
> Vitamin K 1 mg IM
> Hematocrit by warm heel stick within 3 to 8 hr of age; call physician if <50 or >65
> Dextrostix prn; notify physician if <45 mg%; offer early D_5W po
> Feedings: sterile water × 1 by nurse within first 4 hr of life; if tolerated, begin breastfeeding or formula q3 to 4 hr on demand
> Rooming in as desired and infant's condition permits
> Newborn screen for **phenylketonuria** (PKU), **thyroxine** (T_4), and **galactosemia** on day of discharge.

The area used for the examination should be well lighted, warm, and free of drafts. The examiner performs a thorough hand-washing and dons a cover gown as needed before the examination. The infant is undressed as needed and placed on a firm, flat surface. The infant may need to be picked up and cuddled at times for reassurance. The examination is carried out in a systematic manner, beginning with a general evaluation of such characteristics as appearance, maturity, nutritional status, activity, and state of well-being. This general evaluation is followed by more specific observations (see Tables 16-2 and 16-3).

Data are recorded as descriptive notes or are summarized on standard forms. Identifying data are entered first: addressograph; birthdate; weight; length; chest and head circumferences; race; sex; mother's and infant's blood type and Rh; Coombs' test results; and time of examination.

The *general appearance* (posture, maturity, activity, tone, cry, color, edema) and *sleep-wake state* (see Table 16-4) are assessed before disturbing the infant. These observations aid in the interpretations of the findings. Each examiner has a preferred pattern for assessment. One pattern is shown in Tables 16-2 and 16-3. Blood pressure (BP) is not assessed routinely. *Heart and respiratory rates* are easiest to assess when the newborn is quiet. Respirations are counted by observing the chest wall, noting whether the sternum retracts or nares flare and chin lags on inspiration. The examiner notes whether the infant is a normal nose breather (i.e., sleeps with mouth closed, does not have to interrupt feedings to breathe), assesses breath sounds, and notes abnormal sounds—grunting or wheezing—during inspiration or expiration.

The examiner notes the efficiency of the gagging, sneezing, and swallowing reflexes related to maintaining a clear airway.

The examiner watches for bouts of rapid and irregular respirations, gagging, and regurgitation of mucus during "reactivity" periods following birth and after 4 to 6 hours of life (see p. 933).

The infant's *color* is assessed for cyanosis. A pink color over head and trunk and mucous membrane is indicative of adequate oxygenation. Feet and hands may remain slightly cyanotic for 48 hours, especially when they are cold.

On admission and each time the *skin* is exposed while giving care, the infant's skin is assessed for rashes, excoriations (e.g., from fingernails), color (e.g., petechiae, ecchymosis, jaundice, general color, mottling), wounds (e.g., internal fetal monitoring, forceps, scalpel during cesarean birth, circumcision, cord, heel sticks, injections), vernix caseosa, and lanugo. The ax-

Neonatal Health History

Date ______ Infant ______
Date of delivery ______ Sex ______
Time of delivery ______ Age (in hours) now ______

Prenatal data
Maternal age ______ Blood type and Rh ______
Indirect Coombs' ______ EDB via dates ______

Previous obstetric history
Parity (explain all items) ______
Previous pregnancies:
Date ______ Gestational age ______ Sex ______ Weight ______ Delivery ______ Complications ______

Complications of this pregnancy
Preeclampsia ______ Hypertension ______
Diabetes (class) ______ Bleeding ______
Viral/bacterial infection ______
Environmental teratogens ______
Drug use ______
  Over-the-counter ______ Alcohol ______
  Prescription ______ Cocaine ______
  Heroin ______ Methadone ______
Other ______

Results of fetal testing
AFP assay ______
Ultrasound ______ Amniocentesis ______
NST ______ BPS ______

Intrapartum data
Onset of contractions ______
Rupture of membranes (ROM) ______ When? ______
Bloody ______ Meconium stained ______ Foul smell ______
Abnormalities of maternal vital signs ______
Medications during labor ______
Anesthesia/analgesia ______ Time last administered ______
Fetal monitoring (external/internal) ______
Fetal distress ______ Fetal pH ______
Length of stages of labor: 1st ______ 2nd ______ 3rd ______

Delivery
Time ______ Route ______
Reason for operative delivery ______

Resuscitation
Apgar score: 1 minute ______ 5 minute ______
Suction ______ Whiffs of O_2 ______
Positive pressure ______ via mask/endotracheal tube ______
Length ______
Time of first spontaneous breath ______
Medications ______

Other
Voided in delivery room ______ Stool ______
Breastfed ______ Bonding time ______
Observations of bonding behavior ______

In nursery
Time of transfer to nursery if applicable ______
First temperature ______ Placed in warmer/Isolette ______
Eye prophylaxis ______
Vitamin K ______ Time ______ Location ______

Fig. 17-1 Neonatal health history. (From Dickason EJ, Schult MO, and Silverman BL: Maternal-infant nursing care, St Louis, 1990, The CV Mosby Co.)

Table 17-1 Infant State-related Behavior Chart

Behavior/Description of Behavior	Infant State Consideration	Implications for Caregiving
ALERTING Widening and brightening of the eyes. Infants focus attention on stimuli, whether visual, auditory, or objects to be sucked.	From drowsy or active alert to quiet alert.	Infant state and timing are important. When trying to alert infants, try to: 1. Unwrap infant (arms out at least). 2. Place infant in upright position. 3. Talk to infant, putting variation in your pitch and tempo. 4. Show your face to infant. 5. Elicit the rooting, sucking, or grasp reflexes.
VISUAL RESPONSE Newborns have pupillary responses to differences in brightness. Infants can focus on objects or faces about 7-8 inches away. Newborns have preferences for more complex patterns, human faces, and moving objects.	Quiet alert.	Newborn's visual alertness provides opportunities for eye-to-eye contact with caregivers, an important source of beginning caregiver-infant interaction.
AUDITORY RESPONSE Reaction to a variety of sounds, especially in the human voice range. Infants can hear sounds and locate the general direction of the sound, if the source is constant.	Drowsy, quiet alert, active alert.	Enhances communication between infants and caregivers. Crying infants can often be consoled by voice.
IRRITABILITY How easily infants are upset by loud noises, handling by caregivers, temperature changes, removal of blankets or clothes, etc.	From deep sleep, light sleep, drowsy, quiet alert, or active alert to fussing or crying.	Irritable infants need more frequent consoling and more subdued external environments. Parents can be helped to cope with more irritable infants.
READABILITY The cues infants give through motor behavior and activity, looking, listening, and behavior patterns.	All states.	Parents need to learn that newborns' behaviors are part of their individual temperaments and not reflections on their parenting abilities. By observing and understanding an infant's characteristic pattern, parents can respond more appropriately.
SMILE Ranging from a faint grimace to a full-fledged smile. Reflexive.	Drowsy, active alert, quiet alert, light sleep.	Initial smile in the neonatal period is the forerunner of the social smile at 3-4 weeks of age. Important for caregivers to respond to it.
HABITUATION The ability to lessen one's response to repeated stimuli. This is seen where the Moro response is repeatedly elicited. If a noise is continually repeated, infants will usually cease to respond.	Deep sleep, light sleep, also seen in drowsy.	Because of this ability families can carry out normal activities without disturbing infants. Infants who have more difficulty with this will probably not sleep well in active environments.

Modified from Barnard KE et al: Infant state-related behavior chart. In early parent-infant relationships, copyright 1978 by the March of Dimes Birth Defects Foundation, White Plains, N.Y. Reprinted by permission.

Continued.

Table 17-1 **Infant State-related Behavior Chart—cont'd**

Behavior/Description of Behavior	Infant State Consideration	Implications for Caregiving
CUDDLINESS		
Infant's response to being held. Infants nestle and work themselves into the contours of caregivers' bodies.	Primarily in awake states.	Cuddliness is usually rewarding behavior for the caregivers. If infants do not nestle and mold, show the caregivers how to position infants to maximize this response.
CONSOLABILITY		
Measured when infants have been crying for at least 15 seconds. The ability of infants to bring themselves or to be brought by others to a lower state.	From crying to active alert, quiet alert, drowsy, or sleep states.	Crying is the infant behavior that presents the greatest challenge to caregivers. Parents' success or failure in consoling their infants has a significant impact on their feelings of competence as parents.
SELF-CONSOLING		
Maneuvers used by infants to console themselves and move to a lower state: 1. Hand-to-mouth movement. 2. Sucking on fingers, fist, or tongue. 3. Paying attention to voices or faces. 4. Changes in position.	From crying to active alert, quiet alert, drowsy, or sleep states.	If caregivers are aware of these behaviors, they may allow infants the opportunity to gain control of themselves. This does not imply that newborns should be left to cry. Once newborns are crying and do not initiate self-consoling activities, they may need attention from caregivers.
CONSOLING BY CAREGIVERS		
After crying for longer than 15 seconds, the caregivers may try to: 1. Show face to infant. 2. Talk to infant in a steady, soft voice. 3. Hold both infant's arms close to body. 4. Swaddle infant. 5. Pick up infant. 6. Rock infant. 7. Give a pacifier or feed	From crying to active alert, quiet alert, drowsy, or sleep states.	Often parental initial reaction is to pick up infants or feed them when they cry. Parents could be taught to try other soothing maneuvers.
MOTOR BEHAVIOR AND ACTIVITY		
Spontaneous movements of extremities and body when stimulated vs. when left alone. Smooth, rhythmical movements vs. jerky ones.	Quiet alert, active alert.	Smooth, nonjerky movements with periods of inactivity seem most natural. Some parents see jerky movements and startles as negative response to their caregiving and are frightened.

illary *temperature* is measured. Taking the temperature rectally is ordinarily contraindicated. Rectal temperatures may be taken to assess patency of the anus. Waiting for the first stool to appear, however, is the preferable means of assessing anal patency.

The baby's *head* is assessed for skin, hair pattern and distribution, molding, fontanels and sutures, size, shape, symmetry, eyes, nose, mouth, ears, and facies. The neck is inspected and palpated. *Chest assessment* includes measuring the chest circumference and noting the shape of the thorax, the breasts and nipples, and chest movement with respirations. The rate and rhythm of the heart and presence or absence of murmurs are noted. Lung fields are auscultated. The shape of the *abdomen* and the condition of the umbilical cord are assessed. Abdominal circumference may be measured. Bowel sounds and record of stooling behavior are noted. The newborn's *genitals, urinary meatus,* and *anus* are assessed carefully. The *skeletal system* is also inspected.

Neonatal *reflexes* are assessed. The responses reveal the status of the neuromuscular and skeletal systems. The baby's state-related behaviors (Table 17-1) and behavioral patterns and sensory capabilities (Table 17-2) are assessed and documented.

Nursing Diagnoses

Analysis of the significance of findings collected during assessment leads to the establishment of nursing diagnoses. Possible nursing diagnoses *for the newborn* are as follows:

Ineffective breathing pattern related to
- Obstructed airway

Impaired gas exchange related to
- **Hypothermia** (cold stress)

Potential for ineffective thermoregulation related to
- Heat loss to environment

Potential for infection related to
- Environmental factors

Possible nursing diagnoses *for the parent or parents* are as follows:

Altered parenting related to
- Knowledge deficit of newborn's social capabilities
- Knowledge deficit of newborn's dependency needs

Knowledge deficit related to
- Biologic and behavioral characteristics of the newborn

Situational low self-esteem related to
- Misinterpretation of newborn's responses

See the nursing care plan on p. 489.

Planning

Plans for care of the newborn reflect the rapid growth and development during the neonatal period. Changes in biologic and behavioral states are measured in minutes and hours since birth. The neonatal period extends through the first 28 days after birth. By that time the rate of change has slowed enough so that the child's appearance and needs can be referred to in terms of weeks and months.

The focus of care changes between birth and 28 days. During the first 2 hours of life (HOL) the main focus is on the infant's physiologic adaptation. By the end of the neonatal period the infant's socialization needs assume equal importance with physiologic needs.

The care given the neonate during the *first 2 HOL* is part of the care given parents and newborns in the fourth stage of labor (Chapter 15). Care related to *nutritional* needs of infants, including techniques of feeding, is presented in Chapter 18. *Parent-child interactions* are discussed in detail in Chapters 18 and 20.

The information in this section pertains to the maintenance of vital functions, the daily care of infants, and the forms of general therapy carried out routinely in newborn nurseries. Parental education before discharge from the hospital and at the well-baby visit is outlined. An example of an individualized care plan is presented on p 489.

The ***goals*** for newborn care relate to the infant and to the caregiver. The *goals for the infant* include that the infant will:

1. Make the transition from intrauterine to extrauterine life
2. Be free from trauma such as injury and infection
3. Continue the relationship with the primary caregivers begun in the prenatal period

Goals for the parents include that the parents will:

1. Acquire knowledge, skill, and confidence relevant to child care activities
2. Recognize their knowledge of the infant's behavior begun prenatally
3. Reorganize and intensify relationships with their newborn

Implementation

The technical aspects of neonatal care include techniques for health maintenance, detection of disability, and institution of remedial measures. These techniques can be used for teaching purposes. Careful and concise recording of client responses or laboratory results contributes to the continuous supervision vital to mother, newborn, and family.

Protective Environment

The provision of a protective environment is basic to the care of the newborn. The construction, maintenance, and operation of nurseries in accredited hospitals are directed by national professional organizations such as the American Academy of Pediatrics and local or state governing bodies. Detailed information concerning standards of care for newborn nurseries may be obtained from a number of sources (see Appendixes B and I). Prescribed standards cover areas such as the following:

1. *Environmental factors:* provision of adequate lighting, elimination of potential fire hazards, safety of electric appliances, adequate ventilation, and controlled temperature (warm and free of drafts) and humidity (lower than 50%).

Table 17-2 Infant Behavioral Patterns and Sensory Capabilities

Item	Parameters of Normal	Deviations From Normal/Probable Conditions
Behavioral patterns	Cortical control and responsiveness	Central nervous system (CNS) disorders
Feeding	Variations in interest, hunger; usually feeds well within 24 hours of birth	Lethargic, tires easily or may perspire while attempting to feed; poor suck, poor coordination with swallow, cyanosis, choking
Social	Cry is lusty, strong; soon indicative of hunger, pain, attention seeking	Weak or absent; high pitched
	Smiling, focusing evident within first week	Absence; no focusing on person holding him; unconsolable
	Responds by quietness and increased alertness to cuddling, voice	
Sleep-wakefulness	Transitional period with 2 periods of reactivity: at birth and 6-8 hr later (Chapter 16)	Lethargy; drowsiness
	Stabilization with wakeful periods about every 3-4 hr	Disorganized pattern
Elimination	Develops own pattern within first 2 weeks:	See pp. 445 and 446
	Stooling: see p. 446	
	Urination (see "Renal System," p. 445)	Diminished number: dehydration
	First few days: 3-4 times daily	
	End of first week: 5-6 times daily	
	Later: 6-10 times daily with adequate hydration	
Reflex response	Brainstem development and musculoskeletal intactness	Present in anencephalic newborns also
	See "Reflexes," Table 16-3 (p. 475)	Absence; hyperreactive; incomplete; asynchronous
Sensory capabilities		
Vision	Limited accommodation with clearest vision within 18-20 cm (7-8 in)	Absence of these responses may be caused by absence of or diminished acuity or by sensory deprivation
	Detects color by 2 months but attracted by black-white pattern at 5 days or less	
	Focuses and follows by 15 min of age	
	Prefers patterns to plain surfaces	
	Prefers changes in patterns by 2 months	
	At birth, can gaze intently	
Hearing	By 2 min of age, moves eyes in direction of sound	Absence of response: deafness
	Responds to high pitch by "freezing," followed by agitation; to low pitch (crooning) by relaxation	
	Can hear beginning in last trimester of fetal life	
Touch	Sensitivity to pain may be diminished (because of β-endorphins present prenatally)	Unable to be comforted; possible drug dependence
	Soothed by massaging, warmth, weightlessness (as in warm water bath)	
Smell	By days 2 to 7 can distinguish between own mother's used breast pads and those of another woman	
Taste	By 3 days of age, can distinguish between sucrose and glucose and grimaces in response to drop of lemon juice on tongue	
Motor	Coordinates body movement to parent's voice and body movement; imitates parent's actions by 2 weeks of age	Absence

Specific Nursing Care Plan

NEWBORN WITH MUCUS AND "CONE HEAD"

Carol is a 24-year-old, married woman who gave birth to her first child, a term baby girl weighing 3500 g (7 lb 12 oz). Carol's labor progressed smoothly over 12 hours and she had a spontaneous vaginal delivery without complication. The parents were pleased their daughter could remain in Carol's room. The pediatrician's findings were all within normal limits. About 4 hours after delivery, Carol called the nurse because her daughter was "gagging, spitting up, and was a little blue." After the newborn's immediate care was completed, Carol commented about her daughter's "poor little cone head."

ASSESSMENT	NURSING DIAGNOSIS (ND), PLAN/GOAL (P/G)	RATIONALE/ IMPLEMENTATION	EVALUATION
Newborn is gagging and regurgitating mucus.	ND: Ineffective airway clearance (potential) related to excess secretions. P/G: Newborn will maintain open airway.	*A clear airway is essential to maintain respirations:* Hold newborn face downward with head slightly lowered and aspirate mouth and nose with **bulb syringe.** Position newborn on side to facilitate drainage from mouth. Note efficiency of cough, sneeze, gag, and swallow to maintain clear airway. Assess breath sounds. Evaluate for signs of respiratory distress. Comfort newborn after a bout of gagging and regurgitation.	Newborn maintains clear airway. Newborn remains free of respiratory distress.
Parents concerned about newborn's gagging and regurgitation of mucus.	ND: Potential for altered parenting related to lack of understanding of this neonatal characteristic and its management. P/G: Parents will be able to verbalize cause and management of gagging and regurgitation.	*Developing child care skills increases parents' self-confidence:* Explain the physiologic processes (second period of reactivity). Reassure parents that gagging, coughing, and sneezing are normal and expected to clear newborn's airway. Assist parents in positioning child in ways that promote drainage of secretions. Demonstrate and encourage practice with positioning and use of bulb syringe.	Parents verbalize understanding of instruction. Parents demonstrate skill in helping newborn keep a clear airway.
Parents verbalize concern about newborn's "cone head."	ND: Knowledge deficit related to the normal molding during the birth process. P/G: Parents will verbalize understanding of normal molding.	*Knowledge increases parents' self-confidence:* Explain the process of molding and its purpose in a successful vaginal delivery. Reassure parents that the newborn's head will resume its normal shape within a few days.	Parents verbalize understanding of molding. Newborn's head will resume rounded shape within a few days.

2. *Measures to control infection:* adequate floor space to permit positioning bassinets at least 60 cm (24 in) apart, hand-washing facilities, techniques for safe formula preparation and storage, and cleaning and sterilizing of equipment and supplies.

In addition, hospital personnel develop their own policies and procedures directed toward protecting the newborns under their care. For instance:

1. Nursery personnel are restricted to those directly involved in the care of mothers and infants, thereby reducing the opportunities for the introduction of pathogenic organisms. In this respect children born at home are at an advantage because they usually come in contact only with family members. This home environment is somewhat duplicated in hospitals when the infant and mother "room together." The mother and father are active in the care, thereby reducing the number of nursing personnel involved. In many hospitals, nurseries are constructed with anterooms. Physicians carry out examinations and procedures such as circumcisions here. Parents may also come here to feed and hold their infants when the newborn must remain in the hospital for care.

2. Personnel assigned to the nursery wear special uniforms or cover gowns, and before beginning the care of infants, they carry out a *hand-washing technique.* In light of the acquired immunodeficiency syndrome (AIDS) issue the Centers for Disease Control (CDC) in Atlanta recommends the following practice (NAACOG, 1986): ***health care workers must wear gloves when touching mucous membranes or nonintact skin of all patients.*** In addition, masks, eye coverings, and gowns must be used when indicated. Health-care personnel ***must wear gloves and gowns when handling the infant until blood and amniotic fluid have been removed from the infant's skin, when drawing blood (e.g., heel stick), and when caring for a fresh wound (e.g., circumcision).***

3. Anyone coming from "outside" is expected to gown and *wash her or his hands* before coming in contact with infants or equipment. Such people include nurses, physicians, parents, brothers and sisters, department supervisors, electricians, and housekeepers.

4. Individuals with infectious conditions are excluded from contact or must take special precautions when working with newborns; this includes people with upper respiratory tract infections, gastrointestinal tract infections, and infectious skin conditions. Most agencies have now coupled this day-to-day self-screening of personnel with yearly health examinations.

❑ MONITORING THE NEWBORN

After initial assessment, important functions of the nurse are to monitor the condition of the infant, treat deviations from normal, record findings, and report to the physician those findings that require medical intervention.

Maintenance of Body Temperature

On admission to the nursery, initial temperatures as low as 36° C (96.8° F) are not uncommon. The temperature is taken by axilla every hour until stabilized. By the twelfth hour the temperature should stabilize within the normal range.

Cold stress is detrimental to the newborn. It increases the need for oxygen and can upset the acid/base balance. The nurse can help stabilize the infant's temperature by placing the thoroughly dried, unclothed infant under a radiant warmer until the temperature is stabilized. The heater thermostat must be kept plugged into an electrical outlet at all times. It is set to maintain an abdominal skin temperature of 36.5° C (97.6° F). The set point of 36.4° C (97.5° F) is usually chosen for activation of the heater. The alarm is set so that the nurse is warned if the temperature is either below or above the set point.

The **thermistor probe** (metal side next to the infant) is applied with paper tape or nonirritating plastic tape to the abdominal wall between the umbilicus and the xiphoid process of the sternum. It is covered with a small plastic-foam insulator. When applying the probe, bony prominences and placement over the liver (which may generate heat) are to be avoided. The infant is checked frequently to ensure that the probe maintains skin contact.

Other nursing actions that will assist in the stabilization of the temperature are maintaining the ambient temperature in the nursery at 24° C (75° F) and keeping the baby dry and wrapped in warm blankets, with the head covered, while the parent is holding the infant. The initial bath should be postponed until the newborn's skin temperature is stable between 36.5° and 37.2° C (97.6° and 99° F).

Warming Infant with Hypothermia. Even a normal full-term baby in good health can become hypothermic. Birth in a car on the way to the hospital, a cold delivery room, or inadequate drying and wrapping immediately after birth may cause the infant's temperature to fall. Warming the hypothermic baby is accomplished with care. Rapid warming or cooling may cause apneic spells and acidosis in an infant. Therefore the warming process is monitored to progress slowly over a period of 2 to 4 hours.

Maintenance of an Adequate Oxygen Supply

Four conditions are essential for maintenance of an adequate oxygen supply:

1. A clear airway—fundamental to adequate ventilation

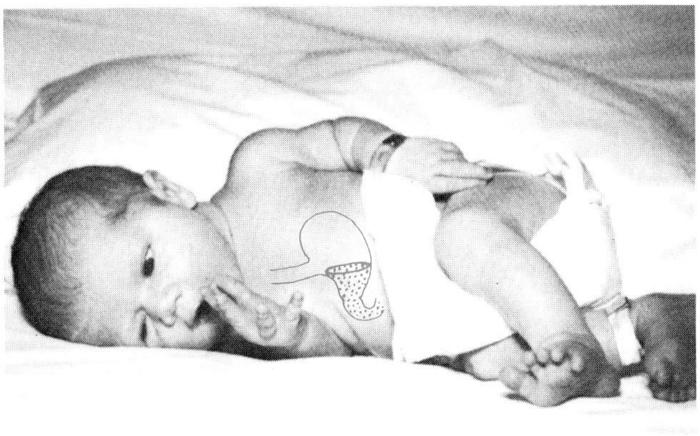

Fig. 17-2 Infant is turned to right side and supported in this position to facilitate drainage from mouth and to promote emptying into the small intestine.

2. Respiratory efforts—necessary to ensure continued ventilation
3. A functioning cardiopulmonary system—essential to maintain oxygen
4. Heat support—necessary because exposure to cold stress increases oxygen needs

Maintenance of Clear Airway. Generally the normal full-term infant born vaginally has little difficulty clearing the air passages. Most secretions are drained by gravity, propelled to the oropharynx by the cough reflex, to be drained or swallowed. The infant is maintained in a side-lying position with a rolled blanket at the back to facilitate drainage (Fig. 17-2). If excessive mucus is present, the foot of the crib may be elevated slightly and the oropharynx is suctioned with a bulb syringe (Fig. 17-3, *A*) or a **DeLee mucus-trap catheter** (Fig. 17-3, *B*) (Procedures 17-1 and 17-2). The bulb syringe is compressed, the tip is placed in the infant's mouth between the gums and the cheek, and then pressure on the bulb is released to suction the secretions. These steps are repeated until excess secretions are removed. The nurse's knowledge and skill in suctioning may be critical in helping both normal and distressed infants establish or maintain adequate respirations. "Milking" the trachea is ineffective. This procedure may injure cartilage and will often delay effective suctioning.

Maintenance of Respiratory Efforts. The normal term infant establishes respirations within minutes of birth, usually without undue difficulty. However, nursery personnel need to be skilled in the techniques for reestablishing respirations and providing increased oxygen in case the need arises (see danger signs box, right). A humidified oxygen source and equipment for the administration of oxygen must be readily available.

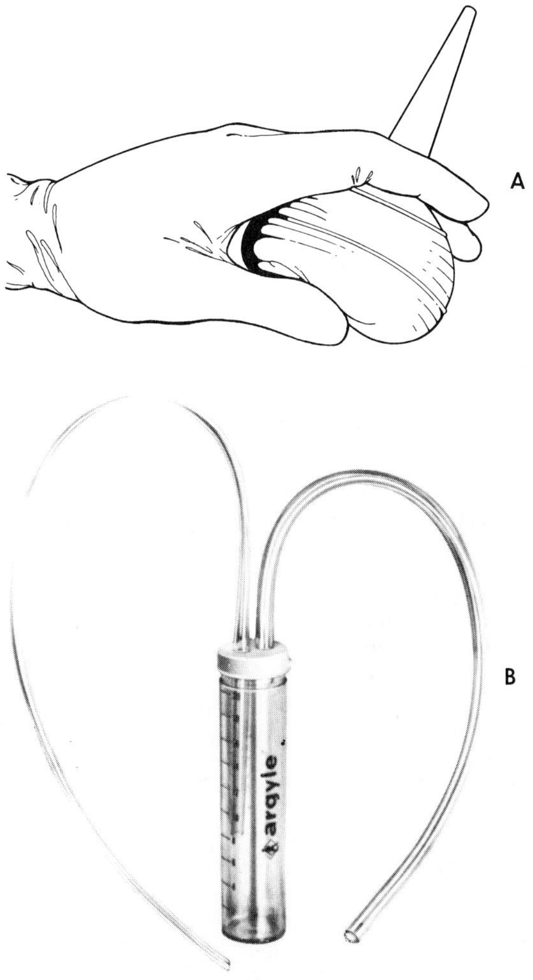

Fig. 17-3 Suctioning devices. **A,** Bulb syringe. Bulb must be compressed before insertion. **B,** DeLee mucus-trap catheter. This should be connected to a mechanical suction source. (**A,** from Smith D: Comprehensive child and family nursing skills, St Louis, 1991, The CV Mosby Co.)

DANGER SIGNS

Abnormal Newborn Breathing

1. **Bradypnea**—respirations ≤ 25 per min
2. **Tachypnea**—respirations ≥ 60 per min
3. Abnormal breath sounds—rales, rhonchi, wheezes, expiratory grunt
4. **Respiratory distress**—nasal flaring, retractions, chin tug, labored breathing

PROCEDURE 17-1

SUCTIONING USING THE DELEE MUCUS TRAP CATHETER (FIG. 17-3, *B*)

DEFINITION

Use of a mucus-trap catheter for removal of secretions.

PURPOSE

To remove mucus or meconium from the nasopharynx and oropharynx.
To remove amniotic fluid from the stomach.

EQUIPMENT

Sterile DeLee mucus-trap catheter (available in reusable glass or disposable plastic) with two-hole tip.
Sterile water. A 120 ml (4 oz) bottle of sterile water for feeding is convenient, already in a sterile container, and decreases risk of contamination possible with large stock bottles.

NURSING ACTIONS	RATIONALE
Wash hands before and after touching baby and equipment. Apply gloves.	Prevents nosocomial infection and implements universal precautions and precautions for intrusive procedures.
Place infant in supine position.	Facilitates suctioning.
Lubricate catheter in sterile water.	Facilitates passage of tube and prevents infection.
Aspirate mouth and throat first, then the nose.	Prevents infant's inhalation of pharyngeal secretions.
Insert catheter:	Decreases risk of laryngeal spasm and reflex.
Orally along base of tongue.	
Nasally horizontally into nares, then raising it to advance it beyond bend at back of nares.	
Avoid forcing catheter.	**Hazard:** Prevents direct tissue trauma or perforation in presence of congenital anomalies such as choanal, esophageal, or intestinal atresia.
Suction is applied by user.	Provides sufficient negative pressure to withdraw mucus or other substances.
Limit suctioning to 10 times or less.	Avoids prolonged suctioning that stimulates laryngospasm and reduces oxygen (O_2) content in airway.
Apply suction only as tube is withdrawn.	Prevents direct tissue trauma.
Rotate catheter when suctioning.	Prevents tissue trauma consequent to tissue's being drawn into eye of catheter.
Discontinue suctioning when: The cry is clear. Air entry into lungs is heard by stethoscope.	Passes the catheter correctly: gagging indicates entrance into esophagus; coughing indicates entrance into trachea.
Cuddle infant.	Reassures infant.
Detach mucus trap catheter and send the enclosed specimen to the laboratory for examination and culture as necessary.	Allows ongoing evaluation of infant's condition.
Record the amount of mucus or amniotic fluid removed.	Ensures communication with other caregivers.

PROCEDURE 17-2

SUCTIONING USING A NASOPHARYNGEAL CATHETER WITH MECHANICAL SUCTION APPARATUS

DEFINITION

Use of mechanical suction apparatus and external suction source for removal of secretions.

PURPOSE

To remove excessive or tenacious mucus from the nasopharynx and oropharynx in resuscitating an infant.

EQUIPMENT

Catheters:
- French, rubber (moderately firm); sizes 10, 12, and 14; two-hole tip French; plastic disposable: sizes 8, 10, and 12; finger control; two-hole tip.

External suction source.

Sterile water. A 120 ml (4 oz) bottle of sterile water for feeding is convenient, is already in sterile container, and reduces risk of contamination possible with large stock bottles.

NURSING ACTIONS	RATIONALE
Wash hands before and after touching baby and equipment. Apply gloves.	Prevents nosocomial infection and implements universal precautions.
Position the infant: Place the infant in supine position. Place a folded towel under the head to move it slightly forward from the neck (as in sniffing).	(1) Separates tongue from pharyngeal wall and (2) prevents obstruction of newborn's normally low palate and macroglossia. (Some physicians prefer to work with the baby on a flat surface with no towel.)
Adjust negative pressure on portable or wall gauges.	Prevents excessive suctioning.
Keep deep suctioning to a minimum.	**Hazard:** Prevents direct trauma to mucosa with edema formation, bleeding, or increased secretions. Prevents stimulation of vagal reflex: bradycardia, cardiac arrhythmias, laryngospasm, and **apnea,** especially if this type of suctioning is done within a few minutes of infant's birth.
Limit each suctioning to 10 seconds or less.	Prevents laryngospasm and oxygen depletion.
If infant is active, an attendant may be needed to stabilize infant's head. Or if there is time, restrain infant by **mummy technique** before this procedure.	Prevents trauma and facilitates suctioning. Both hands are needed to manipulate catheter and finger control of suction pressure.
Lubricate catheter in sterile water.	Facilitates passage of tube and prevents infection.
Turn suction **off** as tube is put into position.	Prevents direct tissue trauma.
Avoid forcing catheter.	**Hazard:** Prevents direct tissue trauma or perforation in presence of congenital anomalies such as choanal, esophageal, or intestinal atresia.
Insert catheter: Orally along base of tongue. Nasally horizontally into nares, then raising it to advance it beyond bend at back of nares.	Decreases risk of laryngeal spasm and reflex apnea.
With catheter in place, put thumb over finger control to create suction. Rotate tubing between fingers while withdrawing catheter.	Prevents direct trauma caused by drawing mucosa into eye of catheter.
Apply suction only as tube is withdrawn.	Prevents direct tissue trauma.
Rotate catheter when suctioning.	Prevents tissue trauma consequent to tissues being drawn into eye of catheter.
Observe infant's response.	Prevents gagging, which indicates entrance into esophagus; coughing indicates entrance into trachea.
Withdraw tube to suction posterior nasopharynx.	
Comfort infant.	Prompts feelings of safety.
Record procedure.	Ensures communication with other caregivers.

Relieving Airway Obstruction. Whaley and Wong (1991) recommend that a choking infant be placed face down over the rescuer's arm with the head lower than the trunk and the head supported. Additional support can be achieved if the rescuer supports his own arm firmly against his thigh (Committee on Accidents and Poison Prevention, 1986). Four quick, sharp back blows are delivered between the infant's shoulder blades with the heel of the rescuer's hand. After delivery of the back blows, the rescuer's free hand is placed flat on the infant's back so that the infant is "sandwiched" between the two hands, making certain the neck and chin are well supported. While the rescuer maintains support with the infant's head lower than the trunk, the infant is turned and placed supine on the rescuer's thigh, where four chest thrusts are applied in rapid succession in the same manner as external chest compressions described for **cardiopulmonary resuscitation (CPR)** (see emergency procedures, p. 495 and p. 497).

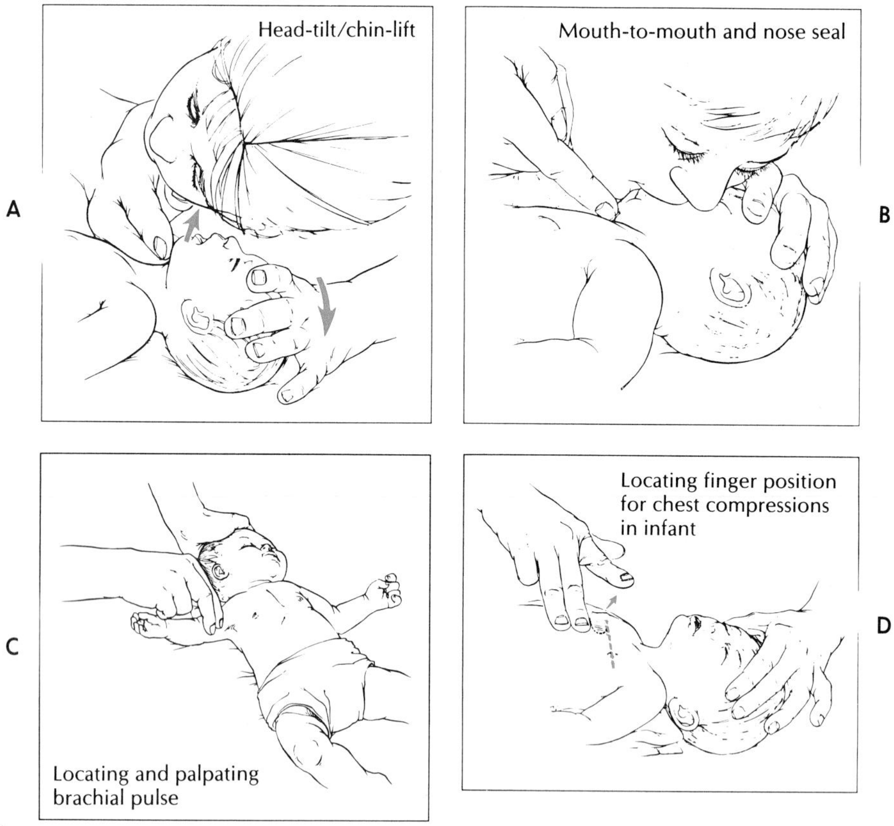

Fig. 17-4 Procedures for cardiopulmonary resuscitation. (From Standards for Cardiopulmonary Resuscitation (CPR) and Emergency Cardiac Care (ECC). IV. Pediatric basic life support, JAMA 225(21):2954, 1986.)

EMERGENCY PROCEDURE

CARDIOPULMONARY RESUSCITATION (CPR) (FIG. 17-4)

DEFINITION

A basic emergency procedure for life support consisting of artificial respiration and manual external cardiac massage.

PURPOSE

To prevent cardiac arrest following cessation of respirations (apnea extending beyond 15 sec).
To restore cardiac function.
To restore respiratory function.

EQUIPMENT

Resuscitation equipment should be readily available in areas in which respiratory arrest might take place, and the status of this equipment should be checked regularly, at least once a day.

NURSING ACTIONS	RATIONALE
Wash hands before and after touching infant and equipment. Glove.	Prevents nosocomial infection and implements universal precautions.
Resuscitation	
Observe color; tap, or gently shake shoulders.	Determines unresponsiveness or respiratory difficulty.
Yell for help; if alone, perform CPR for 1 min before calling for help again.	Brings help.
Turn infant to back, supporting head and neck	Protects neck.
Place on firm, flat surface.	Supports infant's spine; prevents injury during compression of sternum.
Clear airway, prn (see below).	Provides unobstructed ventilation.
Tilt head back gently to "sniffing" or neutral position; use head-tilt/chin-lift maneuver (Fig. 17-4, *A*).	Opens airway.
Do not hyperextend neck.	Prevents kinking of airway.
Assess for evidence of breathing:	Avoids unnecessary intervention.
Observe for chest movement.	
Listen for exhaled air.	
Feel for exhaled air flow.	
Breathe for infant (Fig. 17-4, *B*):	Assists ventilation.
Take a breath.	
Open mouth wide and place over mouth and nose of infant to create seal. (See emergency procedure, mouth-to-mouth resuscitation, p. 497).	Provides mouth-to-mouth and mouth-to-nose resuscitation.
NOTE: Repeat the word *ho* as you gently puff volume of air *in your* cheeks into infant. *Do not* force air.	Permits insufflation under pressure. Reduces risk of gastric distension, regurgitation, and subsequent aspiration.
Infant's chest should rise slightly with each puff; keep fingers on chest wall to sense air entry.	
Give two slow breaths (1 to 1.5 seconds per breath) pausing to inhale between breaths.	
Check pulse of brachial artery (Fig. 17-4, C) while maintaining head tilt.	Determines need for intervention.
If pulse is present, initiate rescue breathing. Continue until spontaneous breathing resumes at rate of every 3 seconds or 20 times per minute.	Avoids unnecessary intervention.
If pulse is not present, initiate chest compressions and coordinate with breathing.	Restores cardiac function.
NOTE: When two people are present, breathing and compressions are shared.	Prevents fatigue.
Provide compressions/breathing:	Coordinates compressions/breathing.
Pause at end of every fifth compression to allow chest to fall by passive recoil.	Allows removal of insufflated air.
Maintain 5:1 ratio for 1 or 2 rescuers.	Maintains arterial P_{O_2} level.
Reassess after 10 cycles, and every few minutes thereafter.	

Continued.

EMERGENCY PROCEDURE—cont'd

NURSING ACTIONS	RATIONALE
Chest compressions:	
Maintain head tilt. With other hand, position fingers for chest compressions.	Restores cardiac function.
Place index finger of hand farthest from infant's head just under imaginary line drawn between nipples (Fig. 17-4, *D*).	
Move index finger to a position one fingerbreadth below this intersection.	Identifies compression area.
Using 2 or 3 fingers, compress sternum to depth of $\frac{1}{2}$ or $\frac{3}{4}$ inch.	
Release pressure without moving fingers from the position.	Minimizes the chance of damage that might occur to the liver or spleen.
Repeat at a rate of at least 100 times per minute; 5 compressions in 3 seconds or less.	Approximates normal neonatal rate.
Perform 10 cycles of 5 compressions and 1 ventilation. (If possible, compressions are accompanied by positive-pressure ventilation at a rate of 40 to 60 per minute). Use this mnemonic: one-two-three-four-five-pause-head tilt-chin lift-ventilate-continue compressions. After cycles, check the brachial pulse to determine pulselessness (Nursing '87 Books).	Assists recall of correct ratio and timing.
Discontinue compressions if the infant's spontaneous heart rate reaches or exceeds 80 beats per minute (bpm).	Prevents disrupting cardiac rhythm that has resumed.
Relieving airway obstruction	
Use no blind finger sweeps.	Avoids pushing obstruction deeper.
Initiate back blows and chest thrusts (Fig. 17-5).	**Hazard:** Avoids the risk of injury to abdominal organs, Heimlich maneuver (abdominal thrusts) should not be used for infants of 1 year of age or less.
Position child prone over forearm with head down and with infant's jaw firmly supported.	Employs gravity to help remove obstruction.
Rest supporting arm on thigh.	Prevents rescuer's fatigue.
Deliver four back blows forcefully between infant's shoulder blades with heel of free hand.	Moves obstructive materials outward.
Place free hand on infant's back to sandwich her/him between both hands: one hand supports the neck, jaw, and chest; the other supports the back.	Avoids injury to infant while turning infant.
Turn infant over and place head down, supporting head and neck. Apply four chest thrusts to same location as chest compressions but use a slower rate.	Forces obstruction outward.
Open the airway with a head-tilt/chin-lift maneuver and attempt to ventilate.	Ventilates infant.
Repeat the sequence until it is effective.	
Alternative position: Place infant face down on your lap with head lower than trunk and head firmly supported. Apply back blows, turn infant, and apply chest thrusts as above.	Employs gravity to remove obstruction.
Continue emergency procedures until signs of recovery occur, as indicated by palpable peripheral pulses, return of pupils to normal size and responsiveness, and the disappearance of mottling and cyanosis.	Continues ventilation. Meets standards of care.
Record time and duration of procedure and effects of intervention.	Ensures communication with other caregivers.
Teach procedure to parents or other caregivers.	Increases parents' knowledge and skill in self-care measure.

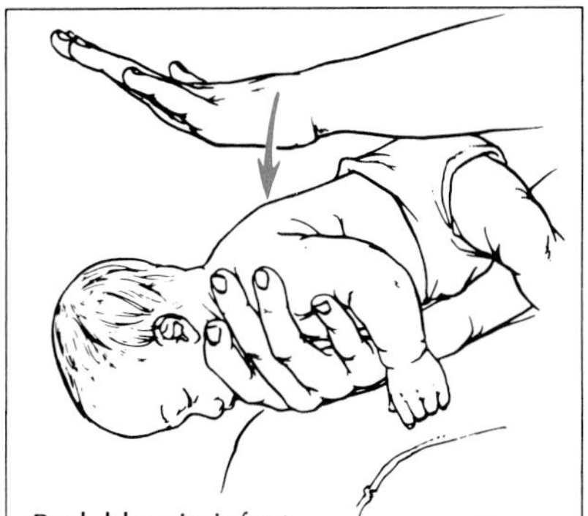

Fig. 17-5 Back blow in infant for clearing airway obstruction. (From Standards for Cardiopulmonary Resuscitation (CPR) and Emergency Cardiac Care (ECC). IV. Pediatric basic life support, JAMA 225(21):2954, 1986.

EMERGENCY PROCEDURE
MOUTH-TO-MOUTH AND MOUTH-TO-NOSE RESUSCITATION

DEFINITION
Artificial resuscitation performed when respirations have ceased.

PURPOSE
To reestablish respiration.

EQUIPMENT
None needed. If available: rolled towel, plastic airway, oxygen, suction.

NURSING ACTIONS	RATIONALE
Wash hands before and after touching infant and equipment. Apply gloves.	Prevents nosocomial infection and to implement universal precautions.
Clear airway of any mucus or debris.	Prevents blowing debris down airway.
Position infant in "sniffing" position by putting rolled towel under head to move it slightly forward from neck, or leave infant on flat surface.	Opens airway by straightening trachea and permitting back of tongue to fall away from posterior pharynx.
Insert plastic airway if available.	Provides unobstructed airway (especially from tongue if infant is flaccid).
Place your mouth over infant's nose and mouth to create seal.	Permits insufflation under pressure.
Repeat the word *ho* as you gently *puff* volume of air *in your cheeks* into infant. *Do not* force air.	Prevents injury to lung tissue (e.g., pneumothorax, pneumomediastinum).
Repeat puffs at rate of 30/min.	Approximates normal respiratory rate.
Infant's chest should rise slightly with each puff; keep fingers on chest wall to sense air entry.	Determines if air is reaching alveolar level.
Allow chest to fall by passive recoil.	Allows removal of insufflated air.
If available, place tubing of oxygen in your mouth as you inhale quickly between puffs.	Increases O_2 content in insufflated air.
Consider airway obstruction. Prepare for laryngoscopy and endotracheal intubation aspiration.	Asesses for obstruction; note if chest wall does not rise and the infant's vital responses do not improve in 30 sec.
Record procedure.	Ensures communication with other caregivers.

❑ HYGIENIC CARE AND SAFETY

Bathing the Infant

Bathing serves a number of purposes. It provides opportunities for complete cleansing of the infant, observation of the infant's condition, promotion of comfort, and parent-child-family socialization. The initial bath is postponed until the infant's temperature stabilizes at 36.5° C (97.6° F) or above.

The temperature of the room should be 24° C (75° F), and the bathing area should be free of drafts to prevent heat loss. Heat loss in the infant is greater than heat loss in the adult because of the relatively large ratio of skin surface to body mass in the newborn. Heat loss must be controlled during the bath period to conserve the infant's energy. Bathing the infant quickly, exposing only a portion of the body at a time, and thorough drying are therefore part of the bathing technique. *Until the initial bath is completed, personnel must wear gloves when handling the newborn.*

Recent Centers for Disease Control (CDC) (1989) regulations related to universal precautions for HIV (see Universal Precautions, p. 668) have increased the use of soap solutions for bathing newborn infants (AAP, 1988). A nonmedicated mild soap may be used for the initial bath. The hair is shampooed, and a brush or comb may be used to remove dried blood and vernix. Cotton balls, not gauze, are used to cleanse the nostrils and ears. Careful drying may decrease the risk of infection (AAP, 1988). The temperature is reassessed 30 minutes after completion of the bath.

After the initial bath, washing with warm water is sufficient for the first week. However, the perineal area should be carefully washed with nonmedicated mild soap and warm water and carefully dried with each diaper change.

The infant's fragile skin can be injured by too vigorous cleansing. Vernix, the white material that looks like cold cream is not removed vigorously as it is attached to the upper layer of the skin. Too vigorous removal results in removal of the protective skin layer. Vernix may be left on for 48 hours; if it persists beyond that time, it may be washed off gently. Some nurses advocate massaging the vernix gently into the skin. To date, no studies have confirmed the benefits or disadvantages of this technique (AAP, 1988).

Guidelines for client teaching are provided for use with mothers who need instruction in the bathing of their infants. The nurse does not need to wear gloves during the bath demonstration for the parent(s) (Fig. 17-6).

Questions have arisen about some routine practices: use of soap, oils, powder, lotion, and sponging. Nursing research can provide needed answers. According to Whaley and Wong (1991):

> One of the most important considerations in skin cleansing is preservation of the skin's pH, which is about 5 soon after birth. The slightly acidic skin surface has bacteriostatic effects. Consequently, only plain warm water should be used for the bath. Alkaline soaps such as Ivory, oils, powder, and lotions are not used because they alter the pH, thus providing a better environment for bacterial growth. Talcum has the added risk of aspiration if applied too close to the infant's face.

Diaper Rash. Treatment of diaper rash involves exposing the rash to warmth and air. Immediately washing and drying the wet and soiled area and changing the diaper after voiding or defecating prevent and help treat diaper rash. The warmth can be achieved with a 25-watt bulb placed 45 cm (18 in) from the affected area.

The most severe type of diaper rash occurs when the area becomes infected, indurated (hardened), and tender. Medical advice should be sought and a specifically ordered medication applied.

A rash on the face may result from the infant's scratching (**excoriation**) or from rubbing the face against the sheets, particularly if regurgitated stomach contents are not washed off promptly.

Care of the Infant's Linens. Care of the infant's clothes and bedding is directed toward minimizing cross infection and removing residues from soap, feces, or urine that may irritate the infant's skin. In the hospital, clothing and bedding are washed separately from other linens and are autoclaved. Some hospitals use disposable shirts and diapers. At home the baby's clothes should be washed separately, with a mild detergent or soap and hot water. A double rinse usually removes traces of the potentially irritating cleansing agent or acid residue from the urine or stool. If possible, the clothing and bedding are dried in the sun to neutralize residues. Parents who have to use coin-operated machines to wash and dry clothes may find it expensive or impossible to wash and rinse the baby's clothes well.

Bedding requires frequent changing. The plastic-coated, firm mattress must be washed daily and the crib or bassinet damp dusted. The infant's toilet articles may be kept separate and convenient for use in a box or basket.

Umbilical Cord Care. The care of the umbilical cord is the same as that for any surgical wound. The goal of care is prevention and early identification of hemorrhage or infection. If bleeding from the blood vessels of the cord is noted, the nurse checks the clamp (or tie) and applies a second clamp next to the first one. If bleeding is not stopped immediately, the nurse calls for physician assistance at once.

Guidelines for Client Teaching

BATHING AN INFANT

ASSESSMENT

1. Woman has just delivered her first child, a boy.
2. She has little experience with the care of children.
3. Woman exhibits a readiness to learn by asking many questions.
4. Woman's culture does not have specific prescription or proscriptions for this activity.

NURSING DIAGNOSES

Knowledge deficit related to bathing an infant. Anxiety, mild, related to care of newborn infant.

GOALS

Short-term

To have woman learn infant bathing technique.

Intermediate

To have woman become skilled in bathing and handling infant.

Long-term

To have woman adjust bathing technique to developing child.

REFERENCES AND TEACHING AIDS

Texts; hospital or clinic-prepared instructions; film or video of parent bathing a baby; and parent's class on bathing a baby.

RATIONALE/CONTENT	TEACHING ACTIONS
Health maintenance of newborn requires parental knowledge of content related to purposes of bathing: It provides opportunities for (1) a complete cleansing of the infant, (2) observing the infant's condition, (3) promoting comfort, and (4) parent-child-family socialization.	Introduction: set tone. Have mother seated comfortably (she may need a pillow or doughnut to sit on). Make sure she can see demonstration. Welcome father (or other family member) if present, and include in the process.
Fitting baths into family's schedule: Initial bath: the initial bath is postponed until the infant's skin temperature stabilizes at 36.5° C (97.6° F) or core temperature stabilizes at 37° (98.6° F) for 2 hours. Daily bath: a daily bath may be given at any time convenient to the parent but not immediately after a feeding period, since the increased handling may cause regurgitation of the feeding.	Ask mother when father and siblings would be available for infant bath. Prevents cold stress.
Preventing heat loss: The temperature of the room should be 24° C (75° F), and the bathing area should be free of drafts. Heat loss in the infant is greater than in the adult because of the relatively large ratio of skin surface to body mass in the newborn. Heat loss must be controlled during the bath period to conserve the infant's energy. Bathing the infant quickly, exposing only a portion of the body at a time, and thorough drying is therefore part of the bathing technique.	Review material pertinent to care before beginning bath to prevent heat loss. Explain that infants do not shiver to increase body temperature, as adults do. Explain mechanism of burning fat for heat maintenance in the infant and the amount of energy it requires. Show a chart depicting this mechanism simplified.
Preventing skin trauma: The fragile skin can be injured by too vigorous cleansing. Vernix, the white, cheesy-looking material on the skin is not removed, since it is attached to the upper layer of the skin. Too vigorous removal results in removal of the protective skin layer. Vernix may be left on for 48 hours; if it persists beyond that time, it may be washed off gently. If stool or other debris has dried and caked on the skin, soak the area to remove it. Do not attempt to rub it off because abrasion may result. Gentleness, patting dry rather than rubbing, and use of a mild soap without perfumes or coloring are recommended. Chemicals in the coloring and perfume can cause rashes in sensitive skin.	Review material pertinent to skin care before beginning bath to prevent heat loss. Review possible sources of skin damage (for all members of family): dyes, perfumes.

Continued.

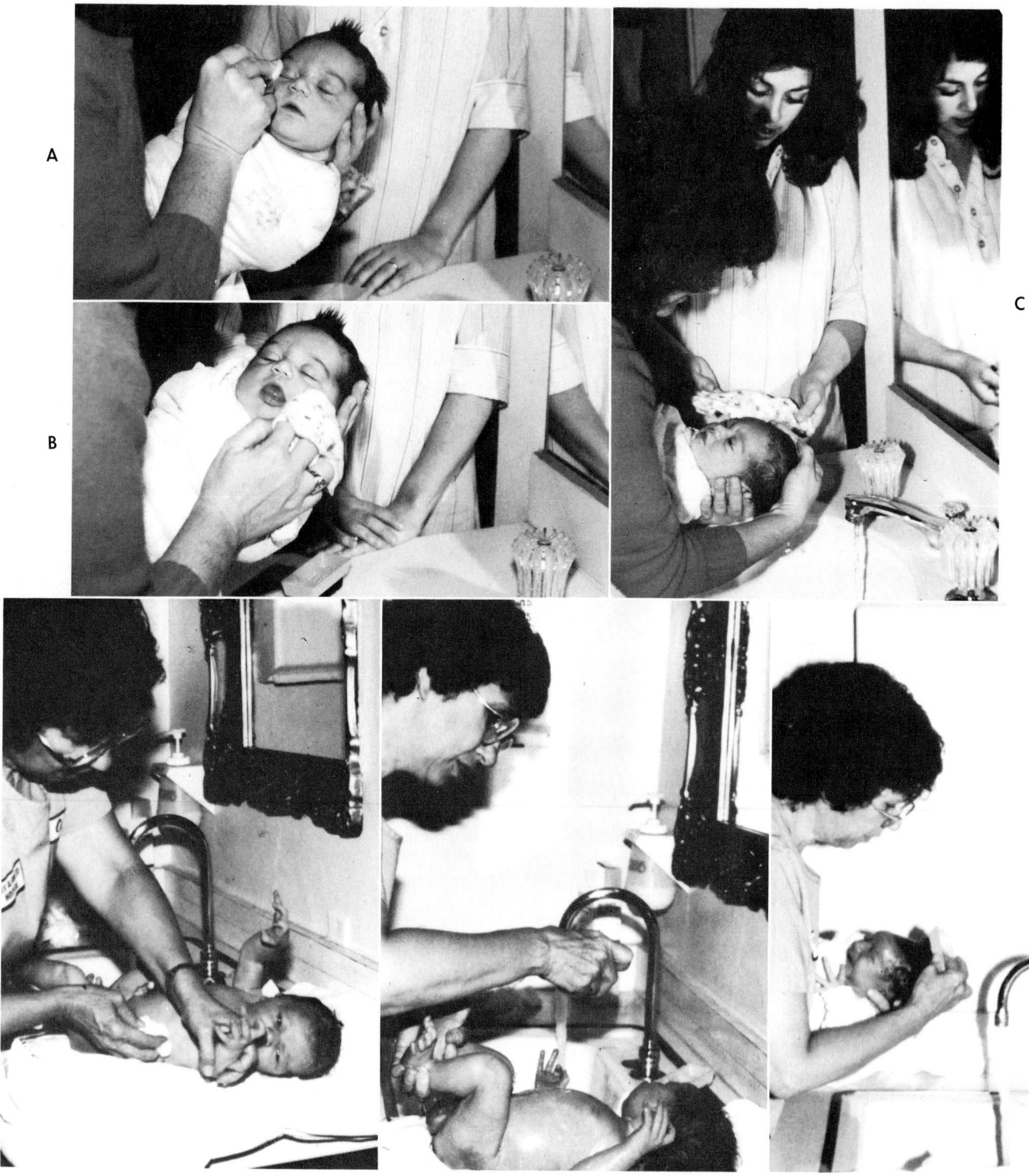

Fig. 17-6 Bathing baby. **A,** Eyes. **B,** Face. **C,** Head and hair. **D,** Sponge-bathing baby. **E,** Rinsing baby. **F,** Brushing hair. Mother in **A, B,** and **C** is being supervised. Note in **D, E,** and **F** that nurse keeps one hand on baby. No gloves required since this is not the first bath. (Courtesy Marjorie Pyle, RNC, Lifecircle, Costa Mesa, Calif.)

Guidelines for Client Teaching—cont'd

RATIONALE/CONTENT	TEACHING ACTIONS
General content: *Developing child care skills increases parents' self-confidence; skill is based on knowledge of the procedure:* Supplies and clothing are made ready.	Arrange work area while explaining process. Comment on equipment and clothing so that mother sees importance of preparing area before child is brought in.
Clothing suitable for wearing indoors: diaper, shirt; stretch suit or nightgown optional.	
Unscented, mild soap.	
Baby lotion, not powder. Baby powder can be inhaled by the infant.	
Pins, if needed for diaper, are placed well out of baby's reach.	Sticking them in a bar of soap lubricates them and keeps them away from the infant.
Cotton balls.	
Towels for drying infant and a clean washcloth.	
Receiving blanket.	
Bring infant to bathing area when all supplies are ready. The infant is never left alone on bath table or in the bath water, not even for a second. If the mother or nurse has to leave, the infant is taken along or put back in the crib.	Model holding and protecting infant with hand (Fig. 17-6). Review major cause of death in small children: drowning.
Test temperature of the water. It should feel pleasantly warm to the inner wrist (about 98 to 99° F).	Demonstrate testing water. Let mother feel.
The infant's head is washed before unwrapping and undressing to prevent heat loss. Cleanse the eyes from the canthus outward, using a **clean** wash-cloth. For the first 2 to 3 days a discharge may result from the reaction of the conjunctiva to the substance (erythromycin) used as a prophylactic measure against infection. Any discharge should be considered abnormal and reported to the physician. When removing eye discharge avoid contamination of one eye with the discharge from the other by using a separate cotton swab and water source (running water from a tap is best) for each eye.	Explain that the infant is washed from head to toe starting with the eyes and ending with the genitals. Demonstrate cleansing the eyes and washing the face (Fig. 17-6, *A* and *B*). Teach general hygiene measure to prevent spread of infection.
The ***scalp*** is washed daily with water and mild soap. It must be rinsed well and dried thoroughly. Scalp desquamation, called ***cradle cap,*** can often be prevented by removing any scales with a fine-toothed comb or brush after washing. If condition persists, the physician may prescribe an ointment to massage into the skin.	Demonstrate washing and drying head. Use football hold (Fig. 17-6, C). Teach mother now (or later) to use football hold.
Creases under the chin and arms and in the groin may need daily cleansing. The crease under the chin may be exposed by elevating the infant's shoulders 5 cm (2 in) and letting the head drop back.	Demonstrate washing creases. Teach potential of warmth, moisture, and unwashed areas for providing an excellent condition for skin break down and infection.
Cleanse ***ears*** and ***nose*** with twists made of moistened cotton.	Demonstrate cleansing of ears and nose. Review reason for the saying, "Do not put anything smaller than your elbow into your ear."
Undress baby and wash body and arms and legs. Pat dry gently. Baby may be tub bathed after the cord drops off.	Demonstrate sponge bath of infant. Rinse well. Pat dry (Fig. 17-6, *C* to *E*).
Care of the cord: Use a cotton swab. Dip swab in solution the physician has ordered and cleanse around base of the cord, where it joins the skin. Notify your physician of any odor, discharge, or skin inflammation around the cord. The clamp is removed when the cord is dry (about 24 to 48 hours) (Fig. 17-7). When you diaper the infant, the diaper should not cover the cord. A wet or soiled diaper will slow or prevent drying of the cord and foster infection. When the cord drops off in a week to 10 days, small drops of blood can be seen when the baby cries. This will heal itself. It is not dangerous.	Demonstrate care of cord. Ask mother what she would report. Ask mother what she has heard about the cord and cord care.

Continued.

Guidelines for Client Teaching—cont'd

RATIONALE/CONTENT	TEACHING ACTIONS
Care of hands and feet: Wash and dry between the fingers and toes daily. Fingernails and toenails are not cut immediately after birth. The nails have to grow out far enough from the skin so that the skin is not cut by mistake. Before the nails can be cut, if the baby scatches himself, you can apply loosely fitted mitts over each hand. Do so as a last resort, however, since it interferes with the baby's ability to console himself. When the nails have grown, the ***fingernails*** and ***toenails*** can be cut more readily with manicure scissors (preferably with rounded tips) when the infant is asleep. Nails are kept short.	Check between fingers and toes. Show picture of mitts. Review safety measures.
Cleansing genitals: Cleanse the ***genitals*** of infants daily and after voiding and defecating. For girls, cleansing of the genitals may be done by separating the labia and gently washing from the pubic area to the anus. For uncircumcised boys, gently pull back (retract) the foreskin. Stop when resistance is felt. Wash the tip (glans) with soap and warm water and replace the foreskin. The foreskin must be returned to its original position to prevent constriction and swelling. In the majority of newborns, the inner layer of the foreskin adheres to the glans. By the age of 3 years, in 90% of boys the foreskin can be retracted easily with pain or trauma. For others, the foreskin is not retractable until the teens. As soon as the foreskin is partly retractable, and the child is old enough, he can be taught self-care.	Demonstrate cleansing of genitals. Review foreskin-purposes, cultural factors, anatomy and physiology—as necessary. Demostrate technique and explain rationale while doing it.
Dressing the infant: When dressing the child, do not pull shirts roughly over the face or catch fingers in shirt sleeves. Bunch up the shirt in both hands and expand the neck opening before placing the neck opening over the face; then slip the shirt over the rest of the head. Diapering the infant may be done before and after feeding. It is not necessary to wake the infant for changing. If cloth diapers are used, absorbency can be increased by bringing the bulk of the diaper in the front for a boy and in the back for a girl. This will help absorb urine so that skin is protected. The diaper between the infant's legs should not be bulky because it can cause outward displacement of the hips. A soaker pad can be placed under the infant as a protection for the blanket. The continued use of plastic or rubber pants may lead to diaper rash.	Demonstrate technique and explain rationale while doing it.
Store infant's towels, wash-cloths, and supplies apart from the family for 2 to 4 months to prevent infection.	Clean and tidy area. Reassure mother you will be with her when she gives the bath tomorrow.

EVALUATION Woman gives return demonstration that shows competence.

Hospital protocol directs the time and technique for routine cord care. The nurse cleanses the cord and skin area around the base of the cord with the prescribed preparation (e.g., erythromycin solution, triple blue dye, or alcohol) and checks daily for signs of infection. The cord clamp is removed after 24 hours (Fig. 17-7).

Positioning and Holding. After feeding, positioning the infant on the right side promotes gastric emptying into the small intestine (Fig. 17-2). Placing the infant in the crib in a side-lying position also permits drainage of mucus from the mouth and applies no pressure to the cord or the sensitive circumcised penis. The infant's position is changed from side to side to help develop even contours of the head and to ease pressure on the other parts of the body.

Anatomically the infant's shape—barrel chest and flat, curveless spine—makes it easy for the child to roll and startle. A folded or rolled blanket against the spine will prevent rolling to the supine position and will promote a feeling of security. Care must be taken to prevent the infant from rolling off of flat, unguarded surfaces. The parent or nurse who must turn away from the infant even for a moment keeps one hand securely on the infant. If left on the parent's bed, the infant is walled in with pillows.

The infant is held securely with support for the head because newborns are unable to maintain an erect head posture for more than a few moments. Fig. 17-8 illustrates various positions for holding an infant with adequate support. Too much stimulation is avoided after feeding and before a sleep period.

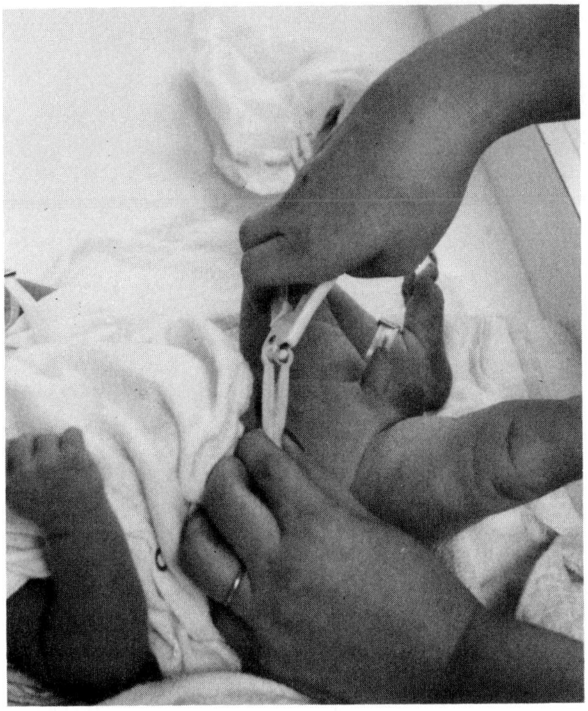

Fig. 17-7 Removal of cord clamp when cord is dry.

Supporting Parents in Care of Their Newborn

Parents' initial contact with their newborn occurs most often in the delivery room. They may hold and initiate breastfeeding while the infant is wide awake during the first period of reactivity (see pp. 441 and 933). The nurse may alert the parents to the newborn infant's mouthing and sucking movements and the responses of the newborn to the sound of their voices and to the visual stimuli of their faces.

After the initial physical examination, administration of the eye prophylaxis and vitamin K, and stabilization of the temperature and initial bath, the newborn infant may be taken to the parents in the bassinet to begin rooming-in. The father is often present in the nursery for the initial nursing care of his newborn. During that time, the nurse can demonstrate the physical and reflex capabilities of the newborn and provide explanations for the medications and care provided.

Each time the newborn is taken into the mother's room, the identification bands on the infant and the mother are matched to be certain the right newborn is taken to the right mother. During the initial acquaintance, the parents should be encouraged to unwrap the newborn infant and inspect it thoroughly.

The parents should be taught how and when to use the bulb syringe (see p. 491) and how to call for the nurse if assistance is needed with the newborn. When the newborn exhibits signs of readiness to begin breastfeeding or bottle feeding, the nurse should provide information and assistance in acquiring these skills. Encouragement and positive reinforcement for parental efforts in caregiving should be liberally bestowed.

Wet diapers provide the impetus for further teaching in how to change the diaper, care of the skin of the newborn, and protecting the umbilical cord from moisture by keeping it outside the diaper. The nurse should look on each wet diaper and feeding episode as an opportunity to provide teaching and encouragement for the new parents.

Swaddling the infant, taking and maintaining the temperature, cleaning the umbilical cord, and bathing and dressing the infant are other skills the nurse may teach the parents. The parents should be made aware of signs of illness in the newborn and what to do if illness occurs. Parents should be provided with the telephone numbers of the pediatrician, the newborn nursery, the Breast Feeding Mothers' Council, the La Leche League, or similar support groups.

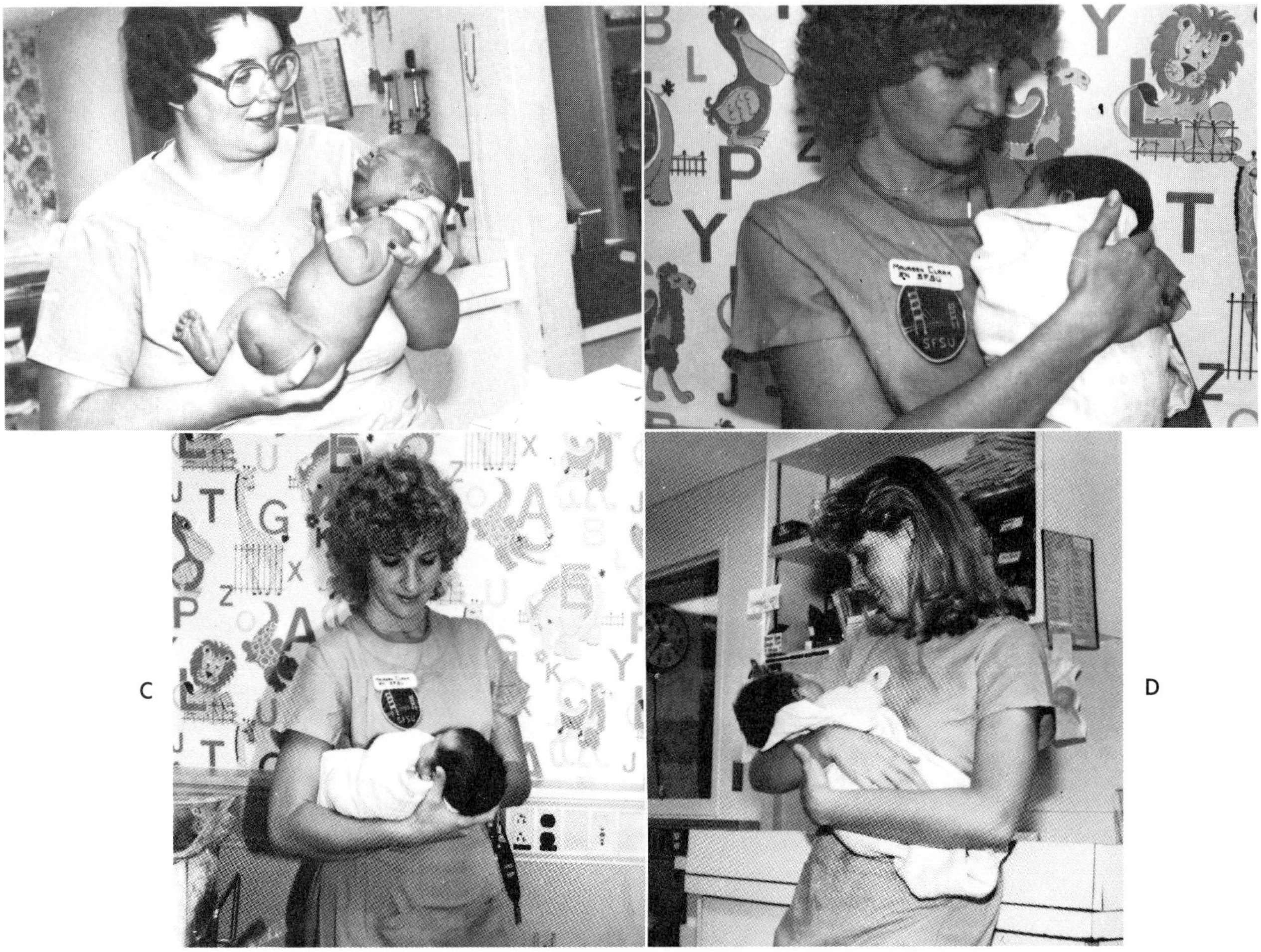

Fig. 17-8 Holding baby securely with support for head. **A,** Holding infant while moving infant from one place to another. Baby (whose temperature is well stabilized in a warm nursery) is undressed to show posture. Note lack of curvature in normal infant's spine and flexion of extremities. **B,** Holding baby upright in "burping" position. **C,** "Football" hold. **D,** Cradling hold.

In many maternity settings, liberal policies permit the parents to have the newborn infant in the room as much or as little as they desire. Anderson (1986) recommended that parents and infants have continuous rooming-in rather than the common practice of separating the newborn from the parents for 3 to 6 hours, having rooming-in during the day and returning the newborn to the nursery at night. Anderson found that newborn infants with continuous rooming-in cried less and mothers slept better with no pain or sleep medication. Mothers were also able to respond promptly to the newborn infants' cues.

Sibling visitation is common in maternity settings. The nurse can assist parents in integrating the newborn into the family by offering suggestions to minimize sibling rivalry.

With the shortened hospital stays so common today, every opportunity must be taken to provide the support and teaching for parents to help them in assuming their parental roles.

Infant's Social Needs

The sensitivity of the caregiver to the social responses of the infant is basic to the development of a mutually satisfying parent-child relationship (Chapters 18 and 20). Sensitivity increases over time as parents' awareness of their infant's social capabilities becomes more acute.

Parental Awareness. The "Mother's assessment of the behavior of her infant" (MABI) assesses how mothers perceive their infants (Field et al, 1978). It was found that mothers perceived their infants in much the same way as the professional examiners did. For example, the mothers noted the postmature infants were not as adaptable or in tune rhythmically with parents.

There was one notable exception: mothers were not as aware of the social capabilities of their infants as were the examiners.

One way nurses can promote parental sensitivity is to share with the parents the process of the Brazelton neonatal behavioral assessment (see p. 453). Examples of comments of parents involved in such teaching about their infants include the following (Edelstein, 1975):

- "After the examination I seemed to notice the various things that were pointed out. Also, I myself tested the baby once we were home. Through the testing I realize more so now that the baby is quite aware of what goes on around him, and since, I've noticed I talk to the baby more now."

  "I was assured that my baby was normal and healthy. Also, it was fascinating to discover all the things he was already aware of. I learned more about him (and babies in general) from participating in the test."

Social Interactions. The activities of daily care during the neonatal period offer the best times for infant and family interaction. While caring for their baby, mother and father can talk to the infant, play baby games, and caress and cuddle the child. In Fig. 17-9, mother, father, and infant engage in arousal, imitation of facial expression, and smiling. Older children's contact with a newborn needs to be supervised for strength of hugs, exploring of eyes and nose, and attempts to feed the baby. Parents often keep baby books that record their infant's progress.

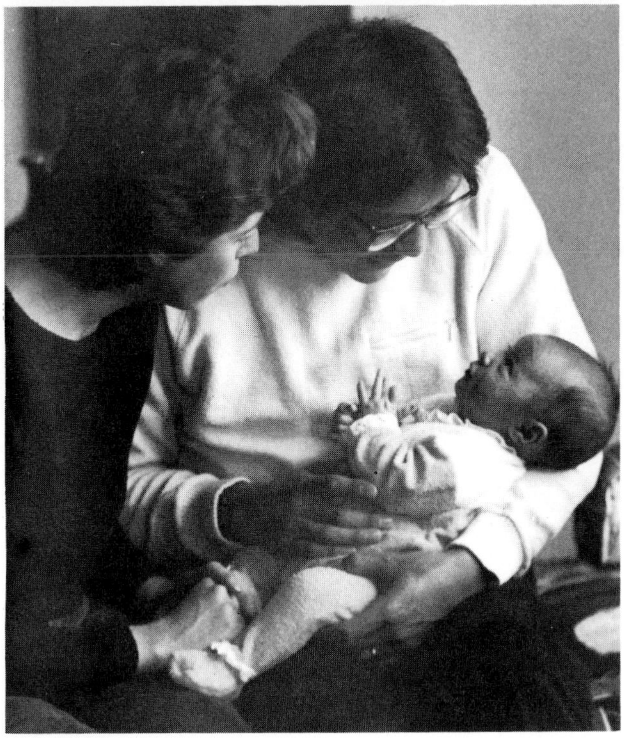

Fig. 17-9 Mother-father-baby interaction. (Courtesy Colleen Stainton.)

THERAPEUTIC INTERVENTIONS IN THE NEWBORN NURSERY

Certain techniques, such as administering vitamin K intramuscularly, are routine in newborn nurseries. Others, such as collection of specimens and the therapy for treatment of hyperbilirubinemia and circumcision, are performed frequently. Infants may need to be restrained during some of these procedures. Nurses must become skilled in the use of therapies to ensure infant safety and therapeutic effectiveness. Parents expect to be told the reasons for the particular therapy and what results to expect.

Intramuscular Injection

Selection of the site for intramuscular injection is important. Injections must be placed in muscles large enough to accommodate the medication, yet major nerves and blood vessels must be avoided. The muscles of newborns may not tolerate more than 0.5 ml. The preferred site for newborns is the vastus lateralis (Fig. 17-10, *A*), although the rectus femoris muscle can also be used. These two muscles, except for the femoral artery on the medial aspect of the thigh, are free of important nerves and blood vessels. The vastus lateralis muscle is the larger of the two and is well developed in the newborn.

The posterior gluteal muscle is very small, poorly developed, and dangerously close to the sciatic nerve, which occupies a larger proportion of space in infants than in older children. Therefore it is not recommended as an injection site until the child has been walking for at least 1 year.

Newborn infants offer little, if any resistance to injections. Although they squirm and may be difficult to hold in position if they are awake, they can usually be restrained without assistance from a second person if the nurse is skilled (Fig. 17-10, *B*). Gloves should be worn when administering injections. The most common injection given in the neonatal period is vitamin K.

Vitamin K. It is recommended that every newborn infant receive a single parenteral dose of 0.5 to 1 mg of vitamin K (AquaMEPHYTON) soon after birth to prevent hemorrhagic disorders. Vitamin K is produced in the gastrointestinal tract starting soon after microorganisms are introduced. By day 8, normal newborns can produce their own Vitamin K.

A
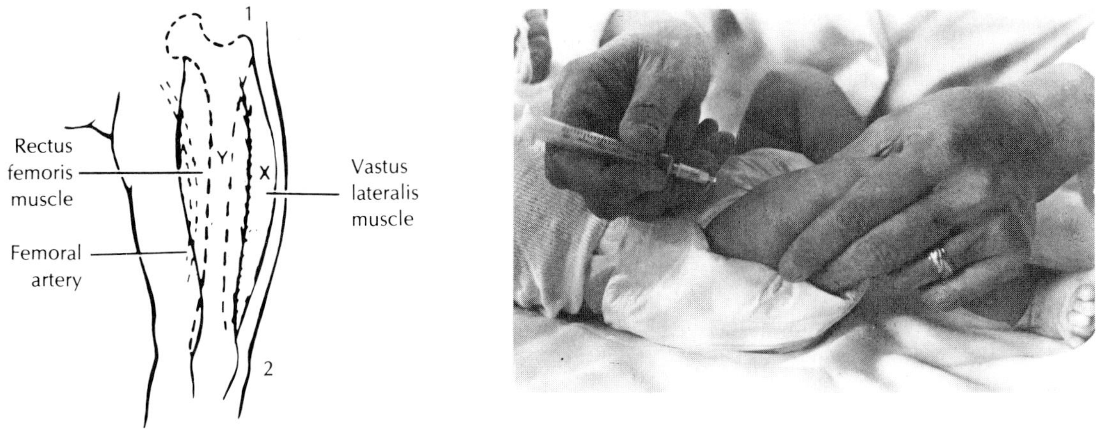

B

Fig. 17-10 **A,** Acceptable intramuscular injection sites for children, X, preferred injection site; Y, alternate injection site. **B,** Infant's leg stabilized for intramuscular injection. Nurse should wear gloves when giving an injection. (From Whaley LF and Wong DL: Nursing care of infants and children, ed 4, St Louis, 1991, The CV Mosby Co.)

A
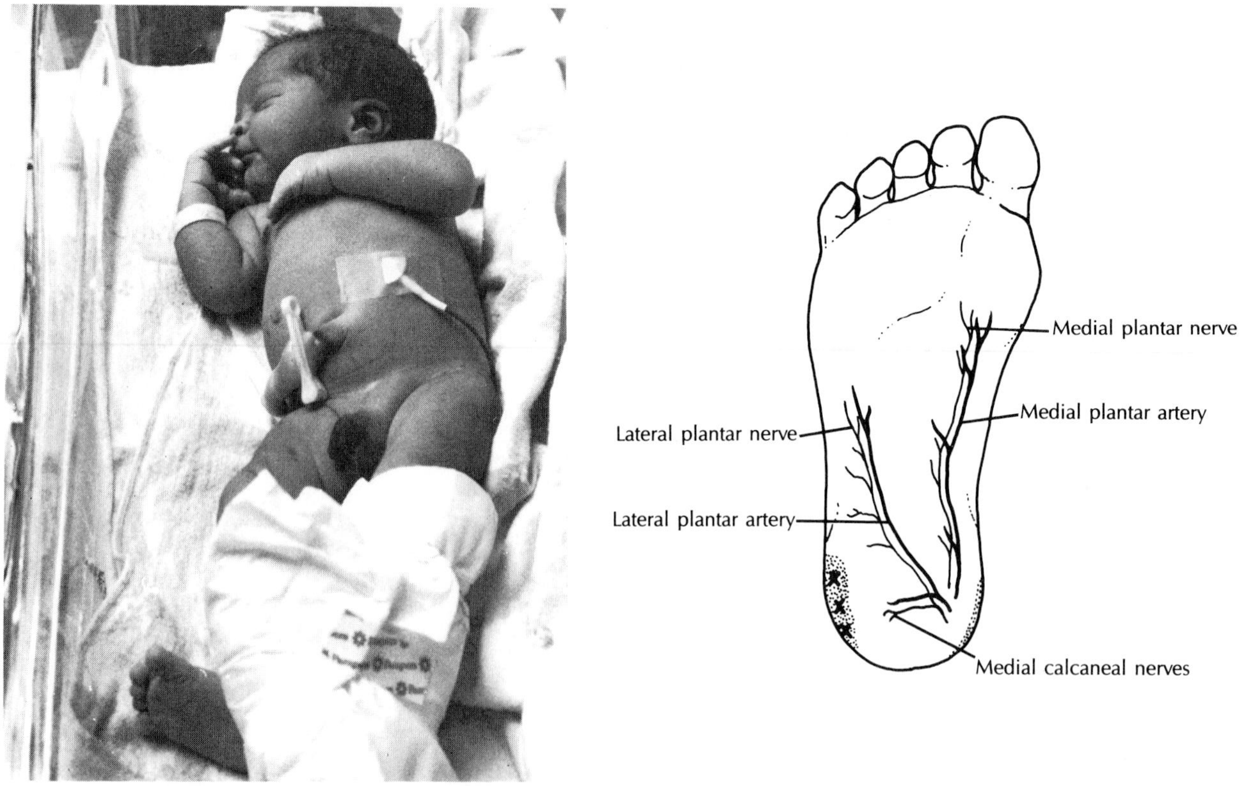

B

Fig. 17-11 **A,** Newborn with foot wrapped for warmth to increase blood flow to extremity before heel stick. **B,** Puncture sites (x) on infant's foot for heel stick samples of capillary blood.

Collection of Specimens

Ongoing evaluation of a newborn requires obtaining blood and urine specimens. The following procedures are used for collecting those specimens: heel stick, assisting with venipuncture, and collection of urine specimen.

Heel Stick. Capillary blood is used for determination of blood glucose level, hematocrit, and to test for phenylketonuria, galactosemia, and hypothyroidism. The nurse commonly draws blood for these tests.

To increase blood flow to the heel, the foot selected for the heel stick is wrapped in a warm wet cloth for approximately 5 minutes (Fig 17-11, *A*). Elevating the head of the bed allows gravity to increase the circulation to the extremity.

The proper site on the heel is selected (Fig. 17-11, *B*). Gloves are worn for the procedure. The heel is cleansed with 70% alcohol and dried with a sterile cotton pledget or gauze square. A Bard-Parker No. 11 blade or a lancet is used to puncture the heel deep enough to obtain free flow of blood. The first drop is discarded and the appropriate capillary tubes are then used to collect the blood. When collection is completed, the site of the puncture is wiped clean with a sterile pledget and covered with a plastic bandage. The infant is rewrapped and picked up and comforted as necessary.

Venipuncture. At times venous blood may be required for laboratory analysis. The nurse assists in collection of venous blood. For external jugular venipuncture, the infant is "mummied" (see p. 513) as necessary (Fig. 17-12, *A*). The infant's head is lowered by placing it over a rolled towel or the edge of a table and stabilized. (Fig. 17-12, *E*). For femoral venipuncture, the infant is positioned in frog posture. The nurse's hands are placed over the infant's knees, avoiding pressure of fingers over the inner aspect of the thigh. When the procedure is completed, firm pressure is applied over the area with sterile gauze for 1 to 3 minutes. The infant is rewrapped and comforted as necessary when the procedure is completed.

After either procedure, site of puncture, amount of blood taken, reason for the specimen, and infant's response are recorded. The specimen is sent to the laboratory for analysis.

Urine Specimens. A variety of urine collection bags are available to collect urine from an infant. The collection device is secured in place over the external genitals with the adhesive backing on the bag. To place the bag, the nurse should separate the infant's legs. The nurse should make sure the pubic and perineal area is clean, dry, and free of mucus. The nurse should not apply powders, oils, or lotion to the skin. The protective paper is removed from the bag, exposing the hypoallergenic adhesive (Fig. 17-13, *A*).

For girls, the perineum is stretched to flatten the skin folds. The adhesive is pressed firmly to the skin all around the urinary meatus and vagina. The nurse should be sure to start at the bridge of skin separating the rectum from the vagina and work upward (Fig. 17-13, *B*).

For boys, the penis and scrotum are tucked through the aperture of the collector before removing the protective paper from the adhesive. The bag is fitted over the penis and the flaps are pressed firmly to the perineum, making sure the entire adhesive coating is firmly attached to the skin with no puckering of the adhesive (Fig. 17-13, *C*).

To drain, the bag is held and tilted so the urine is away from the tab. The tab is removed and the urine is drained into a clean receptacle (Fig. 17-13, *D*).

A 24-hour collection bag can be applied in the same manner. The collection tube can be shortened or capped (Fig. 17-13, *E*). The drainage is directed into a receptacle.

The specimen is sent to the laboratory with a completed laboratory slip. The time and reason for collection of the specimen are recorded.

Therapy for Hyperbilirubinemia

The term infant may have trouble conjugating the increased amount of **bilirubin** derived from disintegrating fetal red blood cells; the serum levels of unconjugated bilirubin rise beyond the limits of normal 12 mg/dl. The goal of **hyperbilirubinemia** treatment is to help the newborn's body reduce serum levels of unconjugated bilirubin. If untreated the levels can continue to rise and the risk of kernicterus increases (Chapter 28).

There are two principal methods for reducing serum bilirubin levels: exchange blood transfusion and **phototherapy.** Exchange transfusion is used to treat infants whose levels of bilirubin cannot be controlled by phototherapy (Chapter 28).

Phototherapy. Research (Speck, 1985) indicates that phototherapy causes a structural isomerization of bilirubin in the skin. During phototherapy infants form lumirubin, a water-soluble product. Lumirubin is formed slowly and excreted rapidly. Lumirubin is excreted both in the urine and feces. Since lumirubin is excreted efficiently by infants, increasing the formation of lumirubin improves the efficacy of phototherapy in the treatment of neonatal jaundice.

The effectiveness of phototherapy is increased by increasing the intensity of the light. An alternative method is to use *green* fluorescent light in place of *blue or white* light. Green fluorescent light does not appear to produce undesirable side effects (Speck, 1985). *Bronze baby syndrome* has occurred in some newborns receiving phototherapy. The serum, urine, and skin

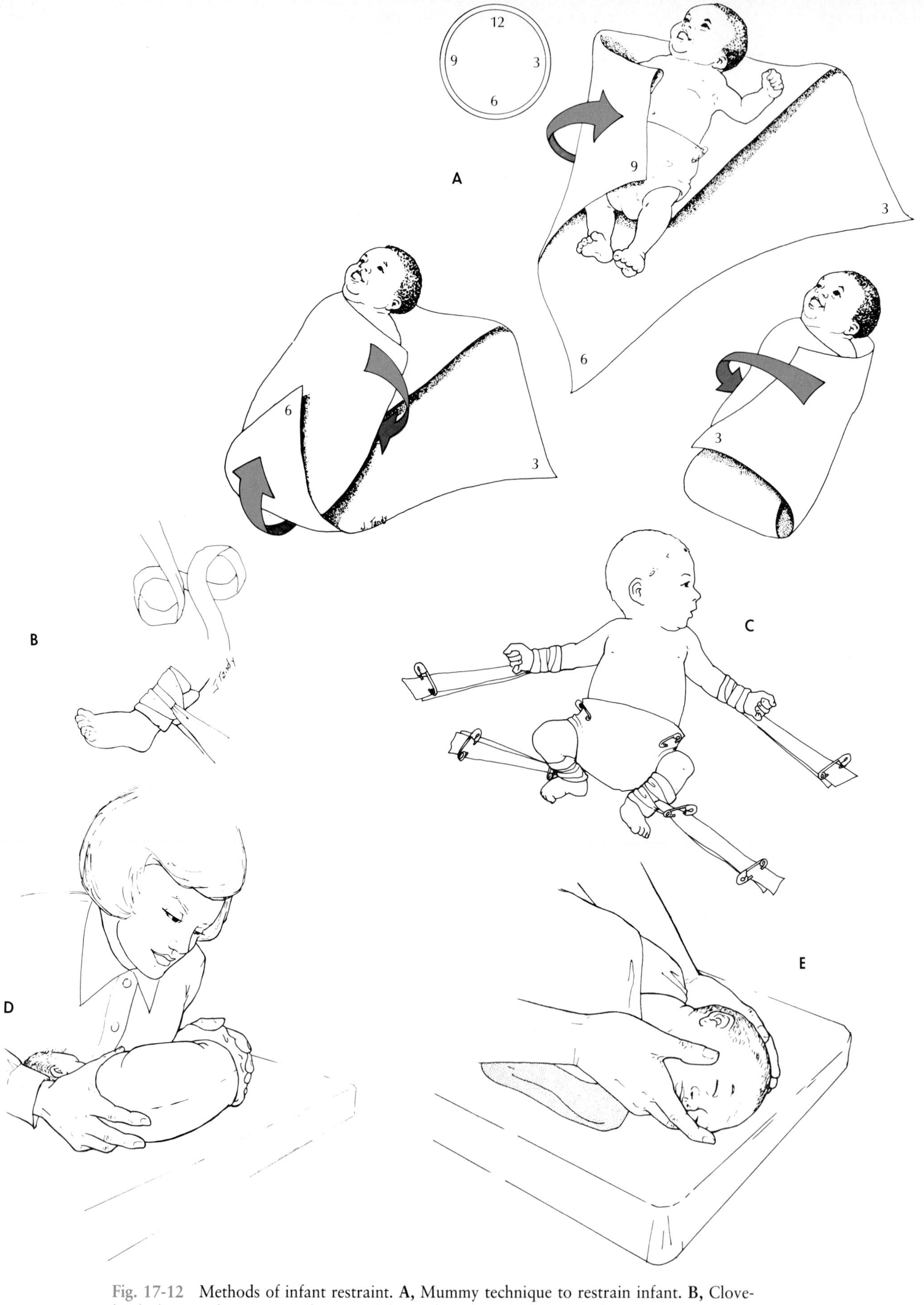

Fig. 17-12 Methods of infant restraint. **A,** Mummy technique to restrain infant. **B,** Clovehitch device. This restraint does not tighten after its application. Apply padding before applying device. **C,** Clovehitch restraints in place. **D,** Position for lumbar puncture. **E,** Position for external jugular venipuncture.

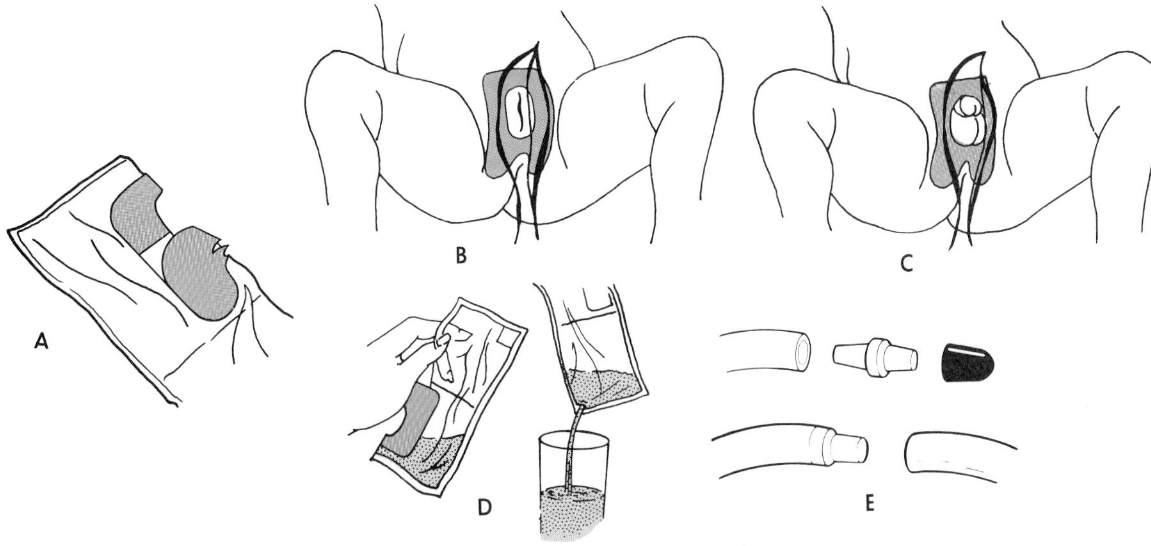

Fig. 17-13 Hollister U-Bag. (Courtesy Hollister, Inc., Chicago.)

turn bronze (brown-black). The cause is unclear. Almost all newborns recover from bronze baby syndrome without sequelae.

The infant is undressed and the infant's eyes are protected with eye patches (Fig. 17-14). To prevent corneal abrasions, the eyes should be closed before placing the eye patches. The eyes are checked for drainage at least once per shift. The infant is removed from the light for feeding. Removal of the eye patch and eye contact are encouraged during feedings.

A paper face mask with the metal strip removed or a disposable diaper may be used to allow optimum skin exposure and protect the genitals and bedding. Loose stools are not uncommon during phototherapy. Infants must have adequate fluid intake during treatment.

After placing the baby under the light, the skin temperature is monitored. If the infant is in an incubator, the temperature dial on the control panel may need to be adjusted to maintain proper temperature.

The time therapy began, the times the infant is removed for care, and the time when the therapy is discontinued are recorded. The infant's response (i.e., stools, temperature, intake) is noted.

Parent Education. Serum levels of bilirubin in the newborn continue to rise until the fifth day of life. Most parents leave the hospital by the second or third day and some as early as 2 hours after delivery. Therefore parents must be able to assess the degree of jaundice the newborn exhibits. They should have written instructions as to whom they should report the infant's condition. Some hospitals have a nurse make a home visit to evaluate the infant's responses. The guidelines for client teaching (p. 510) provide a teaching tool to acquaint parents with the problem of hyperbilirubinemia and its treatment.

A

B

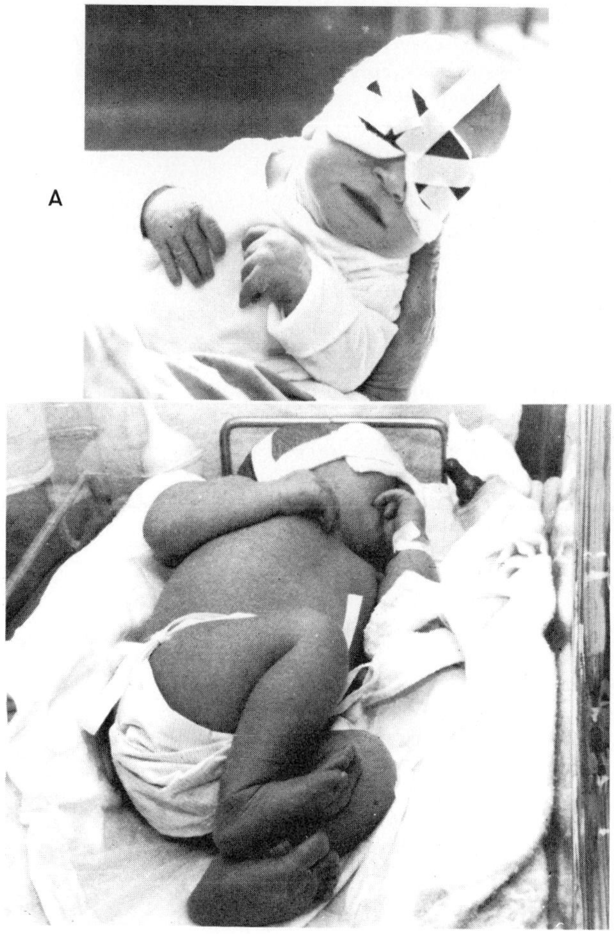

Fig. 17-14 **A,** Placement of eye patches for protection of eyes when infant is receiving phototherapy. Infant is undressed before being put under light. **B,** Under Bililite newborn wears surgical face mask in place of a diaper. (Courtesy Olympic Medical Corp, Seattle.)

Guidelines for Client Teaching
HYPERBILIRUBINEMIA

ASSESSMENT
1. Infant, female term newborn, 8 lb 4 oz, 3 days old.
2. Infant bilirubin level is 13.5 mg/dl.
3. Infant breastfeeding.
4. Physician's orders: serial total bilirubin levels; phototherapy.
5. Parents unaware of causes of jaundice and what phototherapy is.

NURSING DIAGNOSIS
Knowledge deficit (parental) related to hyperbilirubinemia and phototherapy.

GOALS
Short-term

Parents will be able to verbalize what hyperbilirubinemia is and why phototherapy is ordered.

Intermediate

Parents will be able to evaluate their newborn at home for hyperbilirubinemia as evidenced by their description of the process and whom to call with concerns.

Parents' anxiety will be reduced as evidenced by their statements.

Long-term

Parents will experience increased confidence in their caregiving abilities.

REFERENCES AND TEACHING AIDS
Charts, phototherapy equipment, eye mask, paper diaper (or face mask with wire support removed), and printed pamphlets provided by hospital or formula companies for parents to take home and refer to later.

RATIONALE/CONTENT	TEACHING ACTIONS
Knowledge reduces anxiety, therefore review meaning of terms parents will hear: ***Hyperbilirubinemia:*** higher levels of bilirubin than normal. ***Bilirubin:*** end product of red blood cells when they mature and break down. ***Jaundice:*** yellow color of whites of eyes, skin, and mucous membranes caused by circulating bilirubin. ***Phototherapy:*** the use of fluorescent light to break down bilirubin in the skin into substances that can be excreted in the feces (stool) or urine.	Seat parents in a quiet place, where they can see charts and talk easily to the nurse. Have chart made with terms spelled out. If possible, have parents hold their wrapped infant for this part of the class.
Knowledge increases the parents' self-confidence, therefore review process of excreting bilirubin: When red blood cells (RBCs) break down they release bilirubin. Bilirubin circulates in the blood. In the liver it is combined with another substance. In the combined form it goes by way of the blood to the kidneys and the intestines. It gives the yellow color to urine and the brown color to the stool.	Point to chart depicting process as you explain. Ask for questions. Remind parents this is a process difficult for nurses and physicians to learn, so therefore many questions and repeated explanations are expected.
Before the baby was born, her RBCs were more numerous than ours. They also had a shorter life span, 70 to 90 days instead of 120 days. When the RBCs broke down, the baby's blood carried most of the bilirubin by way of the placenta to the mother's liver to be excreted.	Show picture of baby in utero. Trace route of blood from baby to mother's liver.
After the baby was born, her liver began to take care of all the bilirubin. Even though the baby's liver functions well, it cannot handle the whole load. Bilirubin seeps out of the blood and into the tissues, coloring them yellow. The blood level of bilirubin rises quickly up to the fifth day, and then goes down; the jaundice usually clears up by the end of the week.	Point out yellowness of baby's skin. Show chart with approximate amounts of bilirubin and location. Prepare graph illustrating rise and fall of bilirubin over the first week of life.
If the baby is breastfeeding, a certain amount of the jaundice may be caused by the free fatty acids that interfere with the conjugation of bilirubin.	Show chart with contents of breast milk and point out the level of free fatty acids. Refer back to chart depicting process of conjugation.

Guidelines for Client Teaching—cont'd

RATIONALE/CONTENT	TEACHING ACTIONS
Some babies seem to have extra bilirubin to excrete. The amount in the tissues becomes too great when the blood level reaches 12 mg/dl. There is a danger that the bilirubin at high levels will cause damage to the brain. So your doctor wants the baby to be placed under the Bililight for phototherapy. This will help the baby eliminate the extra bilirubin and prevent damage to the baby's brain.	Show Bililight equipment. Let parents feel warmth of the light.
We put eye masks on the baby to keep the light from her eyes.	Demonstrate use of eye mask. Bring infant and place in crib away from Bililight. Apply the eye mask.
We keep the baby undressed so as much light as possible can reach her skin.	Undress baby. Place under Bililight.
We use a paper diaper or the face mask as a small diaper (a "string bikini").	Diaper the infant.
We will take her temperature often so she will not become too hot or too cold.	Take and record temperature. Settle baby comfortably.
We will give her extra water to drink because she will have watery, green stools from the extra bilirubin being excreted.	Return to seats and review care. Distribute pamphlets.
We will be taking her out of the Bililight for feedings and cuddling. We will let you know when to come for feedings and to hold her.	
We will be taking blood tests to check the amount of bilirubin and we will let you know the results.	
Reassure parents that they can have questions answered after discharge.	Leave parents with infant. Tell them they can touch her, but not shield her skin from the light.
If you have any questions, ask us any time. We will give you our phone number and you can call at any hour. It is hard not being able to take her home with you.	Demonstrate stroking baby's hand. Return in about 10 minutes to see if there are any questions. Arrange feeding schedule with mother. Mother can continue to breastfeed or bring breast milk for feedings she will miss.

EVALUATION Parent(s) verbalizes understanding of what has been taught and asks appropriate questions.

Circumcision

Circumcision has been a rite in many cultures for centuries. It continues to be a ritual in religion, for example, the Jewish faith. Circumcision became a common practice in the United States in the early 1870s. About 25% of the world's population circumcise their males sometime between birth and young adulthood.

Recent studies (Witchell, 1985; Cunningham, MacDonald, and Gant, 1989) do not support a connection between circumcision and penile or prostatic cancer and cervical cancer in the female partner. No evidence supports the claim that circumcision decreases the risk to the male for sexually transmitted diseases. Claims that circumcision facilitates hygiene can be refuted by teaching the young child daily cleansing of the penis.

Complications can occur with newborn circumcision. Possible difficulties include urethral fistulas and excessive removal of penile skin. Corrective measures have to be undertaken. They include grafting and the careful use of topical hemostatic agents (Gearhart and Callan, 1986).

Circumcision is an *elective* surgical procedure and as such is a matter of personal choice. The parents' decision to have their newborn circumcised is usually based on one or more of the following factors: hygiene, religious conviction, tradition, culture, or social norms. Some people do not like to touch their infant's genitals. For these parents, circumcision may be the wisest choice.

Regardless of the reason for the decision, it should

be made only after parents have the available facts and sufficient time to review their options. The American Academy of Pediatrics (1975) reaffirmed its position that no medical indications for circumcision of the newborn are valid and that a program of good personal hygiene offers all the advantages of circumcision without the attendant surgical risks. **Phimosis**, tightness of the prepuce, a rare condition, is the only anatomic indication for circumcision. An infant born with hypospadias or epispadias should not be circumcised (Chapter 28). The academy recommended that physicians provide parents with information about the risks of circumcision as well as options regarding this surgical procedure well in advance of delivery.

Procedure. In circumcision the **prepuce** (foreskin) of the glans penis is excised to expose the glans. The operation is performed in the hospital before the infant's discharge. The procedure is no longer done immediately after birth because the cold stress that occurred during the procedure proved detrimental to the infant. Clotting factors drop somewhat immediately after birth and return to prebirth levels by the end of the first week. Therefore performing the circumcision after the baby is a week old has a firmer physiologic basis. The circumcision of a Jewish male is performed on the eighth day after birth unless the infant is unwell.

For the circumcision procedure the infant is positioned on a plastic restraint form so that his movements are restricted (Fig. 17-15). The penis is cleansed with soap and water. The infant is draped to provide warmth and a sterile field. The sterile equipment is readied for use.

Numerous instruments have been designed for circumcision. The Yellen clamp, for instance, may make this an almost bloodless operation. Once the procedure, which takes only a few minutes, is completed, a small petrolatum gauze dressing may be applied for the first day to prevent a cloth diaper from adhering. If a Plastibell is used, the bell applies constant direct pressure to prevent hemorrhage. It also protects against infection, sticking to the diaper, and pain with urination. The bell is fitted over the glans. The suture is tied around the rim of the bell. Excess prepuce is cut away. The plastic rim remains in place for about a week until it falls off, after healing has taken place. Petrolatum gauze is not needed when the bell is used.

Discomfort. If the infant has undergone this surgery without anesthesia, he is comforted until he is quieted. Then he is returned to his crib. These infants usually are fussy for about 2 to 3 hours and may refuse a feeding.

In the Jewish ritual the newborn is given a few drops of wine to relax him in preparation for the surgery. In an article advocating dorsal block for the circumcision, Kirya and Werthmann (1978) wrote:

> Anyone who circumcises a neonate using any of the available techniques senses the pain and stress that the manipulative stages of this procedure generate. During the procedure when the prepuce is clamped with forceps, the infant cries vigorously, trembles, and tries to wiggle out of the restraint. He may eventually become plethoric (flushed), dusky, and mildly cyanotic because of prolonged crying. Occasionally this results in respiratory pauses or regurgitation of feeding.

Pain may not end when the operation is over because the wound requires as long as a week to heal.

Nursing Care. The nurse observes the infant for bleeding. If bleeding is noted from the circumcision,

A

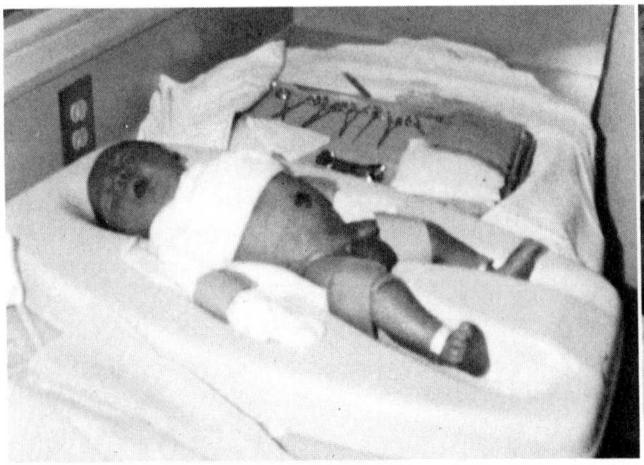

B

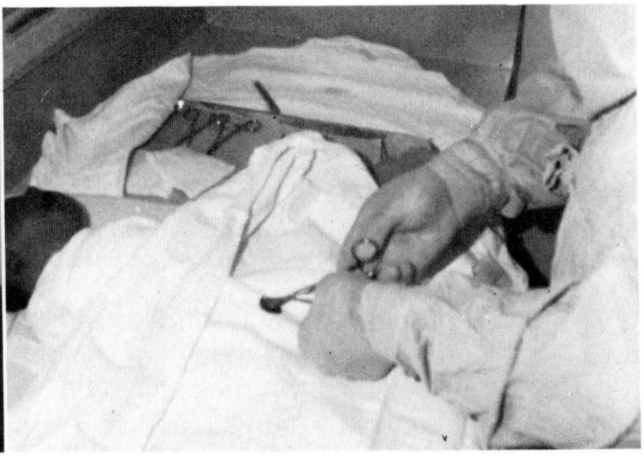

Fig. 17-15 **A,** Proper positioning of infant in Circumstraint. **B,** Physician performing circumcision. Baby is completely covered to prevent cold stress.

the nurse applies gentle pressure to the site of bleeding with a folded sterile gauze pad, 4 in × 4 in. If bleeding is not easily controlled, a blood vessel may need to be ligated. One nurse notifies the physician and prepares equipment (circumcision tray and suture) while the other nurse maintains pressure *intermittently* until the physician arrives. The penis is checked hourly for bleeding for 12 hours; if the parents take the baby home before the end of 12 hours, they have to be taught the actions described previously. Before discharge, the nurse checks to see that the parents have the physician's phone number.

Nursing actions are planned and implemented to prevent infection. The nurse washes the penis gently with water to remove urine and feces and reapplies a fresh (sterile) petrolatum gauze around the glans after each diaper change. The glans penis, normally dark red in appearance during healing, becomes covered with a yellow exudate in 24 hours. This is part of the normal healing process, not an infective process. No attempt is made to remove the exudate, which persists for 2 to 3 days.

Cloth diapers are applied loosely for 2 to 3 days because the incised area at the base of the glans penis remains tender and also because blood absorbed by cloth is easier to see than blood absorbed by a disposable diaper. Cloth diapers are used for about a week or until the glans is completely healed.

Restraining the Infant

Reasons for restraining an infant include protecting the infant from injury, facilitating examinations, and limiting discomfort during tests, procedures, and specimen collections. When restraining an infant, one must keep in mind special considerations:

1. Check the infant frequently.
2. Apply restraints and check them frequently to prevent skin irritation and circulatory impairment.
3. Maintain proper body alignment.
4. Apply restraints without use of knots or pins if possible. If knots are necessary, make the kind that can be released quickly. Use pins with care to prevent puncture wounds and pressure areas—and to prevent the infant's swallowing one of them.
5. The infant in an incubator should be secured to the mattress to protect the extremities, especially when the lid is raised or the mattress moved.

Mummy Technique. The **mummy technique** is used with the stronger, more vigorous newborn. It is used during examinations, treatments, or specimen collections that involve the head and neck.

Equipment includes a blanket and one or two large safety pins (Fig. 17-12, *A*).

The procedure is as follows:

1. Spread blanket on flat surface; crib should suffice.
2. Fold over one corner (12 o'clock position).
3. Lay newborn on blanket so that neck is at fold.
4. Fold corner at 9 o'clock position over right shoulder, tuck this corner securely under infant's left side.
5. Bring corner at 6 o'clock position up over feet and tuck it either under infant's left side or, if long enough, fold it over blanket, crossing it under the infant's chin.
6. Swing corner of 3 o'clock position snugly over infant and fold under infant's right side. Pin this corner into place.

Extremity Restraints. This type of restraint is used to control movements of the infant's arms or legs. It is used during many procedures, such as intubating or gavage feedings. If one extremity is restrained, *all four* extremities must be restrained.

Equipment includes gauze strips or wide strips of soft material and cotton wadding; pins are optional.

The procedure depends on which type of extremity restraints is used. Following are examples:

1. *Pad extremity with cotton wadding.* Fold one end of gauze strip over extremity and pin. Pin other end to mattress.
2. **Clovehitch restraint.** Arrange a long strip of material that is 5 cm (2 in) wide as shown in Fig. 17-12, *B*. Loop device over extremity, which has been padded with cotton; pin loose ends to mattress (Fig. 17-12, *C*). Clovehitch does not tighten even if infant's movements tug on restraint.

Towel Support. Although the towel support is not a true restraint, it controls the infant's position and movement. The towel may be rolled and placed at the infant's back or sides or folded and placed under the neck or upper back. A towel support has the following advantages:

1. It provides comfort and security by stabilizing the infant's position.
2. It maintains positioning to assist respiratory effort and gastrointestinal functions and prevent skin breakdown.
3. It prevents the infant from rolling against the incubator wall, where the child may lose heat by convection.
4. It prevents the infant from falling out of the incubator when the lid is lifted.

The nurse may restrain the infant by using the hands and body. Fig. 17-12, *D*, illustrates restraint of the infant in position for lumbar puncture.

Discharge Planning

For the new parent, child care activities can cause much anxiety. Support from the nursing staff in the mother's beginning efforts can be an important factor in her seeking and accepting help in the future. Whether or not this is the couple's first baby, parents appreciate **anticipatory guidance** in the care of their child. The following topics can be included in discussions with parents. Avoid covering all content at once. The parents can be overwhelmed and become anxious. Follow parental cues to set priorities for teaching. Normal growth and development and the changing needs of the infant (for example, for stimulation, exercise, and social contacts) should be included in discussions with parents, as well as the following topics.

Temperature. Review the following:

1. The causes of elevation in body temperature (such as exercise, cold stress with resultant vasoconstriction, minimum response to infection) and the body's response to extremes in environmental temperature.
2. Symptoms to be reported, such as high or low temperatures with fussiness, stuffy nose, lethargy, irritability, poor feeding, and crying.
3. Ways to reduce body temperature, such as giving a cool tub bath, dressing the infant appropriately for the temperature of the air; protecting the infant from long exposure to sunlight, and using warm wraps in cold weather.

Respirations. Review the following:

1. Normal variations in the rate and rhythm.
2. Reflexes, such as sneezing to clear the air passage.
3. The need to protect the infant from the following:
   a. People with upper respiratory tract infections (an efficient mask can be made by wrapping toilet tissue around the head to cover the mouth and nose if the parent or another has a cold).
   b. Pollution from a smoke-filled environment.
   c. Suffocation from loose bedding, drowning (bath water), entrapment under excessive bedding, anything tied around the infant's neck, poorly constructed playpens, bassinets, or cribs. The pediatrician or pediatric nurse can supply printed directions for making the house safe for an infant.
   d. Aspiration pneumonia: a commonly aspirated substance is baby powder, which is usually a mixture of talc (hydrous magnesium silicate) and other silicates (Whaley and Wong, 1991). Although the use of talc has been discouraged, it is a common baby care product and can cause severe and often fatal aspiration pneumonia. One of the factors involved in talc aspiration is the similar appearance of baby powder containers and nursing bottles. Talc containers often become favorite playthings and are placed in the mouth (Mofenson et al, 1981). Improper use of powder by sprinkling it directly on the skin creates a cloud of talc dust that is easily inhaled. Parents are advised of the danger of baby powder and discouraged from using it. If they prefer to use a powder, a cornstarch preparation can be substituted. Whenever a powder is used, it should be placed in the caregiver's hand and then applied to the skin, never shaken directly from the container to the skin. The container is kept closed and immediately stored in a safe place, especially away from curious toddlers who often imitate caregiving activities and may accidentally shake it on the infant.
4. *Symptoms of the* ***common cold:*** nasal congestion, coughing, sneezing, difficulty in swallowing (sore throat), low-grade fever. Advise the parents on measures to help the infant: for example, feed smaller amounts but feed more frequently to avoid overtiring the infant; hold the baby in an upright position to feed; offer extra sterile water; for sleeping, raise the infant's head and chest by raising the mattress 30 degrees (do not use pillow); avoid drafts; do not overdress the baby; use only medications prescribed by a physician (do not use nose drops, since aspiration may result in lung involvement); cover the upper lip with a light film of petrolatum to minimize excoriation from nasal secretions.

Elimination. Review the following:

1. Changes to be expected in the color of the stool and the number of bowel evacuations, plus the odor of stools for breastfed or bottle-fed infants.
2. The color of normal urine and the number of voidings to expect each day.

Safety. Review the need for the following:

1. Protecting the infant from trauma; for example, keeping objects such as pins and scissors closed and well out of baby's reach. When infant clothes are purchased, the type of closure used should be considered. A front button can easily be pulled off and swallowed. Even though a young infant may not search for buttons or other small objects now, practicing this good habit from the beginning prevents future injuries.
2. Preventing overheating or chilling.
3. Care in transporting infants, particularly in automobiles (Fig. 17-16).
4. Supervising brothers' and sisters' attention to the new baby.

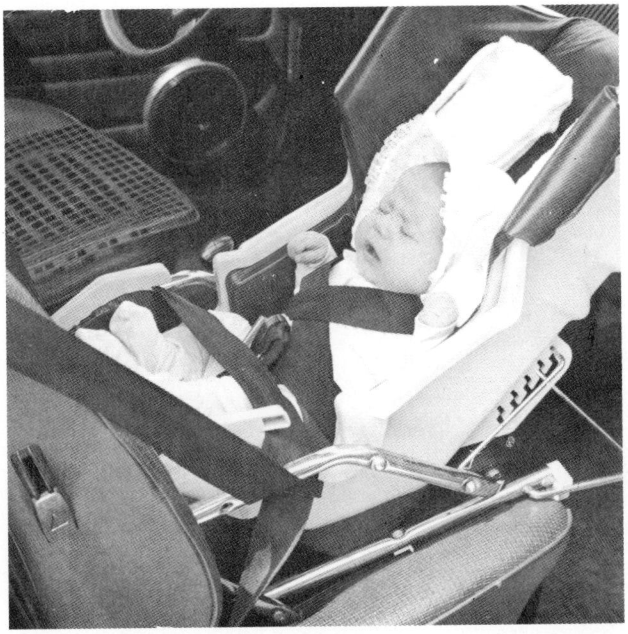

Fig. 17-16 Rearward-facing shell car seat. Infant is placed in car seat when going home from hospital. (From Whaley LF and Wong DL: Nursing care of infants and children, ed 4, St Louis, 1991, The CV Mosby Co.)

Pacifiers/Thumbsucking. Sucking is the infant's chief pleasure. It may not be satisfied by breastfeeding or formula-feeding (Whaley and Wong, 1991). It is such a strong need that infants who are deprived of sucking, such as those with a cleft lip repair, will suck on their tongue. Some newborns are born with sucking pads on their fingers that developed from in utero sucking activity. Several benefits of nonnutritive sucking have been documented, such as increased weight gain in preterm infants and decreased crying (Anderson, 1986).

Problems arise when parents are concerned about sucking of fingers, thumb, or pacifier and attempt to restrain this natural tendency. Before giving advice, nurses investigate the parents' feelings and base guidance on this information. For example, some parents may see no problem with the use of a finger but may find the use of a pacifier repulsive. In general, there is no need to restrain either unless thumb sucking persists past 4 years of age or past the time when the permanent teeth erupt. Parents are advised to work with their pediatrician and pediatric nurse-practitioner about this topic.

To decrease dependence on nonnutritive sucking, sucking pleasure can be increased by prolonging feeding time. A small-holed, firm nipple causes stronger sucking and slower feeding. Also the parent's excessive use of the pacifier to calm the child should be explored. It is not unusual for parents to place a pacifier in the infant's mouth as soon as crying begins, thus reinforcing a pattern of distress-relief (Whaley and Wong, 1991). If the child uses a pacifier, safety considerations in purchasing one must be stressed. A home-made or poorly designed pacifier can be dangerous because the entire object may be aspirated if it is small, or a portion may become detached from the handle and become lodged in the pharynx. Improvised pacifiers, such as those commonly made in hospitals from a padded nipple, also present dangers. The nipple may separate from the plastic collar and be aspirated (Millunchick and McArtor, 1986). In addition, parents may continue to offer this pacifier to the infant at home. Safe pacifiers should be of one-piece construction, have a shield or flange that is large enough to prevent entry into the mouth, and have a handle that can be grasped.

Immunizations. Review schedule for immunizations. The *ability* to protect against antigens by formation of antibodies *develops sequentially* (Chapter 5). The fetus or infant must be developmentally capable of responding to antigens. This is the reason for planning sequential immunizations in infants. A form of passive immunity is present in colostrum and breast milk. It is specific for microbial agents present in the mother's own gastrointestinal tract. As the newborn is being freshly colonized, *these antibodies limit bacterial growth in the gastrointestinal tract and protect against overgrowth.* This information helps health care professionals plan for the use of polio vaccine in breastfed infants. According to Korones (1986):

> Oral polio vaccine depends, for its effectiveness, on multiplication in the intestinal tract. The vaccine fails to immunize babies on breast milk from mothers with high antibody titers to poliovirus because vaccine virus is inactivated in the gut by secretory IgA from breast milk.

Follow-up Care. Plan for infant health follow-up care, that is, at 2 to 4 weeks of age, then every 2 months until 6 to 7 months of age, then every 3 months until 18 months, at 2 years, 3 years, preschool, and every 2 years thereafter.

The newborn's record serves as a documented means of communication among all members of the health-care team. The record contains accurate and complete recordings of the history, physical examination, and laboratory test results, sequential observations, goals, interventions, and the newborn's responses. The record should be readily accessible to the health-care professionals caring for the infant and family. Documentation of the parent's health education, counseling, and responses to information are included. These data provide valuable information for the pediatrician and nurse for the infant's follow-up care and serve as a reservoir for data for future research.

Evaluation

Evaluation is a continuous process. To be effective, it needs to be based on measurable criteria, which reflect the parameters used to measure the goals for care. Parental skill in infant caregiving techniques and their knowledge of their infant's needs and growth patterns form the context in which newborn care is given.

SUMMARY

The care the newborn receives in the first months of life is reflected in the normal growth and development of a healthy infant. The nurse in the various roles as teacher and support person acts as an advocate for the vulnerable infant. The nurse's skills in caring for the newborn and teaching these skills to parents are of paramount importance. Nurses are present during the formative stages of parent-child interactions. From their unique perspective they can do much to help both parents and child.

LEARNING ACTIVITIES

1. Observe or assist in the physical and behavioral assessment of an infant immediately following birth, on admission to the nursery, and during routine assessment.
2. Observe an experienced nurse instruct and explain the behavioral assessment of an infant to the parents.
3. Develop a written plan of care for an infant and her or his parents using a nursing diagnosis as the focus.
4. Practice restraining an infant by several methods.
5. Prepare and teach one class in infant care to parents.
6. Practice the manipulation of various types of equipment found in the newborn nursery.
7. Role play a nurse caring for and educating a mother during a routine assessment of the infant after discharge from the hospital; include proper attention to one of the following problems:
   a. Skin problems show that the infant is not being bathed properly.
   b. Interactions of siblings with the newborn show that they have not accepted the necessity for correct handling and attitudes toward the newborn.
   c. The mother shows a lack of knowledge concerning the newborn's jaundice.
   d. The mother quotes family members regarding proper care of the umbilicus; the infant is wearing a flannel belly band.
8. Practice neonatal CPR and clearing of an airway obstruction in the laboratory setting.

References

American Academy of Pediatrics, Committee on Fetus and Newborn: Report of the Ad Hoc Task Force on Circumcision, Pediatrics 56:610, 1975.
American Academy of Pediatrics: Guidelines for perinatal care, ed 2, p 127, Elk Grove, Ill, 1988.
Anderson G: Pacifiers: the positive side, MCN 11:122, 1986.
Committee on Accidents and Poison Prevention, American Academy Pediatrics: Revised first aid for the choking child, Pediatrics 78:177, 1986.
Cunningham FG, MacDonald PC, and Gant NF: Williams obstetrics, ed 18, Norwalk, Conn, 1989, Appleton & Lange.
Edelstein J: The effect of nursing intervention with the Brazelton Neonatal Behavioral Assessment Scale on postpartum adjustment and maternal perception of the infant, unpublished masters thesis, 1975.
Field T et al: Mothers' assessments of the behavior of their infants, Infant Beh Dev 1:156, 1978.
Gearhart J and Callan N: Complications of newborn circumcision, Contemp OB/GYN 27:57, 1986.
Kirya C and Werthmann M: Neonatal circumcision and penile dorsal nerve block: a painless procedure, J Pediatr 92:998, 1978.
Korones SG: High-risk newborn infants: the basis for intensive nursing care, ed 4, St Louis, 1986, The CV Mosby Co.
Millunchick E and McArtor R: Fatal aspiration of a makeshift pacifier, Pediatrics 77(3):369, 1986.
Mofenson HC et al: Baby powder—a hazard! Pediatrics 68(2):265, 1981.
NAACOG: Neonatal skin care, OGN Nursing Practice Resource 12:3, March, 1985.
NAACOG: CDC reports caution about AIDS virus, NAACOG Newsletter 13(6):June, 1986.
Nursing '87 Books: 1987 Nursing photobook annual, Springhouse, Penn, 1987, Springhouse Corp.
Speck WT: Jaundice and phototherapy: wonder where the yellow went? Paper presented at "The Fetus and the Newborn," Contemporary Forums, San Diego, 1985.
Whaley LF and Wong DL: Nursing care of infants and children, ed 4, St Louis, 1991, The CV Mosby Co.
Witchell M: The circumcision decision and the role of the health provider, ICEA News 24(3):4, 1985.

Bibliography

Anderson CJ: Integration of the Brazelton Neonatal Behavioral Assessment Scale into routine neonatal nursing care, Issues Compr Pediatr Nurs 9:341, 1986.
Anderson GC: Risk in mother-infant separation postbirth, Image J Nurs Sch 21:196, 1989.
Bampton B, Jones J, and Mancini J: Initial mothering patterns of low-income black primiparas, JOGN Nurs 10:174, 1981.
Brown L: Physiologic response to cutaneous pain in neonates, Neonatal Network 6(3):18, 1987.
Brucker MC et al: Neonatal jaundice in the home: assessment with a noninvasive device, JOGN Nurs 16:355, 1987.
Bull M and Lawrence D: Mothers' use of knowledge during the first postpartum weeks, JOGN Nurs 14:315, 1985.
Consullo M et al: An instrument for the measurement of infant-adult synchrony, Nurs Res 36:244, 1987.
Crawford J: A theoretical model of support network conflict experienced by new mothers, Nurs Res 34:100, March/April, 1985.

KEY CONCEPTS

- Assessment of the newborn requires data from the prenatal, intranatal, and postnatal periods.
- Knowledge of the biologic and behavioral characteristics is essential for guiding assessment and interpreting data.
- Providing a protective environment is a key role for the nurse that includes such actions as careful identification procedures, restraining techniques, measures to prevent infection, and support of physiologic functions.
- Maintenance of adequate ventilation includes ensuring an adequate airway and body temperature.
- Each nurse must develop skill in CPR and relieving airway obstruction.
- Parent education is a major role for the nurse and includes involving parents in all phases of the nursing process.
- Circumcision is an elective surgical procedure.
- The newborn has social, as well as physical, needs.
- Whether or not this is the couple's first baby, parents appreciate anticipatory guidance in the care of their child.

Cronenwett LR: Parental network structured and perceived support after birth of first child, Nurs Res 34:347, 1985.

DelGiudice GT: The relationship between sibling jealousy and presence at a sibling's birth, Birth 13(4):250, 1986.

Dodge J: When childbirth is a family affair, RN 48(12):20, 1985.

Fuller RZ: Upper respiratory obstruction in the neonate: a case of neonatal rhinitis, Pediatr Nurs 14(1):30, 1988.

Gibbons MB: Circumcision: the controversy continues, Pediatr Nurs 10(2):103, 1984.

Goodwin BA: Pediatric resuscitation, Crit Care Nurs Q 10(4):69, 1988.

Greer PS: Head coverings for newborns under radiant warmers, JOGN Nurs 17:265, 1988.

Harpin VA and Rutter N: Barrier properties of the newborn infant's skin, J Pediatr 102(3):419, 1983.

Hiser PL: Concerns of multiparas during the second postpartum week, JOGN Nurs 1:195, 1987.

Hutton N and Schreiner R: Urine collection in the neonate: effect of different methods on volume, specific gravity, and glucose, JOGN Nurs 9:165, 1980.

Jaundiced babies bloom with home phototherapy, Clin News 84(7):871, 1984.

Judd JM: Assessing the newborn from head to toe, Nurs '85 15(12):34, 1985.

Kowba MD and Schwirian PM: Direct sibling contact and bacterial colonization in newborns, JOGN Nurs 14:412, Sept/Oct, 1985.

Krozy RE et al: Auto safety, pregnancy and the newborn, JOGN Nurs 14:1, 1985.

Larson E: Trends in neonatal infections, JOGN Nurs 16:404, 1987.

Larson E: Rituals in infection control: what works in the newborn nursery: . . . handwashing and gowning, JOGN Nurs 16:411, 1987.

Leff EW: Comparison of the effectiveness of videotape versus live group infant care classes, JOGN Nurs 17:338, 1988.

Locklin M: Assessing jaundice in full-term newborns, Pediatr Nurs 13(1):15, 1987.

McFadden R: Decreasing the infant's respiratory compromise during suctioning, Am J Nurs 81(12):2148, 1981.

Merrifield EB and Ryberg JW: What parents should know about pacifiers, Child Nurse 3(4):1, 1985.

Moxley S: Neonatal heel puncture, Can Nurse p 25, Jan, 1989.

Orlowski J: Optimum position for external cardiac compression in infants and young children, Ann Emerg Med 15:667, 1986.

Paes B et al: An audit of the effect of two cord-care regimens on bacterial colonization in newborn infants . . . triple dye was more effective than alcohol, QRB 13(3):109, 1987.

Perry D: The umbilical cord: transcultural care and custom, J Nurse Midwife 27(4):25, 1982.

Reid T: Newborn cyanosis, Am J Nurs 82(8):1230, 1982.

Riesch S and Munns S: Promoting awareness: the mother and her baby, Nurs Res 33:271, 1985.

Rutledge DL and Pridham KF: Postpartum mothers' perceptions of competence for infant care, JOGN Nurs 16:185, 1987.

Shibley B: Now newborns can stay home for phototherapy, RN p 69, Feb 1988.

Stang HJ et al: Local anesthesia for neonatal circumcision: effects on distress and cortisol response, JAMA 259(10):1507, 1988.

Strohback ME and Kratina S: Diaper versus bag specimens: a comparison of urine specific gravity values, MCN 7(3):198, 1982.

Tedder JL: Newborn circumcision, JOGN Nurs 16:42, 1987.

Tomlinson PS: Father involvement with first-born infants: interpersonal and situational factors, Pediatr Nurs 13:101, 1987.

Wagner TJ and Hindi-Alexander M: Hazards of baby powder? Pediatr Nurs 10:124, 1984.

Walker LO, Crain H, and Thompson E: Mothering behavior and maternal role attainment during the postpartum period, Nurs Res 35:352, 1986.

CHAPTER

18 Newborn Nutrition and Feeding

Shannon E. Perry and Mary Courtney Moore

Learning Objectives

Correctly define the key terms listed.

Evaluate nutrient needs in relation to infant's growth and development during the first few months of life.

Identify factors that affect parent and newborn readiness for feeding.

Compare nutrition supplements recommended for the breastfed and formula-fed infant.

Review the physiology of lactation in relation to breast development, stages of lactation, and maternal breastfeeding reflexes.

Explore cultural aspects of breastfeeding.

Formulate nursing diagnoses relative to the infant's nutritional status and the parents' needs and preferences.

Examine breastfeeding in relation to advantages, care of breasts, diet and fluids, infant responses, secretion of drugs in milk, maintaining a job, and infant-related and maternal-related concerns.

Discuss formula-feeding in relation to advantages, care of breasts, diet and fluids, infant responses, and formula preparation.

Develop guidelines for client teaching for breastfeeding, formula-feeding, and formula preparation.

Key Terms

breast massage
colostrum
demand feeding
engorgement
extrusion reflex
failure to thrive
feeding reflexes
formula-feeding
formula preparation (terminal heating and aseptic methods)
growth
lactation
lactoferrin
lactogenesis
let-down reflex
manual expression of milk
milk ejection
milk secretion
nipple erection reflex
plugged ducts
prolactin reflex
pumping the breasts
readiness for feeding
rooting reflex
sore nipples
sucking reflex
suckling process
supplemental feedings
swallowing reflex
weaning

Skillful health supervision of infants requires knowledge of their nutritional needs. The adage that "as the twig is bent the tree's inclined" is appropriate when considering nutrition experiences in infancy and possible health consequences in later life. This chapter focuses on nutrition needs for normal growth and development from birth to 3 months. Breastfeeding and bottle-feeding are addressed.

❑ INFANT DEVELOPMENT AND NUTRITION NEEDS

Discussion of the child's **growth** pattern is often the starting point for effective communication with parents regarding proper nutrition for their child.

The full-term infant will generally double the birth weight by the age of 5 months and triple it in 1 year. Most newborn infants experience a 5% to 10% weight loss during the first few days of life. Full-term infants usually regain this weight within 10 days.

Length increases about 50% during the first year. Doubling of birth length does not occur until about 4 years of age. Head circumference also increases rapidly during the first year in conjunction with rapid growth of the brain.

At birth the term infant has a body composed of about 16% fat (by weight). Between 2 and 6 months of age, the increase in adipose tissue is more than twice as great as the increase in muscle mass; fat deposition occurs at a steady pace until about 9 months of age.

Throughout infancy, girls add a greater percentage of weight as fat than boys do; this trend continues throughout the remaining developmental years.

To assist in the clinical evaluation of physical growth of children in the United States, growth "standards," or "norms," have been developed for height or length, body weight, and head circumference.

The rank of an individual child's measurements in relation to American children of the same sex and age can be determined by examining the percentiles of the National Center for Health Statistics (Hamill et al, 1979). Adjustments can be made for children from various segments of the population who might differ based on race, socioeconomic status, and geography. Measurements outside the extreme percentiles may indicate nutritional problems sufficiently severe to affect growth. Measurements within the control or intermediate percentiles indicate that growth is within normal limits by current standards.

Readiness for Feeding

Healthy term neonates are capable of ingesting and digesting selected foods. They also possess the social capabilities necessary to elicit and maintain interest in feeding them.

All the secretions of the infant's digestive tract contain enzymes especially suited to the digestion of human milk. The ability to handle foods other than milk depends on the physiologic development of the infant. The capacities for salivary, gastric, pancreatic, and intestinal digestion increase with age, indicating what may be a natural pattern for introduction of various solid foods (Table 18-1).

At birth, the infant produces little salivary or pancreatic amylase and thus is poorly prepared to digest the complex carbohydrates found in solid foods. Lipase production by the pancreas is lower than in older children or adults. Human milkfat and the vegetable oils used in commercial formulas are fairly well digested, but significant malabsorption of butterfat and other fats occurs. During the first few months of life, rapid maturation occurs so that digestion of the starches found in cereals and vegetables is adequate by about 4 months of age. Therefore introduction of solid foods is practical after this age.

Kidney function of the full-term infant is not completely mature. Well-developed glomeruli filter the blood presented to the kidneys satisfactorily. The tubules, which are functionally less mature, are somewhat limited in their ability to reabsorb water and some solutes. Therefore it is important that the kidneys not be presented with excess solutes (renal solute load) to excrete. For this reason protein beyond that needed for growth and the extra sodium sometimes added to foods as sodium chloride (NaCl, or table salt) should be avoided.

The percentage of body water decreases from 75% at birth to 60% at 1 year of age. This reduction is almost entirely in extracellular water. The ability to re-

Table 18-1 Digestion in Infancy: Birth to 3 Months

Location	Function	Effect on Feeding
Salivary	Amylase not available in significant quantities.	Little digestion of complex carbohydrates (starches).
Gastric	Hydrochloric acid (HCl) and pepsin precipitate casein into curds; separate and acidify whey protein.	Protein digestion begins; lactose ($C_{12}H_{22}O_{11}$) digestion partly begins; fat is not digested in stomach.
Intestinal	Pancreatic and intestinal enzymes digest proteins into amino acids, reduce carbohydrate to monosaccharides, and split fatty acids from triglycerides in the small intestine.	Protein from human milk is 95% digested, and a similar percentage of protein is digested from commercial formulas that are heat treated and sufficiently diluted to produce a soft curd.
	Disaccharidases are present in border of the intestinal mucosa.	Lactose in human milk and lactose or other carbohydrates in commercial formulas are digested in intestinal mucosa.
	Pancreatic amylase is present in small quantities.	Complex carbohydrates are poorly used.
	Pancreatic lipase is present in sufficient quantity.	A total of 80% of human milk fat is digested at birth, and almost 95% is digested by 1 month.
	Lipase, naturally found in human milk, is activated by bile salts.	Digestion of fats from commercial formulas equals that of human milk; fat from other sources (butterfat) is poorly digested.

Modified from Willis NH: Infant nutrition, birth to 3 months: a syllabus, Philadelphia, 1980, JB Lippincott Co.

tain body water through kidney function improves in the early months of life. To the infant this means that risk of dehydration decreases as renal concentrating capacity increases.

The development of feeding behavior depends on the maturation of the central nervous system (CNS). The **rooting, sucking, and swallowing reflexes** are present in the term newborn (Chapter 16). The infant also has an **extrusion reflex** that automatically pushes food out of the mouth when it is placed on the tongue. Between 3 and 6 months of age the extrusion reflex becomes less pronounced.

Early emotional, psychologic, and social attachment of the parent to the infant may influence future aspects of the infant's personality. Feeding is the main means by which the newborn establishes a human relationship with the parent. Development of trust is built on the close relationship between parent and infant. If the infant's needs are satisfied through food and love, a sense of trust is developed between the child and the parent. Food becomes the infant's means of bringing her or his parent and her or his world together. The newborn communicates by vigorous and sustained crying to express hunger, thirst, pain, and discomfort.

Feeding practices from birth, whether by breast or formula, influence the infant's exposure to tactile stimulation. Tactile stimulation is essential to the infant's physical and emotional growth.

Energy Needs (Calories)

The energy requirements of the infant may be considered in three areas: (1) the basal energy requirement that sustains organ metabolic function, (2) the energy needed for physical activity, and (3) the energy needed for growth. During the first 4 months of life, 50% of the infant's energy is expended for basal metabolism, 25% for physical activity and other maintenance functions, and 25% for growth.

The recommended daily dietary allowance (RDA) for energy for the first year is approximately 115 kcal/kg (52 kcal/lb) for the first 6 months and 105 kcal/kg (47 kcal/lb) for the second half of the year (Food and Nutrition Board, 1980). Both human milk and infant formulas supply approximately 67 kcal/dl (20 kcal/oz); thus 720 ml (24 oz) of human milk or formula will supply about 480 kcal.

Fluid Needs

The fluid requirement for normal infants is about 105 ml (3.5 oz)/kg/24 hours. This is usually consumed from the breast or in properly prepared formulas. Infants receiving this amount of water have approximately 100 ml/24 hours available for secretion of urine.

Water intoxication resulting in hyponatremia, weakness, restlessness, nausea, vomiting, diarrhea, polyuria or oliguria, and convulsions can result from excessive feeding of water to infants (David et al, 1981). This also may occur when water is fed as a replacement for milk (Partridge et al, 1981). Diarrhea may also result from excessive fluid intake (Greene and Ghishan, 1983).

Nutrient Needs

Human milk is especially appropriate for meeting almost all of the infant's nutritional needs for the first few months of life. Commercial formulas, most of which are based on skimmed cow's milk, are modified to resemble human milk. Almost all of the nutrients needed for the first 4 to 6 months can be supplied by feedings of human milk or formula.

The protein requirement is greater per unit of body weight in the newborn than at any other time of life. The RDA for protein during the first 6 months is 2.2 g/kg.

The *protein* content of human milk, lower than that of unmodified cow's milk, is sufficient for the newborn. Human milk contains far more lactalbumin in relation to casein, which reduces the amount of potential curd formation in the gut of the infant. Thus human milk is especially digestible. The *amino acid* composition of human milk is ideally suited to the newborn infant's metabolic capabilities. For example, phenylalanine and methionine levels are low and cystine and taurine levels are high. These amino acid patterns are uniquely appropriate for the infant, because the newborn's enzyme systems for metabolism of phenylalanine are immature and therefore function at a diminished rate, when compared with the adult. Furthermore, the infant has a need for cystine and taurine, which are considered nonessential for adults.

For infants to acquire adequate calories from the limited amount of milk or formula they are able to consume, at least 15% of the calories provided must come from fat. The fat must be easily digestible. Fecal loss of fat and therefore of energy may be excessive if whole or evaporated milk without added carbohydrate is fed to infants.

Fat in human milk is easier to digest and absorb than that in cow's milk. This is caused in part by the arrangement of fatty acids on the glycerol molecule. It also is related to the natural lipase activity present in non-heat-treated human milk. The vegetable oils used in preparation of commercial formulas are also well assimilated.

Lactose is the primary carbohydrate of milk and is the most abundant carbohydrate in the diet of infants to 6 months of age. Lactose provides calories in an easily available form. Its slow breakdown and absorption probably benefit calcium absorption. The lactose content in human milk is significantly higher than that in cow's milk. Corn syrup solids or other carbohydrates are added to commercial formulas to provide readily absorbed calories.

Most of the recommended minerals and vitamins are present in appropriate amounts in human milk and formula-feedings. The mineral content of cow's milk is considerably greater than that of human milk, with the exception of iron and fluoride. Both cow's milk and human milk are low in iron. Formulas are available with or without iron fortification. Although iron-fortified formula contains several times more iron than human milk, infants absorb about 48% of the iron from human milk, compared with about 4% from formula (Saarinen, Siimes, and Dallman, 1977). Breastfed infants rarely become iron-deficient before the age of 6 months, both because of the excellent absorption of iron from human milk and because of the stores accrued during the last trimester of pregnancy and the early postnatal period. Human milk is low in fluoride, as is cow's milk and formula. Supplementation is therefore recommended (p. 541).

Another difference is the amount of calcium and phosphorus, minerals especially needed by the rapidly growing infant. Cow's milk contains more of these minerals but a lower calcium:phosphorus ratio (low calcium and high phosphorus). Because of the infant's immature regulatory mechanisms, calcium is excreted, resulting in tetany in young infants fed with whole unmodified cow's milk (Whaley and Wong, 1991). Human milk contains a smaller but more balanced proportion of these minerals and a higher calcium: phosphorus ratio, which are adequate to meet the infant's needs. Formulas are modified so that they have a calcium:phosphorus ratio resembling that of human milk.

Both human and cow's milk contain adequate amounts of zinc, a mineral identified as essential to the human. However, the zinc in human milk is more readily absorbed.

Both human and cow's milk provide adequate amounts of vitamins A and B complex. Vitamin C is low in cow's milk but higher in human milk provided the mother's intake is adequate. Vitamin D is low in human milk but adequate depending on the mother's intake and the infant's exposure to sunlight. Cow's milk and formulas are usually fortified with vitamin D. Human milk contains only one fourth the amount of vitamin K as cow's milk, requiring supplementation at birth (see p. 505). Human milk and formulas are higher in vitamin E and will meet the infant's requirement, whereas cow's milk is low and will not meet the RDA.

❑ LACTATION

Lactation is under the control of numerous endocrine glands, particularly the pituitary hormones prolactin and oxytocin. It is influenced by the **suckling process** and by maternal emotions. The establishment and maintenance of lactation in the human is determined by at least three factors:

1. The anatomic structure of the mammary gland and the development of alveoli, ducts, and nipples
2. The initiation and maintenance of **milk secretion**
3. **Milk ejection** or propulsion of milk from the alveoli to the nipple.

Breast Development

The female human breast, a large exocrine gland, is quiescent during most of the woman's life span. It is composed of about 18 segments embedded in fat and connective tissues and lavishly supplied with blood vessels, lymphatic vessels, and nerves (Chapter 4). The *size of the breast* is related to the amount of fat present and *gives no indication of functional capacity.* The principal feature of mammary growth in pregnancy is a great increase in ducts and alveoli under the influence of many hormones (Chapter 8). Fig. 18-1 shows terminal glandular (alveolar) tissue of each lobule leading into the duct system. The ducts lead into the larger lactifer-

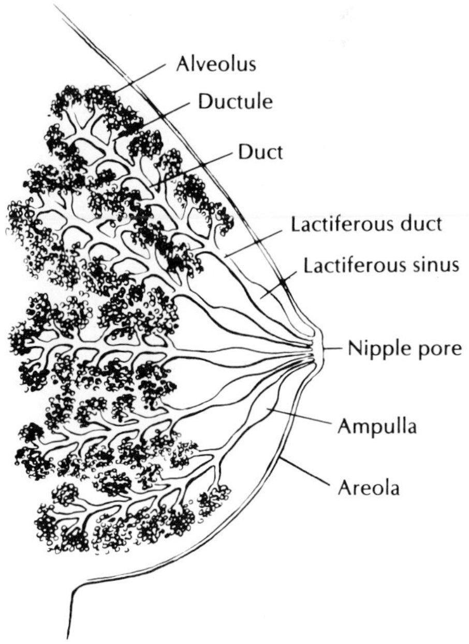

Fig. 18-1 Detailed structural features of human mammary gland. (From Worthington-Roberts B and Williams SR: Nutrition in pregnancy and lactation, ed 4, St Louis, 1989, Times Mirror/Mosby College Publishing.)

ous ducts and sinuses (ampullae). Lactiferous sinuses rest beneath the areola and converge at the nipple pores. Late in pregnancy there is maximum development of the lobuloalveolar system and presumably a sensitization of glandular tissue for action by prolactin. **Colostrum** is secreted in small amounts during the last half of pregnancy.

Stages of Lactation

Lactation, the process of breastfeeding, results from the interplay of hormones and instinctive reflexes and learned behavior of the mother and newborn.

Lactogenesis (milk initiation) commences during the latter part of pregnancy, when secretion of colostrum occurs as a result of stimulation of the mammary alveolar cells by placental lactogen, a prolactin-like substance. It continues after birth as an automatic process.

The continuing secretion of milk is mainly related to sufficient production of the anterior pituitary hormone prolactin and maternal nutrition. Milk secretion occurs by a process of extrusion from the cells.

Movement of milk from alveoli, where it is secreted, to the mouth of the infant is an active process within the breast. This process is brought by the let-down, or milk-ejection, reflex.

The last stage of human lactation is the ingestion of milk by the suckling baby. The full-term, healthy newborn baby possesses three instinctive reflexes needed for successful breastfeeding: the rooting, sucking, and swallowing reflexes (Chapter 16).

Maternal Breastfeeding Reflexes

Three major maternal reflexes involved in breastfeeding are secretion of prolactin (**prolactin reflex**), **nipple erection reflex,** and the **let-down reflex.**

Prolactin is the key lactogenic hormone in initiating and maintaining milk secretion. The sucking stimulus provided by the baby sends a message to the hypothalamus. The hypothalamus stimulates the *anterior* pituitary to release prolactin, the hormone that promotes milk production by the alveolar cells of the mammary glands (Fig. 18-2, *A*). The amount of prolactin secreted, and hence the milk produced, are related to the frequency, intensity, and duration with which the baby breastfeeds.

Stimulation of the nipple by the infant's mouth leads to nipple erection. The stimulation makes the nipple more prominent. This assists the infant to grasp the nipple and aids in the propulsion of milk through the lactiferous sinuses to the nipple pores.

The release of milk from the alveoli and milk ducts occurs as a result of the let-down, or milk-ejection reflex. Fig. 18-2, *B,* illustrates the basic features of the let-down reflex. The sucking stimulus arrives at the hypothalamus, which promotes release of oxytocin from the *posterior* pituitary. Oxytocin stimulates contraction of the myoepithelial cells around the alveoli in the mammary glands. Contraction of these musclelike cells causes milk to be propelled through the duct system and into the lactiferous sinuses, where it becomes available to the breastfeeding infant.

The let-down reflex appears to be sensitive to small

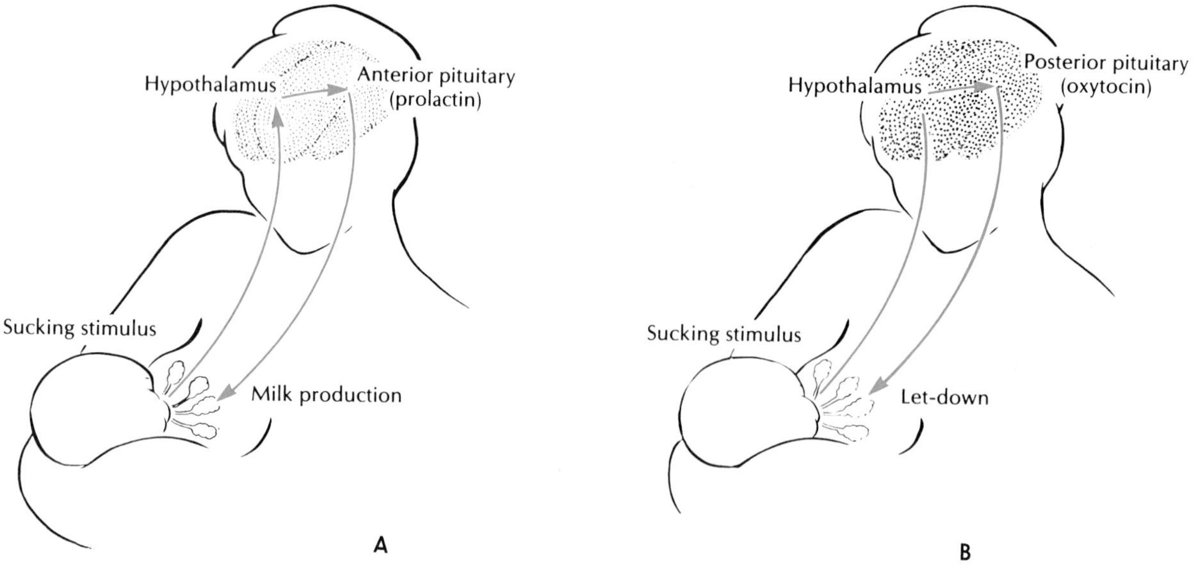

Fig. 18-2 Maternal breastfeeding reflexes. **A,** Milk production. **B,** Let down. (From Worthington-Roberts B and Williams SR: Nutrition in pregnancy and lactation, ed 4, St Louis, 1989, Times Mirror/Mosby College Publishing.)

differences in circulating oxytocin levels. Signs of successful let down are easily recognized by the breastfeeding mother. Common and significant occurrences include milk dripping from the breasts before the baby starts to suckle, milk dripping from the breast opposite to the one being used, and uterine cramps during feeding, caused by the action of oxytocin on the uterus. Minor emotional and psychologic disturbances may influence the ease with which breast milk is released to the baby. The attitude of the mother toward breastfeeding (positive, doubtful, or negative) is a powerful factor in achieving successful lactation, influencing milk production, and facilitating the art of breastfeeding.

Cultural Aspects of Lactation

In the Philippines, if the mother's milk does not flow regularly, a meal of chicken and green papaya boiled in coconut "milk" is suggested (Hart, 1965). According to Hart (1965), the Filipino mother is also advised to eat a soup of boiled clams and ginger. Hart stated that Filipinos use hot applications of special medicinal preparations to stimulate lactation. Furthermore, the Filipino mother believes that raising either arm over her head while lying down will decrease, if not actually stop, lactation. Hart also noted the Filipino women's belief that heavy work will make their milk "hot." Korean mothers eat seaweed soup with rice to increase milk production (Chung, 1977). Currier (1978) reported that Spanish Americans believe that exposing mothers to cold diminishes the flow of milk. Yaqui women massage their breasts to drain them (Shutler, 1977).

In some cultures, colostrum is not fed to the infant. The newborn may be given sterile water until the mother's milk is in. Delay in breastfeeding caused no problems among a group of Vietnamese mothers (Ward et al, 1981). For Hmong women, expressing milk or pumping the breasts is not acceptable (LaDu, 1985). Fat babies are considered healthy among Mexican Americans.

Assessment

Feeding an infant involves the infant and the primary caregiving parent, usually the mother. Therefore both need to be assessed.

Infant

The infant is assessed for developmental **readiness for feeding,** nutritional needs, and success of the feeding program (Owen et al, 1980). Infant factors affecting readiness for feeding (Table 18-2) are assessed

Table 18-2 Newborn Readiness for Feeding

Infant Response	Rationale
Newborn's age in hours or infant's age in days	During reactivity periods, excessive mucus with gagging may occur. Feeding increases the danger of aspiration. In general, reactivity times occur at birth and at 4 to 8 hours of age (p. 441).
Condition at birth	Infants with Apgar scores of 6 or less (depressed) or the infant with low birth weight (2500 g or less) may display a delayed reactivity. This may occur after 12 to 18 hours of age.
Possibility of congenital anomalies of gastrointestinal or respiratory tract; incidence of congenital anomalies higher in preterm infants	With choanal atresia, the newborn is unable to breathe and feed simultaneously. With esophageal atresia, the infant will regurgitate and may aspirate. With tracheoesophageal fistula, feeding may enter trachea directly. With lower gastrointestinal tract obstruction (stenosis, atresia), regurgitation, vomiting, or abdominal distension may compromise respirations.
Gastric capacity	Limited stomach capacity dictates smaller feedings. To provide adequate nutrition, feedings are scheduled more frequently.
CNS maturity	Sucking and swallowing reflexes may not be well developed and synchronized (even in a term baby, the suck and swallow reflex may not be well coordinated during first few hours).
Energy level	Preterm infant or infant with respiratory distress may not have sufficient energy to divert to the process of feeding.
Type of feeding; plain sterile water	Until infant's ability to feed is assessed, danger of aspiration exists. Plain sterile water is less irritating to the respiratory tract. Formula may cause aspiration pneumonia. Glucose water may cause inflammatory response in the respiratory tract similar to response to aspirated formula.

shortly after birth for the breastfed and bottle-fed infant.

As the infant grows and matures, nutrition needs reflect the change. The infant who is obtaining the necessary nutrients and fluid will exhibit a steady increase in weight, good skin and muscle tone, vigorous feeding behavior, and satisfaction. The satisfied newborn sleeps, cries in moderation, and is interested in socializing.

Mother

The mother (couple) is assessed as follows:

1. Physical ability and psychologic readiness for feeding the newborn
2. Knowledge of the advantages of breastfeeding and formula-feeding
3. Knowledge of the infant's nutrition needs and capabilities
4. Knowledge and skill in feeding methods
5. Knowledge of an adequate and safe diet during lactation

The techniques used to assess these areas include primarily interviews, discussions, and observation of skill in feeding methods.

Nursing Diagnoses

When dietary data have been collected and analyzed, nursing diagnoses relative to the infant's nutrition status can be made. Examples include the following:

Knowledge deficit related to
- Normal growth and development of the infant and her or his nutritional needs
- Feeding skills

Situational low self-esteem related to
- Difficulties encountered in feeding

Planning

Teaching and counseling concerning the feeding of infants are part of the daily care plan for maternity clients. The benefits of both breastfeeding and formula-feeding are presented so that the mother can make an intelligent choice as to how to feed her baby. Counseling should begin in the first or second trimester of pregnancy when the mother is unrushed and has time to consider her choices. Women are encouraged to express their opinions and feelings so that they can be discussed and any misinformation can be corrected. During the last months of pregnancy, counseling on the process of lactation is made available to women who have decided to breastfeed. Fathers are encouraged to participate in counseling sessions because their encouragement and emotional support contribute to successful lactation. Many mothers have never seen a woman breastfeeding an infant; they therefore find it especially helpful to have a woman who has successfully breastfed an infant available to answer questions and provide reinforcement.

With the birth of the infant, the parents' choice of feeding method is accepted and supported. Feeding is an emotionally charged area of infant care. Culturally, the size and growth of an infant are equated with excellence and evidence of mothering ability. The infant who is a fussy eater can raise parental anxiety levels. The anxious parent appears to compound the problem, and a vicious cycle can develop. Relatives or friends can take over a feeding period or two. This seems to break the cycle so that the mother can view the feeding session in a more relaxed manner, not as a condemnation of her care. Parents need positive feedback to develop a feeling of confidence in their own ability. Often just listening and praising is the most effective intervention. Tension tends to lessen milk production. The first few days the mother is home with the new baby are often filled with excitement and anxiety about mothering activities, so entertaining company or undertaking extended family commitments may have to be restricted. Many mothers need considerable assistance with infant feeding. Both group and individual teaching are necessary. Hospitals usually provide excellent teaching aids. A sample care plan appears on p. 525.

The ***goals*** for the *infant* include that the infant will:

1. Obtain the levels and types of nutrients necessary to support the infant's body composition, activity, and growth
2. Have a minimum of physiologic stress associated with digestion and metabolism of nutrients and excretion of wastes
3. Obtain sufficient water to maintain adequate body water balance
4. Experience a close and loving feeding interaction

The ***goals*** for the *mother* (parent) include that the mother (parent) will:

1. Obtain knowledge that can be used for sound nutritional selection and feeding practices
2. Become skilled in the feeding method of her (his) choice
3. Achieve closeness and pleasure in the parent-child interaction.

General Nursing Care Plan

NEWBORN NUTRITION AND FEEDING

ASSESSMENT	NURSING DIAGNOSIS (ND), PLAN/GOAL (P/G)	RATIONALE/ IMPLEMENTATION	EVALUATION
Prenatal Assessment of infant feeding preferences. Cultural, religious, social, and financial considerations influencing feeding choice. Practices of woman's friends and her mother. Personal (and father's) goals and preferences.	ND: Knowledge deficit related to newborn feeding. P/G: Woman will make an informed decision about breastfeeding or formula-feeding her newborn.	*Knowledge provides a basis for decision-making:* Evaluate woman's (couple's) goals and preferences for feeding. Discuss the pros and cons of both methods of feeding. Encourage questions, concerns, or feelings surrounding newborn nutrition and feeding. Dispel misconceptions surrounding the feeding option. Encourage the woman to discuss her decision with those members of the family who will be active in child care.	Woman chooses a method of infant feeding suitable to her needs and lifestyle.
First day of life Assess newborn's ability to breastfeed or formula-feed. 1. Reflexes—suck, swallow, gag. 2. No structural abnormalities (e.g. choanal atresia). Assess newborn's readiness for feeding (e.g., rooting reflex, newborn's responsiveness). Assess amount and frequency of feeds.	ND: Ineffective airway clearance related to poor suck, swallow, or gag reflexes. ND: Altered nutrition: less than body requirements, related to infant's lack of interest in feeding or regurgitation. P/G: Newborn will possess readiness to feed and demonstrate intact reflexes.	*Newborns feed more successfully if able and ready:* Have newborn suck on finger. Remove excess mucus from nose and mouth, burp prn. Give newborn sterile water. Initiate and evaluate mother's preferred choice of feeding as soon as possible.	Reflexes (root, suck, swallow, and gag) are present and sufficiently developed to permit feeding by breast or bottle. Newborn accepts, swallows, retains, and assimilates feeding.
Assess woman's ability to feed infant.	ND: Knowledge deficit related to newborn feeding. P/G: Woman will learn how to successfully feed her newborn.	*Competence and confidence increase with practice and assistance:* Encourage the use of wakeful periods for feeding newborn. Assist the mother with the feeding technique she has chosen. Instruct as to feeding techniques and nutritional needs of the newborn. Demonstrate and supervise care needed if newborn chokes, gags, or spits up. Record amounts of formula or time at breast and note newborn's response.	Woman successfully feeds her newborn.

Continued.

ASSESSMENT	NURSING DIAGNOSIS (ND), PLAN/GOAL (P/G)	RATIONALE/ IMPLEMENTATION	EVALUATION
Assess newborn's ability to defecate (stool) and urinate.	ND: Altered bowel or bladder elimination related to a structural or mechanical defect. P/G: Newborn will demonstrate a normal pattern of elimination.	*Elimination is essential for health maintenance:* Record urine amounts and time. Record character of stool and time. Notify physician if no urine within the first 24 hours of life or no stool within the first 48 hours of life. Report and record any structural defects noted (e.g., imperforate anus).	Newborn demonstrates normal pattern of elimination.
Breastfeeding: Parity. First breastfeeding experience? Knowledge about breastfeeding. Support system for breastfeeding experience. Assess breastfeeding problems—mother-related and infant-related.	ND: Knowledge deficit related to breastfeeding and its complications. P/G: Woman will breastfeed successfully and comfortably and will establish a pattern satisfactory to newborn and herself.	*Knowledge and practice increase competence and confidence:* See guidelines for client teaching, p. 528.	Woman successfully and comfortably breastfeeds with a pattern that is satisfying to her and her newborn.
Formula-feeding: Parity. Has she bottle-fed previously? Knowledge about bottle-feeding and amounts of formula required. Financial status.	ND: Knowledge deficit related to preparation of formula and bottle-feeding. P/G: Woman will learn how to prepare formula and bottle-feed her newborn and assess the amount of feeding the newborn requires.	*Knowledge and practice increase competence and confidence:* See guidelines for client teaching, p. 539.	Woman successfully prepares formula and bottle-feeds her newborn and demonstrates an awareness of the newborn's needs (formula, frequency of feeds, etc.).
Follow-up care Assess weight gain. Assess growth pattern. Assess hydration status (weight, skin turgor, sunken eyes or fontanels, moistness of mucous membranes). Assess frequency of feeds, amounts of formula, or breastfeeding time. Assess newborn's satisfaction between feeds. Assess elimination pattern.	ND: Altered health maintenance related to poor nutritional patterns or elimination problems. ND: Altered nutrition: less or more than body requirements related to newborn's feeding pattern. ND: Knowledge deficit related to growing infant's nutritional needs. P/G: Woman will be adept at adjusting feeding process to meet newborn's nutritional needs. P/G: Newborn will grow and gain weight within the normal limits for age. P/G: Newborn will establish a regular elimination pattern.	*Health maintenance requires follow-up care:* Weigh and measure length. Evaluate growth according to age. Note and report poor or excessive growth. Note, report, and seek treatment for dehydration. Discuss feeding pattern and amounts with mother and evaluate newborn's satisfaction. Encourage woman to verbalize feeding problems/concerns. Evaluate and report problems with elimination. Teach woman newborn satisfaction signs.	Woman adjusts feeds according to newborn's needs. Child receives adequate nutrition to grow within the normal limits for age. Child establishes a regular elimination pattern.

Implementation

Nurses act as teachers, counselors, and advocates in helping parents learn about feeding their infants. They act as change agents in motivating parents to adopt healthful eating behaviors for themselves and their families. In doing so they help parents clarify goals and make decisions. Parents need assistance in the techniques of breastfeeding and bottle-feeding. They seek counseling for specific concerns and welcome anticipatory guidance.

Early feeding is feeding within 6 to 8 hours after birth. For the term, nonstressed newborn, early oral or parenteral feeding prevents dehydration, spares the available stores of glycogen, maintains blood glucose levels, and lessens initial weight loss. Serum bilirubin levels within normal limits often follow. Protein catabolism that would result in metabolic acidosis, hyperkalemia, or elevated blood urea nitrogen (BUN) levels is curtailed. Energy is conserved for growth. The sucking response is stimulated.

❑ BREASTFEEDING

Milk from a healthy mother is the food of choice for a healthy infant. Breastfeeding offers many advantages: nutritional, immunologic, and psychologic (Hughes, 1984). The following are some of these advantages:

1. The infant receives immunoglobulins to protect against some infections
2. The infant usually experiences less diarrhea or constipation
3. The type of protein ingested is less likely to cause allergic reactions
4. The infant has fewer problems with overfeeding; the need to "empty the bottle" is eliminated
5. Bottle washing, preparation of formula, and refrigeration are unnecessary
6. Maternal organs return more quickly to their nonpregnant condition (Madgic, 1986)

Guidelines for client teaching regarding breastfeeding are presented on p. 528.

Immunologic Benefits

There is evidence that the newborn infant acquires certain important elements of host resistance from breast milk while maturation of her or his own immune system is taking place. Human milk contains high levels of immunoglobin A (IgA) and affords protection against several bacterial and viral diseases, especially those of the respiratory and gastrointestinal systems (Whaley and Wong, 1991).

Immunoglobulins are believed to function directly in the infant's gastrointestinal tract by diminishing antigen contact with intestinal mucosa until the infant's own antibody responses are developed. **Lactoferrin** is secreted in human milk and is believed to play a role in controlling bacterial growth in the gastrointestinal tract. It works by competing with microorganisms that require iron for replication. The presence of these factors is believed to explain the reduced incidence of illness in breastfed babies that has been reported not only in developing countries but also in the United States.

IgA also probably protects against development of food allergies. In addition, human milk contains numerous other host defense factors, such as macrophages, granulocytes, and T- and B-lymphocytes (Hanson et al, 1985).

Care of Breasts

Daily washing of the breasts with water is sufficient for cleanliness. Nipples should be dry before brassiere flaps are replaced. Air drying for 10 minutes after each feeding is suggested. Nipples are lubricated with a few drops of expressed colostrum or milk, then air dried again. In addition to causing nipples to crack and removing protective secretions, soaps, alcohol, and petrolatum-based preparations may be distasteful to some infants who will then refuse to suckle.

The brassiere needs to be well-fitted, with broad shoulder straps and the flaps over the breasts large enough to release the breasts without discomfort. Milk leaking from the breasts (milk-ejection reflex) can be uncomfortable and embarrassing.

A tingling sensation in the nipple area precedes leaking of the milk. Pressure with the heel of both hands over the nipple areas will often prevent the milk from forming so that leaking from the breasts is forestalled. The brassiere can be padded with folded squares of soft cotton, a perineal pad cut in two, or commercially designed pads. Lining the brassiere cup with plastic material is not recommended, since moisture tends to soften the nipple and predispose it to erosion.

Diet and Fluids

During lactation there is increased need for maternal energy, protein, minerals, and vitamins. This increase covers the cost of secreting milk, provides amounts secreted in milk for nourishment of the infant, and protects the mother's stores. A well-balanced diet containing an extra 640 calories per day (per baby) is necessary for both mother and infant. See Chapter 11 for additional information about nutrition. The breastfeeding mother requires *extra fluids,* as much as 3 L per day. These can be taken routinely before each feeding. Glasses of water, fruit juices, decaffeinated tea, or milk

Guidelines for Client Teaching
BREASTFEEDING

ASSESSMENT

Primipara planning to breastfeed her newborn girl who weighs 3360 g (7½ lb).

NURSING DIAGNOSIS

Knowledge deficit related to breastfeeding and lactation.

GOALS

Short-term

Newborn breastfeeds successfully.

Intermediate

A feeding pattern satisfactory to newborn and mother is established.

Long-term

Mother able to adjust feedings to needs of newborn by recognizing her cues for hunger and satiety. Mother able to breastfeed successfully while maintaining chosen life-style.

REFERENCES AND TEACHING AIDS

Hospital pamphlets about newborn nutrition, films on breastfeeding, posters, booklets, etc.

Texts such as: Pyle M: Breast feeding, a family affair, Costa Mesa, Calif, 1985, Lifecircle; Riordan J: A practical guide to breastfeeding, St Louis, 1983, The CV Mosby Co.

Pamphlets and books available through the La Leche League.

RATIONALE/CONTENT	TEACHING ACTION
Competence and confidence increase with knowledge, therefore the nurse will review the following:	Fill in gaps in knowledge.
Mother may assume any comfortable position. Let the breast fall forward without tension. Leave one hand free to guide the newborn's mouth to the nipple.	Have mother experiment with positions. Have her assume the position that feels most comfortable (Fig. 18-3).
The nipple can be made more prominent by gently rolling it between the fingers. The areolar area will be put in the newborn's mouth with the nipple. This prevents bruising the nipple.	Have woman expose her breast. Have woman prepare her nipple. Point out areolar tissue.
Colostrum is the yellow fluid that can be expressed from the breasts now. It is good for the newborn. It contains some fat and protein and helps newborn resist infections.	Demonstrate technique for expressing milk from the breast. Have woman express some colostrum.
Milk may be expected to appear 48 to 96 hours after delivery. Before the milk comes in, the breasts feel soft to the touch. After the milk comes in, the breasts feel full and warmer.	Have woman touch breasts to feel softness.
Guidance and practice increase competence and confidence:	Demonstrate rooting reflex by touching finger to newborn's lips and cheek.
Have mother hold the newborn so that her cheek touches the breasts. The pressure against the outer angle of the lip begins the rooting reflex (Fig. 18-4). The newborn will turn toward the nipple. She can smell the colostrum and milk and this will also make her turn toward the nipple.	
When newborn opens mouth, move infant's head to breast. Entire nipple and as much of the areola as possible should enter newborn's mouth.	Have the woman practice (Fig. 18-3, *A*). Tell her to avoid holding the breast like a cigarette.
Knowledge of expected newborn responses and maternal sensations increase maternal coping:	Bring newborn to mother. Have her assess her daughter's suck by placing her finger in the infant's mouth with the finger pad touching and stroking the palate. She should be able to feel the tongue cushioning the joint of the finger and stroking the finger, while keeping the gum covered. She should not feel an insecure or loose suction on the finger, or a tapping of the gum on the finger alone or combined with the tongue slipping back and forth across the gum (licking).
At first the newborn sucks in short bursts of three to five sucks followed by single swallows. In 1 to 2 days a sucking pattern evolves. This consists of 10 to 30 sucks followed by swallowing. The newborn's lips and jaws exert pressure on the areola and the tongue "cradles" the nipple so that the tip is not eroded. The pressure combined with negative intraoral pressure brings milk into the mouth (Fig. 18-5).	

Continued.

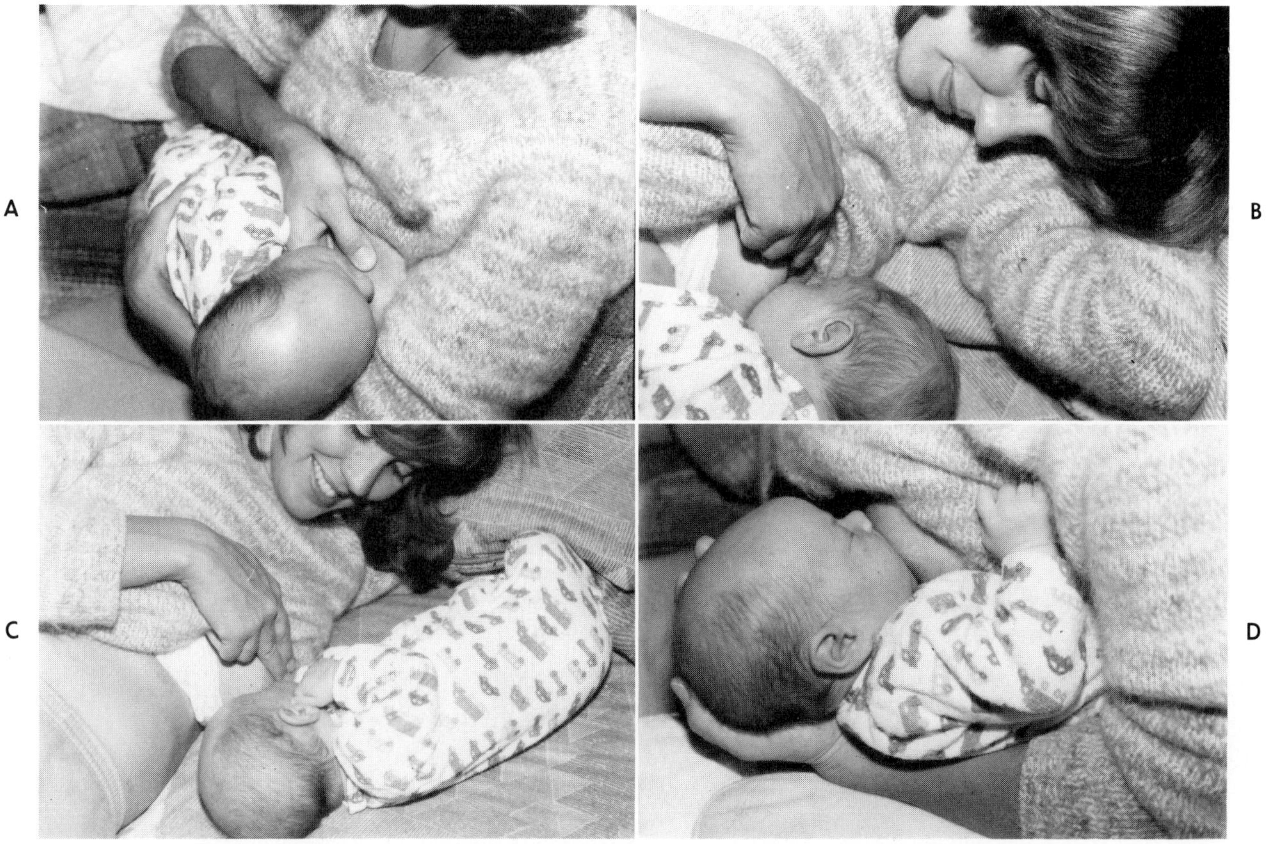

Fig. 18-3 Positioning the baby. **A,** Cradle hold. One arm and hand supports baby. Other hand supports breast (thumb above and fingers below). Breast is guided into baby's mouth. **B,** Side-lying position. Pillows support mother's head. Baby is turned toward mother. Mother depresses breast to facilitate baby's breathing. **C,** Variation on side-lying position. **D,** Football hold. Baby is held in one arm with hand supporting head. (Courtesy Marjorie Pyle, RNC, Lifecircle, Costa Mesa, Calif.)

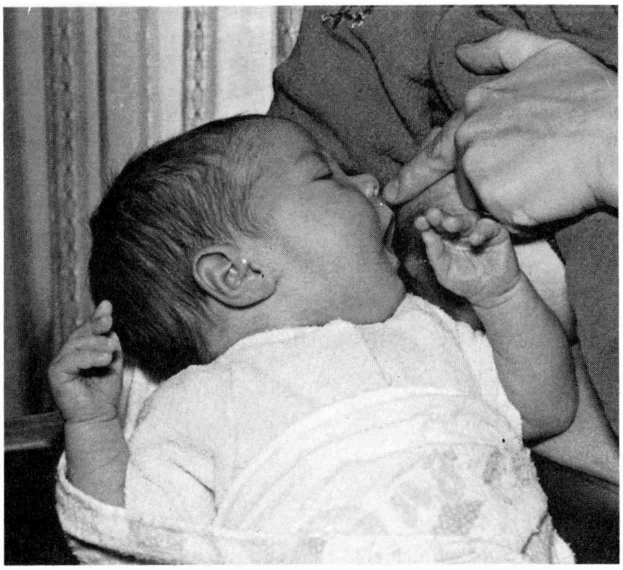

Fig. 18-4 Rooting reflex is apparent when corner of newborn's mouth is touched. Bottom lip lowers on same side; tongue moves toward stimulation. (Courtesy Joan Edelstein and Ralph Levy, San Jose, Calif.)

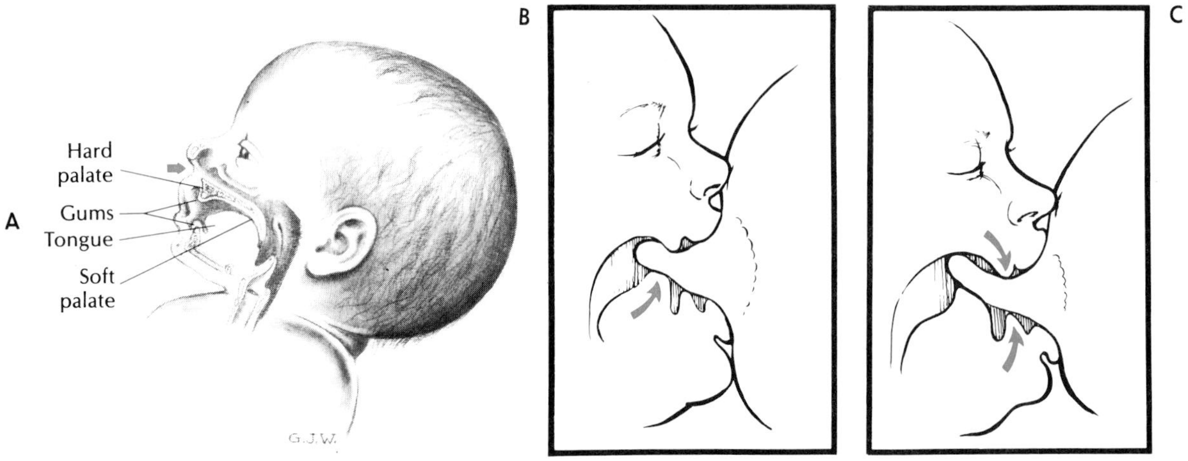

Fig. 18-5 Suckling process: **A,** Infant breathes through nose *(arrow)*. Tongue and palate meet closing esophagus. **B,** Tongue thrusts up and forward to grasp nipple. **C,** Gums compress areola and tongue moves backward creating negative pressure for suction. (**B** and **C** from Riordan J: A practical guide to breastfeeding, St Louis, 1987, The CV Mosby Co.)

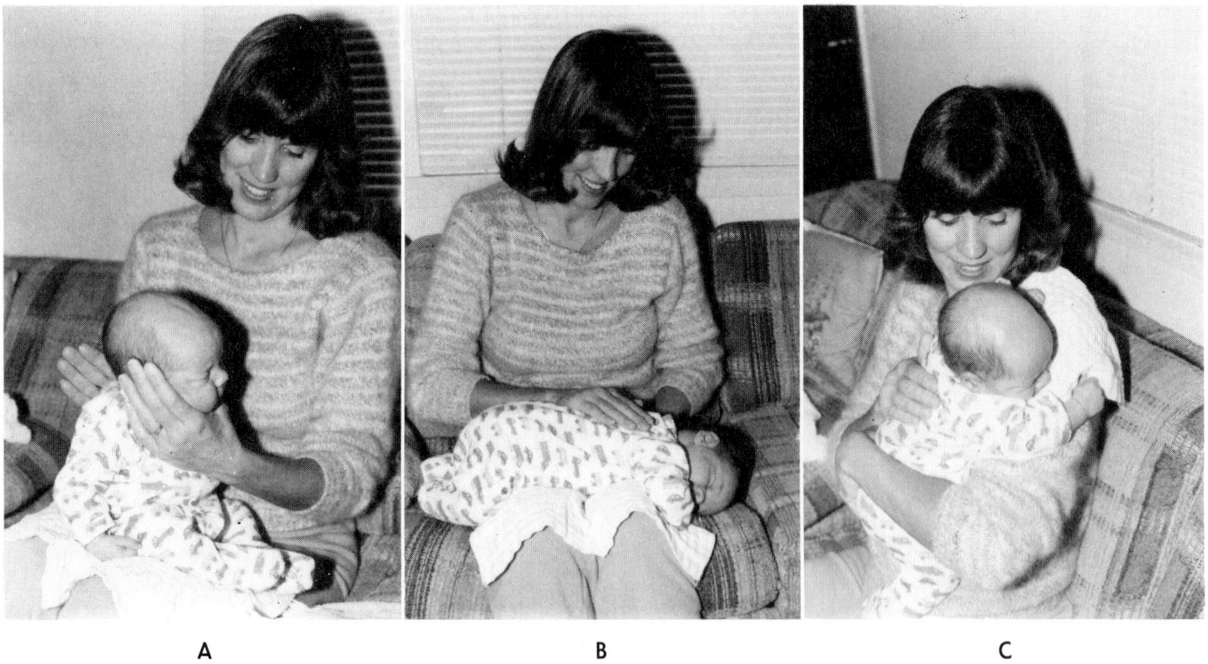

Fig. 18-6 Positions for burping a baby. **A,** Upright. **B,** Across the lap. **C,** Shoulder position. (Courtesy Marjorie Pyle, RNC, Lifecircle, Costa Mesa, Calif.)

Guidelines for Client Teaching—cont'd

RATIONALE/CONTENT	TEACHING ACTIONS
When the newborn is sucking properly, there is no "clicking" noise. This clicking noise means she is sucking on her own tongue in the back of the throat, past the nipple. The rhythmic suck-swallow breathing pattern that indicates milk is flowing can be heard. Some mothers can sense if the newborn has drawn the areolar tissue into the mouth along with the nipple.	Have mother suck her own tongue at the back of the throat to hear the clicking sound.
Get the newborn ready and put her to breast; first making sure she is awake.	If necessary, *waken the newborn* by stroking her cheek, rubbing her feet, and talking to her.
Put her to breast by *bringing the newborn to the breast,* not the breast to the newborn. The newborn's face, chest, abdomen, and knees should all be facing the mother's body. Touch her upper lip with the nipple; the newborn will turn toward the nipple and open her mouth. The newborn is pulled as close to the mother as possible (Fig. 18-3).	Help mother position newborn so that the head is directly facing the breast and the nipple is not pulled to one side. Guide woman through feeding. Point out and explain sensations she is feeling.
Feel how the newborn's jaws fit behind the nipple and the nipple is deep in her mouth.	
If newborn needs more breathing space, lift the breast; or make a "dimple" in the breast for breathing space (Fig. 18-3, *B* and *C*).	Caution woman that making a "dimple" may be done too vigorously and the nipple will be dislodged.
Hold the breast throughout the entire feeding for a few weeks.	Observe technique, degree of relaxation, offer praise.
It is a good idea to use both breasts at each feeding. Once the milk has come in the mother can tell which breast to start with next time by feeling the weight. The heaviest one has the most milk, so start with that one. In the meantime, a safety pin on the bra strap on the side last used will be a reminder for the next feeding.	Review need to empty both breasts since an empty breast signals woman's body to produce more milk.
To remove the newborn from the breast, place a finger in the corner of the newborn's mouth until the suction is broken. The breast can then be comfortably removed. The mother may need assistance to switch breasts. Leave mother to enjoy her newborn.	Return in about 15 minutes to supervise mother removing newborn from the breast. Remind her that *breastfeeding time is not limited* (Slaven, 1981; L'esperance and Frantz, 1985).
Before putting the baby to the other breast, she should be burped. Some newborns never burp, others do frequently. Gently rub or pat the newborn's back.	Demonstrate burping (Fig. 18-6). Supervise mother putting newborn to other breast.
After feeding, place the baby on her right side. This allows air in stomach to come up and not bring the milk with it.	Show woman a picture of a newborn on right side (see Fig. 17-2).

EVALUATION Mother demonstrates competency in breastfeeding.

can be alternated. The mother can keep a pitcher of water close by when breastfeeding, as she often becomes thirsty. The use of beer or wine to aid lactation is *not* recommended (Blume et al, 1987).

Infant Responses

Breastfed babies may wish to feed more often than formula-fed babies. If the baby wants to breastfeed, there is no reason not to do so. Breastfed babies consume what they need and no more. Breastfeeding whenever the baby is hungry is easy to do because the milk is always ready. Some babies may be hungry as frequently as every hour or two on some days, on other days only every 4 hours. The more often the baby nurses, the more milk the breasts produce. Thus whenever a woman's supply is low (e.g., during or after an illness), she should breastfeed more often. If the woman has too much milk, the baby may need to breastfeed on only one side at a feeding for a while.

This will reduce overall stimulation and reduce the milk supply.

Crying does not always mean that the baby is hungry (Chapter 21). The baby may be physically uncomfortable or just want to be held, burped, or changed. Mother can be reassured that she is producing sufficient milk if the infant has 6 to 10 *voidings* of pale, straw-colored urine in 24 hours. In warm weather the baby may be thirsty. The mother can give the baby a bottle of water (preboiled in areas with poor sanitation) (1 to 2 oz) or increase the number of breastfeedings.

The *stools* of breastfed babies are loose. Some infants have a bowel movement at each feeding, whereas others may go up to 5 days without one. Babies who are fed only breast milk do not become constipated, although they may strain considerably in passing the stool. The stool is not irritating to the skin.

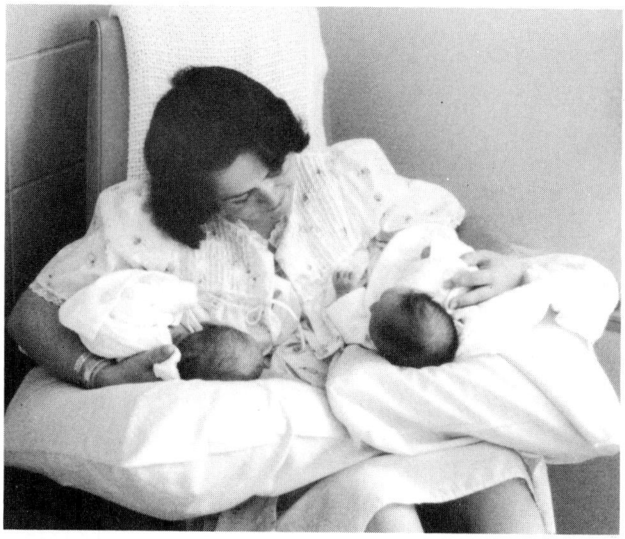

Fig. 18-7 Breastfeeding twins. Note support with pillows. Infants in "football hold" position. (Courtesy Colleen Stainton.)

Special Considerations in Breastfeeding

Breastfeeding Twins. Breastfeeding twins takes planning and patience. If the mother elects the rooming-in regimen, the added care of two infants may prove too taxing to her strength. However, many mothers have stated that the early adjustment made going home easier. It is suggested that these mothers remain longer in the hospital unless there is help at home. It is important to establish a feeding schedule as soon as possible. The mother may use a modified **demand feeding** schedule. She can feed the first baby who wakes up, then wake up the second baby. She may decide to breastfeed them simultaneously (Fig. 18-7).

A record of the feeding times, which breast was used by which baby, and which side was used first is useful during the early weeks. If one twin feeds more readily than the other, an effort should be made to have that twin feed on alternate breasts to equalize stimulation. If feeding simultaneously, the mother should experiment with positions. Each baby may be supported on pillows and in the football hold. One may be held in the football hold and the other in the cradle hold. Obviously the mother with twins will need extra assistance from her family, extra nourishment (500 calories per day per baby), and extra rest. She will need sufficient energy not only to care for and breastfeed each baby but also to provide the mothering each child needs.

Breastfeeding in Diabetic Women. Breastfeeding is encouraged in diabetic women not only for its psychologic benefits and its advantages for the infant but also for its antidiabetogenic effect. Breastfeeding decreases the insulin dosage for insulin-dependent women. The insulin dosage must be readjusted at the time of weaning. (See Fig. 24-1, *F* to *G*.)

Effect of Oral Contraceptives. If *oral contraceptives* are taken sooner than 6 weeks after delivery, the amount of milk a woman produces may be diminished. Experience indicates that most women will not have difficulty producing an adequate amount of milk if they do not use oral contraceptives until after weaning the infant.

Effect of Menstruation. If menstruation occurs, the mother can continue to breastfeed. Although some babies may act fussy, the quality and quantity of the milk are not affected.

Maternal Commitments. On occasions when the mother needs to be away from the infant at feeding time, a bottle of breast milk, expressed earlier, can be substituted. If the mother returns to work, she can continue to breastfeed (Price and Bamford, 1983; MacLaughlin and Strelnick, 1984). The length of time a woman breastfeeds her infant will depend on her own feelings and situation. Milk will continue to be produced as long as it is taken from the breast.

Concerns. The inexperienced breastfeeding mother is likely to encounter major or minor problems in the course of adjusting to breastfeeding (Chapman et al, 1985). Success or failure at the breastfeeding effort may depend largely on the availability of help in the early weeks and the support of a clinician or friend who provides useful tips. Mother-related problems in breastfeeding are presented in Table 18-3. Problems relating to the infant are presented in Table 18-4.

Table 18-3 **Mother-related Problems in Breastfeeding**

Problem	Nursing Action
ENGORGED BREASTS If feeding has been on demand since birth, painful **engorgement** of the breasts is not likely to occur. However, because of the lag between the production of milk and the efficiency of the ejection reflexes, engorgement of the breasts may occur for up to 48 hours after the milk comes in. The mother often complains that the breast is tender and that the tenderness extends into the axilla. The breasts usually feel firm, tense, and warm as a result of the increased blood supply, and the skin may appear shiny and taut. The unyielding areolae makes it difficult for the infant to grasp the nipple. Breastfeeding can be uncomfortable to the mother and frustrating for both mother and infant.	1. Application of moist heat: apply wet cloths as hot as can be endured to the whole breast and, at the same time, express milk from the nipple. As the wet cloth cools, replace with another one. Shower and direct the hot water to the breasts. 2. **Breast massage** (Fig. 18-8): **A,** Begin by placing one hand over the other above the breast. **B,** Gently, but firmly, exert pressure evenly with the thumbs across the top and fingers underneath the breast. **C,** Come together with the heel of the hand on each side and release at the areola, being careful not to touch the areola and nipple. **D,** Then gently lift the breast from beneath and drop lightly. Repeat 4 to 5 times with each breast. 3. **Manual expression of milk** (Fig. 18-9) **A,** Place the thumb and forefinger on opposite sides of the breast just outside the areola, press downward into the rib cage, and then **B,** gently squeeze together and downward; the nipple should not be pulled outward. Repeat the procedure moving the thumb and forefinger around the nipple until as much milk as desired has been expressed. If the milk is to be used later, *it should be expressed into a sterile bottle and frozen.* Milk expression is not easy for some women at first, but persistence usually brings success if the mother takes the time.
SORE NIPPLES The nipples may become sore during the early days of breastfeeding. **Sore nipples** may be prevented or limited by using a correct position and avoiding undue breast engorgement. If soreness occurs, it is usually temporary until the nipples become accustomed to the baby's sucking (Borovies, 1984). Some mothers report soreness for up to 3 months (Chapman et al, 1985).	1. Expose the nipples to air. 2. Use a heat lamp to dry the nipples after the feeding (40-watt bulb in a desk lamp, positioned 45 cm [18 in] from breast). 3. If soreness occurs, limit sucking time to 5 minutes on each breast, the time it takes to empty the breasts of milk. 4. Use a pacifier if the infant's sucking needs have not been met. 5. Use a nipple shield. 6. Discontinue breastfeeding for 48 hours. During this time the milk is expressed manually or with a breast pump, collected in a sterilized glass, and given to the baby by bottle. Precautions for maintaining the milk in a safe condition must be followed. Bottles and nipples must be sterilized by immersing them in water and boiling for 10 minutes; any milk not immediately consumed must be refrigerated or frozen.
PLUGGED DUCTS Occasionally a milk duct will become plugged, creating a tender spot on the breast, which may appear lumpy and hot. **Plugged ducts** might result from inadequate emptying of the milk ducts or from wearing a brassiere that is too tight.	1. Offer the sore breast first so that it will be emptied more completely. 2. Nurse longer and more often; if the breast gets too full, the plugged duct becomes worse and infection may develop. 3. Change positions at every feeding so that the pressure of the feeding will be applied to different places on the breast. 4. Apply warm compresses to the breasts between feedings to reduce the risk of infection by keeping the ducts open.

Continued.

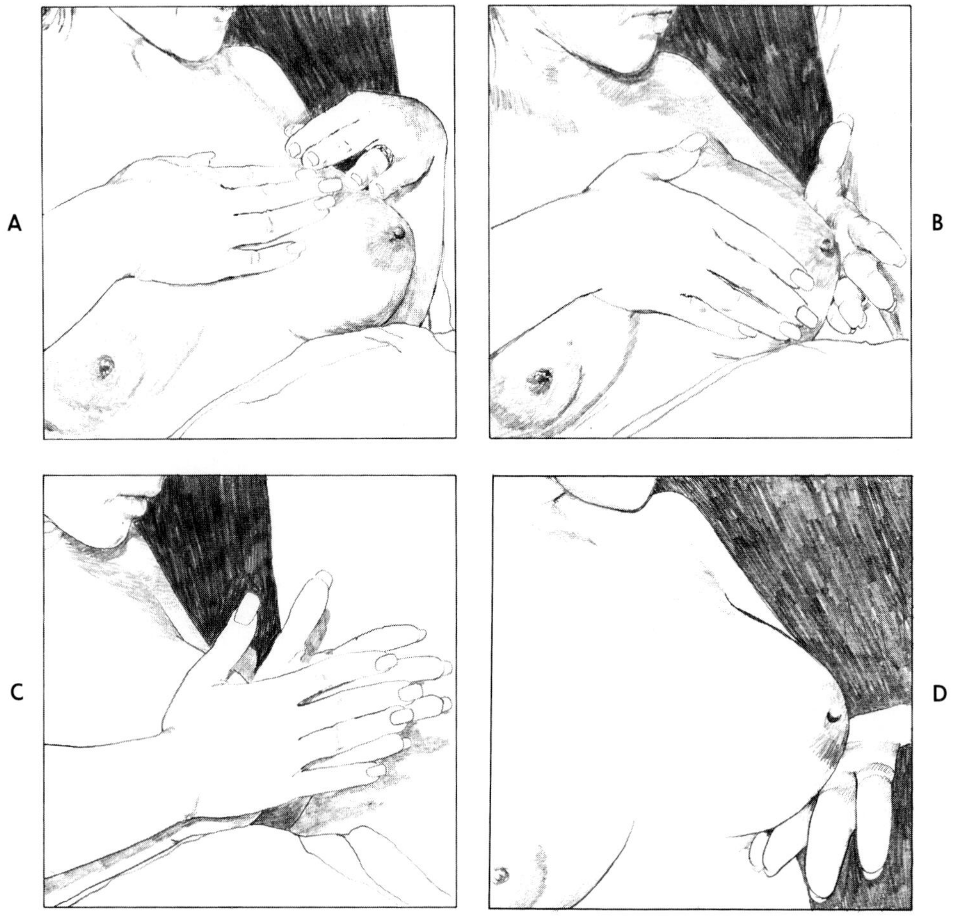

Fig. 18-8 Breast massage. (Courtesy Marjorie Pyle, RNC, Lifecircle, Costa Mesa, Calif.)

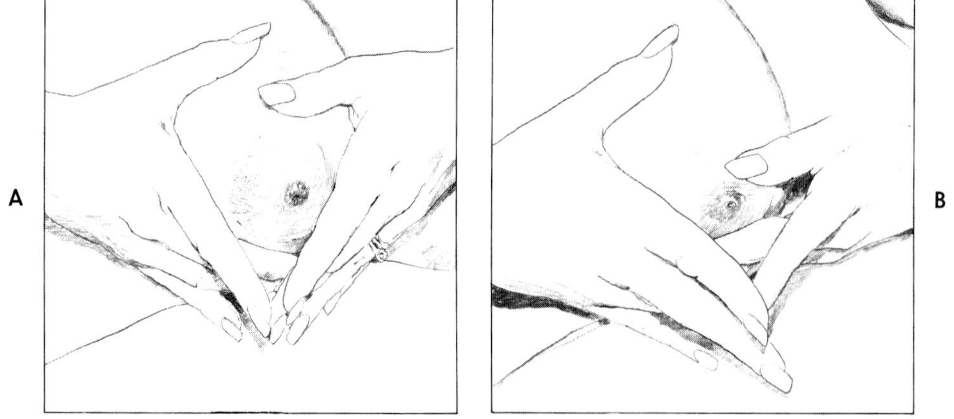

Fig. 18-9 Manual expression of human milk. (Courtesy Marjorie Pyle, RNC, Lifecircle, Costa Mesa, Calif.)

Table 18-3 Mother-related Problems in Breastfeeding—cont'd

Problem	Nursing Action
INCREASED LOCHIAL FLOW	
The breastfeeding mother may note an increase in lochial flow once feeding begins. At times afterpains are intensified to such a degree that the mother becomes uncomfortable, and her tension interferes with feeding the infant.	Offer a mild analgesic for pain 40 minutes before the feeding period. The mother may be reassured that this discomfort is transitory and will be gone in about 2 days.
PERCEPTION OF INADEQUATE AMOUNT OF MILK	
Insufficient milk supply is rarely a problem for the well-nourished mother. Since sucking stimulates the flow of milk, feeding on demand for adequate duration should supply ample amounts of milk.	1. Increase frequency of feedings to increase supply. 2. Note frequency of infant urination; 6 to 10 voidings every 24 hours is adequate. 3. Weight gain of ½ oz/day indicates adequate intake. 4. Reassure mother if infant seems satisfied.
FAILURE OF INFANT TO THRIVE	
Occasionally, an infant will experience **failure to thrive** (have an inadequate weight gain) while seemingly feeding properly.	1. Assist in the explanation of potential problems. 2. Encourage mother to turn to commercial infant formula for at least partial nutrition support of the infant, if the cause of the problem cannot be identified or the defined problem cannot be corrected. 3. Refer the mother to a pediatrician if condition continues, or prn.
BREAST PUMPING	
For a number of reasons, mothers may wish to remove milk from their breasts and save it for a later feeding, take it to their hospitalized newborn, or donate it to a milk bank. Under such circumstances, milk can be expressed by hand; and for some women **pumping the breasts** by hand is satisfactory. For many women, however, a manual or electric breast pump provides a better stimulus for milk flow and a more efficient mode of milk collection.	Instruct the mother in the use of the breast pump (Fig. 18-10).
MATERNAL INFECTION	
If breast tenderness is accompanied by fever and a general flulike feeling, a breast infection is probably present (Chapter 23).	Instruct the mother to notify her physician immediately.
SEXUAL SENSATIONS	
For some women the rhythmic uterine contractions occurring while breastfeeding are akin to those experienced during orgasm. These unexpected sexual sensations within the context of child care may be disturbing.	Reassure as to normalcy of such feelings.
RELACTATION AND LACTATION AFTER ADOPTING	
Occasionally a mother starts breastfeeding late or discontinues it but decides at a much later date that she would like to begin again. ***After adopting an infant,*** a minority of women decide to attempt lactation even though they have never done so before or, at best, have breastfed a previous baby of their own. With much sucking stimulus, lactation can be induced but only with great perseverance and in most cases only if a woman has once carried a pregnancy well into the second trimester. Since the mammary glands complete their development for lactation during the first 6 months of pregnancy, a woman who has never been pregnant or never carried a pregnancy beyond the first trimester is a poor candidate for successful induction of lactation.	Instruct the mother to attempt relactation or induced lactation through providing the infant substantial opportunities to suck at the breast. With much sucking stimulus over several days' time many patient and persistent women can initiate the lactation process late or once again. Their volume of milk production may be less than the infant demands, in which case a supplemental feeding following breastfeeding may be necessary. Alternatively, some women find the Lact-Aid Nursing Trainer to complement their own milk production (Fig. 18-11). While the baby sucks at the breast she or he also obtains milk via suction through a small tube leading to a bag of fresh formula that is clipped to the mother's brassiere. While the infant sucks, the mother's milk supply is built up and the infant receives adequate nutrition through the Lact-Aid feeding device.

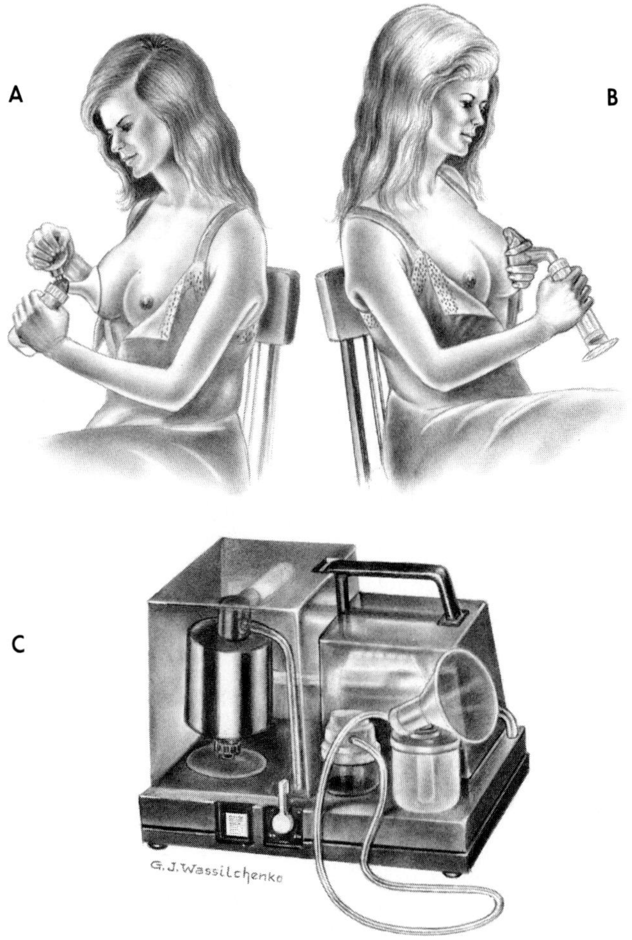

Fig. 18-10 Commonly used breast pumps. **A,** Swedish pump. **B,** Syringe pump. **C,** Electric pump.

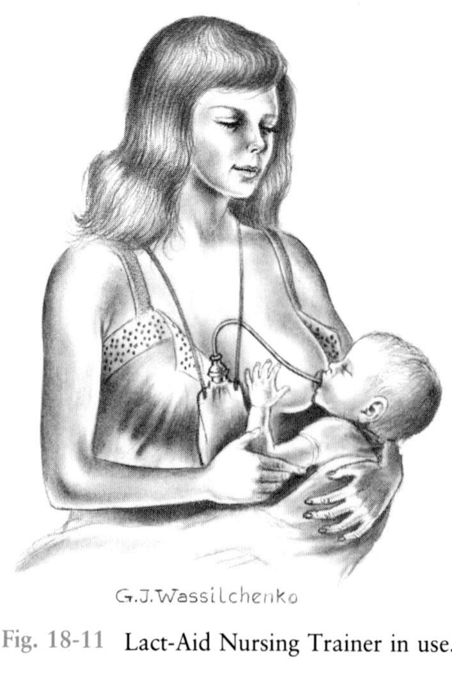

Fig. 18-11 Lact-Aid Nursing Trainer in use.

Table 18-4 Infant-related Concerns in the Initiation of Breastfeeding

Concern	Nursing Action
The infant does not open wide enough to grasp the nipple.	Help the mother depress the infant's lower jaw with one finger as she guides the nipple into the mouth.
The infant grasps the nipple and areolar tissue correctly but will not suck.	Help the mother *stimulate sucking motions* by pressing upward under the baby's chin. Expression of colostrum results, and the infant is stimulated by the taste to begin sucking.
The infant makes frantic rooting, mouthing motions but will not grasp the nipple and eventually begins to cry and stiffen her or his body in apparent frustration.	Help the mother interrupt the feeding, comfort the infant, and take time to relax herself, and then she may begin again.
The infant may suck for a few minutes and then fall asleep.	Help the mother interrupt the feeding and take time to *awaken the infant*. Stimulation may include loosening the wraps, holding the baby upright, talking to the baby, or gently rubbing her or his back or the soles of the feet. A sleepy infant will not nurse satisfactorily. If it is impossible to wake the baby, it is better to postpone the feeding.
The infant starts by sucking vigorously and, as the milk flows freely, develops a long, slow, rhythmic sucking. The sucking then changes to a short, rapid sucking with frequent rest periods. This behavior indicates a slowing of the flow of milk.	Help the mother massage the breasts toward the nipple. This starts the milk flowing freely again, and the infant will revert to the slow, rhythmic sucking. As soon as sucking resumes, the massage is discontinued so that the infant will not be overwhelmed and choked by the milk flowing too rapidly.

Contaminants in Maternal Milk. Nonnutrients enter human milk from the bloodstream of the lactating mother. Such compounds include environmental pollutants, nicotine, methadone, marijuana, caffeine, and alcohol (see Appendix H and Chapter 25). The distribution of a compound across the membrane between plasma and milk is influenced by its solubility in fat, its degree of ionization, its degree of protein binding, and active vs. passive transport.

Effect of Maternal Substance Abuse. Comments on advising substance abusers who choose to breastfeed are made in Chapter 25.

Substance abuse poses significant concern for the nursing infant. Regular use of *alcohol* is common in our society. However, during both pregnancy and lactation, even moderate drinking can pose problems for the unborn child or infant. *Smoking* by the lactating woman can cause a decrease in her milk supply. Another reason not to smoke is the second-hand smoke in the baby's atmosphere. This smoke can aggravate or even trigger asthma symptoms, and babies of parents who smoke have a higher incidence of lung disease. *Caffeine* should be taken in moderation by the breastfeeding mother. While only 1% of the mother's ingested caffeine passes through to the milk, the baby's immature system cannot get rid of the caffeine as effectively.

❑ FORMULA-FEEDING

Formula-feeding has proven a successful substitute for breastfeeding in certain instances. These include the following:

1. The family decides against breastfeeding or the mother is unable to breastfeed because of disease or anomalies.
2. The mother's schedule does not permit her to breastfeed.
3. Special formula is required because of infant allergies or special dietary needs.
4. Supplemental feedings are required.
5. The infant is adopted.

Formulas are recommended by physicians based on the infant's nutrition needs, cost, need for refrigeration, convenience, and the mother's ability to prepare the formula accurately and safely.

Inexperienced mothers who are formula-feeding their infants need the same teaching, counseling, and support as do the mothers who are breastfeeding. They need assistance with the feeding process and with problems they experience. Some mothers who elect formula-feeding express concern that the baby will suffer as a result of their decision. They need assurance that knowledge of their infant's nutrition needs and skill in use of formula-feeding can be an acceptable substitute for breastfeeding. Emphasis on the beneficial use of the feeding time for close contact with their infant can help relieve their tensions. Guidelines for client teaching regarding formula-feeding are presented on p. 539.

Care of Breasts. The breasts should be washed daily with clear water or a mild soap. A well-fitting brassiere provides needed support. During the early postpartum period, a tight binder, ice packs, and a mild analgesic may be necessary to relieve discomfort caused by pressure if the milk comes in. Nipple stimulation should be avoided. An antilactogenic medication (e.g., Parlodel) may be ordered to suppress lactation. Rebound production of milk infrequently occurs when the medication is discontinued (Chapter 21).

Diet and Fluids. A formula-feeding mother needs a well-balanced diet to restore maternal energy, provide protein for healing, and provide minerals and vitamins. An adequate fluid intake is important to maintain renal function and bowel regularity.

Infant Responses. Since cow's milk formula forms a larger curd, stomach emptying time is slower than with breast milk. Formula-fed babies eat every 3 to 5 hours. The physician provides instructions as to the amounts of formula to be fed the infant over 24 hours and when to increase the amounts to ensure meeting the growing infant's nutrition needs. Formula may be fed at room temperature or warmed until the milk feels warm when tested on the caregiver's inner arm. The infant may need extra water in warm weather.

Infants swallow more air when fed from a bottle and should be burped after every ½ to 1 ounce of formula. Unused formula should be discarded after a feeding. Bottles, nipples, water, and formula need not be sterilized unless the water is not safe.

The stools of formula-fed babies are firmer than those of breastfed babies and have a characteristic odor. Infants may have one to two stools per day. The diaper should be changed and the skin thoroughly cleaned to prevent irritation to the skin.

Formula Preparation

Hospitals today use commercially prepared formula. It comes prepackaged and can be stored at room temperature. Many parents elect to use similar brands. One consideration in the use of commercially prepared formulas is their cost. It is wise to advise parents to do comparison shopping, since one preparation can be considerably more expensive than another. Also there are a variety of bottles and nipples from which to choose.

Commercial Formulas. The Committee on Nutrition of the American Academy of Pediatrics proposed standards for infant formulas in 1976. Recommendations for minimum desirable concentrations of major nutrients were largely based on levels found in mature human milk.

Commercial formulas prepared from nonfat cow's milk are readily available and generally are used for feeding in early infancy. Most commercial formulas provide 20 kcal/oz. Several brands are marketed, with and without added iron. Commercial formulas supply all the known vitamins. Commercial formulas are also modified in one or more of the following ways:

1. Butterfat is removed and vegetable oils are added to increase the amount of unsaturated fatty acid, particularly linoleic acid, an essential fatty acid. This makes the cow's milk formula more like human milk in essential fatty acid content. Fat in this form is better digested by the infant.
2. Protein is treated to produce a softer, more flocculent curd that is more easily digested by the infant.
3. Protein and mineral concentrations are adjusted to more nearly resemble those in human milk. To achieve adequate levels of calories, sugar is added. This is usually in the form of lactose or corn syrup solids.

Most formulas are available in the following forms:

1. Concentrated: requires dilution with water
2. Ready-to-use (bulk): requires measuring into bottles
3. Ready-to-use (individual feedings): sold in disposable bottles; is generally the most expensive
4. Dry powder form: requires mixing with water according to label instructions; is least bulky and requires no refrigeration unless it is reconstituted well before the time it is to be served.

Instructions for mixing powdered or concentrated formulas should be followed accurately to prevent overdilution or underdilution. When formulas are underdiluted with water, the renal solute load is increased and may lead to dehydration of the infant. If overdilution occurs, inadequate calories and nutrients are provided, and failure to thrive may result. When the safety of the community or home water supply is in doubt, water sterilized by boiling for 15 minutes is recommended for diluting formulas and feeding the infant.

CAUTION: *Honey* is sometimes used as a sweetener for home-prepared infant foods or formula, and occasionally it is recommended for use on pacifiers to promote sucking in hypotonic babies. Use of honey for any of these purposes, however, is discouraged because some sources contain spores of *Clostridium botulinum* (Arnon et al, 1979; Whaley and Wong, 1991). These spores are extremely resistant to heat and therefore are not destroyed in the processing of honey. If ingested by an infant, spores may germinate, and lethal toxin may be released into the lumen of the bowel. Infant botu-

Guidelines for Client Teaching
FORMULA-FEEDING

ASSESSMENT

Sharon, age 17, delivered her daughter 6 hours ago. The newborn is a healthy term baby weighing 2912 g (6 ½ lb). The nurse fed the newborn (sterile water) initially at 2 hours of age. Her sucking and swallowing reflexes were normal. The mother is anxious about bottle-feeding her newborn. Up to now she has had no contact with newborns.

NURSING DIAGNOSES

Knowledge deficit related to bottle-feeding a newborn.
Anxiety, mild, related to being a new parent.

GOALS

Short-term

Sharon will bottle-feed her newborn successfully.

Intermediate

Sharon is able to assess the amount of feeding her daughter requires.
Sharon is able to prepare the formula.

Long-term

Sharon's awareness of her daughter's needs increases.

REFERENCES AND TEACHING AIDS

Posters, films, and hospital and commercial booklets from formula companies related to formula/bottle-feeding a newborn. Bottle, nipple; cork and needle.
Cans of formula; ready to feed, and that which has to be mixed with water.

RATIONALE/CONTENT	TEACHING ACTIONS
Knowledge and practice increase competence and self-confidence, therefore the nurse will review general content with the mother:	Give newborn to the mother to hold while the discussion goes on.
Newborn needs to be wide awake. These are hospital bottles of formula. They can be stored at room temperature. You may use this brand or the one your pediatrician recommends. They contain 4 oz of formula (120 ml). Your baby will probably drink 2 to 3 oz (60 to 90 ml) at a feeding for a few days and then increase. If you do not use all the formula, throw the remainder away, since it spoils once opened.	Show Sharon a sample bottle of formula.
You can keep track of how many ounces your daughter drinks in 1 day by writing it down. When you take her for a check-up, your physician or nurse will ask you the amount of intake.	Show Sharon how to note time and amount.
Your daughter will probably be hungry every 2½ to 3 hours. If she fusses or cries in between feedings, check her diaper or her need to be picked up and cuddled. As she gets older, she may be thirsty. Check with the pediatrician concerning water supplementation.	
Test the temperature of the formula by letting a few drops fall on the inside of your wrist. If the formula feels comfortably warm to you, it is the correct temperature. If the formula is refrigerated, warm it by placing the bottle in a pan of hot water. Check it often for correct temperature. *Do not use microwave oven.*	Shake a few drops of formula on Sharon's inside wrist. Dry her wrist with a facial tissue. Explain that microwaving may affect nutrient quality of milk and does cause "hot spots" in the fluid, which can burn the baby's mouth.
Test the size of the nipple hole by holding the bottle and nipple upside down. The formula should drip from the nipple. If it runs in a stream, the hole is too big. If it has to be shaken for the formula to come out, the hole is too small. To correct this you can try a softer nipple or enlarge the hole in the nipple or both. To enlarge hole, heat a needle stuck into a cork (used as a handle) and insert the hot needle into the nipple. New nipples may be softened by boiling for 5 minutes before using. If nipple collapses, unscrew bottle lid to let air in.	Demonstrate how to check nipple hole. Demonstrate with needle embedded in cork. Heat over match flame and enlarge the hole on the sample nipple.

Continued.

Guidelines for Client Teaching—cont'd

RATIONALE/CONTENT	TEACHING ACTIONS
Some newborns need burping. They tend to swallow air when sucking. Burp her before feeding, if she has been crying, then after every ounce of formula. As she gets older and you get more experienced, you will know when to burp her.	Show pictures of mother burping baby (see Fig. 18-6). Demonstrate burping technique with Sharon's baby.
To feed her, place the nipple in her mouth over her tongue. It should rest against the roof of her mouth. This stimulates sucking reflex.	Show Sharon picture (Fig. 18-12). Have her practice.
Hold the bottle like a pencil. Keep nipple filled with milk so she doesn't suck air.	Point out on picture (Fig. 18-12). Demonstrate.
Start out with her away from you until nipple is in her mouth. If she is too close, she will turn toward you and not the nipple; this is the rooting reflex.	Have Sharon hold her daughter away from herself.
After she starts feeding then you can hold her close.	Help Sharon start feeding.
Some newborns take longer to feed than others. Slow, patient feeding, keeping her awake and encouraging her to take more may be necessary.	Reassure Sharon that this is a characteristic of newborn feeding and not poor mothering.
The stools of a formula-fed newborn are soft but formed. They will be yellow with a characteristic odor. She will probably defecate either during the feeding or after. Change the diaper immediately since the composition of the stool is irritating to the skin.	Show picture of type of stool newborns will have once meconium has passed.
Knowledge regarding safety aids in prevention, therefore the nurse will review safety measures, including:	Use poster to show dangers. Ask Sharon to demonstrate what to do if newborn chokes. Place bulb syringe.
Don't prop the bottle, the nipple may fall against the throat and block the air, or she could drown in her formula or aspirate any that was regurgitated.	
Newborns should never be left alone while feeding until they are old enough to remove bottle from their mouth.	
Bottles taken to bed can lead to early dental problems in young children (baby bottle syndrome).	
Practice how to hold newborn and use the bulb syringe in case she should choke.	
After she is finished, place her in her crib on her right side so air can come up easily.	Check amount of formula for hospital record. Supervise burping the newborn. Show picture (Fig. 17-2).

EVALUATION Sharon demonstrates competence and skill in formula/bottle-feeding her daughter and asks appropriate questions.

lism may ultimately develop, and in some cases it is known to be fatal.

Home-prepared Formulas. Some parents wish to prepare their own formulas. Instruction in the preparation of formula includes methods for sterilizing and storing it. The guidelines for client teaching on formula-feeding can be used as an instruction guide to help the inexperienced mother.

The two traditional ways of **formula preparation** are the **terminal heating method** and the **aseptic method.** In the terminal heating method all the utensils and formula are boiled together for 25 minutes. In the aseptic method the equipment is boiled separately, after which the formula is poured into the bottles. Under improved sanitary conditions, neither of these methods is essential. The clean technique is satisfactory. The nurse must be aware when sanitation in any community warrants the use of a traditional method of formula preparation.

Recent recommendations for labeling commercial infant formulas require that the directions for preparation and use of the formula include pictures and symbols for nonreading individuals. In addition manufacturers are translating the directions into foreign languages, such as Spanish and Vietnamese, to prevent misunderstanding and errors in formula preparation. It

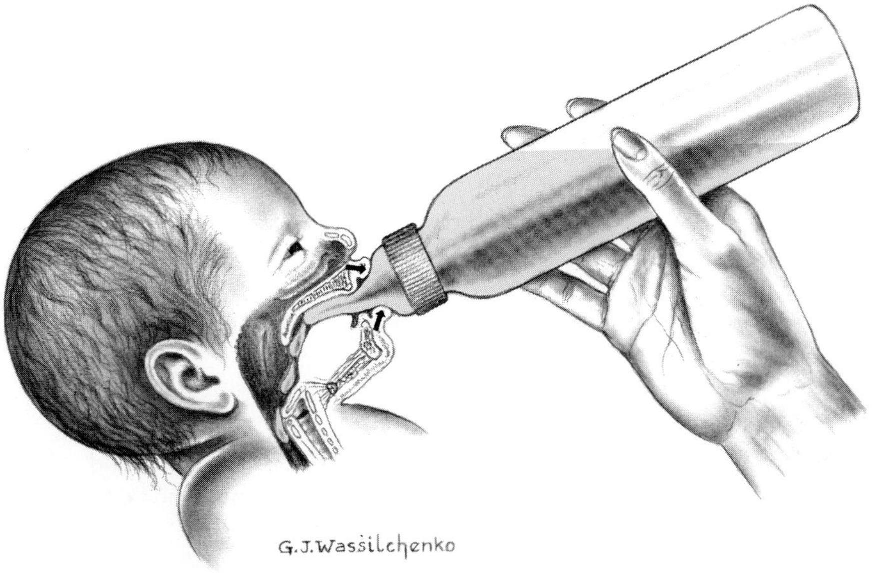

Fig. 18-12 Bottle-feeding. Bottle is held in hand like a pencil. Note milk covers nipple area so infant will not suck in air.

is important to impress upon families that the proportions *must not be altered*—neither diluted to extend the amount of formula nor concentrated to provide more calories (Whaley and Wong, 1991).

Mineral and Vitamin Supplementation

Shortly after birth, vitamin K is administered intramuscularly to prevent hemorrhagic disease of the newborn (Chapter 17). Normally, vitamin K is synthesized by the intestinal flora. However, since the infant's intestine is sterile at birth, and since breast milk contains low levels of vitamin K, the supply is inadequate for at least the first 3 to 4 days.

The normal infant receiving breast milk from a well-nourished mother needs no specific vitamin and mineral supplements, with the exceptions of fluoride in a dose of 0.25 mg daily (regardless of the fluoride content of the local water supply) and iron by 6 months of age (when fetal iron stores are depleted). Supplements of 400 IU of vitamin D daily may be indicated if the mother's vitamin D intake is inadequate or if the infant does not benefit from adequate ultraviolet light because of dark skin color or little exposure to light (American Academy of Pediatrics, 1980 a,b).

Milk from strict vegetarian mothers (those who include no animal products in their diet) may be too low in vitamin B_{12} to meet the infant's needs. These infants (and/or mothers) require a supplement (Specker et al, 1988). Like human milk, commercial iron-fortified formula supplies all the nutrients needed by the infant for the first 6 months. The only supplementation required is 0.25 mg of fluoride if the local water supply is not fluoridated or if the infant is given ready-to-feed formula, which eliminates the use of fluoridated tap water (American Academy of Pediatrics, Committee on Nutrition, 1986).

❑ DISCHARGE PLANNING

Anticipatory guidance can be given before the mother leaves the hospital or at the well baby checkups if the mother elects early discharge. Knowledge such as the following is helpful to the parent (Pyle, 1985).

Frequency of Feeding

During the daytime, awaken and feed the infant so that she or he is not sleeping more than 3 hours at a time. At night, let baby sleep and only feed if baby awakens. Make the night feedings businesslike so that baby learns that nights are not play time. At the beginning, most mothers prefer to take the baby to bed to breastfeed or formula-feed. Mothers also find that baby will sleep better if laid across her upper abdomen, so that baby hears her heartbeat and has the warm body contact.

Ideally for the newborn, feeding schedules are determined by the infant's hunger. Feeding infants when they signal readiness is called *demand feeding*. *Scheduled feedings* are arranged at predetermined intervals to meet family routines. The newborn will feed every

1½ to 3 hours during the daytime, and usually every 3 to 5 hours at night. Breastfed infants need to feed *at least every 3 hours* during the daytime. "Good" babies who rarely cry, sleep, and only awaken to nurse every 4 to 6 hours, usually do not have an adequate weight gain, and the mother may not maintain an adequate milk supply. Most babies will average 10 feedings during a 24-hour period. The following provides a guide for formula-fed infants' average intake of formula:

Age	Quantity per Feeding	Number of Feedings per 24 Hours
Birth to 3 weeks	2 to 3 oz (60-90 ml)	6 to 10
3 weeks to 2 months	5 oz (150 ml)	5 to 8
2 to 3 months	5 to 7 oz (150-210 ml)	5 to 6

Mothers will notice spurts in the infant's appetite between 10 days and 2 weeks; 6 weeks and 9 weeks; and 3 months and 6 months. These appetite spurts correspond to growth spurts. The infant wants to breastfeed more frequently and for longer periods. For the breastfeeding baby, increasing the feedings results in a greater production of milk. The satisfied infant then tapers off her or his demands. For the formula-fed baby, the amount of formula offered can be increased by 2 to 4 oz (60 to 120 ml).

Supplemental Feedings for Breastfed Babies

Supplemental feedings should *not* be offered to breastfed infants in the nursery because, if satiated, they will not suck vigorously at the breast (Whaley and Wong, 1991). Lactation depends on emptying the breast at each feeding. If milk is allowed to accumulate in the ducts, breast engorgement and ischemia result, suppressing the activity of the acini (milk-secreting cells). Consequently milk production is reduced. In addition, the process of sucking from a bottle is different from breast-nipple compression. The relatively inflexible rubber nipple prevents the tongue from its usual rhythmic action. Infants learn to put the tongue against the nipple holes to slow down the more rapid flow of fluid. When infants use these same tongue movements during breastfeeding, they may push the human nipple out of the mouth and may not grasp the areola properly (Lawrence, 1985).

Usually by 3 to 4 weeks of age, lactation is well established and a feeding schedule has been formed. Formula-fed infants ingest about 2 to 3 ounces of formula at each feeding and are fed about 6 times a day. Breastfed infants may feed as frequently as 10 to 12 times daily. Larger infants are able to retain increased amounts because of greater stomach capacity; as a result they generally sleep through the night sooner than smaller infants. After the milk supply is established, an occasional bottle will not affect lactation and breastfeeding.

Weaning. **Weaning** may take place because the infant has signified a desire to drink from a cup or because the mother will be absent. Some infants wean themselves, gradually refusing more and more feedings until only the early morning and night feedings are left. Others resist attempts to wean them, and mothers have to substitute other social times to compensate them for their loss. Ideally the process is a gradual one extending over several weeks.

Introducing Solid Foods. The infant receives the right balance of nutrients from breast milk or formula during the first 4 to 6 months (Broussard, 1984). It is not true that when solids are given it will help the baby sleep through the night. Introduction of solid foods before the infant is 4 to 6 months of age may result in overfeeding and decreased intake of breast milk or formula (Madgic, 1986). The infant cannot communicate feeling full like an older child can by turning her or his head away. The proper balance of carbohydrate, protein, and fat for an infant to grow properly is in breast milk or formula.

The infant's individual growth pattern should help determine the right time to start solids. The physician will advise when to introduce solid foods. The schedule for introducing solid foods and the types of foods to serve will be discussed during well-baby supervision visits with the pediatrician and pediatric nurse (American Academy of Pediatrics, 1980 b, 1983 a, b).

Referrals. Referral procedures provide an opportunity for individuals and groups to take advantage of services available from other sources. A properly coordinated health service delivery for infants and children that includes a registered dietitian can contribute to a sense of continuity and to consistency of care and advice. The mother is encouraged to contact the local association that assists with breastfeeding (Appendix I).

Evaluation

The process of evaluation is continuous. As the infant matures, the norms for nutritional intake are adjusted to meet growth needs. The criteria are measurable in terms of the infant's growth, energy levels, and appearance. Parental knowledge is a key factor in infant nutrition and feeding. Parental knowledge and infant well-being and the findings that represent normal response form the basis for selecting appropriate nursing actions and evaluating their effectiveness.

SUMMARY

Providing nutrition services to parents and their infants and assistance with feeding is a function of the health care team. Physicians, nurses, registered dietitians, social workers, and health educators are major contributors to the care. One of the most important contributors, the nurse, can assist with nutrition assessment and provide education and counseling. Nurses can help interpret dietary prescriptions and make appropriate referrals of more complicated problems to nutritional personnel. Nurses can provide needed teaching and support in the early postpartum period when feeding is being established.

LEARNING ACTIVITIES

1. Teach a new mothers class on breastfeeding, including:
   a. Technique
   b. Care of breasts
   c. Common problems and treatments

   Use charts or visual aids when appropriate.
2. Prepare a nutritional diary for an infant. Describe factors that may be problem areas and develop a counseling plan to meet the needs of the infant and mother.
3. Conduct a group discussion of feelings and cultural conditioning regarding breastfeeding. At a later meeting, ask a lecturer from the LaLeche League or a similar support group to speak, and follow the presentation with another discussion of how or why your feelings have or have not changed on the subject.
4. Observe new mothers breast-feed and formula-feed their infants. Report on the clients' responses and any prejudices expressed and observe for the interaction between mother and baby.
5. Research vegetarian diets. Bring findings to a discussion of the influence of such diets on the nutrition of a breastfed infant.

KEY CONCEPTS

- Healthy term babies are developmentally ready for feeding.
- Teaching and counseling concerning the feeding of infants are important aspects of the daily care plan for maternity clients.
- The mother (parent) is presented with the benefits of both breastfeeding and formula-feeding as a basis for decision making.
- Feeding is an emotionally charged area of infant care.
- Most parents benefit from teaching related to chosen method of feeding.
- The attitude of the mother (and spouse) toward breastfeeding is a powerful factor in achieving successful lactation.
- The size of the breast gives no indication of its functional capacity.
- Limiting of breastfeeding time does not prevent nipple soreness.
- The composition and characteristics of commercial formulas are based on those of mature human milk.
- Use of honey in home-prepared formulas can be fatal in some cases; parents should be warned.
- Unmodified cow's milk is not suitable for infants less than 6 months of age, and 2% or skim milk is unsuitable for infants less than 12 months of age.

References

American Academy of Pediatrics, Committee on Nutrition: Commentary on breast-feeding and infant formulas, including proposed standards for formulas, Pediatrics 57:278, 1976.

American Academy of Pediatrics, Committee on Nutrition: Vitamin and mineral supplement needs in normal children in the United States, Pediatrics 66(6):1015, 1980a.

American Academy of Pediatrics, Committee on Nutrition: On the feeding of supplemental foods to infants, Pediatrics 65(6):1178, 1980b.

American Academy of Pediatrics, Committee on Nutrition: The use of whole cow's milk in infancy, Pediatrics 72(2):253, 1983a.

American Academy of Pediatrics, Committee on Nutrition: Toward a prudent diet for children, Pediatrics 71(1):78, 1983b.

American Academy of Pediatrics, Committee on Nutrition: Imitation and substitute milks, Pediatrics 73(6):876, 1984.

American Academy of Pediatrics, Committee on Nutrition: Fluoride supplementation, Pediatrics 77:758, 1986.

Arnon SS et al: Honey and other environmental risk factors for infant botulism, J Pediatr 95:331, 1979.

Blume S et al: Beer and breast-feeding mom, JAMA 258(15):2126, 1987.

Borovies D: Assessing and managing pain in breast-feeding mothers, MCN 9:272, 1984.

Broussard A: Anticipatory guidance: adding solids to the infant's diet, JOGN Nurs 13:239, 1984.

Chapman J et al: Concerns of breast-feeding mothers from birth to 4 months, Nurs Res 34:374, 1985.

Chung HJ: Understanding the Oriental maternity patient, Nurs Clin North Am 12:67, 1977.

Currier RL: The hot-cold syndrome and symbolic balance in Mexican and Spanish-American folk medicine. In Martinez RA, editor: Hispanic culture and health care: fact, fiction, folklore, St Louis, 1978, The CV Mosby Co.

David R et al: Water intoxication in normal infants: role of antidiuretic hormone in pathogenesis, Pediatrics 68:349, 1981.

Food and Nutrition Board: Recommended dietary allowances, Washington, DC, 1980, National Academy of Sciences.

Greene HL and Ghishan FK: Excessive fluid intake as a cause of chronic diarrhea of young children, J Pediatr 102:836, 1983.

Hamill PVV et al: Physical growth: national center for health statistics percentiles, Am J Clin Nutr 32:607, 1979 (data from the Fels Research Institute, Wright State University School of Medicine, Yellow Springs, Ohio).

Hanson LA et al: Protective factors in milk and the development of the immune system, Pediatrics 75(suppl):172, 1985.

Hart DV: From pregnancy through birth in a Bisavan Filipino village. In Hart DV, Rajadhon PA, and Coughlin RJ, editors: Southeast Asian birth customs: three studies in reproduction, New Haven, Conn, 1965, Human Relations Area Files.

Hughes R: Satisfaction with one's body and success in breast feeding, Issues in Comprehensive Pediatric Nursing 7:141, 1984.

LaDu EB: Childbirth care for Hmong families, Am J Mat Child Nurs 10:382, 1985.

Lawrence R: Breast-feeding: a guide for the medical profession, ed 2, St Louis, 1985, The CV Mosby Co.

L'Esperance C and Frantz K: Time limitation for early breast-feeding JOGN Nurs 14(2):114, 1985.

Madgic D: Nutrition notes for new mothers, Stanford, Calif, 1986, Department of Dietetics, Stanford University Hospital.

MacLauglin S and Strelnick E: Breastfeeding and working outside the home, Issues in Comprehensive Pediatric Nursing 7:67, 1984.

Owen AL et al: Infant feeding guide, Bloomfield, NJ, 1980, Health Learning System.

Partridge JC et al: Water intoxication secondary to feeding mismanagement, Am J Dis Child 135:38, 1981.

Price A and Bamford N: The breast feeding guide for the working woman, New York, 1983, Simon and Schuster.

Pyle M: Breast feeding is a family affair, Costa Mesa, Calif, 1985, Lifecircle.

Riordan J: A practical guide to breastfeeding, St Louis, 1983, The CV Mosby Co.

Saarinen UM, Siimes MA, and Dallman PR: Iron absorption in infants: high bioavailability of breast milk iron as indicated by the extrinsic tag method of iron absorption and by the concentration of serum ferritin, J Pediatr 91:36, 1977.

Shutler ME: Disease and curing in a Yaqui community. In Spicer EH, editor: Ethnic medicine in the Southwest, Tucson, Ariz, 1977, The University of Arizona Press.

Slaven S: Unlimited sucking time improves breastfeeding, Lancet 8216:392, 1981.

Specker BL et al: Increased urinary methylmalonic acid excretion in breast-fed infants of vegetarian mothers and identification of an acceptable dietary source of vitamin B_{12}, Am J Clin Nutr 47:89, 1988.

Ward BG et al: Vietnamese refugees in Adelaide: an obstetric analysis, Med J Aust 1:72, 1981.

Whaley LF and Wong DL: Nursing care of infants and children, ed 4, St Louis, 1991, The CV Mosby Co.

Williams SR: Nutrition and diet therapy, ed 6, St Louis, 1989, The CV Mosby Co.

Bibliography

Aberman S et al: Infant feeding practices, mother's decision-making, JOGN Nurs 14:394, Sept/Oct, 1985.

Anderson GC: Pacifiers: the positive side, MCN 11:122, 1986.

Balkam JA: Guidelines for drug therapy during lactation, JOGN Nurs 15(1):65, 1986.

Breastfeeding Your Twins, 1984, *Health* Education Associates, 520 School House Lane, Willow Grove, PA 09190.

Chase HP et al: Kwashiorkor in the United States, Pediatrics 66:972, 1980.

Dilts CL: Nursing management of mastitis due to breastfeeding, JOGN Nurs 14(4):286, 1985.

Evans CJ, Lyons NB, and Killien MG: The effect of infant formula samples on breastfeeding practice, JOGN Nurs 15(5):401, 1986.

Frank DA et al: Commercial discharge packs and breastfeeding counseling: effects on infant-feeding practices in a randomized trial, Pediatrics 80:845, 1987.

Gaull GE, Wright CE, and Isaacs CE: Significance of growth modulators in human milk, Pediatrics 75(suppl):142, 1985.

Hughes RB et al: Outcome of teaching clean vs. terminal methods of formula preparation, Pediatr Nurs 13(4):275, 1987.

Jordan PL: Breastfeeding as a risk factor for fathers, JOGN Nurs 15(2):94, 1986.

Kearney MH: Identifying psychosocial obstacles to breastfeeding success, JOGN Nurs 17(2):98, 1988.
Lauwers J and Woessner C: Pain—more than discomfort to breastfeeding women, Int J Childbirth Ed 2(2):30, 1987.
Martone DJ et al: Initial differences in postpartum attachment behavior in breastfeeding and bottlefeeding mothers, JOGN Nurs 17:212, 1988.
McKay S and Mahan C: Ways to upgrade postpartal care, Contemp OB/GYN 27:6:63, Nov, 1985.
Menchin M: Infant formula: a mass, uncontrolled trial in perinatal care . . . claims of nutritional adequacy, Birth 14:25, 1987.
Morse JM et al: Minimal breastfeeding, JOGN Nurs 15:333, 1986.
Morse JM et al: Leaking: a problem of lactation, J Nurse Midwife 34:15, 1989.
Niebyl JR: Making the breastfeeding decision, Contemp OB/GYN 28(3):43, 1986.
Pittard WB, III, et al: Bacteriostatic qualities of human milk, J Pediatr 107(2):240, 1985.
Ream S et al: Infant nutrition and supplements, JOGN Nurs 14:371, 1985.
Reiff MI and Essock-Vitale SM: Hospital influences on early infant-feeding practices, Pediatrics 76(6):872, 1985.
Reifsnider E and Myers ST: Employed mothers can breastfeed too! MCN 10(4):256, 1985.
Schafer O: The impact of culture on breastfeeding patterns, J Perinat 6(1):62, 1986.
Virden SF: The relationship between infant feeding method and maternal role adjustment, J Nurse Midwife 33:31, 1988.
Walker M: How to evaluate breast pumps, MCN 12(4):270, 1987.
Williams SR: Basic nutrition and diet therapy, ed 8, St Louis, 1988, The CV Mosby Co.
Wolf DM and Coachman-Moore VE: The consulting nutritionist in perinatal health care, J Perinat 6:335, 1986.
Wong S, and Stepp-Gilbert, E: Lactation suppression: nonpharmaceutical versus pharmaceutical method, JOGN Nurs 14:302, 1985.
Worthington-Roberts B and Williams SR: Nutrition in pregnancy and lactation, ed 4, St Louis, 1989, Times Mirror/Mosby College Publishing.
Zinaman MJ: Breast pumps: ensuring mothers' success, Contemp OB/GYN, 30:Oct, 1987 (special issue).

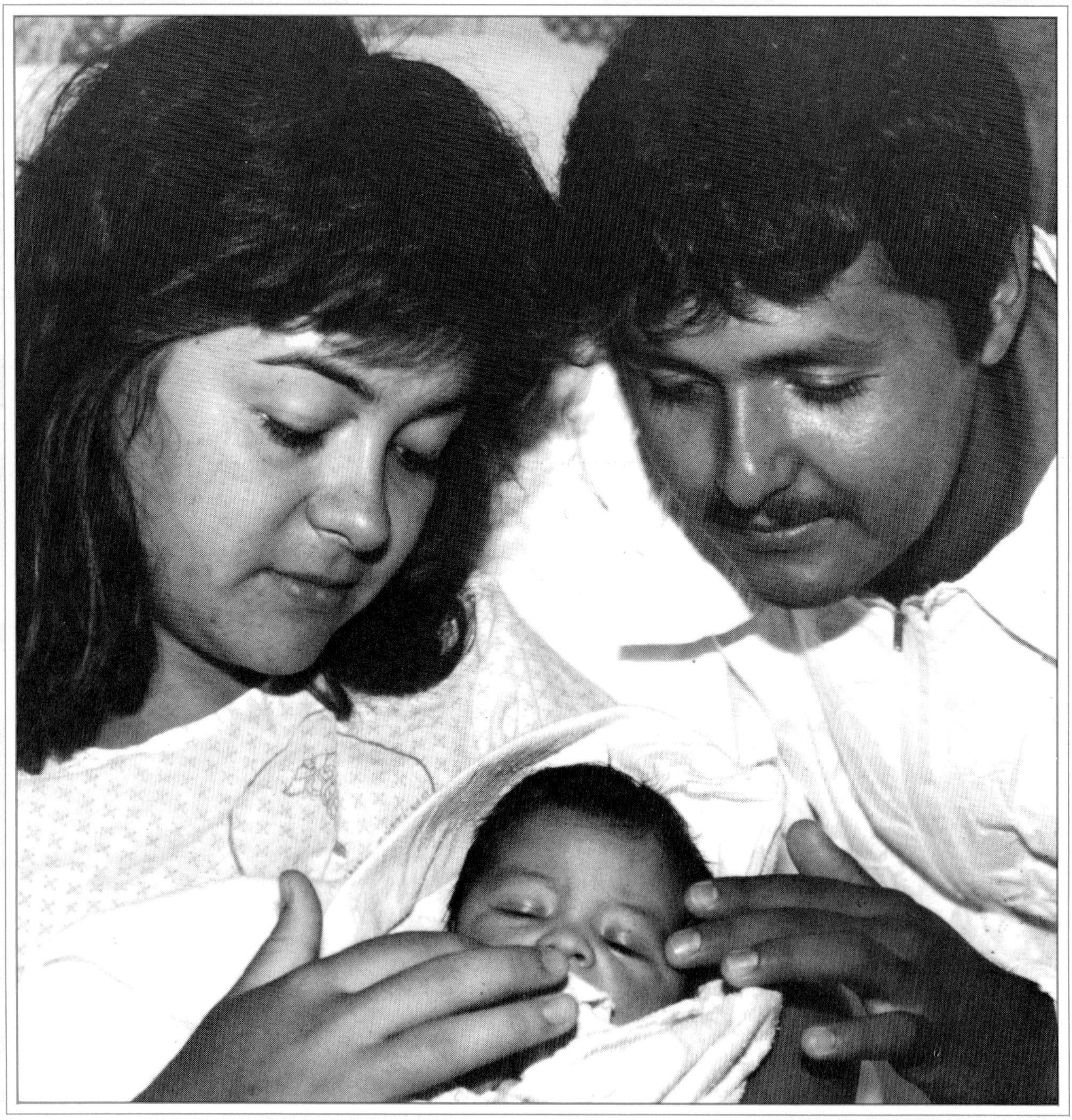

UNIT

V

NORMAL POSTPARTUM PERIOD

CHAPTER

19 Maternal Physiology During the Postpartum Period

Deitra Leonard Lowdermilk

Learning Objectives

Correctly define the key terms listed.

Identify characteristics and measurement of normal uterine involution and lochia.

Describe maternal anatomic and physiologic changes during the postpartum recovery and return to the nonpregnant state.

Recognize expected values for vital signs and blood pressure, deviations from normal findings, and probable causes.

Key Terms

adynamic ileus
afterpains
anovulatory cycle
bradycardia
colostrum
diaphoresis
diastasis recti abdominis
diuresis
engorgement (breast)
fourth trimester
hemorrhoids
human placental lactogen (hPL)
involution
lochia: rubra, serosa, alba
oxytocic medication
prolactin
puerperium (early and late)
thromboembolism

The postpartum period is the six-week interval between the delivery of the newborn and the return of the reproductive organs to their normal nonpregnant state. This period is commonly referred to as the **fourth trimester** of pregnancy. The physiologic changes that occur are distinctive, although considered normal as the processes of pregnancy are reversed. Many factors, including energy level, degree of comfort, health of the newborn, and care and encouragement given by the health professionals, contribute to the mother's response to her infant during this time. To provide care beneficial to the mother, her infant, and her family, the nurse must synthesize knowledge from maternal anatomy and physiology of the recovery period, the newborn's physical and behavioral characteristics, infant care activities, and family response to the birth of the child. In short, the nurse must use a holistic approach to nursing care. This chapter focuses on anatomic and physiologic changes of the woman after delivery.

❏ REPRODUCTIVE SYSTEM AND ASSOCIATED STRUCTURES

Uterine Involution

At the end of the third stage of labor the uterus is in the midline, about 2 cm *below* the level of the umbilicus with the fundus resting on the sacral promontory. At this time, uterine size approximates the size at 16 weeks of gestation (about the size of a grapefruit). The uterus is about 14 cm (5½ in) long, 12 cm (4¾ in) wide, and 10 cm (4 in) thick and weighs about 1000 g (2 lb). When relaxed, the uterus is discoid; when contracted, it is globular.

Within 12 hours the fundus may be approximately 1 cm *above* the umbilicus (Fig. 19-1). From then on, **involution** progresses rapidly, and with the improved tone of the uterine supports, the fundus descends about 1 to 2 cm every 24 hours. By the sixth postpartum day the fundus normally will be half the distance from the symphysis pubis to the umbilicus. The uterus should not be palpable abdominally after the ninth postpartum day.

The uterus, which at full term weighs about 11 times its prepregnant weight, rapidly involutes to about 500 g (1 lb) 1 week after delivery and 350 g (11 to 12 oz) 2 weeks after delivery. A week after delivery the

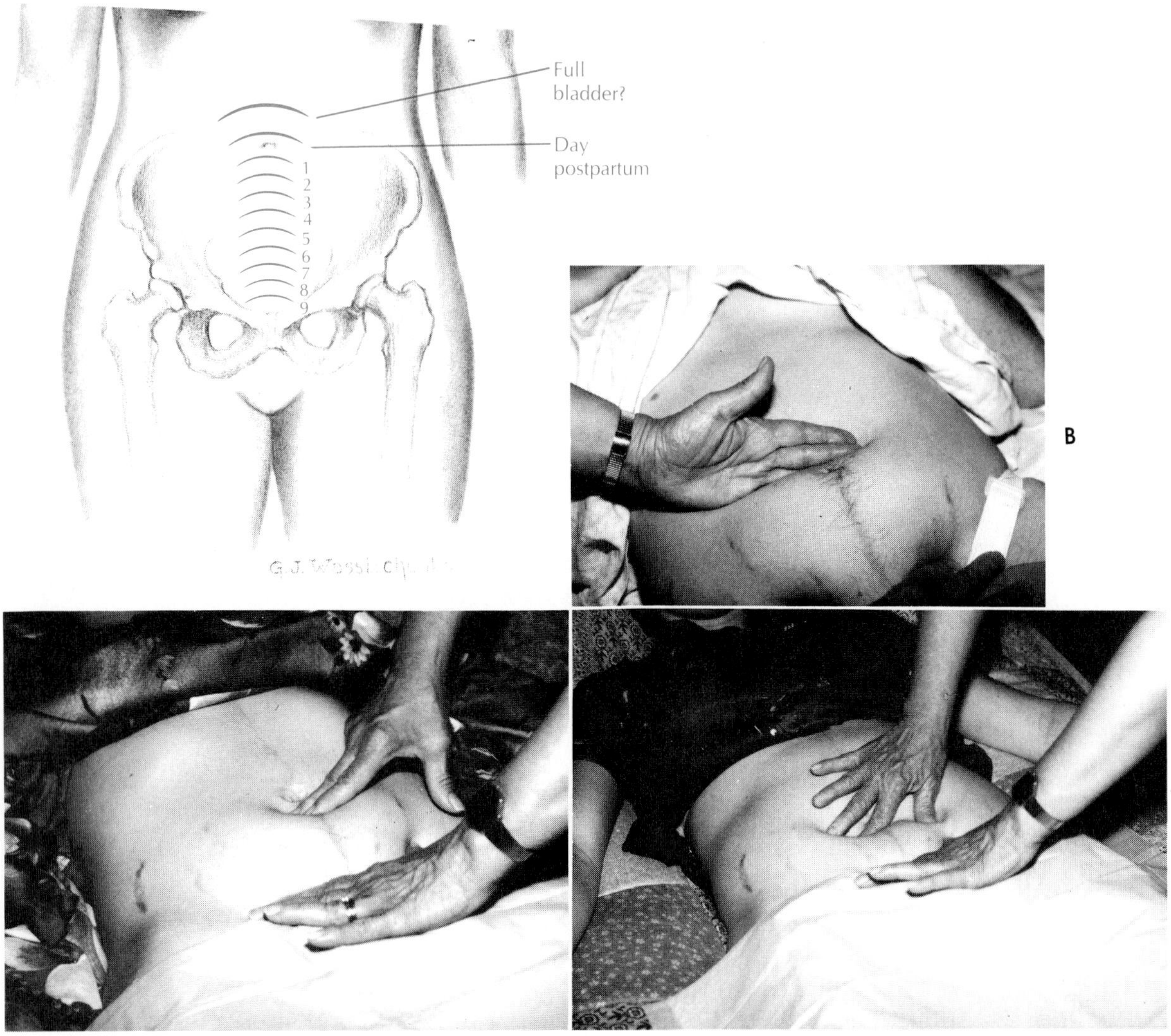

Fig. 19-1 Assessment of involution of uterus after delivery. **A,** Normal progress, days 1 through 9. **B,** Size and position of uterus 2 hours after delivery. **C,** 2 days after delivery. **D,** 4 days after delivery. (**B, C,** and **D** Courtesy Marjorie Pyle, RNC, Lifecircle, Costa Mesa, Calif.)

uterus lies in the true pelvis once again. At 6 weeks it weighs 50 to 60 g (Figs. 19-1 and 19-2).

The level of estrogen, which stimulated myometrial growth, and the level of progesterone, which was responsible for much of the increased uterine weight and collagen formation during gestation, drop rapidly after delivery. Uterine involution within 4 to 6 weeks occurs principally by a decrease in the size of individual myometrial cells. However, the augmentation of connective tissue and elastin in the myometrium and blood vessels and the increase in the total uterine cell number are permanent. Hence uterine size is increased slightly after each pregnancy.

Uterine Contractions

The intensity of uterine contractions increases significantly immediately after delivery, presumably in response to the greatly diminished intrauterine volume. During the first 1 to 2 postpartum hours, uterine activity decreases smoothly and progressively and stabilizes. Uterine contractions become uncoordinated unless coordination is reestablished with exogenous (injected) oxytocin or endogenous oxytocin (released in response to nipple stimulation from suckling, for example). Uterine myometrial activity contributes to hemostasis by compressing the intramural blood vessels.

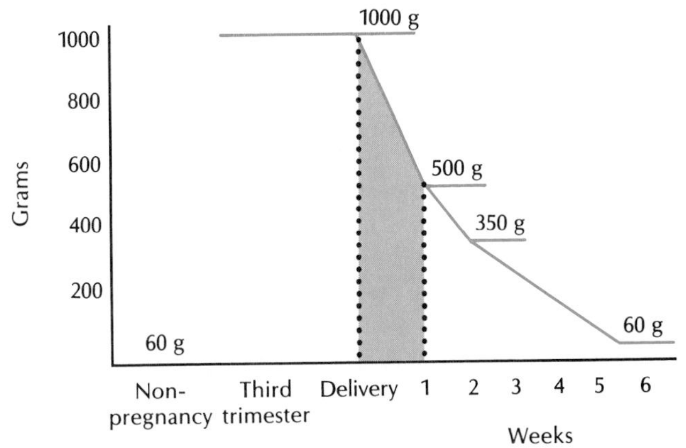

Fig. 19-2 Uterine weight before, during, and after pregnancy. Greatest change is in first week after childbirth. (Redrawn from Wiggins JD: Childbearing: physiology, experiences, needs, St Louis, 1979, The CV Mosby Co.)

Afterpains

In primiparas the tone of the uterus is increased so that the fundus generally remains firm. Periodic relaxation and contraction are more common for multiparas and may cause uncomfortable **afterpains** that persist throughout the **early puerperium.** Afterpains are more noticeable after deliveries where the uterus was overdistended (e.g., large baby, twins). Breastfeeding usually intensifies these afterpains because oxytocin is released by the posterior pituitary gland in response to nipple stimulation. Increased intensity also may occur after administration of **oxytocic medication.**

Placental Site

Immediately after the placenta and membranes are delivered, the placental site is elevated, irregular, and partially obliterated by vascular constriction and thrombosis. Upward growth of the endometrium prevents scar formation that is characteristic of normal wound healing. This unique healing process enables the endometrium to resume its usual cycle of changes and to permit implantation and placentation in future pregnancies. Endometrial regeneration is completed by the end of the third postpartum week except at the placental site. Regeneration at the placental site usually is not complete until 6 weeks after delivery.

Failure of the placental site to heal completely is called *subinvolution* of the placental site (Chapter 23). Women with this condition have persistent lochia and episodes of brisk, painless bleeding. Curettage usually is required.

Lochia

Postdelivery uterine discharge initially is bright red, changing to dark red or reddish brown; it may contain small clots. Lochia refers only to uterine discharge. The blood seen on the peripad or bed linens may be from a different source (Table 19-1). Regardless of the source of bleeding, if the peripad is soaked through in 15 minutes or less, the flow is considered excessive.

Lochia rubra consists mainly of blood, and decidual and trophoblastic debris. The flow pales, becoming pink or brown after 3 to 4 days (lochia serosa). **Lochia serosa** consists of old blood, serum, leukocytes, and tissue debris. About 10 days after delivery, the drainage becomes yellow to white (lochia alba). **Lochia alba** consists of numerous leukocytes, decidua, epithelial cells, mucus, serum, and bacteria. Lochia alba may continue until about 2 to 6 weeks after delivery.

The amount of lochia is described as scant, light, moderate, and heavy (Jacobson, 1985):

scant Blood only on tissue when wiped or less than 2.5 cm (1 in) on a peripad (see Fig. 15-37).
light Less than 10 cm (4 in) stain on a peripad.
moderate Less than 15 cm (6 in) stain on peripad.
heavy Saturated peripad within 1 hour.

If the woman receives an oxytocic medication, regardless of the route of administration, the flow of lochia is usually scant until the effects of the medication wear off. Flow of lochia usually increases with ambulation and breastfeeding. After lying in bed for a prolonged period, the woman may experience a gush of blood upon standing, which is not to be confused with hemorrhage.

Table 19-1 **Lochia and Nonlochia Bleeding**

Lochia	Nonlochia Bleeding
Lochia usually trickles from the vaginal opening. The steady flow is greater as the uterus contracts.	If the bloody discharge spurts from the vagina, there may be cervical or vaginal tears in addition to the normal lochia.
A gush of lochia may result as the uterus is massaged. If it is dark in color, it has been pooled in the relaxed vagina, and the amount soon lessens to a trickle of bright red lochia (in the early puerperium).	If the amount of bleeding continues to be excessive and bright red, a tear may be the source.

Persistence of lochia rubra early in the postpartum period suggests continued bleeding as a result of retained fragments of the placenta or membranes. Recurrence of bleeding about 10 days after delivery indicates bleeding from the placental site, which is healing. However, after 3 to 4 weeks bleeding may be caused by infection or subinvolution of the placental site. Continued lochia serosa or lochia alba may indicate endometritis, particularly if fever, pain, or tenderness is associated with the discharge. Lochia should smell like normal menstrual flow; an offensive odor usually indicates infection (Chapter 23).

Cervix

The cervix up to the lower uterine segment remains edematous, thin, and fragile for several days after delivery. The ectocervix (portion of the cervix that protrudes into the vagina) is soft, appears bruised, and has some small lacerations—optimum conditions for the development of infection. The cervical os, dilated to 10 cm during labor, closes gradually. Two fingers may still be introduced into the cervical os for the first 4 to 6 days after delivery; however, only the smallest curette may be introduced by the end of 2 weeks. By the eighteenth hour the cervix has shortened, has a firm consistency, and has regained its form. By the end of the first week, recovery is almost complete. The external os, however, does not regain its prepregnant appearance; it is no longer shaped like a circle but appears as a jagged slit often described as "fish mouth" (see Fig. 8-6). Production of cervical and other estrogen-influenced mucus and mucosal characteristics may be delayed in the lactating woman.

Vagina and Perineum

Postpartum estrogen deprivation is responsible for the thinness of the *vaginal mucosa* and the absence of rugae. The greatly distended, smooth-walled vagina gradually returns to its nonpregnant size by 6 to 8 weeks after delivery. Rugae reappear by about the fourth week, although they are never as prominent as they are in the nulliparous woman. Most rugae may be permanently flattened. The mucosa remains atrophic in the lactating woman at least until menstruation begins again. Thickening of the vaginal mucosa occurs with the return of ovarian function. Profuse vaginal discharge is usually not present at 4 to 6 weeks after delivery unless there is an associated vaginitis. The estrogen deficiency is responsible for the decreased amount of vaginal lubrication and thinner vaginal mucosa. Localized dryness and coital discomfort (dyspareunia) may persist until ovarian function returns and menstruation resumes. Use of a water-soluble lubricant during intercourse is usually recommended, since it is helpful in reducing discomfort.

Initially the *introitus* is erythematous and edematous, especially in the area of the episiotomy or laceration repair. Careful repair, prevention or early treatment of hematomas, and good hygiene during the first 2 weeks after delivery usually result in an introitus barely distinguishable from that of a nulliparous woman.

Most *episiotomies* are visible only if the woman is lying on her side and her buttock is raised. A good light source is essential for visualization of some episiotomies. The healing process of an episiotomy is the same as for any surgical incision. Signs of infection (pain, redness, warmth, swelling, or discharge) or loss of approximation (separation) of the incision edges may occur.

Hemorrhoids (anal varicosities) are commonly seen. The women often experience associated symptoms such as itching, discomfort, and bright red bleeding with defecation.

Pelvic Muscular Support

Injury of the supporting structures of the uterus and vagina may occur during childbirth and may become gynecologic problems later in life. The term *relaxation* refers to the lengthening and weakening of the fascial supports of pelvic structures. These include the uterus, upper posterior vaginal wall, urethra, bladder, and rectum. Although relaxations can occur in any woman, most are direct but delayed complications to childbirth.

Abdominal Wall

When the woman stands up during the first days after delivery, abdominal muscles cannot retain abdominal contents. The abdomen protrudes and gives the woman a still-pregnant appearance (Fig. 19-3). During the first 2 weeks after delivery, the abdominal wall is relaxed. About 6 weeks are required before the abdominal wall returns to its nonparous state. The skin regains most of its previous elasticity, but some striae persist. The return of muscle tone depends on previous tone, proper exercise, and amount of adipose tissue. On occasion, with or without overdistension because of a large fetus or multiple fetuses, the abdominal wall muscles separate, a condition termed **diastasis recti abdominis** (see Fig. 8-11). Persistence of this defect may be disturbing to the woman, but surgical correction is rarely necessary. With time, the defect becomes less apparent.

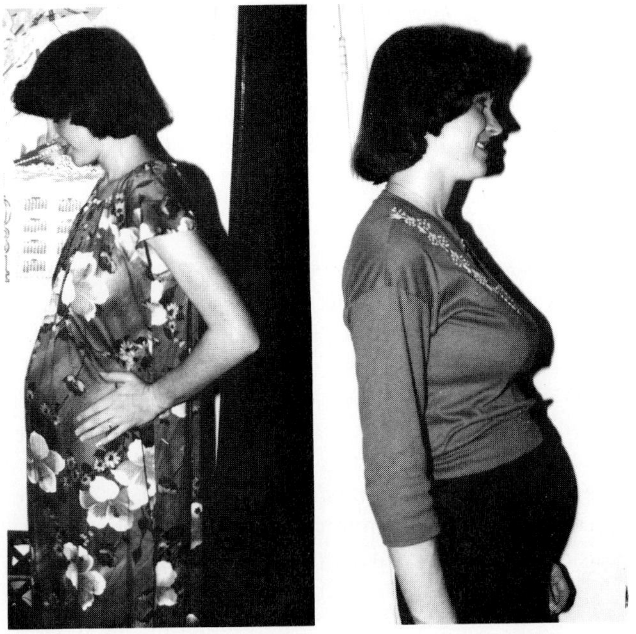

Fig. 19-3 Abdomen after delivery. **A,** Two hours after delivery. **B,** Eight days after delivery. (Courtesy Marjorie Pyle, RNC, Lifecircle, Costa Mesa, Calif.)

Breasts

The concentrations of hormones that stimulated breast development during pregnancy (estrogen, progesterone, human chorionic gonadotropin, prolactin, cortisol, and insulin) decrease promptly after delivery. The time it takes for the return of these hormones to prepregnancy levels is determined in part by whether the mother breastfeeds her infant.

Nonbreastfeeding Mothers. The breasts feel generally nodular (in nonpregnant women they feel granular). The nodularity is bilateral and diffuse.

If the woman chooses not to breastfeed and no antilactogenic medication is taken, prolactin levels drop rapidly. **Colostrum** secretion and excretion persist for the first few days after delivery. Palpation of the breast on the second or third day, as milk production begins, may reveal tissue tenderness in some women. On the third or fourth postpartum day, **engorgement** of the breasts may occur. They are distended (swollen), firm, tender, and warm to the touch (vasocongestion makes them feel warm). Milk can be expressed from the nipples. Axillary breast tissue (the tail of Spence) and any accessory breast or nipple tissue along the milk line may be involved. Breast distension is primarily caused by temporary congestion of veins and lymphatics rather than from an accumulation of milk. Engorgement resolves spontaneously, and discomfort decreases usually within 24 to 36 hours. If suckling is never begun (or is discontinued), lactation ceases within a few days to a week.

Breastfeeding Mothers. As lactation is established, a mass (lump) may be felt; however, a filled milk sac will shift position from day to day. Before lactation begins, the breasts feel soft and a yellowish fluid, colostrum, can be expressed from the nipples. After lactation begins, the breasts feel warm to the touch and firm. Tenderness persists for about 48 hours. Bluish white milk (skim-milk appearance) can be expressed from the nipples. The nipples are examined for erectility as opposed to inversion and for cracks or fissures.

For a discussion of breast changes associated with lactation, see Chapter 18.

❑ ENDOCRINE SYSTEM

Numerous changes occur in the endocrine system during the puerperium. These changes are summarized in Table 19-2.

Placental Hormones

Plasma levels of placental hormones fall rapidly after delivery. **Human placental lactogen (hPL)** levels reach undetectable levels within 24 hours (see also discussions of growth hormone and carbohydrate metabolism). *Human chorionic gonadotropin* (hCG) declines rapidly and remains low until ovulation occurs.

Estrogen levels in plasma fall to 10% of the prenatal value within 3 hours after delivery; the lowest levels occur about day 7. The significant decline in estrogen is

Table 19-2 **Endocrine Changes in the Puerperium**

Hormone	Change Lowest Level
Human placental lactogen (hPL)	Decreases <24 hours
Estrogen	Decreases Day 7
Progesterone	Decreases Day 7
Follicle-stimulating hormone (FSH)	Decreases Day 10-12
Luteinizing hormone (LH)	Decreases Day 10-12
Prolactin	Decreases Day 14
Growth hormone	Stays low through day 3
Thyroid	No change
Corticosteroids	Decreases Day 7
Plasma renin	Decreases <2 hours
Angiotensin II	Decreases <2 hours

accompanied by the onset of breast engorgement on about postpartum day 3. Plasma levels of estrogen do not increase to follicular levels until 19 to 21 days after delivery. In lactating women, return to normal estrogen levels is somewhat delayed.

Progesterone levels in plasma fall below luteal levels by the third postpartum day and cannot be detected in serum after the first postdelivery week. Progesterone production begins with the first ovulation.

Pituitary Hormones

Prolactin levels in blood rise progressively throughout pregnancy. After delivery, in nonlactating women, prolactin levels decline, reaching the prepregnant range within 2 weeks. Initially, suckling and lactation are accompanied by dramatic increases in prolactin concentration. Serum prolactin levels are influenced by the number of times per day breastfeeding occurs. Normal basal values of prolactin are reached by 6 months if breastfeeding occurs only 1 to 3 times per day. High prolactin levels persist for more than a year if suckling occurs more than 6 times per day.

Levels of *follicle-stimulating hormone* (FSH) and *luteinizing hormone* (LH) are low in all women for 10 to 12 days after delivery. FSH levels rise to follicular phase concentration by the third postpartum week, while LH levels remain low until after ovulation occurs.

Hypothalamic-Pituitary-Ovarian Function

Little is known about the physiology of the hypothalamus, the pituitary gland, and the ovaries during the puerperium after term gestation. The exact nature of the changing endocrine function is unclear at this time (Scott et al, 1990). However, considerable information is available on the time of appearance of the first ovulation and the reestablishment of menstruation for lactating and nonlactating women. For all women, the first menses *usually* follows an **anovulatory cycle** or a cycle associated with inadequate corpus luteum function (low LH and progesterone).

Among lactating women, 15% have resumed menstruation by 6 weeks, and 45% by 12 weeks. Among nonlactating women, 40% menstruate by 6 weeks, 65% by 12 weeks, and 90% by 24 weeks. For lactating women, 80% of first menstrual cycles are anovulatory; for nonlactating women 50% of first cycles are anovulatory (Scott et al, 1990).

Much of the variability in the reestablishment of menstruation and ovulation observed in lactating women may result from individual differences in the strength of the infant's suckling stimulus and the number of feedings per day. This emphasizes the fact that *breastfeeding is not a reliable form of birth control.*

The first menstrual flow is usually heavier than normal. Within 3 to 4 cycles the amount of menstrual flow has returned to the woman's prepregnant volume.

Other Endocrine Changes

Growth hormone secretion remains depressed during late pregnancy and the early puerperium. The low level of growth hormone and the rapid decline in the hormones hPL, estrogens, and cortisol and in the placental enzyme, insulinase, *reduce the antiinsulin factors* in the early puerperium. Therefore new mothers have low fasting plasma glucose levels, and insulin requirements for insulin-dependent diabetic women usually fall after delivery (Chapter 24). Normal hormonal alterations render the early puerperium a transitional period for *carbohydrate metabolism* so that interpretation of glucose tolerance tests is difficult at this time.

Thyroid function is difficult to evaluate during the early puerperium because of the rapid fluctuation in many endocrine hormones. Postpartum hypothyroidism is suspected if the woman fails to lactate or recovery from childbirth is delayed.

A progressive increase of plasma levels of *corticosteroids* during pregnancy and labor is followed by a decline to nonpregnant values by the end of the first week after delivery. Within 2 hours after delivery, *plasma renin* and *angiotensin II* levels drop to within the normal nonpregnant range. This finding may indicate that the fetoplacental unit is one source of maternal plasma renin.

The *basal metabolic rate* remains elevated for 7 to 14 days after delivery. Normal nonpregnant values for respiratory system function are given in Appendix E.

Fatigue is customary during the first few days after delivery. Extra rest and sleep are required. The underlying cause is unclear, but may be related to the rapid endocrine changes.

❑ CARDIOVASCULAR SYSTEM

Blood Volume

Changes in blood volume depend on several factors, for example, blood loss during delivery, and mobilization and subsequent excretion of extravascular water (physiologic edema). Blood loss results in immediate but limited decrease in total blood volume. Thereafter, normal shifts in body water result in a slow decline in blood volume. By the third to fourth week after delivery the blood volume usually has regressed to nonpregnant values (Fig. 19-4).

Pregnancy-induced hypervolemia (increase of at

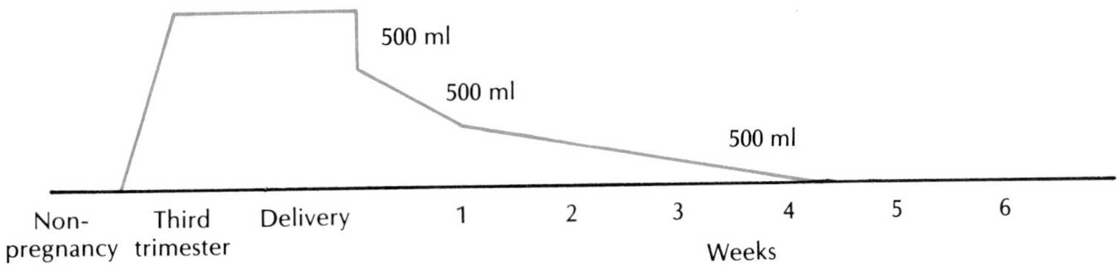

Fig. 19-4 Rate of loss of 1500 ml in blood volume during first postdelivery month. Greatest change at delivery, then in week after childbirth. (From Wiggins JD: Childbearing: physiology, experiences, needs, St Louis, 1979, The CV Mosby Co.)

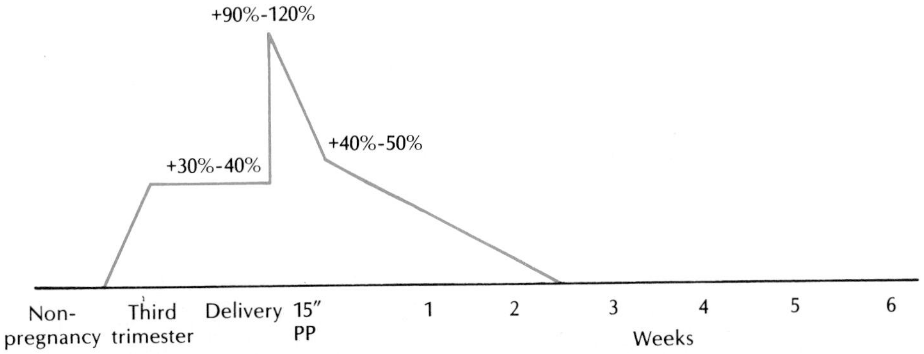

Fig. 19-5 Cardiac output. Work of heart increases during labor and decreases significantly immediately after birth of baby. (From Wiggins JD: Childbearing: physiology, experiences, needs, St Louis, 1979, The CV Mosby Co.)

least 40% from 1 to 2 L near term) allows most women to tolerate a considerable blood loss at delivery. Many women lose 300 to 400 ml of blood during vaginal delivery of a single fetus and about twice this amount during cesarean delivery.

Readjustments in the maternal vasculature after delivery are dramatic and rapid. The woman's response to blood loss during the early puerperium differs from that in a nonpregnant woman. Three postpartum physiologic changes protect the woman: (1) elimination of uteroplacental circulation reduces the size of the maternal vascular bed by 10% to 15%, (2) loss of placental endocrine function removes the stimulus for vasodilatation, and (3) mobilization of extravascular water stored during pregnancy occurs. Thus hypovolemic shock usually does not occur with normal blood loss.

Cardiac Output

The cardiac output continues to increase during the first and second stages of labor. It peaks during the puerperium regardless of the type of delivery or use of conduction anesthesia (Fig. 19-5). Cardiac output remains elevated for up to 48 hours postpartum, but returns to nonpregnant levels within 2 or 3 weeks (Robson, Dunlop, and Hunter, 1987).

Vital Signs and Blood Pressure

Few alterations in vital signs and blood pressure are seen under normal circumstances (Table 19-3). Respiratory function returns to nonpregnant levels by 6 months after delivery. After the uterus is emptied, the diaphragm descends, the normal cardiac axis is restored, and cardiologic features (point of maximum impulse [PMI], ECG) are normalized.

Blood Constituents

During the first 72 hours after delivery, there is a greater loss in plasma volume than in blood cells. The decrease in plasma volume plus the increase in red blood cell (RBC) mass of pregnancy is associated with a rise in hematocrit by the third to seventh day after delivery. There is no RBC destruction during the puerperium, but any gain will disappear gradually in accordance with the life span of the RBC. In uncomplicated cases the hematocrit will have returned to the normal

Table 19-3 Vital Signs and Blood Pressure After Delivery

Normal Findings	Deviations from Normal Findings and Probable Causes
TEMPERATURE	
During first 24 hours, may rise to 38° C (100.4° F) as a result of dehydrating effects of labor. After 24 hours the woman should be afebrile.	A diagnosis of puerperal sepsis is suggested if a rise in maternal temperature to 38° C (100.4° F) is noted after the first 24 hours after delivery and recurs or persists for 2 days. Other possibilities are mastitis, endometritis, urinary tract infections, and other systemic infections.
PULSE	
Bradycardia is a common finding for the first 6 to 8 days after delivery. Bradycardia is a consequence of increased cardiac output and stroke volume. The pulse returns to nonpregnant levels by 3 months after delivery. A pulse rate of between 50 and 70 beats per minute (bpm) may be considered normal.	A rapid pulse rate or one that is increasing may indicate hypovolemia as a result of hemorrhage.
RESPIRATIONS	
Respirations should fall to within the woman's normal predelivery range.	Hypoventilation may follow an unusually high subarachnoid (spinal) block.
BLOOD PRESSURE	
Blood pressure is altered *slightly* if at all. Orthostatic hypotension, as indicated by feelings of faintness or dizziness immediately after standing up, can develop in the first 48 hours as a result of the splanchnic engorgement that may occur after delivery.	A low or falling blood pressure may reflect hypovolemia secondary to hemorrhage. However, it is a late sign, and other symptoms of hemorrhage usually alert the staff. An increased reading may result from excessive use of vasopressor or oxytocic medications. Since pregnancy-induced hypertension (PIH) can persist into or occur first in the postpartum period, routine evaluation of blood pressure is needed. If a woman complains of headache, hypertension must be ruled out as a cause before analgesics are administered. If the blood pressure is elevated, the woman is confined to bed and the physician notified. (See also Chapter 23).

nonpregnant range by the fourth or fifth postdelivery week.

Normal leukocytosis of pregnancy averages about 12,000/mm^3. During the first 10 to 12 days after delivery, values between 20,000 to 25,000/mm^3 are common. Neutrophils are the most numerous WBCs. Leukocytosis coupled with the normal increase in erythrocyte sedimentation rate may confuse the interpretation of acute infections at this time.

An extensive activation of blood-clotting factors occurs after delivery. This activation, together with immobility, trauma, or sepsis, encourages thromboembolism. Factors I, II, VIII, IX, and X decrease within a few days to prepregnant levels. The elevated levels of fibrin split products are probably the result of their release from the placental site.

Thromboembolism. To avoid the formation of a **thromboembolism,** the woman's legs are examined daily for signs of thrombosis (pain, warmth, and tenderness; swollen reddened vein that feels hard or solid to touch). There may or may not be a positive Homans' sign (dorsiflexion of foot, similar to that done to relieve leg cramps [see Fig. 10-17], which causes calf muscles to compress tibial veins and produce pain if thrombosis is present). It is important to remember that deep venous thrombosis may be silent, that is, not cause pain.

Varicosities. Varicosities of the legs and around the anus (hemorrhoids) are common during pregnancy. Varices, even the less common vulvar varices, empty rapidly immediately after delivery. Surgical correction of varicosities is not considered during pregnancy. Total or the nearly total regression is anticipated after delivery.

URINARY SYSTEM

The hormonal changes of pregnancy (high steroid levels) contribute to the increase in renal function, and conversely the diminishing steroid levels after delivery may partly explain the reduced renal function during the puerperium. Kidney function returns to normal within a month after delivery. About 6 weeks are required for the pregnancy-induced hypotonia and dilatation of the ureters and renal pelves to subside. In a small percentage of women, dilatation of the urinary tract may persist for 3 months.

The renal glycosuria induced by pregnancy disappears. *Lactosuria* may be expected in lactating women. However, it cannot be detected by use of the Clinitest, since this test is specific for the presence of glucose, not lactose, in urine. As a result of the catalytic processes of involution, the *blood urea nitrogen (BUN)* is increased. *Mild proteinuria* (+1) is also a normal finding for 1 to 2 days after delivery in about 50% of women. *Acetonuria* may even occur in women after an uncomplicated delivery or after a prolonged labor with dehydration.

Profuse **diaphoresis,** especially at night (night sweats), is not unusual for 2 to 3 days after delivery. Diaphoresis is a mechanism to reduce the retained fluids of pregnancy and usually is not a symptom of infection.

The renal plasma flow and glomerular filtration rate (GFR) that increased by 25% to 50% during pregnancy remain elevated for at least the first postpartum week. Normally a marked **diuresis** begins within 12 hours after delivery. The volume of urinary output along with loss through perspiration accounts for a large portion of the weight loss during the early puerperium. This weight loss is approximately 5.5 kg (12 lb) after delivery of the fetus, placenta, and amniotic fluid and an additional 4 kg (9 lb) during the puerperium because of excretion of fluids and electrolytes accumulated during pregnancy. The mechanism that facilitates elimination of the excess tissue fluid accumulated during pregnancy is often referred to as the *reversal of the water metabolism of pregnancy.*

Trauma occurs to the urethra and bladder as the infant passes through the pelvis. The bladder wall is hyperemic and edematous, often with small areas of hemorrhage. Clean-catch or catheterized urine specimens after delivery often reveal hematuria from bladder trauma. In the **late puerperium,** hematuria may be a sign of urinary tract infection. The urethra and urinary meatus may be edematous. Birth-induced trauma and the effects of analgesia, especially conduction anesthesia, cause relative insensitivity that depresses the urge to void. In addition, pelvic soreness caused by the forces of labor, vaginal lacerations, or the episiotomy reduces or alters the voiding reflex. This alteration, together with postpartum diuresis, may allow rapid filling of the bladder.

Distension of the bladder can readily occur as the water metabolism of pregnancy is reversed and fluids are mobilized in the elimination of end products of protein catabolism. Overdistension can make the bladder more susceptible to infection as well as impede the resumption of normal voiding. If prolonged bladder overdistension occurs, further damage to the bladder wall (atony) may result.

Bladder tone is usually restored within 5 to 7 days after delivery with adequate emptying of the bladder.

GASTROINTESTINAL SYSTEM

The mother is usually hungry shortly after delivery and can tolerate a light diet. After full recovery from analgesia, anesthesia, and fatigue, most new mothers are ravenously hungry. Requests for double portions of food and frequent snacks are not uncommon. For a discussion of diet during lactation, see Chapter 18.

Typically, decreased muscle tone and motility of the gastrointestinal tract persists for only a short time after delivery. Excess analgesia and anesthesia could delay a return to normal tonicity and motility.

A spontaneous bowel evacuation may be delayed until 2 to 3 days after delivery. This can be explained by decreased muscle tone (**adynamic ileus**) in the intestines during labor and the immediate puerperium, prelabor diarrhea or a predelivery enema, lack of food, and possible dehydration. The mother is often concerned about discomfort during the bowel movement because of perineal tenderness as a result of episiotomy, lacerations, or hemorrhoids. Regular bowel habits need to be established when bowel tone returns.

NEUROLOGIC SYSTEM

Neurologic changes during the puerperium are those resulting from a reversal of maternal adaptations to pregnancy and those resulting from trauma during labor and delivery.

Pregnancy-induced neurologic discomforts abate after delivery. Elimination of physiologic edema through the diuresis that follows delivery relieves *carpal tunnel syndrome* by easing the compression of the median nerve. The periodic numbness and tingling of fingers that afflict 5% of gravidas usually disappear after delivery unless lifting and carrying the baby aggravates the condition. For a discussion of nerve injury incurred during childbirth, see Chapter 24. *Headache* requires careful assessment. Postpartum headaches may be caused by various conditions, including pregnancy-induced hypertension, stress, and leakage of cerebrospinal fluid into the extradural space during placement of the needle for spinal anesthesia. Duration of the headaches varies from 1 to 3 days to several weeks, depending on the cause and effectiveness of the treatment.

❑ MUSCULOSKELETAL SYSTEM

Adaptations in the mother's musculoskeletal system are reversed in the puerperium. The adaptations include those that contribute to relaxation and subsequent hypermobility of the joints and in the change in the mother's center of gravity because of the enlarging uterus. *Stabilization of joints* is complete by 6 to 8 weeks after delivery. However, although all other joints return to their normal prepregnant position before restabilization, those in the parous woman's feet do not; the new mother may notice a permanent increase in shoe size.

❑ INTEGUMENTARY SYSTEM

Chloasma of pregnancy usually disappears at the termination of pregnancy. *Hyperpigmentation* of the areolae and *linea nigra* may not regress completely after delivery, and some women will have permanent darker pigmentation of these areas.

Vascular abnormalities such as spider angiomas (nevi), palmar erythema, and epulis generally regress in response to the rapid decline in estrogens after termination of pregnancy. For some women, spider nevi persist indefinitely.

The abundance of fine *hair* seen during pregnancy usually disappears after delivery; however, any coarse or bristly hair that appears during pregnancy usually remains. *Fingernails* return to their nonpregnant characteristics of consistency and strength.

Diaphoresis is the most noticeable change in the integumentary system (see reversal of water metabolism of pregnancy, p. 557).

❑ IMMUNE SYSTEM

The mother's need for *rubella vaccination* or for prevention of Rh isoimmunization is determined.

For discussion of acquired immunodeficiency syndrome (AIDS) and other questions concerning immunology, see Chapter 5.

SUMMARY

The maternity nurse needs a solid understanding of normal physiologic responses during the postpartum period. This enables the nurse to provide quality nursing care. Knowledge of normal findings will allow the nurse to plan for care and encourage client participation. Women and their families will be better able to anticipate and adjust to postpartum changes if they have been provided with adequate health information. The nurse is in a key role to provide health education to women and their families. The nurse can help ease the transition from pregnancy to motherhood.

LEARNING ACTIVITIES

1. Develop a class for new mothers that will cover all aspects of the postpartum anatomic and physiologic changes and correlate discussion with prenatal adaptations. Research available audiovisual aids.
2. Assess individual multiparous and primiparous women and use findings as the basis of a group discussion of similarities and differences.
3. Observe the return visit of a postpartum client to the clinic and note especially assessment of involution progress, laboratory tests, and physical problems.
4. Compare the vital signs and blood pressure of a woman during labor and the first postpartum day. Explain the changes, if any.
5. Review a blood work report on a postpartum woman. Compare the results with the normal findings for the postpartum period.
6. In a group conference, answer and give rationale for the following questions:
   a. Women who breastfeed often ask whether one can become pregnant while breastfeeding. What should the nurse answer?
   b. Early ambulation of the mother following delivery promotes what normal functions?

KEY CONCEPTS

- The uterus involutes rapidly after delivery, returning to the true pelvis within 1 week.
- The rapid drop in estrogen and progesterone following delivery of the placenta is responsible for many of the anatomic and physiologic changes in the puerperium.
- Assessment of lochia and fundal height is essential to monitoring the progress of normal involution and identifying potential problems.
- Breastfeeding is a *not* a reliable form of birth control.
- Bradycardia is a common finding for the first 6 to 8 days.
- Activation of blood clotting factors, immobility, and sepsis predispose the woman to thromboembolism.
- Marked diuresis, decreased bladder sensitivity, and overdistension of the bladder can lead to problems with urinary elimination.
- Postpartum physiologic changes allow the woman to tolerate considerable blood loss at delivery.

References

Jacobson H: A standard for assessing lochia volume, MCN 10(3):174, 1985.

Robson SC, Dunlop W, and Hunter S: Haemodynamic changes during the early puerperium, Br Med J 294:1065, 1987.

Scott JR et al: Danforth's obstetrics and gynecology, ed 6, Philadelphia, 1990, JB Lippincott Co.

Bibliography

Brewer MM et al: Postpartum change in maternal weight and body fat deposits in lactating vs. non-lactating women, Am J Clin Nutr 49(2):259, 1989.

Butters L et al: The influence of breast and bottlefeeding on blood pressure, Midwifery 4(3):130, 1988.

Cunningham FG, MacDonald PC, and Gant NF: Williams obstetrics, ed 18, Norwalk, Conn, 1989, Appleton & Lange.

Dougherty MC et al: The effect of exercise on the circumvaginal muscles in postpartum women, J Nurse Midwife 34(1):8, 1989.

Drake ML et al: Physical and psychological symptoms experienced by Canadian women and their husbands during pregnancy and the postpartum, J Adv Nurs 13(4):436, 1988.

Ferguson H: Planning letter-perfect postpartum care, Nurs '87 17(5):50, 1987.

Fischman SH et al: Changes in sexual relationships in postpartum couples, JOGN Nurs 15(1):58, 1986.

Gorrie TM: Postpartal nursing diagnosis, JOGN Nurs 15(1):52, 1986.

Greene GW et al: Postpartum weight change: how much of the weight gained in pregnancy will be lost after delivery? Obstet Gynecol 71(51):701, 1988.

Hans A: Postpartum assessment: the psychological component, JOGN Nurs 15(1):49, 1986.

McKay S and Mahan CS: Ways to upgrade postpartal care, Contemp OB/GYN 27:63, 1985.

Myles MF: Textbook for midwives with modern concepts of obstetric and neonatal care, ed 9, New York, 1981, Churchill Livingstone, Inc.

Oxorn H: Oxorn-Foote human labor and birth, ed 5, Norwalk, Conn, 1986, Appleton-Century-Crofts.

Quistad C: How to smooth mom's postpartum path, RN 47:40, April, 1984.

Tulman LJ: Recovery from childbirth—does the "postpartum period" last only 6 weeks? NJ Nurse 19(1):11, 1989.

Tulman LJ and Fawcett J: Return of functional ability after childbirth, Nurs Res 37(2):77, 1988.

Willson JR and Carrington ER: Obstetrics and gynecology, ed 8, St Louis, 1987, The CV Mosby Co.

CHAPTER

20 Family Dynamics After Childbirth

Deitra Leonard Lowdermilk

Learning Objectives

Correctly define the key terms listed.
Describe the two components of the parenting process.
Discuss five preconditions that influence attachment.
List the sensual responses that strengthen attachment.
Differentiate the three periods in parental role change following childbirth.
List six parental tasks and responsibilities.
Identify infant behaviors that facilitate and inhibit parental attachment.
Identify behaviors of the three phases of maternal adjustment.
Discuss maternal age over 35 as a factor influencing parental response.
Explain paternal adjustment.
List three ways to facilitate parent-infant adjustment.
Explain effects of a parent's sensory impairment on the attachment process.
List three activities that facilitate sibling attachment.
Describe grandparent adjustment.

Key Terms

attachment
biorhythmicity
claiming process
cognitive-affective skills
cognitive-motor skills
en face
engrossment
entrainment
executive behaviors
fingertip exploration
habituation
infant-parent interaction
  rhythm
  behavioral repertoires
  responsivity
maternal adjustment
  dependent phase
  dependent-independent phase
  interdependent phase
maternal age over 35
mothering function
mutuality
positive feedback
postpartum depression ("baby blues")
sibling rivalry
signaling behaviors
significant other
taking-hold phase
taking-in phase

The birth of a child poses a fundamental challenge to the existing interactional structure of the family. Becoming a parent creates a period of instability that requires behaviors that promote the transition to parenthood. Parents must explore their relationship with the infant as well as redefine the relationship between themselves. If there are other children, parents must adjust their own life space to include another child, and the older children must adjust to the infant's claim on parental time and love (Walz and Rich, 1983). This chapter reviews the parenting process, including adjustments of parents, siblings, and grandparents.

❑ PARENTING PROCESS

Biologic parenthood for both parents begins with the union of ovum and sperm. During the prenatal period the mother is the primary agent in providing an environment in which the unborn child may develop and grow. This close symbiotic union of mother and child ends with birth. Others may then assume partial or complete involvement in the infant's care. Whoever—whether biologic or substitute parent, woman or man—assumes the parental role enters into a crucial relationship with a child that will persist throughout the life of each. Men and women, of course, may exist without a child; thus, in essence, parenthood is optional. Parenthood may serve as a maturation factor in the life of a man and woman regardless of whether it is biologically based. For children, parenthood is all important; their continued existence depends on the quality of care they receive.

The tasks, responsibilities, and attitudes that make up parenting care have been designated by Steele and Pollack (1968) as the **"mothering function."** It is a process in which an adult (a mature, caring, capable, self-sufficient person) assumes the care of an infant (an immature, helpless, dependent person). Either parent may exhibit "motherliness." Motherliness is now recognized to be a non-gender-related ability. The ability to show gentleness, love, and understanding and to place another's welfare above one's own is not limited to women—it is a human characteristic.

Steele and Pollack (1968) describe parenting as one process with two components. The first, being practical or mechanical in nature, involves cognitive and motor skills; the second, emotional in nature, involves cognitive and affective skills. Both components are essential to the infant's well-being and future development.

Cognitive-motor Skills

The first component in the process of parenting includes childcare activities such as "feeding, holding, clothing, and cleaning the infant, protecting it from harm, and providing mobility for it" (Steele and Pollack, 1968). These task-oriented activities, or **cognitive-motor skills,** do not appear automatically as efficient caregiving behaviors at the birth of one's child. The parents' abilities in these respects have been influenced by cultural and personal experiences. Many parents have to learn how to do these tasks, and this learning process can be difficult. However, almost all parents with the desire to learn and with the support of others become adept in caregiving activities.

Cognitive-affective Skills

The psychologic component in childcare, motherliness or fatherliness, appears to stem from the *parents'* earliest experiences with a loving, accepting mother figure. In this sense parents may be said to "inherit" the ability to show concern and tenderness and to pass on this ability to the next generation by repeating the kind of parent-child relationship they experienced. The **cognitive-affective skills** of parenting include an attitude of tenderness, awareness, and concern for the child's needs and desires. This component of parenting has a profound effect on the manner in which the practical aspects of childcare are performed and on the emotional response of the child to the care. Benedek (1950) describes a positive parent-child relationship as mutually rewarding. This relationship is fundamental to a person's development of confidence in the expectations that others will be willing to help and that the person is worth helping. Erikson's concept (1959, 1964) of "basic trust" is similar. He claims that development of a sense of trust determines the infant's responses to others throughout life. Persons who experienced a positive parent-child relationship tend to be social or outgoing and able to seek and accept assistance from others. In contrast, those deficient in a sense of trust tend to be alienated and isolated. They are most likely to have crises because of their inability to make use of situational supports in times of stress.

❑ PARENTAL ATTACHMENT

Although much research has been directed toward unraveling the process by which a parent comes to love and accept a child and a child comes to love and accept a parent, we still do not know what motivates and commits them to decades of supportive and nurturing care of each other. We do know that it begins as a process of **attachment** (Fig. 20-1). The attachment process has been described as linear, beginning during pregnancy, intensifying during the early postdelivery period, and being constant and consistent once established. It is critical to mental and physical health across the life span (Parkes and Stevenson-Hinde, 1982).

Mercer (1982) lists *five preconditions that influence attachment:*

1. A parent's emotional health (including the ability to trust another person)
2. A social support system encompassing mate, friends, and family
3. A competent level of communication and caregiving skills
4. Parental proximity to the infant
5. Parent-infant fit (including infant state, temperament, and sex)

If any of these preconditions is not present or is distorted, skilled intervention is necessary to ensure the attachment process.

According to Stainton (1983b), attachment is a mutual exchange of feelings predicated by attractiveness,

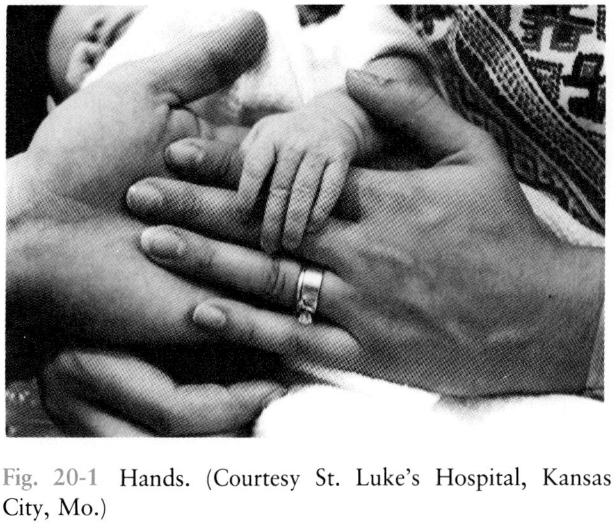

Fig. 20-1 Hands. (Courtesy St. Luke's Hospital, Kansas City, Mo.)

responsiveness, and satisfaction and is subject to changes in intensity as circumstances change over time. Attachment is developed and maintained by proximity and interaction. As with any developmental process, it is characterized by periods of progress and regression, and temporary or permanent withdrawal from attachment figures can occur.

Mercer (1982) notes that attachment is facilitated by **positive feedback.** "Positive feedback includes the social, verbal and nonverbal responses, either real or perceived, that indicate acceptance of one partner by the other." She goes on to say that attachment occurs through "a mutually satisfying experience." The newborn infant grasps a finger or a strand of hair, becoming attached to the parent. A mother commented on her son's grasp reflex, "I put my finger in his hand, and he grabbed right on. It is just a reflex, I know, but it felt good anyway."

Various theories have attempted to explain the basis for attachment. Freudian psychoanalytic theory emphasizes the development of a bond between child and mother as a result of the mother's satisfying the infant's innate needs to socialize with another and the physical needs for survival. Social learning theory contributed the principles of reinforcement to the attachment process. As discomfort is reduced or removed by the mother (or other caregiver) and pleasure substituted, the mother becomes associated with the pleasurable feeling of being satisfied. She becomes important to the infant, is loved, and can therefore act as a reinforcing agent or event. The mother becomes a **significant other** in the infant's life.

Bowlby (1958) and others (Ainsworth, 1969, 1970; Ainsworth and Bell, 1970; Brazelton, 1963, 1973) have extended the concept of attachment to include **mutuality;** that is, the infant's behaviors and characteristics call forth a corresponding set of maternal behaviors and characteristics. The infant displays **signaling behaviors** such as crying, smiling, and cooing that initiate the contact and bring the mother near the child. These behaviors are followed by **executive behaviors** such as rooting, grasping, and postural adjustments that maintain the contact. The caregiver is attracted to an alert, responsive, cuddly infant and repelled by an irritable, apparently disinterested infant. Attachment occurs more readily with the infant whose temperament, social capabilities, appearance, and gender fit the parent's expectations. If the child does not meet these expectations, resolution of disappointment can delay the attachment process.

An important part of attachment is the family identification of the new baby (Fig. 20-2) through the **claiming process.** The child is first identified in terms of "likeness" to other family members, then in terms of "differences," and finally in terms of "uniqueness." The unique newcomer is thus *incorporated* into the family. Mothers and fathers scrutinize an infant carefully. They point out characteristics that the child shares with other family members and indicate recognition of a relationship between them. Mothers make

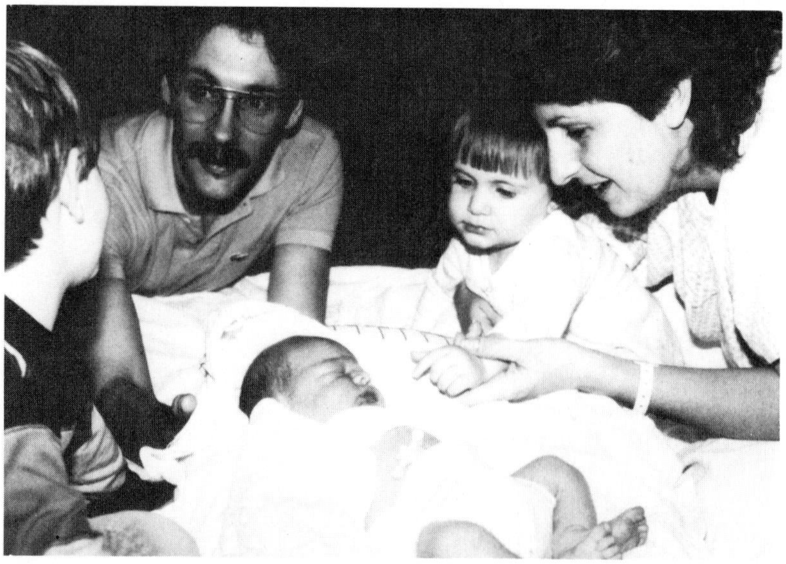

Fig. 20-2 The family examines the new baby. They discuss her appearance and admire her. (Courtesy Marjorie Pyle, RNC, Lifecircle, Costa Mesa, Calif.)

comments such as the following that reveal the claiming process: "Russ held him close and said, 'He's the image of his father,' but I found one part like me—his toes are shaped like mine. Look, he's smiling; he likes his mother's jokes."

On the other hand, some mothers react negatively. They "claim" the infant in terms of the discomfort or pain the baby causes the mother. The mother interprets the infant's normal responses as being negative toward the mother. The mother reacts to her child with dislike or indifference. She does not hold the child close or touch the child to be comforting; for example, "The nurse put the baby into Marie's arms. She promptly laid him across her knees and glanced up at the television. 'Stay still 'til I finish watching—you've been enough trouble already.' "

Parental responses have direct implications for nursing. Nurses can establish an environment that enhances positive parent-child contacts. They can encourage parental awareness of infant responses and ability to communicate, provide support and encouragement as parents attempt to become competent and loving in their role, and enhance the attachment process.

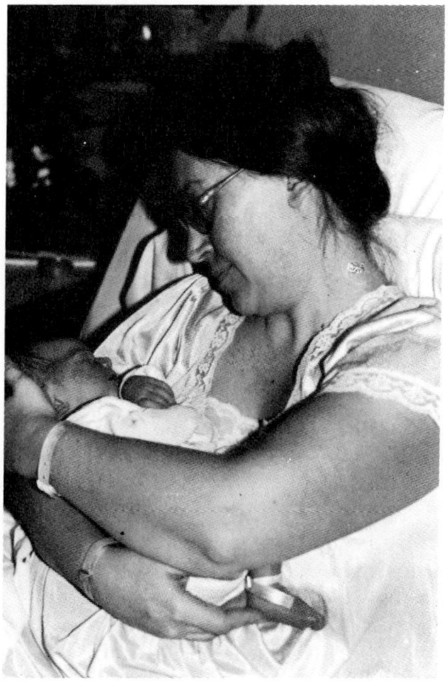

Fig. 20-3 Mother interacts with daughter through touching infant's head and feet. (Courtesy Judy Bamber, San Jose, Calif.)

Sensual Responses

Attachment is strengthened through the use of sensual responses or abilities by both partners in the parent-child interaction. The sensual responses and abilities include the following.

Touch. Touch, or the tactile sense, is used extensively by parents and other caregivers as a means of becoming acquainted with the newborn. The fingertip, one of the most touch-sensitive areas of the body, is used to explore the infant's head, face, and body surfaces. The open palms and arms are used to handle the infant (Tulman, 1985). Many mothers reach out for their infants as soon as they are born and the cord is cut. They lift them to their breasts, enfold them in their arms, and cradle them. Once the child is close to them they begin the exploration process with their fingertips. For some other mothers and other caregivers (fathers, nursing and medical students) studies have depicted a predictable pattern of touch behavior (Rubin, 1963; Klaus and Kennell, 1982; Tulman, 1985). The caregiver begins with a **fingertip exploration** of the infant's head and extremities. Within a short time the caregiver uses the palm to caress the baby's trunk and eventually enfolds the infant in her or his arms. Gentle stroking motions are used to soothe and quiet the infant. Mothers pat or gently rub their infant's back after feedings. Infants pat the mother's breast as they nurse. Mothers and fathers want to touch, pick up, and hold their infant (Fig. 20-3). Parents and child seem to enjoy sharing each other's body warmth. Mothers will say, "I love her warm little body against mine."

Parents can be helped to recognize and respond to the similarities of their child's responses before and after birth. Prenatal strategies that have been used to promote intrauterine attachment include having the mother feel for fetal parts abdominally, massaging and rubbing the abdomen, and noting what maternal activities cause changes in fetal activity. Studies have found the fetus is more active when the mother engages in activities like jogging and will become quiet when the mother relaxes, as when taking a warm shower (Davis and Akridge, 1987). Increasing sensitivity to the infant's like and dislike of types of touch can bring parents closer to their babies.

Eye-to-Eye Contact. Interest in having eye contact is demonstrated again and again. Some mothers remark that once their babies have looked at them, they feel much closer to them (Klaus and Kennell, 1982). Others have also noted this response: "I was a mother and looked into his eyes so clear; fell into his eyes, and in love" (Lang, 1972). Parents spend much time getting their babies to open their eyes and look at them. In our culture eye contact appears to have a cementing effect on the development of a beginning and trusting relationship and is an important factor in human relationships at all ages.

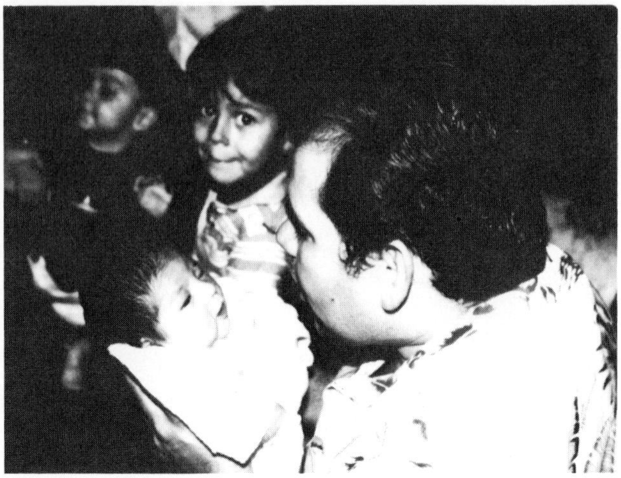

Fig. 20-4 Father and new baby make eye contact in *en face* position. (Courtesy Marjorie Pyle, RNC, Lifecircle, Costa Mesa, Calif.)

As newborns become functionally able to sustain eye contact, parents and child spend much time gazing at one another (Fig. 20-4). We need to implement medical and nursing practices that encourage this exchange. Instillation of protective eye drops can be withheld until the infant and parents have some time together. Lights can be dimmed so that the child's eyes will open. Newborns can be held close enough to see the parents' faces.

Voice. The shared response of parents and infant to each other's voice is also remarkable. Parents wait tensely for the first cry. Once it has reassured them of the baby's health, they begin comforting behaviors. As the parents talk in high-pitched voices, the infant is alerted and turns toward them.

Odor. Another behavior shared by parents and infant is responsive to each other's odor. Mothers comment on the smell of their babies when first born and have noted that each child has a unique odor. Infants learn rapidly to distinguish the odor of their own mother's breast milk (Stainton, 1985).

Entrainment. Newborns have been found to move in time with the structure of adult speech (Condon and Sander, 1974). They wave their arms, lift their heads, kick their legs, seemingly "dancing in tune" to their parent's voice. This means that the infant has developed *culturally determined rhythms* of speech long before using the spoken language in communicating. A *carryover* (**entrainment**) occurs once the child begins to talk. This shared rhythm also acts to give the parent positive feedback and to establish a positive setting for effective communication.

Biorhythmicity. The unborn child can be said to be in tune with the mother's natural rhythms, such as heartbeats. After birth, a crying infant may be soothed by being held in a position in the mother's arms where her heartbeat can be heard or by hearing a recording of a heartbeat. One of the newborn's tasks is to establish a personal rhythm (**biorhythmicity**). Parents can help in this process by giving consistent loving care and by using their infant's alert state to develop responsive behavior and thereby increase social interactions and opportunities for learning. The more quickly parents become competent in child-care activities, the more quickly their psychologic energy can be directed toward observing the communication cues the infant gives them.

Early Contact

Research with mammals other than humans indicates that early contact between mother and offspring is important in developing future relationships. *To date,* ***no*** *scientific evidence has demonstrated that* ***immediate contact*** *after birth is essential for the human parent-child relationship.* According to Siegel (1982), findings from carefully controlled replicated investigations appear to document that:

> Early contact, irrespective of its supplementation by extended contact, favorably affects maternal affectional behavior during the first postpartum days. The results are consistent across low and middle socioeconomic status mother-infant pairs as well as in developed and less developed countries.

He also notes that early contact has a positive effect on the duration of breastfeeding. However, long-range effects of early contact have yet to be documented (Lamb, 1982).

The physiologic benefits of early contact between mother and infant have been documented (Klaus and Kennell, 1982). For the mother, levels of oxytocin and prolactin rise; for the infant, sucking reflexes are employed early. The process of developing active immunity begins as the infant inhales flora from the mother's skin.

The first hours or days after birth may be a sensitive time for parent infant interaction. Early close contact may *facilitate* the attachment process between parent and child. This is not to say a delay will inhibit this process (humans are too resilient for that), but additional psychologic energy may be needed to accomplish the same effect. For parents unable or unwilling to expend this energy the delay may affect the infant's future well-being.

In one of the first texts on newborn disorders, Budin

(1907) notes that "mothers separated from their young soon lost all interest in those whom they were unable to nurse or cherish." Subsequent investigators have brought to light similar behaviors when interactions between parent and child meet interference. Bowlby's work (1958, 1969) emphasizes the attachment process between infant and mother and details the effects of loss of that attachment to the infant. Research in the area of child abuse documents the greater percentage of neglect, abuse, and failure to thrive among infants separated from parents for relatively long periods because of illness or preterm birth (Hefler and Kempe, 1965; Barnett et al, 1970; Leifer et al, 1972; Klaus and Kennell, 1982).

Parents who desire but are unable to have early contact with their newborn infant *can be reassured that such contact is not essential for optimum parent-child interactions.* Otherwise, ***adopted infants*** would not form the usual affectional ties with their parents. Nor does the mode of infant-mother contact after delivery (skin-to-skin versus wrapped) appear to have any important effect. Nurses need to counsel mothers to allay fears that their emotional bond to their infant is not necessarily weaker because they missed early contact or because the contact was not skin to skin (Curry, 1979). Women who have experienced a long and difficult labor often are too exhausted to respond other than in a perfunctory way to the newborn. They may welcome the attention of others and be grateful that the infant is healthy, but their primary need centers on recovery from the physical and emotional aspects of pregnancy and childbirth. Infants born at risk as a result of either fetal or maternal disabilities, usually are transferred to the intensive care nursery as quickly as possible. Concerns for their need for intensive medical and nursing care supersede concerns about providing close contact between the infant and the mother or father. Opportunities to be with the infant in the intensive care nursery, to touch or hold her or him if at all possible, and to receive reports of the infant's progress must be part of the nursing care plan.

Extended Contact

Since the early 1970s, consumers have worked toward childbirth practices that promoted the family as the focus of care. The alternatives of homebirth, birthing centers, and family-centered maternity care units reflect this desire by parents to share in the birth process and to have more contact with their infants.

One widely used method of family-centered care is the provision of rooming-in facilities for the mother and her baby. The infant is transferred to the area from the transitional nursery after evidencing satisfactory postdelivery adjustment. The father is encouraged to visit and to participate in the care of the infant. Siblings and grandparents are also encouraged to visit and become acquainted with the infant. Some hospitals have established family birth units. The mother is accompanied by the father during the delivery of the infant, and all three may remain together until discharged. Medical and nursing personnel are available for any care necessary for the mother and child. Other hospitals arrange for the discharge of mother and infant any time from 2 to 24 hours after delivery if the condition of the mother and that of the child warrants it. Follow-up care with nursing personnel from a health agency is part of this plan.

Mother-baby care is another form of family-centered care. Care for the mother and baby is provided by a primary nurse, fostering family unity (Fig. 20-5). Parents are more likely to be more self-confident in care and maternal attachment and maternal role attainment is promoted (NAACOG, 1989).

Extended contact with the infant should be available for all parents, but especially for those at risk for parenting inadequacies, such as adolescents and low-income women. Any activity that optimizes family-centered care is worthy of serious consideration by postpartum nurses.

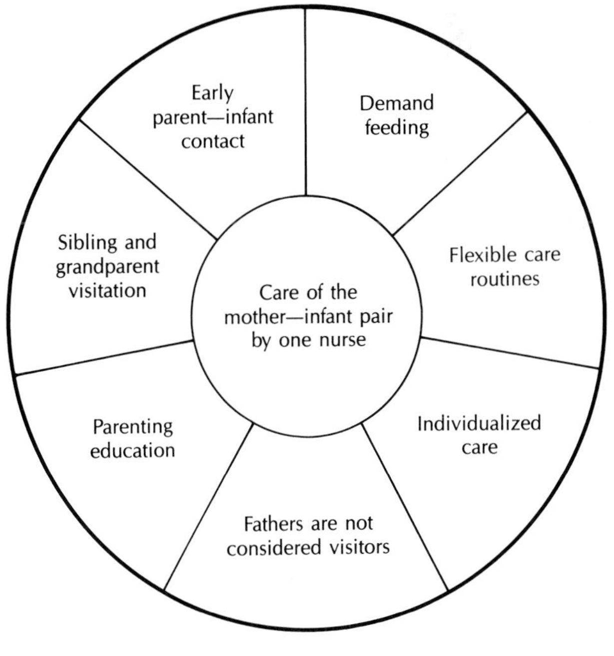

Fig. 20-5 The wheel of family-centered postpartum and newborn care. (Adapted from Watter NE: JOGN Nurs 6:480, 1985.)

❑ PARENTAL ROLE AFTER CHILDBIRTH

For the biologic parent the parental role does not begin at birth but rather enlarges and intensifies. Care and nurturing of the child is not initiated in the postdelivery period. Before birth the mother who carried out the dictates of health (e.g., diet, rest, exercise) for the "good of her baby," the father who supported and sheltered her, and the parents who became aware of and attached to their unborn child were already functioning in the parental role.

During the postdelivery period, new tasks and responsibilities arise and old behaviors need to be modified or new ones added. Mothers' and fathers' responses to the parental role change over time and tend to follow a predictable course.

During the early period parents have to reorganize their relationship with their child. The child's needs for shelter, nourishment, protection, and socializing continue. What was accomplished through the biologic process of pregnancy now requires an array of caregiving activities. This period is characterized by intense learning and need for nurturing. The family structure and functioning as a system has been forever altered. The duration of this period varies with people but lasts about 4 weeks.

The next period represents a time of drawing together and uniting the family unit. This consolidation period involves negotiations as to roles (wife-husband, mother-father, parent-child, sibling-sibling). It involves a stabilizing of tasks, a coming to terms with commitments. Parents demonstrate growing competence in child-care activities and become sensitive to the meaning of their infant's behavior. This period lasts approximately 2 months and in conjunction with the early period forms what is now termed the ***fourth trimester.***

Parents and children grow in their roles until separated by death. The most outstanding feature of the lifelong process of parent-child interaction is change, consistent evolution over time. The people involved deal not only with the present but also with the future. They need support and care in the here and now and anticipatory guidance for coming changes.

Parental Tasks and Responsibilities

Parents need to reconcile the actual child with the fantasy and dream child. This means coming to terms with the infant's physical appearance, sex, innate temperament, and physical status. If the real child differs greatly from the fantasy child, parents may delay acceptance for a period. In some instances they may never accept the child. Mothers describe the differences between the real and the imagined child as follows (Stainton, 1983a):

■ In the words of one mother, "I was surprised that she seemed to me to be a complete person with a personality of her own. I expected a blank tablet, a piece of clay for me to mold or a sponge for me to fill." Another, "I could not believe how determined and demanding he could be. I was going to control him and get him fitted into our life-style."

Some parents are startled by the appearance of the infant—size, color, molding of the head, or bowed appearance of the legs (Chapter 16). Many fathers have commented that they thought the odd shape of the child's head (molding) meant the child would be mentally retarded.

Disappointment over the sex of the infant can take time to resolve. The mother or father may be able to give adequate physical mothering but may find it difficult to be sincerely involved with the infant until these feelings have been resolved.

Parents need to establish the newborn as a person separate from themselves, that is, as someone having many dependency needs and requiring much nurturing.

Parents need to become adept in the care of the infant. This includes caregiving activities, noting the communication cues given by the infant to indicate needs, and responding appropriately to the infant's needs.

Parents need to establish reasonable evaluative criteria to use in assessing the success or failure of the care given the infant. Parents are surprisingly sensitive to infant responses. One father told of his first attempt to give his child a kiss. At that moment the child turned her head. The father felt hurt, although he understood that the baby was totally unaware of her own movements. How the infant responds to the parental care and attention is interpreted by the parent as a comment on the quality of the care being given. These responses may include crying, weight gain or loss, or sleeping at a designated time. Continued responses deemed negative by the parent can result in alienation of parent and child to the infant's detriment (Table 20-1).

Self-esteem grows with competence. Mothers of preterm infants have noted that the adept handling of their infants by nurses made their own efforts to sustain their child appear inadequate. Mothers who have supplied breast milk for their infant comment that this makes them feel they are contributing in a unique way to the welfare of their child.

Criticism, real or imagined, of new parents' ability to provide adequate physical care, nutrition, or social stimulation for their infant can prove devastating. These "critics" may need constructive direction. Assistance, including advice by husbands, wives, mothers,

Table 20-1 Infant Behaviors Affecting Parental Attachment

Facilitating Behaviors	Inhibiting Behaviors
Visually alert; eye-to-eye contact; tracking or following of parent's face	Sleepy; eyes closed most of the time; gaze aversion
Appealing facial appearance; randomness of body movements reflecting helplessness	Resemblance to person parent dislikes; hyperirritability or jerky body movements when touched
Smiles	Bland facial expression; infrequent smiles
Vocalization; crying only when hungry or wet	Crying for hours on end; colicky
Grasp reflex	Exaggerated motor reflex
Anticipatory approach behaviors for feedings; sucks well; feeds easily	Feeds poorly; regurgitates; vomits often
Enjoys being cuddled, held	Resists holding and cuddling by crying, stiffening body
Easily consolable	Inconsolable; unresponsive to parenting, caretaking tasks
Activity and regularity somewhat predictable	Unpredictable feeding and sleeping schedule
Attention span sufficient to focus on parents	Inability to attend to parent's face or offered stimulation
Differential crying, smiling, and vocalizing; recognizes and prefers parents	Shows no preference for parents over others
Approaches through locomotion	Unresponsive to parent's approaches
Clings to parent; puts arms around parent's neck	Seeks attention from any adult in room
Lifts arms to parents in greeting	Ignores parents

From Gerson E: Infant behavior in the first year of life, New York, 1973; Raven Press, Copyright © 1973. With permission.

mothers-in-law, and professional workers, can be seen as supportive. Conversely, it can be seen as an indication of how inept these persons have judged the new parent to be.

Parents must establish a place for the newborn within the family group. Whether the infant is the first born or last born, all family members must adjust their roles to accommodate the newcomer. An only child needs support to accept a rival to parental affections. An older child needs support when losing a favored position. The parents are expected to negotiate these changes.

Parents need to establish the primacy of their adult relationships to maintain the family as a group. Since this includes reorganizing many roles, for example, sexual roles, child-care roles, career roles, and community roles, time and energy must be provided for this vital task.

Maternal Adjustment

Three phases are discernible as the mother adjusts to her version of the parental role. These phases of **maternal adjustment** are characterized by dependent behavior, dependent-independent behavior, and interdependent behavior.

Dependent Phase. During the first 1 to 2 days after delivery the mother's dependency needs predominate. To the extent that these needs are met by others, the mother is able to divert her psychologic energy to her child rather than to herself. She needs "mothering" to "mother." Rubin (1961) has aptly described these few days as the "**taking-in phase**": a time when nurturing and protective care are required by the new mother.

For a few days following birth, mature and apparently healthy women appear to suspend involvement in everyday responsibilities. They rely on others to respond to their needs for comfort, rest, nourishment, and closeness to their families and newborn.

The **dependent phase** is a time of great excitement, and most parents are extremely talkative. They need to verbalize their experience of pregnancy and birth. Focusing on, analyzing, and accepting these experiences help the parents move on to the next phase. Some parents are able to use the staff or other mothers as an "audience." Others are unable to do this and need the opportunity to be with family or friends.

Since anxiety and preoccupation with her new role often narrow a mother's perceptual field, information may have to be repeated. The new mother may require reminders to rest, or conversely, to ambulate enough to promote recovery. Ward routine does not necessarily loom large in the new mother's order of priorities; showers are taken when examinations are scheduled, and telephone conversations preclude "being ready" for the baby. Regulations seem cumbersome, and sometimes mothers and their families have difficulty accepting rules that interfere with their needs to share reactions about their child.

Physical discomfort arising from an episiotomy, sore

nipples, hemorrhoids, afterpains, and occasionally a sprained coccygeal joint can interfere with the mother's need for rest and relaxation. The judicious use of comfort measures and medication depends on the nurse. Many women hesitate to ask for medication, believing that any pain they experience is normal and to be expected; few have a knowledge of the use of heat or cold to relieve local pain.

Dependent-Independent Phase. If the mother has received adequate nurturing in the first few days, by the third day her desire for independent action reasserts itself. In the **dependent-independent phase,** the mother alternates between a need for extensive nurturing and acceptance by others and the desire "to take charge" once again. She responds enthusiastically to opportunities to learn and practice the care of the baby or, if she is an accomplished mother, to carry out or direct this care.

The reality of parenthood must be experienced to be understood fully regardless of the desire for the baby and the amount of prenatal preparation undertaken. One young mother expressed it as follows (Lang, 1972):

> ■ But then in my second week, as my strength began to return, my energies began to focus on the overwhelming task of motherhood that stood before me. And I realized then that I faced that task alone. Not that my husband wouldn't stand by me, not that my friends would not share experiences with me, but I stood alone with the realization that only I could be the child's mother.

In the period of 6 to 8 weeks after delivery the mastery of the tasks of parenthood are crucial. Realistic expectations facilitate the subsequent functioning of the family as a unit.

Some women adjust with considerable difficulty to the isolation of themselves with their babies and resent the endless coping with home and child-care responsibilities. The mothers who appear to need additional supportive counseling include:

1. Primiparas inexperienced in child care
2. Women whose careers had provided outside stimulation
3. Women who lack friends or family members with whom to share delights and concerns
4. Adolescent mothers

Depressive states are not uncommon during this phase. *Feelings of extreme vulnerability* may arise from a number of factors. Psychologically the mother may be overwhelmed by the actuality of parental responsibilities. She may feel deprived of the pregnant state, with its concomitant supportive care of family members and friends. Some mothers regret the loss of the mother-unborn child relationship and mourn its passing. Still others experience a letdown feeling when labor and birth are complete. They had prepared themselves for an elemental experience, a walk "through the shadows," and now it is safely over.

Once immediate tasks and adjustments have been undertaken and brought under control, a plateau is reached. At this time the life-long effects of the parents' new responsibilities come into focus. Some parents experience a feeling of being trapped and wonder what life is all about.

Occasionally the mother becomes increasingly fatigued during the last month of pregnancy, when sleep is interrupted by shortness of breath and urinary frequency. Leg cramps, or inability to lie in a comfortable position can disturb sleep. *Fatigue* following delivery is compounded by around-the-clock demands of the new baby and can accentuate the feelings of depression. It has been suggested that a lowered level of circulating glucocorticoids or a condition of subclinical hypothyroidism may exist during the puerperium. This physiologic state could explain some minor degrees of **postpartum depression ("baby blues").**

Depressive reactions are not necessarily expressed verbally. A depressive state signified by typical behaviors (withdrawal, loss of interest in surroundings, and crying) can be manifested (p. 600).

It is hoped that toward the end of the dependent-independent phase the tasks and adjustments of daily routine will begin to follow a pattern. The baby begins to take an established position in the family. Many of the feeding problems, whether related to breastfeeding or bottle-feeding, have been largely resolved. The mother's physical energy and strength return; the **"taking-hold phase"** (Rubin, 1961) is ending. By the fifth week the infant has been examined by the physician and the mother also has been examined or has made arrangements for a checkup. It is time to move on to the next phase of adjustment.

Interdependent Phase. In this phase interdependent behavior reasserts itself, and the mother and her family move forward as a system with interacting members. The relationship of husband and wife, although altered by the introduction of a child, resumes many of its former characteristics. A primary need is to establish a life-style that includes, but in some respects excludes, the child. Husband and wife must share interest and activities that are adult in scope.

Most couples begin intercourse by the third or fourth week after the child is born; some begin earlier, as soon as it can be accomplished without discomfort for the woman. Sexual intimacy increases the man-woman aspect of the family, and the adult pair shares a closeness denied to other family members. Many new fathers speak of the alienation experienced when they observe the intimate mother-child relationship, and some are frank in expressing feelings of jealousy toward the infant. The resumption of the marital relationship seems to bring the parents' relationship back into focus.

The **interdependent phase** is often one of stress for the parental pair. Career patterns of men from their 20s through their 40s show intense activity centering around advancement in their profession or job. This often necessitates long hours away from the home or moving from one locality to another. Meanwhile the women are engrossed in home activities directed toward the care of the young children. Interests and needs diverge, and there may be a gradual estrangement, which is glossed over for the time being because of the individual needs of each. A special effort must be undertaken to strengthen the adult-adult relationship as a basis for the family unit.

Paternal Adjustment

During the last decade a growing interest in the relationship of the father and the child has become evident. It is now recognized that the mother-child relationship does not exist in a vacuum but within the context of the family system. Parent's attitudes toward and expectations of one another's parental behavior affect the behavior of each dyad. In our culture the newborn has been found to have a powerful impact on the father. Fathers have demonstrated intense involvement with their babies. Greenberg and Morris (1976) named the father's absorption, preoccupation, and interest in the infant **engrossment.** These researchers delineate a number of characteristics of engrossment. Some of the sensual responses relating to touch and eye-to-eye contact are the same as discussed earlier. The father's keen awareness of features both unique and similar to himself is another characteristic related to the father's need to claim the infant. An outstanding response is one of *strong attraction* to the newborn. Much time is spent "communicating" with the infant and taking delight in the infant's response to the father. Fathers feel a sense of increased self-esteem, a sense of being "proud, bigger, more mature, and older" after seeing their baby for the first time. Studies have shown a difference in father-infant relationships. Fathers tend to take the lead in initiating play and other social situations. Mothers tend to take the lead in caregiving activities (Clarke-Stewart, 1978). The subtle and more overt differences in stimulation from two sources, mother and father, provide a wider social experience for the child. In addition the child has improved chances of developing at least one good parenting relationship (Kunst-Wilson and Cronenwett, 1981).

Much has still to be learned about the relationships between fathers and their offspring. The mother's biologic relationship with the child can be a basis for predicting behaviors in the mother-child relationship. But the knowledge that a man is the father of a child gives us no clues as to his relationships or behaviors with the child.

There is no evidence as yet as to what effect individual styles have on the father's actual experience with this child. Despite their active involvement in the perinatal period, fathers tend to gravitate toward more traditional roles as they become more involved in job-related activities and less in child-care activities. However, if the father does involve himself in caregiving, he responds much as the mother in talking to the infant (Field, 1978a).

Infant-Parent Adjustment

The **infant-parent interaction** is characterized by a "set of rhythms, behavioral repertoires, and responsivity or response styles" (Field, 1978a). These traits are unique to each partner. Interactions can be facilitated in any of three ways: (1) modulation of **rhythm,** (2) modification of **behavioral repertoires,** and (3) mutual **responsivity.**

Rhythm. To modulate the rhythm, both parent and infant must be able to interact. Therefore the infant must be in the alert state, one of the most difficult of the sleep-wake states to maintain. The alert state occurs most often during a feeding or in face-to-face play. The parent must work hard to help the infant maintain the alert state long enough and often enough for interactions to take place. The ***en face*** position (parent positions face in same plane as that of newborn) is usually assumed (Fig. 20-6). Evidently mothers learn how to do this: multiparous mothers show particular sensitivity and responsiveness to their infant's feeding rhythms. The mother who is sensitive to feeding rhythms reserves stimulation for pauses in sucking activity. For example, the mother learns not to talk or smile excessively while the infant is sucking because the infant will stop feeding to interact with her (Field, 1978b). With maturity the infant can sustain longer interactions by modulating activity rhythms, that is, limb movement, sucking, gaze alternation, and **habituation** (Fig. 20-7). "In the interim, the adult learns to attend to these rhythms, modulate her or his own rhythms, and thereby facilitate a rhythmical turn-taking interaction" (Field, 1978a).

Repertoires. Both contributors to the infant-parent interaction have a repertoire of behaviors they can use to facilitate interactions. Fathers and mothers engage in these behaviors depending on the amount of contact and caregiving of the infant.

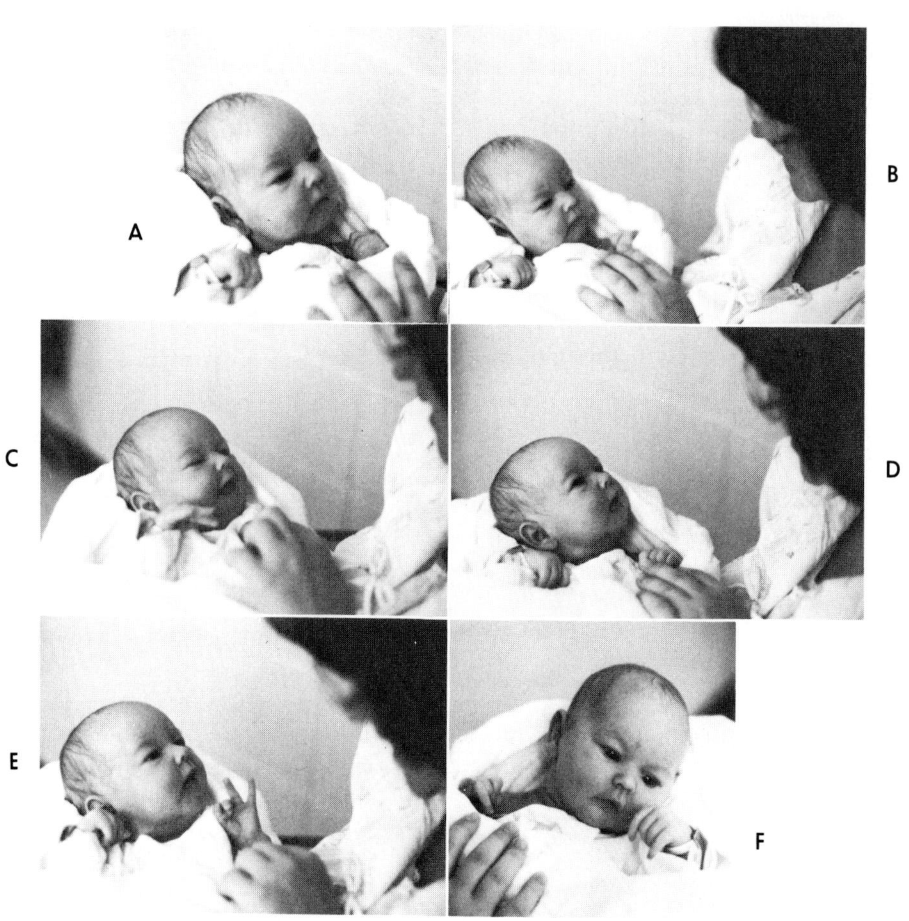

Fig. 20-6 Holding newborn in *en face* position, mother works to alert her daughter, 6 hours old. **A,** Infant is quiet and alert. **B,** Mother begins talking to daughter. Note frown of concentration. **C,** Infant responds, opens mouth like her mother. **D,** Infant gazes at her mother. **E,** Infant waves hand, opens mouth. **F,** Infant glances away, resting. Hand relaxes. (Courtesy Colleen Stainton.)

The *infant's repertoire* includes gaze behaviors, vocalizing, and facial expressions. The infant is able to focus and follow the human face from birth. The infant is also able to use gaze alternation. These abilities are under voluntary control. "The infant appears to look away from the mother's face when under- or overaroused to modulate his or her arousal level and process the stimulation he or she is receiving" (Field, 1978a). Brazelton et al (1974) suggest that one of the key responses for the parents to learn is *sensitivity to the infant's capacity for attention and inattention.* Developing this sensitivity is especially important in interacting with premature infants (Sammons and Lewis, 1985). Field (1978b) states, "Mothers who are more active or 'overstimulating' and less sensitive or responsive to their infant's pauses or turning away during the conversation are less able to elicit or hold their infants' gaze."

Body gestures form a part of the infant's "early language." Babies greet parents with waving hands or with a reaching out of hands. They can raise an eyebrow or soften their expression to elicit loving attention. They can be stimulated to smile or laugh with game playing. To end an interaction they use pouting or crying, arching of the back, and general squirming.

The parents' repertoire includes various behaviors for interacting with their infant. One of these behaviors is constantly looking at the infant and noting the infant's behavior. New parents often remark that they are exhausted from looking at the baby and smiling. Adults also infantilize their speech to help the infant "listen." They do this by slowing the tempo, speaking loudly and rhythmically, and by emphasizing key words. They repeat phrases frequently. Infantilizing does not mean using "baby talk," which involves distortion of sounds.

A

B

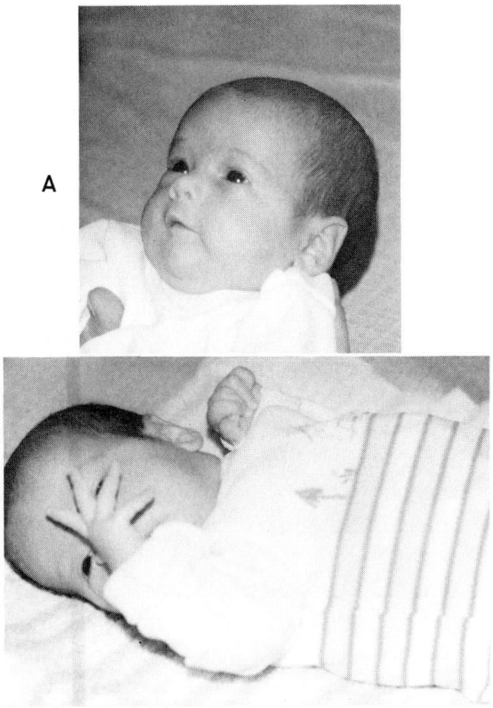

Fig. 20-7 **A**, Alerting. **B**, Habituating. (Courtesy Colleen Stainton.)

Parents will also use facial expressions as a means of interaction. They may slow and exaggerate expressions such as surprise, happiness, and confusion to communicate them to the infant. Playing games, such as "peek-a-boo," is another means of interaction. Parents can also be observed imitating the infant's behaviors. If the baby smiles, the parent will also smile. If the baby frowns, the parent responds in kind.

Responsivity. Contingent responses are those that occur within a specific time and are similar in form to a stimulus behavior. They elicit a feeling in the person originating the behavior of having an influence on the interaction. In other words, they act as positive feedback. Adults view infant behaviors such as smiling, cooing, and sustained eye contact, usually in *en face* position, as contingent responses. The adults are encouraged to continue the same game when the infant responds in such a way. These responses act as rewards to the initiator. When the adult imitates the infant, the infant appears to enjoy the responses. The infant in turn imitates behaviors of adults soon after birth. The parent shows progression in presenting behaviors for the baby to imitate; for example, in early interactions the parent will grimace rather than laugh, which is in keeping with the infant's developmental level. Such "turnabout" behaviors sustain interactions and promote harmony in the relationship.

Factors Influencing Parental Responses

How the parents respond to the birth of their child is influenced by various factors, including age, social networks, socioeconomic conditions, and personal aspirations for the future.

Maternal Age Over 35. Maternal age has a definite effect on pregnancy outcome. The mother and fetus are both at highest risk when the mother is an adolescent or **over** 35 years old. Adolescent pregnancy is a significant issue in North America and is addressed in Chapter 27.

Issues and concerns related to the over-35 age group have become increasingly more prominent in the last decade (p. 206). There have always been women over 35 who have continued their childbearing either by choice or because of lack or failure of contraception during the perimenopausal years. Added to this group are women who have postponed pregnancy because of careers or other reasons, and women with infertility problems who have become pregnant because of new technology that has expanded alternatives for couples desiring children.

Studies have identified certain factors that can influence parental responses in this older group. *Fatigue and the need for more rest* seem to be the major concerns of older parents with newborns (Queenan, 1987; Winslow, 1987). Many of these mothers, being less resilient than younger women, may need to stay in the hospital longer, rather than be forced to an early discharge, as some third party payers are requiring.

Measures designed to assist the mother in regaining strength and muscle tone (e.g., prenatal and postdelivery exercises) are emphasized. Some older mothers may find that the care of the newborn infant exhausts their physical capabilities. Many women might benefit from referral to supportive resources in the community (Scott, Meredith, and Angwin, 1986).

Social Networks. Primiparas and multiparas may have different needs. Multiparas may be more realistic in anticipating their physical limitations and can adjust to changes in roles and relationships more easily. Primiparas may need more supportive care and follow-up for parenting, including referral to community resources. The families and friends of the parents and their newborn child form an important dimension of the parent's social network. Social networks provide a support system on which parents can rely for assistance (Cronenwett, 1985a, b; Crawford, 1985). Positive emotional and affectional relationships appear critical to the enhancement of parenting skills and nurturance of children (Gottlieb, 1980; Schornkoff, 1984). Social networks promote the growth potential of children and the prevention of their maltreatment. Mercer (1982) and Crawford (1985) found that social networks provided support but were also a source of conflict. Parents or in-laws who assisted with household responsibilities and who did not intrude into the parents' privacy or critically judge them were most appreciated. Sometimes a large network caused problems in that it generated conflicting advice to the new parents.

Socioeconomic Conditions. Parents whose economic condition is made worse with the birth of each child and who are unable to use an effective method of fertility management may find childbirth compounded by concern for their own health and a sense of helplessness. Mothers who are alone, deserted by husband, family, and friends, or who are in an untenable economic state may view the birth of the child with dread. The difficulties in which they find themselves may overcome any desire for mothering the infant (Chapter 25).

Nursing measures designed to help persons in these circumstances involve social and economic community agencies as well as health agencies. Satisfactory outcomes of such problems often require long-term commitments from both the woman or couple and the community. Adequate situational supports need to be instituted in the prenatal period.

Personal Aspirations. For some women parenthood interferes with or curtails their plans for personal freedom or advancement in their career. Resentment concerning their loss may not have been resolved during the prenatal period. If this resentment is not resolved, it will spill over into caregiving activities and may result in indifference and neglect. Or, conversely, it may result in oversolicitousness and the setting of impossibly high standards by the mother for her behavior or the child's performance (Shainess, 1970).

Nursing intervention includes providing opportunities for parents to vent their feelings freely to an objective listener; to discuss measures to permit personal growth of the parent, for example, by parttime employment, volunteer work, and use of agencies that provide babysitting care or mother substitutes during parents' vacations; and to learn about the care of the child.

PARENTAL SENSORY IMPAIRMENT

In the early dialogue between parent and child, all senses—sight, hearing, touch, taste, and smell—are used by both to initiate and sustain the *attachment process.* A parent who is deprived of one of the senses needs to develop an enriched use of the remaining sensory sources.

Blind Parent

Although parents who are blind need the presence as well as the support of another responsible person, they can become adept in some child-care activities, as the following report indicates:

> We had always planned to have a child. My family and Dick's both wanted us to have the happiness of children and were willing to help us with the baby care. First I bathed and changed a doll; then I practiced caring for my sister's baby. I would feel in all the creases with my finger to see if they were clean and dry. We used disposable diapers that do not need pins. My mother made baby clothes with fastenings of press cloth (Velcro) so I would not have to fiddle with buttons. I feel really confident now. I know I can't do everything for her, but I can do enough to feel like a "mother," and I know she will have all the love she needs.

One of the major difficulties blind parents experience is the skepticism, overt or covert, of the professional worker. Blind persons sense a reluctance on the part of others to concede that they have a right to be parents. One blind mother-to-be noted that the best approach by the nurse is for the nurse to assess the mother's capabilities (Asrael, 1983). From that basis the nurse can make plans to assist the woman (i.e., the same as for a sighted mother). Another mother talked about the shyness, fear, or reluctance she sensed in nurses that resulted in her being left alone or being involved in awkward conversations.

Another mother expressed how sensitive the blind can become to other sensory output. She remarked that she could tell when her infant was facing her because she could feel his breath on her face.

Three mothers who are blind volunteered the following suggestions for providing care for the needs of women such as themselves during childbearing:

1. Clients who are blind need verbal teaching from health care providers because maternity information is not accessible to blind people.
2. Clients need an orientation to the hospital room that allows the client to move about the room independently. For example, "Go to the left of the bed and trail the wall until you feel the first door. That is the bathroom."
3. Clients need explanations of routines.
4. Clients need opportunities to feel devices (e.g., monitors, pelvic models) and to hear descriptions of the devices.
5. Clients need "a chance to ask questions!"
6. Clients need the opportunity to hold and touch their baby after delivery.
7. Nurses need to demonstrate baby care by touch and to follow with, "Now let me see you do it."
8. Nurses need to give instructions such as "I'm going to give you the baby. The head is on the left side."

Eye-to-eye contact is considered important in our culture. With a parent who is blind, this critical component in the parent-child attachment process is obviously missing. However, since the blind parent may have no experience in using this strategy to promote relationships, he or she cannot be said to miss it. The infant will need other sensory input from the blind parent. Perhaps an infant looking into the eyes of a mother who is blind is not conscious that the eyes are unseeing. Other persons in the newborn's environment can participate in active eye-to-eye contact to supply this lack. Another problem may arise if the parent who is blind has an impassive facial expression. One observer noticed an infant making repeated attempts to engage in face play with his mother, who was blind. After repeated failure of his efforts, he abandoned the behavior with his mother and intensified it with his father. This problem might be overcome by the person's learning to accompany talking and cooing to the infant with head nodding and smiling.

Deaf Parent

The parent who has a hearing impairment faces another set of problems, particularly if the deafness dates from birth or early childhood. The mother and her partner are likely to have established an independent household. A number of devices that transform sound into light flashes are now marketed. The infant's room can be fitted with such a device to permit immediate detection of crying. Even if the parent(s) is not speech trained, her or his vocalizing can serve as both stimulus and response to the infant's early vocalizing. Deaf parents can provide additional vocal training by use of records and television so that from birth onward the child is aware of the full range of the human voice. Sign language is acquired readily by the young child, and the first sign used as varied as the first word.

Baranowski (1983) described childbirth education classes for expectant deaf parents: "The students were attentive, asked questions, and readily participated in discussions. Their regular attendance indicated that they were interested in the classes."

Section 504 of the Rehabilitation Act of 1973 requires that hospitals and other institutions receiving funds from the U.S. Department of Health and Human Services use various communication techniques and resources with the deaf, including staff members or a certified interpreter who are proficient in sign language. The nurse who is bilingual has an advantage in providing care for clients.

❑ SIBLING ADAPTATION

Introduction of the infant into a family with one or more children may pose problems for the parents. They are faced with the task of caring for a new child while not neglecting the others. Parents need to distribute their attention in a manner that they consider fair.

Older children have to assume new positions within the family hierarchy. The older child's goal is to maintain a leading position. The child who is next in birth order to the infant has to gain a superior position over the newcomer (Kreppner et al, 1982). As the infant develops and begins to assert herself or himself, the older child works toward dominance. "He or she takes away toys and other objects the younger child is grasping for, thereby demonstrating that he or she has control over the situation. The older child also intervenes more openly when parents are interacting with the younger child" (Kreppner et al, 1982). One 3-year-old child encouraged his mother to put the new baby "out with the garbage because we've seen enough of her."

Regression to an infantile level of behavior may be seen in some children. They may revert to bed-wetting, whining, or refusing to feed themselves. An older child who is still young wavers between thinking "I'm big now" and thinking "I'm still a baby, so look after me." Jealous reactions are to be expected once the initial excitement of having a new baby in the home is over, since the baby absorbs the time and attention of the important persons in the other children's lives.

Parents, especially mothers, spend much time and energy promoting sibling acceptance of a new baby. Older children are involved actively in preparation for the infant, and involvement intensifies after the birth of the child. Mother and father face a number of tasks related to **sibling rivalry** and adjustment. The tasks include the following:

1. Making the older child feel loved and wanted.
2. Managing guilt arising from feelings that older children are being deprived of parental time and attention.
3. Developing feelings of confidence in her or his ability to nurture more than one child.
4. Adjusting time and space to accommodate the new baby.
5. Monitoring behavior of older children toward the more vulnerable infant and diverting aggressive behavior.

The new parent can learn many innovative techniques by listening to other parents describe their efforts to ease the older siblings' acceptance of the new child (see guidelines for client teaching: sibling preparation, p. 224). Walz and Rich (1983) have described a number of creative parental interventions.

1. A mother took her firstborn on a tour of her hospital room and pointed out similarities to the first child. "This is the same room I was in with you, and I think the baby is in the same cot that you were in."
2. The newborn was described as a "special gift" for the older child.
3. The children were in the *first* group (grandparents, sister) to see the newborn (Fig. 20-8).

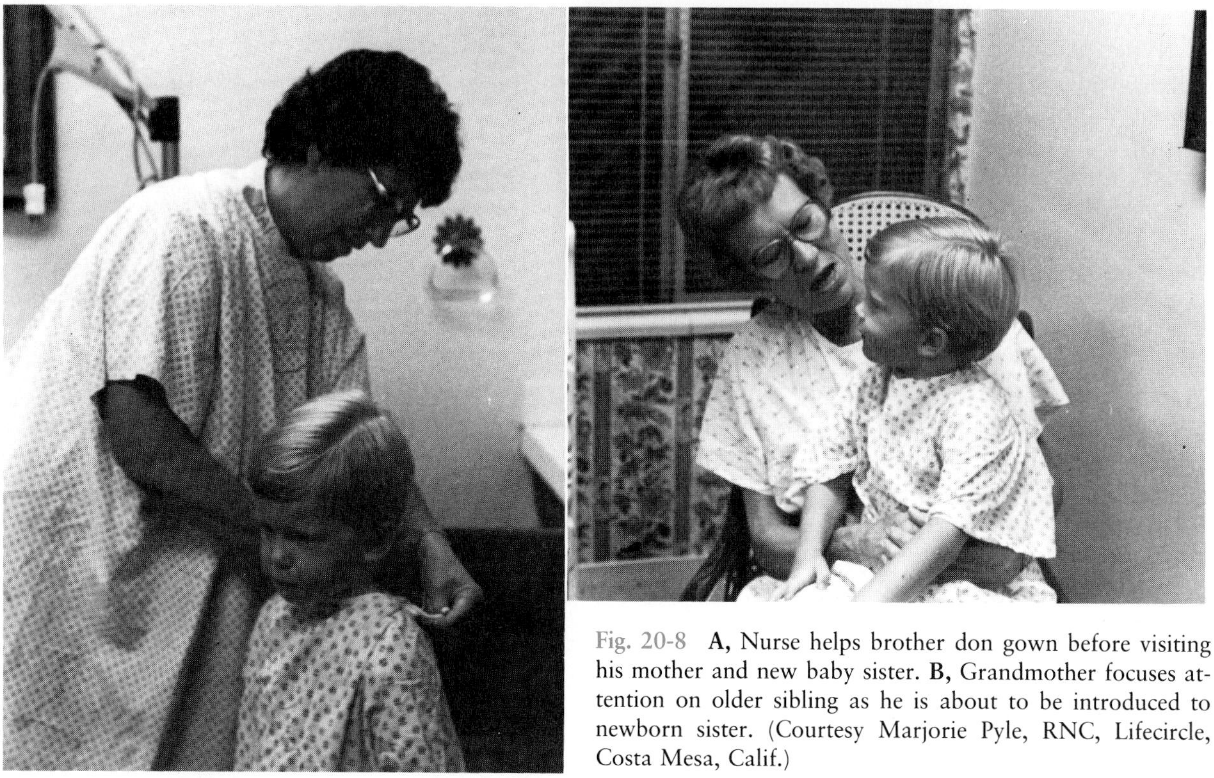

A

B

Fig. 20-8 **A,** Nurse helps brother don gown before visiting his mother and new baby sister. **B,** Grandmother focuses attention on older sibling as he is about to be introduced to newborn sister. (Courtesy Marjorie Pyle, RNC, Lifecircle, Costa Mesa, Calif.)

4. Time was planned for both children. A mother remarked, "When I get home, I'll arrange my day so that I can have the baby's care done in the morning while Sam (first child) is at school. Maybe the baby will sleep part of the afternoon and I can spend some time with Sam."

Fathers were enlisted as the main support for mothers reallocating time to include older children. "My husband will take care of Becca (first child) and I will have the baby, because he can do things with Becca she will enjoy. I will give the baby things my husband can't." Other husbands were expected to help with the care of the newborn to permit the mother to spend more time with the older child. Studies (Umphenour, 1980; Kowba et al, 1985; and Wranesh, 1982) have demonstrated that healthy newborns who have direct sibling contact are not at risk for exposure to pathogenic organisms. Therefore separation of newborns and older siblings does not appear to be warranted.

Acquaintance behaviors of siblings with the newborn have been described by Marecki et al, 1985, and Anderberg, 1988. The acquaintance process depends on the information given to the child before the baby is born and on the cognitive developmental level of the child. The initial behaviors of siblings with the newborn include looking at the infant and touching the head.

The initial adjustment of older children to a newborn takes time. Children should be allowed to interact at their own pace rather than being forced. To expect a young child to accept and love a rival for the parents' affection assumes a too-mature response. Sibling love grows as does other love, that is, by being with another person and sharing experiences (Fig. 20-9).

❑ GRANDPARENT ADAPTATION

The amount of involvement of grandparents in the care of the newborn depends on many factors, for example, willingness of the grandparents to become involved, proximity of the grandparents, and ethnic and cultural expectations of the role grandparents play (Grosso et al, 1981).

The woman's mother is an important model for child-rearing practices (Rubin, 1975). She acts as a source of knowledge and as a support person. Grandchildren are tangible evidence of continuity, of immortality. Often grandparents comment that the presence of grandchildren helps relieve loneliness and boredom (Fig. 20-10).

"There are many ways to encourage new parents to include the grandparents, enriching their child's life and benefiting from the extended family themselves" (Olson, 1981). As parents are assisted in working

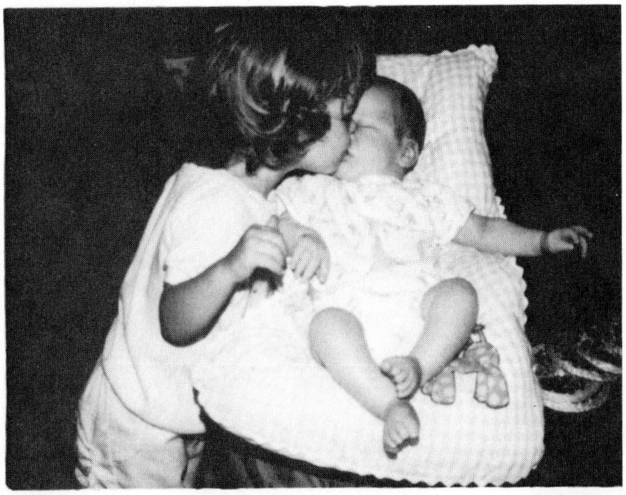

Fig. 20-9 Sister kisses her new brother. Family contacts are important for newborn and siblings. (Courtesy Marjorie Pyle, RNC, Lifecircle, Costa Mesa, Calif.)

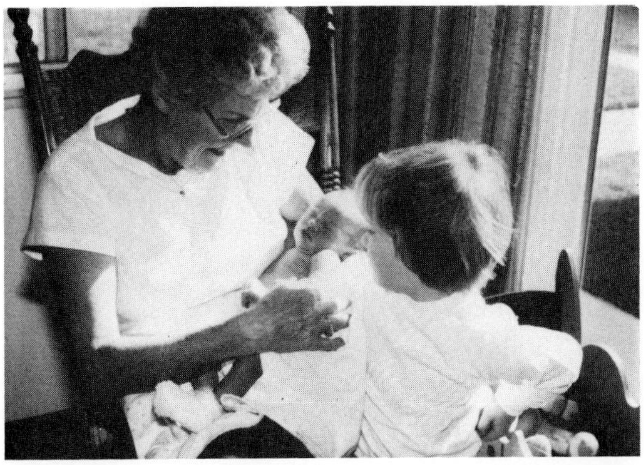

Fig. 20-10 Grandmother holds new baby as older brother looks on. (Courtesy Marjorie Pyle, RNC, Lifecircle, Costa Mesa, Calif.)

through differing opinions and unresolved conflicts (e.g., dependency, control) between themselves and their parents, they can move toward mastery of the developmental tasks of adulthood. Grandparental support can be a stabilizing influence for families undergoing developmental crises such as childbearing and new parenthood (Newell, 1984). Grandparents can foster the learning of parental skills and preserve tradition. One simple technique to help people span the generation gap is through a printed "letter to new parents" (written from the grandparents' perspective), which can be included in prenatal kits distributed in childbirth preparation classes and made available to all family members on the postpartum unit (Olson, 1981). Another way to help grandparents bridge the generation gap and help them understand parenting concepts that their adult children are using is to offer classes (Maloni, McIndue, and Rubenstein, 1987). Included in these classes would be information about up-to-date childbearing practices, especially family-centered care; infant care, feeding, and safety (car seats); and exploration of roles grandparents play in the family unit. Both techniques can foster open discussion between the generations about feelings and needs of parents and grandparents.

Grandparents can do things that no one else can do. They can tell their grandchildren about their roots and stories about their parents. They contribute to a sense of family continuity and provide for maintenance of cultural traditions.

Grandparents who are free to love the grandchild crazily, blindly, lavishly, and without reservation (LeShan, 1975) can have a significant positive influence on the child's life. Praise and encouragement from a significant person fosters the development of a positive self-image and a sense of being worthy (see Fig. 20-8, *B*).

SUMMARY

The childbearing family faces a constant challenge of maintaining balance between the integration of new family members and changing established interaction patterns and problem-solving strategies. The family's ability to meet the challenge is critical for parents and children. Nursing actions designed to strengthen family bonds and facilitate the mother's and father's attainment of parental roles serve an important social purpose.

LEARNING ACTIVITIES

1. Observe different mothers and fathers with their infants. In clinical conference, discuss the types of attachment behaviors observed, including differences between mothers and fathers. Discuss the rationale for these responses. Discuss possible interventions to facilitate attachment.
2. Take turns role-playing a blind or deaf mother interacting both with her newborn and with the nurse who is attempting to provide client education. Follow with a discussion of the responses and frustrations experienced by each party.
3. Develop a client teaching program that explains the reasons for sibling rivalry or jealousy and provides possible interventions the parents might employ to counteract the problem.
4. In the group setting, discuss own relationships with grandparents and how these experiences compare with the text discussion of the grandparent role.

KEY CONCEPTS

- The birth of a child poses a fundamental challenge to the existing interactional structure of a family.
- Either parent may exhibit "motherliness."
- Attachment is the process by which parent and child come to love and accept each other.
- Attachment is strengthened through the use of sensual responses or abilities by both partners in the parent-child interaction.
- Early contact with the newborn is not essential for optimum parent-child interactions.
- For the biologic parent, the parental role does not begin at birth, but rather enlarges and intensifies.
- In adjusting to the parental role, the mother moves from a dependent state to an interdependent state.
- Mothers may be overwhelmed by the actuality of parenting responsibilities and may exhibit signs of postpartum depression ("baby blues").
- A primary need of parents is to establish a lifestyle that includes, but in some respects excludes, the child.
- In Western culture the newborn has been found to have a powerful impact on the father.
- Modulation of rhythm, modification of behavioral repertoires, and mutual responsivity facilitate infant-parent adjustment.
- Many factors influence parental responses (e.g., their age, socioeconomic level, and their expectations of what their child will be like).
- Parents face a number of tasks related to sibling adjustment that require creative parental interventions.
- As parents work through differing opinions and unresolved conflicts between themselves and their parents, they can move toward mastery of the developmental tasks of adulthood.

References

Anderberg GJ: Initial acquaintance and attachment behavior of siblings with the newborn, JOGN Nurs 17(1):49, 1988.

Ainsworth MD: Object relations, dependency, and attachment: a theoretical review of the infant-mother relationship, Child Dev 40:969, 1969.

Ainsworth MD: The development of infant-mother attachment. In Caldwell BM and Reccurti HN, editors: Review of child development research, vol 3, New York, 1970, Russell Sage Foundation.

Ainsworth MD and Bell SM: Attachment, exploration and separation: illustrated by the behavior of one-year-olds in a strange situation, Child Dev 41:49, 1970.

Asrael W: Disabled women and childbearing: the nurse's role, NAACOG Update series, 1 (lesson 8), 1983.

Baranowski E: Childbirth education classes for expectant deaf parents, MCN 8:143, 1983.

Barnett CR et al: Neonatal separation: the maternal side of interactional deprivation, Pediatrics 54:197, 1970.

Benedek T: Adaptation to reality in early infancy, Psychoanal Q 7:200, 1950.

Bowlby J: The nature of the child's tie to his mother, Int J Psychoanal 39:350, 1958.

Bowlby J: Attachment and loss, vol 1: Attachment, New York, 1969, Basic Books, Inc, Publishers.

Brazelton TB: The early mother-infant adjustment, Pediatrics 32:931, 1963.

Brazelton TB: Effect of maternal expectations on early infant behavior, Early Child Dev Care 2:259, 1973.

Brazelton TB et al: The origins of reciprocity: the early mother-infant interaction. In Lewis M and Rosenblum LA, editors: The effect of the infant on its caregiver, New York, 1974, John Wiley & Sons, Inc.

Budin P: The nursling, London, 1907, Caxton Publishing Co.

Clarke-Stewart K: And daddy makes three: the father's impact on mother and young child, Child Dev 49:466, 1978.

Condon W and Sander L: Neonate movement is synchronized with adult speech: interactional participation and language acquisition, Science 183:99, 1974.

Crawford J: A theoretical model of support network conflict experienced by new mothers, Nurs Res 34:100, March/April, 1985.

Cronenwett LR: Network structure, social support, and psychological outcomes of pregnancy, Nurs Res 34:93, March/April, 1985a.

Cronenwett LR: Parental network structured and perceived support after birth of first child, Nurs Res 34:347, Nov/Dec, 1985b.

Curry MS: Contact during first hour with the wrapped or naked newborn: effect on maternal attachment behaviors at 36 hours and three months, Birth Fam J 6:4, Winter, 1979.

Davis MI and Akridge KM: The effect of promoting intrauterine attachment in primiparas on postdelivery attachment, JOGN Nurs 16(6):430, 1987.

Erikson EH: Identity and the life cycle: selected papers. In Psychological issues, vol 1, no 1, New York, 1959, International Universities Press, Inc.

Erikson EH: Childhood and society, New York, 1964, WW Norton & Co, Inc.

Field T: The three Rs of infant-adult interactions: rhythms, repertoires, and responsibility, J Pediatr Psychol 3:131, 1978a.

Field T: Visual and cardiac responses to animate and inanimate faces by young term and preterm infants, Child Dev vol 49, 1978b.

Gottlieb BH: The role of individual and social support in preventing child maltreatment. In Garbarino J and Stocking S, editors: Protecting children from abuse/neglect, San Francisco, 1980, Jossey-Bass, Inc, Publishers.

Greenberg M and Morris N: Engrossment: the newborn's impact on the father, Nurs Digest 4:19, Jan/Feb, 1976.

Grosso C et al: The Vietnamese American family . . . and grandma makes three, MCN 6:177, 1981.

Hefler RE and Kempe CH: The battered child, Chicago, 1965, University of Chicago Press.

Klaus MH, and Kennell, JH: Parent-infant bonding, ed 2, St Louis, 1982, The CV Mosby Co.

Kowba MD et al: Direct sibling contact and bacterial colonization in newborns, JOGN Nurs 14:412, Sept/Oct, 1985.

Kreppner, K, and others: Infant and family development from triads to tetrads, Hum. Dev. 25:373, 1982.

Kunst-Wilson W and Cronenwett L: Nursing care for the emerging family: promoting paternal behavior, Res Nurs Health 4:201, 1981.

Lamb M: Early contact and maternal-infant bonding: one decade later, Pediatrics 70:325, 1982.

Lang R: Birth book, Ben Lomond, Calif, 1972, Genesis Press.

Leifer AD et al: Effects of mother-infant separation on maternal attachment behavior, Child Dev 43:1203, 1972.

LeShan E: The wonderful crisis of middle age, New York, 1975, Warner Books, Inc.

Maloni JA, McIndoe JE, and Rubenstein G: Expectant grandparents classes, JOGN Nurs 16(1):26, 1987.

Marecki M, et al: Early sibling attachment, JOGN Nurs 14(5):418, 1985.

Mercer RT: Parent-infant attachment. In Sonstegard LJ et al: editors: Women's health, vol 2: Childbearing, New York, 1982, Grune & Stratton, Inc.

NAACOG Committee on Practice: Mother-baby care, NAACOG OGN Nursing Practice Resource, Washington, DC, 1989, The Committee.

Newell NJ: Grandparents, the overlooked support system for new parents during the fourth trimester, NAACOG Update Series 1 (lesson 21), 1984.

Olson ML: Fitting grandparents into new families, MCN 6:419, 1981.

Parkes CM and Stevenson-Hinde J: The place of attachment in human behavior, New York, 1982, Basic Books, Inc, Publishers.

Queenan JT, moderator: Managing pregnancy in patients over 35, Contemp OB/GYN 29(5):180, 1987.

Rubin R: Maternal behavior, Nurs Outlook 9:682, 1961.

Rubin R: Maternal touch at first contact with the newborn infant, Nurs Outlook 11:828, 1963.

Rubin R: Maternal tasks in pregnancy, Matern Child Nurs J 4:143, Fall, 1975.

Sammons WA and Lewis JM: Premature babies: a different beginning, St Louis, 1985, The CV Mosby Co.

Schornkoff JP: Social support and the development of vulnerable children, Am J Public Health 74:310, 1980.

Scott L, Meredith A, and Angwin, J: Time out for motherhood: a guide for today's working woman to the financial, emotional and career aspects of having a baby, Los Angelos, 1986, Jeremy P Tarcher, Inc.

Shainess N: Abortion is no man's business, Psychology Today, p. 18, March, 1970.

Siegel E: A critical examination of studies of parent-infant bonding. In Klaus M and Robertson M, editors: Birth, interaction and attachment, Evansville, Inc, 1982, Johnson & Johnson Baby Products Co.

Stainton MC: A comparison of prenatal and postnatal perceptions of their babies by parents, Paper presented to the First International Congress on Pre- and Para-natal Psychology, Toronto, July 8, 1983a.

Stainton MC: Maternal newborn attachment origins and processes. III. Interactional synchrony: the prelude to attachment, doctoral thesis, University of California, San Francisco, 1983b.

Stainton MC: Origins of attachment: Culture and cue sensitivity. Dissertation Abstracts International, *46*, 3786-B. (University Microfilms No. 8600606), 1985.

Steele B and Pollock C: A psychiatric study of parents who abuse infants and small children. In Helfer RE and Kempe C, editors: The battered child, Chicago, 1968, University of Chicago Press.

Tulman L: Mothers and unrelated persons' initial handling of newborn infants, Nurs Res 34:205, July/Aug, 1985.

Umphenour JH: Bacterial colonization in neonates with sibling visitation, JOGN Nurs 9:73, 1980.

Walz B and Rich O: Maternal tasks of taking on a second child in the postpartum period, Matern Child Nurs J 12:3, Fall, 1983.

Winslow W: First pregnancy after 35: what is the experience? MCN 12(2):92, 1987.

Wranesh BL: The effect of sibling visitation on bacterial colonization rate in neonates, JOGN Nurs 11:211, 1982.

Bibliography

Booth CL, Johnson-Crowley N, and Bernard KE: Infant massage and exercise: worth the effort? MCN 10(3):184, 1985.

Dormire SL, Strauss SS, and Clarke BA: Social support and adaptation to the parent role in first-time adolescent mothers, JOGN Nurs 18(4):327, 1989.

Fawcett J and York R: Spouses' physical and psychological symptoms during pregnancy and the postpartum, Nurs Res 35(3):144, 1986.

Fawcett J et al: Spouses' body image changes during and after pregnancy: a replication and extension, Nurs Res 36(4):220, 1986.

Fortier JC: The relationship of vaginal and cesarean births to father-infant attachment, JOGN Nurs 17(2):128, 1988.

Gay JT, Edgil AE, and Douglass AB: Reva Rubin Revisited, JOGN Nurs 17(6):394, 1988.

Hans H: Postpartum assessment: the psychological component, JOGN Nurs 15(1):49, 1986.

Humenick SS and Bugen LA: Parenting roles: expectation versus reality, MCN 12(1):36, 1987.

Majewski J: Social support and the transition to the maternal role, Health Care Women Int 8(5):397, 1987.

Martell LK: Postpartum depression as a family problem, MCN 15(2):90, 1990.

Martone DJ and Nash BR: Initial differences in postpartum attachment behavior in breastfeeding and bottle-feeding mothers, JOGN Nurs 17(3):212, 1988.

Mercer RT and Stainton MC: Perceptions of the birth experience: a cross-cultural comparison, Health Care Women Int 5:29, 1984.

Norr KF, Roberts JE, and Freese U: Early postpartum rooming-in and maternal attachment behaviors in a group of medically indigent primiparas, J Nurse Midwife 34(2):85, 1989.

Palkovitz R: Sources of father-infant bonding beliefs: implications for childbirth education, Matern Child Nurs J 17(2):101, 1988.

Sherwen, LN: Psychosocial Dimensions of the Pregnant Family, New York, 1987, Springer Publishing Co, Inc.

Stein A: Pregnancy in gravidas over age 35 years, J Nurse Midwife 28(1):17, 1983.

Tulman L: Initial handling of newborn infants by vaginally and cesarean-delivered mothers, Nurs Res 35:296, 1986.

Wilkerson NN and Barrows TL: Synchronizing care with mother-baby rhythms, MCN 13(4):264, 1988.

CHAPTER

21 Nursing Care During the Postpartum Period

Vicki Akin

Learning Objectives

Correctly define the key terms listed.

Review the components of the postpartum interview, physical examination, and laboratory tests.

Outline the normal progression of puerperal changes and schedule of assessment from day 1 through day 3.

Formulate examples of potential nursing diagnoses for physical and emotional care.

Identify goals for postpartum physical and emotional care.

Summarize general care for rest, ambulation and exercise, bed rest, immunizations, comfort, and safety.

Compare and contrast parental responses to the birth of a child focusing on adaptive and maladaptive behaviors of the mother, infant, and family.

Explain mother's need to integrate the birth experience.

Examine crisis prevention as a component of postpartum emotional care.

Explore the cultural aspects of postpartum care, both physical and emotional.

List physical danger signs during the postpartum period.

Determine the nurse's responsibilities related to discharge.

Key Terms

adaptive behaviors
boggy uterus
cultural proscriptions
depressive states ("the baby blues")
hemorrhoids
Homans' sign
infant massage
"living ligature"
lochia
maladaptive behaviors
oxytocic medications
parenting difficulties
parenting disorders
perineum
pollution state
$Rh_0(D)$ immune globulin
rubella vaccination
self-care
sibling rivalry
sitz bath
"spinal" headache
suppression of lactation
"taking-hold"
"taking-in"
thromboembolism
thrombosis

The approach to care of women during the postpartum (puerperal) period has changed from one modeled on the concept of sick care to one that is *wellness oriented*. Women are concerned about their comfort and recovery, desirous of having contact with their infants, motivated to learn about newborn care and self-care, and eager to share their experiences with their families and friends. Their health care is now a collaborative effort on the part of all involved—mother, nurse, physician, and family—to achieve health awareness goals.

Knowledge of physiologic changes in the mother and emotional changes in the entire family are essential in appropriately evaluating assessment findings. Nursing diagnoses, planning, and implementation consider the need of the mother and family to participate with the nurse in learning **self-care**. Early discharge, within 24 hours after delivery, is the preference for some. For others, early discharge is a necessity for reasons such as minimal insurance coverage. The teaching-learning process is initiated in the fourth stage of labor and is continued throughout the postpartum period, with ongoing evaluation and modifications. Effects of learning may not be evident because of the short-term contact with childbearing families after delivery. Long-term effects are yet to be identified through nursing research.

This chapter focuses both on the mother's physiologic needs and on the family's emotional needs. The first portion of the chapter provides the nurse with several procedures for care and guidelines for client teaching. The second portion addresses the emotional needs and care of the family. The nurse makes a significant contribution to providing total care to the woman and her family. Kunst-Wilson and Cronenwett (1981) make the following comment:

> [Nurses'] unique ability to deal with both the physical and psychological spheres, and the interactions of each on the other, especially important in childbearing, makes nursing's potential contribution more comprehensive than that of related disciplines. The nurse has the professional skills to deliver services personally in the office, home, or hospital setting, depending on the family's needs. Thus no major aspect of the normal childbearing experience is beyond the bounds of the nurse's skills.

❑ PHYSICAL CARE

Assessment

The initial assessment includes the report from the nurse in the labor unit. The admitting nurse is given a brief description of all pertinent information (p. 434). The woman's record is reviewed for information from the prenatal and labor records that is necessary for her nursing care plan.

During the assessment the nurse can determine the mother's emotional status, energy level, degree and location of physical discomfort, hunger, and thirst. To some degree, her knowledge level concerning self-care and infant care can also be determined. If appropriate, ethnic and cultural expectations are assessed regarding postpartum recovery patterns. The nursing care plan must consider individual variations in maternal behaviors and degree of participation in self-care and in infant care.

Physical/Psychosocial Examination

Postpartum assessment is based on expected maternal changes. A head-to-toe assessment is performed when the client is admitted to the unit and at least daily throughout her hospital stay to determine any potential problems.

The length of the fourth stage and the time of transfer to the postpartum unit varies with each institution. Included in the daily assessments are vital signs, reproductive/genitourinary concerns, cardiovascular/gastrointestinal function, routine laboratory tests, and psychosocial factors. The following discussion will provide guidelines for the type and frequency of these assessments.

Vital Signs. The blood pressure, pulse, and respirations are assessed every 15 minutes for the first hour after delivery (p. 424), every 30 minutes for the next 2 hours, and then every hour for the next 2 hours. Vital signs continue to be monitored every 4 hours for the first 24 hours after birth and then once every 8 hours. When admitting the mother to the recovery area her temperature is assessed. The temperature is assessed 1 hour later, then every 4 hours for the first 24 hours, then every 8 hours unless problems develop.

Reproductive/Genitourinary. During the first hour after delivery the fundus, lochia, and bladder are assessed every 15 minutes. The fundus is assessed for firmness, location, and position. Massage may be necessary to firm up a boggy uterus. At the same time the suprapubic area should be palpated for bladder fullness. The peripad is examined for color, amount, and any odor of the lochia. Clots may also be expelled during this time and should be carefully assessed for amount and documented. Also the linens under the buttocks should be checked for any pooling of blood. These assessments should be performed twice in the second hour, and then once in the third and fourth hours after delivery. Assessments continue for the next 24 hours, along with vital signs.

The 2 hours after delivery are also an excellent time to encourage the mother to breastfeed if she desires (Chapter 11). The infant is in an alert state and ready to breastfeed, which will aid in the contraction of the uterus and prevention of hemorrhage. This is a wonderful opportunity for the nurse to demonstrate and instruct the mother in breastfeeding and to assess the physical appearance of the breasts.

If the woman has chosen not to breastfeed, instructions should be given for nonpharmacologic **suppression of lactation.** Some suggestions include wearing a tight-fitting bra, applying ice packs, and avoiding any stimulation of the breasts. In either instance, the breasts should be assessed every 8 hours throughout the hospital stay for nipple soreness, fissures, redness, tenderness, or engorgement.

Cardiovascular/Gastrointestinal. The woman's legs are inspected every 8 hours throughout the hospital stay for evidence of edema or thrombophlebitis. Each foot is flexed with the leg extended (see Fig 10-17, *A*) to assess for pain in the calf area along with inspection for redness or swelling and palpation for increased warmth. Evidence of pain in the calf is a positive **Homan's sign.** Pulses may be absent in the presence of thrombophlebitis.

The woman should be asked daily if she has had a

bowel movement. Stool softeners or laxatives may be part of the physician's regimen. The anal area should be assessed for **hemorrhoids** while performing the reproductive examination.

Routine Laboratory Tests. Hemoglobin and hematocrit may be performed on the first postpartum day for assessment of blood loss during delivery. The prenatal record will provide information about the woman's rubella and Rh status and possible treatments that are needed. A clean-catch or catheterized urine specimen may be obtained and sent for routine urinalysis or culture and sensitivity.

Psychosocial Factors. During the first hours after delivery, as physical parameters are monitored, the nurse will also observe the mother and family for healthy bonding (attachment) behaviors (p. 561). The family interactions should continue to be monitored and documented every 4 to 8 hours throughout the hospital stay. The nurse should also be familiar with the different cultural behaviors of families so that normal cultural practices are not confused with abnormal bonding behaviors. The nurse must be able to intervene or refer the family to appropriate resources as indicated.

Nursing Diagnoses

Although women experience similar problems during the postpartum period, certain factors act to make each woman's experience unique. The labor a woman experienced (whether it was long or short), whether she plans to bottle-feed or breastfeed, whether she had an episiotomy, and whether she has other children are some factors to consider. Nursing diagnoses lend direction to types of nursing actions needed to implement a plan of care. Examples of nursing diagnoses follow:

Potential for infection related to
- Childbirth trauma to tissues

Constipation or urinary retention related to
- Post-childbirth discomfort
- Childbirth trauma to tissues

Sleep pattern disturbance related to
- Discomforts of postpartum period
- Long labor process

Pain related to
- Childbirth discomforts

Potential for injury related to
- Postpartum hemorrhage
- Effects of anesthesia

Knowledge deficit related to
- Importance of voiding as deterrent to hemorrhage

Situational low self-esteem related to
- Actual vs. expected birth experience

Ineffective breastfeeding related to
- Maternal discomfort
- Infant positioning
- Normal physiologic response

Planning

The nursing plan is individualized for the postpartum woman and the infant, even if the nursery retains primary responsibility for the infant. Once the nursing diagnoses are formulated, the nurse decides what nursing measures would be appropriate and which are to be given priority. The organization of care must take the newborn into consideration. The day actually revolves around the baby's feeding and care times.

The mother assumes increasing responsibility for her own self-care. The nurse is responsible for consistent assessment of actual or potential problems. In some areas "couple nursing" (mother and baby) has been introduced. The nurse has been educated in mother and infant care and acts as the primary nurse for both mother and infant even if the newborn is kept in the central nursery. This approach is a variation of rooming-in, in which mother and child room together and mother and nurse share the care of the infant.

The nursing care plan will include assessments to detect deviations from normal physical and psychosocial status, comfort measures to relieve discomfort or pain, and safety measures to prevent injury or infection. The nurse also will provide teaching and counseling measures designed to promote a mother's (and father's) feeling of competence in the care of herself and newly born child. The nurse evaluates continuously and is ready to change the plan if indicated. The nurse's ability to adapt the care plan to specific medical and nursing diagnoses results in individualized client care.

Standardized care plans are used by almost all facilities and health care providers (Fig. 21-1) and are found in many nursing textbooks. A standard care plan is an aid for students and new graduates in grasping concepts or setting priorities and selecting appropriate actions for real or potential problems (see nursing care plans in this chapter). In addition, it can be used as a checklist for giving general direction for implementing the nursing process with a client. Caution is advised against total reliance on a standardized plan: the uniqueness of the individual may be overlooked.

Goals during the postpartum period include that the woman will:

1. Remain infection free
2. Demonstrate normal involution, lochia changes without hemorrhage
3. Verbalize adequate comfort levels and be free from injury
4. Demonstrate normal bowel and bladder patterns

Name:	Grav: Para: Ab: Stb:	Infant	Family:
	Marital status:	Sex: Wt: Length:	Adults:
Room:	Occupation:	Time: Day: Date:	
		Pediatrician: Feeding:	Siblings:
	Rh: Type:	Baby's Rh: Type: Coombs:	
	Rubella antibody titer:	Condition of baby: Date:	

Short-term goal:

Long-term goal:

Emergency number: Person: Relationship: Address:

Date	Nursing diagnoses	Evaluative criteria	Nursing actions

Client teaching: **Mother**
Breast care
Perineal care; hemorrhoids
Lochia flow norms
Postpartum nutrition and fluid needs
Exercise/rest
Family schedules
Sexual relations
Emotional adjustments
Cesarean delivery
Tubal occlusion

Infant
Characteristics
Bathing
Cord/circumcision
Thermometer use
Bulb syringe
Breast feeding
Storage of milk
Formula feeding
Positioning/handling
Clothing; Diapering
Signs of illness
Safety/poison control
Car seats; CPR
Family planning options
Importance of follow-up care for self and infant

Discharge planning

1. Mother will have follow-up care for self and infant arranged prior to discharge.
2. Mother has received and verbalized understanding of discharge instructions re: care of breasts, perineum, stitches, nutrition, rest/exercise, resumption of sexual activity, danger signs to report to physician.
3. Mother demonstrates comfort and competence in caregiver skills with own infant.

Return visit:

Referrals: ( ) social work
( ) home care

Date/ resolution	Client problem(s)	Expected outcome (short/long-term goals)	Date outcome to be reached	Nursing action	Signature
/	Potential postpartum hemorrhage	Will verbalize lochia flow norms, how to report abnormal signs.		Teach lochia flow norms: color, amount, odor, length of flow, and how to report to nurse/physician.	
/				Assess fundal tone, height, position q15 min first hour postpartum, massage uterus prn.	
/				Assess q½h x 2, then q shift and prn.	
/				Teach mother how to massage fundus.	
/	Potential infection	Will verbalize lochia flow norms, how to report abnormal signs.		Alert woman to report temp. of 100.4° F, foul-smelling lochia, abdominal pain, general feeling of not being well.	
/		Will demonstrate appropriate hygiene and care of perineum, stitches.		Teach use of surgigator, squeeze bottle, sitz bath, avoidance of tampons, intercourse, swimming until postpartum checkup.	
/	Potential anxiety secondary to lack of knowledge/experience in care taking of infant, feeding.	Will demonstrate competence in infant care taking and feeding techniques.		Provide early contact with infant and encourage eye-to-eye, skin-to-skin contact.	
/				Assess readiness for learning, provide frequent opportunity for observing/practicing infant care skills, feedings.	
/				Provide emotional support and positive reinforcement with learned skills.	

Fig. 21-1 Plan of nursing care for woman after normal delivery. (Adapted from Fountain Valley Community Hospital, Fountain Valley Calif.)

5. Verbalize and demonstrate self-care and infant care skills
6. Verbalize knowledge of community agencies available for assistance
7. Verbalize understanding of postpartum complications
8. Demonstrate knowledge of type of infant feeding of choice

Implementation

The first step in providing individualized care is to confirm the client's identity by checking her arm band. At the same time, the infant's identification number is matched with the corresponding band on the mother's wrist. The nurse demonstrates caring and respect by determining how the mother wishes to be addressed and then notes her preference in her record and on the card index (Kardex).

Orientation to Environment

The woman and her family are oriented to their surroundings. Familiarity with the unit, routines, resources, and personnel reduces one potential source of anxiety—the unknown. The mother is reassured through knowing whom and how she can call for assistance and what she can expect in the way of supplies and services. If the woman's usual daily routine before admission differs from the facility's routine, the nurse works with the woman to develop a mutually acceptable and workable routine.

Ethnic and cultural variations in care of the woman after delivery can be discussed and plans for modifying nursing actions made (see pp. 605 to 608). An example of a cultural variation follows:

■ A Vietnamese woman who had been in the United States for 4 years requested rooming-in facilities following delivery. Instead of participating in the care of her infant, she refused to do so, remained in bed, wore a woolen cap, and appeared distressed and angry. The staff were nonplussed by her behavior. One nurse decided to put newly learned concepts concerning cross-cultural nursing into effect. She began by praising the woman's ability to speak English and after eliciting a smile, remarked, "Every country has developed good ways to look after mothers and babies. Would you tell me about the care in Vietnam?" There was an immediate response. The woman explained that in her country women remained in bed for 10 days after delivery and the biggest danger to their health was getting a cold. The baby was kept in the room with his mother, but either a grandmother or nurse took complete charge of the care.

Evidently the woman was operating in tune with her cultural expectations, and the nurses were operating within theirs. This rather simple approach to resolving a nursing problem also proved successful in subsequent cases.

Prevention of Infection

Facilities (unit kitchens, bathroom, and bed units) and supplies (linens) must be kept scrupulously clean. Frequent changes of draw sheet and a daily change of linen are recommended. Supervision of use of facilities to prevent cross infection among women is necessary (e.g., common sitz bath must be scrubbed after each woman's use, ventilation system is monitored). Personnel must be conscientious about their hand-washing techniques to prevent cross infection. Personnel with colds, coughs, or skin infections (e.g., a cold sore on the lips [herpes simplex virus, type 1]) must follow hospital protocol when in contact with women during the puerperium.

Daily assessment for signs and symptoms of infection include monitoring temperature, inspecting perineum and breasts, ascultating lungs, and inspecting skin integrity (i.e., intravenous [IV] site). To completely assess the **perineum,** the woman must be turned onto her side. After donning gloves, the nurse spreads the woman's buttocks to check for redness, swelling, and intactness of the suture line. The woman is informed of the status of her perineum.

Education of the woman is important to maintain cleanliness and prevent infection. Teaching the woman to wipe from front to back (vagina to anus) is the first step in preventing contamination of the vaginal and genitourinary areas. In many hospitals a squeeze bottle filled with warm water or a Surgi-Gator or Hygienic is used after each voiding to cleanse the perineal area. The woman is also taught to change her peripad with each voiding and to avoid inserting anything (i.e., tampons) into the vagina.

Rest, Ambulation, and Exercise

The excitement and exhilaration experienced after the birth of the infant may make rest difficult. The new mother, who is often anxious about her ability to care for her infant or is uncomfortable, may also have difficulty sleeping. Backrubs, other comfort measures, and medication for sleep for the first few nights may be necessary. The nurse may also assist the family to limit visitors and provide a comfortable chair or bed for the father.

Early ambulation has proved successful in reducing the incidence of thromboembolism and in promoting women's more rapid recovery of strength. Confinement

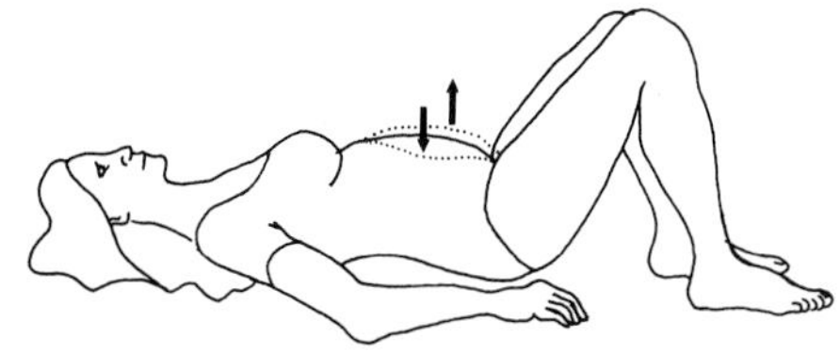

Abdominal Breathing. Lie on back with knees bent. Inhale deeply through nose. Keep ribs stationary and allow abdomen to expand upwards. Exhale slowly but forcefully while contracting the abdominal muscles; hold for 3 to 5 seconds while exhaling. Relax.

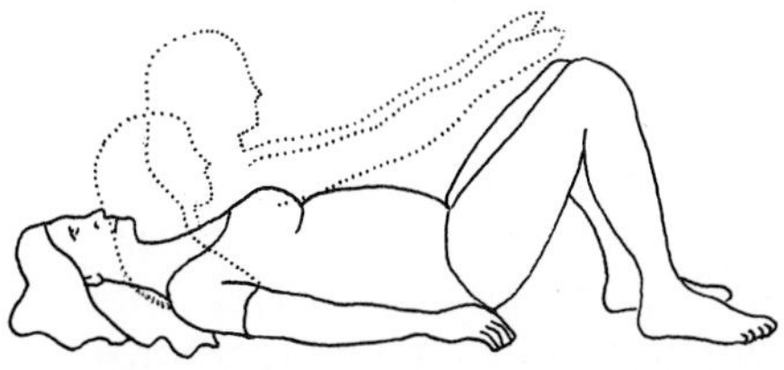

Reach for the Knees. Lie on back with knees bent. While inhaling deeply lower chin onto chest. While exhaling, raise head and shoulders slowly and smoothly and reach for knees with arms outstretched. The body should only rise as far as the back will naturally bend while waist remains on floor or bed (about 6 to 8 inches). Slowly and smoothly lower head and shoulders back to starting position. Relax.

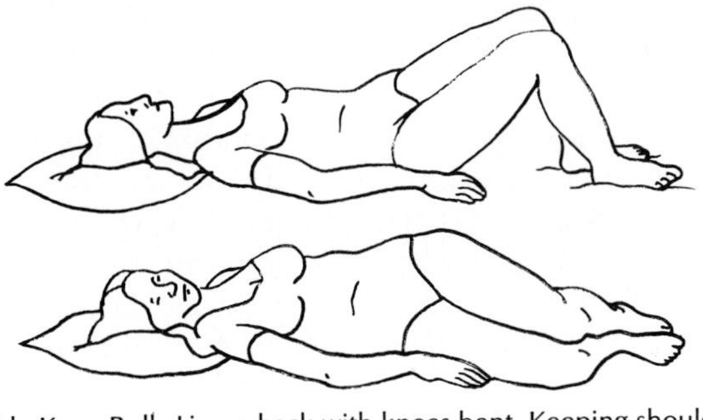

Double Knee Roll. Lie on back with knees bent. Keeping shoulders flat and feet stationary, slowly and smoothly roll knees over to the left to touch floor or bed. Maintaining a smooth motion, roll knees back over to the right until they touch floor or bed. Return to starting position and relax.

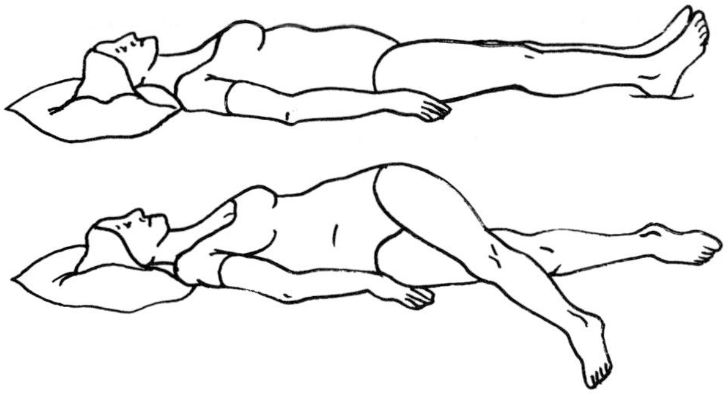

Leg Roll. Lie on back with legs straight. Keeping shoulders flat and legs straight, slowly and smoothly lift left leg and roll it over to touch the right side of floor or bed and return to starting position. Repeat, rolling right leg over to touch left side of floor or bed. Relax.

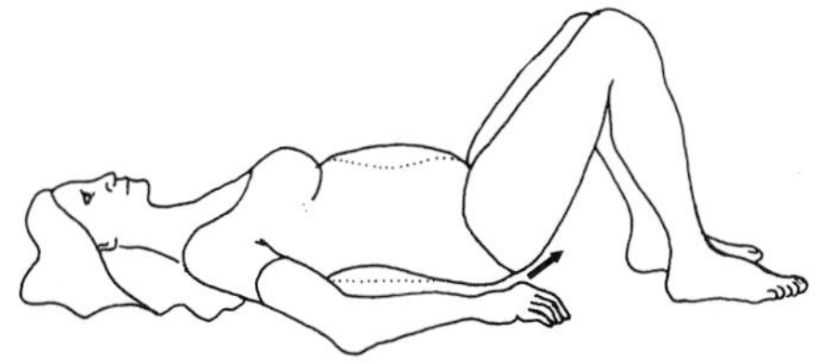

Combined Abdominal Breathing and Supine Pelvic Tilt (Pelvic Rock). Lie on back with knees bent. While inhaling deeply, roll pelvis back by flattening lower back on floor or bed. Exhale slowly but forcefully while contracting abdominal muscles and tightening buttocks. Hold for 3 to 5 seconds while exhaling. Relax.

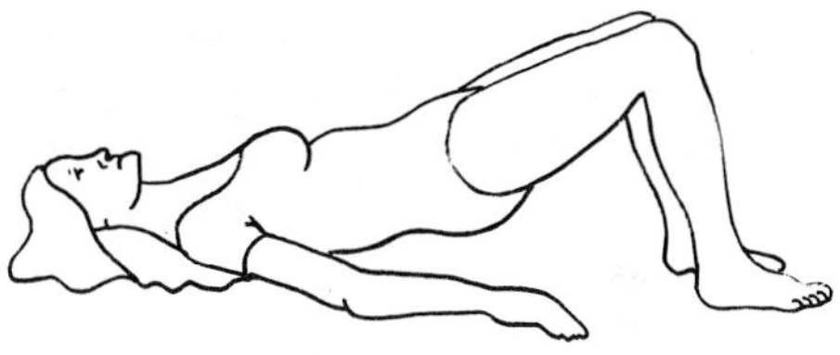

Buttocks Lift. Lie on back with arms at sides, knees bent and feet flat. Slowly raise buttocks and arch back. Return slowly to starting position.

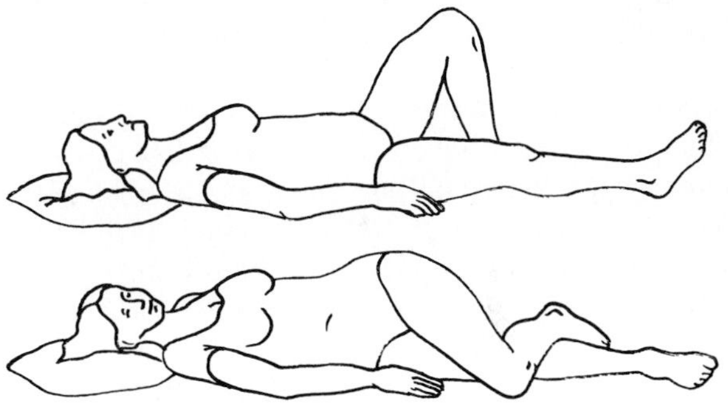

Single Knee Roll. Lie on back with with right leg straight and left leg bent at the knee. Keeping shoulders flat, slowly and smoothly roll left knee over to the right to touch floor or bed and then back to starting position. Reverse position of legs. Roll right knee over to the left to touch floor or bed and return to starting position. Relax.

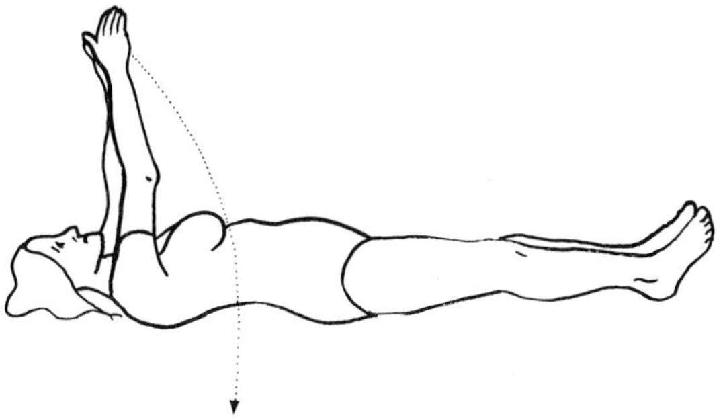

Arm Raises. Lie on back with arms extended at 90° angle from body. Raise arms so they are perpendicular and hands touch. Lower slowly.

Fig. 21-2 Postpartum exercise should begin as soon as possible. The woman should start with simple exercises and gradually progress to more strenuous ones.

to bed is not required for women who had general anesthesia, who had *epidural* or *caudal anesthesia,* or who had local anesthesia such as paracervical or pudendal block. Free movement is permitted once the anesthetic wears off unless an analgesic has been administered. After the first vital rest period is over (usually about 2 to 8 hours), the mother is encouraged to ambulate frequently. Postpartum exercises are begun as soon as the woman indicates readiness (Fig. 21-2). Exercise also promotes rest.

Parturients who received *intrathecal subarachnoid spinal anesthesia* should remain flat in bed with one flat pillow to align the head with the shoulders for at least 8 hours before they are allowed to ambulate. This position prevents leakage of spinal fluid through the dural membrane at the site of the needle puncture (a potential fistula tract), which causes a severe **"spinal" headache.** Since mothers automatically raise their heads to view their infants, the nurse needs to warn the mother to remain flat in bed. The nurse then positions or holds the infant so that the mother can see the child. Infant feeding by the mother may be delayed until she is able to sit up (check hospital protocol). The mother is encouraged to increase her intake of oral fluids (Chapter 13) but will require a bedpan or possible catheterization.

Prevention of **thrombosis** is part of the nursing care plan. If a woman is confined to bed longer than 8 hours (e.g., after spinal anesthesia or cesarean birth), exercise to promote circulation in the legs is indicated:

1. Alternate flexion and extension of feet
2. Rotate feet
3. Alternate flexion and extension of legs
4. Press back of knee to bed surface; relax

If the woman is susceptible to **thromboembolism,** the physician may avoid use of estrogens to inhibit or suppress lactation. Women with varicosities are encouraged to wear support hose. The woman is encouraged to walk about actively for true ambulation and discouraged from sitting immobile in a chair. If a thrombus is suspected (as evidenced by a positive Homans' sign, warmth, redness, or tenderness in the suspected leg), the physician should be notified immediately; meanwhile the woman should be confined to bed, with the affected limb elevated on pillows.

Immunizations

Rubella vaccination and $Rh_0(D)$ immune globulin are administered during the puerperium as necessary. For a detailed discussion of the Rh factor and isoimmunization, see Chapter 28; for a general discussion of the immune system, see Chapter 5.

During the puerperium the nurse apprises the mother of the recommended schedule of immunizations for the infant.

Rubella Vaccination. For women who have not had rubella (10% to 20% of all women) or women who are serologically negative (i.e., titer of 1:8 or less), **rubella vaccination** is recommended in the immediate postdelivery period to prevent fetal anomalies in future pregnancies. Seroconversion occurs in approximately 90% of women vaccinated after delivery. The live attenuated rubella virus is not communicable; therefore nursing mothers can be vaccinated. However, the live attenuated rubella vaccine is made from duck eggs, so women who have allergies to these eggs may develop a hypersensitivity reaction to the vaccine, for which they will need adrenalin. A transient arthralgia or rash is common in vaccinated women but is benign. Since the vaccine may be teratogenic the client should sign an informed consent and should receive written information about the vaccine, its side effects and risks, and the necessity for practicing contraception to avoid pregnancy for a period of 2 to 3 months after vaccination.

Prevention of Rh Isoimmunization. Injection of **$Rh_0(D)$ immune globulin** within 72 hours of delivery will prevent sensitization in the Rh-negative woman who has had a fetomaternal transfusion of Rh-positive fetal red blood cells (RBCs). The administration of 300 μg of $Rh_0(D)$ immune globulin is usually sufficient to prevent maternal sensitization. $Rh_0(D)$ immune globulin promotes lysis of fetal Rh-positive RBCs circulating in the maternal bloodstream before the mother forms her own antibodies against them. If a large fetomaternal transfusion is suspected, the dose needed can be assessed by either the Betke-Kleihauer or the D^u test, which detects 20 ml or more of Rh-positive fetal blood in the maternal circulation. The $Rh_0(D)$ immune globulin is administered after all known abortions (gestational age of 8 weeks or more), since the risk of sensitization after abortion is about half the risk after a full-term pregnancy.* *It is administered after delivery to any woman who meets the following three criteria:* (1) the mother must be $Rh_0(D)$ negative with no Rh antibodies (i.e., indirect Coombs' test is negative), (2) the infant must be $Rh_0(D)$-positive, or D^u-positive, and (3) results of direct Coombs' test on the cord blood must be negative. If the woman meets these criteria, a 1:1000 dilution of $Rh_0(D)$ immune globulin† is crossmatched to the mother's red cells to ensure compatibility. The same precautions are followed when administering a blood transfusion to ensure that the immune

*For prenatal prophylaxis, see Chapters 10 and 28.

†A blood product. Certain religions proscribe use of blood or blood products.

globulin is administered to the correct woman. *If administered to an Rh-positive person, immune globulin will act to promote lysis of the Rh-positive RBCs.* The dose is administered to the mother intramuscularly (*never* intravenously or to the infant).

Comfort

Most women during the early postpartum period need occasional pharmacologic analgesia for general muscle aches, perineal discomfort, incision or episiotomy pain, afterpains, engorgement, or mild tension headaches. Most physicians routinely order a variety of prn analgesics, including both narcotic and nonnarcotic choices, and dosage and time frequency ranges. When administering an analgesic the nurse must make a clinical judgment on the type, dosage, and frequency from the medications ordered. Research has shown that nurses, as well as physicians, underestimate the woman's pain and usually undermedicate.

The woman's description of the type and severity of her pain is the nurse's best guide in choosing between analgesics. One method used to quantify pain is to have the woman rate her pain on a 10-point scale with 10 being the most severe pain she can imagine. To confirm the location and extent of discomfort the nurse inspects and palpates areas of pain as appropriate for redness, swelling, discharge, and heat and observes for body tension, guarded movements, and facial tension. Blood pressure, pulse, and respiration may be elevated in response to acute pain. Diaphoresis may accompany severe pain. A lack of objective symptoms does not necessarily mean there is no pain, since there may also be a cultural component to the expression of pain.

Nursing actions are chosen so that the pain sensation is eliminated or reduced to a tolerable level that allows the woman to perform self-care activities and begin infant care. Individuals vary in their attitudes about involvement in their own care. Many women will want to participate in decisions about analgesia and have many concerns about the effects on the infant if they are breastfeeding. Severe pain also interferes with active participation in choosing pain-relief measures.

If an analgesic is to be given, the nurse informs the client of the prescribed analgesic, its common side effects, and presence in breast milk if she is breastfeeding. A woman may prefer another analgesic or pain control measure if a side effect is felt to be unacceptable. For example, a new mother planning to keep her infant at her bedside may not be comfortable with an analgesic that may make her drowsy. Pain is a frightening, lonely experience and a woman should feel confident that her needs for pain relief will be attended to. Therefore the nurse evaluates the effectiveness of the analgesic every 15 minutes until acceptable pain relief is achieved.

If evaluation reveals there is no improvement in reported pain in 30 minutes, to enhance the analgesic, the nurse institutes appropriate *nonpharmacologic pain measures* that were not previously instituted, such as ice packs, warm compresses, distraction, imagery, therapeutic touch, relaxation, and bonding with the infant. Pain relief is enhanced by using more than one method or route.

If acceptable pain relief has not been achieved in 1 hour and there has not been a change in the initial assessment, the nurse may need to contact the physician for additional pain relief orders or directions. Unrelieved pain results in fatigue, anxiety, and worsening perception of pain. Once pain has become severe, a larger dose or stronger analgesia is required.

When acceptable analgesia has been achieved the nurse evaluates with the woman her pain relief and her expectation and desire to participate in pain control. The nurse identifies any changes the mother desires in her regimen and adds changes to the care plan. *A woman's belief regarding what is helpful to achieve pain relief is vital to the success of any pain regimen.*

❑ NURSING CARE RELATED TO PHYSICAL ADAPTATION

The nurse has many roles when caring for the postpartum client. These include providing physical care, teaching self-care, and providing anticipatory guidance and counseling. Nursing priorities during the postpartum period include uterine atony; full urinary bladder; care of episiotomy, laceration, or hemorrhoids; and suppression of lactation in non-breastfeeding women. The general nursing care plan at the end of this section (p. 591) assists the nurse in providing comprehensive physical care for the woman.

Uterine Atony

The nursing process begins with collection of assessment data. This data includes palpation of a relaxed ("boggy") **uterus** and an increase in the amount of **lochia** (see Figs. 15-36 and 15-37). Nursing diagnoses and a plan of care are then developed. Nursing diagnoses may include altered tissue perfusion related to hemorrhage; potential fluid volume deficit related to hemorrhage, knowledge deficit related to lack of experience; and anxiety or fear related to concern for safety of self. The goals of care are for the woman's uterus to remain firm and that she experience no further hemorrhage.

Setting priorities in nursing interventions is important. The first intervention is stimulation of uterine tone (**living ligature**) by gently massaging the fundus until firm. Clots may also be expelled. While massaging the fundus, the nurse palpates for a full bladder. Frequent monitoring for a full bladder and uterine atony may be the only interventions needed at this time.

Education of the woman is also important to maintain uterine tone. Fundal massage can be a very uncomfortable procedure. Teaching the woman about the procedure enables her to maintain some control. The teaching plan should include a demonstration of self-fundal palpation and massage, information regarding the importance of voiding at regular intervals, and possibly breastfeeding or nipple stimulation to release oxytocin. The woman and her family may also want to know why uterine atony occurs. The nurse must be aware of the physiologic events that precipitate hemorrhage.

The uterus may remain atonic (boggy) even with massage and expulsion of clots. If this occurs, it is important that the nurse remain with the woman and summon help. Some hospitals may have standard protocols for postpartum hemorrhage. The protocol may specify IV therapy, medication (p. 587), and contacting the physician for possible surgical intervention. The primary nurse should keep the mother and family informed and assist them to remain calm. Efforts of the other health team members are coordinated by the primary nurse. Pharmacologic measures to stimulate uterine tone are presented in Table 21-1.

Evaluation of the woman's responses to interventions is an ongoing part of the nursing process. All responses to interventions should be carefully recorded. If goals are not met or new needs emerge, the woman's plan of care is modified accordingly.

Full Urinary Bladder

The assessment for a full bladder may include palpation of the bladder concurrent with palpation of fundal tone. The fundus may be displaced to the side or well above the umbilicus. The nurse will also note an increase in the amount of lochia. Other data may include unequal input and output. The woman may indicate that she has the urge to void but is unable to do so.

Nursing diagnoses for full urinary bladder may include altered patterns of urinary elimination related to tissue trauma and/or effects of anesthesia; or pain related to the sensation of the full bladder. The goals for care include that the woman will spontaneously empty her bladder and resume her normal voiding patterns.

Nursing interventions focus on helping the woman spontaneously empty her bladder as soon as possible. The first priority is to assist the woman to the bathroom or onto a bedpan if she is unable to ambulate. Running water in the sink, placing the woman's hands in warm water, or pouring water from a squeeze bottle over the perineum may stimulate voiding. Other techniques include assisting the woman into the shower or sitz bath (see Fig. 21-3) and encouraging her to void; or placing oil of peppermint (wintergreen) in a bedpan under the woman. The vapors may trigger spontaneous voiding. Fluid intake should be encouraged. Cranberry juice is often recommended as a deterrent to urinary tract infection.

If these measures are unsuccessful, a sterile catheter may be inserted to drain the urine. Care must be taken not to drain too much urine at once. If the bladder appears to be overdistended, a Foley (retention) catheter should be inserted, 800 ml removed, and the tube clamped. Additional urine should be removed at intervals. Many hospitals have standard orders for this condition. In some institutions the physician must be informed.

Evaluation should be ongoing, and the plan of care should be revised as indicated by the woman's response. All responses are carefully recorded and reported.

Care of Episiotomy, Lacerations, and Hemorrhoids

Assessment begins with a review of the woman's chart to determine if an episiotomy was performed or if a laceration occurred during the birth process. The nurse then asks the woman to turn onto her side, dons gloves, and inspects the perineal area for an intact suture line, redness, swelling, or the presence of hemorrhoids.

Any of these conditions would lead the nurse to diagnoses that may include impaired tissue integrity related to birth trauma; constipation related to hemorrhoids; pain related to trauma; and potential for infection related to effects of episiotomy or laceration. The goals for care include promotion of healing, prevention of infection, and minimum discomfort for the woman.

A variety of interventions aid the healing process and enhance comfort. Simple measures include encouraging the woman to lie on her side or to use a pillow while sitting. Other interventions include application of an ice pack, topical applications, dry heat, cleansing with a squeeze bottle or Surgi-Gator (Fig. 21-4), and a cleansing shower or **sitz bath** (Procedure 21-1). Many of these interventions are also effective for hemorrhoids, especially ice packs, sitz baths, and topical applications. Some women may complain that their hemorrhoids are more bothersome than their episiotomy.

The nurse needs to evaluate the various options and

Table 21-1 Pharmacologic Measures to Stimulate Uterine Tone

Intervention	Action, Uses During Puerperium	Onset of Effect, Duration, Usual Dose	Contraindications, Precautions	Comments
Oxytocin injection, USP (10 U/ml) (Pitocin, Syntocinon, Uteracon), oxytocic, synthetic posterior pituitary hormone	Stimulates phasic uterine muscle contraction, promotes milk-ejection (let-down) reflex, facilitates flow of milk during engorgement.	IV injection, 10 U; onset in 1 min. IV infusion, 10-40 U/1000 ml 5% dextrose or physiologic electrolyte solution. IM injection, 3-10 U; onset in 3-7 min; duration 30-60 min.	Hypersensitivity; return of atony when effect wears off. May cause severe hypertension if client is also receiving ephedrine, methoxamine, or other vasopressors.	**Alert:** Assess for return of atony; store in cool place.
Ergonovine, USP, NF (Ergotrate Maleate); oxytocic, ergot alkaloid	Stimulates prolonged, nonphasic uterine contractions.	Oral: 0.2-0.4 mg every 6-12 hr for 48 hr; onset in 6-15 min. IM injection: 0.2 mg (1 ml) if nausea precludes oral preparation, onset "in a few minutes." Initial response: firm, tetanic contraction. Subsequent response: alternating minor relaxations and contractions for 1½ hr; then vigorous rhythmic contractions for 3-4 hr after injection.	Severe hypertensive episodes may occur if given to hypertensive clients or those receiving vasoconstrictors; hypersensitivity; nausea, vomiting; sudden change in blood pressure or pulse.	**Alert:** Assess for changes in blood pressure, pulse; store in cool place.
Methylergonovine, NF (Methergine); oxytocic, ergot alkaloid and congener of lysergic acid (LSD)	Stimulates rapid, sustained tetanic uterine contractions; used in treatment of subinvolution; has only minimum vasoconstrictive effect.	Oral: 0.2 mg tab, every 6-8 hr for maximum of 1 wk; onset in 5-10 min. IM injection 0.2 mg (1 ml) every 2-4 hr; onset in 2-5 min. IV infusion *(emergency only)*: 0.2 mg (1 ml) *slowly over 60 sec;* onset immediate.	Nausea, vomiting; transient hypertension; dizziness, headache; tinnitus; diaphoresis; palpitations; temporary chest pains.	**Alert:** Do not administer with Percodan—may result in hallucinations; assess blood pressure; store in cold place, away from light.
Carboprost (Prostin/M15); oxytocic, prostaglandin	Stimulates rapid, sustained uterine contractions; used for treatment of uterine atony and uterine inversion.	IM injection 1 ampule (250 μg), onset within minutes; intramyometrial injection (by physician only), ½-2 ampules (125-500 μg) diluted with 10 ml saline (injected transabdominally into anterior wall of uterus); onset within minutes.	Severe hypertension (systolic >170 mm Hg or diastolic >100 mm Hg) and in clients with severe symptomatic asthma. Diarrhea is commonly seen with dosage above 1 ampule; there is usually a rise in systolic and diastolic blood pressure; bronchoconstriction and wheezing are concerns.	**Alert:** Monitor blood pressure and for adverse reactions; store in refrigerator.

PROCEDURE 21-1

CARE AFTER REPAIR OF EPISIOTOMY OR LACERATION

DEFINITION

Treatment of the surgical incision of the perineum, done electively to facilitate delivery of the baby and prevent perineal lacerations (a torn, jagged wound)

PURPOSE

To promote healing, increase comfort, teach mother self-care techniques, and identify and treat complications.

EQUIPMENT

Ice pack with cover; squeeze bottle; sitz bath and thermometer (see Fig. 21-3), or Surgi-Gator (if available) (see Fig. 21-4); towels, as necessary; anesthetic cream or spray; witch hazel pads (Tucks); clean gloves.

NURSING ACTIONS	RATIONALE
Wash hands and don gloves before and after touching woman and equipment.	Prevents nosocomial infection and implements universal precautions.
Gather equipment.	Improves efficiency.
Explain procedure to woman.	Decreases anxiety and elicits cooperation.
ICE PACK	
Apply a covered ice pack to perineum.	Decreases chance of "burn" from cold pack.
1. During first 2 hours after delivery.	Decreases edema formation and increases comfort.
2. After the first 2 hours after delivery.	Provides anesthetic effect.
SITZ BATH	
Built-in type (see Fig. 21-3):	

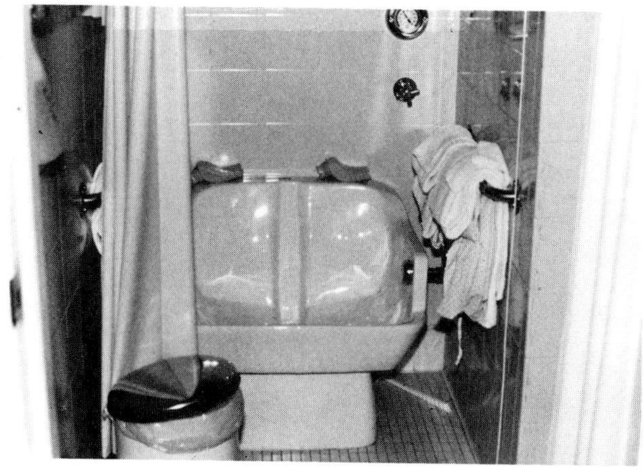

Fig. 21-3 Sitz bath. (Courtesy Marjorie Pyle, RNC, Lifecircle, Costa Mesa, Calif.)

NURSING ACTIONS	RATIONALE
Prepare bath by thoroughly scrubbing with cleaning agent and rinsing.	Decreases possibility of infection from another woman; prevents irritation from cleaning agent.
Pad with towel before filling.	Promotes comfort and keeps woman from slipping (padding before filling keeps towel from floating).
Fill ½ to ⅓ full with water of correct temperature 38° to 40.6° C, or 45° C (100.4° to 105° F, or 113° F).	Provides soothing temperature. The increased blood flow to area is thought by some to facilitate healing; others think that this causes swelling and adds to discomfort.*
Encourage woman to use at least twice a day for 20 minutes.	Provides comfort and aids healing.
Place call bell within easy reach.	Ensures safety since the warm water and other factors may cause woman to feel faint and need assistance.
Teach woman to enter bath by tightening gluteal muscles and keeping them tightened and then relaxing them after she is in the bath.	Decreases perineal discomfort while sitting down. Allows water to reach perineum.
Place dry towels within reach.	Increases comfort and ensures safety.
Ensure privacy.	Shows respect for woman.
Check woman in 15 min; assess pulse as needed.	Ensures safety. Increased or irregular pulse may indicate cardiovascular stress; assist woman back to bed.
	Decreases perineal discomfort.
Disposable type:	
Clamp tubing and fill bag with warm water.	Prevents spillage.

*Other authors propose cool sitz bath (Droegemueller, 1980; Ramler and Roberts, 1986).

PROCEDURE 21-1—cont'd

NURSING ACTIONS	RATIONALE
Raise toilet seat, place bath in bowl with overflow opening directed toward back of toilet.	Allows water to drain into toilet bowl.
Place container above toilet bowl.	Drains water bag by gravity.
Attach tube into groove at front of bath.	Situates tubing below level of water.
Loosen tube clamp to regulate rate of flow; fill bath to about ½ full; continue as above for built-in sitz bath.	See rationale for built-in sitz bath.
SQUEEZE BOTTLE	
Demonstrate for and assist woman; explain rationale.	Cleanses perineum after voiding. Encourages self-care.
Fill bottle with tap water warmed to approximately 38° C (100° F) (comfortably warm on the wrist).	Provides comfortable temperatures.
Instruct woman to position nozzle between her legs so that squirts of water reach perineum as she sits on toilet seat.	Cleanses and soothes perineum.
Explain that it will take whole bottle of water over perineum.	Cleanses perineum well.
Remind her to blot dry with toilet paper or clean wipes.	Avoids tissue trauma and promotes comfort.
Remind her to avoid contamination from anal area.	Prevents infection.
Apply new clean pad.	Prevents infection.
SURGI-GATOR	
Assemble Surgi-Gator (see Fig. 21-4).	Cleanses and provides comfort to perineum.
Instruct woman regarding use and rationale.	Encourages self-care.
Follow package directions.	Promotes maximum benefit of appliance.
Instruct woman to sit on toilet with legs apart and to put nozzle so tip is just past the perineum, adjusting placement as needed.	Provides the jets of water to the perineal area.
Remind her to return her applicator to her bedside stand.	Prevents loss or cross infection; each client is provided with her own applicator.
DRY HEAT	
Inspect lamp for defects.	Prevents fires or burns.
Cover lamp with towels.	Prevents burns if lamp touches skin.
Position lamp 50 cm (20 in) from perineum; use 3 times a day for 20 min periods.	Provides comfortable warmth. Promotes comfort, keeps area dry, and promotes healing.
Teach regarding use of 40-watt bulb at home.	Provides effective "heat" lamp in the home.
Provide draping over woman.	Promotes privacy. Demonstrates respect and caring.
If same lamp is being used by several woman, clean it carefully between uses.	Prevents cross infection.
TOPICAL APPLICATIONS	
Apply anesthetic cream or spray; use sparingly 3 to 4 times per day.	Promotes comfort.
Offer witch hazel pads (Tucks) after voiding or defecating; woman pats perineum dry from front to back, then applies witch hazel pads.	Decreases swelling and promotes healing.
CLEANSING	
Wash perineum with mild soap and warm water at least once daily.	Minimizes fear of "breaking the stiches" or pain, which deters women from washing perineum.
Cleanse from symphysis pubis to anal area.	Prevents contamination of the vagina and urethra with fecal material.
Apply peripad from front to back, protecting inner surface of pad from contamination.	Prevents infection from contamination.
Wrap soiled pad and place in covered waste container.	
Change pad every time she voids or defecates or at least 4 times per day.	Prevents infection.
Wash hands before and after changing pads.	Prevents infection.
Assess amount and character of lochia with each pad change.	Identifies possible complications early.

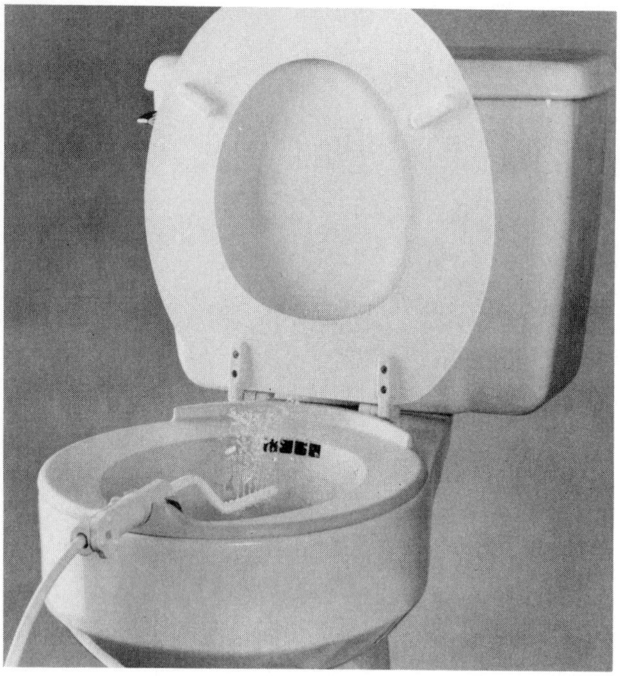

Fig. 21-4 Hygienic sitz bath (Surgi-Gator) for perineal care. (Courtesy Andermac, Inc, Yuba City, Calif.)

determine, along with each woman, the care method that is most effective. The plan of care should be developed with the woman's assistance and should focus on her preferences and priorities. Documentation of the plan provides a guide for other members of the health care team.

Supression of Lactation

Suppression of lactation is undergone when the woman (couple) has decided not to breastfeed or in the case of neonatal death. Nursing diagnoses appropriate for these women may include altered tissue perfusion related to breast engorgement; knowledge deficit related to inexperience with suppression techniques; and pain related to engorged breasts. The goals of care are for the woman to experience no breast engorgement, to learn suppression techniques (see general nursing care plan, p. 593), and to experience minimum, if any, discomfort.

Nursing interventions may include mechanical (nonpharmacologic) suppression techniques or pharmacologic therapies as prescribed by a physician. The first priority in mechanical suppression is the wearing of a snug support bra or a breast binder for at least 72 hours after delivery. The woman should avoid any breast stimulation, including running warm water over the breasts, breastfeeding, or pumping of the breasts.

Should engorgement occur, the nurse should assure the woman that it is temporary and that ice packs and analgesia will decrease the symptoms. The woman is instructed to maintain an adequate fluid intake and to avoid taking diuretics.

The most commonly prescribed medication for suppression of lactation is bromocriptine (Parlodel). This nonestrogen medication suppresses lactation by preventing the secretion of prolactin. The drug is taken twice a day for 14 days. There may be a rebound breast engorgement when the medication is discontinued. These symptoms are usually mild and mechanical suppression may be helpful. Some physicians may prescribe estrogens (Tace or Deladumone) to suppress lactation. The nurse should follow the hospital protocols to obtain informed consent and provide literature included with the drug package regarding estrogen and its possible association with cancer. Women who receive these estrogen-containing antilactogenics have an increased incidence of thrombus formation and should be observed closely.

▪ ▪ ▪

The general nursing care plan that follows summarizes nursing actions appropriate to physical care in the early postpartum period. The nurse must be sure to individualize each care plan to meet the particular needs of each client.

Evaluation

The nurse can be reasonably assured that care was effective when the goals for care have been met; that is: normal involution is progressing; comfort is maintained; bowel and bladder patterns are normal; no infection occurs; self-care measures are learned; and community resources are identified as needed.

NURSING CARE RELATED TO PSYCHOSOCIAL ADAPTATION

Nurses have a leadership role in efforts to provide holistic client care in the postpartum period. Interventions intended to establish healthy early family relationships can be the unique contribution of nursing. Healthy family relationships promote the growth potential of the newborn and other family members. Caregivers need to be alert to parents who have positive family circumstances, as well as to those who exhibit warning signs during the postdelivery period.

General Nursing Care Plan

EARLY POSTPARTUM

ASSESSMENT	NURSING DIAGNOSIS (ND), PLAN/GOAL (P/G)	RATIONALE/ IMPLEMENTATION	EVALUATION
Vital signs Temperature Increased pulse Record of blood loss or anemia Rupture of membranes >24 hr	ND: Potential for infection related to problems that can arise during labor, delivery, and postpartum. ND: Potential knowledge deficit related to signs and symptoms of infection. P/G: Woman does not develop signs and symptoms of infection. Woman verbalizes understanding of infection and fever.	*Early identification of risk factors for infection enhances the treatment regimen, therefore the nurse will assess for:* Chills or fever of 38° C (100.4° F) or more. Localized redness, heat, pain anywhere on body. Urinary frequency, *pain,* or *burning* on urination. Foul-smelling lochia.	Woman reports any symptoms she experiences immediately. Woman is aware of normal ranges of vital signs. Woman does not develop infection; or if she does, identification and resolution are timely.
	ND: Potential for hyperthermia related to infection. P/G: Woman understands and uses temperature reduction techniques; temperature returns to within normal limits.	*Hyperthermia increases maternal discomfort:* Report fever to physician. Encourage oral fluids or continue IV fluids as ordered. Decrease environmental temperature, remove blankets or heavy clothing. Administer antipyretic medication as ordered.	Woman uses same temperature reduction techniques at home. Woman understands information presented. Woman's temperature returns to within normal range.
Increased blood pressure History of hypertension Decreased blood pressure Estimated blood loss after delivery	ND: Potential for injury, maternal, related to hypertension/ hypotension. P/G: Woman will remain normotensive.	*Injury may result from increase or decrease in blood pressure:* Give anticipatory guidance for prevention (i.e., diet, exercise, medication). Teach woman about orthostatic hypotension related to splanchnic engorgement. Monitor every 4-8 hr.	Woman aware of normal range. Woman implements preventive measures. Woman takes precautions against fainting during first ambulation; calls for assistance.
Headache Spinal anesthesia Stress Hypertension	ND: Pain: headache related to stress, increased blood pressure, spinal anesthesia. P/G: Woman will not have headache; or, if headache develops, she receives prompt relief.	*Reduction of pain enhances ability to deal with psychosocial concerns:* Teach relaxation and stress reduction techniques. Have woman lie down on left side. Keep woman recovering from spinal anesthesia flat as prescribed. Administer medications as ordered. Increase fluid intake. Prepare for blood patch procedure.	Woman knows and uses relaxation techniques. Woman knows importance of taking antihypertensive medications. Woman understands reason for headache and complies with prevention or treatment.

Continued.

ASSESSMENT	NURSING DIAGNOSIS (ND), PLAN/GOAL (P/G)	RATIONALE/ IMPLEMENTATION	EVALUATION
Uterus Position, size Tone Response to gentle massage Rate of involution Afterpains	ND: Potential for injury related to hemorrhage from an atonic uterus postdelivery. P/G: Fundus remains firm, lochia moderate without evidence of hemorrhage. P/G: Woman states that afterpains are tolerable and she is satisfied with measures used.	*Prompt identification and treatment of hemorrhage prevents complications:* Assess tone and response to gentle massage. Use appropriate measures to maintain tone and relieve discomfort of afterpains. Teach woman how to assess fundus. Teach woman how to massage uterus.	Woman understands purpose of firm uterus and follows through with self-massage. Woman's fundus remains firm. Woman experiences no hemorrhage.
Lochia Color and character Amount Size, number of clots Odor ("fleshy")	ND: Potential for infection/hemorrhage related to conditions causing abnormal lochia. P/G: Woman's lochia remains within normal limits.	*Prevention, recognition, and prompt treatment of infection minimize complications:* Monitor amount and character of lochia when massaging fundus. If heavy, reassess source of bleeding, uterine tone, and degree of bladder distension. Record size and amount of expelled clots. Teach expected regression (color and amount) during involution. Teach woman about atony of the uterus and subsequent hemorrhage.	Woman verbalizes understanding and reports any unusual symptoms. Lochia is moderate or less with no clots or just a few small clots.
Perineum Healing of episiotomy/ laceration Swelling, bruising Hematoma Size, number of hemorrhoids	ND: Impaired skin integrity related to episiotomy/lacerations acquired during delivery. P/G: Woman's childbirth-related tissue trauma heals without difficulty. ND: Pain, related to episiotomy, laceration, hemorrhoids, swelling, bruising, or hematoma. P/G: Woman indicates pain has decreased.	*Assessment and interventions to promote tissue healing prevent complications:* Monitor perineal healing. Wash hands before and after care of perineum. Teach woman comfort measures. Give woman opportunity to look at perineum and its repair (if interested). Describe to woman what to expect while perineum is healing and hemorrhoids are regressing. Teach woman how to avoid contamination of perineum and vulva.	Perineum heals well. Hemorrhoids regress. Woman employs comfort measures. Comfort is maintained. Woman verbalizes understanding of information presented, uses proper pericare.

ASSESSMENT	NURSING DIAGNOSIS (ND), PLAN/GOAL (P/G)	RATIONALE/ IMPLEMENTATION	EVALUATION
Urinary tract Symptoms of infection Distension Completeness of emptying Ability to void Total amount in 24 hours	ND: Potential for infection related to bladder trauma during delivery, or retention and stasis of urine. P/G: Woman does not experience bladder distension or infection.	*It is preferable to prevent, rather than treat urinary tract infection:* Teach woman to wipe from front to back. Use strict aseptic technique when catheterization is necessary. Help woman void and empty bladder frequently. Teach woman symptoms of urinary tract infection.	Woman does not develop urinary infection. Woman understands symptoms and reports their development.
	ND: Urinary retention related to anesthesia and bladder trauma. P/G: Woman resumes normal pattern of urine elimination.	*Regular voiding patterns decrease potential complications:* Encourage oral fluids. Assist to bathroom, if possible, or provide bedpan. Run water in sink. Pour warm water down perineum or immerse in warm sitz bath. Use spirit of peppermint. Catheterize if ordered. Teach Credé's method (use of manual pressure on bladder to express urine).	Woman voids and empties bladder completely at least every 4 hours. Bladder distension does not occur. If catheterization is necessary, infection or loss of self-esteem does not occur.
Bowels Bowel sounds Passing flatus Abdominal distension Bowel movement Constipation Diarrhea Hemorrhoids	ND: Constipation related to fear of tearing stitches or pain, medications, decreased peristalsis, hemorrhoids. P/G: Woman returns to normal bowel elimination patterns.	*Constipation may lead to straining or impaction:* Encourage and assist with early ambulation, fluids, foods with roughage. Encourage immediate response to urge to defecate. Administer stool softeners as prescribed. Counsel woman on: fluids, foods; exercise; bowel habits; hygiene after defecation. Check chart for record of last bowel movement during labor and delivery.	Woman's bowel elimination pattern restored. Woman has minimum discomfort. Woman continues to use preventive and comfort measures learned during hospitalization.
Breasts Soft, filling, firm Engorged Painful Mastitis Breastfeeding or bottle-feeding	ND: Pain of engorged breasts related to lactation or suppression. ND: Ineffective breastfeeding related to engorgement, poor infant sucking, or inexperience. P/G: Woman's goal of lactation or suppression is met with little if any discomfort. P/G: Woman expresses satisfaction with breastfeeding attempts.	*Prevention of breast engorgement promotes comfort:* Teach newborn nutrition and feeding. Tell woman to wear a good supporting bra or provide a binder. Place ice packs to breasts for engorgement as ordered. Give medications as prescribed.	Lactation initiated successfully with minimum or no discomfort. Woman is satisfied with breastfeeding experience. Lactation is suppressed with minimum discomfort.

Continued.

General Nursing Care Plan—cont'd

ASSESSMENT	NURSING DIAGNOSIS (ND), PLAN/GOAL (P/G)	RATIONALE/ IMPLEMENTATION	EVALUATION
Nipples Protruding Inverted Sore or tender Cracked or bleeding	ND: Impaired skin integrity related to learning to breastfeed and take care of nipples. P/G: Woman learns feeding techniques and care of nipples.	*Proper care of breasts and correct positioning of infant decrease nipple soreness:* Assist woman with breastfeeding. Employ preventive and comfort measures: Teach hygiene: use warm water, no soap; wash breasts first with fresh washcloth. Teach use of breast pump and manual expression. Teach positioning for breastfeeding. Give information on breastfeeding support groups	Woman learns feeding techniques and care of nipples. Nipples are not injured or uncomfortable.
Hemoglobin and hematocrit May be decreased at this time Estimated blood loss	ND: Altered cardiopulmonary tissue perfusion related to anemia. P/G: Anemia is detected if present and corrective measures are initiated. ND: Knowledge deficit related to anemia. P/G: Woman's anemia is resolved; future occurrence is prevented.	*Decreased hemoglobin or hematocrit may lead to serious complications:* Evaluate laboratory reports. Alert physician to low levels and implement orders (i.e., blood transfusion). Protect woman from falls. Explain rationale for tests. Explain significance of woman's test results. Teach importance of nutrition. Counsel regarding iron supplementation.	Values are within normal limits. Woman learns self-care through nutrition. Woman prevents anemia in self and family.
Coagulation factors Thrombus formation Intravascular coagulation: local or disseminated (DIC) Positive Homans' sign Redness, pain Swelling of leg Laboratory results	ND: Pain from thrombus formation related to alterations in coagulation process. ND: Potential for injury related to development of DIC. P/G: Woman develops no problem related to coagulation.	*Thrombus formation and further complications threaten woman's health:* Encourage early ambulation. Monitor for and teach woman symptomatology of thrombus formation (Homans' sign). Monitor for and teach woman problems with ambulation and exercise, redness or swelling of calf or leg. Monitor for symptoms of DIC. Teach woman rationale for assessment and measures to take should symptomatology of thrombus occur.	No coagulation problems occur. Woman recognizes and seeks therapy for symptomatology of thrombus formation.

Assessment

Women indicate a need to review the birth experience (Konrad, 1987). The mother's critical self-evaluation of her intrapartum behavior is indicative of one of the important psychologic tasks of the postpartum period. The nurse needs to identify the mother's perception of the fit between her prenatal expectation for her behavior and the intrapartum reality.

Parental Responses

Parental responses to the birth of a child include behaviors that are either adaptive or maladaptive. Both mother and father exhibit these behaviors, although to date most research has centered on the mother. Parents who are faced with the crisis of a severe life stress may not be able to provide supportive parenting for their child. Life stress reduces both psychologic well-being and physical health. These are two important factors in establishing and maintaining relationships with others. Another critical factor is a feeling of personal control.

Many new mothers will experience **parenting difficulties** until their skills become established. Once they feel confidence in their skills, the increase in self-esteem promotes a positive affective response to the child. However, some parents will exhibit **parenting disorders** (a matter of degree) that place the child in jeopardy and at risk. Protocols for the physical screening of high-risk gravidas and fetuses have been developed and confirmed. However, tools predicting high-risk parenting behaviors require more replication over larger population samples before they can be used with the same precision.

The quality of motherliness or fatherliness in parent's behavior prompts nurturing and protection as opposed to neglect or abuse of the child. Cues indicating the presence or absence of this quality appear early in the postdelivery period as parents react to the newborn child and continue the process of establishing a relationship (Table 21-2).

Adaptive Behavior. Adaptive behaviors stem from the parents' realistic perception and acceptance of their newborn's needs and her or his limited abilities, immature social responses, and helplessness (Steele and Pollock, 1968). Parental unity can be said to be satisfactory when parents can find pleasure in their infant and in the tasks done for and with him; when they understand their infant's emotional states and provide comfort; and when they read the infant's cues for new experience and can sense the infant's fatigue level.

Maladaptive Behavior. Maladaptive behaviors are exhibited when parents respond inappropriately to the needs of their infant. They expect responses from the infant far in excess of the infant's ability to perform. They interpret inadequate responses as defiance or as negative judgment of parental capabilities. They obtain no pleasure from physical contact with their child. Such infants tend to be handled roughly. They are held in a manner that allows the head to dangle without support, and are not cuddled. The parents see the child as unattractive. The child caring tasks of bathing and changing are viewed with disgust or annoyance. There is a lack of discrimination in responding to the infant's signals relative to hunger, fatigue, need for soothing or stimulating speech, and need for comforting body or eye contact. The parents of these infants often show excessive concern over the health of their child and cannot distinguish between the expected minor illnesses of childhood and serious disabilities. It appears difficult for them to accept their child as healthy and happy.

Interpretation of Infant Behaviors. The parents' response is profoundly affected by their interpretation of the infant's behaviors. Feedback is an important component in any relationship. Mothers and fathers make value judgments about their infant's behavior and respond as though the baby had either "praised" or "criticized" them. Table 21-3 provides a listing of infant behaviors and their evaluation by parents as either adaptive (positive feedback) or maladaptive (negative feedback) (Mercer, 1982).

Parent-Infant Interactions

To assess parent and child relationships and competency in child care, the nurse observes parental attitudes toward themselves and their responsibilities. She assesses the mother's perceptual acuity and the amount of physical and psychic energy the mother possesses. Cultural or ethnic variations in maternal and paternal roles are also noted. This information provides the context within which the parents will give care to their child. Competency in child care can be determined during feeding periods or when the mother or father is giving general care to the infant (Fig. 21-5).

Nursing Diagnoses

After analyzing the data obtained from assessment, the nurse establishes nursing diagnoses that will act as guides to action. The following are examples of diagnoses made for specific clients:

Altered family processes related to
- Unexpected birth of twins

Impaired verbal communication related to
- Client's deafness
- Client's language not same as nurse's

Table 21-2 Mothering Behaviors*

Adaptive Behaviors	Maladaptive Behaviors
FEEDING	
Offers appropriate amount and type of food to infant	Provides inadequate type or amount of food for infant
Holds infant in comfortable position during feeding	Does not hold infant, or holds in uncomfortable position during feeding
Burps baby during and after feeding	Does not burp infant
Prepares food appropriately	Prepares food inappropriately
Offers food at comfortable pace for infant	Offers food at pace too rapid or slow for infant's comfort
INFANT STIMULATION	
Provides appropriate verbal stimulation for infant during visit	Provides no, or only aggressive, verbal stimulation for infant during visit
Provides tactile stimulation for infant at times other than during feeding or moving infant away from danger	Does not provide tactile stimulation or only that of aggressive handling of infant
Provides age-appropriate toys	No evidence of age-appropriate toys
Interacts with infant in a way that provides for infant's satisfaction	Frustrates infant during interactions
INFANT REST	
Provides quiet or relaxed environment for infant's rest, including scheduled rest periods	Does not provide quiet environment or consistent schedule for rest periods
Ensures that infant's needs for food, warmth, and dryness are met before sleep	Does not attend to infant's needs for food, warmth, and dryness before sleep
PERCEPTION	
Demonstrates realistic perception of infant's condition in accordance with medical and nursing diagnoses	Shows unrealistic perception of infant's condition
Has realistic expectations for infant	Demonstrates unrealistic expectations of infant
Recognizes infant's unfolding skills or behavior	Has no awareness of infant's development
Shows realistic perception of own mothering behavior	Shows unrealistic perception of own mothering
INITIATIVE	
Shows initiative in attempts to manage infant's problems, including actively seeking information about infants	Shows no initiative in attempts to meet infant's needs or to manage problems; does not follow through with plans
RECREATION	
Provides positive outlets for own recreation or relaxation	Does not provide positive outlets for own recreation or relaxation
INTERACTION WITH OTHER CHILDREN	
Demonstrates positive interaction with other children in home	Demonstrates hostile-aggressive interaction with other children in home
MOTHERING ROLE	
Expresses satisfaction with mothering	Expresses dissatisfaction with mothering

Reprinted by permission from Mercer RT: In Sonstegard LJ et al, editors: Women's health: childbearing, vol 2, New York, 1982, Grune & Stratton, Inc.
*These describe paternal as well as maternal behaviors.

Table 21-3 Infant Behaviors

Adaptive Behaviors	Maladaptive Behaviors
SLEEPING	
Receives adequate sleep for normal growth—at least 17 hours each day without restless sleep patterns or prolonged crying at nap or bedtime after other needs have been met	Receives inadequate sleep for normal growth—less than 16 hours each day; shows restless sleep patterns or prolonged crying at nap or bedtime
FEEDING	
Actively seeks food offered	Resists food offered
Actively sucks and swallows food	Does not suck effectively
Demonstrates pleasurable relief after eating	Remains fussy after adequate amount of feeding—no pleasurable relief
RESPONSE TO ENVIRONMENT	
Demonstrates active response to environment by ignoring or reaching-out behavior	Seems apathetic to environment
VOCALIZING	
Demonstrates vocalizations when alert if developmentally ready	Makes infrequent or no vocalizations during visit although developmentally ready
SMILING	
Demonstrates smiling behavior if older than 2 months	Does not demonstrate smiling behavior during visit
CUDDLING	
Cuddles when held	Resists being held or stiffens when held

Reprinted by permission from Mercer RT: In Sonstegard LJ et al, editors: Women's health: childbearing, vol 2, New York, 1982, Grune & Stratton, Inc.

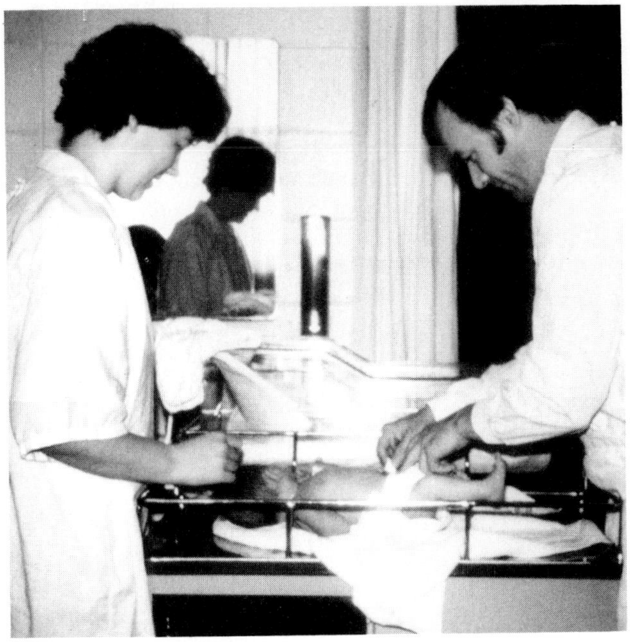

Fig. 21-5 Father bathes his infant with support of nursing student. (Courtesy Colleen Stainton.)

Altered parenting related to
- Long, difficult labor

Knowledge/skill deficit related to
- Usual infant behaviors
- Holding, cuddling, interacting with infant

Anxiety related to
- Newness of parenting role, sibling rivalry, or grandparental response

Potential for situational low self-esteem related to
- Lack of knowledge of infant characteristics or of care-giving skills
- Grandparental responses

Planning

The postnatal period is a crucial one for the family. It contains the potential for crisis in family adjustment. Developing a plan of care that recognizes family strengths and provides support for family weaknesses does much to help family members take on new tasks and responsibilities.

Goals may include that the parents will:

1. Express a healthy self-esteem, self-concept
2. Demonstrate a healthy parent-child relationship

3. Participate in the care of the infant through class attendance and return demonstrations
4. Meet their cultural expectations of themselves and their experiences.

Implementation

Adaptation to the parental role is a complex process. The nurse's application of knowledge in the care of new parents can help them with this role transition. One of the new mother's first psychologic tasks is to integrate the birth experience.

Integration of the Birth Experience

The nurse who interviews a new mother about her birth experience in a thoughtful, sensitive manner has already intervened therapeutically. Inviting the new mother to review the events and describe how she felt helps her understand what happened and begin the integration process. The new mother usually initiates this portion of the interview with such statements as, "I'm sorry I . . ."; "You should have seen how I screamed. . ." "I just can't remember some things." Feelings of anger and resentment and vocalizing are understandable, temporary responses to an acute, stressful situation. The normalcy of these reactions can be validated by the nurse. However, statements such as "everyone does it" puts all women in the same category and may be perceived as a lack of regard for the individual (Konrad, 1987). Restating or rephrasing are useful communication techniques (Chapter 1). These techniques help the woman fill in the whole picture for herself, reflect on her meaning behind her words, and identify connections between this experience and previous ones. The need for input regarding the birth experience is consistent with Rubin's (1961) **"taking-in"** phase seen in the early postpartum period. Assisting the new mother with this postpartum psychologic task is a valuable function of the nurse. The labor and delivery nurse can be instrumental in this process by taking time for a follow-up visit to the new mother. She can best help the mother put in perspective the events that occurred during the labor and delivery process.

❑ CRISIS PREVENTION

Nursing is directed toward increasing the mother's mastery of the "art of motherhood," thereby increasing or sustaining her self-esteem. Nursing care encompasses measures that encourage assertive, self-reliant behaviors in family members. Nursing interventions may be grouped under those pertaining to the crisis intervention theory: perception, situational supports, and coping mechanisms (Chapter 1).

Perception

One of the main concepts to be stressed repeatedly is that parenthood is a learned role. As with any other learned role, it takes time to master, improves with experience, and evolves gradually and continually as the needs of the parents and child change. Rubin (1961) proposed that for 2 or 3 days after the birth of a child, a mother is receptive to learning about her new role. Rubin termed this the **"taking-hold"** phase. Most mothers are discharged within 24 to 48 hours, so follow-up is difficult. Teaching today must take place during this period when the mother may have difficulty absorbing a great deal of new information.

Caplan (1957) noted that intervention during the early peurperium had a much greater influence on the attitudes of family members than it did at periods of stability of emotional functioning. Care during the early puerperium needs to reflect the mother's and father's psychologic readiness for learning new skills.

Parents have been found to be receptive to information regarding their infant's interactive capabilities during the early puerperium. During this time the parents' awareness of their own behavioral responses toward their infant can be enhanced. Parents' anxiety levels must be addressed, because anxiety can reduce their ability to learn.

Care of the newborn may be limited to feeding during the first few days. When the mother's strength returns, she also may wish to bathe and change the infant. Demonstrations and discussions of these techniques with the parents and supervision of their efforts are incorporated into the nursing care. Through the loving and attentive manner nurses exhibit while providing physical care, they act as role models. As one nurse described it:

■ I found the mother crying and distraught as she wrapped and unwrapped her baby. She said, "I don't seem to be able to do anything right." I took the baby from her and talked to him. "What are you doing to your mother? You've got her all upset!" The baby alerted to my voice and looked at me. Then I said to the mother, "Now, you talk to him." She said, "You're a big lovely boy, don't cry so much." The baby hearing her voice promptly turned his head from me to look at her. I said, "You see, he knows his mother's voice and prefers it to mine." The mother was surprised and seemed very pleased and excited. We then reviewed how to wrap a baby snugly.

Recognition and praise of her successes increase the mother's feeling of competence and control in her ability to mother. Feelings of self-esteem in the mother are increased through positive feedback. Fig. 21-6 shows a feedback circle in which the left side presents an exam-

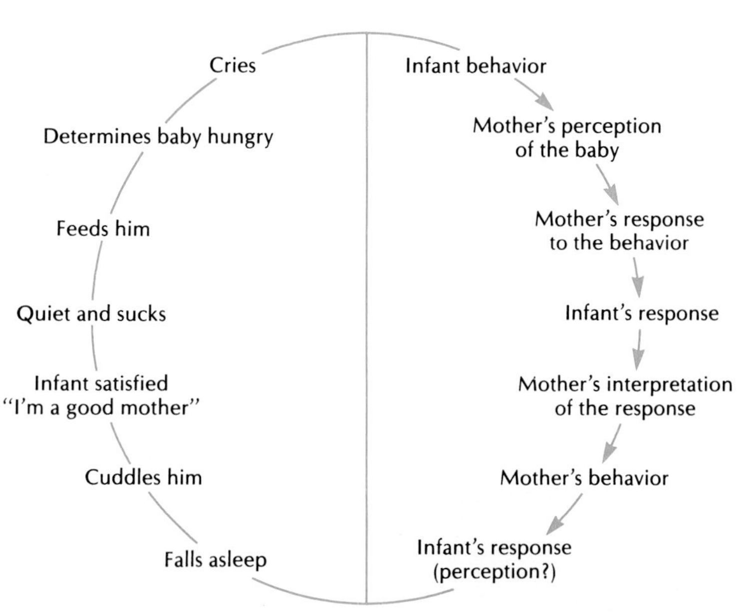

Fig. 21-6 Maternal-infant feedback mechanisms. (From Stainton MC: Assessment and support of healthy parent-child relationships, Proceedings of POGP: Pediatrics, Obstetrics and Gynecology Workshop for Nurses, Saskatoon, 1977, University of Saskatchewan.)

ple of a positive mother-infant interaction based on the sequence outlined on the right side.

Researchers in their studies of mother-infant interactions have used various techniques to promote the mother's awareness of the behavioral and social capabilities of their newborns. In one of Field's early studies (1977) mothers were asked to imitate their babies rather than attempt to keep their babies' attention. By doing this the mothers decreased their activities and increased responsiveness to infant behavior. By advising mothers to repeat phrases and to be silent during gaze aversion, Field noted mothers were increasingly sensitive to their infants' behavioral cues and responsive to their signals. Anderson (1981) combined providing information to the mother about neonatal behavior with a demonstration of the infant's behavior as a means of enhancing the quality of mother-infant interaction. Riesch and Munns (1985) provided an audiotape with accompanying text for the mothers to listen to privately. They reported the following:

> Mothers who received the intervention to inform them of the neonate's social capabilities and of the maternal behaviors to enhance and support their infants reported significantly more of their own behavior than did mothers who did not receive the treatment. Awareness of one's own behavior undoubtedly was a significant factor in the mother's reporting of her own behavior that her infant noticed. The new mother is concerned about how she will perform her new role; she needs to meet her own expectations and those of others in the performance of her maternal role (Humenick and Bugen, 1987). The mother's expectations may or may not be realistic. Unrealistic expectations may serve as a detriment to a mother's accomplishments. Informing the mother of the responses she can initiate in order to enhance or support her particular infant may relieve some of her role uncertainty, thus allowing her to interact freely with her infant.

Because of the sheltered environment provided after delivery, women may misjudge the actual amount of physical and psychic energy they possess. They may expect to resume tasks too soon and then feel discouraged when they are not able to do so. Their still-pregnant look prompts well-meaning people to ask them when they expect their baby (Fig. 21-7). These remarks can add to the mother's feelings of discouragement. In addition, the baby's behavior does not always meet expectations. Sore nipples, worry about adequate milk supply, or even lack of sensations anticipated with breastfeeding can lead to a mother's disappointment. Some babies cry more than expected or do not seem satisfied with their feedings. Many babies have fussy periods that do not respond to any ministrations:

> But my husband, too, was disconcerted at first, for the intense, unending plaintive cries of our firstborn reached to the very depths of our hearts. And we both had really believed that, somehow, a baby born naturally at home and never separated from his mother would not be so fretful. However, it becomes apparent that all babies cry (Lang, 1972).

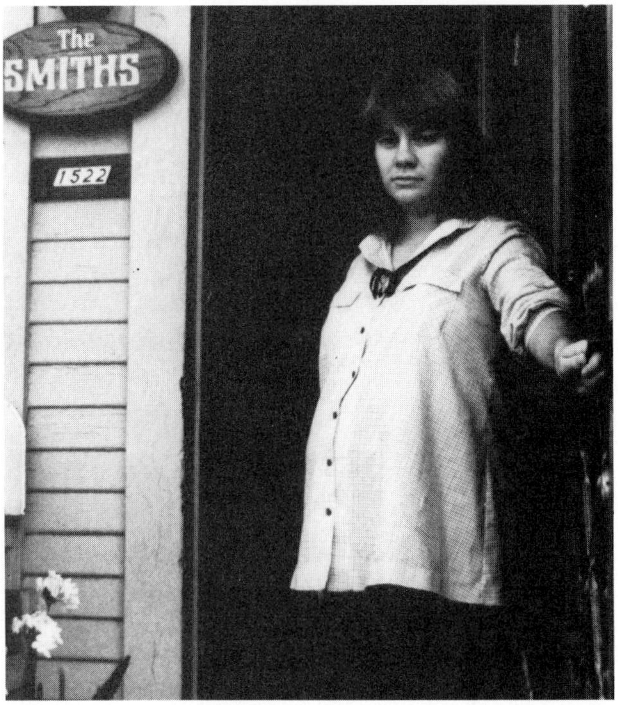

Fig. 21-7 Lack of abdominal muscle tone shortly after delivery gives mother still-pregnant appearance. (Courtesy Marjorie Pyle, RNC, Lifecircle, Costa Mesa, Calif.)

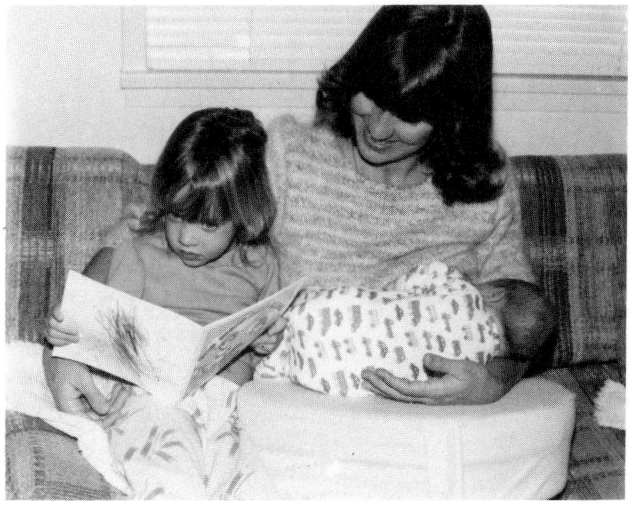

Fig. 21-8 Mother shares feeding time of newborn with older sibling. Baby is supported on an adjustable pad (Keiki Designs). (Courtesy Marjorie Pyle, RNC, Lifecircle, Costa Mesa, Calif.)

Mothers also are faced with the need to help siblings adjust to the new sister or brother (see guidelines for client teaching, Chapter 9; p. 573). **Sibling rivalry** may require parental time and attention to be handled successfully (Fig. 21-8). Even if the children have participated in planning for the new baby, they may be unable to accept the reality of diminished parental attention. Their behavior may reflect their feelings of frustration (see specific nursing care plan, p. 602).

Forewarning about the possibility of such happenings even in the best regulated homes permits the parents to judge themselves less harshly. They are better prepared to seek assistance, change routine, or accept the happening as a passing phase.

Postpartum Depression

Depressive states, often called **"the baby blues,"** may occur after delivery and are not dismissed lightly. Symptoms begin 2 or 3 days after delivery and usually disappear within a week or two. The woman experiences a letdown feeling accompanied by irritability. She may cry easily, lose her appetite, have trouble sleeping, and feel anxious. Mothers of preterm infants have been found to initially experience higher levels of anxiety and depression (Gennaro, 1988). Severe depressive psychosis occurs rarely (Chapter 25).

The nurse can best assist the woman and family by assuring them that this depression is both normal and temporary. Recognizing the state, helping the woman verbalize her feelings, and providing support and understanding are important nursing actions. The nurse can explain to the woman and family that the depression may be caused by hormonal changes, emotional reaction to the role transition, discomfort, or fatigue. Setting up tasks the woman can accomplish easily and successfully are interventions that can help counteract the feelings of depression. It is also important to encourage adequate rest and nutrition. Since the woman will likely continue to experience symptoms after discharge, the nurse should always include the woman's partner in all interventions to support the woman and express concerns.

Support Systems

The North American culture emphasizes the instinctual components of motherhood. As a result, many parents hesitate to seek help from nurses, physicians, family, and friends. Long-term support by nurses or physicians is a positive factor in the ultimate adjustment of the family. Besides providing emotional support, families and friends can assist with housework, and baby-sitting with older children, and eventually, the new baby. Being able to share experiences verbally with others who are interested and experienced also tends to reassure the new mother. A mother, in discussing visits by the family to see the new baby, commented as follows:

■ I want the family to come. You people praise him so and think he is the most wonderful baby. All my friends have their own babies and are too busy trying to get compliments for them to give us any. All babies need aunties and grandmothers!

Being given information about the availability of health facilities and how to get in touch with the nurse or physician relieves new parents of feeling total responsibility for the health of the new baby.

Home visits by nurses can be used to relieve stress and help parents anticipate and prepare for other possible stresses. Hospital stays are short; the parents leave the hospital in the "honeymoon" phase of transition. The realities of recovery and the parenting role become evident quickly, especially for those without assistance in the home. Rubin (1961) defines this as *letting go*. Parental expectations of each other, even if discussed thoroughly prenatally, usually do not go as expected by either partner (Humenick and Bugen, 1987). Parents need to be encouraged to communicate openly with each other regarding their stresses. Some anticipatory guidance before discharge and during the home visit may enable new parents to negotiate constructively any role dissonance they may experience and to have more realistic expectations of each other and the baby and baby care. Visits may be spaced to take into account potential stress times, such as 2 or 3 days after coming home from the hospital and the third and sixth weeks at home (Fig. 21-9).

The supportive care given at such times includes care for the entire family. Parents are as concerned with the ups and downs of other family members as they are with those of mother and child. The nurse may give supportive care by listening to (1) accounts of successes and failures, (2) individuals' feelings about the new baby, and (3) individuals' comments about what they expect of others (e.g., family members and friends) in their new roles. One prime requisite is to set up a climate for the safe expression of doubts and anger, as well as happiness. The family will test the nurse's intent and knowledge, and the nurse must recognize and accept this.

The following specific nursing care plan on p. 602 demonstrates how home care can be tailored to the unique needs of the postpartum family.

Nursing Strategies to Meet Changing Parental Needs. The infant, parents, and family must pass through three distinct periods as the parents learn more about the infant, themselves, and their relationship to the family. These three periods are known as the early, consolidation, and growth periods.

Early Period. The nurse encourages infant contact during the early period by timing the contact with the newborn's normal wake/sleep cycles. The parents are encouraged to care for the infant and to examine the infant as the nurse describes any normal variations. The parents are given a demonstration of infant care, beginning with the use of a bulb syringe. Videotapes and written materials may supplement actual demonstrations. The family is introduced to the infant with reassurance provided to the siblings as appropriate for their age.

Consolidation Period. This is the time when the infant, parents, and family are working together to incorporate the new person into the family. Parents should be praised for their successes in caring for the infant. They need to discuss their role as parents and their response to the complexities of the role. Support people, such as social service workers, may be contacted to provide additional support if the family expresses a need. The nurse should discuss typical sibling reactions and explore with the parents methods of coping with difficult family situations.

Growth Period. This period may not begin until weeks after the birth, when the family can absorb more

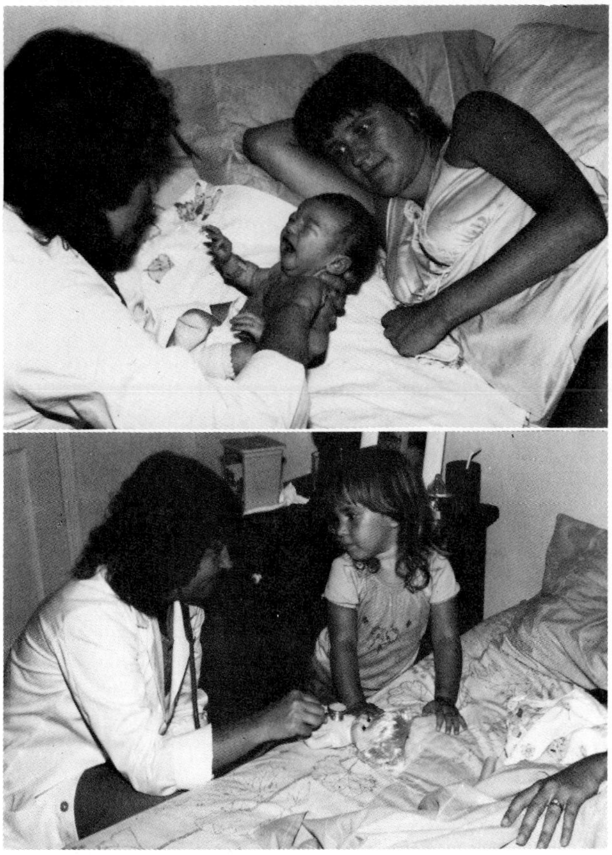

A

B

Fig. 21-9 **A,** Nurse-midwife assesses newborn with mother watching. **B,** Nurse-midwife reviews assessment of newborn for older sister using sister's doll. (Courtesy Marjorie Pyle, RNC, Lifecircle, Costa Mesa, Calif.)

Specific Nursing Care Plan

NURSING CARE DURING POSTPARTUM PERIOD

Laura and Jim had their second child, a girl, 4 days ago. The first child, Scott, is now 3 years old. Laura's HMO insurance promotes early discharge with a home health nurse that visits 24 hours after her return home. When the home health nurse arrives, Laura reports two problems to her:

1. She is having trouble with her first bowel movement. She had had an episiotomy and has hemorrhoids. She is concerned about being hurt and uncomfortable.
2. The 3-year-old son, Scott, is jealous of the new baby. He is whiny and fretful. He has begun to wet his pants again.

Jim's mother is staying with them to help out. She is annoyed with Scott. She says "He is very spoiled. If he were mine, I'd spank his bottom." She has taken Scott with her to the grocery store. The baby is asleep when the nurse arrives.

Laura reports that she has been taking fluids well and has eaten well-balanced meals with plenty of fresh fruits and vegetables.

ASSESSMENT	NURSING DIAGNOSIS (ND), PLAN/GOAL (P/G)	RATIONALE/ IMPLEMENTATION	EVALUATION
Elimination Gave birth 4 days ago. Had a midline episiotomy that is now intact and healing. Has three moderate-sized hemorrhoids that hurt and itch. Last bowel movement was the day of delivery. Laura states she knows little about care of hemorrhoids.	ND: Constipation, related to fear of injury and pain at episiotomy site. P/G: Laura experiences a bowel movement without injury to episiotomy. ND: Pain, related to constipation, episiotomy, and hemorrhoids. P/G: Laura experiences no aggravation of hemorrhoids or discomfort. ND: Knowledge deficit related to care of hemorrhoids. P/G: Laura reports confidence in self-care for hemorrhoids.	*Constipation may lead to straining and pain:* Share assessment data. By physician's order; prepare Laura for and administer a commercially available physiologic enema solution. Stay within shouting distance as enema is expelled. Note results. Reassess perineum and share findings with Laura. Review care of hemorrhoids with Laura.	Laura states she feels so much better having a nurse available at this time. Laura states the enema was not as uncomfortable as expected. Laura states she is glad there was a nurse to "explain things." Laura states she understands care of hemorrhoids.
Coping—stress tolerance Three-year-old sibling jealous of new baby and has regressed, is now wetting pants again.	ND: Anxiety (Scott) related to fear of losing his mother's attention. P/G: Scott is less anxious regarding his status in family.	*Sibling anxiety can cause problems for all family members, therefore the nurse will encourage Laura to:* Plan time with Scott alone. Plan playing "older level" games with child. Involve father with son.	Scott's anxiety lessens as shown by his returning to his pattern of remaining dry and being away from mother for longer periods.
Grandmother intolerant of Scott's response to new sister.	ND: Ineffective family coping; compromised, related to conflict in method of supporting and disciplining child. P/G: Family will develop a plan that is mutually satisfying; spanking will not be used as a means of discipline.	*Coping skills differ among family members; the nurse can assist them to work together by:* Suggesting that grandmother care for newborn during time Scott is usually fretful. Praising grandmother for help she is providing to the family. Suggesting an outing for father, grandmother, and Scott.	Grandmother becomes more understanding of Scott's acting out. Grandmother verbalizes pleasure with outing and this time to get better acquainted with the men and boys in her life.

information regarding growth and development of the infant and family. The parents are taught normal physical and psychosocial growth and development patterns. This may include concrete information about adding solids to the infant's diet or the type of toy appropriate to stimulate the baby. The parents are encouraged to discuss any problems in child care (i.e., feeding problems) and how they react to the infant. Parents may be referred to telephone crisis centers or social service agencies if problems are identified. The nurse will also discuss with the parents and families their reactions, including sibling reaction or demands placed on other family members.

Coping Mechanisms

Family commitments involve having both time and energy for individual family members—mother, father, and children. In addition to new parents learning the techniques for care of themselves and their babies, other suggestions have proved helpful to parents in coping with readjusting their lives. A list of these suggestions can be given to new parents, but discussion of specific ways of handling them is also necessary. Discussion with the parents should include the following suggestions:

- *Set priorities for tasks.* Many tasks can be left for a later period or done by others. Be adamant about not taking on extra tasks for family, friends, or community. Try not to schedule a move to a new location soon after giving birth.
- *Do not become overly concerned with appearances*—tidiness in the home is not as important as time spent with the family. Taking up the role of "super housekeeper" can be postponed until other adjustments are made.

  Sometimes new mothers become overburdened with visits from relatives eager "to take over the baby." The husband can help his wife redirect these wellmeaning people toward helping with housework and cooking. This leaves the parent free to interact with the child.
- *Get plenty of rest and sleep;* rearrange schedules if necessary. Since naps may not be possible if there are other children in the family, going to bed early is recommended; let friends know when to visit.
- *Do not undertake the care of another incapacitated relative* at this point; such responsibilities should be undertaken by other family members.
- *Arrange for some time away from the baby;* enlist the help of friends, family, or others for baby-sitting. Relaxation for both husband and wife is necessary. Baby-sitting, if at all possible, must be planned and a regular schedule developed. This includes time off for the mother during the day so that she can get away from the home and its responsibilities. In some localities, churches or other agencies have developed programs attuned to the needs of mothers. The young children are cared for while the mothers take part in activities with other mothers. This helps them establish relationships with others who are also involved in the care of young children. A mutual sharing of successes and failures in this regard helps the new mother maintain a feeling of equilibrium.

  At the very least the mother needs to plan to get out of the house at least once each day. Access to a car and being able to drive are assets. Taking the baby out for a walk or shopping helps break up the daily routine.
- *Make plans regarding fertility management* before intercourse is resumed and the possibility of pregnancy arises.
- *Be open in your communication with others.* Share incidents of delight or of worry with others. Be open in your requests for support. Discussions with other mothers are helpful. The multiparous mother provides practical advice for the primiparous mother.
- *Learn what health facilities are available,* for example, well-baby centers, immunization clinics, mother-infant classes (i.e., exercise, massage) and how to get in touch with the physician or nurse. If you have questions, remember that the hospital is open all day and night and you can call the emergency or maternity department at any time.
- *Prepare for returning to work.* Most women are physically able to return to work by the end of the sixth week. If plans for child care were not made before the birth, adjustments for child care must be made. Ideally a substitute parent would be one who could come to the home and provide love, as well as care, for the child. Some parents are fortunate enough to have grandparents or other relatives willing and able to fill such a role. Others must take the child to another person's home or a day-care center early in the morning and pick the child up at night. The care provided by day-care centers is needed by some children whose mothers must work to help support them or who are the sole support of the child. For families who require this type of service, assistance in locating such help can be obtained from the local health department and parent referrals. Unfortunately there are not enough quality places available for all children requiring day care.
- *Include the father in caregiving activities.* Research shows that most fathers participate in infant care to the extent that the mother allows (Stainton, 1985).

Crisis Prevention: Infant's Crying

Babies cry because they are hungry or wet, too hot or too cold, because they are ill, or simply because they want attention. And, if the baby is crying just to be held, who is to say that this is not a legitimate reason to cry? The way babies cry seems to contain the message they want to convey. Parents soon recognize the difference between cries. When parents want to respond to their baby's cry, they need to be encouraged not to be put off by friends or relatives who say they are spoiling the child. *A tiny infant cannot be spoiled.* Bell and Ainsworth (1972) found that "Mothers who ignore and delay in responding to the crying of an infant when he is tiny have babies who cry more frequently and persistently later on." A baby's cry requires an investigation to identify the specific need.

Nurses, and often knowledgeable grandparents, have a special role in helping parents and baby synchronize (Darbyshire, 1985). Reciprocal signaling and responding is an important part of parenting (Lamb, 1981). Attachment is greatly enhanced for the mother (parent) who is able to detect and respond to the baby's distress signals and who can comfort and console the baby effectively (Darbyshire, 1985). Conversely, the effect on a mother (parent) faced with a crying, fussing, irritable, and unconsolable baby can be devastating for all concerned (Kirkland, 1985; Mortimer and Kevill, 1985).

Life with a crying baby is a crisis situation. Eventually, parents are "ground down," worrying that something is wrong, facing guilt and loss of self-esteem about their inability to comfort a crying baby. Physical and emotional fatigue compound the crisis.

Parents benefit from concrete suggestions. Knowing that "all parents go through this" is not helpful. If the crying signal is not yet set, several possibilities are explored and tested—hunger, cold, wet diaper. Pain is suspected if there are areas of redness or diaper rash. Loneliness, the need to make contact, may be the sole cause. First the cold, hunger, wet diaper, and pain are treated. Then other comforting techniques are used—*carrying and rocking, sounds, non-nutritive sucking, swaddling, and* ***infant massage.***

People who care for newborns soon become aware that rocking a crying baby vertically and intermittently promotes a "bright-alert" state, whereas continuous horizontal rocking induces the baby to sleep (Byrne and Horowitz, 1981). Studies have also shown that the ideal rate to rock a baby is around 60 to 90 rocks a minute (Pederson, 1975).

The sound of a human voice or soft music can be an effective means to soothe a baby. The old practice of swaddling (wrapping snugly) has been found to pacify some infants. Nonnutritive sucking on a pacifier is another effective method. (See Chapter 17 about the use of safe pacifiers.) Infant massage has benefits for both parent and child (Chapter 17).

Crisis Prevention: Siblings and Grandparents

Preparation of siblings and of parents for the reactions of siblings begins before childbirth. Preparation of siblings and grandparents is discussed in Chapter 9.

Classes for grandparents-to-be are designed to help the givers and receivers of advice understand one another (Chapter 9) and update the grandparents to contemporary thinking. Examples of contemporary childrearing theories with which grandparents may be unfamiliar are that one cannot spoil a newborn, breastfeeding is superior to formula-feeding, and bright colors are better than pastels for the baby's room since they are more stimulating. Safer infant car seats and disposable diapers are advances that most grandparents readily appreciate.

Few people move gracefully or fearlessly into new identities. Nurses support the grandparents who are the role models and support network for the new parents. Nurses also help new parents bridge the generation gap by keeping communication open. On occasion, the nurse suggests the scripts parents need to work toward to have the kind of loving relationship they would like to have. Many hospitals distribute pamphlets to grandparents concerning the topic of helping the new parents "without interfering." Several publications on the topic are available at local bookstores.

Care after Multifetal Birth

The mother with a multifetal pregnancy (e.g., twins) requires the same physical care as any other new mother. She is more prone to develop postdelivery hemorrhage because of excessive uterine distension. Therefore she must be carefully assessed.

Psychologically, however, even the most willing of mothers can find their coping mechanisms overwhelmed by both the idea and reality of caring for two or more newborns. Mother-child attachment takes longer because the mother attaches first to one newborn and then to the other. Parents must organize simplified and flexible plans of care. The almost constant attention required until the infants' schedule of care can be synchronized may prove exhausting. If possible, help is obtained, particularly to guarantee sufficient rest for the mother. The added expense can also be burdensome to a young family. One mother expressed anger at the surprise birth of twins. The explanation of such errors did not placate her. She needed time to vent these feelings before she could be helped with changing her anticipated plan for care. Some communities have support groups for parents of twins, and these can be a great resource for new parents. Another resource that may be available is a list of community agencies or retail operations that provide services to parents of twins; this may be useful in easing added financial needs.

Most parents are anxious to know if their children are identical or fraternal. Gross examination of the placenta at birth cannot prove whether twins are identical. Therefore it is best to tell parents differentiation in the type of twinning cannot be made at this time.

If the infants are born prematurely or are small for gestational age, their prolonged hospital stay can cause parental separation anxiety. If this is the case, the mother may be encouraged to visit or care for the infants in the hospital. She can use this waiting time to recover as much physical strength as possible. It provides time for the family to prepare for the infants' homecoming. Introduction of multiple siblings into a family also can result in intense rivalry. All children compete for the mother's attention. Substitute mothering by interested relatives can do much to ease the strain.

❑ CULTURAL ASPECTS OF POSTPARTUM CARE

The greatest conflict between Western and non-Western beliefs and practices in childbearing occurs in the postpartum period (Fig. 21-10). If a woman delivers in the hospital, she and her family are directly confronted with culturally related problems that are not as easily resolved as those encountered in the prenatal and labor and delivery stages (Fig. 21-11). Moreover, the

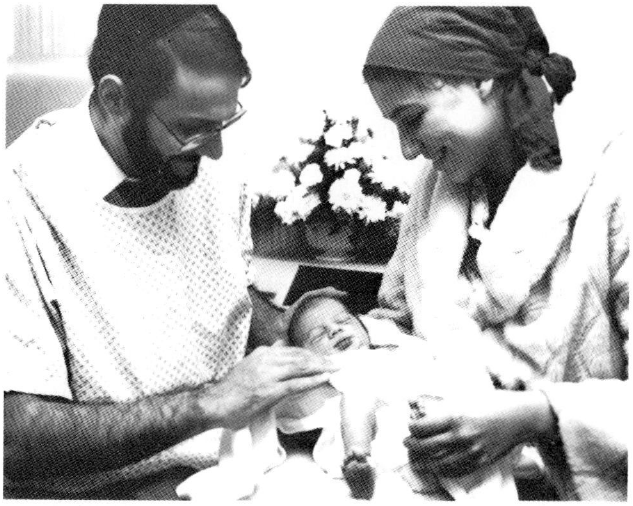

Fig. 21-10 Parents admire their new baby.

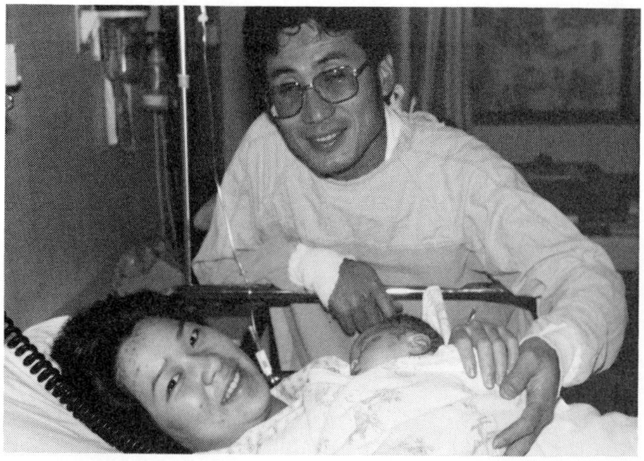

Fig. 21-11 New parents after the cesarean birth of their daughter.

nurses caring for these mothers may view the woman's behavior as totally incomprehensible since it varies so dramatically from Western health care provider's expectations.

Cultural proscriptions during the postdelivery period exist to hasten the recovery of the mother, to assist her physically and emotionally in her assumption of her new maternal role, and to protect and care for the newborn child.

The behavior patterns for many cultures include a period of seclusion for women lasting from 7 to 40 days with a minimum of activity allowed for mothers. These practices are based on two beliefs: that delivery has upset the balance of the mother's body and that the mother, infant, and those caring for them are in a **pollution state.**

Maintenance of a State of Balance

Cultures that subscribe to a belief in the necessity of body balance believe that the body has lost a great deal of heat during the labor and delivery process and that the mother is therefore subject to a number of illnesses. Thus certain practices must be followed to restore the balance of heat and cold. Adherents of both humoral and yin and yang theories have prescriptions and proscriptions for restoration of balance of heat and cold (Currier, 1978).

After delivery, hot and cold restrictions prevail. The mother must remain on strict bed rest without a pillow. Hot or steam baths (but not showers) are permitted only after the second postpartum day. Heat—such as a hot water bottle on the abdomen—helps involution. Physical warmth is essential; blankets may be added even on the warmest day. Liquids must be served without ice.

Food

Food is one way in which heat can be restored and cold diminished. The classic Chinese diet (Campbell and Chang, 1975) represents an effort to decrease yin forces, which are cold. Included are an abundance of hot foods. The quality of heat and cold cannot always be measured by actual temperature. The essence of cold might be in a food even if the food is heated. Pillsbury (1978) notes that some foods are considered cold because they are grown in the damp earth or in watery places. Green vegetables, fruits, meats, and fish are commonly considered cold foods. Asians rank rice, eggs, and chicken high on the heat scale and thus believe they should be eaten frequently. It is obvious that many, if not most, of the foods served on hospital trays, such as meats, vegetables, fruits, and fruit juices, are considered cold. These will probably not be eaten by many Asian, Southeast Asian, and Spanish-speaking women.

However, if a hot substance is added to boiled water, it may counteract the coldness. For example, the chicken soup is so powerful that the cold quality of the water with which it is made is counteracted. Ginger added to hot water that has been boiled may cause the same effect. It is obvious then, that ice water, used frequently in hospitals, is forbidden.

Clark (1970) wrote that Mexican-American women are forbidden to eat "cold" foods such as hot chilies, pickles, any food prepared with vinegar, tomatoes, spinach, any pork product, and most fruits. Fruits such as bananas and grapefruit and other citrus fruits must be avoided because of their acidity and because they are believed to cause varicose veins in mothers. Although fruits and vegetables are also prohibited in the pregnant Vietnamese woman's diet, pork legs and knuckles are allowed because pork is believed to improve the secretion of milk (Coughlin, 1965). Hart (1965) reported that to prevent stomachaches, Filipino women avoid "cold" foods such as eels, oysters, squash, and uncooked fruits and vegetables. Filipino women also refrain from eating sour foods because they supposedly cause the mother's milk to curdle. "Tasty" foods with strong, rich flavor, such as peanuts, canned fish, and fatty meats, are avoided because they are believed to cause lactation to stop. The nurse should also understand that Filipino and Chinese women prefer to drink warm water instead of ice water (Campbell and Chang, 1975; Hart, 1965). According to Campbell and Chang, two possible reasons for this preference are (1) the belief that drinking ice water "shocks" the body and (2) the history of poor sanitation in the Philippines and China, which has made it a custom for people in these countries to boil drinking water.

Since, according to Hart (1969), disagreement occurs among Latin Americans and Filipinos about the classifications of basic foods into hot and cold categories, *nurses should use clients as their major cultural informants.* With flexibility and creativity, the nurse can plan with clients and with other health team members nutritious and culturally acceptable diets. With little difficulty the nurse can advise the pregnant woman in selecting those foods in the hospital that are healthy, as well as those that the woman considers culturally appropriate. Similarly, the nurse can allow, as much as possible, family members to bring foods to the mother that are not readily available in the hospital but are highly recommended in the woman's culture.

Lactation

In the Philippines, if the mother's milk does not flow regularly, a meal of chicken and green papaya, boiled in coconut "milk" is suggested (Hart, 1965). Chicken soup is also believed important in the production of a nursing mother's milk. According to Hart (1965), the Filipino mother is also advised to eat a soup of boiled clams and ginger. Hart stated that Filipinos use hot applications of special medicinal preparations to stimulate lactation. Furthermore, the Filipino mother believes that raising either arm over her head while lying down will decrease, if not actually stop, lactation. Hart (1965) also noted the Filipino women's belief that heavy work will make their milk "hot." Korean mothers eat seaweed soup with rice to increase milk production (Chung, 1977). Currier (1978) reported that Spanish-Americans believe that exposing mothers to cold diminishes the flow of milk. Asian mothers may believe that they must refrain from breastfeeding until their milk is in. Offering the breast to the infant before the milk comes in is thought to further deplete the mother of vital heat and fluids during this perilous time (Lee, 1989).

Activities of Daily Living

In addition to food, contact with air and wind is proscribed by Asians, Filipinos, Mexican-Americans, and southern blacks. Cold must be prevented from entering the body, to counteract further imbalance. Air is considered cold, whatever the temperature, and thus windows and doors must be kept closed. The Chinese belief that a woman's pores are open for 30 days after delivering a baby coincides with the period in which they believe the mother has an excess of cold (Campbell and Chang, 1973; Pillsbury, 1978). Air conditioners are a source of fear for women in the hospital. Fans are to be avoided. New mothers will keep themselves totally covered with blankets despite how hot the temperature of the room may be. The Chinese believe that for these 30 days after birth, cold air can enter the body through the vagina (Campbell and Chang, 1975). This is consistent with the Chinese belief that during the postdelivery period some balance of the yang, or "hot" air, should be returned by decreasing the yin energy forces, or "cold" air in the body. Similarly, Spanish women believe that during the 40-day postdelivery period they should avoid exposing themselves to any condition that could cause bad air *(malaire)* to enter the vagina (Baca, 1973).

Water is considered cold at all times, even if it is heated. Therefore not bathing for a period of time is a widely held belief. Recognizing these beliefs, the nurse can encourage the mother to take frequent sponge baths and emphasize perineal care, breast care, and other hygienic and comfort measures. Some mothers will take all kinds of measures to avoid the daily shower but will not directly refuse, complying by going to the shower room, turning on the water, and remaining in such a position that the water will not touch them. Pillsbury (1978) notes that Chinese women who have been westernized in so many ways still adhere to the postpartum practice of avoiding water. They must not wash themselves, their dishes, or their clothes. To the Chinese and other Asians, contact with water, considered cold, causes wind to enter the body and will result in future years in asthma, arthritis, and chronic aches and pains.

In some cultures women use abdominal binders during the pregnancy, as well as during the postdelivery period. Some Mexican-Americans use binders during the first 40 days of the puerperium (Clark, 1970). It is believed by these persons that binders help organs in the stomach return to their normal positions, push the hips together, and firm up the stomach muscles. Binders are used in conjunction with massage to help the woman with the "slipped" uterus (Hart, 1965). According to Hart (1965), in some regions in the Philippines, binders are worn by women both during pregnancy and after delivery to prevent *buhî-buhî. Buhî-buhî* is a syndrome in which ascending gas, starting under the lower left rib, produces symptoms ascribed to postdelivery hemorrhage, such as tachycardia, vertigo, partial blindness, and impaired respiration. The use of the binder is also thought to prevent the postdelivery expansion of the uterus. Another reason this practice is followed by Filipino women is the notion that the "cold" womb should be protected.

Pollution State

In addition to an imbalance of hot and cold, several cultures consider that the mother and infant are in a state of pollution after delivery. A certain time must elapse and certain rituals must be performed before purity is restored. A state of seclusion is commonly compulsory, during which time the mother is encouraged to limit her activities. This is in contrast to the hospital practice of early ambulation following delivery, early infant care responsibilities, and early discharge from the hospital. Mexican-Americans may observe *la cuarentina* for 40 days after birth of babies (Clark, 1970). For the Chinese mother, going out during the first month after birth will offend the gods because dirty birth blood remains throughout the month (Pillsbury, 1978). The Filipino mother (Stern et al, 1980) is commonly misunderstood as lazy and not caring when she refuses to do what is requested in the hospital and at home. Recently, in a personal communication from a group of Cambodian women, concern was expressed about how they will manage after the baby is born because they do not have an extended family to assist during the required time of seclusion and limited activity. The fear of subsequent illness, especially arthritis, in later years is very real to them. Homemaker services are not available to them because according to the Western view, they are able bodied and assistance cannot be justified. Their hope for the future is based on the belief that counteracting the bad effects of not carrying out cultural proscriptions for the postpartum period can be accomplished only by going through a follow-up pregnancy correctly. Their chances of doing future pregnancies "correctly" are remote, however. The cultural quandary for these women is clear.

The cultural knowledge of childbearing Cambodian women was studied (Kulin, 1988). A number of unique beliefs were identified: birthmarks are attributed to a mark made by soot in the person's previous life; and activities such as jumping could cause the umbilical cord to break. Herbal medicines are used prenatally to ensure a fast and short labor and to prevent the birth of a baby with vernix (Kulin, 1988). Vernix is believed to be sperm. Since sexual activity is not sanctioned after 6 months of pregnancy, the presence of vernix would indicate to others the woman's transgression of this restriction.

Snow (1974) described the view of southern blacks that blood is a pollutant that carries contaminants from the body. Southern blacks and others believe that an adequate lochia flow is essential and going outside in the wind or air could thicken and halt the flow of blood, extending the time of pollution. Some Filipino mothers may remain bedfast for 2 weeks, after which time a special bath is taken to further remove the debris of pregnancy believed to be found in perspiration.

"Mother roasting" is a Southeast Asian custom (Hart, 1965). In this practice the mother sits on a cane-bottom (or bamboo-slat) chair draped in a blanket from head to floor, while a bowl of glowing hot coals is placed under her (Nydegger and Nydegger, 1963).

There she "roasts" until the coals are cold. This is repeated daily for 11 to 30 days. According to Stern et al (1980), "roasting" is practiced by Filipinos in the most remote provinces only (Chapter 11). The purpose of this is to hasten the healing process, much like perineal heat lamps used in recent times.

Filipinos believe that this practice stops the blood, fixes the uterus in position, and alleviates birth soreness (Hart, 1965). Vietnamese women practice roasting for the following reasons: (1) the mother's blood must be kept "warm," (2) the mother's uterus will contract properly and consequently prevent unhealthy distortion of the woman's figure, and (3) steam baths will prevent the woman from having a bad body odor during her entire life (Coughlin, 1965). At the end of the 30 to 40 days, the woman usually takes a cleansing bath. Then she resumes her normal activities in the community. Since she has been "cleansed," members of the community need not avoid contacts with a formerly pregnant woman.

Horn (1982) supplies a recent example of acculturated behavior. After the birth of her first child, a Greek-American mother followed the ancient proscription of participation in church activities for 40 days. While her husband attended the church wedding of a friend, this woman did her weekly shopping at the local supermarket. In most cultural groups sexual relations are prohibited until after the seclusion period and sometimes throughout lactation.

Some cultural groups have unique practices. For example, the women of Northern Thailand bind their wrists with string. The purpose of wrist binding is to prevent the loss of the soul, which may lead to wind disease, a specific complex of symptoms indicating a state of humoral imbalance characterized by weakness, nausea, and hypersensitivity to odors (Kundstadter, 1978). Northern Thai women giving birth will most likely have their wrists bound and would be extremely frightened and upset if the strings were removed.

The preceding examples indicate that, from the time of delivery to a certain designated time afterward, mothers in many cultures are considered highly susceptible to ensuing illness, either immediately or at an unspecified time in the future. Furthermore, their state of pollution requires that only certain persons contact them during the specified time they remain in seclusion. Most of their activities are carried on by others, usually members of the extended family or friends. The end of the time of seclusion is often marked by a ceremony and includes ritual cleansing of the woman, child, and place of seclusion (Brownlee, 1978). It is important for nurses to understand these factors, assist women in carrying out their beliefs and practices insofar as is possible, and assist them with necessary adjustments when their expectations are not feasible. The nurse *never* assumes conformance to cultural practices by ethnic origin. Many young women who are first or second generation American follow their cultural traditions when their grandmother is present, but request a shower and cold drink when the family leaves. The nurse uses discretion to assist the woman to integrate her cultural beliefs into her life-style.

❑ DISCHARGE FROM HOSPITAL

Discharge Planning. Discharge planning begins with the first contact with the client, when the client's physical, emotional, social, and economic profiles start to emerge. The goals listed on pp. 580, 582, and 597 and in the nursing care plans in this chapter serve as guidelines for assessing the client's needs at discharge. In the preparation of a client for discharge, the nurse does the following:

1. Identifies gaps in knowledge and reviews these points, if necessary:
   (a) Self-care activities and infant-care activities
   (b) Danger signs (see box below)
   (c) Return of ovulation and menstruation
   (d) Lactation and weaning or suppression of lactation
   (e) Resumption of sexual intercourse and fertility management
   (f) Medications that have been prescribed for the client
2. Helps the client develop a support system for help with cooking, cleaning, child care, shopping, and so on
3. Identifies the need for referral to community resources (e.g., homemaker or child care services, food stamps) and initiates communication with the proper agency or person (social worker), when appropriate

DANGER SIGNS

Postpartum (Physical)

1. Fever, with or without chills
2. Foul-smelling or irritating vaginal discharge
3. Excessive lochia or vaginal discharge
4. Recurrence of bright red vaginal bleeding after the lochia has changed to rust color
5. A swollen area on the leg that is painful, red, or hot to the touch
6. Localized swelling or a painful, hot area on the breast
7. A burning sensation during urination or an inability to urinate
8. Pelvic or perineal pain

4. Provides the client with a printed instruction sheet that includes phone numbers to call day and night in case of questions or problems.

Early Discharge. The duration of hospitalization and the subsequent convalescence at home are still under debate. Most women who do not experience complications return home before the third postdelivery day. Some women who are carefully screened by the nurse, obstetrician, and pediatrician leave much earlier—anywhere from 8 to 24 hours after delivery. Because these clients are in particular need of follow-up care for themselves and their infants, hospitals have established early discharge programs to assist with such care. These programs provide an alternative mode of mother-infant care.

Planning for early discharge begins in the prenatal period and involves the nurse, physician, pediatrician, and other appropriate members of the health care team. The families who participate should meet the following criteria: (1) live within a reasonable distance of the hospital, (2) have taken preparation-for-parenthood classes that include content related to assessment of the mother's recovery, care of the mother during the puerperium, and identification and reporting of possible complications, (3) have someone at home to assist in the care of the infant and mother, and (4) have no major medical problems. If a family is interested in early discharge, they are asked to notify the attending physician and nursing staff at the beginning of prenatal care. Opportunities are provided to meet the nurse who will be making home visits during the puerperium for health assessment and any teaching that is necessary. Women with complications, however, should be asymptomatic for at least 24 hours and capable of personal care before leaving the hospital.

Return Visit. Since biblical times, the puerperium has been considered to last 6 weeks. Hence a return visit and examination have been scheduled traditionally 6 weeks after delivery. This is illogical because many problems, such as leukorrhea, may be identified and successfully treated earlier. Individualization is important, therefore, but a more logical date for return examination would be 2 to 4 weeks after delivery.

It is also necessary to discuss methods of birth control with the woman and her partner. Approximately 40% of non-breastfeeding women will menstruate within 6 weeks. Of these, half will ovulate during their first menstrual cycle. Women who are breastfeeding will resume menstruation within 12 weeks of delivery. Most of these women will have one or more anovulatory cycles before they ovulate, but this must not be considered as an effective method of birth control (Easterling and Herbert, 1990).

Closing the Client's Chart. Just before the time when the client would be leaving the maternity unit, the nurse reviews the client's chart (audits the chart) to see that laboratory reports, medications, signatures, and so on are in order. Some hospitals have a checklist to follow before the client's discharge. The nurse verifies that medications, if ordered, have arrived on the unit, that any valuables kept secured during the client's stay have been returned to her and that she has signed a receipt for them, and that the infant is ready to be discharged.

Escorting the Client from the Hospital. The nurse is careful not to administer any medication that would make the mother sleepy if she is the one who will be holding the baby on the way out of the hospital. In most instances, the woman is seated in a wheelchair and is usually given the baby to hold. Some families leave unescorted and ambulatory, depending on hospital protocol. The woman's possessions are gathered and taken out with her and her family; usually they are placed on some type of cart or carried by family members. Of course, *the woman's and the baby's identification bands have been carefully checked.* As the client and the baby are assisted into the car, the nurse should make sure that there is a car seat in which to secure the baby. If there is not, the nurse should return both to the unit and arrange with a social worker, if necessary to provide one for the trip home.

CAUTION: Whether or not the woman and her family have chosen early discharge, the nurse and the physician are held responsible if the woman is discharged before her condition has stabilized within normal limits. If complications occur, the medical and nursing staff could be sued for "abandonment."

Evaluation

Evaluation is a continuous process. Parental, infant, and family relationships are consistently assessed as indicators of healthy family adjustments after the birth of a child. The nurse can be reasonably assured that care was effective to the extent that the goals for care have been met; that is, the parents express a healthy self-esteem, demonstrate a healthy parent-child relationship, participate in the care of the newborn, and meet their cultural expectations of themselves and their experience (Fig. 21-12).

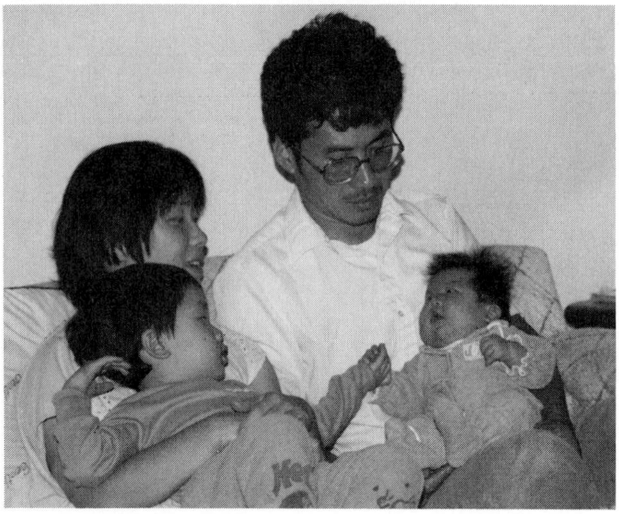

Fig. 21-12 Healthy family relationships promote the growth potential of the newborn and other family members.

SUMMARY

The normal postpartum period is a time of rapid change. Change takes place in the physiologic and psychosocial dimensions of the woman, the newborn, and their family. The nurse who makes pertinent assessments, plans and implements client-centered care, and evaluates the effectiveness of the care is enacting an important role in the health of the child-bearing family.

LEARNING ACTIVITIES

1. Research in depth one culture that interests you (perhaps your own ethnic background). Talk with clients and health care workers and do library research to obtain data about general and childbearing and childrearing customs. Share your findings in a group setting.
2. Formulate a nursing care plan comparing and contrasting nursing care for a multipara and primipara.
3. Using the parent-infant interaction assessment tool in this chapter, assess a client during the hospital stay and, if possible, during a home visit. Discuss findings with the group.
4. Assess own attitudes and concepts regarding parenting. Use these reports as the basis for group discussion and self-disclosure that works toward a better understanding of lack of parental attachment.
5. In the newborn nursery, select a baby that you "really like" and one that you "can't stand." Identify those characteristics of the newborn that influence your response to the babies; process record a 3 to 5 minute interaction with each one. Reflect on what you would do if *your* baby had the characteristics of the one you "can't stand." Devise strategies for intervention for the mother (or father) whose baby does not meet their expectations.
6. Role play a client discharge including teaching, follow-up medication, and documentation. Discharge at least one client, review with group strengths and weaknesses of experience.

KEY CONCEPTS

- Postpartum care is modeled on the concept of health.
- The nursing care plan includes assessments to detect deviations from normal, comfort measures to relieve discomfort or pain, and safety measures to prevent injury or infection.
- The nurse provides teaching and counseling measures designed to promote a mother's (and father's) feeling of competence and control in the care of herself and newly born child.
- The nurse's clinical expertise is required to implement many therapeutic measures for physical care including care of the boggy uterus, the full urinary bladder, the need for pharmacologic relief of discomfort, care after repair of episiotomy or laceration, care of hemorrhoids, and suppression of lactation.
- Nurses have a leadership role in helping clients establish healthy early family relationships.
- The parents' response is profoundly affected by their interpretation of the infant's response.
- Crisis prevention is an important function of the nurse and includes anticipatory guidance for infant's crying, sibling responses, and interactions with the grandparents.
- Mothers (and fathers) often misjudge the actual amount of physical and emotional energy required for the role transition to parenthood.
- The behaviors of self, the infant, the spouse, and others may not always meet expectations.
- Family commitments involve having time and energy for individual family members—mother, father, and children—and for the couple, away from the child (or children).
- The greatest conflict between Western and non-Western beliefs and practices in childbearing occurs in the postpartum period.

References

Anderson CJ: Enhancing reciprocity between mother and neonate, Nurs Res 30:89, 1981.

Baca J: Some health beliefs of the Spanish-speaking. In Reinhardt AM and Quinn MD, editors: Family-centered community nursing, St Louis, 1973, The CV Mosby Co.

Bell RQ and Ainsworth MDS: Infant crying and maternal responsiveness, Child Dev 43:1171, 1972.

Brownlee AT: Community, culture, and care: a cross-cultural guide for health workers, St Louis, 1978, The CV Mosby Co.

Byrne JM and Horowitz FS: Rocking as a soothing intervention: The influence of direction and type of movement, Infant Behav Dev 4:207, 1981.

Campbell T and Chang B: Health care of the Chinese in America. In Spradley BW, editor: Contemporary community Nursing, Boston, 1975, Little, Brown & Co, Inc.

Caplan G: Psychological aspects of maternity care, Am J Public Health 47:25, 1957.

Catanzarite VA and Aisenbrey C: Prostaglandins: mundane and visionary applications, Contemp OB/GYN 30(4):21, 1987.

Chung HJ: Understanding the Oriental maternity patient, Nurs Clin North Am 12:67, 1977.

Clark M: Health in the Mexican-American culture: a community study, Berkely, Calif, 1970, University of California Press.

Coughlin R: Pregnancy and birth in Vietnam. In Hart D, Rajadhon PA, and Coughlin RJ, editors: Southeast Asian birth customs: three studies in human reproduction, New Haven, Conn, 1965, Human Relations Area Files, pp 205-273.

Cunningham FG, MacDonald PC, and Gant NF: Williams obstetrics, ed 18, Norwalk, Conn, 1989, Appleton & Lange.

Currier RL: The hot-cold syndrome and symbolic balance in Mexican and Spanish-American folk medicine. In Martinez RA, editor: Hispanic culture and health care: fact, fiction, folklore, St Louis, 1978, The CV Mosby Co.

Darbyshire P: Comfort for the crying child, Nurs Times, p 59, Sept 11, 1985.

Droegemueller W: Cold sitz bath for relief of postpartum perineal pain, Clin Obstet Gynecol 23:1039, 1980.

Easterling WE and Herbert WNP: The puerperium. In Scott JR et al: Danforth's obstetrics and gynecology, ed 6, Philadelphia, 1990, JB Lippincott Co.

Field TM: Effects of early separation, interactive deficits, and experimental manipulation on infant-mother face-to-face interaction, Child Dev 48:763, 1977.

Gennaro S: Postpartal anxiety and depression in mothers of term and preterm infants, Nurs Res 37(2):82, 1988.

Hart DV: From pregnancy through birth in a Bisayan Filipino village. In Hart DV, Rajadhon PA, and Coughlin RJ, editors: Southeast Asian birth customs; three studies in reproduction, New Haven, Conn, 1965, Human Relations Area Files, pp 1-113.

Hart DV: Bisayan Filipino and Malayan humoral pathologies: folk medicine and ethnohistory in Southeast Asia, New York, 1969, Cornell University Southeast Asia Program, pp. 43, 46.

Herron MA: One approach to preventing preterm birth, J Perinat Neonat Nurs 2(1):33, 1988.

Hill D: Effects of heat and cold on the perineum after episiotomy/laceration, JOGN Nurs 18(2):124, 1989.

Horn BM: Northwest coast Indians: the Muchleshoot. In Kay MA, editors: Anthropology of human births, Philadelphia, 1982, FA Davis Co.

Humenick SS, and Bugen LA: Parenting roles: expectation versus reality, MCN 12(1):36, 1987.

Kirkland J: Crying and babies: helping families cope, Kent, 1985, Croom Helm Ltd.

Konrad CJ: Helping mothers integrate the birth experience, MCN 12(4):268, 1987.

Kulin J: Childbearing Cambodian refugee women, Can Nurse, p 46, June, 1988.

Kundstadter P: Do cultural differences make any difference? Choice points in medical systems available in Northwestern Thailand. In Kleinman A et al, editors: Culture and healing in Asian societies, Cambridge, Mass, 1978, Schenkman Books, Inc.

Kunst-Wilson W and Cronenwett LR: Nursery care for the emerging family: promoting paternal behavior, Res Nurs Health 4:201, 1981.

Lamb ME: The development of social expectations in the first year of life. In Lamb M and Sherrod L, editors: Infant social cognition, Hillside, New Jersey, 1981, Lawrence Erlbaum Associates, Inc.

Lang R: Birth book, Ben Lomond, Calif, 1972, Genesis Press.

Lee RV et al: Southeast Asian folklore about pregnancy and parturition, Obstet Gynecol 71:243, 1988.

Lee RV: Understanding Southeast Asian mothers-to-be, Childbirth Educ 8(3):32, 1989.

Mortimer P and Kevill F: Infant care: frustration and despair, Nurs Times, Community Outlook, p 19, May, 1985.

NPA Bulletin: increasing culturally relevant practice with Hispanic clients, 3(4):23, 1988.

Nydegger WF and Nydegger C: Tarong: an Ilocos barrio in the Philippines. In Whiting BB, editor: Six cultures: studies of child rearing, New York, 1963, John Wiley & Sons, Inc.

Pederson DR: The soothing effects of rocking as determined by the direction and frequency of movement, Can J Behav Sci 7:237, 1975.

Pillsbury BLK: "Doing the month": confinement and convalescence of Chinese women after childbirth, Soc Sci Med 12:11, 1978.

Ramler D and Roberts J: A comparison of cold and warm sitz baths for relief of postpartum perineal pain, JOGN Nurs 15(6):471, 1986.

Riesch S and Munns S: Promoting awareness: the mother and her baby, Nurs Res 33:271, Sept/Oct, 1985.

Rubin R: Puerperal change, Nurs Outlook 9:753, 1961.

Schornkoff JP: Social support and the development of vulnerable children, Am J Public Health 74:310, 1984.

Snow L: Folk medical beliefs and their implications for care of patients, Ann Intern Med 81:82, 1974.

Stainton MC: Parent-infant interaction: putting theory into practice, Calgary, Alberta, Canada, 1981, University of Calgary Faculty of Nursing.

Stainton MC: Maternal newborn attachment origins and processes. III. Interactional synchony: the prelude to attachment, doctoral thesis, University of California, San Francisco, 1985.

Steele B and Pollock C: A psychiatric study of parents who abuse infants and small children. In Helfer RE and Kempe C, editors: The battered child, Chicago, 1968, University of Chicago Press.

Stern PN et al: Culturally induced stress during childbearing: the Filipino-American experience, Issues Health Care Women 2(3-4):67, 1980.

Bibliography

Booth CL, Johnson-Crowly, and Barnard KE: Infant massage and exercise: worth the effort? MCN 10(3):184, 1985.

Bull M and Lawrence D: Mother's use of knowledge during the first postpartum weeks, JOGN Nurs 14:315, July/Aug, 1985.

Davis JH et al: A study of mothers' postpartum teaching priorities, Matern Child Nurs J p 41-50, 1989.

Degenhart-Leskosky SM: Health education needs of adolescent and nonadolescent mothers, JOGN Nurs 18(3):238, 1989.

Fawcett J and York R: Spouses' physical and psychological symptoms during pregnancy and the postpartum, Nurs Res 35(3):144, 1986.

Fischman SH et al: Changes in sexual relationships in postpartum couples, JOGN Nurs 15:58, Jan/Feb, 1986.

Gorrie TM: Postpartal nursing diagnoses, JOGN Nurs 15:52, Jan/Feb, 1986.

Gosha J and Brucker MC: A self-help group for new mothers: an evaluation, MCN 11:20, Jan/Feb, 1986.

Hans A: Postpartum assessment: the psychological component, JOGN Nurs 15:49, Jan/Feb, 1986.

Hiser PL: Concerns of multiparas during the second postpartum week, JOGN Nurs 16(5):195, 1987.

Horn M and Manion J: Creative grandparenting: bonding the generations, JOGN Nurs 14(3):233, 1985.

Jankowski H and Wells S: Self-administered medications for obstetric patients, MCN (12):199, 1987.

Johnstone HA and Marcinak JF: Candidiasis in the breastfeeding mother and infant, JOGN Nurs 19(2):171, 1990.

Keefe MR: The impact of infant rooming-in on maternal sleep at night, JOGN Nurs 17(2):122, 1988.

Knorr ER: Decision making in obstetrical nursing, Toronto, 1987, BC Decker, Inc.

Leininger M: Transcultural nursing: an essential knowledge and practice field for today, Can Nurse 80:41, Dec, 1984.

Marecki M et al: Early sibling attachment, JOGN Nurs 14:418, Sept/Oct 1985.

Martell LK: Postpartum depression as a family problem, MCN 15(2):90, 1990.

McCaffery M: Patient-controlled analgesia: more than a machine, Nurs '87 17(11):62, 1987.

Mead-Bennett E: The relationship of primigravid sleep experience and select moods on the first postpartum day, JOGN Nurs 19(2):146, 1990.

Mueller LS: Pregnancy and sexuality, JOGN Nurs 14(4):289, 1985.

NAACOG: Nurses offer home health-care alternatives, NAACOG Newsletter 15(5):4, 1988.

Norr KF et al: Early discharge with home follow-up: impact on low income mother and infants, JOGN Nurs 18(2):133, 1989.

Nurses Association of the American College of Obstetricians and Gynecologists: Standards for obstetric gynecologic and neonatal nursing, ed 3, Washington, DC, 1986, The Association.

Petrick JM: Postpartum depression identification of high-risk moms, JOGN Nurs 13(1):37, 1984.

Stolte K: Postpartum 'missing pieces': sequela of a passing obstetrical era? Birth 13(2):100, 1986.

Storr GB: Prevention of nipple tenderness and breast engorgement in the postpartal period, JOGN Nurs 17(3):203, 1988.

Strang VR and Sullivan PL: Body image attitudes during pregnancy and the postpartum period, JOGN Nurs 14:332, July/Aug, 1985.

Tilkian SM: Clinical implications of laboratory tests, ed 4, St Louis, 1987, The CV Mosby Co.

Tribotti S et al: Nursing diagnoses for the postpartum woman, JOGN Nurs 17(6):410, 1988.

Tucker SM et al: Patient care standards: nursing process, diagnosis and outcome, ed 4, St Louis, 1988, The CV Mosby Co.

Tulman L and Fawcett J: Return of functional ability after childbirth, Nurs Res 37(2):77, 1988.

Tulman L et al: Changes in functional status after childbirth, Nurs Res 39(2):70, 1990.

Zalar MK: Sexual counseling for pregnant couples, MCN 1:176, 1976.

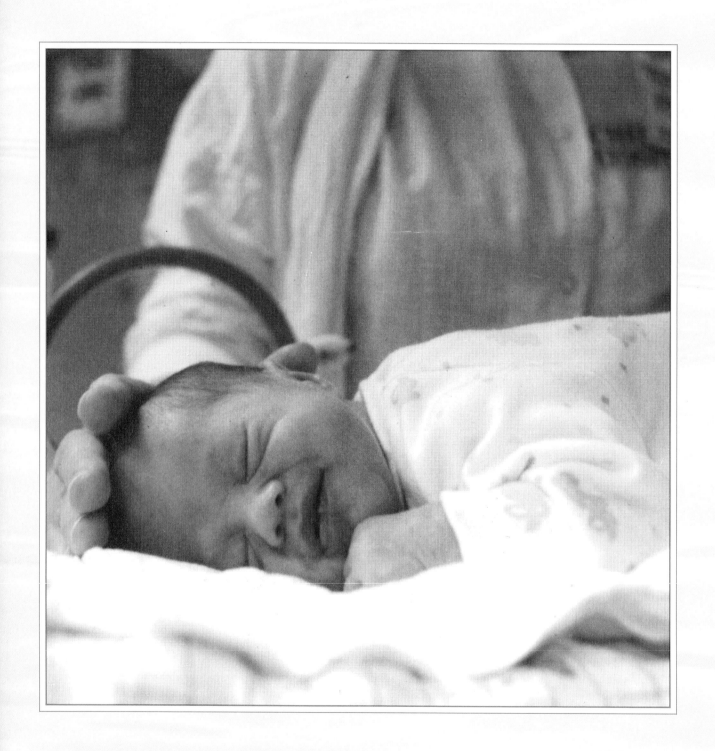

UNIT

VI

COMPLICATIONS OF CHILDBEARING

CHAPTER

22 Assessment for Risk Factors

Irene M. Bobak

Learning Objectives

Correctly define the key terms listed.

Explore the scope of high-risk pregnancy.

List risk factors identified through interview, physical examination, and diagnostic techniques.

Understand the various diagnostic modalities and implications of findings.

Explain diagnostic techniques to clients and their families.

Explain client teaching for antenatal monitoring.

Key Terms

acoustic stimulation
alpha-fetoprotein (aFP)
amniocentesis
amniotic fluid assessment
Apt test
biophysical profile
biparietal diameter (BPD)
chorionic villi sampling (CVS)
contraction stress test (CST)
Coombs' test
daily fetal movement count (DFMC)
fetal activity-acceleration determination (FAD)
fetal breathing movements (FBMs)
intrauterine growth retardation (IUGR)
lecithin/sphingomyelin (L/S) ratio
magnetic resonance imaging (MRI)
meconium-stained amniotic fluid
neonatal respiratory distress
nonstress test (NST)
percutaneous umbilical (cord) blood sampling (PUBS)
phosphatidylglycerol (PGL)
shake test
ultrasonography

Of the approximately 3 million births that occur in the United States each year, 500,000 will be categorized as high risk because of maternal or fetal complications. The united efforts of all members of the obstetric team and close collaboration with other medical personnel are required to adequately care for the high-risk client. In this chapter the high-risk client and the factors associated with diagnosis of high risk are identified. Techniques of biophysical monitoring of fetal health are emphasized.

❑ SCOPE OF THE PROBLEM

A high-risk pregnancy is one in which the life or health of the mother or offspring is jeopardized by a disorder coincidental with or unique to pregnancy. For the mother the high-risk status extends (arbitrarily) through the puerperium, that is, until 29 days after delivery. Postdelivery maternal complications are usually resolved within a month of birth, but perinatal morbidity may continue for months or years.

A better understanding of human reproduction has greatly reduced maternal morbidity and mortality. Knowledge of the fetus and neonatal disorders has increased dramatically in the last 10 to 15 years. This has led to a gratifying drop in perinatal morbidity and mortality during this period. Since 1969, when the perinatal death rate dropped below 30 per 1000 live births for the first time, the rate has steadily declined. In 1985, the death rate was estimated to be 14.7 per 1000 live births.

Maternal Health Problems

Different parts of the world have different leading causes of maternal death attributable to pregnancy. In general three major causes have persisted for the last 35 years: hypertensive disorders, infection, and hemorrhage.

Causes of Mortality	Percent
Hypertensive disorders	21
Infection	18
Hemorrhage	14
Other (cardiac, diabetes mellitus, trauma)	46

In the United States, maternal mortality for white women is still less than for all other women, although the gap that existed 30 years ago has been narrowed dramatically. Today the mortality ratio for white women and all others is 2:3. This decline is attributed to changes in social and economic factors and to availability of health care.

Fetal and Neonatal Health Problems

Fetal death (demise) is defined as the death in utero before complete expulsion of the product of human conception. It does not result from therapeutic or elective abortion. Fetal death is also called intrauterine death and results in stillbirth.

Neonatal death is the death of a liveborn neonate at 20 weeks' gestation or more. A liveborn neonate is one who shows any evidence of life after birth, even if only momentary (respiration, heartbeat, voluntary muscle movement, or pulsation within the umbilical cord), and who dies within 28 days.

Perinatal death rate is defined as the sum of fetal and neonatal death rates. This statistic is considered the most sensitive indicator of the effectiveness of perinatal care.

The incidence of ***infant mortality*** is expressed as the number of deaths per 100,000 live births. Infant mortality includes the neonatal death rate. As Table 22-1 demonstrates, the majority of the 10 leading causes of death during infancy continue to occur during the perinatal period; almost 75% of all infant deaths occur within the first 20 days of life. Although a number of perinatal problems have benefited from improved treatment, congenital anomalies continue to be the leading cause of infant mortality, accounting for about 22% of those deaths. The incidence of most birth defects has neither substantially decreased nor increased. Problems related to low birth weight and preterm birth are chiefly responsible for deaths during the first 4 weeks of life.

When infant mortality is categorized according to race, a disturbing difference is seen. The infant mortality for whites is considerably lower than for all other races in the United States, with blacks having almost twice the rate for whites. Although the birth rate of both groups has declined, the gap has remained fairly constant (Cunningham, MacDonald, Gant, 1989).

Table 22-1 Leading Causes of Death in Infants Under 1 Year of Age, United States, 1984 (Estimated Rates per 100,000 Live Births)

Rank	Causes of Death	Rate
1	Other conditions originating in the perinatal period	272.7
2	Congenital anomalies	228.1
3	All other causes	170.2
4	Sudden infant death syndrome	131.7
5	Respiratory distress syndrome	103.9
6	Disorders relating to short gestation and unspecified low birth weight	93.3
7	Intrauterine hypoxia and birth asphyxia	26.2
8	Pneumonia and influenza	17.0
9	Birth trauma	8.9
10	Certain gastrointestinal diseases	7.6

From National Center for Health Statistics: Annual summary of births, marriages, divorces, and deaths: United States, 1984. Monthly vital statistics report 33(13):8, DHHS Pub No (PHS) 85-1120, Sept 26, 1985.

❏ RISK FACTORS

Research and experience have led to the identification of factors that jeopardize the pregnant and postdelivery woman and the fetus/neonate. This knowledge has permitted the development of increasingly effective preventive and therapeutic measures that can minimize the incidence of morbidity, disability, and death of the mother or infant. Commonly it is the alert nurse, conversant and familiar with deviations from normal, who notes and reports potential or actual high-risk factors. The interrelationship of risk factors that influence pregnancy outcome are summarized schematically in Fig. 22-1.

Several factors place the pregnancy at high risk. A careful health assessment alerts the caregiver to preexisting or current factors. Poverty, inadequate nutrition, infection (e.g., toxoplasmosis, other, rubella, cytomeg-

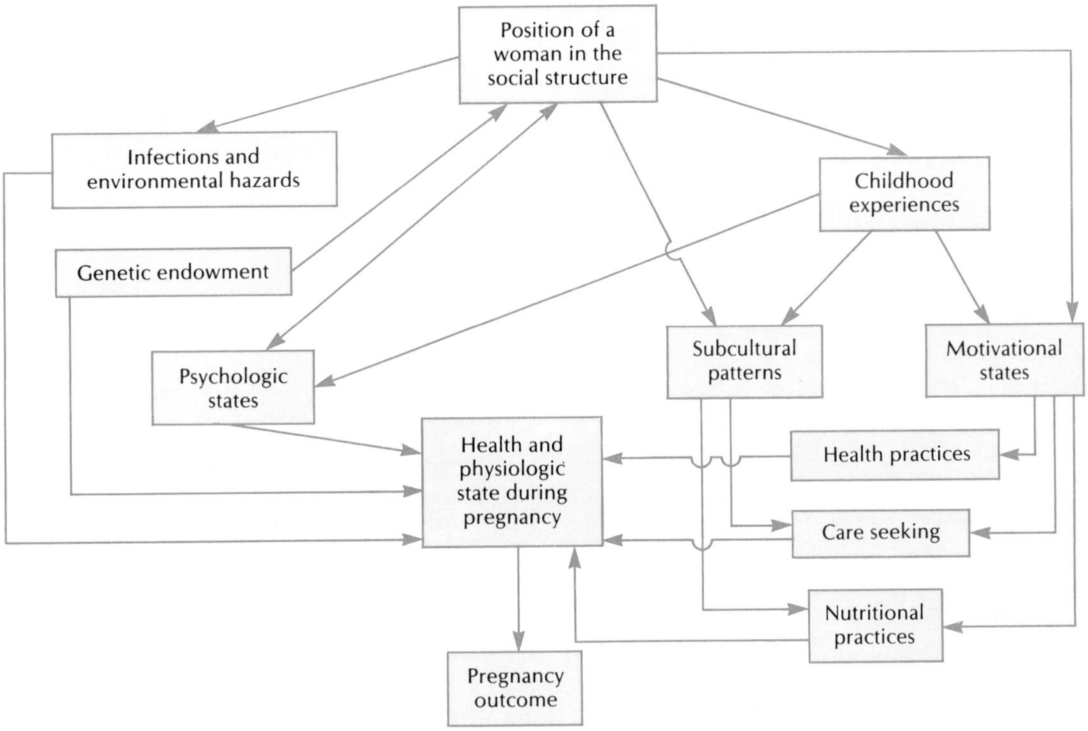

Fig. 22-1 Summary of risk factors that may affect pregnancy outcome. (From Fogel CI and Woods DF: Health care of women, St Louis, 1981, The CV Mosby Co.)

alovirus, herpes [TORCH], sexually transmitted diseases [STDs]), medical conditions, and use of substances such as tobacco, alcohol, and other drugs jeopardize the entire childbearing experience for the mother, fetus/neonate, and family.

Early in pregnancy abnormalities in the mother's reproductive or endocrine systems may lead to spontaneous abortion (miscarriage). Problems of implantation or genetic defect often result in spontaneous abortion. During the *second trimester,* maternal and fetal conditions may lead to late abortion or preterm labor. Uterine abnormalities or incompetent cervical os, cyanotic heart disease, Rh incompatibility, and hypertension are among maternal conditions that may complicate pregnancy and its outcome. Gross abnormality of the fetus and multifetal gestation are two fetal risk factors. Additional risk factors may occur during the *third trimester.* Fetal malformations or malpresentations, umbilical cord complications, placenta previa, abruptio placentae, preterm rupture of membranes, preterm labor, postterm labor, hydramnios, or oligohydramnios may jeopardize maternal and fetal/neonatal well-being. Risk factors during *labor* are discussed in Chapter 26. Several categories of high-risk pregnancy are presented in the box on p. 620.

Hemorrhage, infection, abnormal vital signs, traumatic labor or delivery, and some psychosocial events are specific factors that place the new mother at risk during the *early puerperium.*

Risks in the Workplace and Environment

Hazards to reproductive health in the environment and workplace affect everyone. The hazards exist whether the pregnant woman works in or outside the home. Pollution with chemicals, fumes, and noise and direct and indirect effects from equipment, furniture, buildings, and grounds have become major health concerns.

Substances that can be inhaled from the air are the most common concern. Also worrisome are materials that can be absorbed through the skin and those that can enter the body by mouth, such as lead dust that has settled on the fingers. Other potential threats arise from *physical forces:* eye stress from working at a video display terminal (VDT) all day, temperature, atmospheric pressure, oxygen content of the air, noise, vibration, acceleration, and ionizing radiation.

Whether or not a substance or condition produces detectable effects depends in part on exposure level, dose, or length of exposure. Some individuals are more susceptible than others. Genetic factors, general health,

CATEGORIES OF HIGH-RISK PREGNANCY

MATERNAL AGE AND PARITY FACTORS

1. Age 16 years or under
2. Nullipara 35 years or over
3. Multipara 40 years or over
4. Interval of 8 years or more since last pregnancy
5. High parity (5 or more)
6. Pregnancy occurring 3 months or less after last delivery

NONMARITAL PREGNANCY

PREGNANCY-INDUCED HYPERTENSION (PIH), HYPERTENSION, KIDNEY DISEASE

1. Preeclampsia with hospitalization before labor
2. Eclampsia
3. Kidney disease—pyelonephritis, nephritis, nephrosis, etc.
4. Chronic hypertension, severe (160/100 mm Hg or over)
5. Blood pressure 140/90 mm Hg or above on 2 readings 30 minutes apart

ANEMIA AND HEMORRHAGE

1. Hematocrit 30% or below in pregnancy
2. Hemorrhage (previous pregnancy)—severe, requiring transfusion
3. Hemorrhage (present pregnancy)
4. Anemia (hemoglobin below 10 g) for which treatment other than oral iron preparations is required (hemolytic, macrocytic, anemias, etc.)
5. Sickle cell trait or disease
6. History of bleeding or clotting disorder at any time

FETAL FACTORS

1. Two or more previous preterm deliveries (twins = one delivery)
2. Two or more consecutive spontaneous abortions (miscarriages)
3. One or more stillbirths at term gestation
4. One or more gross anomalies
5. Rh incompatibility or ABO immunization problems
6. History of previous birth defects—cerebral palsy, brain damage, mental retardation, metabolic disorders such as phenylketonuria (PKU)
7. History of large infants (over 4032 g [9 lb])

PATERNAL AGE (?) AND OTHER FACTORS (?)

DYSTOCIA (HISTORY OF OR ANTICIPATED)

1. Contracted pelvis or cephalopelvic disproportion (CPD)
2. Multifetal pregnancy in current pregnancy
3. Two or more breech deliveries
4. Previous operative deliveries (e.g., cesarean or midforceps delivery)
5. History of prolonged labor (more than 18 hours for nullipara; more than 12 hours for multipara)
6. Previously diagnosed genital tract anomalies (incompetent cervix, cervical or uterine malformation, solitary ovary or tube) or problem (ovarian mass, endometriosis)
7. Short stature (1.5 m [60 in] or less)

HISTORY OF OR CONCURRENT CONDITIONS

1. Diabetes mellitus; gestational diabetes
2. Hyperemesis gravidarum
3. Thyroid disease (hypothyroidism or hyperthyroidism)
4. Malnutrition or extreme obesity (20% over ideal weight for height; 15% under ideal weight for height)
5. Organic heart disease
6. Syphilis and TORCH infections: toxoplasmosis, rubella in first 10 weeks of *this* pregnancy, cytomegalovirus (CMV), and herpes simplex; acquired immunodeficiency syndrome (AIDS); chlamydia; human papilloma virus (HPV)
7. Tuberculosis or other serious pulmonary pathologic condition (e.g., emphysema, asthma)
8. Malignant or premalignant tumors (including hydatidiform mole)
9. Alcoholism, substance dependency
10. Psychiatric disease or epilepsy (documented)
11. Mental retardation

THOSE WITH PREVIOUS HISTORY OF

1. Late registration, or poor clinic attendance
2. Family violence including battery; rape, incest
3. Home situation making clinic attendance and hospitalization difficult
4. Mothers, including minors, without family resources (including desertions, adoptions, injuries, separations, family withdrawals, sole support)

Modified from Fogel CI and Woods NF: Health care of women: a nursing perspective, St Louis, 1981, The CV Mosby Co.

physical exertion, and life-style (including smoking and diet) can also affect susceptibility to chemicals and conditions in the environment.

Nonionizing radiation in microwave ovens and ultrasound have different characteristics and biologic effects than ionizing radiation (e.g., x-rays). Nonionizing radiation in microwaves and ultrasound diagnostic equipment does *not* have sufficient energy to ionize molecules and disrupt cellular deoxyribonucleic acid (DNA) (Jankowski, 1986). There is no evidence of mutagenic or carcinogenic effects from properly constructed microwave ovens or from diagnostic ultrasound (Brent, 1980; NIOSH, 1981; ACOG, 1984; Bond, 1986). Magnetic resonance imagery (MRI) and VDTs* also do *not* represent reproductive health hazards (Budinger, 1981; Thomas and Morris, 1981; Hirning and Aitken, 1982; Bond, 1986; Droegemueller et al, 1987).

The chemicals to worry about are those that come

*Controversy continues regarding the safety of VDTs.

from industrial waste, landfill seepage, agricultural herbicides and pesticides, gasoline and oil, and common household solvents and cleaners (Ferguson, 1986; Shavelson, 1987). Methylene chloride is a liquid paint and grease remover. It is a common component of aerosol propellents in such products as hair spray, pesticides, paints, and lubricants. It is used in the electronic industry to clean printed circuit boards and is the solvent of choice for decaffeinating coffee. Absorbed in the body, it generates carbon monoxide, which interferes with the body's ability to pick up and deliver oxygen. Inhalation of low levels for short periods (minutes to hours) may cause dizziness, nausea, headache, and confusion. At high levels, it may cause unconsciousness and death (Hazards, 1986).

Drinking water may contain arsenic, benzene, cadmium, carbon tetrachloride, dioxin, lead, and vinyl chloride among others. Certain geographic areas contain greater concentrations of these pollutants than others. Under-the-sink filtering systems filter out some of the substances (How, 1987).

Women are exposed to potentially hazardous substances in their homes and workplaces. Homemakers and domestic workers are exposed to alkalis, bleaches, detergents, and solvents that emit fumes. Fresh paint increases levels of hydrocarbons in the environment especially if ventilation is poor. Sealers used to prevent plumbing leaks at joints often contain arsenic to retard growth of mold. This arsenic and other chemicals may be leached from plumbing systems and coat dishes and silverware.

Noise is everywhere. Sound is a form of energy with the potential to damage tissues (Noise, 1986). Women report fetal startle responses to loud noises such as telephone rings and some forms of music. Some women experience excessive and extremely uncomfortable fetal movements in response to hard rock music. Newborns in intensive care nurseries show better weight gain when the noise level is controlled. Long-term damage has not been identified.

Hospital staff are exposed to gases, x-rays, antineoplastic medications, needle accidents, and weight-related and other accidents (Munley et al, 1986; Moses, 1987). Vehicle drivers breathe carbon monoxide and other combustion products of gasoline, as well as polynuclear aromatics. They are also subjected to physical stress, vibration, and accidents. Electronics assemblers are exposed to trichloroethylene, lead, tin, methylene chloride, antimony, epoxy resins, and methyl ethyl ketones. Hairdressers work with acetone, aerosol propellents (e.g., freon), benzyl alcohol, ethyl alcohol, and hair dyes. Cigarette smoke is encountered commonly. Animal handlers, including meat cutters, inspectors, and teachers, are exposed to infections and flea and tick preparations.

Lead is a potential hazard to potters, artists, ceramists, and glass workers. Lead poisoning is still a threat (Lead, 1988). Lead poisoning is responsible for menstrual abnormalities, spontaneous abortion, decreased fertility in females and males, stillbirths, infants of low birth weight (LBW), and poor neurobehavioral development in children (Bellinger et al, 1987).

Nursing Management

Findings from the woman's present health status, including an extensive reproductive health history, are accumulated. Nonoccupational exposure to drugs (smoking, alcohol, "recreational" chemicals) and infection, geographic location and proximity to toxic disposal sites and industries, and spouse's occupation are noted. The woman's and her partner's current and past occupational histories are vital to detection of hazards to the reproductive system. The time, length of exposure, work conditions, and symptomatology related to work are identified.

A toxicology screen is ordered if it is indicated. The presence and level of toxins, and the number and condition of blood components may need to be assessed. If exposure of either parent to a mutagen is suspected, a karyotype may be ordered. Investigation of the cause of a defect includes a search for possible environmental agents. A retrospective approach often yields data that are difficult to validate so that an association may be suspected but not conclusive.

Prevention should be the focus of care. Cleanliness, ventilation, adherence to manufacturer's directions for use and disposal of materials, use of protective gear to shield against known and unknown hazards, and avoidance of exposure are examples of strategies to reduce risk.

In some instances safer materials can be substituted for potentially hazardous ones. Most household cleaning needs can be met with baking soda, table salt, distilled white vinegar, lemon juice, trisodium phosphate (TSP) (which does not emit fumes), a plunger, and some common sense. These substances clean drains, wash windows, degrease, prevent mold and mildew, disinfect, and scour (Dadd, 1987).

❑ DIAGNOSTIC MODALITIES

A variety of diagnostic modalities are available today to monitor the well-being of the fetus and the mother. These tests can alert the health care team to actual or potential problems. Many of these problems can be effectively treated if identified in the early stage. Others will require skillful and supportive care to minimize morbidity and mortality and to help the woman and family cope with the problem.

Each diagnostic procedure involves some degree of risk. In addition, the cost of the procedures varies, with some tests being quite costly. These factors must be weighed and discussed with the woman and family to determine whether the advantages of the test outweigh the potential risks and additional expense. Since these tests have limitations in terms of diagnostic accuracy and applicability, no one test should be used as the basis for determining health status or planning care.

Ultrasonography

When directional beams of sound strike an object, an echo is returned. The time delay between the emission of the sound and the return of the echo is noted as well as the direction from which the echo comes. From these data the object's distance and location can be calculated. Sonar (underwater) and radar (air) are familiar uses of very high frequency sound. First introduced in the 1960s, diagnostic ultrasound (ultrasonography) has developed rapidly to enjoy a principal position in medical imaging today.

Ultrasound is sound having a frequency higher than that of normal human hearing. The range of human hearing extends from 20 Hz to 20 kHz (20,000 Hz). Bats and some insects use ultrasound in the range of about 100 kHz to navigate. Diagnostic ultrasound is beyond audible range but well below that used by sonar and radar. Medical diagnostic ultrasound covers the range from approximately 1 to 10 MHz; 2.25 MHz (2,250,000 Hz) is generally used in obstetric and gynecologic imaging.

Table 22-2 presents a summary of modalities, imaging, and principal uses of diagnostic ultrasound. Static image scanners are useful for gynecologic, as well as obstetric, diagnosis. Dynamic image scanners provide direct visualization of indicators of fetal viability—fetal cardiac and body movement. The usual examination takes only about 5 minutes. Since the scanner can be moved about, it can be taken directly into labor and delivery rooms for directing amniocentesis or evaluating the source of vaginal bleeding.

Applications in Pregnancy. When carefully performed and accurately interpreted, ultrasonography can supply vital information. During the ***first trimester,*** ultrasound examination is performed to obtain the following information: (1) number, size, and location of gestational sacs (Fig. 22-2), (2) presence or absence of fetal cardiac and body movement, (3) presence or absence of uterine abnormalities (e.g., bicornuate uterus, fibroids) or adnexal masses (e.g., ovarian cysts, ectopic pregnancy), (4) pregnancy dating (e.g., **biparietal diameter [BPD]**, crown-rump length), and (5) coexistence and location of an intrauterine device (IUD).

During the ***second*** and ***third trimesters*** the following information is sought: (1) fetal viability, number, position, gestational age, growth pattern, and anomalies such as conjoined (Siamese) twins, (2) amniotic fluid volume, (3) placental location, maturity, or anomolous development, (4) uterine fibroids and anomalies, and (5) adnexal masses. An example of the application of the findings is presented in Table 22-3. Ultrasound is routinely used in conjunction with amniocentesis. In general, the use of ultrasound has hastened diagnoses

Table 22-2 Diagnostic Ultrasound: Operational Modes

Modality	Product	Principal Use
Pulsed wave*	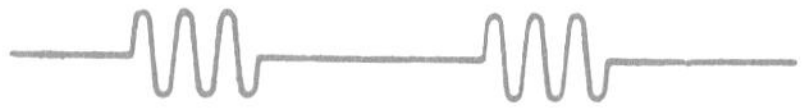	
A mode	Static image	Diagnostic evaluation of brain
B mode (gray scale)†	Static image	Images of abdominal and pelvic structures
M mode	Dynamic imaging	Monitoring of heart and measuring of heart wall displacement
Real time†	Static image and dynamic imaging	Provides dynamic imaging and static images
Continuous wave	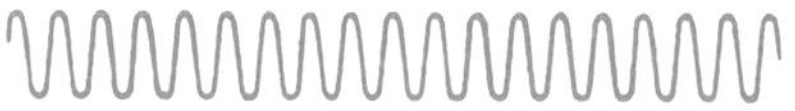	
Doppler mode†	Ranging mode	Fetal heart monitoring

*Pulsed wave—sound emitted at intervals; continuous wave—sound emitted continuously; A mode—one-dimensional image that appears as spikes on a horizontal base; distance between spikes can be measured (e.g., BPD); B mode (gray scale)—rough, two-dimensional image of various tissue densities for visualizing tissue texture and contour; M mode—time-related tracings showing straight lines for motionless structures and wiggly lines for structural motion (e.g., atrial septal defects and patent ductus arteriosus); static—stationary; dynamic—moving; Doppler mode—detection of change in frequency (wavelength) of structures in motion (e.g., blood flow in umbilical cord and placenta, closure of fetal cardiac valves); real time—dynamic imaging (limb and respiratory movements), as well as static images (BPD, placental location).

†Used extensively in obstetrics and gynecology.

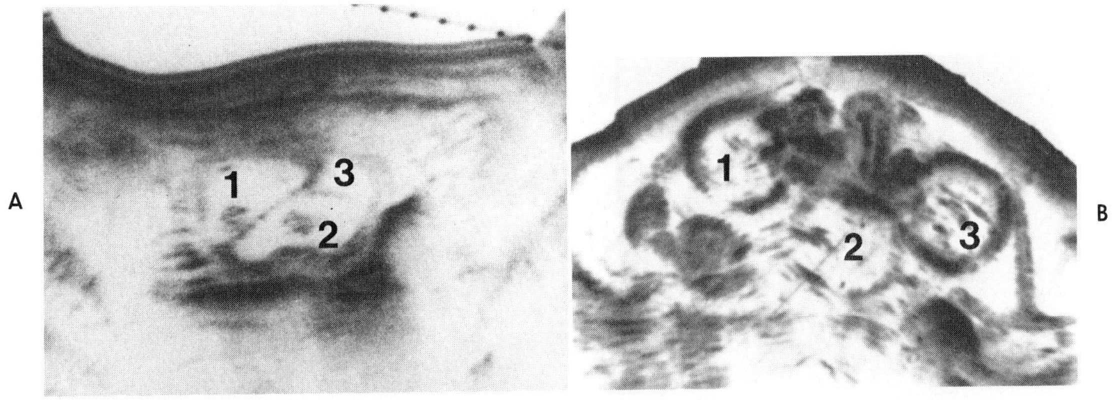

Fig. 22-2 **A,** Transverse static image scan demonstrates three well-formed gestational sacs. **B,** Subsequent static image scan demonstrates three well-defined fetal heads in this woman carrying triplets. (From Athey PA and Hadlock FP: Ultrasound in obstetrics and gynecology, ed 2, St Louis, 1985, The CV Mosby Co.)

Table 22-3 Application of Ultrasonography During Pregnancy

Condition	Ultrasonographic Evidence	Intervention
Impending abortion (before eighth menstrual week)	Poorly formed or "sagging" gestational sac	Eliminate time trying to save pregnancy; possibly decrease blood loss and sequelae of blood loss or of treatment for blood loss
Fetal death (after eighth menstrual week)	No cardiac activity	Empty uterus before development of *retained dead fetus syndrome*
Ectopic pregnancy	Adnexal mass	Early surgical intervention to prevent emergency situation
Molar pregnancy (hydatidiform mole)	"Snow storm" appearance within enlarged uterus (Fig. 22-3)	Terminate pregnancy to decrease morbidity from preeclampsia and begin surveillance of hCG* levels
Developmental uterine abnormalities	Resembles coexistent solid neoplasm; variable appearance	Avoid misdiagnosis with inappropriate therapy; provide time to consider type of delivery
IUD	Locate site	
	Imbedded in myometrial wall apart from gestational sac and placenta	Pregnancy usually goes to term with no IUD-related problem
	Located partially or totally within gestational sac or within placenta	Pregnancy usually ends in spontaneous abortion and may be associated with generalized sepsis

*Human chorionic gonadotropin.

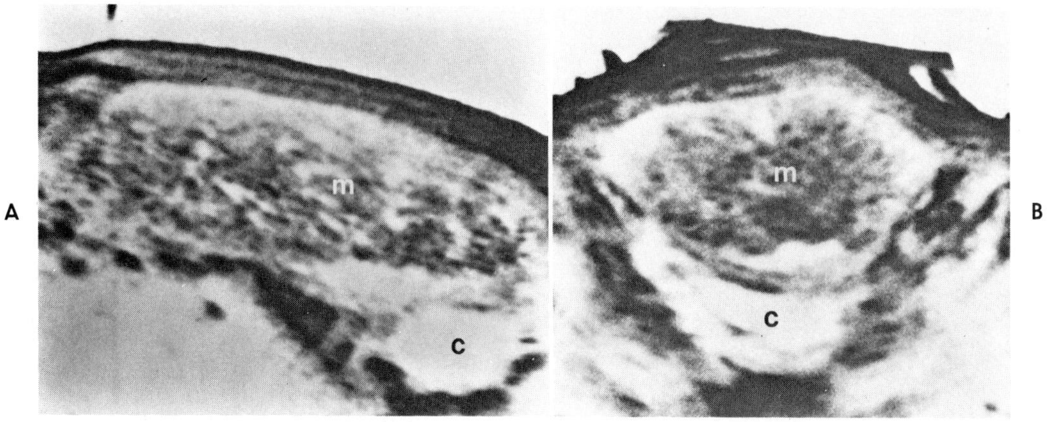

Fig. 22-3 **A,** Longitudinal and **B,** transverse scans of molar pregnancy *(m)*. Note typical vesicular (grapelike) pattern. Also demonstrated are multiloculated lutein ovarian cysts *(c)* in cul-de-sac. (From Athey PA and Hadlock FP: Ultrasound in obstetrics and gynecology, ed 2, St Louis, 1985, The CV Mosby Co.)

so that appropriate therapy can be instituted early in the pregnancy. Early therapy may decrease the severity and duration of morbidity, both physical and emotional, of the mother (family). Early diagnosis of fetal anomaly, for instance, makes possible choices such as intrauterine surgery or other therapy for the fetus, discontinuation of the pregnancy, and preparation of the family for the care of a child with a disorder or planning for placement of child after birth.

Findings

Fetal Viability. Fetal heart activity can be demonstrated as early as 6 to 7 weeks by real-time echo scanners and at 10 to 12 weeks by Doppler mode. This information assists in management when the woman experiences vaginal bleeding; incomplete, complete, and missed abortion can be differentiated. By 9 to 10 weeks, molar pregnancy (hydatidiform mole) can be diagnosed (Fig. 22-3).

Gestational Age. Not all women are candidates for the use of ultrasound to determine gestational age. Several indicators have been established for need. Indications for ultrasonographic estimation of fetal age include uncertain dates for the last menstrual period (LMP) or last normal menstrual period (LNMP), recent discontinuation of oral hormonal suppression of ovulation (birth control pills), bleeding episode during the first trimester, amenorrhea of at least 3 months' duration, uterine size that does not agree with dates, previous cesarean birth, and other high-risk conditions. Four methods of estimation of fetal age are used: (1) determination of gestational sac dimensions (about 8 weeks), (2) measurement of crown-rump length (between 7 and 14 weeks), (3) measurement of femur length (after 12 weeks), and (4) measurement of the BPD starting at about 12 weeks.

Fetal BPD at 36 weeks should be approximately 8.7 cm. Term pregnancy and fetal maturity can be diagnosed with some confidence if the biparietal cephalometry by ultrasonography is greater than 9.8 cm (Fig. 22-4). An estimate of fetal weight is based on BPD. With a BPD of 9.8 cm, fetal weight is estimated at over 3180 g (7 lb).

Fetal Growth and Anatomy. Fetal growth may be jeopardized under certain conditions. Some of the conditions that serve as indicators for ultrasound assessment of fetal growth include the following: poor maternal weight gain or pattern of weight gain; previous **intrauterine growth retardation (IUGR)**; chronic infections (especially urinary tract infections); ingestion of drugs such as anticonvulsants or heroin; diabetes mellitus; pregnancy-induced or other hypertension; multifetal pregnancy; and other medical or surgical complications. Serial evaluations of BPD and limb length can differentiate between wrong dates and true IUGR. IUGR may be symmetric (the fetus is small in all parameters) or asymmetric (head and body growth vary). Symmetric IUGR may be caused by low genetic growth potential, intrauterine infection, maternal undernutrition or heavy smoking, or chromosomal aberration. Asymmetric IUGR may reflect placental insufficiency secondary to hypertension, renal disease, or cardiovascular disease. Therapy varies with the probable cause.

The BPD, head circumference, abdominal circumference, and estimated fetal weight for a normal 32-week fetus are illustrated in Fig. 22-5.

Depending on the gestational age, the following structures may be identified: head (including ventricles

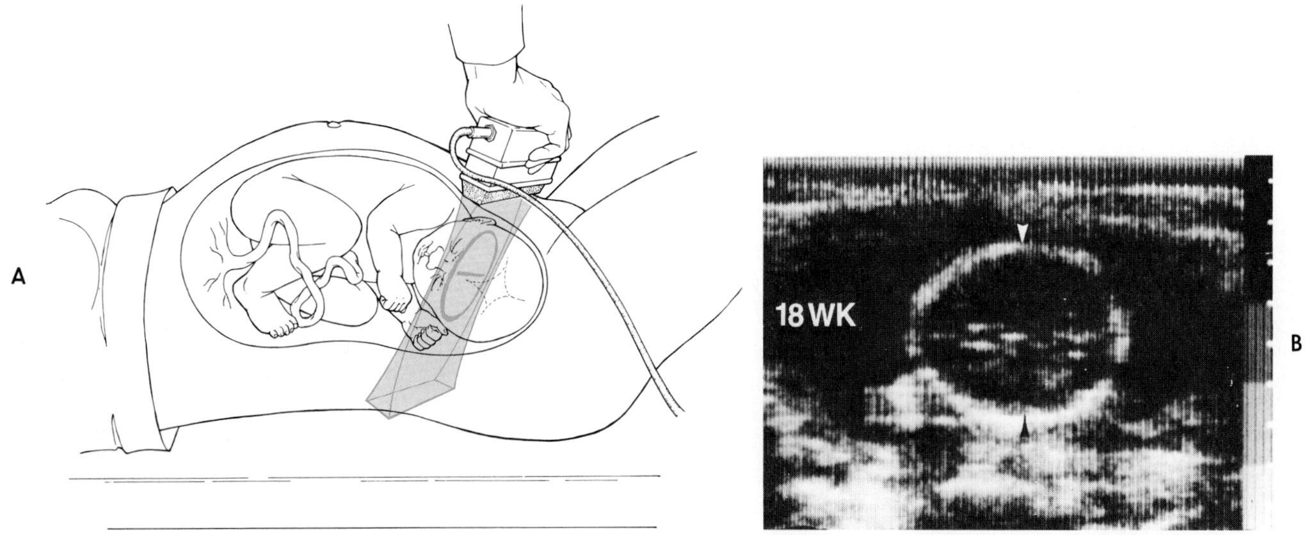

Fig. 22-4 **A,** Biparietal *(arrow)* cephalometry by ultrasound. **B,** Linear-array, real-time image demonstrates fetal BPD *(arrow)* at 18 weeks. (**B,** From Athey PA and Hadlock FP: Ultrasound in obstetrics and gynecology, ed 2, St Louis, 1985, The CV Mosby Co.)

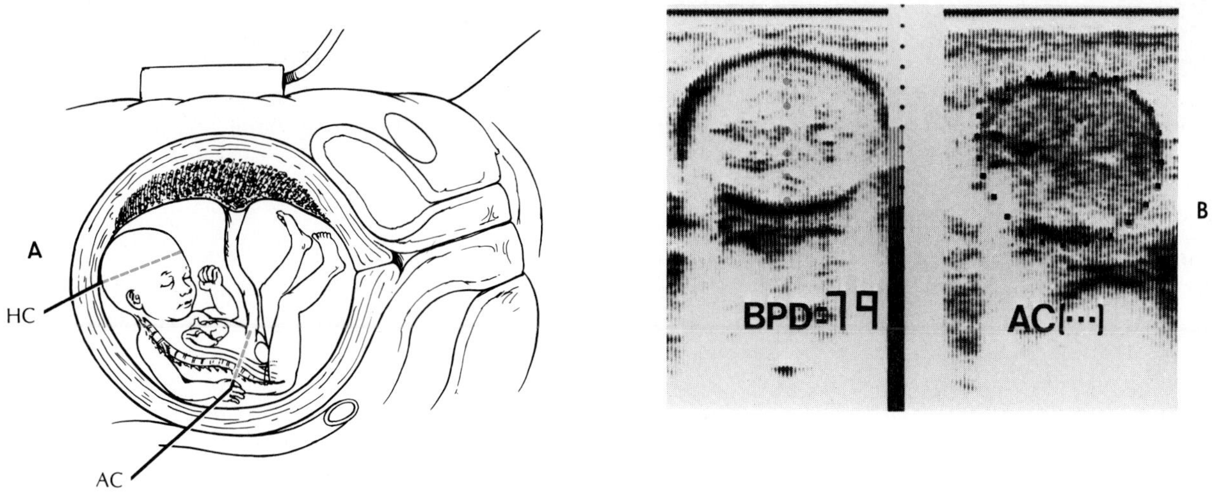

Fig. 22-5 **A,** Schematic presentation of appropriate planes of sections *(dotted lines)* for head circumference *(HC),* and abdominal circumference *(AC).* **B,** Real-time ultrasound image demonstrates typical head and body images that correspond to planes in **A.** Using these two images, one can determine BPD (7.9 cm), HC (30 cm), AC (28 cm), and estimated fetal weight *(EFW)* (1840 g) in this normal 32-week fetus. (From Athey PA and Hadlock FP: Ultrasound in obstetrics and gynecology, ed 2, St Louis, 1985, The CV Mosby Co.)

and blood vessels), neck, spine, heart, stomach, small bowel, liver, kidneys, bladder and limbs. Structural defects may be identified before delivery. Advances in technology may make fetal surgery and genetic engineering a reality for many conditions in the next few years.

Placental Position and Function. The pattern of uterine and placental growth and the fullness of the bladder influence the apparent location of the placenta. During the first trimester, differentiation of the endometrium and the small placenta is difficult and adds to the difficulty of performing an amniocentesis. During the middle of the second trimester the placenta can be clearly defined, but if it is seen to be low lying, its relationship to the internal cervical os can sometimes be altered dramatically by changing the *degree of fullness of the maternal bladder.* In approximately 15% to 20% of all pregnancies in which ultrasound scanning is done in the second trimester, the placenta seems to be overlying the os; at term the incidence of placenta previa is only 0.5%. Three factors may be responsible for the seeming "migration" of the placenta: (1) the maternal bladder can distort the uterine cavity, (2) the lower uterine segment elongates as pregnancy progresses, and (3) poor imaging or misinterpretation of the image can result in an inappropriate diagnosis. The diagnosis of *placenta previa* can seldom be confirmed until the third trimester.

Fetal Well-being. Among the many physiologic measurements that can be accomplished with ultrasound are the following: heart motion, beat-to-beat variability, **fetal breathing movements (FBMs),** fetal urine production (following serial measurements of bladder volume), fetal limb and head movements, and analysis of vascular waveforms from the fetal circulation (McCallum, 1984). It has been noted that FBMs are decreased with maternal smoking and alcohol ingestion and increased with hyperglycemia. Fetal limb and head movements serve as an index of neurologic development.

Biophysical Profile. Manning et al (1985) developed a tool for fetal assessment based on fetal biophysical profile scoring (p. 635). Ultrasound is used to assess fetal breathing movements, gross body movements, fetal tone, reactive fetal heart rate, and qualitative amniotic fluid volume. Numerical scores are assigned to each parameter. High scores indicate fetal well-being, whereas low scores indicate the need for further evaluation.

Preparation of the Woman. The woman is directed to come for the examination with a full bladder. The full bladder supports the uterus in position for the imaging. If her bladder is empty, the test may be delayed for about 1 hour until she is able to fill her bladder; it takes only a few moments to empty the bladder if this is needed for the examination. If transvaginal ultrasound is used, the urinary bladder need not be full (Modica and Timor-Tritsch, 1988). The woman is positioned comfortably with small pillows under her head and knees. The display panel should be positioned so that the woman can observe the images on the screen if she wishes (Fig 22-6). Some women do *not* want to watch.

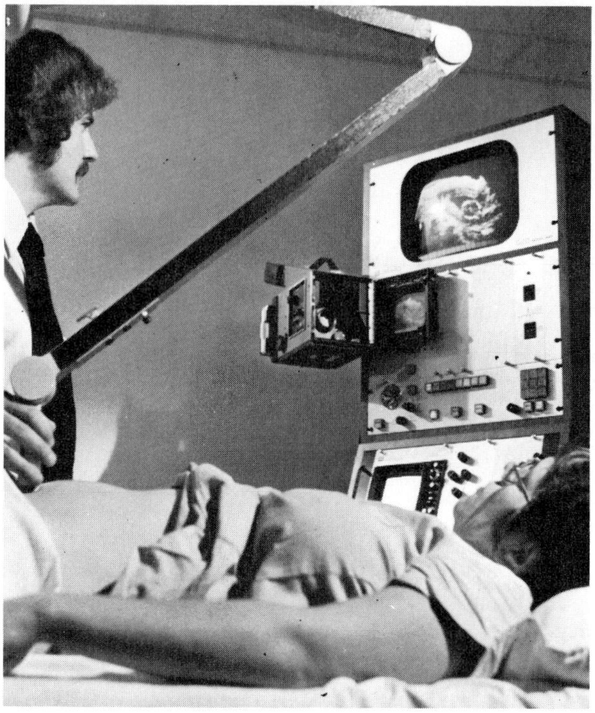

Fig. 22-6 Ultrasonography. (Courtesy March of Dimes.)

There is no conclusive evidence that humans have been harmed by diagnostic ultrasound during the 25 years it has been used (Athey and Hadlock, 1985; Cunningham, MacDonald, Gant, 1989). No detrimental effects have been observed to date on the fetus or mother either histologically, functionally, or embryologically in experimental work; however, there is a hypothetical risk that cannot be ignored or overlooked. Benefit must be weighed against hypothetical risk. Gravidas should be informed of the clinical indication for ultrasound, specific benefit, potential risk, and alternatives, if any.

Magnetic Resonance Imaging

Magnetic resonance imaging (MRI) is a noninvasive tool that can be used for obstetric diagnosis. In a relatively brief time, MRI has progressed from a primitive imaging modality to one whose image quality and diagnostic abilities rival or surpass all other imaging procedures (Kanal and Wolf, 1986). Like computerized tomography (CT), MRI provides excellent pictures of soft tissue; unlike CT, ionizing radiation is not used. After MRI signals are generated and analyzed, they are displayed on an oscilloscope screen.

In utero imaging during first-, second-, and third-trimester pregnancies in Europe has produced excellent visualization of fetal anatomy. Direct scanning of the placenta with or without paramagnetic contrast agents may further increase the capacity to evaluate placental positioning or fetal maturity. In North America, most MRI has been confined to second- or third-trimester pregnancies because of unproved concerns about the effects of this modality on fetal development. Fetal growth and fetal subcutaneous fat thickness can be directly measured, and studies are being performed to assess a possible role for MRI in such disorders as IUGR (Kanal and Wolf, 1986).

Fetal Blood Sampling

Fetal scalp blood sampling is dependent on ruptured membranes and cervical dilatation. Therefore it is used only for intrapartum fetal surveillance. During pregnancy *percutaneous umbilical [cord] blood sampling-(PUBS)* provides a simple, relatively safe method of obtaining fetal blood for prenatal diagnosis and therapy. In PUBS, the placenta and cord insertion site are localized with a high-resolution sector ultrasound scanner after 18 weeks' gestation. Mother (and fetus) is anesthetized with intravenous (IV) sedation. A local anesthetic is used at the insertion site. A long (9 cm [3½ in]) spinal needle is used to obtain 1 to 2 ml of heparinized fetal blood for analysis. Indications include the need for chromosomal analysis and identification of hemoglobinopathies, coagulopathies, and intrauterine infections. Current complications include fetal loss, prematurity, and infection; no statistics are available. While genetic indications are expanding most rapidly, the diagnosis and treatment of fetal hypoxia and isoimmunization also are being implemented (Goldberg, 1987; Cunningham, MacDonald, and Gant, 1989).

Chorionic Villi Sampling

Chorionic villi sampling (CVS) could partially replace amniocentesis for genetic diagnosis. Although there are risks to the fetus, the greatest advantage in this new technique (Fig. 22-7) is that genetic diagnosis can be moved ahead from the second to the first trimester—as early as the eighth week—and can produce results rapidly. This increases the potential for improving fetal treatment by allowing earlier intervention (Golbus, 1987). Earlier diagnosis also reduces a couple's waiting period, imposes less social and psychologic stress, permits the couple "privacy" because the

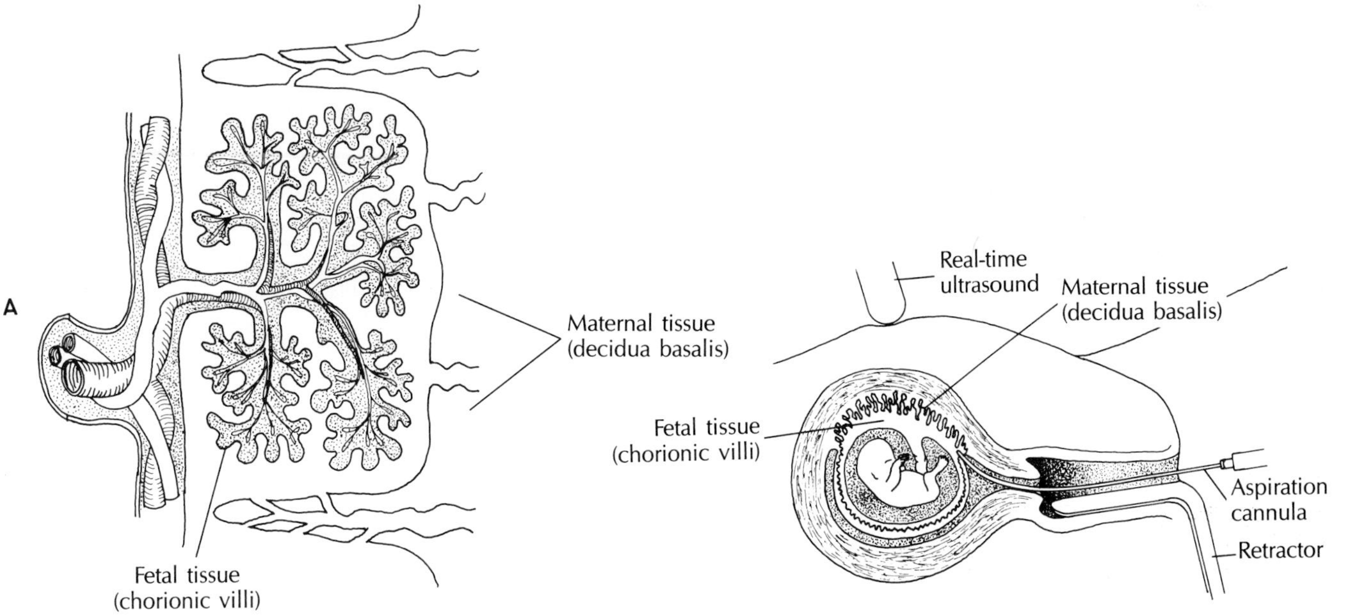

Fig. 22-7 Chorionic villi sampling. **A,** Chorionic villi at time of sampling (between 8 and 14 weeks). **B,** Taking sample by transcervical method.

pregnancy is not obvious as yet, and allows for an earlier and safer abortion if the couple so chooses.

This procedure is done between weeks 8 and 14 (see Fig. 22-7) and involves the removal of a small tissue specimen from the fetal portion of the placenta. Since chorionic villi originate in the zygote, that tissue reflects the genetic makeup of the fetus. The specimen is removed either from the chorion frondosum or the chorion laeve.

Real-time ultrasound is used to guide the procedure. The aspiration cannula and obturator must negotiate the cervical canal, must be placed at a suitable site, and must avoid rupturing the amniotic sac.

Two other techniques used in CVS are direct vision biopsy using a hysteroscope and transabdominal aspiration guided by ultrasound. The magnitude of the procedure-related risk in CVS is around 2% (Jackson, 1988), but the types of complications (e.g., spontaneous abortion, infection, hematoma, intrauterine death, growth retardation, Rh isoimmunization, and trauma) are predictable. At present, if the risk of a fetal genetic disorder (e.g., hemoglobinopathies) is 25% or more, CVS is one possible diagnostic alternative.

Maternal Blood Assessments. Human chorionic gonadotropin (hCG) is normally produced by the trophoblast of pregnancy. It is of clinical value for diagnosing early pregnancy. hCG is measured to identify persistent trophoblastic neoplasia (gestational trophoblastic disease [GTD]).

Coombs' test for Rh incompatibility is discussed at length in Chapter 28. If Coombs' titer is greater than 1:8 to 1:16, amniocentesis for delta optical density (ΔOD) is indicated to determine need for intrauterine transfusion (Table 22-4).

Amniocentesis

An **amniocentesis** is performed when there is an indication of problems with the pregnancy or fetus. The test is commonly used to diagnose genetic problems, to estimate fetal maturity, and to diagnose fetal hemolytic disease (e.g., Rh incompatibility). Amniocentesis is possible after the fourteenth week, when the uterus becomes an abdominal organ and when there is sufficient amniotic fluid for this procedure (Fig. 22-8).

The mother and family are informed of the need for the surgical procedure and appraised of the risks. An informed consent statement and a surgical permit are signed by the woman (Chapter 3). Ultrasonography is performed to determine the exact location of the fetus, placenta, and pockets of amniotic fluid. Using ultrasonography for this purpose has greatly reduced risks previously associated with amniocentesis. If the pregnancy is less than 20 weeks, a full bladder helps brace

Table 22-4 **Summary of Biochemical Monitoring Techniques**

Test	Possible Findings	Clinical Significance
MATERNAL BLOOD		
Coombs' test	Titer of 1:8 and rising	Significant Rh incompatibility
Alpha-fetoprotein	See below	
AMNIOTIC FLUID ANALYSIS		
Color	Meconium	Possible hypoxia or asphyxia
Lung profile		Fetal lung maturity
Lecithin/sphingomyelin (L/S) ratio	>2	
Phosphatidylglycerol (PGL)	Present	
Creatinine	>2 mg/dl	Gestational age >36 weeks
Billirubin (ΔOD 450/nm)	<0.015	Gestational age >36 weeks, normal pregnancy
	High levels	Fetal hemolytic disease in Rh isoimmunized pregnancies
Lipid cells	>10%	Gestational age >35 weeks
Alpha-fetoprotein	High levels after 15-week gestation	Open neural tube or other defect
Osmolality	Decline after 20-week gestation	Advancing nonspecific gestational age
Genetic disorders	Dependent on cultured cells for karyotype and enzymatic activity	Counseling may be required
Sex-linked		
Chromosomal		
Metabolic		

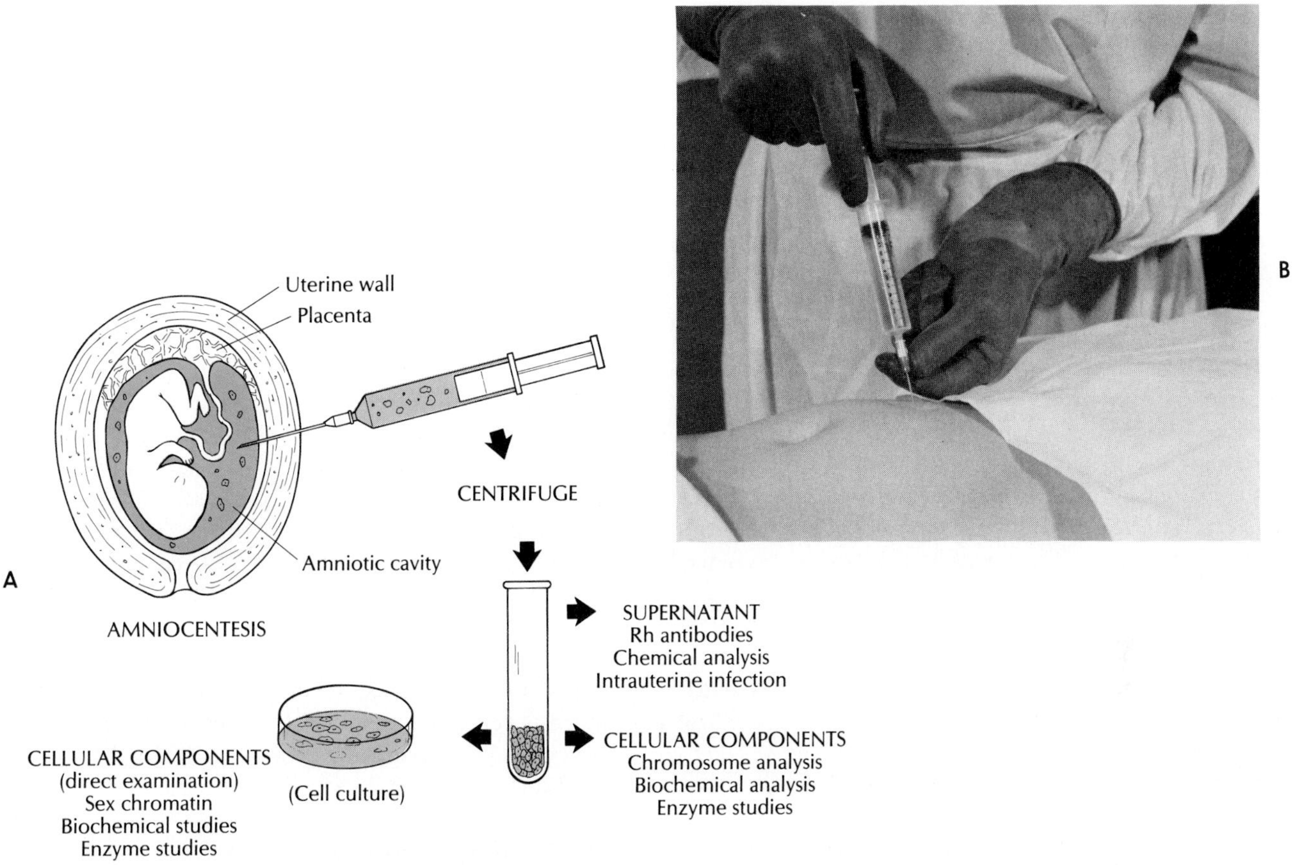

Fig. 22-8 **A,** Amniocentesis and laboratory utilization of amniotic fluid aspirant. **B,** Transabdominal amniocentesis. (**A,** From Whaley LF: Understanding inherited disorders, St Louis, 1974, The CV Mosby Co. **B,** Courtesy March of Dimes.)

the uterus (see bladder preparation under ultrasonography, p. 626).

Complications. Overall complications are less than 1% for both mother and fetus.

Maternal complications include hemorrhage, fetomaternal hemorrhage with possible maternal Rh isoimmunization, infection, labor, abruptio placentae, inadvertent damage to the intestines or bladder, and amniotic fluid embolism.

Fetal complications include death, hemorrhage, infection (amnionitis), direct injury from the needle, abortion or preterm labor, and leakage of amniotic fluid.

Identifying Genetic Problems. Cells are cultured for *karyotyping* of chromosomes (see Fig. 7-1). Chromosomal aberrations appear in fetuses of 1% to 2% of women between 35 and 38 years of age, 2% of women between 39 and 40 years of age, and 10% of women over 45 years of age. Down's syndrome (trisomy 21) is a noted example.

Fetal cells are assessed for *sex chromatin*. Sex determination is important if a sex-linked disorder (especially in the male fetus) is suspected. *Biochemical analysis* of enzymes produced from a cell culture is done to detect inborn errors of metabolism (over 60 types can be detected). Examples of inborn errors of metabolism that can be diagnosed prenatally include the following: galactosemia (deficient ceramidase activity in cultured cells), maple syrup urine disease (deficient branched chain keto acid decarboxylase in cultured cells), and Tay-Sachs disease (deficient β-N-acetyl-hexosaminidase A and B activity in cultured cells). Biochemical analysis can also identify cystic fibrosis and Duchenne's muscular dystrophy. *DNA analysis* of fetal cells from **amniotic fluid assessment** and fetal blood sampling identifies sickle cell anemia and thalassemia.

Alpha-fetoprotein (AFP). The normal source of **alpha-fetoprotein (AFP)** in amniotic fluid is fetal urine. Some of the protein crosses fetal membranes into maternal circulation. Correct interpretation of concentration of AFP requires precise knowledge of gestational age. AFP levels may be elevated in the presence of a variety of conditions in which fetal integument is not intact and the protein leaks from the capillaries into the amniotic fluid. Elevated levels are associated with neural tube defects, such as spina bifida and anencephaly (Table 22-4). The recurrence risk of neural tube defects after one affected fetus is 2%; after two affected fetuses, 6% to 8% (Anderson, 1987). AFP may also be elevated with severe fetal hemolytic disease, esophageal atresia, congenital nephrosis, omphalocele, fetal hemorrhage into amniotic fluid, oligohydramnios, low birth weight, and fetal death. Levels may also be elevated in a normal multifetal pregnancy. Low levels may be associated with chromosomal trisomies (e.g., Down's syndrome), gestational trophoblastic disease, fetal death, increased maternal weight, and overestimation of gestational age (Cunningham, MacDonald, Gant, 1989). ***It must be remembered that this screening test is not perfect. There will be false positives as well as false negatives.***

Fetal Maturity. Greater accuracy in estimating fetal maturity is now possible through use of amniotic fluid or its exfoliated cellular content. Term pregnancy and fetal maturity can be demonstrated by the following laboratory studies.

A **lecithin/sphingomyelin (L/S) ratio** greater than 2 indicates adequate lung maturity for extrauterine life (Chapter 7 and Table 22-4). This is generally achieved by 36 weeks' gestational age. A practical means of determining the L/S ratio is the rapid surfactant test, also known as the **shake test** or foam stabilization test. Equal parts of fresh amniotic fluid and normal saline solution are added to two parts 95% ethyl alcohol. The mixture is shaken vigorously for 30 seconds. If bubbles are still present at the meniscus 15 minutes after shaking, the fetal lung is judged to be mature. See Chapters 7 and 28 for discussions of other phospholipids and lung maturity.

An L/S ratio of 2 does not necessarily mean that the neonate will not develop respiratory distress syndrome (RDS). This is especially true with certain pregnancy complications. The conditions in which an L/S ratio of 2 is not reassuring include the following: maternal diabetes mellitus (Quirk and Bleasdale, 1986), erythroblastosis fetalis, and fetal/neonatal sepsis (Cunningham, MacDonald, and Gant, 1989).

Phosphatidylglycerol (PGL) enhances the surface-active properties of lecithin. An L/S ratio of 2 is insufficient to prevent RDS if PGL is lacking. In the absence of PGL, the **neonatal respiratory distress** syndrome may develop. Amniostat-FLM is a 15-minute immunologic agglutination test to identify PGL in amniotic fluid. If PGL is present, it is *improbable* that the neonate will develop RDS (Saad et al, 1988).

A ΔOD of *bilirubinoid pigments* of 450 nm <0.01 indicates a gestational age of greater than 38 weeks. Bilirubin disappears after 36 weeks.

When the *creatinine* (estimate of renal maturity) value is greater than 1.8 mg/dl, the gestational age is greater than 36 weeks in the absence of maternal renal disease and dehydration or of fetal anomaly.

After *fetal lipid-containing exfoliated cells* are stained with Nile blue sulfate, a finding of more than 20% orange-staining cells indicates a gestational age of greater than 35 weeks; the fetus probably weighs 2500 g. (For information regarding the use of amniocentesis in estimating fetal health, see Procedure 22-1.)

Fetal Hemolytic Disease. Identification and follow-up of fetal hemolytic disease in isoimmunized pregnancies is another indication for amniocentesis. The first ΔOD analysis for amount of bilirubin in amniotic fluid is postponed until 24 to 25 weeks. Therapy by intrauterine transfusion of packed, Rh-negative, type O red blood cells is not possible before that time (Chapter 28).

Apt Test. The **Apt test** is used to differentiate maternal and fetal blood when there is vaginal bleeding during pregnancy or labor. It is performed as follows: Add 0.5 ml bloody fluid to 4.5 ml distilled water. Shake. Add 1 ml 0.25N sodium hydroxide. Fetal and cord blood remain pink for 1 or 2 minutes. Maternal blood becomes brown in 30 seconds.

Meconium in Amniotic Fluid. There are three possible reasons for the passage of meconium during the intrapartum period: (1) it is a normal physiologic function that occurs with maturity; (2) it is the result of hypoxia-induced peristalsis and sphincter relaxation, and (3) it may be a sequela to umbilical cord compression–induced vagal stimulation in mature fetuses (meconium passage is infrequent before weeks 32 to 34, with an increased incidence after 38 weeks).

The appearance of **meconium-stained amniotic fluid** is an indication for careful evaluation. The following criteria are proposed for evaluating meconium passage during the intrapartum period (Scott et al, 1990):

1. Consistency: "old and thin" vs. "new and thick." A new and thick consistency is more likely to be the result of fetal stress.
2. Timing: thick, fresh meconium passed for the first time in late labor, associated with nonremediable severe variable or late FHR decelerations, is an omninous sign. However, *the presence of meconium alone is not necessarily a sign of fetal distress.*
3. Presence of other indicators: meconium passage and nonremediable severe variable or late decelerations (especially with poor baseline variability) with or without acidosis confirmed by scalp-blood sampling are ominous signs.

PROCEDURE 22-1

AMNIOCENTESIS

DEFINITION
The removal of a small amount of amniotic fluid for laboratory analysis and prenatal diagnosis.

PURPOSE
To establish prenatal diagnosis of genetic problems, estimate gestational age, identify and monitor isoimmune disease, accomplish amniography and fetography, perform second-trimester elective abortion (see Chapter 6), estimate fetal lung maturity (L/S ratio and phosphatidylglycerol).

EQUIPMENT
Amniocentesis tray; electronic fetal monitor; flashlight; amber-colored test tubes (or test tubes wrapped in aluminum foil); bandage; antibacterial cleanser; sterile gowns, masks, and gloves; ultrasound machine and conductive gel.

NURSING ACTIONS	RATIONALE
Wash hands before and after touching woman and equipment. Glove, prn.	Prevents nosocomial infection and implements universal precautions.
Prepare woman for procedure:	Collaborative effort facilitates procedure.
Take baseline vital signs and fetal heart rate (FHR).	Assesses subsequent values.
Premedicate (if ordered).	Assists woman in relaxing.
Place woman in supine position with her hands under her head or across her chest.	Positions woman in a way that facilitates procedure.
Prepare the abdomen with a shave and a scrub with povidone-iodine (Betadine), if ordered by physician.	Minimizes possibility of infection.
Draw blood sample.	Compares with postprocedure blood sample for assessing probable fetomaternal hemorrhage. Assesses levels of AFP.
Act as a support person during procedure:	As with any surgical procedure, the woman and family will be tense and anxious as to the outcome.
Explain reason for such a long needle.	The needle passes through layers of fat and muscle before reaching the uterus. Actually only a small portion of the needle enters the uterus.
Show woman that the ultrasound guides the doctor in placement of the needle.	
Reinforce the physician's explanation for not using local anesthetic.	The physician will not use a local anesthetic for two reasons: (1) It "stings" and (2) it would mean two needles. Once the skin is pierced, there is a sensation of pressure, but not pain.
Assist the physician:	Collaborates in the completion of the procedure accurately and with least potential for injury to maternal-placental-fetal unit.
Label three sterile tubes.	Identifies specimen.
If bilirubin determination is needed, darken the room, use a flashlight, and immediately cover the filled amber-colored or aluminum foil-wrapped tube.	Prevents light from altering bilirubin, since a true reading cannot be obtained if the fluid is exposed to light.
After fluid is withdrawn, wash all povidone-iodine off the abdomen and apply a bandage.	Prevents skin burn.
Assist with or draw blood sample.	Assesses for the presence of fetomaternal hemorrhage. Assesses AFP level.
Continue monitoring the FHR for 30 minutes and assess for uterine contractions.	Identifies complications.

The presence of meconium in amniotic fluid should not be considered the sole basis for intervention. Electronic fetal monitoring and fetal scalp blood sampling are valuable tools to further assess fetal status.

❑ BIOPHYSICAL MONITORING

Evaluation of fetal well-being and maturity is essential in the management of the high-risk pregnancy. The **nonstress test** (NST), or **fetal activity-acceleration determination** (FAD), the **contraction stress test** (CST), and the **biophysical profile** have been widely employed for the determination of fetal well-being. In addition, **daily fetal movement count** (DFMC), as recorded by the expectant mother, has proved to be an additional method of assessing fetal well-being.

The desired goals of antepartum monitoring are to prevent intrauterine fetal death and avoid unnecessary premature intervention.

Indications for both the NST and the CST include:

Maternal diabetes mellitus
Chronic hypertension
Hypertensive disorders in pregnancy
IUGR
Sickle cell disease
Maternal cyanotic heart disease
Suspected postmaturity
History of previous stillbirth
Rh sensitization (isoimmunization)
Meconium-stained amniotic fluid (at amniocentesis)
Abnormal estriol excretion pattern
Hyperthyroidism
Collagen diseases
Older gravida
≥40 weeks' gestation
Chronic renal disease

There are no contraindications for the NST. Absolute contraindications for the CST are rupture of membranes and previous classical cesarean delivery. The following are considered relative contraindications for the CST: multifetal pregnancy, previous preterm labor, placenta previa, hydramnios, and previous low transverse cesarean delivery. As a rule, reactive patterns with the NST or negative results with the CST are associated with favorable outcomes. In general, biophysical assessment is considered reliable, but false negatives and false positives do occur (Haesslein, 1987; Scott et al, 1990).

Nonstress Test

The basis for the NST, or FAD, is that the normal fetus will produce characteristic heart rate patterns. Acceleration of FHR in response to fetal movement is the desired outcome of the NST. This then allows most high-risk pregnancies to continue, with the test being repeated twice a week. A ***reactive pattern suggests fetal well-being*** with an associated good perinatal outcome.

The nurse observes the strip chart for signs of *fetal activity* and a concurrent acceleration of FHR. If evidence of fetal movement is not apparent on the chart paper, the woman is asked to depress a button on a handheld event marker that is connected into the appropriate outlet on the monitor when she feels fetal movement. The "event" of fetal movement is then noted by a spike or arrow printed by the stylus on the uterine activity panel of the strip chart. The test usually takes 20 to 30 minutes but may take longer if the fetus needs to be moved or awakened because of a sleep state (Fig. 22-9).

The **acoustic stimulation** test is another method of testing antepartum FHR response. The test takes approximately 10 minutes to complete, with the fetus monitored for 5 minutes before fetal acoustic stimulation to obtain a baseline FHR. The sound source is then applied on the maternal abdomen over the fetal head. Monitoring continues for another 5 minutes, and the strip chart is assessed.

A guide for interpretation of the acoustic stimulation test follows:

Reactive acoustic stimulation test	FHR acceleration of at least 15 bpm for at least 120 seconds or two accelerations of at least 15 bpm for at least 15 seconds within 5 minutes of stimulus
Nonreactive acoustic stimulation test	Inability to fulfill either criterion for reactivity as described above within 5 minutes

Contraction Stress Tests

The basis for the CST is that a healthy fetus can withstand a decreased oxygen supply during the physiologic stress of an oxytocin-stimulated contraction, whereas a compromised fetus will demonstrate late decelerations that are nonreassuring and indicative of uteroplacental insufficiency. ***A negative test suggests fetal well-being.***

Contraindications include the following: threatened preterm labor, placenta previa, hydramnios, multiple fetuses, rupture of membranes, previous preterm labor, and previous classical cesarean delivery (Cunningham, MacDonald, and Gant, 1989).

Nipple-stimulated Contraction Stress Test. The woman is monitored indirectly, and the nurse observes

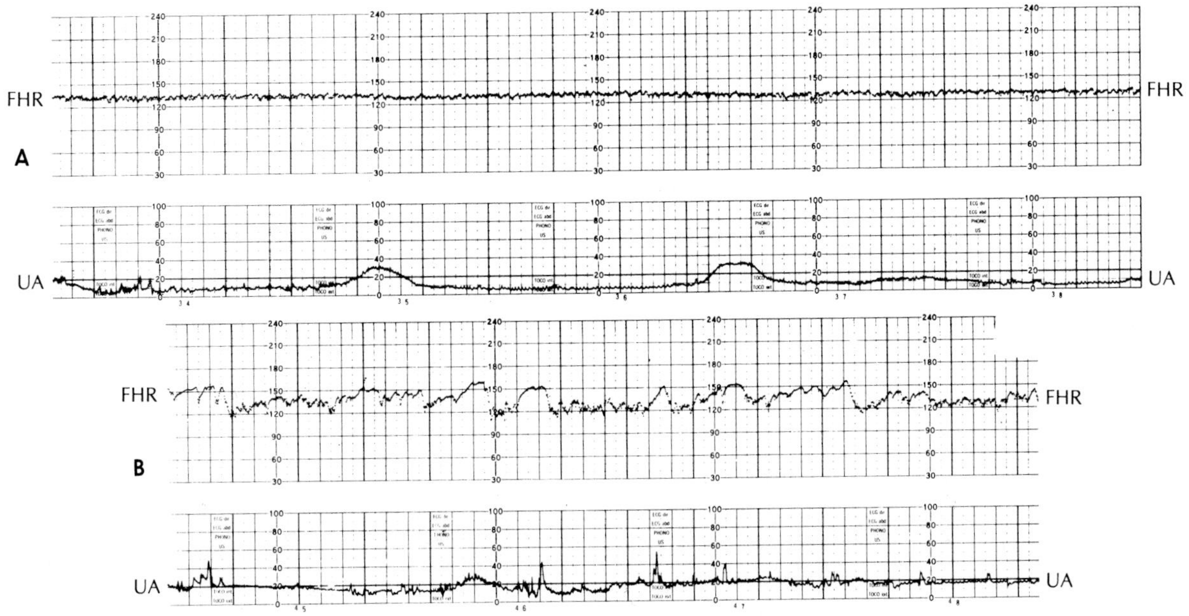

Fig. 22-9 Nonstress test. **A,** Decreased variability caused by fetal sleep cycle. **B,** Reactive nonstress test, indicative of fetal well-being, 15 minutes later. (From Perez RH: Protocols for perinatal nursing practice, St Louis, 1981, The CV Mosby Co.)

the strip chart for 10 minutes before initiating nipple-stimulated contractions. If the woman has three or more spontaneous contractions within a 10-minute period, the nipple-stimulated contractions need not be initiated. If less than three spontaneous contractions occur within the period, and if late decelerations do not occur with intermittent spontaneous contractions, nipple stimulation can be initiated. The nurse explains the procedure to the woman and then proceeds by applying warm, moist washcloths to both breasts for several minutes. The woman is instructed to massage or roll the nipple of one breast for 10 minutes. If uterine contractions do not occur, both breasts should be stimulated for 10 minutes. The breasts should be restimulated intermittently as needed to maintain uterine contractions. If nipple stimulation does not produce the desired uterine activity, the nurse should proceed with an oxytocin-stimulated CST.

Oxytocin-stimulated Contraction Stress Test. The physician orders the dosage, which usually starts at 0.5 mU/min.* The oxytocin is always diluted in an IV solution and piggybacked into the tubing of the main IV. The infusion is usually delivered by an infusion pump or controller to ensure accurate dosage. The oxytocin infusion is usually increased by 0.5 mU/min at 15- to 20-minute intervals until three uterine contractions of good quality are observed within a 10-minute period. The FHR pattern is then interpreted. The oxytocin infusion is discontinued and the maintenance IV solution infused until such time as uterine activity has returned to the preoxytocin infusion level. The IV is then removed, and the fetal monitor is discontinued. The woman can be sent home on the physician's orders.

Interpretation of Results. A guide for the interpretation of the CST follows:

Result	Interpretation
Negative	No late decelerations with a minimum of three uterine contractions lasting 40 to 60 seconds within a 10-minute period (Fig. 22-10)
Positive	Persistent and consistent late decelerations occurring with more than half the contractions (Fig. 22-11)
Suspicious	Late decelerations occurring with less than half the uterine contractions once an adequate contraction pattern has been established
Hyperstimulation	Late decelerations occurring with excessive uterine activity (contractions more often than every 2 minutes or lasting longer than 90 seconds) or a persistent increase in uterine tone
Unsatisfactory	Inadequate uterine contraction pattern or tracing too poor to interpret

*See Chapter 26 for calculating dosage of oxytocin (Pitocin) and drops per minute.

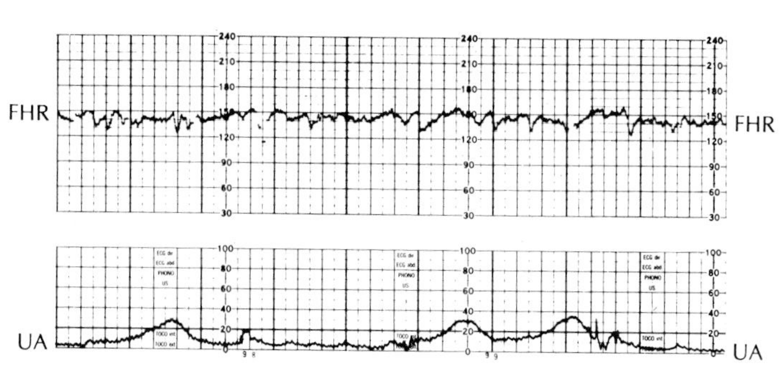

Fig. 22-10 Negative CST: fetal well-being.

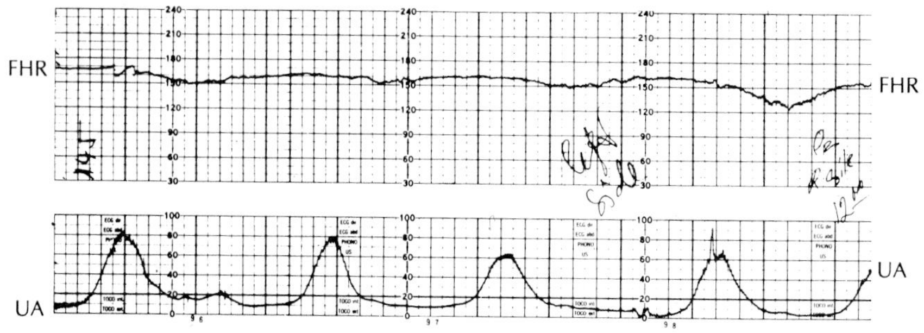

Fig. 22-11 Positive CST: compromised fetus. (From Perez RH: Protocols for perinatal nursing practice, St Louis, 1981, The CV Mosby Co.)

The clinical significance of the CST is as follows:

Result	Interpretation
Negative	Reassurance that the fetus is likely to survive labor, should it occur within 1 week; more frequent testing may be indicated by the clinical situation
Positive	Management lies between use of other tools of fetal assessment and termination of pregnancy; a positive test indicates that the fetus is at increased risk for perinatal morbidity and mortality; the physician may perform an expeditious vaginal delivery following a successful induction or may proceed directly to cesarean delivery
Suspicious, hyperstimulation, or unsatisfactory	NST and CST should be repeated within 24 hours; if interpretable data cannot be achieved, other methods of fetal assessment must be used

Daily Fetal Movement Count (DFMC)

Frequent movements of the fetus, as perceived by the mother, have been reassuring signs for centuries. Various investigators have recently reported a marked decrease in fetal movement before an episode of fetal distress or fetal death.

DFMCs, as reported by the mother, have been compared with movements recorded electronically, revealing that almost 90% of all fetal movements can be identified by the mother. This simple, inexpensive, readily applied "test" is continuously available away from the clinical area and relatively easy for the woman to do accurately. Maternal perception of a minimum of 10 movements during the daylight hours is considered reassuring (Haesslein, 1987).

Should a woman complain of decreased fetal movement, she may be asked by the physician to lie down for a period of 1 hour and count all the fetal movements. If she feels three or more during that time, she can be reassured. However, she is cautioned to continue to be aware of fetal movements and report the hourly observations should the problem recur. An immediate NST is usually performed if only one or two movements are felt. If the NST is reactive, no further testing is done unless there are some other risk factors. A nonreactive NST would be followed by a CST, the potential outcomes and significance of which have been previously described.

Biophysical Profile

The central nervous system (CNS) regulates fetal movements, breathing, tone, and heart rate variability. Therefore these are acute biophysical variables, which can be used to develop a **biophysical profile.** If one is abnormal, others are likely to be abnormal as well. However, decreased amniotic fluid volume probably reflects a chronic condition associated with fetal stress. When the fetus is stressed (e.g., chronic hypoxia), blood flow is shunted away from the kidneys. Decreased urine volume and, in turn, a decreased amniotic fluid volume result (Cunningham, MacDonald, Gant, 1989).

In 1980, Manning, Platt, and Supos were the first to report the use of the biophysical profile to assess fetal well-being. Their profile included five components. The five components and normal findings are presented in Table 22-5. Rupture of membranes should not alter the biophysical activity of a healthy fetus or the observed volume of amniotic fluid. All components, except for reactive FHR, are assessed by ultrasonography in about 30 minutes' time.

Baskett (1988) stressed that in preterm neonates, falsely abnormal tests are more common. Postterm pregnancy and fetal growth retardation are associated

Table 22-5 Biophysical Profile

Variables	Normal (score = 2)	Abnormal (score = 0)
Fetal breathing movements	One or more episodes in 30 min, each lasting ≥30 sec	Episodes absent or no episode of ≥30 sec in 30 min
Gross body movements	Three or more discrete body/limb movements in 30 min (episodes of active continuous movement considered as a single movement)	Less than three episodes of body/limb movements in 30 min
Fetal tone	One or more episodes of active extension with return to flexion of fetal limb(s) or trunk; opening and closing of hand considered normal tone	Slow extension with return to flexion; movement of limb in full extension, or fetal movement absent
Reactive fetal heart rate	Two or more episodes of acceleration (≥15 bpm) in 20 min, each lasting ≥15 sec and associated with fetal movement	Less than two episodes of acceleration or acceleration of <15 bpm in 20 min
Qualitative amniotic fluid volume	One or more pockets of fluid measuring ≥1 cm in two perpendicular planes	Pockets absent or pocket <1 cm in two perpendicular planes

Score	Interpretation	Recommended Management
10	Normal infant, low risk for chronic asphyxia	Repeat testing at weekly intervals; repeat twice weekly in diabetic women and women ≥42 weeks
8	Normal infant, low risk for chronic asphyxia	Repeat testing at weekly intervals; repeat twice weekly in diabetic women and women ≥42 weeks; oligohydramnios is indication for delivery
6	Suspected chronic asphyxia	Repeat testing within 24 hr; oligohydramnios or repeat score ≤6 is indication for delivery
4	Suspected chronic asphyxia	Indications for delivery are ≥36 weeks and favorable cervix; if <36 weeks and lecithin/sphingomyelin ratio <2.0, repeat test in 24 hr; repeat score ≤6 or oligohydramnios is indication for delivery
2	Strong suspicion of chronic asphyxia	Extend testing time to 120 min; persistent score ≤4, regardless of gestational age, is indication for delivery

Reprinted with permission from Manning FA et al: Fetal assessment based on fetal biophysical profile scoring: experience in 12,620 referred high risk pregnancies, Am J Obstet Gynecol 151:345, 1985.

with oligohydramnios (Cunningham, MacDonald, Gant, 1989). If a pregnancy is postterm and decreased amniotic fluid volume is observed, despite normal findings for all other parameters, cesarean delivery is advocated (Platt, 1989). With decreased amniotic fluid volume, there is an increased risk of cord compression. Early manifestations of fetal infection may be a nonreactive NST and the absence of fetal breathing. Loss of fetal movement and poor fetal tone are late signs. Therefore biophysical profile scores may assist in the diagnosis of babies at risk for perinatal sepsis (Vintzileos et al, 1985).

By 1987, Manning et al modified their original profile. If the other four parameters are observed to be normal, they do not perform the NST. Platt et al (1985) concluded that the biophysical profile had a markedly higher positive predictive value than the NST in determining overall abnormal fetal condition. Divon et al (1988) found that the identification of spontaneous late decelerations (Chapter 14) during the biophysical profile testing was associated with significant fetal morbidity regardless of the score.

Variations of the original biophysical profile have been reported. Shime et al (1984) omitted observation of fetal tone. Vintzileos et al (1983) added a sixth factor—placental grading.

SUMMARY

Assessment of risk is the focus of this chapter. Assessment through interview, physical examination, and diagnostic techniques is discussed. Risk assessment identifies a population that requires special attention. Early identification of risk facilitates prospective planning and implementation of client and family care management throughout the childbearing cycle.

LEARNING ACTIVITIES

1. Observe an ultrasound test being performed. Have the examiner or interpreter explain the results.
2. Assist with an amniocentesis and obtain copies of the results. Have a physician assist you in interpreting the results and their implications.
3. Role-play a nurse attending a woman undergoing amniocentesis for determination of the possibility of genetic defect. Discuss the nurse's responsibilities for client education in this situation.
4. Review several clients' charts. Identify risk factors and give rationale for each choice.
5. Assist with a CST or NST. Evaluate the fetal monitor strip and determine if it is an example of a reactive NST or a nonreactive NST; a positive oxytocin challenge test or a negative oxytocin challenge test.
6. Make a list of the household chemicals used in your home. In a group seminar compile a master list. Select some examples from the list, identify their purpose, describe why they are hazardous, and list what alternatives can be substituted to accomplish the same purpose.

References

ACOG American College of Obstetricians and Gynecologists: Video display terminals and reproductive health—a statement to the US House of Representatives' Subcommittee on Health and Safety, Washington, DC, 1984.

Athey PA and Hadlock FP: Ultrasound in obstetrics and gynecology, ed 2, St Louis, 1985, The CV Mosby Co.

Anderson RL: Maternal serum alpha-fetoprotein screening, Paper presented at UCSF antepartum and intrapartum management conference, San Francisco, June, 1987.

Baskett TF: Gestational age and fetal biophysical assessment, Am J Obstet Gynecol 158:332, 1988.

Bellinger D et al: Longitudinal analyses of prenatal and postnatal lead exposure and early cognitive development, N Engl J Med 316(7):1037, 1987.

Bond MB: Reproductive hazards in the workplace, Contemp OB/GYN 28(3):57, 1986.

Brent RL: X-ray, microwave and ultrasound: the real and unreal hazards, Pediatr Ann 9:469, Dec, 1980.

Budinger TF: Nuclear magnetic resonance (NMR) in vivo studies: known thresholds for health effects, J Comput Assist Tomogr 5:800, Dec, 1981.

Cunningham FG, MacDonald PC, and Gant NF: Williams obstetrics, ed 18, Norwalk, Conn, 1989, Appleton & Lange.

Dadd DL: Nontoxic cleaners for your home, San Francisco Chronicle, p C8, April 1, 1987.

Dauphinee JD: Antepartum testing: a challenge for nursing, J Perinat and Neonat Nurs 1(1):29, 1987.

Divon MY, et al: Fetal biophysical profile scoring: the significance of fetal heart rate late decelerations. Abstract No 199. Presented at the 35th Annual Meeting of the Society of Gynecologic Investigation, March 17-20, 1988.

Droegemueller W et al: Comprehensive gynecology, St Louis, 1987, The CV Mosby Co.

Ferguson S: Birth defects and the environment—finding the connection, CBE Environmental Rev, p 8, Fall, 1986.

Goldberg JD: Antepartum fetal blood sampling, Paper presented at UCSF antepartum and intrapartum management conference, San Francisco, June, 1987.

Golbus MS: Chorionic villus sampling or amniocentesis? Paper presented at UCSF antepartum and intrapartum management conference, San Francisco, June, 1987.

Green D and Malin J: Prenatal diagnosis: when reality shatters parents' dreams, Nurs '88 18(2):61, 1988.

Haesslein HC: Antepartum fetal assessment, Paper presented at USCF antepartum and intrapartum management conference, San Francisco, June, 1987.

Hazards of methylene chloride, Harvard Medical School Health Letter 11(10):5, 1986.

Hirning CR and Aitken JH: Cathode-ray tube x-ray emission standard for video display terminals, Health Phys 43:727, Nov, 1982.

How to tell if your water is pure, San Francisco Chronicle, p C1, Feb 4, 1987.

Jackson L: CVS Newsletter, No. 24, Feb. 14, 1988.

Jankowski CF: The risks of radiation during pregnancy, Am J Nurs 86(3):260, 1986.

Kanal E and Wolf GL: Magnetic resonance imaging: an overview, Fam Pract recertification 8(9):35, 1986.

KEY CONCEPTS

- A high-risk pregnancy is one in which the life or well-being of the mother or offspring is jeopardized by a biophysical or psychosocial disorder coincidental with or unique to pregnancy.
- Factors that place the pregnancy and fetus/neonate at risk include anatomic, physiologic, therapeutic, environmental, and idiopathic events.
- Pollution of the environment is a serious and growing hazard to reproductive health.
- Psychosocial perinatal warning indicators include characteristics of the parents, the child, their support systems, and family circumstances.
- Diagnostic techniques include ultrasonography, MRI, PUBS, CVS, EFM, and biophysical profile.
- Biochemical monitoring techniques involve assessment of maternal urine and blood, and of amniotic fluid and its components.
- Maternal and perinatal mortality for whites is considerably lower than for all other races in the United States.
- There is excellent evidence that mortality decreases when high risk is identified early and intensive care applied.
- CVS could partially replace amniocentesis for genetic diagnosis.
- Evaluation of fetal well-being and maturity, essential in the management of the high-risk pregnancy, requires the knowledgeable and willing cooperation of the gravida and her family.
- A *reactive* NST and a *negative* CST suggest fetal well-being.

Lead poisoning still a threat, state says, San Francisco Chronicle, p A2, Feb 6, 1988.

Manning FA, Platt LD, and Supos L: Antepartum fetal evaluation: development of a fetal biophysical profile, Am J Obstet Gynecol 136:787, 1980.

Manning FA et al: Fetal assessment based on fetal biophysical profile scoring: experience in 12,620 referred high risk pregnancies, Am J Obstet Gynecol 151:343, 1985.

Manning FA et al: Fetal biophysical profile scoring: selective use of the nonstress test, Am J Obstet Gynecol 156:709, 1987.

McCallum WD: Ultrasound applications in pregnancy, Midcoastal California Perinatal Outreach Program, Jan, 1984.

Modica MM and Timor-Tritsch IE: Transvaginal sonography provides a sharper view into the pelvis, JOGN Nurs 17(2):89, 1988.

Moses M: Reproductive health in the workplace: health workers and reproductive hazards, BIRTH 14(3):153, 1987.

Munley AJ et al: Exposure of midwives to nitrous oxide in four hospitals, Br Med J 293:1063, 1986.

National Institute for Occupational Safety and Health: Potential health hazards of video display terminals, US Department of Health and Human Services, 1981, NIOSH Pub #81-129.

Noise pollution: irritant or hazard? Harvard Medical School Health Newsletter 11(8):1, 1986.

Platt LD: Predicting fetal health with the biophysical profile, Contemp OB/GYN 33(2):105, 1989.

Platt LD et al: A prospective trial of the fetal biophysical profile versus the nonstress test in the management of high-risk pregnancies, Am J Obstet Gynecol 153:624, 1985.

Quirk JG and Bleasdale JE: Fetal lung maturation in the pregnancy complicated by diabetes mellitus. In DiRenzo GC and Hawkins PR, editors: Perinatal medicine: updates and controversies, New York, 1986, Cortina Learning International, Inc.

Saad SA et al: The reliability and clinical use of a rapid phosphatidylglycerol assay in normal and diabetic pregnancies, Am J Obstet Gynecol 157:1516, 1988.

Scott JR et al: Danforth's obstetrics and gynecology, ed 6, Philadelphia, 1990, JB Lippincott Co.

Shavelson L: Poisoned lives: six stories from toxic California, Image, p 22, July 26, 1987.

Shime J et al: Prolonged pregnancy: surveillance of the fetus and the neonate and the course of labor and delivery, Am J Obstet Gynecol 148:547, 1984.

Thomas A and Morris PG: The effects of NMR exposure in living organisms. I. A microbial assay, Br J Radiol 54:615, July, 1981.

Vintzileos AM et al: The fetal biophysical profile and its predictive value, Obstet Gynecol 62:271, 1983.

Vintzileos AM et al: The fetal biophysical profile in patients with premature rupture of membranes: an early predictor of fetal infection, Am J Obstet Gynecol 152:510, 1985.

Bibliography

Anonymous. OSHA work-practice guidelines for personnel dealing with cytotoxic (antineoplastic) drugs, Am J Hosp Pharm 43:1193, 1986.

Bingol N et al: Terotogenicity of cocaine in humans, J Pediatr 110:93, 1987.

Blank JJ: Electronic fetal monitoring: Nursing management defined, J Obstet Gynecol Neonatal Nurs 14:463, 1985.

Brucker MC and MacMullen NJ: CVS: counseling your patient, Nurse Pract 12(8):34, 1987.

Dahlberg NL: A perinatal center based antepartum homecare program, JOGN Nurs 17(1):30, 1988.

Dunn PA, Weiner S, and Ludomirski A: Percutaneous umbilical blood sampling, JOGN Nurs 17(5):308, 1988.

Dupre L: Safety in the workplace. I. Handling chemotherapy drugs, Calif Nurs Rev 10(2):12, 1988.

Eden R: Standards of care for the postdate pregnancy, Contemp OB/GYN 34(2):308, 1989.

Engstrom JL: Measurement of fundal height, JOGN Nurs 17(3):172, 1988.
Estok P and Rudy E: Marathon running: comparison of physical and psychosocial risks for men and women, Res Nurs Health 10(2):79, 1987.
Ferguson HW: Biophysical profile scoring: the fetal Apgar, Am J Nurs 88(5):662, 1988.
Foster SD: MCN patient teaching, MCN 12(2):131, 1987.
Freitas CA, Helmer FT, and Cousins N: The development and management uses of a patient classification system for a high-risk perinatal center, JOGN Nurs 16(5):330, 1987.
Freivogel W: High court upholds special pregnancy benefits, St Louis Post Dispatch, Jan 14, 1987.
Green D: Prenatal diagnosis: when reality shatters parents' dreams, Nurs '88 18(2):61, 1988.
Health status of Vietnam veterans. III. Reproductive outcomes and child health, JAMA 259(18):2715, 1988.
Hogge WA: Prenatal diagnosis of thalassemias, Contemp OB/GYN 34(2):23, 1989.
Jaffe MS and Melson KA: Laboratory and diagnostic cards: clinical implications and teaching, St Louis, 1988, The CV Mosby Co.
Krakoff IH: Cancer chemotherapeutic agents, Cancer 37:93, 1987.
Kyba FN, Ogburn-Russell L, and Rutledge JN: Magnetic resonance imaging: the latest in diagnostic technology, RN 17(1):44, 1987.
Ledger KE and Williams DL: Parents at risk: an instructional program for perinatal assessment and preventive intervention, Victoria, BC, Canada, 1981, Ministry of Health, Province of British Columbia, and Queen Alexandra Solarium for Crippled Children Society (Queen Alexandra Hospital, 2400 Arbutus Rd, Victoria, BC, Canada V8N IV7).
Lewis C and Mocarski V: Obstetric ultrasound: application in a clinic setting, JOGN Nurs 16(1):56, 1987.
McDonald AD et al: Visual display units and pregnancy: evidence from the Montreal survey, J Occup Med 28(12):1226, 1986.
McDonald AD et al: Spontaneous abortion and occupation, J Occup Med 28(12):1232, 1986.
McKee D: New Milner-Fenwick Program addresses pregnant working woman, Patientvision Update, p 8, Summer, 1987.
Miller SA: Chemotherapy drug handling safety, Calif Nurs Review 10(2):12, 1988.
Moenning RK and Hill WC: A randomized study comparing two methods of performing the breast stimulation stress test, JOGN Nurs 16(4):253, 1987.
NAACOG: Reproductive health hazards: women in the workplace, 11:issue, Feb, 1985.
Nurses' Association of the American College of Obstetricians and Gynecologists: Electronic fetal monitoring: nursing practice competencies and educational guidelines, Washington, DC, 1986, NAACOG.
O'Brien GD: Limits of ultrasound screening for anomalies, Contemp OB/GYN 34(1):51, 1989.
Platt LD: How to use the latest vaginal ultrasound equipment, Contemp OB/GYN, Technology 32 (special issue), p 129, 1989.
Scialli AR and Lione A: Major environmental toxicants, Contemp OB/GYN 34(2):120, 1989.
Stockwell H and Lyman G: Cigarette smoking and the risk of female reproductive cancer, Am J Obstet Gynecol 157(1):35, 1987.
Stringer MR: Chorionic villi sampling: a nursing perspective, JOGN Nurs 17(1):19, 1988.

CHAPTER

23 Hypertensive States, Maternal Infections, and Hemorrhagic Disorders

Irene M. Bobak and Vicki Akin

Learning Objectives

Correctly define the key terms listed.

Describe the assessment techniques and formulate a nursing plan of care for the woman with preeclampsia.

Describe the HELLP syndrome and list appropriate nursing actions.

Summarize care of women with selected infections.

Review infection control to minimize nosocomial infections and occupational risk for infection.

Compare and contrast abruptio placentae and placenta previa.

Discuss clotting disorders in pregnancy with emphasis on disseminated intravascular coagulation (DIC).

Review postdelivery hemorrhage causes, signs and symptoms, possible complications, and management.

Describe hemorrhagic shock and its management; discuss hazards of therapy.

Key Terms

abruptio placentae
bacteremic shock
cerclage
clonus (ankle)
Cullen's sign
deep tendon reflexes (DTRs)
dependent edema
disseminated intravascular coagulation (DIC)
eclampsia
ectopic pregnancy
embolism
fomites
gestational hypertension
HELLP syndrome
hematomas
hemorrhagic shock
hydatidiform mole
hyperreflexia
incompetent cervix
magnesium sulfate
nosocomial
pitting edema
placenta previa
preeclampsia
puerperal infection
roll-over test
sexually transmitted diseases (STDs)
spontaneous abortion
TORCH infections
toxic shock syndrome (TSS)
trophoblastic disease
universal precautions
uterine atony

Providing safe and effective care for the high-risk client requires a joint effort from all members of the health care team, with each member contributing his or her unique skills and talents to provide maximum outcome for mother and infant. This chapter reviews major maternal conditions that predispose or commit the woman and fetus to an abnormal response to pregnancy. The three major maternal conditions presented are hypertensive states, infection, and hemorrhage.

Hypertensive States in Pregnancy

Hypertensive states complicate approximately 5% to 7% of pregnancies in otherwise normal primigravid women, and as many as 20% to 40% of pregnancies in women with chronic renal disease or vascular disorders such as essential hypertension, diabetes mellitus, and lupus erythematosus (Scott, et al, 1990). In many regions of North America and in many parts of the world, hypertension complicating pregnancy is the leading cause of maternal and infant morbidity and mortality. Diminished placental perfusion resulting from arteriolar vasospasm places the fetus at risk. Eclampsia (seizures) from profound cerebral effects is the major maternal hazard. Early recognition and timely intervention are vital to arrest the progression of the disorder when possible, to prevent injury to the mother, to prevent eclampsia, and to effect a safe delivery of the infant.

Gestational Hypertension. **Gestational hypertension** is hypertension that develops after 20 weeks of gestation in a previously normotensive woman. It is defined as an elevation of systolic and diastolic pressures equal to or exceeding 140/90 mm Hg. An alternative definition that is more sensitive to individual variations is a rise in systolic pressure of 30 mm Hg or a rise in diastolic pressure of 15 mm Hg above the woman's baseline values. The latter definition is useful because blood pressure varies with age, race, physiologic state, dietary habits, and heredity. Gestational hypertension is not accompanied by other evidence of preeclampsia (e.g., proteinuria) or hypertensive vascular disease. This condition, sometimes referred to as **pregnancy-induced hypertension (PIH), disappears within 10 postpartum days (Iams and Zuspan, 1990).**

The blood pressure elevation must be present on two occasions 6 hours apart. Techniques of measurement must be standardized, for instance, always taken with the woman sitting *or* in a lateral position. The technique used must be noted in the client's record to provide data to guide interpretation of previous, present, and future readings.

Preeclampsia. The presence of ***proteinuria*** distinguishes **preeclampsia** from gestational hypertension. Preeclampsia may be accompanied by ***edema,*** which is a generalized accumulation of interstitial fluid (face, hands, abdomen, sacrum, tibia, ankles) after 12 hours of bed rest or a *weight gain* of more than 2 kg (4 to 4½ lb) per week. Edema, however, no longer enters into the diagnosis of preeclampsia (Iams and Zuspan, 1990). In the presence of trophoblastic disease (e.g., hydatidiform mole), preeclampsia can develop before week 20 of gestation.

Preeclampsia is a syndrome of *unknown etiology.* It is somehow related to the physiologic changes of pregnancy, because it disappears after the termination of pregnancy. It is much more likely to develop in the woman who is exposed to *chorionic villi* for the first time, as in a primigravida, or is exposed to a superabundance of chorionic villi, as with twins or hydatidiform mole. Common theories implicate nutritional deficiency, especially protein and calories; immunologic dysfunction; genetic predisposition; uterine ischemia; or vasospasm.

The higher incidence of preeclampsia in daughters of mothers who experienced the disorder supports the theory of hereditary tendency.

Uterine ischemia, insufficient blood flow through the uterus, may initiate a vasospastic response. Ischemia may explain the increased incidence in primigravidas and in gravidas with multifetal gestation when uterine growth and development do not keep pace with increased demands for blood flow.

Eclampsia. **Eclampsia** includes the symptoms of severe preeclampsia and one or more of the following: (1) tonic and clonic ***convulsions or coma,*** with the coma possibly following an unobserved seizure related to other seizure disorders, (2) ***hypertensive crisis,*** or (3) ***shock.***

Concurrent Hypertension and Pregnancy (CHP). Concurrent hypertension and pregnancy (CHP) is hypertension that develops before pregnancy or before week 20 of gestation that is not pregnancy associated.

Pathophysiology

In some pregnant women vascular sensitivity to angiotensin II increases. This increased vascular sensitivity occurs before the onset of *hypertension* (see rollover test, p. 642). Vasospasm results. Vasospasm decreases the diameters of blood vessels, impeding blood flow, and raising blood pressure. Blood flow to all body organs is decreased. Function in organs such as the placenta, kidneys, liver, and brain is depressed by 40% to 60%. Many pathophysiologic sequelae are seen.

Impaired placental perfusion leads to early degenerative aging of the placenta and possible intrauterine growth retardation (IUGR) of the fetus. The theory that impaired prostaglandin synthesis (p. 77) may be a factor in PIH is important to recall. Uterine activity and sensitivity to oxytocin is increased. ***Therefore increased sensitivity to the effects of oxytocin must be taken into account when the drug is used for induction or augmentation of labor.***

Reduced kidney perfusion decreases the glomerular filtration rate (GFR) and leads to degenerative glomerular changes. *Protein, primarily albumin, is lost in the urine.* Uric acid clearance is decreased. Sodium and water are retained. Plasma colloid osmotic pressure decreases as serum albumin levels fall. Fluid moves out of the intravascular compartment, resulting in *hemoconcentration,* increased blood viscosity, and tissue *edema.* The hematocrit increases as fluid leaves the intravascular space (Cunningham, MacDonald, and Gant, 1989). Therefore a rising hematocrit is seen as the condition worsens; a falling hematocrit (to normal levels) accompanies improvement of the condition. In severe preeclampsia, blood volume may fall to or below nonpregnant levels, severe edema develops, and *rapid weight gain* is seen (Scott et al, 1990).

Decreased perfusion of the liver leads to impaired function. Hepatic edema and subcapsular hemorrhage, experienced by the gravida as *epigastric or right upper quadrant pain,* is one sign of impending eclampsia (convulsion). Rupture of the liver is a rare but catastrophic complication (Cunningham, MacDonald, and Gant, 1989). Liver enzyme levels (e.g., SGOT) rise in the wake of liver damage.

Arteriolar vasospasms and decreased blood flow to the retina lead to *visual symptoms* such as scotoma (blind spots) and blurring. The same pathologic condition leads to cerebral edema and hemorrhages, and increased *central nervous system (CNS) irritability.* CNS irritability is expressed as headache, hyperreflexia, positive ankle clonus, and occasionally convulsions (pp. 645 and 650). Affectual changes are often seen.

Debate continues whether preeclampsia contributes to or is the result of **disseminated intravascular coagulation (DIC)** or whether DIC occurs with preeclampsia.

If the hypertension is difficult to bring under control, cardiac and pulmonary complications can occur. Heart failure, a common cause of maternal death attributed to preeclampsia, is rare in young, otherwise healthy women (Scott et al, 1990). Sudden circulatory collapse and shock may occur in women with a history of repeated hypertensive pregnancies. A rapid fall in systolic blood pressure by 70 mm Hg or more is most often seen *a few hours after delivery* although it may occur before or during labor.

Typically, pulmonary edema caused by preeclampsia is associated with severe generalized edema. Intravenous (IV) fluid infusion is an iatrogenic cause of fluid overload. Pulmonary edema and congestive heart failure are virtually the only accepted indications for diuretic therapy during pregnancy (Scott et al, 1990).

Morbidity and Mortality

Placental abruption with or without hypofibrinogenemia or DIC may occur with eclampsia. During a convulsion the woman may bite her tongue or lips; ribs or vertebrae may be fractured; and retinal detachments may occur. Eclampsia occurs in 0.05% to 0.2% of all pregnancies and in 1.5% of twin gestations (Anderson, 1987). About 8% of women with eclampsia die of the disease or its complications. The most common causes of death are intracranial hemorrhage and congestive heart failure.

Perinatal morbidity is high, because most women with preeclampsia deliver before the thirty-seventh week of gestation. The fetal outcome of maternal hypertension is questionable because of placental insufficiency. Generally the fetus is small-for-gestational age (SGA). However, these infants generally do better than other preterm infants of the same weight and gestational age born of nonhypertensive mothers. This is probably because of intrauterine stress that increases the rapidity of fetal lung maturation.

In many parts of North America the *perinatal mortality* is at least 20% with eclampsia. This is mainly because of the effects of hypoxia, prematurity, or acidosis during maternal convulsions. A single maternal convulsion increases the prospect of perinatal death at least fivefold.

The HELLP Syndrome

The **HELLP syndrome** (H: hemolysis, EL: elevated liver enzymes, and LP: low platelet count) represents an extension of the pathology of severe preeclampsia–eclampsia (Scott et al, 1990). The initial symptoms of the HELLP syndrome usually appear early in the third trimester. A circulating immunologic component may be the underlying cause.

For a woman to be diagnosed as having the HELLP syndrome, her platelet count must be $<100,000/mm^3$, her liver enzyme levels must be elevated (SGOT/SGPT), and some evidence for intravascular hemolysis must be present (schistocytes or burr cells on peripheral smear). The hemolysis that occurs accounts for the large drop in hematocrit out of proportion to blood loss that is found in the majority of new mothers with HELLP syndrome during the postpartum period (Weinstein, 1986). A unique form of coagulopathy (not DIC) occurs with the HELLP syndrome.

Recognition of the clinical and laboratory findings of the HELLP syndrome is important if early, aggressive therapy is to be initiated to prevent maternal and neonatal mortality (Weinstein, 1986; Anderson, 1987).

The unfavorable cervix and the aggressive nature of this disorder support cesarean delivery. Prolonged induction of labor could increase maternal morbidity. Fresh-frozen plasma may be needed if bleeding persists. The major laboratory manifestations of the disease, however, may not appear until the early postpartum period (48 to 72 hours). Delayed transfusion of packed red blood cells (RBCs) is often necessary because of the continued hemolysis. It is important to attempt to lower the blood pressure if the diastolic pressure is consistently greater than 110 mm Hg. ***Blood pressure may be normal or slightly elevated, so it is not an adequate indicator of the severity of the disease. Hypoglycemia*** may be present in the woman with the HELLP syndrome and, when the blood sugar is <40 mg/dl, is associated with a high maternal mortality (Egley, Gutliph, and Bowes, 1985).

It is possible that some immunologic component crossing the placenta is responsible for the leukopenia seen in some newborns (Weinstein, 1986). Similar findings of the thrombocytopenia and leukopenia of the newborn from the mother with the HELLP syndrome have been reported by Brazie, Gumm, and Little (1982).

Assessment

Interview and Physical Examination

Preeclampsia can occur without warning or with the gradual development of symptoms. Therefore each woman is assessed for etiologic factors during the first prenatal visit. During each subsequent visit the woman is assessed for symptomatology that suggests the onset or presence of preeclampsia (Table 23-1).

In addition to the determination of the systolic and diastolic pressures, the *blood pressure* may be evaluated by two other methods: by the mean arterial pressure (MAP) and by the roll-over test. A blood pressure of 140/90 represents an *MAP* of 107 mm Hg. (MAP is calculated by adding the diastolic pressure to one third of the pulse pressure.

The **roll-over test** may be of some predictive value to detect women at risk for preeclampsia (O'Brien, 1990). To perform this test, the nurse measures the blood pressure with the woman in the lateral recumbent position until the pressure is stable. The woman is rolled to the supine position and the blood pressure is measured

Table 23-1 Differentiation of Mild and Severe Preeclampsia

	Mild Preeclampsia*	Severe Preeclampsia
MATERNAL EFFECTS		
Blood pressure	Rise in systolic blood pressure of 30 mm Hg or more. A rise in diastolic blood pressure of 15 mm Hg or more or a reading of 140/90 mm Hg × 2, 6 hours apart.	Rise to 160/110 mm Hg or more on two separate occasions 6 hours apart with pregnant woman on bed rest.
MAP	140/90 = 107.	160/110 = 127.
Weight gain	Weight gain of more than 1.4 kg (3 lb)/month during the second trimester, more than 0.5 kg (1 lb)/week during the third trimester, or a sudden weight gain of 2 kg (4-4½ lb)/week at any time.	Same as mild preeclampsia.
Proteinuria Qualitative dipstick Quantitative 24-hour analysis	Proteinuria of 300 mg/L in a 24-hour specimen or greater than 1 g/L in a random daytime specimen of 2 or more occasions 6 hours apart as protein loss is variable. With dipstick, values vary from trace to 1+.	Proteinuria of 5-10 g/L in 24 hours or 2+ or more protein on dipstick.
Edema	Dependent edema, some puffiness of eyes, face, fingers; pulmonary rales absent.	Generalized edema, noticeable puffiness of eyes, face, fingers. Pulmonary edema → crackles (rales).
Reflexes	Hyperreflexia 3+ No ankle clonus.	Hyperreflexia 3+ or more. Ankle clonus.
Urine output	Output matches intake.	Oliguria: less than 100 ml/4 hr output.
Headache	Transient	Severe.
Visual problems	Absent.	Blurred, photophobia, blind spots on funduscopy.
Irritability	Transient.	Severe.
Serum creatinine	Normal.	Elevated.
Thrombocytopenia	Absent.	Present.
SGOT elevation	Minimal.	Marked.
FETAL EFFECTS		
Placental perfusion	Reduced.	Decreased perfusion expressed as IUGR in fetus. FHR: late decelerations.
Premature placental aging	Not apparent.	At birth placenta appears smaller than normal for the duration of the pregnancy. Premature aging is apparent with numerous areas of broken syncytia. Ischemic necroses (white infarcts) are numerous, and intervillous fibrin deposition (red infarcts) may be recorded.

*No preeclampsia should be considered "mild" (Knuppel and Drukker, 1986; Scott et al, 1990).

immediately; the blood pressure measurement is repeated in 5 minutes. A *positive test* is defined as an increase of 20 mm Hg or more in diastolic pressure at the 5-minute reading. A *negative test* is defined as less than a 20 mm Hg rise in the diastolic pressure at the 5-minute reading (Knuppel and Drukker, 1986). The mechanism by which the supine position effects a rise in blood pressure is not clear, but it is another manifestation of intrinsic vascular hypersensitivity in women destined to develop preeclampsia (Reiss, 1987; Cunningham, MacDonald, and Gant, 1989).

Although it is not a simple test to perform and not absolutely accurate, the roll-over test may indicate most women who are in danger of developing preeclampsia.

One intent of the assessment of the blood pressure, weight, and urine in pregnant women is the prompt identification of complications such as preeclampsia. Observation of edema plus assessment findings warrant additional investigation. *Edema* is assessed for distribution, degree, and pitting. If periorbital or facial edema is not obvious, the gravida is asked if it was present when she awoke. As the day progresses, gravity is responsible for movement of fluid to dependent body parts. In more severe preeclampsia, facial edema is obvious. Edema may be described as dependent or pitting (Kozier and Erb, 1987).

Dependent edema is edema of the lowest or most dependent parts of the body, where hydrostatic pressure is greatest. If a person is ambulatory, this edema may first be evident in the feet and ankles. If the person is confined to bed, the edema is more likely to occur in the sacral region.

Pitting edema is edema that leaves a small depression or pit after finger pressure is applied to the swollen area. The pit is caused by movement of fluid to adjacent tissue, away from the point of pressure. Within 10 to 30 seconds the pit normally disappears.

Although the amount of edema is difficult to quantitate, the following method may be used to record relative degrees of edema formation:

+1 Minimum (2 mm) edema of the pedal and pretibial areas
+2 Marked (4 mm) edema of the lower extremities
+3 Edema of the face and hands, lower abdominal walls, and sacrum (depth of 6 mm)
+4 Anasarca (generalized massive edema) with ascites (depth of 8 mm)

Deep tendon reflexes (DTRs) are evaluated if preeclampsia is suspected. The biceps and patellar reflexes and ankle clonus are assessed and the findings recorded (Fig. 23-1; Table 23-2). To elicit the biceps reflex a downward blow is struck over the thumb, which is situated over the biceps tendon. *Normal response is flexion of the arm at the elbow* or +2 (Table 23-2). The ***patellar reflex*** is elicited with the woman's legs hanging freely over the end of the examining table, or with the woman lying on her left side with the knee slightly flexed. A blow with a percussion hammer is dealt directly to the patellar tendon, inferior to the patella. *Normal response is the extension or kicking out of the leg.* To assess for hyperactive reflexes (**clonus**) at the ankle joint, the leg should be supported with the knee flexed. With one hand, the foot is sharply dorsiflexed and the position maintained for a moment. The foot is then released. *Normal (negative clonus) response* is

Table 23-2 **Assessing Deep Tendon Reflexes (DTRs)**

Degree	Grading	Clinical Significance and Nursing Actions
Brisk with sustained clonus	5+	Woman not responding to medications as desired; may be accompanied by apprehension, restlessness, excitability; notify physician
Hyperactive response (brisk with transient clonus)	4+	Woman not responding to medications as desired; may be accompanied by apprehension, restlessness, excitability; notify physician
More than normal (brisk)	3+	Woman responding; however, important to assess frequently
Normal, active	2+	Safe dosage level, therapeutic effect
Low response (sluggish or dull)	1+	Notify physician for medical directives
No response	0	Turn off magnesium sulfate drip; change to "keep open" solution; notify physician for immediate care; prepare antidote (calcium chloride [Iams and Zuspan, 1990] *or* calcium gluconate [Scott et al, 1990], 1 g for IV injection to be given over 3 min)

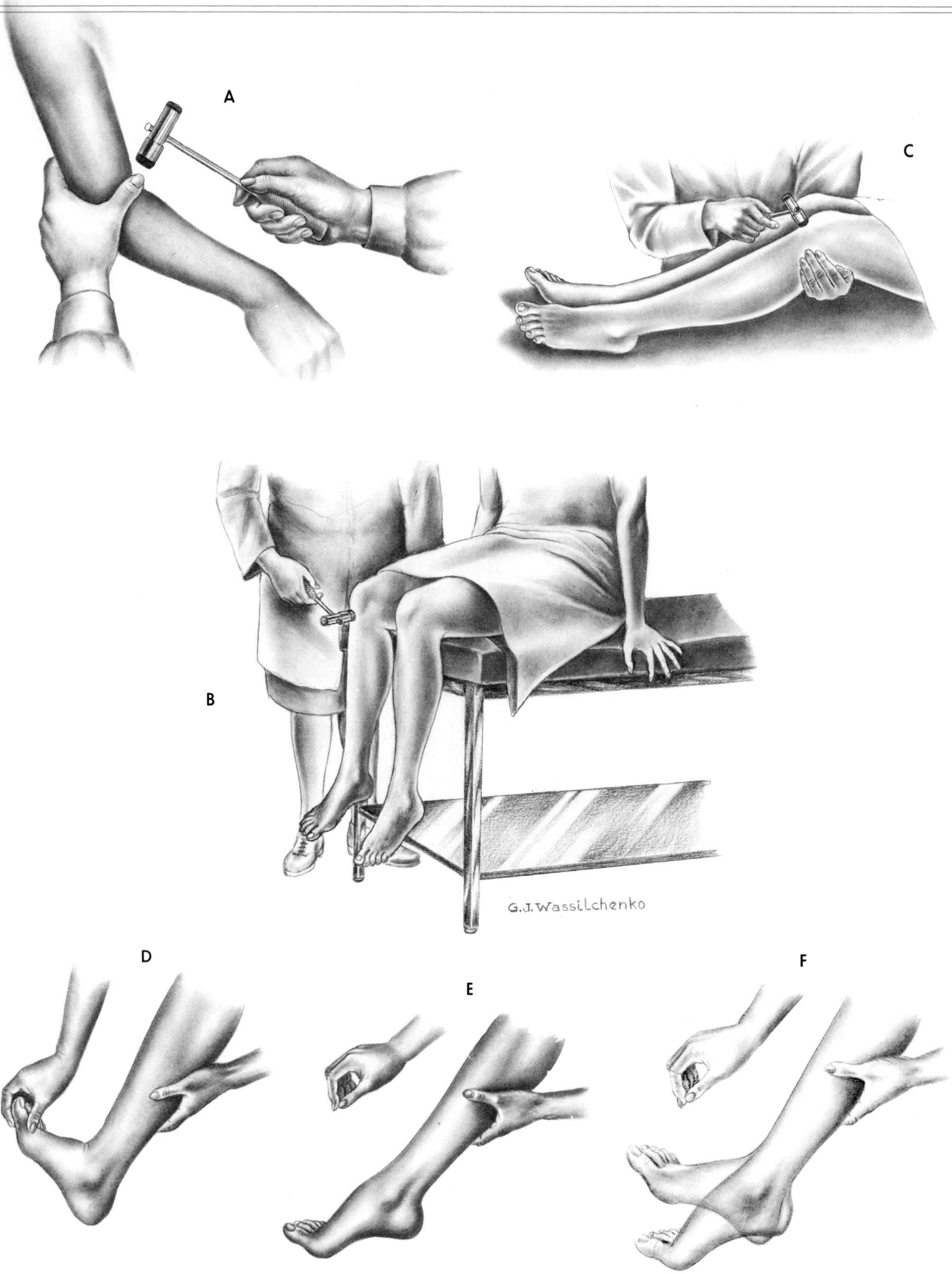

Fig. 23-1 **A,** Biceps reflex. **B,** Patellar reflex with client's legs hanging freely over end of examining table, **C,** with client in supine position. **D,** Hyperactive reflexes (clonus) at ankle joint. **E,** Normal (negative clonus) response. **F,** Abnormal (positive clonus) response.

elicited when, while the foot is held in dorsiflexion, no rhythmic oscillations (jerking) are felt. When the foot is released, no oscillations are seen as foot drops to plantar flexed position. *Abnormal (positive clonus)* response is recognized by rhythmic oscillations of one or more "beats" felt when the foot is in dorsiflexion and seen as foot drops to the plantar flexed position.

The fetal heart rate (FHR) and rhythm are assessed. Fetal movement and growth are determined by Leopold's maneuvers (Chapter 15). Fundal height is measured. Biophysical or biochemical monitoring for fetal well-being may be ordered (Chapter 14).

Uterine tonicity is evaluated for signs of labor and abruptio placentae. If labor is suspected, a vaginal examination for cervical changes is indicated.

During the physical examination, the gravida is scrutinized for signs of thrombocytopenia (decreased platelets). Ecchymotic areas, history of bruising with mild trauma, and bleeding from gums may manifest coagulopathy.

Danger signs of preeclampsia are summarized in the box below.

Eclampsia is usually preceded by various premonitory symptoms and signs, including headache, severe epigastric pain, hyperreflexia, and hemoconcentration; but convulsions can appear suddenly and without warning in a seemingly stable woman with only minimum blood-pressure elevations (Cunningham, MacDonald, and Gant, 1989).

The convulsions that occur in eclampsia are an awesome, frightening sequence to observe. Increased hypertension and tonic contraction of all body muscles (e.g., arms flexed, hands clenched, legs inverted) precedes the tonic-clonic convulsions. During this stage muscles relax and contract alternately. Respirations are halted and then begin again with long, deep, stertorous inhalation. Hypotension follows and coma ensues in 2 to 3 minutes to hours. Nystagmus and muscular twitching persist for a time. Disorientation and amnesia cloud the immediate recovery. Oliguria and anuria are notable. The seizure can recur within minutes of the first convulsion or the woman may never experience another.

DANGER SIGNS

Preeclampsia

1. Rapid rise in blood pressure
2. Rapid gain in weight
3. Generalized edema
4. Quantitative increase in proteinuria
5. Epigastric pain
6. Marked hyperreflexia; especially transient or sustained ankle clonus
7. Severe headache
8. Visual disturbances
9. Oliguria with urinary output of less than 100 ml in 4 hours
10. Drowsiness, listlessness (dulled sensorium)
11. Nausea and vomiting, severe

Laboratory Tests

The nurse assists in obtaining a number of blood and urine specimens to aid in the diagnosis of preeclampsia, HELLP syndrome, or chronic hypertension. An initial specimen of blood will be analyzed for the following:

- CBC (including a platelet count)
- Clotting studies (including bleeding time, PT, PTT, and fibrinogen)
- Liver enzymes (SGOT or AST, SGPT or ALT)
- Chemistry panel (BUN, creatinine, and glucose)
- Type and screen, possible cross-match

The hematocrit, platelets, and glucose will be monitored closely for changes in these values and appropriate interventions.

Urine specimens may be obtained as single random specimens or 24-hour collections. Random specimens are obtained to measure proteinuria. Specimens should be clean-catch and show greater than +2 on two samples at least 6 hours apart (or a single specimen from catheter collection). Protein readings are designated as follows:

0	
Trace	
+1	30 mg/dl (equivalent to 300 mg/L)
+2	100 mg/dl
+3	300 mg/dl
+4	Over 1000 mg (1 g)/dl

Urine output is assessed for volume of at least 100 ml/4 hours. A 24-hour specimen is collected to measure creatinine and protein clearance

Nursing Diagnoses

Medical management of preeclampsia requires the coordinated efforts of the entire health care team. Nursing actions will be derived from medical management, physician's directives, and nursing diagnoses. Examples of relevant nursing diagnoses include the following:

"Mild" Preeclampsia

Knowledge deficit related to

- Preeclampsia and its effects on mother and infant
- Management (diet, bed rest)

Ineffective individual/family coping related to
- Mother's restricted activity and concern over a complicated pregnancy
- Mother's inability to work outside the home

Moderate and Severe Preeclampsia

Sensory/perceptual alterations related to
- Preeclampsia

Potential for injury to mother or fetus related to
- Therapy or eclampsia

Altered cardiopulmonary tissue perfusion related to
- Preeclampsia or its complications (DIC, pulmonary edema, seizures)

Planning

Planning care follows medical diagnosis, choice of home or hospital management, and the woman's and family's resources. A plan is developed mutually with the client, if possible, and should be individualized and related specifically to the needs of the client and her family.

Goals for care include the following:

1. Woman will receive early adequate prenatal care and nutrition to minimize chances of developing preeclampsia and eclampsia
2. Woman and newborn will suffer no adverse sequelae to preeclampsia or its management

Implementation

The development of preeclampsia causes anxiety in the woman and her family. There is a threat to the well-being of the mother and her unborn child, and the family's expectations about pregnancy and delivery must be altered. Such disruption in a family constitutes a crisis. The physical nature of the crisis requires the beneficial use of modern technology. The woman and her family's perception of the disease process, the reasons for it, and the care received will affect their compliance with and participation in therapy. The family will need to use coping mechanisms and support systems to help them through the experience. A plan of care for the woman suffering from severe preeclampsia is superimposed on the nursing care all women need during labor and delivery.

Teacher/Counselor/Advocate

The most effective therapy is ***prevention.*** Sachs et al (1987) "observed an association between the receipt of little or no antenatal care and higher maternal (morbidity and) mortality rates. Measures should be taken to improve public education and access to antenatal care." Nutrition counseling, referral to community resources, mobilization of support systems, and information about normal adaptations to pregnancy are essential components of care.

Encouragement of ***early identification*** and reporting of symptomatology of physical danger signs during pregnancy (Chapter 10, p. 253) is an essential component of client teaching during pregnancy. The nurse's skills in health assessment for etiologic factors and symptomatology of preeclampsia cannot be overestimated.

Home Management

The most effective therapy for preeclampsia is preventing progression of the condition. Management at home can be satisfactory if the preeclampsia is mild and fetal growth retardation is not a problem. Home therapy includes twice-weekly medical and nursing assessment, encouraging the client to participate in the care, dietary modifications, and bed rest. Application of the nursing process to at-home care of a woman with mild preeclampsia is presented in the general nursing care plan that follows on p. 647. This care is given in addition to the general care needed in pregnancy.

❑ HOSPITAL CARE FOR SEVERE PREECLAMPSIA

Severe preeclampsia is diagnosed when one or more of the following are present (Weinstein, 1986): (1) blood pressure of at least 160 mm Hg systolic or 110 mm Hg (MAP 127 or more) diastolic on two readings 6 hours apart; (2) proteinuria of ≥ 5 g/24 hours; (3) oliguria (<400 ml in 24 hours); (4) cerebral or visual disturbances; and (5) pulmonary edema or cyanosis.

The woman may also be hospitalized for lesser degrees of hypertension but with any of the following: (1) proteinuria of 1+ or more; (2) increasing edema, (3) persistent or severe headache; (4) nausea and vomiting; and (5) epigastric pain.

Severe preeclampsia represents an obstetric emergency. Immediate and continuous care by the obstetric team is mandatory to prevent maternal and fetal morbidity or mortality.

The woman is admitted to either the delivery suite or to a private room on the antepartum or postpartum unit. The room must be close to staff and emergency drugs, supplies, and equipment. Noise and external stimuli must be minimized.

The extensiveness of health assessment on admission is governed by the severity of the woman's condition.

General Nursing Care Plan

HOME MANAGEMENT OF PREECLAMPSIA

ASSESSMENT	NURSING DIAGNOSIS (ND), PLAN/GOAL (P/G)	RATIONALE/ IMPLEMENTATION	EVALUATION
Risk factors: Primigravida (<15 to >35). Multifetal gestation. Diabetes mellitus. Rh incompatibility. Renal disease. Chronic hypertension. Over 20 weeks gestation. Diet deficient in protein and calories.	ND: Knowledge deficit related to condition. P/G: Woman does not develop preeclampsia.	*Knowledge about condition allows the woman and her family to become participants in care and to reduce stress:* Assess risk factors at initial and subsequent prenatal visits. Include support person or family in discussions of problems and rationale for treatment	Woman verbalizes understanding of information presented. Woman states she will come to all prenatal visits as scheduled.
Symptomatology: Sudden weight gain. Generalized edema. Increase in blood pressure *over baseline:* Systolic: 30 mm Hg. Diastolic: 15 mm Hg. Proteinuria.	ND: Potential for injury: fetus and mother related to hypertension, vasospasm, decreased GFR, and edema. P/G: Woman's preeclampsia remains in control.	*Knowledge increases woman's and family's ability to assess and monitor the condition, therefore the nurse will teach her to:* Assess weight every day—watch for an increase of 2 or more pounds per week. Monitor fluid intake and urine output. Observe for pitting edema of lower extremities, tight rings, shoes, facial puffiness. Use dipstick for assessment of proteinuria.	Woman reports weight, urine output, results of urine dipstick, and edema to nurse every day.
Knowledge of symptomatology. Readiness to learn. Ability to learn content (as influenced by effects of illness on medications, language barrier, age, or experience, or innate intelligence).	ND: Knowledge deficit related to severity of preeclampsia and effects on mother and fetus. P/G: Woman knows signs and symptoms and has a printed list readily available to her and her family members; promptly reports symptomatology to health care provider.	*Recognize central nervous system (CNS) symptomatology:* Blurred vision. Headaches. Nausea and vomiting. Hyperreflexia. Convulsions. *Hepatic symptoms:* Epigastric pain (right upper quadrant). *Urinary output:* Proteinuria >2+. Oliguria. *Fetal distress:* Decreased fetal activity. Changes in fetal activity. *Abruptio placentae:* Vaginal bleeding or spotting. Uterine tenderness. Change in fetal activity. Abdominal pain.	Woman (family) demonstrates understanding of information presented. Woman (family) tests urine several times per day. Woman experiences diuresis. Fetal kick count is ≥6/hr on two 1-hour evaluations each day. Woman keeps scheduled appointments. Woman verbalizes understanding of information presented. Woman reports any problems immediately.

General Nursing Care Plan—cont'd

ASSESSMENT	NURSING DIAGNOSIS (ND), PLAN/GOAL (P/G)	RATIONALE/ IMPLEMENTATION	EVALUATION
Woman overweight or undernourished. Excessive sodium intake. Inadequate protein and caloric intake. Financial status. Cultural/religious influences. Pitting edema.	ND: Altered nutrition: less than or more than body requirements. P/G: Woman follows prescribed diet. ND: Potential intravascular fluid volume deficit related to protein loss and fluid shifts to the extravascular space. P/G: Woman maintains adequate intravascular fluid volume.	*Nutritional status is a therapeutic measure:* Provide nutrition counseling re: intake of sodium chloride ("salt"), protein, calories; re: physician's orders; re: personal and family preferences, budget, and storage and preparation facilities.	Woman keeps a diet history. Woman verbalizes understanding of limiting excessively salty foods. Woman follows prescribed diet. Woman's hematocrit remains within normal limits (i.e., no evidence of hemoconcentration).
Home situation: resources that would permit woman to be on bed rest and to restrict activity. Woman needs help around house. Knowledge of stress reduction techniques. Other children in the home.	ND: Activity intolerance related to the disease process. P/G: Woman (family) implements home care as prescribed.	*Bed rest is a therapeutic measure:* Teach woman importance of remaining in bed. Teach relaxation. Act as a client advocate and put family in touch with community support systems. Assess family and internal support systems.	Woman remains on bed rest, left side as much as possible. Woman uses relaxation techniques with success. Arrangements are made for help with house and any other children in family.

An assessment guide appears in the box below. Weight is taken on admittance and every day thereafter. An indwelling urinary catheter facilitates monitoring of renal function and effectiveness of therapy. If appropriate, vaginal examination reveals the state of the cervix. Abdominal palpation establishes uterine tonicity and fetal size, activity, and position. Electronic monitoring of the mother and fetus is initiated to determine fetal status. The nurse's skill in implementing the techniques described can be reassuring to the woman and her family.

CLINICAL ASSESSMENT GUIDE FOR PREECLAMPSIA

Record woman's response to "How do you feel?"
Complete head-to-toe assessment
Describe facies, affect, and level of consciousness (LOC)
Auscultate chest; listen for moist respirations or cough
Observe and note location of edema
Record temperature, blood pressure, and weight
Auscultate FHR; assess rhythm and quality
Assess fetal activity
Check urine amount and protein level
Test and record DTRs
Assess onset of labor
Record amount of fluid intake and urinary output
Record medication, dosage, and time of administration
Assess cardiac status (murmur, circulation)

Commonly bed rest is ordered. The nurse's ingenuity may be called on to help the woman cope physically and psychologically with the side effects of immobility. Thromboembolic events, which are a risk factor during normal pregnancy, pose an even greater risk with preeclampsia.

Control of Blood Pressure. The diastolic blood pressure should not be permitted to consistently exceed 100 mm Hg (Iams, 1990). If this occurs, IV hydralazine in 2.5 to 5 mg IV-bolus doses is given. If additional hydralazine is needed after two doses, it is administered by a constant infusion pump in which 100 mg of hydralazine is instilled into a plastic bag containing 200 ml of saline. Infusion rate is dictated by the blood-pressure level and should be monitored by a pulse Doppler blood pressure cuff. If a blood pressure cuff is used for an obese woman, use a thigh cuff.

The *standard of care in the United States* is the use of magnesium sulfate to control convulsions and the use of hydralazine (Apresoline, Neopresol) to control blood pressure.

Other drugs can also be used in pregnancy hypertension. These include methyldopa (Aldomet) and propranolol (Inderal). Diuretic agents are not used because they may adversely effect the fetus. No evidence exists that either diuretics or antihypertensive agents prevent the development of preeclampsia.

Prevention of Eclampsia and Use of Magnesium Sulfate

One of the important goals of care for the woman with severe preeclampsia is preventing or controlling convulsions. **Magnesium sulfate,** an anticonvulsant and smooth muscle relaxant, is given to prevent convulsions. It is not a hypotensive drug. Benefits include an increase in uterine blood flow to protect the fetus and an increase in prostacyclins to prevent uterine vasoconstriction (Iams and Zuspan, 1990).

Magnesium sulfate may be given intravenously (IV) or intramuscularly (IM). Various dosage schedules are used. For example, an initial IV dose of 4 g of magnesium sulfate in 250 ml of 5% dextrose in water may be given (infused *slowly* at a rate of 5 ml/30 sec). Then, 4 to 5 g IM may be given in each buttock (1% procaine may be ordered added to the solution to reduce the pain of injection). When magnesium sulfate is given *intramuscularly,* levels are adequate during the first 1 to 2 hours of administration, but inadequate for the next 3 to 4 hours (Sibai, 1987). The IM dose can be followed at 4-hour intervals with IM doses of 4 to 5 g.

When magnesium sulfate is given *intravenously,* the effect is immediate. A therapeutic serum level (4 to 8 mg/dl) is usually maintained by a constant infusion of 2 g/hr (Anderson, 1987; Sibai, 1987). Early symptomatology of toxicity includes nausea, feeling of warmth, flushing, muscle weakness, and slurred speech.

Magnesium sulfate interferes with neuromuscular impulse transmission, resulting in muscle relaxation. It reduces blood pressure by splanchnic vasodilatation; therefore severe hypotension can occur. The woman's blood pressure should be monitored continuously while the drug is being administered intravenously and every 15 minutes at other times.

Urinary output must be closely monitored because magnesium sulfate both increases sodium retention and is excreted by the kidneys. Hourly urinary output must be measured when magnesium sulfate is administered intravenously. ***The woman's urinary output must total at least 100 ml every 4 hours.*** If output is less, the physician should be notified. Toxic drug levels can occur. If adequate output is not maintained the dose should not be repeated.

A retention catheter is inserted if accurate hourly determination of urinary output is warranted. Hourly measurement is necessary when the woman is receiving a medication such as magnesium sulfate or when decreasing urinary output is suspected or actual.

Diuresis within 24 to 48 hours is an excellent prognostic sign. It is considered evidence that perfusion of the kidney is improved as a result of relaxation of arteriolar spasm. With improved perfusion, fluid moves from interstitial spaces to the intravascular bed, and edema is reduced. Diuresis results in weight loss. In the presence of a large urinary output, the dosage of magnesium sulfate may need to be increased to 3 g/hr IV. If the volume of urine is under 100 ml/4 hr, the dosage of magnesium sulfate is reduced. The physician is notified.

Adverse effects of magnesium sulfate also include respiratory paralysis. ***Maternal toxicity has been reached when respirations are fewer than 12/min.*** The drug is withheld if respirations are fewer than 12/min. The woman receiving magnesium sulfate therapy ***should never be left unattended*** because magnesium sulfate toxicity with respiratory arrest may occur.

Maternal toxicity has been reached when reflex activity is absent. It is imperative that the reflexes be checked before and after each injection of magnesium sulfate (see Table 23-2 and Fig. 23-1). If the mother is receiving a continuous IV infusion of magnesium sulfate, patellar and brachial reflexes are assessed every hour (Anderson, 1987; Sibai, 1987).

A response to rise in serum levels of magnesium occurs:

4-8 mg/dl: Therapeutic level
10-12 mg/dl: Reflexes disappear
15-17 mg/dl: Respirations slow (below 12) or respiratory arrest
30-35 mg/dl: Cardiac arrest is possible; total paralysis

The absence of reflexes is a clear sign of toxicity. The drug should be discontinued immediately (Sibai, 1987). Serum levels are obtained every 4 to 6 hours and as needed.

Toxic levels in the fetus cause marked slowing of respirations and hyporeflexia after birth. Sibai (1987) reports that neonatal toxic effects are rare in the healthy term newborn whose weight is within normal range for gestational age. The danger signs for both fetus and mother that are associated with magnesium sulfate toxicity are summarized in the box on p. 650.

Antidote. The antidote for magnesium sulfate toxicity is a calcium salt such as ***calcium gluconate*** or ***calcium chloride.*** A 10 ml vial of the antidote should be kept at the bedside. If needed, it is administered over 3 minutes intravenously and repeated every hour until the respiratory, urinary, and neurologic depression has been alleviated. *The maximum number of injections of a calcium salt is eight injections in a 24-hour period.*

If improvement occurs therapy is continued until labor begins spontaneously. If the fetal age is greater

DANGER SIGNS

Magnesium sulfate Toxicity

1. Sudden hypotension
2. Urinary output less than 25 ml/hr
3. Respiration less than 12/min
4. Hyporeflexia, absence of reflexes
5. Toxic serum levels (p. 649)
6. Sudden decrease in FHR

than 38 weeks with a lecithin/sphingomyelin (L/S) ratio of 2:1 and other indications of fetal maturity, labor may be induced (Chapter 22 and 26). If improvement does not occur or the fetus shows signs of stress, the care for severe preeclampsia–eclampsia is initiated.

Immediate Care of Eclampsia

The immediate care during a convulsion is to ensure a patent airway. Once this has been attained, adequate oxygenation must be provided. If convulsions occur, turn woman onto left side to prevent aspiration of vomitus and supine hypotension syndrome. Insert folded towel, plastic airway, or padded tongue blade into *side* of mouth to prevent biting of lips or tongue and to maintain airway.* Do not insert object to back of throat, since it will initiate the gag reflex. Do not put fingers into woman's mouth; she may bite them involuntarily. Suction food and fluid from glottis or trachea after convulsion ceases. Give $MgSO_4$ (and amobarbital sodium for recurrent convulsions) as ordered (Anderson, 1987). Start an IV with large bore needle if not in position. Administer oxygen by means of face mask or tent after convulsion ceases (masks and nasal catheters cause excessive stimulation) and suctioning is done. Oxygen rate may be up to 10 L/min (as opposed to 3 L/min advocated for continuous O_2 in chronic conditions). Record time and duration of convulsions; include description. Note any urinary or fecal incontinence. Monitor fetus for adverse effects. A transient bradycardia and decreased fetal heart rate variability may be present.

Have the woman's blood typed and matched. Keep the blood available for emergency transfusion; women with eclampsia often develop premature separation of the placenta, hemorrhage, and shock.

Give fluids as directed; record the time, the amount, and the woman's response. Central venous pressure (CVP) or pulmonary arterial wedge pressure (PAWP) (Swan-Ganz catheter) may be required for accurate fluid monitoring in the presence of pulmonary edema or acute renal failure. Hospital protocols vary. Permit nothing by mouth (NPO) if woman is convulsing, or has symptoms of severe preeclampsia. Insert indwelling catheter for accurate measurement of urinary output if one is not in place. Evaluate blood sugar by bedside fingerstick or venous draw every 1 to 8 hours as ordered. Administer glucose solutions as ordered. To correct hypovolemia, crystalloids (0.9% saline or Ringer's lactated solution) are infused intravenously at a rate that maintains a urine output of 30 ml/hr. Record maternal response.

Give medications (e.g., magnesium sulfate) as directed. Monitor and record the woman's response, drugs, dosages, and times given.

A rapid assessment of uterine activity, cervical status, and fetal status is performed. During the convulsion, membranes may have ruptured, the cervix may have dilated, and delivery may be imminent. If delivery is not imminent, once the woman's seizure tendency and blood pressure are controlled, a decision should be made as to whether delivery should take place. The more serious the condition of the woman, the greater the need to proceed to delivery. Delivery is the definitive cure for the disease, and all medications and therapy are merely temporary measures (Iams and Zuspan, 1990). If fetal lungs are not mature and delivery can be delayed for 48 hours, steroids such as betamethasone (Chapter 26) may be given. Induction of labor and vaginal birth or cesarean delivery may be implemented, depending on the mother's and fetus's conditions.

Laboratory tests are ordered to assess for the HELLP syndrome and to have blood typed and cross-matched for packed cells. Other tests include electrolytes, liver function battery, and complete hemogram and clotting profile, including platelets and fibrin split products (to assess for DIC).

The woman may have been incontinent of urine and stool or the membranes may have ruptured during the convulsion; she will need assistance with hygiene and a change of gown. Oral care with a soft toothbrush may be of comfort to her.

The physician or nurse explains procedures briefly and quietly. The woman is never left alone if the condition is severe or if she is receiving magnesium sulfate therapy. The family is also kept informed of management, rationale, and the woman's progress.

Delivery. Preeclampsia–eclampsia and severe hypertensive or renal disease are intensified by the continuation of pregnancy. Termination of gestation is the only practical treatment. The fetus may therefore be premature or otherwise compromised. Eclampsia is controlled before induction of labor is attempted; then

*Check hospital protocol. Many facilities no longer advocate inserting anything into the mouth at this time.

labor is induced (Chapter 26). Analgesia with meperidine (Demerol), 25 to 50 mg, is suggested (Anderson, 1987).

Anesthesia for delivery could be any modality except spinal anesthesia. A spinal anesthetic is contraindicated because of the deranged maternal physiology. Epidural anesthesia under good conditions is possible after adequate hydration, as is general anesthesia. If delivery is vaginal, local anesthesia or pudendal block is satisfactory. If labor cannot be readily induced, cesarean delivery should be performed. Abruptio placentae is associated with 20% of women with preeclampsia. Pediatric staff should be on standby in case the newborn needs resuscitation.

A general nursing care plan for hospital management of severe preeclampsia follows.

General Nursing Care Plan

HOSPITAL MANAGEMENT OF SEVERE PREECLAMPSIA

ASSESSMENT	NURSING DIAGNOSIS (ND), PLAN/GOAL (P/G)	RATIONALE/ IMPLEMENTATION	EVALUATION
Blood pressure, 160/110 or more. Proteinuria, 3 +, 4+. Urinary output, scant, dark color. Weight gain, 2 kg (4 lb) in less than a week. Hematocrit increases (hemoconcentration). Generalized edema.	ND: Potential for injury: maternal and fetal, related to edema, proteinuria, hypertension. P/G: Mother and fetus suffer no adverse sequelae.	*Prompt identification and appropriate treatment will decrease complications:* Keep woman on absolute bed rest in left lateral position with side rails up. Start IV and maintain rate to keep line open. Insert indwelling urinary catheter. Monitor intake and output every hour. Have woman select people she wishes to stay with her; limit other visitors. Maintain calm unhurried approach to care. Give rationale for care.	Woman's symptomatology of preeclampsia regresses. Woman's (family's) stress and anxiety kept to a minimum. Family members are kept informed.
	ND: Altered cardiopulmonary tissue perfusion related to edema and expansion of extravascular fluid. P/G: The woman's intravascular volume and tissue perfusion return to normal.	*Maintenance of cardiac output is essential for maternal and fetal health:* Continue surveillance of blood pressure every hour or more, check for generalized edema, weight, and urinary output, hematocrit, platelets, and SGOT daily or as ordered. Report deviations immediately. Implement physician-ordered therapies.	Woman's hematocrit and other lab values return to within normal limits. Woman experiences diuresis.

Continued.

General Nursing Care Plan—cont'd

ASSESSMENT	NURSING DIAGNOSIS (ND), PLAN/GOAL (P/G)	RATIONALE/ IMPLEMENTATION	EVALUATION
Platelets decrease.	ND: Potential for injury: maternal and fetal, related to undetected hemoconcentration and clotting disturbances. P/G: Woman does not develop coagulopathy.	*Blood clotting factors are necessary to prevent hemorrhage:* Check gums, area around blood pressure cuff for petechiae. Monitor lab work. Prepare to administer blood products. Keep side rails up and padded.	Symptoms improve. Woman does not develop complications.
Epigastric or right upper quadrant pain. Nausea and vomiting. Headaches. Blurred vision. Hyperreflexia. Changes in LOC. Seizures. Retinal detachment. Blindness.	ND: Pain related to stretching of the hepatic capsule or cerebral edema. ND: Potential for injury, maternal and fetal, related to possible seizure activity or aspiration of stomach contents. ND: Sensory/perceptual alterations related to edema, proteinuria, hypertension. P/G: Woman and fetus suffer no adverse sequelae.	*Early identification of complications assists in revising treatment plan:* Control amount of external stimuli. Monitor symptoms. Assess LOC. Assess reflexes and clonus. Report any changes. Implement physician-ordered therapy. Monitor fetus continually.	Seizures are prevented. Woman rests comfortably. Symptoms improve. Woman remains lucid. Eyegrounds do not change.
Presence of crackles (rales). Pulmonary edema. Fetal distress. Late decelerations of FHR.	ND: Impaired gas exchange related to pulmonary edema. P/G: Woman's respiratory function remains within normal limits. ND: Potential for injury: fetus, related to inadequate placental perfusion. P/G: FHR remains stable; fetus born healthy.	Listen periodically to lung sounds. Monitor intake and output closely. Prevent supine hypotensive syndrome: place woman on left side; when on back, raise headrest and place a wedge under right hip. Transfer to perinatal center.	Breath sounds remain within normal limits. Woman remains on side. FHR remains stable.
Levels of creatinine and urea increase. Oliguria (<100 ml/4 hr). Increased proteinuria. Generalized edema. Sudden weight gain.	ND: Altered patterns of urinary elimination related to decreased renal perfusion and GFR. P/G: Woman's urinary elimination remains within normal limits. Diuresis occurs. Proteinuria decreases/stops.	*Renal functions are essential for homeostasis:* Report output of <100 ml/4 hr. Keep accurate intake and output records every hour. Check urine for protein every 4 hours. Send blood specimen to laboratory for measurement of creatinine; check results against previous tests.	Urinary elimination remains within normal limits. Diuresis occurs. Proteinuria decreases. Creatinine remains within normal limits.

General Nursing Care Plan—cont'd

ASSESSMENT	NURSING DIAGNOSIS (ND), PLAN/GOAL (P/G)	RATIONALE/ IMPLEMENTATION	EVALUATION
Administration of magnesium sulfate.	ND: Potential for injury: maternal and fetal, related to magnesium sulfate side effects/toxicity. P/G: Woman suffers no side effects/toxicity.	*Magnesium sulfate is the preferred drug for treatment:* Follow hospital protocol. Check blood levels of magnesium sulfate periodically. Assess reflexes, LOC, and respiratory rate frequently. Keep antidote (calcium salt) on hand.	Further complications from magnesium sulfate administration do not occur.
Woman (couple) anxious. Fearful of injury to fetus. Transferred to perinatal center.	ND: Anxiety related to sudden change in condition. P/G: Woman's (family's) anxiety is minimized. ND: Ineffective individual and family coping related to stress of disease process. P/G: Woman (family) develop increased coping skills.	*Coping mechanisms are individual to the woman and family:* Assess affect, restlessness, anxiety. Assess response to support person. Observe for adverse behavior. Keep woman (couple) informed of progress in simple language. Make sure instructions are consistent.	Woman feels free to express concerns. Support person does not make woman more anxious.
Preterm labor; maternal and fetal condition is otherwise stable.	ND: Potential for injury: fetus, related to preterm birth. P/G: Woman's pregnancy and labor result in a healthy mother and newborn.	*Stress may initiate labor:* Observe woman for progress of labor. Prepare for delivery. Prepare woman (couple) for delivery by answering questions, supplying information and reinforcing information given to her by the physician.	Preterm labor does not occur; or, labor progresses normally. Healthy mother and newborn result.

Evaluation

Care could be evaluated as effective if the following are noted: the woman's condition improves; CNS irritability is reduced; convulsions (if any) are terminated; hypertension is reduced; water imbalance, acid-base imbalance, and other electrolyte imbalances are corrected; proteinuria is reduced, and serum protein level is increased; fetal well-being continues; and placental complications are absent or controlled, and delivery proceeds as previously planned whether vaginal, induced, or cesarean. If the outcome for the mother or newborn is unfavorable, the family is assisted to cope with loss and grief (Chapter 29).

POSTDELIVERY NURSING CARE

The nursing care of the woman who experiences hypertensive disease differs from that required in a normal postpartum period in a number of respects. The following content emphasizes the specific nursing strategies needed by these women.

Assessment

Blood pressure is measured every 4 hours for 48 hours or more frequently as the woman's condition warrants. *Even if no convulsions occurred before delivery, they may occur within this period.* Magnesium sulfate infusion may continue 12 to 48 hours after delivery. The same assessments continue until the drug is discontinued. The woman may also have a boggy uterus and a large lochia flow secondary to the magnesium sulfate therapy. This needs to be closely monitored. Diuresis should occur within 72 hours after birth.

The woman is asked to report headaches, blurred vision, etc. The nurse assesses affect, alertness, or dullness. Blood pressure is reassessed before giving analgesic for headache. NOTE: No ergot products (see Table 21-1) are given because they increase blood pressure.

The woman's and family's responses to labor are monitored. Regular postpartum assessment is performed.

Nursing Diagnoses

Examples might include the following:

Situational low self-esteem related to
- Inability to accept high-risk nature of delivery

Potential anxiety of mother related to
- Initial occurrence of hypertension during puerperium

Potential altered family processes related to
- Stress during high-risk postdelivery period
- Separation from newborn if in newborn intensive care unit.

Planning/Implementation

Postpartum care for the woman with hypertensive disease includes care related to normal involution. The woman may need to continue with medication if her diastolic blood pressure exceeds 100 mm Hg at the time of discharge. In addition the woman and her family need opportunities to discuss their emotional response to complications. The nurse also provides information concerning the prognosis. Preeclampsia–eclampsia does not necessarily recur in subsequent pregnancies, but careful prenatal care is essential.

The nurse reaffirms the physician's advice that evaluation must be thorough during the postdelivery examination to rule out chronic hypertension. The woman needs family planning information (the next pregnancy should be delayed for 2 years; the woman may not be a candidate for oral contraceptive use) (Chapter 6).

Evaluation

The nurse may consider that care was effective if the following are noted: the woman's recovery from preeclampsia is complete *or* woman begins therapy for chronic hypertension not related to pregnancy; her self-concept is not impaired; and the infant is healthy *or* has minimum impairment. The evaluation is recorded on the woman's record so that care remains consistent after discharge.

Maternal Infections

Sexually transmitted diseases and other infections are responsible for significant morbidity. Financial costs are substantial. However, the personal costs of suffering imposed by the disease process and its sequelae cannot be measured. Some consequences persist for a lifetime, such as congenital infection that compromises a child's quality of life, and infertility and sterility. The latter problems are discussed in Chapter 6.

Pregnancy confers no immunity against infection and both mother and fetus must be considered when the pregnant woman carries an infection.

Prevention is particularly important in maternity nursing. Many tragedies can be averted by informed anticipation. For example, vaccination against rubella before pregnancy currently is the only means to control this disorder since there is no cure. Women are becoming more knowledgeable about factors such as infections, which can jeopardize their fertility or fetal development. The large number of infections, the varying responses of the fetus or newborn, and the range of nursing and medical actions necessitate a readily available resource (see also Chapter 28).

❑ SEXUALLY TRANSMITTED DISEASE

Venereal diseases (named after Venus, the goddess of love), now termed **sexually transmitted diseases (STDs)**, often share common characteristics. They have a predilection for genital and perigenital sites, perhaps because of genital pH, temperature, moisture, and hormonal influences. The causative organisms are relatively unstable when removed from their natural habitat. They are either completely or predominantly transferred from one person to another through sexual contact.

Chlamydia Trachomatis

Chlamydial infections are epidemic in the United States. These infections are 3 times more prevalent than gonorrhea and 30 times more prevalent than syphilis. *Chlamydia trachomatis* is the most common sexually transmitted bacterial pathogen in the United States. This pathogen is responsible for substantial morbidity, personal suffering, and heavy economic burden (Washington et al, 1987a,b).

Maternal effects are usually mild. Infection of the cervix may be asymptomatic or evident by appearance of congestion, edema, mucopurulent discharge, dyspareunia, and bleeding. Lymphogranuloma venereum, urethritis, dysuria, acute salpingitis with symptoms of pelvic inflammatory disease (PID), sterility, or infertility may occur. Other conditions include conjunctivitis, sore throat, and perihepatitis.

Fetal or neonatal effects are common. Stillbirth and neonatal death are 10 times more common than in noninfected women. Preterm birth may result. The newborn may acquire the infection by direct contact with an infected birth canal. Newborn infection may be asymptomatic. ***Inclusion conjunctivitis*** occurs in one third of exposed newborns. Conjunctivitis appears after 3 to 4 days. Chronic follicular conjunctivitis with conjunctival scarring and corneal neovascularization contributes to vision sequelae. About 25% of newborns with *Chlamydia* ***pneumonia*** can exhibit symptoms of serious tachypnea, dyspnea, or apnea that require hospitalization (Schachter et al, 1986).

This infection is implicated in *cervical dysplasia* on Papanicolaou smear, in ectopic pregnancy, and in sterility in the female; as well as in genital inflammation and damage to the prostate and sperm in the male.

Populations at risk have been identified (Corbett and Meyer, 1987; Marvin and Slevin, 1987). The sexually active female under 20 years of age is 2 to 3 times more likely to become infected than women between 20 and 29. Women over 30 have the lowest rate. Women and men with multiple sexual partners are at highest risk. People who *do not* use barrier methods of birth control (condom, spermicide, diaphragm) have a higher incidence. In men, the infection is linked to nongonococcal urethritis (NGU).

Ceftriaxone (or amoxicillin with probenecid) initially and tetracycline subsequently is the treatment of choice. Erythromycin is substituted if the woman is sensitive to penicillin or if she is pregnant.

Human Papillomavirus

Condylomata acuminata are sexually transmitted lesions caused by human papillomavirus (HPV). The incidence has increased dramatically in the last few years. There are over 46 HPVs that infect skin and mucosal surfaces. HPV-6 and HPV-11 are among the 15 HPVs known to infect the genital tract. Disease occurs at the site of entry of the virus after an incubation period of 1 to 6 months. *HPV is not disseminated through the bloodstream.* HPV is clinically significant because various types are associated with congenitally derived respiratory papillomatosis in children (Chapter 28) and cervical carcinoma in adult women.

Condylomata acuminata are dry, wartlike growths on the vulva, vagina, cervix, or rectum. They may be small or large, single or multiple, or have a cauliflower appearance. Chronic vaginal discharge, pruritus, or dyspareunia can occur. Diagnosis is by colposcopy and direct visualization of the growths, biopsy, or presence of koilocytes (nuclear abnormalities in squamous cervical epithelium) seen in Papanicolaou smears.

In the immunocompetent person, condylomata acuminata may regress spontaneously. The condition is difficult to treat in many people, however. Available therapy is primarily cytotoxic or destructive. *Cytotoxic* agents are podophyllin (podophyllum resin) and 5-fluorouracil (5-FU). Podophyllin, 20% to 30% in tincture of benzoin, is used for lesions 2 cm or less in diameter, but not in the vagina or on the cervix. Petrolatum is used to protect surrounding skin because podophyllin is caustic and cytotoxic. The woman must wash the medication off after 4 hours or sooner if burning occurs. She is treated weekly for 6 weeks. Therapy may not produce a cure. The recurrence rate is 70%. ***Podophyllin is not to be used during pregnancy.*** The use of podophyllin during pregnancy is associated with fetal death and preterm labor. The more effective cytotoxic agent is 5-FU in 5% cream. This highly toxic agent is used for resistant condylomata. The cure rate approaches 90%. Local pain and epithelial erosions are side effects of local application. Treatment with 5-FU is most effective when used in conjunction with laser therapy.

The most effective *destructive* method utilizes a laser with local anesthesia. It is precise and sterile, and is accompanied by minimum bleeding and trauma. The treated area does not regain its normal pigmentation for several years. Post-laser-therapy instruction follows:

1. Keep area clean by irrigating with warm water twice a day; dry with electric hair dryer.
2. Apply antibacterial cream twice a day.
3. Use gauze dressing to prevent rubbing against clothing.
4. Use lidocaine ointment 5% for discomfort.
5. Return to clinic as instructed.
6. Use latex condoms until disease is cured in the woman. Condoms are dense enough to prevent passage of viruses (500 A° = size of HPV).

Trichloroacetic acid, 50% solution, is a destructive therapy that is somewhat safer to use than podophyllin. It can be self-applied with a cotton swab and does not need to be washed off.

Therapy during pregnancy is determined on an individual basis. About 30% of pregnant women harbor HPV in the genital tract (Ferenczy, 1987). Large, outward-growing lesions on the vulva that may interfere with delivery or episiotomy are usually treated. Laser treatment has been used to treat genital warts between

30 and 32 weeks gestation. Treatment is usually followed by vaginal delivery with no complications (Ferenczy, 1987). Flat lesions do not pose mechanical problems for vaginal delivery. However, they too may be associated with transmission of the virus to the newborn (Chapter 28). The woman is advised of the risk that if she delivers vaginally, her child may be one of the 300 children per year who are diagnosed with recurrent juvenile respiratory papillomatosis (Ferenczy, 1987; Huffman and Blanco, 1987). The woman can make an informed decision concerning vaginal or abdominal birth.

Gardnerella Vaginalis

Gardnerella vaginalis is the type of bacteria implicated in bacterial vaginosis. Diagnosis is based on clinical signs. The vaginal fluid pH is elevated (usually ≥4.5), thus altering the flora. The homogeneous vaginal discharge has an amine (fishy) odor when mixed with 10% potassium hydroxide. "Clue cells" are seen on microscopic examination of vaginal discharge.

The *maternal effect* of infection with this bacteria is usually a mild illness. The bacterial vaginosis is expressed by a milklike discharge. Itching, burning, and pain may be present in the vagina and around the introitus. Obstetric complications can occur, especially in untreated cases. Amniotic fluid infection, premature rupture of membranes (PROM), preterm labor and delivery, and postpartum endometritis have been linked to this infection. *Fetal and neonatal effects* include septicemia and death.

G. vaginalis is transmitted through sexual contact, especially when estrogen levels are high. It is often seen with other infections of the vagina. Because therapy is often a sulfa-based medication (suppository, cream), each woman is assessed for sensitivity to sulfonamides before medication is prescribed.

An 85% to 95% cure rate is achieved with oral metronidazole 500 mg 2 times per day for 7 days. Best results are obtained if the woman and her partner(s) are treated at the same time. Adjunctive topical medication may include metronidazole, sulfonamides, povidone-iodine, or chlorhexidine.

Gonorrhea

Gonorrhea ("clap," "drip") is caused by *Neisseria gonorrhoeae,* a type of diplococci bacteria. Although gonorrhea is an STD, it is also spread by direct contact with infected lesions and **fomites.** Self-inoculation with contaminated hands is common. Secretions on fomites such as washcloths, towels, bed linens, and clothing are often implicated. Thus this bean-shaped gram-negative organism is responsible for genitourinary, anorectal, oropharyngeal, and systemic infections.

Gonorrhea often is only mildly symptomatic in women, or the diplococci may persist unsuspected in the lower genital tract. Symptomatology of lower urogenital tract infection includes dysuria and frequency, heavy green-yellow purulent discharge at the cervical os, cervical tenderness, vulvovaginitis, bartholinitis, dyspareunia, and postcoital bleeding. Swollen and painful Bartholin's glands and tenderness in the lymph nodes in the groin usually accompany infection. In 10% to 15% of cases, the upper urogenital tract is affected in the later stage of infection. Lower abdominal pain, cervical tenderness, fever, nausea, and vomiting are accompanying symptoms. Adnexal abscess and pelvic tenderness indicate PID. PID is implicated in ectopic pregnancy or sterility. Chronic pelvic pain and low backache may be seen. Anorectal infection is diagnosed by local inflammation, burning, and pruritus. Oropharyngeal infection may be asymptomatic or result in inflammation and sore throat. Systemic infection results in gonococcemia, skin rashes, arthritis, pericarditis, and meningitis. Gonococcal perihepatitis (Fitz-Hugh and Curtis syndrome) is discussed in Chapter 24.

Maternal effects are seen. After the third month of pregnancy, gonorrheal salpingitis rarely occurs. Postdelivery maternal complications of untreated gonorrhea include gonococcal endometritis, acute salpingitis, dermatitis, and arthritis.

Neonatal effects include ***ophthalmia neonatorum*** and pneumonia. Ophthalmitis with partial or total blindness can occur. Neonatal sepsis is characterized by temperature instability, hypotonia, poor feeding, and jaundice.

Prevention is achieved by limiting the number of sexual partners; using barrier contraception, including nonoxynol-9 spermicide; and avoiding oral-genital sexual activity. The incubation period is 2 to 5 days. In the woman, the early stage may be asymptomatic. In addition, 5% of women with gonorrhea also have syphilis.

The woman and her sexual partner(s) must be treated simultaneously to prevent reinfection (the ping-pong effect). Gravid women allergic to penicillin can be given erythromycin or spectinomycin; nongravid women can be given cephalosporins and kanamycin. Erythromycin is contraindicated in women with liver disease.

After therapy the woman is advised to abstain from sexual intercourse or to have her partner(s) use condoms until cultures are negative at two consecutive follow-up visits. Oral-genital sex especially should be avoided.

Syphilis

Syphilis ("lues") is caused by the spirochete, *Treponema pallidum,* after an incubation period of several weeks. The spirochete is responsible for chancre, condylomata lata, cardiovascular disease, neurologic disease, and congenital syphilis.

Nonspecific serologic tests for nontreponemal antigens used for screening purposes are of two types: complement fixation (Kolmer, Wasserman) and flocculation (Kahn, RPR [rapid plasma reagin], VDRL [Venereal Disease Research Laboratories]). Any test for antibodies may be negative in the presence of active infection because it takes time for the body's immune system to develop antibodies to any antigen.

Fetal and neonatal effects are seen. Syphilis probably continues to be a major cause of late abortion throughout the world, despite widespread success of diagnosis and treatment of this disease. Primary and secondary stages of untreated syphilis lead to stillbirth. Latent and tertiary stages of untreated syphilis lead to secondary syphilis (congenital syphilis) in the newborn.

Congenital syphilis occurs when the spirochetes cross the placenta after the sixteenth to eighteenth week of gestation. The following sequelae are seen: snuffles (rhinitis), rhagades (cracks, fissures around the mouth), hydrocephaly, and corneal opacity. A symmetric rash may appear anywhere over the body, including palms of hands and soles of feet. Later, saddle nose, saber shin, Hutchinson's teeth (notched, tapered canines), and diabetes develop in untreated children. There are no residual effects if the mother is treated adequately before the fifth month of gestation. Destruction of tissue that occurs before treatment cannot be reversed, but additional tissue destruction is prevented by adequate treatment.

Therapy for syphilis includes the following possible regimens (Corbett and Meyer, 1987; Tramont, 1987): penicillin G benzathine, tetracycline if allergic to penicillin, or erythromycin if unable to take penicillin or tetracycline. However, there is a steady flow of treatment failures. One possible reason may be developing organism resistance (Guinan, 1987). A second reason may be an alteration in the immune status of the infected person (Tramont, 1987). Neurologic complications of syphilis have developed in persons infected with acquired immunodeficiency syndrome (AIDS).

TORCH Infections

Toxoplasmosis, other infections (e.g., hepatitis), rubella virus, cytomegalovirus, and herpes simplex viruses, known collectively as **TORCH infections,** comprise a group of organisms capable of crossing the placenta and adversely affecting the development of the fetus.

Toxoplasmosis manifests itself as an acute infection similar to influenza. During the initial interview, the nurse asks if the woman has been exposed to cats and possibly infected litter boxes; or eats poorly cooked meats (e.g., lamb, beef, pork). If so, a serum titer is drawn to determine infection. Should the titer continue to rise, the woman may wish to consider therapeutic abortion. Newborn effects may include parasitemia if the mother has an acute infection.

Hepatitis B virus is passed through contaminated needles or blood transfusion. Because of potential adverse effects on the mother and fetus/neonate, it is suggested that all pregnant women be routinely screened in the prenatal period for hepatitis B surface antigen (HB_SAG). The results will indicate if the woman has active disease, is a carrier, or has developed immunity. If the fetus is exposed to hepatitis in the first trimester, anomalies may develop. If no treatment is received, up to 90% of newborns may become chronic carriers (Towers, 1987). The treatment consists of hepatitis B immune globulin (HBIG) and hepatitis B vaccine (Heptavax-B) given intramuscularly soon after birth. The newborn must be washed thoroughly before any injections are given to prevent infection from surface contaminants. Although HB_SAG has been found in human milk, breastfeeding is considered safe as long as the newborn has received the above treatment. Vaccination is recommended for any population at risk, including health care workers.

Rubella, or German measles, still poses a significant risk to both mother and newborn. A detailed discussion of this infection can be found in Chapters 5 and 28.

The fourth TORCH infection is ***cytomegalovirus (CMV).*** This disease is transmitted sexually or via the respiratory tract. The mother may show no symptoms or a mononucleosis-like syndrome. The fetus suffers more damage. Fetal death or severe generalized disease may result. This includes hemolytic anemias, hydrocephalus or microcephalus, and pneumonitis.

Herpes Simplex Virus

Herpes simplex completes the list of TORCH infections. Herpes simplex virus type 1 (HSV-1) infections predominate during childhood. The virus is transmitted primarily by contact with *oral* secretions and causes cold sores and fever blisters. HSV-2 infections usually occur after puberty with sexual activity. HSV-2 is transmitted primarily by contact with *genital* secretions. Although it has been shown that HSV can survive for many hours on objects like doorknobs, faucets, and toilets, people are not likely to be infected by contact with such objects.

HSV interacts with epithelial or neuroepithelial cells and neurons. The incubation period is between 2 and 4 weeks. During the initial infection, HSV migrates to one or more sensory nerve ganglia, where it remains latent and dormant indefinitely (Fig. 23-2 *A*). An intact immune system cures the infection at the portal (place of entry). The *primary* infection involves mucocutaneous cells; recurrent infection involves stratified epithelial cells. Stressor stimuli trigger recurrent infection (Fig. 23-2, *B*). Fever, another infection, emotions, menstruation, and ultraviolet light are some common stressors. Infections seem to be more severe in the woman during pregnancy.

HSV is diagnosed by cytologic testing and microscopic examination of cells obtained from a Papanicolaou smear.

HSV infections may involve external genitals, the vagina, and cervix. Symptomatology is more pronounced with first infections of HSV. Painful blisters form, rupture, and then drain, leaving shallow ulcers that crust over and disappear after 2 to 6 weeks. A vaginal discharge is seen if the cervix or vaginal mucosa is involved. The woman may experience fever, malaise, anorexia, painful inguinal lymphadenopathy, dysuria, and dyspareunia.

Recurrences are sometimes preceded by itching, a burning sensation in the genital area, tingling in the legs, or a slight increase in vaginal discharge. Repeated recurrence may result in keratitis, encephalitis, and possibly cervical carcinoma. Symptomatic therapy is available. No specific cure has been identified.

Maternal effects include preterm labor and the possibility of cesarean delivery. The Committee on Fetus, Newborn and Infectious Diseases of the American Academy of Pediatrics proposed guidelines for delivery of women with HSV (Table 23-3). For asymptomatic women, vaginal samples can be taken at birth. Test results are available in a few days. If results are positive, staff and parents can be vigilent for signs of neonatal illness. Early intervention in the disease greatly boosts chances of survival.

Fetal and neonatal effects are serious. Abortion and preterm birth occur. Transplacental infection is rare but the consequences are serious. Microcephaly, men-

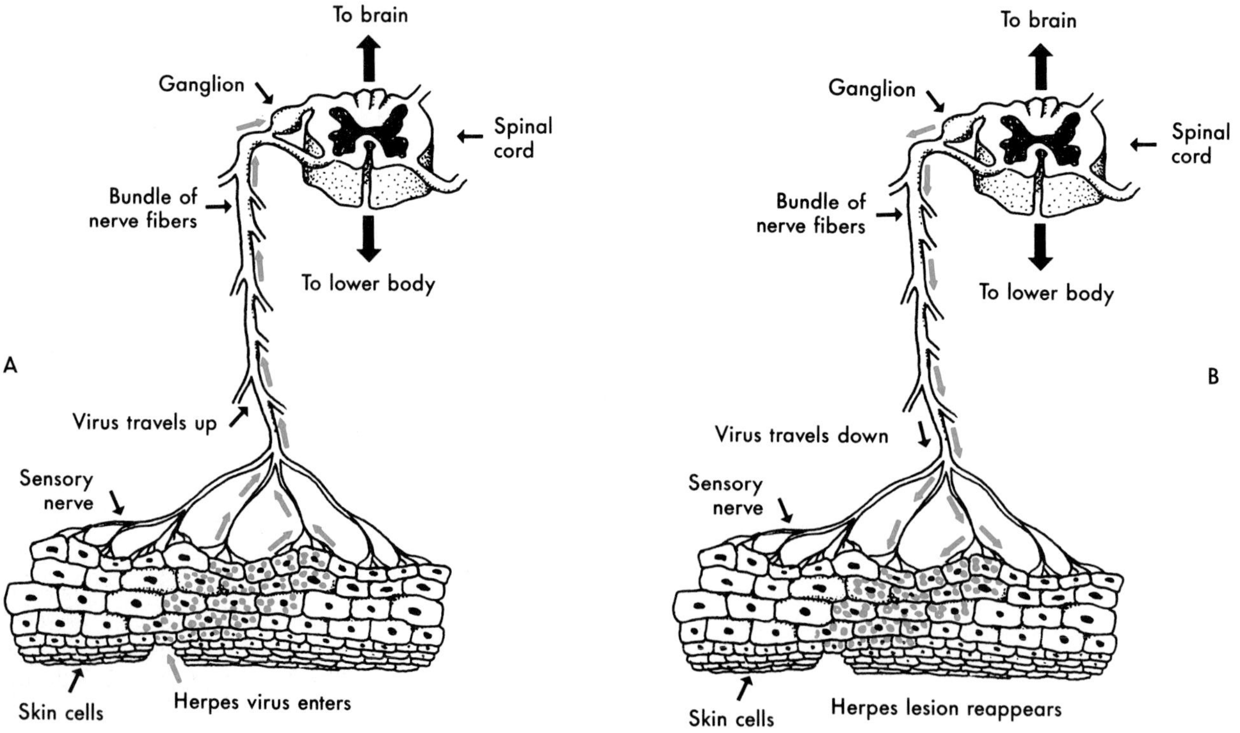

Fig. 23-2 **A,** Initial herpes infection takes place when virus (colored dots) enters cells of mucous membranes, eyes, or skin. They reproduce and travel up (colored arrows) the sensory nerves until they reach a ganglion (cluster of nerve cell bodies). There they are protected from the body's immune system, which overcomes the infection at the place of entry. **B,** Though the entry wound soon heals, when conditions allow, the virus may later travel back down the nerve pathway to reinfect skin cells again.

Table 23-3 Guidelines for Delivery of Women with Herpes genitalis

Maternal Condition	Risk of Transmission	Mode of Delivery	Postpartum Placement: Mother	Postpartum Placement: Newborn
Virologic or cytologic studies are negative 1 week before delivery	Low	Vaginal	Private room	Nursery permissible
Cervical lesion present *or* culture is positive *and* membranes intact or ruptured less than 4 hours before	Low	Abdominal (cesarean)	Private room	Room-in with mother
Cervical lesion present or culture is positive and membranes ruptured more than 4 hours before	High (regardless of mode of delivery)	Vaginal	Private room	Room-in with mother

tal retardation, retinal dysplasia, patent ductus arteriosus, and intracranial calcification are sequelae. After intranatal infection, signs appear in 4 to 7 days. The signs include lethargy, poor feeding, jaundice, bleeding, pneumonia, convulsions, opisthotonus, bulging fontanels, and skin and mouth lesions. Neonatal infection with disseminated disease results in 82% mortality. Survivors suffer central nervous system (CNS) or ocular sequelae and usually have a recurrence in the first 5 years of life. According to the Centers for Disease Control (CDC) (1986) substantial numbers of intrauterine or postpartum infections occur and cannot be prevented by cesarean delivery.

Counseling. Good hygiene and prevention of transmission of infection are of extreme importance. The woman should also be taught comfort measures to deal with the pain of outbreaks. Pouring warm water over the urethra and vulva or urinating through an empty toilet paper tube is helpful in preventing pain during urination. Comfort can be increased with warm sitz baths for 15 minutes at a time with a drying agent such as Domeboro (two packets or tablets to a shallow tub of warm water) 3 to 5 times daily or cold milk baths or soaks with aluminum acetate (Burow's Solution) 1:20. Strong deodorant soaps, creams, and ointments should be avoided. Drying the genital area with a blow dryer after washing is useful. Only 100% cotton underwear should be worn. The woman is advised to avoid tight-fitting jeans and pants or pantyhose with nylon inserts. Physical and mental health is important. Being rundown makes anyone more vulnerable to infection.

Frequent intercourse with numerous male partners without using a barrier contraceptive exposes the cervix to multiple sperm specimens and infections with HSV or HPV. The combination of these events is thought to be carcinogenic, therefore yearly Papanicolaou smears are advisable. Any sexual contact should be avoided during the entire time that lesions are present. Using condoms and spermicides for 6 weeks after the lesions disappear will help prevent the spread of HSV (p. 667).

Drug therapy is limited. Acyclovir (Zovirax) is the first drug approved by the Food and Drug Administration (FDA) for treatment of HSV. It may be administered orally, intravenously, or as a topical ointment. It is most effective for primary lesions. Researchers are seeking a herpes vaccine.

Infection control measures start with good handwashing by the nurse and family. Gloves should be worn when touching lesions or their secretions. Hospital and home areas occupied by the mother need routine cleaning. A family member with an oral lesion is cautioned against kissing the newborn; masks may be appropriate. The family is reassured that strict personnel policies are used. Any health care provider or family member with an oral HSV lesion or skin lesion (herpetic whitlow) should not give care to a mother or newborn until the lesion is dried and crusted to avoid **nosocomial** (hospital-acquired) infection.

❑ VAGINAL INFECTIONS

Any irritating vaginal discharge should be evaluated promptly and appropriate treatment initiated immediately. Management of vaginal infections becomes more complicated if multiple organisms or agents are involved. Pediculosis pubis, threadworm, varicosities, and allergic response to perineal deodorants may obstruct the differential diagnosis and management. The discomforts imposed by these conditions challenge the woman's emotional, as well as her physical, well-being.

Infections must be distinguished from the normal vaginal discharge, leukorrhea. ***Leukorrhea*** is a whitish discharge. It consists of mucus and exfoliated vaginal epithelial cells secondary to hyperplasia of the vaginal mucosa such as occurs during pregnancy, at the time of ovulation, and just before menstruation. If it is copious, it can cause discomfort from maceration.

Vaginal infections may be sexually transmitted. Trichomonal vaginitis and monilial vaginitis are considered to be sexually transmitted in most, but not all cases. Simple vaginitis may be attributed to faulty hygiene, tight clothing, or emotional stress.

Simple Vaginitis

Infectious organisms such as *E. coli*, staphylococci, and streptococci change the normal acidity of the vagina. A pH of 3.5 to 4.5 is needed to support Döderlein's bacilli, the vagina's main line of defense. The proximity of the urethra to the vagina predisposes the woman with vaginitis to a concurrent urethritis.

Burning, pruritus (itching), redness, and edema of surrounding tissues are characteristic of simple vaginitis. These symptoms are particularly discomforting during voiding and defecating.

Objectives of management of simple vaginitis are to relieve discomfort, to foster growth of Döderlein's bacilli, to eradicate offending organisms, and to prevent recurrence. Interventions may include maintaining scrupulous cleanliness, especially after elimination, and taking (or applying) medications as ordered.

Cervicitis

Abnormal discharge may be the result of an infection of the cervix and not due to vaginitis. Spotting of blood between periods or after intercourse, and cramping during intercourse are characteristic. Sexually transmitted gonorrhea, chlamydia, trichomoniasis, or herpetic infection is the usual infection implicated. Therapy is specific to the causative microbe.

Monilial Vaginitis

Candida albicans, a fungus (yeast) normally found in the intestinal tract, contaminates and infects the vagina. Infection with *C. albicans* is also known as moniliasis, thrush, or candidiasis. This infection is seen commonly in women with poorly controlled diabetes mellitus, since the organism thrives in a carbohydrate-rich milieu. Antibiotic or steroid therapy will reduce the number of Döderlein's bacilli and thus can cause monilial vaginitis. Döderlein's bacilli help maintain an acidic pH.

The thick vaginal discharge is irritating and pruritic (severe itching). Commonly dysuria and dyspareunia (painful intercourse) are complaints. Speculum examination reveals thick, white, tenacious cheese-like patches adhering to the pale, dry, and sometimes cyanotic vaginal mucosa.

Scrupulous cleanliness, especially after elimination, is essential. Miconazole nitrate 2% vaginal cream is preferred during pregnancy. Cotton underwear or pantyhose with a cotton crotch should be used. Nylon fabric retains too much heat and stops air from circulating; this supports growth of the fungus. The woman is advised to abstain from intercourse or use a condom until the infection is cured. Women with recurrent infection should be checked for diabetes mellitus, and control of diabetes should be instituted if required (Chapter 24).

C. albicans also causes thrush in the newborn. Infection may occur by direct contact with an infected birth canal or from the contaminated hands of those who take care of the newborn.

Trichomonas Vaginitis

Trichomonas vaginalis (trichomoniasis) is a hearty protozoan that thrives in an alkaline milieu. In symptom-free individuals the infection may be identified during a routine examination or with a Papanicolaou smear.

The profuse, bubbly (foamy), white leukorrhea characteristic of this infection causes irritation, hyperemia, edema of the vulva, and dyspareunia (painful intercourse). Urinary frequency and dysuria may occur. In the male partner the protozoan may be harbored in the urogenital tract (without symptoms) and remain a source of reinfection for his mate.

❑ GENERAL INFECTIONS

Many infections place the woman at risk during the childbearing cycle. Following are some maternal infections the nurse may encounter.

Parvovirus. Parvovirus is a deoxyribonucleic acid (DNA) virus that is common in 30% to 50% of the adult population and has been shown to increase fetal mortality (Samra, Obhrai, and Constantine, 1989). Transmission is possibly by respiratory secretions, blood, and blood products (CDC, 1989). The common form is known as erythema infectiosum, fifth disease, or B19 infection (Helmstrom, 1990). In adults it may cause headache, sore throat, and a rubella-like rash, or it can induce aplastic crisis in people with sickle cell disease.

Since women may ignore the symptoms at first, this diagnosis may be difficult to determine. The virus does cross the placenta and infect the fetus. The disease can lead to severe anemia in the fetus, congestive heart failure, fetal hydrops, and death (Thurn, 1988; Chorba and Anderson, 1989). Bernstein and Capeless (1989) have found that monitoring the maternal serum alphafetoprotein and serial ultrasound determinations may identify fetal problems. No vaccine to prevent it or medication to treat it is available (Mead, 1989). Treatment for the mother is symptomatic to relieve general discomfort; the fetus may require an intrauterine blood transfusion to treat the anemia.

Coxsackievirus B. This virus may cause mild illness in the *mother*. It is responsible for death, cardiovascular anomalies, myocarditis, and meningoencephalitis in the *fetus*.

Chickenpox (Varicella). *Maternal effects* vary. The infection may appear as herpes zoster (shingles). The severe disseminated epidemic type of varicella during pregnancy may be fatal for the mother (and fetus) because of necrotizing angitis (inflammation of blood and lymph vessels). Mothers may be screened at the initial prenatal visit for antibodies to varicella. If negative (passive immunity), varicella zoster immune globulin (VZIg) may be given, although the expense may outweigh the benefits (Gershon, 1988).

Fetal and neonatal effects are also seen. Abortion or fetal death may occur. Infected newborns may exhibit defects of skin, bone, and muscle; chorioretinitis; or hydrocephalus. Newborn effects are rare, although approximately 2% of those infants exposed in utero will have congenital varicella (Gershon, 1988); other infants may develop chickenpox if maternal chickenpox rash occurred 5 days or less before delivery. The infant can be treated with VZ1g vaccine and sent home with careful instruction to the mother and close follow-up for the next 5 to 10 days. A vaccine of live attenuated varicella to provide active immunity is now available.

Group B β-hemolytic Streptococcus. Group B β-hemolytic streptococcus is a type of bacteria that can cause *maternal effects* of septicemia, cellulitis (erysipelas), fever, puerperal infection, impetigo, scarlet fever, and abortion. It is estimated that 20% of pregnant women are colonized with group B β-hemolytic streptococcus (Gotoff, 1988). The organism is acquired by the newborn via ascending infection from the infected vagina. Early detection and treatment of the disease may prevent newborn consequences such as sepsis or death (Gotoff, 1988).

Listeriosis. Listeriosis is caused by a gram-positive bacterium, *Listeria monocytogenes*. This organism is harbored in the vagina or cervix by 4% of pregnant women. The woman with listeriosis may exhibit influenza-like symptoms. It occurs most commonly in summer or fall. Other symptoms include vaginitis, urinary tract infection, and enteritis. *Fetal and neonatal effects* are serious. This infection may result in preterm delivery or abortion. Amnionitis or placentitis is evidenced by dirty brown amniotic fluid. With neonatal infection, generalized skin rash and meningitis are seen. Pneumonia carries a 50% mortality. Meningitis, which appears most often in term males, may appear later in the neonatal period. Treatment with penicillin or erythromycin is usually successful. Unfortunately the diagnosis of listeriosis is often obscure or delayed; hence the prognosis for the fetus or newborn generally is poor. Effects may include death within 2 to 12 hours of birth, blindness, deafness, spinal meningitis, mental retardation, and learning or behavior problems in survivors. Penicillin is the drug of choice.

Influenza. Influenza is caused by a virus. *Maternal effects* can be serious if complicated by pneumonia. Abortion and preterm labor may result. *Fetal and neonatal effects* include death, preterm birth, and occasionally, anencephaly or meningomyelocele. If the woman is not pregnant, she may be given polyvalent influenza virus (attenuated live virus) vaccine.

Lyme Disease. Lyme disease is spread by tick bites. The disease, caused by a spirochete *Borrelia burgdorferi*, is a multisystem inflammatory disease. It may damage the fetus if maternal infection is not diagnosed and treated (Williams and Strobino, 1990). Three documented cases of maternal-fetal transmission resulted in stillbirth (1) or neonatal deaths (2) within 39 hours of birth. The Centers for Disease Control reported a study of 19 women who had Lyme disease during pregnancy. Five (26%) of the 19 pregnancies had an adverse outcome: stillbirth, preterm birth, syndactyly, cortical blindness with developmental delay, and rash. Although none of these outcomes could definitely be linked to Lyme disease, no other causes were implicated (Markowitz et al, 1986). Most obstetricians treat pregnant women who have tick bites and suggestive symptoms (skin lesion, arthritis, arthralgia, neurologic and cardiac manifestations) agressively with an antibiotic regimen lasting several weeks (Williams and Strobino, 1990).

Tick repellents containing diethyltoluamide (DEET) should be used only after careful consideration and then with great caution, because they have been associated with convulsions in children who've had repeated application to the skin. Use during pregnancy should be based on assessment of both risks and benefits and avoided if possible, just as one attempts to minimize exposure to any toxic products. If temporary protection is essential, spraying the repellent on clothing alone is advised (Williams and Strobino, 1990). Further information may be obtained from the National Lyme Borreliosis Foundation, Box 462, Tolland, CT, 06084 (203)871-1900.

❑ URINARY TRACT INFECTIONS

Urinary tract infection (UTI) affects about 10% of pregnant women, most of these in the prenatal period. Approximately one third of those who have had UTIs previously will develop them again during pregnancy. Cervicitis, vaginitis, obstruction of the flaccid ureters (particularly on the right because of pressure by the pregnant uterus against the slightly dilated flaccid ureters), vesicoureteral reflux, and the trauma of delivery predispose pregnant women to UTI, generally from *E. coli.* Asymptomatic bacteriuria occurs in about 5% to 15% of all pregnant women. If untreated, pyelonephritis during gestation will develop in approximately 30% of these women. UTI has been implicated as an etiologic factor in preterm labor and birth.

Urine culture and sensitivity tests should be obtained early in pregnancy, preferably at the first visit, from a clean-catch urine specimen. Catheterization should be avoided if possible. If infection is diagnosed, treatment with an appropriate antibiotic drug for 2 to 3 weeks, together with forced fluids and urinary tract antispasmodic medication (e.g., belladonna derivatives) is recommended. Infections caused by the colon aerogenic organisms generally respond well to sulfisoxazole (Gantrisin) or nitrofurantoin. Treatment should be continued for 2 to 3 weeks until two negative cultures are obtained, and the infant, when born, should be observed for hyperbilirubinemia (Chapter 28). Retreatment of the mother may be necessary if there is a recurrence.

Pyelonephritis

Pyelonephritis is caused by a bacterium. Some maternal infections are asymptomatic. Acute pyelonephritis is distinguished by urinary frequency, urgency, pyuria, dysuria, chills, fever, backache, nausea, and vomiting. Costovertebral angle tenderness and tenderness over the affected kidney are experienced. *Fetal and neonatal effects* are serious. Acute pyelonephritis commonly is associated with preterm labor (Scott et al, 1990). The newborn is then exposed to the hazards of prematurity.

Treatment with penicillin or cephalosporin and adequate hydration are warranted. Therapy with sulfonamides may cause icterus, hemolytic anemia, and kernicterus. The newborn may also be at risk as a result of intrauterine growth retardation (IUGR). Nitrofurantoin therapy for the mother during pregnancy may lead to megaloblastic anemia or glucose-6-phosphate dehydrogenase (G6PD) deficiency in the newborn. The women who are most vulnerable to UTI are primigravidas, women with difficult labors, and women with diabetes or sickle cell disease.

❑ PUERPERAL INFECTION

Puerperal infection (puerperal sepsis or "childbed fever") is any clinical infection of the genital canal that occurs within 28 days after abortion or delivery. Puerperal sepsis occurs after about 6% of deliveries in the United States.

An episiotomy or lacerations of the vagina or cervix may open avenues for sepsis. Even more formidable, however, may be the large placental site. Here the denuded endometrium (decidua basalis) and residual blood after parturition make the uterus an ideal site for a wound infection. The virulence of infecting organisms, the woman's resistance to them, and the rapidity and specificity of therapy determine the efficacy of treatment. Fortunately body defenses generally limit the disease in most instances. Puerperal infection probably is the major cause of maternal morbidity and mortality throughout the world.

The most common infecting organisms are the numerous streptococcal and anaerobic organisms. Fulminating epidemic puerperal sepsis classically is caused by the group B β-hemolytic streptococcus. The less virulent anaerobic streptococci may be responsible for other puerperal infections, however. *Staphylococcus aureus,* gonococci, coliform bacteria, and clostridia are less common but serious pathogenic organisms causing puerperal infection.

Commonly the infection is complicated by medical disorders such as anemia, malnutrition, or diabetes mellitus. Obstetric problems, including premature rupture of membranes (PROM), a long, exhausting labor, instrument delivery, hemorrhage, and retention of the products of conception, increase the likelihood and severity of puerperal sepsis.

An *endometritis,* usually at the placental site, permits infection to begin. Localized infection may be followed by salpingitis, peritonitis, and pelvic abscess formation. (Tubal occlusion after salpingitis is a common cause of infertility.) Septicemia may develop. Secondary abscesses may arise in distant sites such as the lungs or liver. Pulmonary embolism or septic shock, often with disseminated intravascular coagulation (DIC), from any serious genital infection may prove fatal. Postdelivery femoral thrombophlebitis ("milk leg") may result in a swollen, painful leg.

Clinical Findings. The symptomatology of puerperal infection may be mild or fulminating. Any fever, that is, ***a temperature of 38° C (100.4° F) or more on 2 successive days, not counting the first 24 hours after delivery,*** must be considered caused by puerperal infection in the absence of proof of another cause.

General malaise, anorexia, chills, or fever may begin as early as the second postdelivery day. Perineal discomfort or lower abdominal distress, nausea, and vomiting may soon develop. Foul or profuse lochia, hectic fever, tachycardia, ileus, pelvic pain, and tenderness characterize critical puerperal sepsis. Without improvement, bacteremic shock or death may ensue.

Laboratory Findings. Considerable ***leukocytosis, a shift to the left*** of the differential white blood cell (WBC) count and a markedly increased red blood cell (RBC) sedimentation rate are typical of puerperal infections. Anemia, often an accompaniment, is evidenced by reduced RBC, hemoglobin, and hematocrit values. Intracervical or intrauterine bacterial cultures (aerobic and anerobic) should reveal the offending pathogens within 36 to 48 hours.

The physician must distinguish nongenital from genital sepsis. Mastitis, respiratory and urinary tract infections, and enteritis are considered in that order of probability.

Management

The most effective and cheapest treatment of puerperal infection is prevention. Preventive measures might include good prenatal nutrition to control anemia and intranatal control of hemorrhage. Good maternal hygiene is essential. Strict adherence by all medical personnel to the best aseptic techniques during the entire hospital and delivery period is mandatory. Coitus after rupture of membranes is contraindicated. Dystocia or prolonged labor should be avoided, especially after leaking of amniotic fluid. Traumatic vaginal delivery must be avoided, blood loss replaced, and fluid-electrolyte balance maintained.

Infection measures for cure and comfort are instituted. Fluid and electrolyte balance is vital. Broad-spectrum antibiotics are administered intravenously until the infecting organism is identified. Then organism-specific antibiotic therapy is begun. The mother and infant are separated during the febrile period. Other members of the family are encouraged to nurture the newborn. Isolation protocol of the agency is warranted.

Surgical measures may be required. These include surgical procedures such as curettage to remove the retained products of conception, hysterectomy (if the uterus is ruptured), colpotomy to drain a pelvic abscess, or ligation or clipping of the vena cava and ovarian veins to prevent septic embolism.

The virulence of the organisms, the resistance of the woman, and her likely response to treatment are the intangibles of prognosis. Prevention, supportive therapy, and prompt massive antibiotic administration have reduced the maternal mortality in the United States to less than 0.4%. Regrettably, in developing countries the death rate may be more than 10 to 20 times this figure.

❑ MASTITIS

Mastitis, or breast infection, affects about 1% of recently delivered women, most of whom are primiparas who are breastfeeding. Mastitis is almost always unilateral and develops well after the flow of milk has been established. The infecting organism generally is the hemolytic *S. aureus*. An infected nipple fissure usually is the initial lesion, but the ductal system is involved next. Inflammatory edema and engorgement of the breasts soon obstruct the flow of milk in a lobe; regional, then generalized mastitis follows. If prompt resolution of the septic process does not occur, a breast abscess is virtually inevitable. Almost all instances of acute mastitis can be avoided by proper breastfeeding technique.

Chills, fever, malaise, and local breast tenderness are noted first. Eventual localization of sepsis and axillary adenopathy are delayed developments. Intensive antibiotic therapy (such as cephalosporins and vancomycin, which are particularly useful in staphylococcal infections), support of breasts, local heat (or cold), and analgesics are required. Breastfeeding may continue. If an abscess develops, wide incision and drainage must be done. Lactation is maintained (if desired) by emptying the breasts every 4 hours by manual expression or breast pump. Most women respond to treatment, and an abscess can be prevented.

A general nursing care plan for maternal infections follows on p. 664.

❑ TOXIC SHOCK SYNDROME

Toxic shock syndrome (TSS) is a potentially life-threatening systemic disorder that has three principal clinical manifestations: ***fever of sudden onset*** (over 38.9° C [102° F]), ***hypotension*** (systolic pressure <90 mm Hg; orthostatic dizziness; disorientation), and ***rash*** (diffuse, macular erythroderma). The erythematous macular desquamating rash is most prominent on palms and soles. The acute phase to TSS lasts about 4 to 5 days; the convalescent phase, about 1 to 2 weeks.

A toxin secreted by strains of *S. aureus* is the causative factor in TSS. About 9% of women harbor the organism normally in their vaginas. Poor perineal hygiene and lack of handwashing before touching the perineal area may increase risk. Commonly associated conditions that may predispose the person to TSS by providing a portal of entry into systemic circulation include menstruation, chronic vaginal infection (e.g., herpes), puerperal endometritis, and use of high-absorbency tampons or barrier contraceptives (e.g., sponge, diaphragm) (Berkley et al, 1987; Wolf et al, 1987).

Mortality is associated with TSS. In order of incidence the three causes of mortality are (1) adult respi-

General Nursing Care Plan

MATERNAL INFECTION

ASSESSMENT	NURSING DIAGNOSIS (ND), PLAN/GOAL (P/G)	RATIONALE/ IMPLEMENTATION	EVALUATION
Prenatal: History of UTIs, vaginal infections. Assess whether the woman has any specific risk factors for infection (population, geographical). Physical assessment: 1. Fever, malaise. 2. General affect. 3. Signs and symptoms of infection: rash. Laboratory tests: 1. Urinalysis. 2. Blood tests (Hgb, Hct, antibody titers, syphilis, HIV antibodies, diabetes). 3. Cultures: gonorrhea, etc.	ND: Potential for injury related to infection (maternal and fetal). ND: Altered patterns of urinary elimination related to UTI. ND: Altered skin integrity related to introduction of infection. P/G: Woman will seek prompt treatment for signs and symptoms of infection. P/G: Woman will follow treatment regimen.	*Early identification and treatment of the disease will help protect mother and fetus:* Note and evaluate any complaints suggestive of infection (past and present). Implement universal precautions to protect self and others from spread of infection. Assist physician and support woman and family during tests and when test results are explained. Explain necessity of taking all antibiotic tablets as ordered. Viral infections are treated symptomatically. Suggest comfort measures that will help relieve discomfort. All over-the-counter (OTC) preparations must be approved by a physician. Explain preterm labor precautions and effects on fetus.	Infection is prevented or treated promptly with no or minimum sequelae to mother or newborn.
Assess woman's knowledge about infection, its signs and symptoms, treatment and potential sequelae.	ND: Knowledge deficit related to infection, its treatment, and possible sequelae. ND: Altered family processes related to interruption of sexual relations. ND: Body image disturbance, situational low self-esteem, altered role performance, and personal identity disturbance related to contagious infection. ND: Anxiety related to spread of infection.	*Education will help the woman understand the infectious process and provide self-care:* Review the signs and symptoms of infection. Explain general care issues: 1. Adequate hydration. 2. Rest. 3. Adherence to medication regimen. 4. Control of fever with fluids, cool bath, and acetaminophen (Tylenol). 5. Well-balanced diet. 6. Personal hygiene.	Woman learns the signs and symptoms of infection. Woman learns how to treat and manage her infection. Woman learns how to prevent spread of infection to others. Woman verbalizes understanding of necessary isolation precautions.

General Nursing Care Plan—cont'd

ASSESSMENT	NURSING DIAGNOSIS (ND), PLAN/GOAL (P/G)	RATIONALE/ IMPLEMENTATION	EVALUATION
	ND: Fear related to possible fetal sequelae. P/G: Woman will verbalize signs and symptoms, treatment, and possible sequelae of infection. P/G: Woman will verbalize how to prevent spread of infection to others. P/G: Woman and family will verbalize change in relationship relative to disease and express positive self-image.	Clarify misconceptions. Help woman formulate questions for physician. Assist woman in preparation to inform partner of infection and any necessary treatment. Teach woman how to prevent spread of infection. Explain any isolation precautions necessary by the health care team to prevent spread of infection. Encourage verbalization of concerns and fears. Assist with counseling before proposed therapeutic abortion.	
Postnatal: Assess all prenatal and intrapartal data. Physical assessment: 1. Newborn—assess for symptomatology of infection. 2. Mother—vital signs, general affect, malaise, rash, lymph gland enlargement; redness, tenderness, warmth, pain over a specific area. Laboratory tests: culture of any exudate, blood tests for infection, urinalysis.	ND: Potential for injury related to infection. ND: Altered patterns of urinary elimination related to UTI. P/G: Woman and infant will experience minimum or no sequelae after treatment of infection.	*Interventions are interdependent with the physician:* Obtain specimens ordered for laboratory testing. Administer medications as ordered (medications for symptomatic relief or antibiotics). Ensure adequate rest, nutrition, and fluids. Provide high-risk care to infant.	Infection is treated promptly with no or minimum sequelae for mother and infant.
Assess knowledge regarding infection: prevention, identification, treatment.	ND: Knowledge deficit related to infection. P/G: Woman will learn how her infection is identified and managed.	*Education will help the woman understand the infectious process and implications for herself and her newborn:* Review possible sequelae from infection that she or her newborn might experience. Counsel regarding breastfeeding (some infections are transmitted in breast milk). Encourage questions and clarify misconceptions. Teach woman the importance of following the treatment regimen and the need for follow-up. Assist woman and family with grieving if indicated.	Woman learns about prevention, identification, and management of infection.

Continued.

General Nursing Care Plan—cont'd

ASSESSMENT	NURSING DIAGNOSIS (ND), PLAN/GOAL (P/G)	RATIONALE/ IMPLEMENTATION	EVALUATION
Assess need for isolation precautions for mother and newborn.	ND: Potential for injury related to possible spread of infection to others. ND: Altered parenting related to fear of spreading infection to newborn. P/G: Woman will remain in isolation to prevent potential spread of infection.	*It is the nurse's responsibility to help prevent spread of infection to others via cross-contamination:* Isolate mother and newborn if necessary. Teach mother how to prevent the spread of infection to her newborn. Encourage mother-infant interaction while reinforcing isolation guidelines. Institute universal precautions and strict handwashing technique. Screen visitors for possible infections (chickenpox, measles, etc.) and restrict as needed.	Spread of infection is prevented. Mother interacts with child while maintaining isolation protocol.

ratory distress syndrome (ARDS), (2) uncontrollable hypotension, and (3) DIC. Survivors may suffer adverse sequelae. Some women have persistent abnormalities in intellectual function. Persistent problems include impaired memory, concentration, and calculation ability; abnormal electrocardiogram (ECG); and impaired cerebellar function (**hyperreflexia**). For a few women sequelae are more serious. Impaired renal function, neuromuscular function (vocal cord paralysis), and peripheral perfusion, especially of the hands and feet, may persist after the infection is cured.

❑ BACTEREMIC SHOCK

Critical infections, particularly by bacteria that liberate endotoxin, such as enteric gram-negative bacilli, may cause **bacteremic** (septic) **shock.** Pregnant women, especially those with diabetes mellitus, or women who are receiving immunosuppressive drugs, are at increased risk of having this disorder.

High spiking fever and chills are evidence of serious sepsis. Anxiety is followed by apathy. Concomitantly the temperature often falls to slightly subnormal levels. The skin then becomes pale, cool, and moist. The pulse will be rapid and thready. Marked hypotension and peripheral cyanosis develop. Oliguria occurs.

Laboratory studies reveal marked evidence of infection (blood culture may reveal bacteremia later). Hemoconcentration, acidosis, and DIC may develop. Central venous pressure (CVP) generally is low. Electrocardiogram (ECG) may reveal changes indicative of myocardial insufficiency. Evidence of cardiac, pulmonary, and renal failure will be notable. Hypoxia is the major problem, however. Hypoxia is especially noxious to the CNS, myocardium, and lungs.

The physician will initiate antishock therapy. Massive doses of antibiotics and corticosteroids are given intravenously if possible. The woman may be given digitalis. Heart function and urinary output are monitored closely. The infected area is drained or the focus of infection is removed (for example, by hysterectomy or abortion) if the woman's condition will permit.

Prompt diagnosis and intensive treatment afford a fairly good prognosis. Encouraging signs include increasing alertness and the establishment of good urinary flow.

❑ ACQUIRED IMMUNODEFICIENCY SYNDROME (AIDS)

Transmission of human immunodeficiency virus (HIV), a retrovirus, occurs primarily through the exchange of body fluids (e.g., blood, semen, perinatal events) (Friedland and Klein, 1987; Hecht, 1987;

Laudesman et al, 1987). Severe depression of the cellular immune system characterizes acquired immunodeficiency syndrome (AIDS) (Chapter 5). Although the populations at high risk have been well-documented, *all* women should be assessed for the possibility of having been exposed to HIV. AIDS in women is commonly reported at a later stage in the disease and they usually enter the hospital for initiation of treatment when the illness is more severe. The delay may be due in part because women may have symptoms different from those of men (Shaw, 1986). Chronic vaginitis is a common presenting problem.

Delay in diagnosis must be avoided when the woman is pregnant. Exposure to the virus has a significant impact on the woman's pregnancy and newborn feeding method and on the newborn's health status (Klug, 1986). The HIV from infected women is transmitted in three ways (Friedland and Klein, 1987; Landesman et al, 1987):

1. To the fetus as early as the first trimester through maternal circulation
2. To the fetus/neonate during labor and delivery by inoculation or ingestion of maternal blood and other infected fluids
3. To the infant through breast milk

Regardless of whether AIDS is diagnosed, the nursing process is implemented in a culturally sensitive and humane manner. "HIV infection is a biologic event, not a moral comment. It is vital to remember, to model, and to teach that (personal) reactions to particular life-styles, practices, or behaviors must not influence (the nurse's) ability to provide objective, compassionate, and effective health care to all" (Keeling, 1987).

Prenatal Period

The incidence of AIDS in pregnant women is expected to increase (Minkoff, 1987a). The health history, physical examination, and laboratory testing must reflect this expectation if women and their newborns are to receive appropriate care. Women who fall into the high-risk category for AIDS should be retested for HIV antibodies late in the third trimester (Minkoff, 1987a). Prenatal testing for conditions associated with AIDS may help identify the woman with AIDS (Foster, 1987; Minkoff, 1987a; Rhoads et al, 1987): gonorrhea, syphilis, prolonged and persistent episodes of herpes, *C. Trachomatis,* hepatitis B, *Mycobacterium tuberculosis,* candidiasis (oropharyngeal or chronic vaginal infection), CMV, and toxoplasmosis. About half of AIDS sufferers have elevated CMV titers. Because CMV inclusion disease poses a serious hazard to the fetus, pregnant women are advised to avoid direct contact with AIDS sufferers.

History of vaccinations and immune status is documented. The titers for chickenpox and rubella are determined, and tuberculosis skin testing (purified protein derivative [PPD]) is done. Previous vaccination with Recombivax HB vaccine (Merck) is noted. (This vaccine is now free of association with human blood or blood products.)

The woman may be a candidate for receiving *Rh_oD immune globulin.* Transmission of HIV has not been traced to the Rh vaccine. The preparation process involves ethyl alcohol, which inactivates the virus. The vaccine is made from blood drawn from an identified group of regular donors. New blood tests that can detect evidence of HIV are used on blood used to produce the vaccine (Francis and Chin, 1987; MMWR, 1987).

Some prenatal discomforts (e.g., fatigue, anorexia, and weight loss) mimic signs and symptoms of HIV infection. Differential diagnosis of *all* "pregnancy-induced" complaints and symptomatology of infections is warranted.

To support any pregnant woman's immune system, appropriate counseling is provided for optimum nutrition; sleep, rest, exercise; and stress reduction. If AIDS is diagnosed, the woman is advised of the possible consequences for her infant. The woman is supported in her decision. Should she choose to continue the pregnancy, she is counseled regarding ***"safe sex"*** techniques. Use of condoms and nonoxynol-9 spermicide is encouraged to minimize further exposure to HIV if her partner(s) is the source. Orogenital sex is discouraged. Cates and Lloyd-Schulz (1988) have found that 67% of AIDS in women are related to the use of drugs by the woman or her partner. As necessary, the woman is referred for drug rehabilitation to discontinue substance abuse. Abuse of alcohol, amphetamines (speed, crack), marijuana, nitrites (poppers, amyl), or other drugs compromises the body's immune system and increases the risk for AIDS and associated conditions:

1. HIV may require the presence of an already damaged immune system before it can cause disease
2. Alcohol and drugs interfere with many medical and alternative therapies for AIDS
3. Alcohol and drugs affect the judgment of the user, who may become more prone to engage in activities that put people at high risk for AIDS or increase exposure to HIV
4. Alcohol and drug abuse causes stress, including sleep problems, which harms immune system functioning

Intrapartum Period

Care of the parturient is not substantially altered by asymptomatic infection with HIV (Minkoff, 1987a).

The mode of delivery is based on obstetric considerations. The mode of delivery is not an issue because the virus crosses the placenta early in pregnancy.

The primary focus is the prevention of nosocomial spread of HIV and the protection of care providers. The risk of transmission of HIV is considered to be low during vaginal delivery despite the exposure to the infected woman's blood, amniotic fluid, and vaginal secretions. (See precautions for invasive procedures, p. 671).

External electronic fetal monitoring (EFM) is preferred if EFM is needed. There is a possibility of inoculation of the virus into the newborn if fetal scalp blood sampling is done or if a fetal scalp electrode is applied. In addition, the one who performs either of these procedures, is put at risk by accidental sticks to the finger.

Postpartum Period

Little is known of the clinical course of the postpartum period for the woman infected with HIV. While the immediate postpartum period has not been noted to be remarkable (Update, 1987), longer follow-up has revealed a high frequency of clinical illness in mothers whose children develop disease (Scott, 1985; Minkoff et al, 1987b,c).

The newborn can be with the mother, but breastfeeding is contraindicated. Universal precautions are implemented for mother and newborn, as they are with all clients. The woman and her infant are referred to physicians who are experienced in the treatment of AIDS and associated conditions. See specific nursing care plan, p. 669.

❑ INFECTION CONTROL

Infection control measures are essential to protect care providers and prevent nosocomial infection of clients, regardless of the infectious agent. The risk of occupational transmission varies with the disease. Even if that risk is low, as it is with HIV, that any risk exists is significant to warrant *reasonable* precautions.

Precautions against airborne disease transmission are available in all health care agencies. **Universal precautions** from the CDC follow.

Universal Precautions

Since medical history and examination cannot reliably identify all people infected with HIV or other blood-borne pathogens, blood and body-fluid precautions should be consistently used for all people. This approach, previously recommended by CDC and referred to as "universal blood and body-fluid precautions" or "universal precautions," should be used in the care of ***all*** people, especially including those in emergency-care settings in which the risk of blood exposure is increased and the infection status of the person is usually unknown.

1. All health care workers should routinely use appropriate ***barrier precautions*** to prevent skin and mucous-membrane exposure when contact with blood or other body fluids of any person is anticipated. *Gloves* should be worn for touching blood and body fluids, mucous membranes, or non-intact skin of all persons, for handling items or surfaces soiled with blood or body fluids, and for performing venipuncture and other vascular access procedures. *Gloves should be changed after contact with each client. Masks and protective eyewear or face shields should be worn during procedures that are likely to generate droplets of blood or other body fluids to prevent exposure of mucous membranes of the mouth, nose, and eyes. Gowns or aprons* should be worn during procedures that are likely to generate splashes of blood or other body fluids.

2. Hands and other skin surfaces should be ***washed*** immediately and thoroughly if contaminated with blood or other body fluids. Hands should be washed before and immediately after gloves are removed.

3. All health care workers should take precautions to ***prevent injuries*** caused by needles, scalpels, and other sharp instruments or devices during procedures; when cleaning used instruments; during disposal of used needles; and when handling sharp instruments after procedures. *To prevent needlestick injuries,* needles should not be recapped, purposely bent or broken by hand, removed from disposable syringes, or otherwise manipulated by hand. After they are used, disposable syringes and needles, scalpel blades, and other sharp items should be placed in puncture-resistant containers for disposal; the puncture-resistant containers should be located as close as practical to the use area. Large-bore reusable needles should be placed in a puncture-resistant container for transport to the reprocessing area.

4. Although saliva has not been implicated in HIV transmission, to minimize the need for ***emergency mouth-to-mouth resuscitation,*** mouthpieces, resuscitation bags, or other ventilation devices should be available for use in areas in which the need for resuscitation is predictable.

5. ***Health care workers*** who have exudative lesions or weeping dermatitis should refrain from all direct client care and from handling client care equipment until the condition resolves.

6. ***Pregnant health care workers*** are not known to be at greater risk of contracting HIV infection than health care workers who are not pregnant; however, if a health care worker develops HIV infection during preg-

Specific Nursing Care Plan

POSTPARTUM WOMAN WITH HEPATITIS B, POSSIBLY AIDS, AND A URINARY TRACT INFECTION (UTI)

Ann is a 26-year-old, single female who is admitted to the postpartum unit after delivering a 2464 g (5½ lb) boy with Apgar scores of 7^1, 8^5 via an uncomplicated spontaneous vaginal delivery. Ann admits to a history of IV drug abuse and was hospitalized at 20 weeks gestation for hepatitis B. On that admission, Ann stated that she had been sharing needles for her drug habit. Ann denies the use of any drugs since her last hospitalization and is currently active in a drug rehabilitation program.

During Ann's initial interview to the labor floor, she complained of having recent night sweats, as well as frequency and urgency of urination. HIV—pending; drug screen—pending; urine culture—pending; urinalysis—specific gravity 1.015; pH 8.0; glucose—negative; protein—negative; blood—large; ketone—negative; WBC—many; bacteria—many.

ASSESSMENT	NURSING DIAGNOSIS (ND), PLAN/GOAL (P/G)	RATIONALE/ IMPLEMENTATION	EVALUATION
Former IV drug abuser (or present?) Hepatitis B at 20 weeks gestation. Night sweats. Assess knowledge of isolation precautions.	ND: Potential for injury related to spread of infection. ND: Knowledge deficit related to isolation guidelines. ND: Situational low self-esteem related to isolation precautions and infection. P/G: Ann will be treated without spread of infection to others. P/G: Ann will verbalize understanding of isolation precautions.	*Protection of Ann, family, and staff from risks of potential infection is essential to prevent further spread of infection:* Implement universal precautions. Stress hand washing. Prevent needle/sharps injury. For blood spills, use sodium hydrochloride solution (household bleach). Ann may visit child in special care nursery. Ann may not breastfeed at this time as a result of suspected AIDS. Explain the isolation precautions implemented and answer any questions or concerns Ann might have. Blood and specimens should be double bagged or sealed in an impervious container labeled "blood/body fluids precautions." Equipment and linens soiled with body fluid should be discarded or double bagged and labeled before being sent for decontamination. Immunologically-compromised staff should not care for Ann.	Spread of infection is prevented. Ann verbalizes understanding of isolation procedures and their purpose. Ann demonstrates understanding and acceptance of isolation. Ann learns appropriate methods for feeding and caring for her infant. Ann demonstrates no loss of self-esteem or self-worth. Family supports Ann.

Continued.

Specific Nursing Care Plan—cont'd

ASSESSMENT	NURSING DIAGNOSIS (ND), PLAN/GOAL (P/G)	RATIONALE/ IMPLEMENTATION	EVALUATION
		Provide education and support for family and staff.	
Complains of frequency and urgency during urination. Urine culture pending. Urinalysis: alkaline and concentrated; hematuria; WBC—many; bacteria—many. Assess knowledge about identification and treatment of a UTI. Assess knowledge about prevention of UTI.	ND: Potential for injury related to UTI. ND: Altered patterns of urinary elimination related to UTI. ND: Knowledge deficit related to identification and treatment of a UTI. P/G: Ann's UTI will be resolved by discharge. P/G: Ann will adhere to treatment regimen. P/G: Ann will void 300 to 400 ml every 3 hours.	*If left untreated, UTIs may lead to further complications:* Encourage fluids (especially cranberry juice, if she is not being treated with sulfa-based medications.) Administer medications as ordered and evaluate results. Evaluate for systemic symptoms (malaise, fever, etc.) Note and report flank pain to physician. Explain importance of taking all prescribed medications. Encourage Ann to seek follow-up care if frequency and urgency persist or recur after discharge. Teach preventive measures.	Ann's UTI is treated promptly and she does not experience any potential sequelae. Ann resumes normal pattern of urinary elimination. Ann verbalizes understanding of importance of following treatment regimen for a UTI. Ann does not experience recurrence of UTI.
Assess Ann's understanding and acceptance of her infections and needed therapy. Newborn status.	ND: Spiritual distress related to infections and possible consequences. P/G: Ann will come to terms with her condition.	*Emotional support combined with physical support assist the healing process:* Teach Ann about her infections, their course, identification, treatment or possible sequelae. Answer questions Ann has regarding her diagnosis, condition of her infant, or any concerns or feelings she wishes to express. Refer to follow-up care agency if seropositive for HIV. Assess Ann's relationship with infant and short- and long-term family plans.	Ann retains or develops a sense of self-esteem and self-worth. At subsequent visits in clinic or home Ann continues to demonstrate: Use of appropriate precautions for control of and prevention of spread of infection. Self-esteem and self-worth.

nancy, the newborn is at risk of infection resulting from perinatal transmission. Other infections that are associated with HIV (i.e., CMV) can be contracted and cause harm to the fetus. Because of this risk, pregnant health care workers should be especially familiar with and strictly adhere to precautions to minimize the risk of HIV transmission.

Precautions for Invasive Procedures

An invasive procedure is defined as surgical entry into tissues, cavities, or organs or repair of major traumatic injuries (1) in an operating or delivery room, emergency department, or out-of-hospital setting; including both physicians' and dentists' offices; and (2) a vaginal or cesarean delivery or other invasive obstetric procedure during which bleeding may occur. The universal blood and body-fluid precautions listed above, combined with the precautions listed below, should be the minimum precautions for ***all*** such invasive procedures.

1. All health care workers who participate in invasive procedures must routinely use appropriate barrier precautions to prevent skin and mucous-membrane contact with blood and other body fluids of all clients. Gloves and surgical masks must be worn for all invasive procedures. Protective eyewear or face shields should be worn for procedures that commonly result in the generation of droplets, splashing of blood or other body fluids, or the generation of bone chips. Gowns or aprons made of materials that provide an effective barrier should be worn during invasive procedures that are likely to result in the splashing of blood or other body fluids. *All health care workers who perform or assist in vaginal or cesarean deliveries should wear gloves and gowns when handling the placenta or the newborn until blood and amniotic fluid have been removed from the infant's skin. They should also wear gloves during post-delivery care of the umbilical cord.*

2. If a glove is torn or a needlestick or other injury occurs, the glove should be removed and a new glove used as promptly as client safety permits; the needle or instrument involved in the incident should also be removed from the sterile field.

According to staff members in the AIDS unit at San Francisco General Hospital, treatment precautions by health care providers are the same as those for the care of people with hepatitis B (p. 657). These precautions for health care providers and the nonpregnant people who come in contact with AIDS sufferers support those described above. In addition the following is appropriate: wash washable surfaces and used equipment with a solution of sodium hypochlorite (household bleach) and water—1 cup of household bleach to 9 cups of water. Remove blood or other fluids before disinfection to avoid neutralizing the bleach solution.

Maternal Hemorrhagic Disorders

Hemorrhagic disorders in pregnancy are medical emergencies. They require expert teamwork on the part of physician and nurse to minimize the deleterious effects.

The nurse must be alert to the symptoms of hemorrhage and shock and be prepared to act quickly to minimize blood loss and hasten return to normal state.

Early in pregnancy, abortion or ectopic pregnancy is the most common cause of excessive bleeding. Later, premature separation of the normally implanted placenta or placenta previa may be the cause of hemorrhage.

Postdelivery hemorrhage is a possibility during any childbirth experience. Specific problems that result in hemorrhage are uterine atony, lacerations of the birth canal, hematomas, episiotomy dehiscence, retained placenta, inversion of the uterus, and subinvolution of the uterus. Postdelivery anterior pituitary necrosis (Sheehan's syndrome) secondary to hypovolemic shock is also discussed.

❑ EARLY PREGNANCY

Spontaneous Abortion

Spontaneous abortion is the termination of pregnancy, before viability, from natural causes. Viability is reached at about 24 weeks gestation, when the fetus weighs 600 g (1lb 5oz) or more. With today's technology for newborn care, such an infant has at least a chance to survive. An ***early spontaneous abortion,*** or miscarriage, is one that occurs before 16 weeks gestation; a ***late abortion*** is one occurring between 16 and 24 weeks gestation. About three fourths of these abortions occur before the sixteenth week of pregnancy, and the majority of these take place before the eighth week. More than half of all spontaneous abortions are caused by fetoplacental developmental defects. Most of the other spontaneous abortions result from maternal causes; the reasons for the remainder are speculative. Many early pregnancies are lost for unknown reasons before the diagnosis of pregnancy is even made.

Recurrent (habitual) spontaneous ***abortion*** is the loss of three or more previable pregnancies. The causes of recurrent early abortion may include (1) endocrine imbalance (e.g., diabetes mellitus), (2) infections (e.g., bacteriuria, and *C. trachomatis*), (3) systemic disorders (e.g., lupus erythematosus), (4) psychologic factors (but proof is lacking), (5) genetic factors (about 60% of early abortions display an abnormal chromosomal makeup), and (6) cocaine use, which recently has been linked to spontaneous abortion and preterm labor (Cocaine, 1987). An increase in maternal blood pressure and a reduction in uterine blood flow may be etiologic factors (Cole, 1987; Woods, Plessinger, and Clark, 1987). (See chapter 6 for management of infertility.)

Anomalies of the reproductive tract cause second- or third-trimester pregnancy loss. Little can be done to avoid genetic causes of pregnancy loss, but prepregnancy correction of maternal disorders, immunization against infectious diseases, proper early prenatal care, and treatment of pregnancy complications will do much to prevent abortion.

There are five types of spontaneous abortion—threatened, inevitable, incomplete, complete, septic—and missed (Fig. 23-3). Symptoms of a ***threatened abortion*** (Fig. 23-3, *A*) may include spotting of blood, but the cervical os is closed. Management includes bed

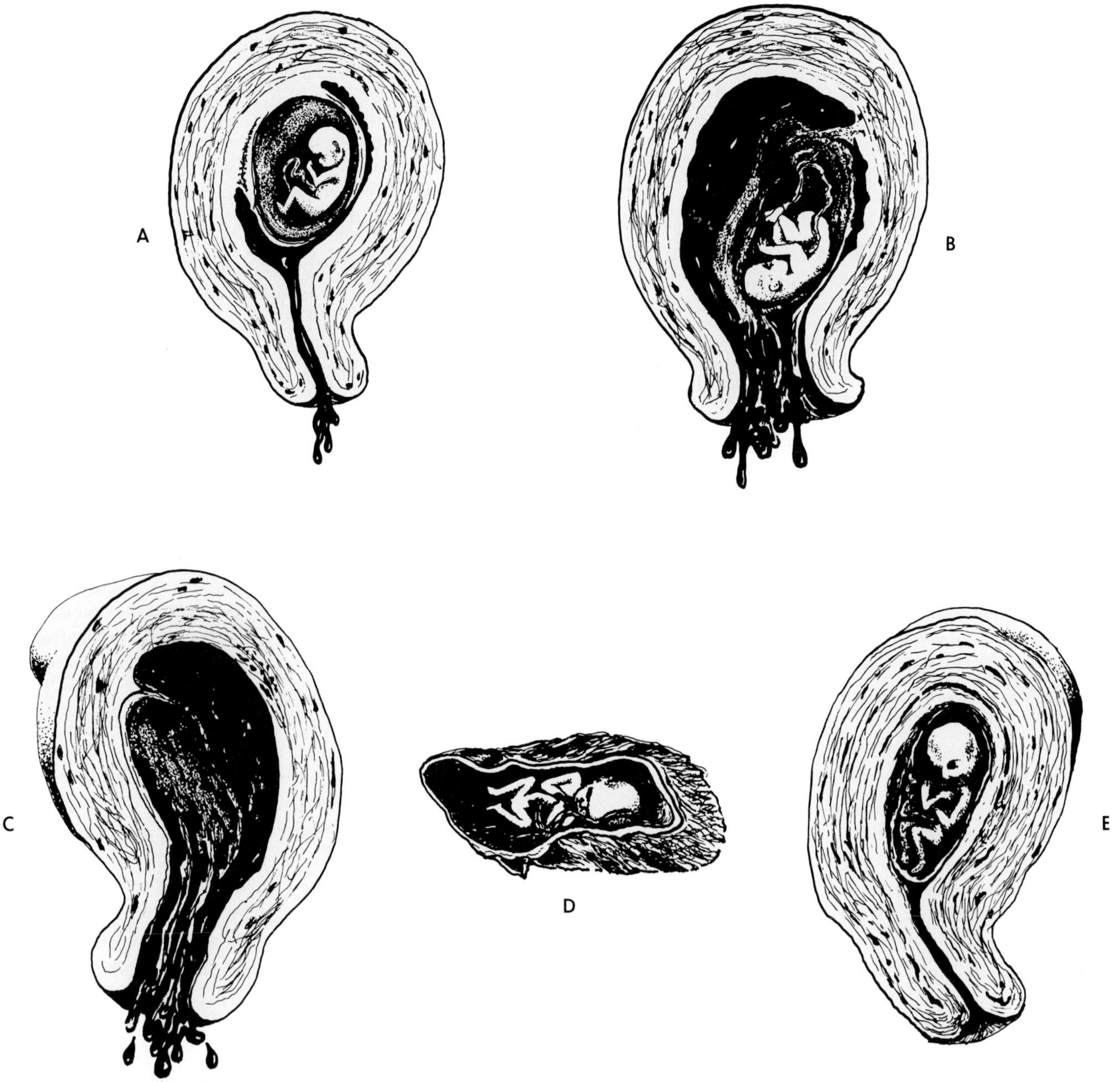

Fig. 23-3 Spontaneous abortion. **A**, Threatened. **B**, Inevitable. **C**, Incomplete. **D**, Complete. **E**, Missed.

rest and avoidance of stress and orgasm. Follow-up treatment is individualized to the woman's course.

Inevitable (Fig. 23-3, *B*) and ***incomplete*** (Fig. 23-3, *C*) abortions involve a moderate to heavy amount of bleeding with an open cervical os. Tissue may also be present. Prompt termination of the pregnancy, usually by curettage, is the suggested treatment.

In a ***complete abortion*** (Fig. 23-3, *D*) all of the fetal tissue has been passed, the cervix is closed, and there may be slight bleeding. There is no need for further treatment.

Presenting symptoms of a ***septic abortion*** include fever and abdominal tenderness. There is usually an odor to the vaginal bleeding, which may be slight to heavy. Termination of the pregnancy, antibiotic therapy, and treatment of septic shock are initiated.

A ***missed abortion*** (Fig. 23-3, *E*) refers to a pregnancy in which the products of conception have died but spontaneous abortion does not occur. It may be diagnosed when the uterus is smaller than expected for the duration of pregnancy. There may be no bleeding or cramping and the cervical os is closed. Treatment may include waiting up to 1 month for spontaneous abortion with frequent monitoring of the woman's clotting factors. If spontaneous abortion does not occur, the physician will terminate the pregnancy to prevent DIC in the mother.

Complications of abortion include the following:

1. *Uterine lithopedion, or "womb stone."* A missed abortion is retained for months or years, and the products of conception have calcified (see Fig. 23-3, *E*).
2. *Hemorrhage or sepsis.* Hemorrhage and sepsis (e.g., salpingitis, peritonitis) occur especially in induced abortion under septic conditions and in instances of neglected care. Death may follow instrumentation and perforation of the soft, slightly enlarged uterus, or septicemia or septic emboli may follow spontaneous incomplete abortion. Even mild infection may be followed by tubal occlusion and infertility.

Signs and symptoms depend on the duration of pregnancy. The woman may feel she is experiencing a heavy menstrual flow if abortion occurs before the sixth week of pregnancy. Abortion that occurs between the sixth and twelfth weeks of pregnancy will cause moderate discomfort and blood loss. After the twelfth week, abortion is typified by severe pain, similar to that of labor, because the fetus must be expelled.

The following *laboratory findings* are characteristic of abortion. A negative or weakly positive *urine* pregnancy test is characteristic of abortion. With considerable or persistent blood loss, *anemia* is likely (hemoglobin level less than 10.5 g/dl). *Sepsis* may develop with incomplete or missed abortion. Temperature is greater than 38° C (100.4° F), and *white blood cell count* (WBC) is greater than 12,000/μl. An increased sedimentation rate is the rule with pregnancy, anemia, or infection. Therefore sedimentation rate is not helpful for differential diagnostic purposes. *Endocrine studies* show that human chorionic gonadotropin (hCG), estrogen, and progesterone titers are minimal or absent in established abortions.

Management depends on the classification of spontaneous abortion.

General preoperative and postoperative care is appropriate for the woman requiring surgical intervention for spontaneous abortion. Before the procedure a full history and a general and pelvic examination should be performed. Laboratory tests include a complete blood count (CBC), blood typing for group and Rh factor and cross-matching, and urinalysis. Chest x-ray films and ECG evaluation are obtained if necessary. Blood, fluid, and electrolyte imbalances are corrected as soon as possible.

Analgesics, or anesthesia appropriate to the procedure, or both are used. Intravenous (IV) administration of oxytocin, 1 ml (10 U) in 500 ml of infusate may be needed to induce abortion. After evacuation of the uterus, 10 to 20 U in 1000 ml of infusate may be given to prevent hemorrhage.

Ergot products such as ergonovine (see Table 21-1), which contract the uterus and cervix, are contraindicated until the uterus is emptied to avoid retention of fragments of tissue. Retained fragments of fetal or placental tissue predispose the woman to uterine relaxation and puerperal infection. Three or four doses of ergonovine, 0.2 mg orally or intramuscularly (IM) every 4 hours, should be given if the woman is normotensive. Antibiotics are given as necessary. Transfusion may be required for shock or anemia. If the woman is Rh negative and has not developed isoimmunization (i.e., she is Coombs negative), she is given an IM injection of $Rh_0(D)$ immune globulin within 72 hours of the abortion.

Incompetent Cervix

An **incompetent cervix** is characterized by painless dilatation of the cervical os without labor or contractions of the uterus. Miscarriage or preterm delivery may result. Etiologic factors include a prior traumatic delivery, forceful dilatation and curettage (D&C) of the cervix, or mother (of woman) took diethylstilbestrol (DES) while pregnant. Other instances may result from a congenitally short cervix or anomalous uterus.

Correction of the weakened cervix is possible by wedge trachelorrhaphy (removal of a wedge from the anterior segment of the cervix with closure) in the nonpregnant woman. During gestation, a **cerclage,** band of homologous fascia, or nonabsorbable ribbon (Mersilene) may be placed around the cervix beneath the

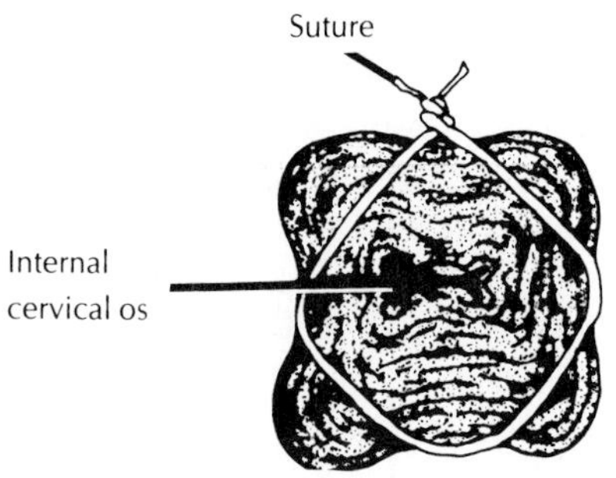

Fig. 23-4 Correction of incompetent cervical os: McDonald operation. Cross-section view of closed internal os.

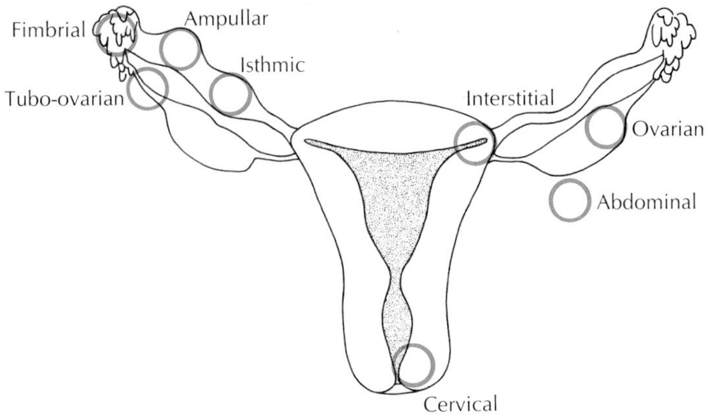

Fig. 23-5 Sites of implantation of ectopic pregnancies. Order of frequency of occurrence is ampulla, isthmus, interstitium, fimbria, tuboovarian ligament, ovary, abdominal cavity, and cervix (external os).

mucosa to constrict the internal os of the cervix (Fig. 23-4). Successful continuation of the pregnancy to viability or beyond occurs in the majority of women, provided the membranes remain intact and the cervix is not more than 3 cm dilated or more than 50% effaced at the time of correction.

Ectopic Pregnancy

Ectopic pregnancy is one in which the fetus is implanted outside the uterine cavity (Fig. 23-5). Fully 90% of ectopic pregnancies occur in the fallopian tube, most of these on the right side, for undetermined reasons. Approximately 1 of every 200 pregnancies is ectopic, and at least three fourths of these become symptomatic and are diagnosed during the first trimester. Ectopic pregnancy is a significant cause of maternal morbidity and mortality even in developed countries.

Most extrauterine pregnancies result from abnormalities that impede or prevent the transit of the fertilized ovum through the fallopian tube (e.g., peritubal adhesions following PID). On occasion, an ovum is fertilized within the ovary or soon after ovulation.

Ectopic pregnancy is classified according to the site of implantation (e.g., tubal, ovarian). The uterus is the only organ capable of containing and sustaining a term pregnancy. However, the rare abdominal pregnancy, with delivery by laparotomy, may result in a living newborn.

There are no *signs or symptoms* diagnostic of early ectopic pregnancy. A missed period, adnexal fullness, and tenderness may suggest an unruptured tubal pregnancy. In contrast, the following triad is associated with *early* ruptured extrauterine pregnancy in almost 50% of cases: amenorrhea or an abnormal menstrual period followed by slight uterine bleeding, adnexal or cul-de-sac mass, and unilateral pelvic pain over the mass. Decidua but no placental villi may be found on curettage.

Additional findings of *acute* rupture may include shock, referred shoulder pain, or evidence of acute blood loss in chronic ruptured tubal pregnancy.

In *chronic* ruptured tubal pregnancy, which represents slightly more than half the total of ectopic pregnancies, internal bleeding usually has been slow and the symptoms atypical or inconclusive. In addition to slight, dark, vaginal bleeding, a sense of pelvic pressure or fullness; lower abdominal tenderness; flatulence; and a tense, sensitive, semicystic, perhaps crepitant, cul-de-sac mass may be felt. Slight fever, leukocytosis, and a falling hematocrit or hemoglobin level may be noted. An ecchymotic blueness of the umbilicus (**Cullen's sign**), which is indicative of hematoperitoneum, may develop in a neglected ruptured intraabdominal ectopic pregnancy.

The addition of *ultrasound* as an aid in the management of a woman with an ectopic pregnancy has allowed improved accuracy in the preoperative diagnosis and has reduced the number of unnecessary laparoscopies being performed. An appropriately timed ultrasound examination for the at-risk woman allows earlier diagnosis and a resultant reduction in the mortality and morbidity resulting from this condition (de Crespigny, 1987).

Prevention of ectopic pregnancy per se is impossible. The major *management* problem in ectopic pregnancy is hemorrhage; bleeding must be quickly and effectively controlled. Blood transfusions must be available. Laparotomy may be done immediately after the diagnosis of ectopic pregnancy is made. Blood and clots are evacuated, and bleeding vessels are controlled. Excision of the cornua and fallopian tube is recommended if the tube is grossly involved; the ovary is conserved if possible. Hysterectomy usually is necessary for ruptured

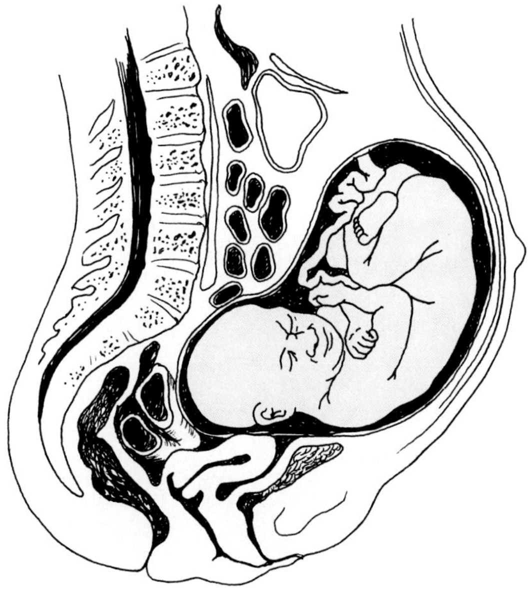

Fig. 23-6 Ectopic pregnancy, abdominal.

cornual or interstitial pregnancy. Ovarian pregnancy always requires loss of the ovary.

Microsurgical techniques permit linear incision of the tube. Salpingostomy and evacuation of a small tubal pregnancy may be feasible in rare instances (Diamond and DeCherney, 1987).

Advanced ***ectopic abdominal pregnancy*** requires laparotomy as soon as the woman is fit for surgery (Fig. 23-6). If the placenta of a second- or third-trimester abdominal pregnancy is attached to a vital organ, such as the liver, no attempt at separation and removal should be made. The cord should be cut flush with the placenta and the afterbirth left in situ. Degeneration and absorption of the placenta usually occur without complications.

Prognosis varies. Maternal death from ectopic pregnancy is about 1 in 800 in North America. Maternal morbidity and secondary surgery are high, however, principally because of inaccurate or delayed diagnosis of ectopic pregnancy. The perinatal mortality in ectopic pregnancy is virtually 100%. Ectopic pregnancy recurs in approximately 10% of women, but more than 50% of women who have had an ectopic pregnancy achieve at least one normal pregnancy thereafter.

Hydatidiform Mole

Gestational trophoblastic neoplasms are divided into three groups: **hydatidiform mole** (H. mole), invasive mole (chorioadenoma destruens), and choriocarcinoma.

The ***complete mole*** or classic mole, results from fertilization of an egg whose nucleus has been lost or inactivated (Fig. 23-7, *A*). The nucleus of a sperm (23X) duplicates, resulting in the diploid number, 46XX. The mole resembles a bunch of white grapes (Fig. 23-7, *B*). The hydropic (fluid-filled) vesicles grow rapidly, causing the uterus to be larger than expected for duration of pregnancy. Usually, the mole contains no fetus, no placenta, and no amniotic membranes or fluid. Maternal blood has no placenta to receive it. Therefore hemorrhage into the uterine cavity results, and vaginal bleeding is seen. In about 90% of the 46XX diploid H. moles, a progression toward choriocarcinoma occurs. The *incidence* of complete H. mole in the United States is 1 in 1500 pregnancies. The risk of developing a second mole is 4 to 5 times higher than the risk of the first.

The karyotype of the ***partial mole*** is normal diploid, trisomic, or triploid (Fig. 23-8). There is evidence of an embryo or fetus. Embryonic membranes are present. The potential for malignant transformation is much less than that associated with the complete H. mole (Scott et al, 1990).

Approximately 80% of partial H. moles regress spontaneously; 15% continue as nonmetastatic gestational trophoblastic disease, and 5% become metastatic gestational trophoblastic disease. Of women with metastatic **trophoblastic disease,** 50% develop the neoplasms as sequelae of a molar pregnancy (Scott et al, 1990).

In the early stages the *signs and symptoms* of H. mole cannot be distinguished from normal pregnancy. Later, vaginal bleeding occurs in almost every case. The vaginal discharge may be dark brown (resembling prune juice) or bright red, scant, or profuse. It may continue for only a few days or intermittently for weeks. Early in pregnancy about half the women have a uterus significantly larger than expected from the menstrual dates. The percentage of women with an excessively enlarged uterus increases as the length of time from the last menstrual period (LMP) increases. Approximately 25% of women will have a uterus smaller than would be expected from the menstrual dates.

Anemia from blood loss, excessive nausea and vomiting (hyperemesis gravidarum), and abdominal cramps caused by uterine distension are relatively common findings. Anemia results from intrauterine bleeding. Preeclampsia occurs in about 15% of cases, usually between 9 and 12 gestational weeks. In addition, symptoms of true preeclampsia-eclampsia may occur even though it is well before the twentieth week of pregnancy (p. 640). Hyperthyroidism and pulmonary embolization of trophoblastic elements occur less commonly but are serious complications of H. mole.

Many moles abort spontaneously. When hydropic

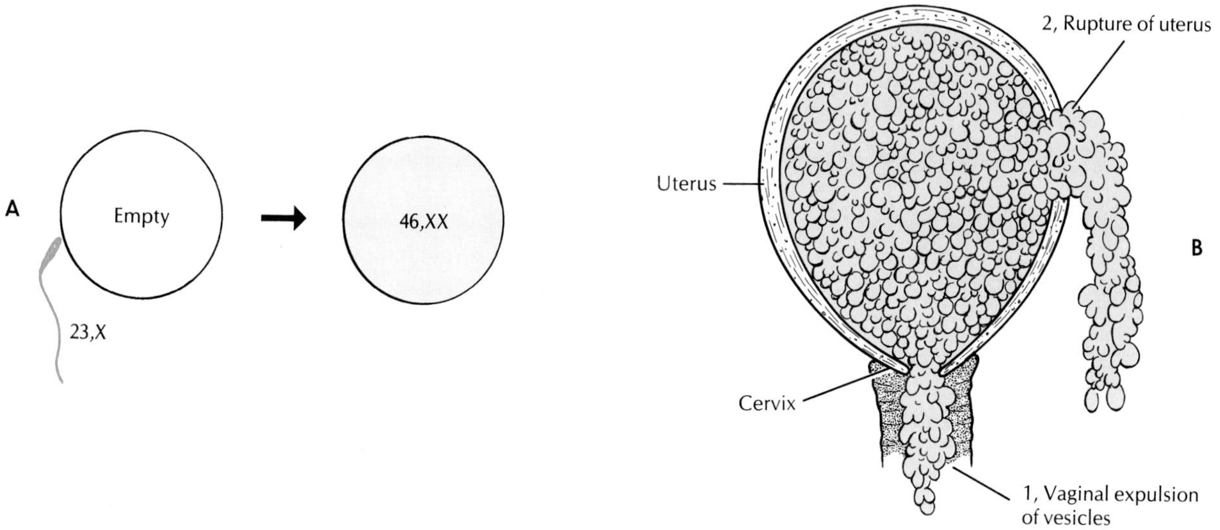

Fig. 23-7 **A,** Chromosomal origin of a complete mole. A single sperm (blue) fertilizes an "empty" ovum. Reduplication of the sperm's 23,X set gives a completely homozygous diploid 46,XX. A similar process follows fertilization of an empty ovum by two sperms with two independently drawn sets of 23,X or 23,Y; therefore both karyotypes of 46,XX and 46,XY can result. **B,** Uterine rupture with hydatidiform mole. *1,* Evacuation of mole through cervix. *2,* Rupture of uterus and spillage of mole into peritoneal cavity (rare).

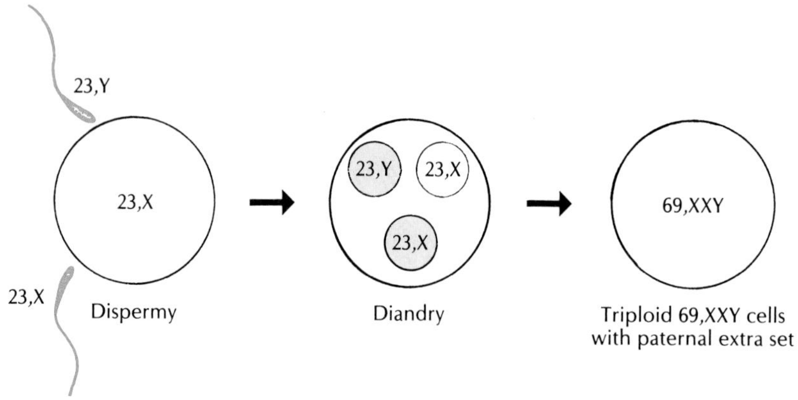

Fig. 23-8 Chromosomal origin of the triploid, partial mole. A normal ovum with a 23,X haploid set is fertilized by two sperms (blue) to give a total of 69 chromosomes. A sex configuration of XXY, XXX, or XYY, is possible.

vesicles are passed vaginally and the woman saves the specimen, the *diagnosis* can be established with certainty. The sonographic pattern of a molar pregnancy is characterized by a diffuse "snowstorm" pattern (see Fig. 22-3) (Athey and Hadlock, 1985). Any uncertainty in diagnosis is usually clarified by an accurate clinical history, an accurate hCG titer (although even a high titer is not considered diagnostic), and, if necessary, a repeat sonogram in 2 weeks.

Suction curettage (D&C) offers a safe, rapid, and effective method of evacuation of hydatidiform mole in almost all women (Scott et al, 1990). Women who do not desire preservation of reproductive function may benefit from primary hysterectomy as the method of choice for evacuation of H. mole and concurrent sterilization. Induction of labor with oxytocic agents or prostaglandins is not recommended.

Follow-up management includes frequent physical and pelvic examinations along with measurement of serum hCG levels for at least 1 year. A rising titer and an enlarging uterus may indicate ***choriocarcinoma.*** This malignant condition is treated with anti-cancer drugs. Therefore, to avoid confusion with signs of pregnancy, pregnancy should be avoided for 1 year. Pregnancy can then be attempted with a low probability of recurrence of a molar pregnancy. Cure of the malignant condition is defined as complete absence of all clinical and hormonal evidence of disease for 5 years.

❑ LATE PREGNANCY

Premature Separation of Placenta

Premature separation of the placenta, also termed **abruptio placentae,** is the detachment of part or all of the placenta from its implantation site (Fig. 23-9). Separation occurs in the area of the decidua basalis after the twentieth week of pregnancy, before the birth of the baby.

Premature separation of the placenta is a serious disorder and accounts for about 15% of all perinatal deaths. Approximately one third of infants of women with premature separation of the placenta die. More than 50% of these die as a result of preterm delivery, and many others die of intrauterine hypoxia.

Premature separation of the placenta occurs in about 1% of all pregnancies. The cause of premature separation of the placenta is unknown in most cases. This problem is much more common in women with hypertension of any cause and is 3 times greater in women with a gravidity of more than five. Abdominal trauma is a factor in less than 5% of cases, and short cord is identified in less than 1%. Women who use cocaine during their pregnancy significantly increase the incidence of abruptio placentae (Scott et al, 1990).

Clinical Manifestations and Differential Diagnosis. The separation may be partial or complete, or only the margin of the placenta may be involved. Bleeding from the placental site may dissect (separate) the membranes from the decidua basalis and flow out through the vagina; it may remain concealed (retroplacental hemorrhage); or it may do both (see Fig. 23-9). Clinical symptoms vary with the degree of separation.

Symptoms include *uterine bleeding* with a small to moderate amount of dark-red vaginal bleeding in 80% to 85% of cases. Bleeding may result in hypovolemia (shock; oliguria, anuria) and coagulopathy. *Uterine hypertonicity* (mild to severe) and pain are present. *Pain* is mild to severe, localized over one region of the uterus, or diffuse over the uterus with a boardlike abdomen. Couvelaire uterus (see below and p. 678) may occur.

Laboratory findings include a positive Apt test

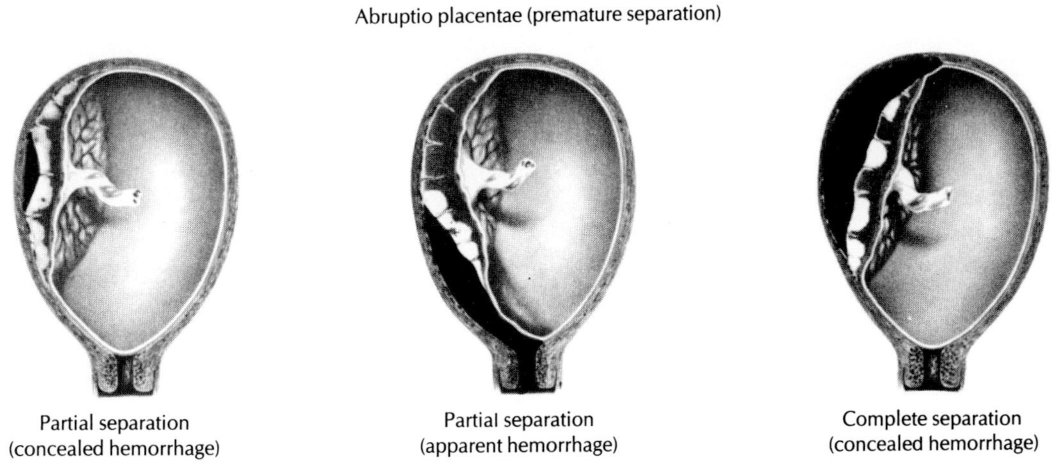

Fig. 23-9 Abruptio placentae. Premature separation of normally implanted placenta. (Courtesy Ross Laboratories, Columbus, Ohio.)

(Chapter 22) of amniotic fluid (indicates presence of maternal blood); a fall in hemoglobin and hematocrit (may appear later); and a fall in coagulation factors. From 10% to 30% of clients will develop clotting defects (e.g., DIC) (the majority within 8 hours of hospital admission) and increased clot retraction.

Ultrasonography reveals that the implantation site of the placenta is normal. Initially, a retroplacental blood clot may not be visible, but the enlarging clot may be seen when the sonogram is repeated.

Significant complications accompany moderate to severe abruptio placentae. *Hypovolemic shock* can result in renal failure and pituitary necrosis (Sheehan's syndrome). *Fetal hypoxia or anoxia* with possible fetal death may occur. Clotting defects (DIC) develop. Bleeding into the myometrium causes Couvelaire uterus. *Couvelaire uterus* has several sequelae: myometrial tissue is damaged, uterine tonicity increases, uterus becomes more irritable, and the ability of the uterus to relax between contractions diminishes or is lost. Electronic fetal monitoring (EFM) reflects the increasing fetal distress that may finally end in fetal death. After delivery, the uterus may feel firm, but may not be able to efficiently contract and close off bleeding sinuses; *postpartum hemorrhage* should be anticipated.

Management. The nurse assists the physician in implementing therapeutic measures. Side-lying position with a wedge placed under the supine woman's right hip facilitates adequate uterine-placental perfusion. Blood lost is restored. If shock is present or appears imminent *and* clotting mechanism is intact, hemodynamic assessment with central venous pressure (CVP) or Swan-Ganz catheter is started to monitor blood and fluid replacement accurately. A retention catheter is placed to monitor urinary output accurately for volume and proteinuria. Oliguria and proteinuria are ominous signs. Coagulopathy is anticipated and corrected. The fetus is monitored and delivered when indicated. Hysterectomy may be necessary to control bleeding or if Couvelaire uterus occurs. The woman and her family need emotional support.

Prognosis. Maternal mortality approaches 1% in premature separation of the placenta; this condition remains a leading cause of maternal death. The mother's prognosis depends on the extent of the placental detachment, overall blood loss, degree of DIC, and time between the placental "accident" and delivery. Fortunately, 80% to 90% of all premature separations of the placenta only involve two or three cotyledons, and therefore the prognosis is generally not grave.

Fetal prognosis is poor. At least one third of babies of mothers with premature placental separation die before, during, or soon after birth. Of those who survive, there is an increase in the absolute numbers of neurologically damaged infants.

Placenta Previa

In **placenta previa** the placenta is implanted in the lower uterine segment. The degree to which the internal cervical os is covered by the placenta determines how placenta previa is classified. Placenta previa (Fig. 23-10) often is described as ***complete, total,*** or ***central*** if the internal os is entirely covered by the placenta, when the cervix is fully dilated. ***Partial placenta previa*** implies incomplete coverage. ***Marginal placenta previa*** indicates that only an edge of the placenta approaches the internal os. The term ***low-lying (low) implantation*** is used when the placenta is situated in the lower uterine segment but away from the os.

In the second trimester approximately 45% of all placentas are implanted in the lower uterine segment. As the lower uterine segment elongates, the placenta seems to move upward (p. 626). By term only 1 placenta in 200 is still a previa (Scott et al, 1990). Those placentas most likely to remain unchanged are the ones classified as central (complete).

The cause of placenta previa is uncertain. Reduced vascularity of the upper segment subsequent to scarring from uterine surgery (abortion, cesarean delivery), molar pregnancy, and tumor necessitating lower implantation of the placenta are plausible theories. Multifetal gestation that requires a larger surface area for placental implantation may be a factor. Vessels of the endometrium involved in previous sites of implantation undergo changes that may reduce the blood supply to those regions, thus predisposing the woman to low implantation in subsequent pregnancies.

The site of implantation and size of the placenta are related. Specifically, because the circulation of the lower uterine segment is less favorable than that of the fundus, placenta previa may need to cover a larger area for adequate efficiency. In placenta previa the surface area may be at least 30% greater than the average placenta implanted in the fundus.

Clinical Manifestations and Differential Diagnosis. *Painless uterine bleeding,* especially during the third trimester, characterizes placenta previa. Rarely is the first episode life-threatening or a cause of hypovolemic shock. Approximately 7% of placenta previas are without symptoms and are an incidental finding on ultrasonic scans. A few are manifest for the first time at term, when the lower uterine segment stretches and thins; at that time tearing and bleeding occur at the lower implantation site. About 3% of all cases of placenta previa are accompanied by placenta accreta, increta, or percreta (p. 684).

The *bright-red bleeding* may be intermittent, may occur in gushes, or, more rarely, may be continuous. It may start while the woman is resting or in the midst of any activity. Fortunately, severe hemorrhage almost never occurs unless vaginal or rectal examination ini-

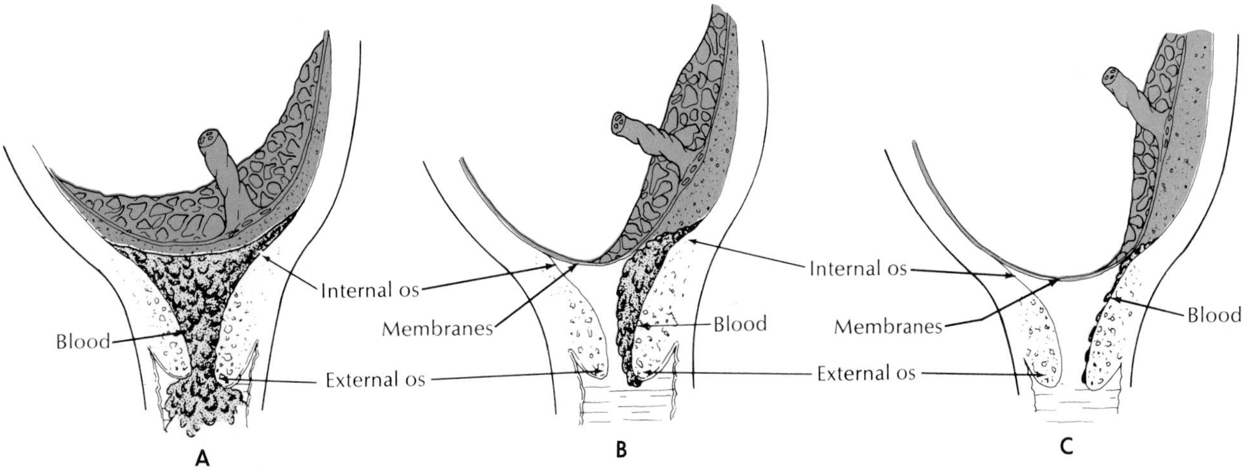

Fig. 23-10 Types of placenta previa after onset of labor. **A**, Complete, or total. **B**, Incomplete or partial. **C**, Marginal, or low lying.

tiates violent bleeding before or during early labor.

The detachment of placenta previa is painless. However, if the first bleeding coincides with the onset of labor, the woman may experience discomfort because of uterine contractions.

Abdominal examination usually reveals a *soft (relaxed), nontender uterus* of normal tone. If the fetus is in a longitudinal lie, the fundal height is usually greater than expected for gestational age because the low placenta hinders descent of the presenting fetal part. Leopold's maneuvers may reveal a fetus in an oblique or breech position or transverse lie because of the abnormal site of placental implantation.

As a rule, fetal distress or fetal death occurs only if a significant portion of the placenta previa becomes detached from the decidua basalis or if the mother suffers hypovolemic shock.

Obstetric ultrasound, with either real-time (linear or sector) or static imaging, is the diagnostic method of choice. If ultrasound reveals a normally implanted placenta, a speculum examination is performed to rule out local causes of bleeding (e.g., cervicitis, polyps, or carcinoma of the cervix), and a coagulation profile is obtained to rule out other causes of bleeding.

If possible, sterile vaginal speculum examination by the physician for diagnosing placenta previa should be postponed until viability has been reached (preferably after the thirty-fourth week), and after the ultrasound report is available. The vaginal examination, known as the ***double-setup procedure,*** is a serious undertaking; it is attempted only if the physician is prepared for delivery. In a double setup a sterile vaginal examination is performed in an operating room with staff and equipment ready to effect an immediate vaginal or cesarean delivery. Since manipulation of the lower uterine segment or cervix may result in profound hemorrhage, preparation for immediate delivery is essential.

Management. When fetal maturity is near, conservative management (e.g., bed rest to extend the period of gestation) is usually possible because initial spontaneous critical bleeding almost never occurs in placenta previa. When fetal lung maturity (L/S ratio of at least 2:1) is achieved and survival is likely, then delivery is accomplished.

After the diagnosis of placenta previa has been made, the woman should remain in the hospital under close supervision. At least two units of blood, typed and cross-matched, must be available for emergency use. A hematocrit of at least 30% is maintained (Scott et al, 1990). The duration of pregnancy should be confirmed and, except in an emergency, delivery postponed until after the thirty-sixth week. If the woman has greater than a 30% placenta previa or if bleeding is excessive, cesarean delivery is indicated, preferably with the woman under light general inhalation anesthesia. Under certain conditions, vaginal delivery may be possible (e.g., placenta previa is marginal or partial). However, the woman is kept NPO since operative delivery is a possibility.

Blood loss may not cease with the delivery of the infant. The large vascular channels in the lower uterine segment may continue to bleed because of the diminished muscle content of the lower uterine segment. The natural mechanism to control bleeding—the interlacing muscle bundles (the "living ligature") contracting around open vessels—so characteristic of the upper part of the uterus is absent in the lower part of the uterus. *Therefore postpartum hemorrhage may occur even if the fundus is contracted firmly.*

The location of the placental site close to the cervical os renders it more accessible to ascending infection from the vagina. *Hemorrhage and anemia increase the predisposition to* antenatal *infection* (placentitis) and postpartum (puerperal) infection.

If uterine bleeding cannot be controlled with oxytocic drugs, ligation of the hypogastric (internal iliac) arteries (see Fig. 4-12, *A*) or even hysterectomy may be necessary.

Hypovolemia must be treated without overtransfusion or overinfusion. Precise control of blood and fluid replacement necessitates continuous hemodynamic monitoring (p. 684).

Prognosis. Maternal morbidity may occur from the placenta previa itself, the management, or the birth. Antenatal hemorrhage may be fatal or nearly fatal.

Complications associated with the management of placenta previa include sepsis, surgery-related trauma to structures adjacent to the uterus, anesthesia complications, blood transfusion reactions, or overinfusion of fluids.

Maternal mortality in placenta previa has dropped almost 50%, to about 0.6%, during the past decade in larger centers in North America because of conservative therapy. The perinatal mortality (resulting primarily from preterm birth) still approaches 20% in most hospitals.

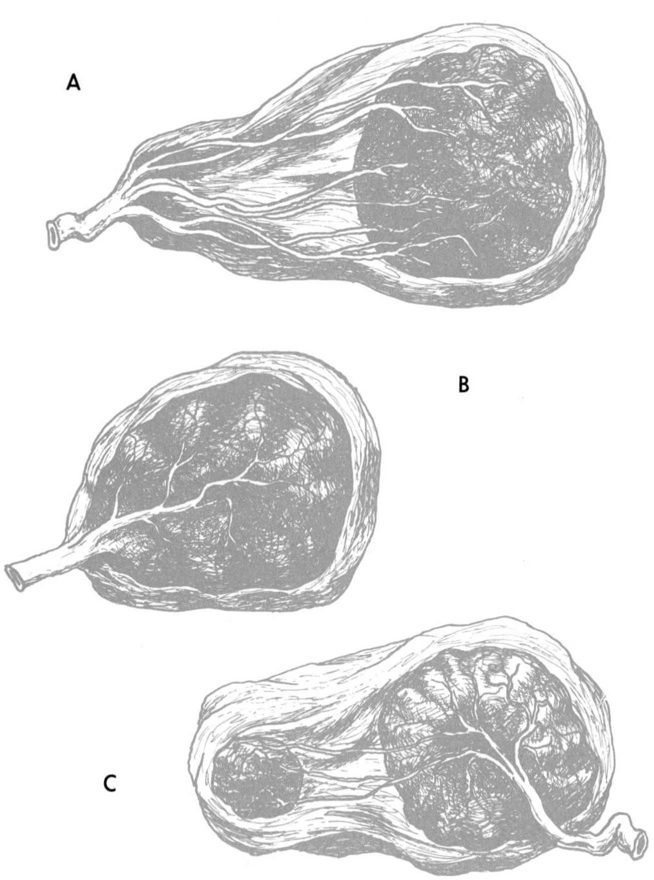

Fig. 23-11 Cord insertion and placental variations. **A,** Velamentous insertion of cord. **B,** Battledore placenta. **C,** Placenta succenturiate.

Cord Insertion and Placental Variations

A ***velamentous insertion of the cord*** is a rare placental anomaly in which the cord vessels begin to branch at the membranes and then course onto the placenta (Fig. 23-11, *A*). Rupture of the membranes or traction on the cord may tear one or more of the fetal vessels. As a result the fetus may quickly exsanguinate (bleed to death). *Battledore* (marginal) (Fig. 23-11, *B*) insertion of the cord increases the risk of fetal hemorrhage, especially following marginal separation of the placenta.

Rarely, the placenta may be divided into two or more separate lobes, resulting in ***succenturiate placenta*** (Fig. 23-11, *C*). Each lobe has a distinct circulation; the vessels collect at the periphery, and the main trunks unite eventually to form the vessels of the cord. Blood vessels joining the lobes may be supported only by the fetal membranes and are therefore in danger of tearing during labor or during the birth of the baby or of the placenta. During delivery of the placenta, one or more of the separate lobes may remain attached to the decidua basalis, preventing uterine contraction.

❑ CLOTTING DISORDERS IN PREGNANCY

Normally there is a delicate balance (homeostasis) maintained between two opposing systems, the *hemostatic* system and the fibrinolytic system. The hemostatic system is involved in the life-saving process; this system stops the flow of blood from injured vessels, in part through the formation of insoluble fibrin that acts as a hemostatic platelet plug. The phases of the coagulation process involve an interaction of the coagulation factors (e.g., fibrinogen; prothrombin; platelet factor 3; thromboplastin; calcium) in which each factor sequentially activates the factor next in line in the so-called cascade effect sequence. The *fibrinolytic* system refers to the process by which the fibrin is split into fibrinolytic degradation products (FDP) and circulation is restored.

A history of abnormal bleeding, inheritance of unusual bleeding tendencies, and a report of significant aberrations of laboratory findings indicate a bleeding or clotting problem. The comprehension of useful tests of hemostasis is based on the usual mechanisms for the control of bleeding, that is, the function of platelets and the necessary clotting factors.

Disseminated Intravascular Coagulation

Disseminated intravascular coagulation (DIC, defibrination syndrome, defibrination coagulopathy) is a pathologic form of clotting that is diffuse and consumes large amounts of clotting factors causing widespread external and/or internal bleeding.

Unanticipated, profuse, locally uncontrollable uterine hemorrhage; bleeding from the episiotomy, lacerations or needle puncture sites; amniotic fluid embolism; or shock often initiates the DIC syndrome in the woman (ecchymosis or bleeding from mucous membranes or gastrointestinal tract may be apparent in the infant). Unless DIC is treated immediately and effectively, death often results.

Physical examination reveals unusual bleeding. Spontaneous bleeding from the woman's gums or nose may be noted. Petechiae may appear around the blood pressure cuff on her arm. Excessive bleeding may occur from the site of a slight trauma (e.g., venipuncture sites, IM or subcutaneous injection sites, nicks from shaving of perineum or abdomen, injury from insertion of urinary catheter). Maternal symptoms may include tachycardia and diaphoresis. *Laboratory tests* reveal reduced platelets, fibrinogen, proaccelerin, antihemophilic factor, and prothrombin (the factors consumed during coagulation). Other factors should be normal. Fibrinolysis is first increased but later is severely depressed. Degradation of fibrin leads to the accumulation of fibrin-split products in the blood. Fibrin split-products have anticoagulant properties and thus prolong the prothrombin time (PT). Bleeding time is normal; coagulation time shows no clot; clot retraction time shows no clot; and partial thromboplastin time (PTT) is increased. DIC must be distinguished from other clotting disorders before initiating therapy.

Management. The primary *management* of all cases of DIC involves correction of the underlying cause, replacement of coagulation factors, and maintenance of physiologic functioning. Removal of the underlying cause may include delivery of the dead fetus; treatment of existing infection or preeclampsia-eclampsia; or removal of abrupted placenta. Packed red blood cells may be transfused to correct anemia. Deficiencies secondary to DIC primarily involve platelets, factors V and VIII, fibrinogen, and prothrombin. Administration of *fresh-frozen plasma* in combination with *platelet concentrates* is effective in all these conditions when replacement therapy is warranted (Scott et al, 1990). Adequate fibrinogen levels can be obtained by infusion of *cryoprecipitate* with significantly less risk of hepatitis transmission. Each bag of cryoprecipitate contains an average of 250 mg fibrinogen; 16 to 20 bags are required for replacement therapy. Heparin therapy may be ordered to control coagulation. It is usually administered by continuous infusion pump.

CVP monitoring is begun to attempt to maintain CVP within normal limits: 6 to 12 cm H_2O (Fig. 23-12). Since renal failure is one consequence of DIC, urinary output is monitored. Output must be maintained at more than 30 ml/hr. Supportive measures also include keeping the woman's right hip elevated to prevent hypotensive syndrome. Oxygen is administered by a tight-fitting mask at 10 to 12 L/min. The emotional needs of the family are recognized and supported. *Prognosis* depends on the degree and extent of the underlying disorder as well as the response of the woman to prompt and proper treatment.

Autoimmune Thrombocytopenic Purpura

Autoimmune thrombocytopenic purpura (ATP) is an autoimmune disorder in which antiplatelet antibodies decrease the life span of the platelets. Thrombocytopenia, capillary fragility, and increased bleeding time are diagnostic.

ATP may result in severe hemorrhage after cesarean delivery or from cervical or vaginal lacerations. The incidence of postdelivery uterine bleeding or vaginal **hematomas** is also increased in ATP.

Neonatal thrombocytopenia occurs in about 50% of the cases and is associated with a high mortality. Platelet transfusions are given to maintain the platelet count at 100,000/cu mm. Corticosteroids are given if the diagnosis is made before or during pregnancy. Splenectomy, if needed, is deferred until after the puerperium.

von Willebrand's Disease

This type of hemophilia is probably the most common of all hereditary bleeding disorders (Rigby, 1987). It results from a factor VIII deficiency and platelet dysfunction. It is transmitted as an incomplete autosomal-dominant trait to both sexes. Although von Willebrand's disease is rare, it is one of the most common congenital clotting defects in American women of childbearing age. The symptoms include a familial bleeding tendency, previous bleeding episodes, prolonged bleeding time (most important test), factor VIII deficiency (mild to moderate), and bleeding from mucous membranes. Since factor VIII increases during pregnancy, this increase may be sufficient to offset danger from hemorrhage during childbirth. However, the woman should be observed for at least 1 week postpartum.

Treatment of von Willebrand's disease consists of replacement of factor VIII, if it is less than 30%, through administration of cryoprecipitate or fresh frozen plasma.

Measurement of CVP with manometer.

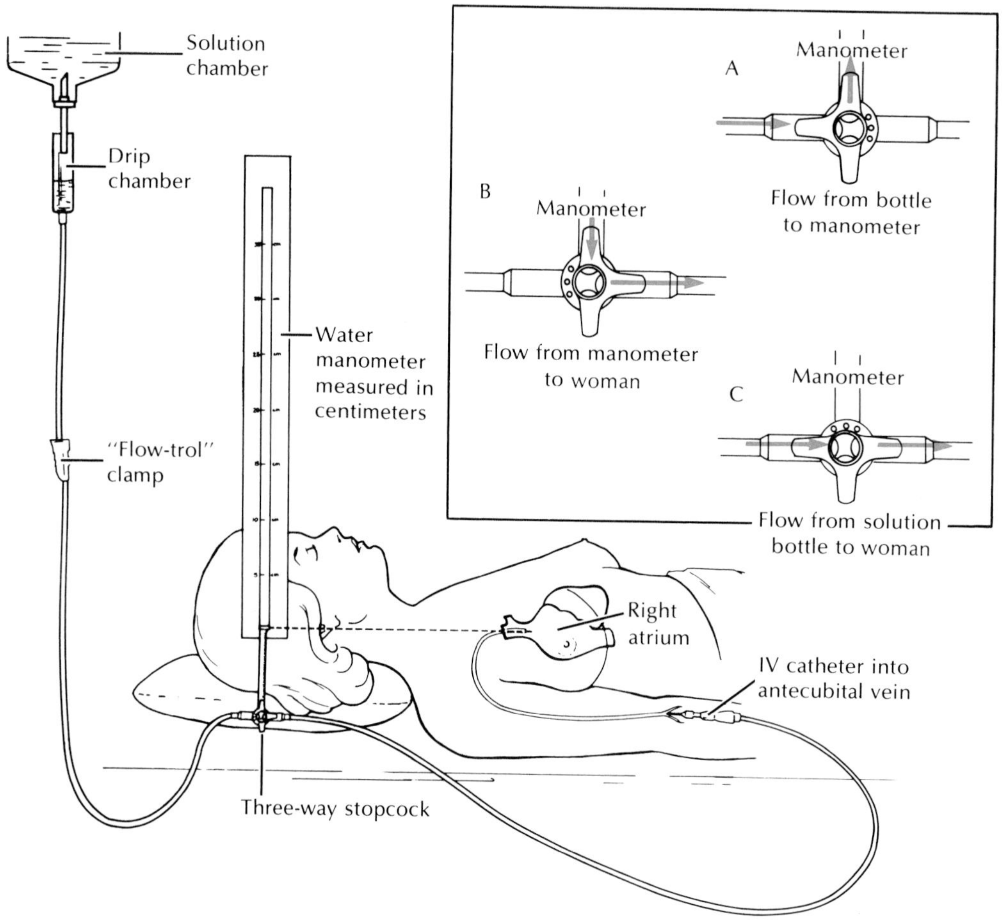

Fig. 23-12 Measurement of CVP with manometer.

❑ POSTDELIVERY HEMORRHAGE

Hemorrhage is a leading cause of maternal death world-wide. Postdelivery hemorrhage, traditionally the loss of 500 ml of blood or more after delivery, is the most common and most serious type of excessive obstetric blood loss. At least 5% of women suffer postdelivery hemorrhage.

A small woman is less able to withstand the loss of blood than a larger one. It has been noted that the average maternal blood loss can be as much as 10% of the woman's blood volume without immediate critical consequence. Therefore a more meaningful definition of postdelivery hemorrhage is the loss of 1% or more of body weight, a figure easily referable to blood volume because 1 ml of blood weighs 1 g.

Postdelivery hemorrhage may be sudden and even exsanguinating. Moderate but persistent bleeding may continue for days or weeks. Postdelivery hemorrhage may be early, within the first 24 hours after delivery, or late, from 24 hours after delivery until the twenty-eighth day.

Control of bleeding from the placental site is accomplished by prolonged contraction and retraction of interlacing strands of myometrium, the ***living ligature.*** A firm or contracted uterus does not normally bleed after delivery unless placenta previa had existed. Therefore careful assessment of uterine tone and the maintenance of uterine contractions through manual massage or oxytocic stimulation are important parts of postdelivery care.

The most common causes of postdelivery hemorrhage, in approximate order of frequency, are mismanagement of the third stage of labor, uterine atony, and lacerations of the birth canal. Hematologic disorders (e.g., DIC) or complications of pregnancy (e.g., inversion of the uterus, placenta accreta) may be factors in postdelivery hemorrhage. Other factors may include tumors of the cervix or uterus (e.g., fibroids), medical complications of pregnancy (e.g., hyperthyroidism), or infections of the genital tract (e.g., endometritis).

Early postdelivery hemorrhage almost invariably is caused by uterine atony, lacerations of the birth canal, or DIC. ***Late postdelivery hemorrhage*** most commonly is the result of subinvolution of the uterus, retained placental tissue, or infection.

It is helpful to consider the problem of excessive bleeding with reference to the stages of labor. From delivery of the fetus until separation of the placenta the character and quantity of blood passed may suggest excessive bleeding. For example, *dark blood* is probably of venous origin, perhaps from varices or superficial lacerations of the birth canal. *Bright blood* is arterial and indicates, for example, deep lacerations of the cervix. *Spurts of blood* with clots may indicate partial placental separation. *Failure of blood to clot* or remain clotted is indicative of coagulopathy.

The period from the separation of the placenta to its delivery may be when excessive bleeding occurs. Commonly this is the result of incomplete placental separation, often caused by poor management of the third stage of labor (e.g., undue manipulation of the fundus). After the placenta has been recovered, persistent or excessive blood loss usually is the result of atony of the uterus (i.e., its failure to contract well or maintain its contraction) or prolapse of the uterus into the pelvis. Late hemorrhage may be the result of partial involution of the uterus and unrecognized lacerations of the birth canal.

Complications of postdelivery hemorrhage are either immediate or delayed. Hemorrhagic (hypovolemic) shock (p. 684) and death may occur from sudden, exsanguinating hemorrhage. Delayed complications provoked by postdelivery hemorrhage include anemia, puerperal infection, and thromboembolism.

Uterine Atony

Uterine atony is the principal cause of postdelivery hemorrhage. Uterine atony is marked hypotonia of the uterus. Uterine atony occurs in at least 5% of deliveries, particularly when the woman is a grand multipara; with hydramnios; when the fetus is large; or after the delivery of twins or triplets. In such conditions, the uterus is "overstretched" and contracts poorly.

Uterine atony may be an undesirable side-effect of analgesics or anesthesia administered during labor. Mismanagement of the third stage of labor, allowing only partial separation of the placenta or retention of placental fragments, may be associated with uterine atony. In the postdelivery period, a filling urinary bladder may result in hemorrhage. See Chapter 15 for the management of uterine atony.

Lacerations of the Birth Canal

Lacerations of the birth canal are second only to uterine atony as a major cause of postdelivery hemorrhage. Therefore prevention, recognition, and prompt, effective treatment of birth canal lacerations are vitally important.

Continued bleeding despite efficient postdelivery uterine contractions demands inspection or reinspection of the birth passage. Continuous bleeding from so-called minor sources may be just as dangerous as a sudden loss of a large amount of blood, although often it is ignored until shock develops. Birth canal lacerations may include injuries to the labia, perineum, vagina, and cervix.

Extreme vascularity in the *labial* and periclitoral areas often results in profuse bleeding if laceration occurs. Immediate repair, by means of fine (e.g., 4-0 chromic) suture on an atraumatic needle, is required.

Lacerations of the *perineum* are the most common of all injuries in the lower genital tract. These are classified as first, second, third, and fourth degree (Chapter 15). An episiotomy may extend to become either a third- or fourth-degree laceration. The care of the woman who has suffered lacerations of the perineum is similar to that advocated for episiotomies, that is, analgesia as needed for pain, and heat or cold applications as necessary. *To avoid injury to the suture line, a woman with third- or fourth-degree lacerations is not given routine postdelivery rectal suppositories or enemas.* Attention to diet and intake of fluids is emphasized, as well as oral stool softeners to assist her in reestablishing bowel habits.

Prolonged pressure of the fetal head on the vaginal mucosa ultimately will interfere with the circulation and may produce ischemic or pressure necrosis. The state of the tissues, therefore, together with the type of delivery, may result in deep *vaginal lacerations* and may predispose to *vaginal hematomas*.

Vaginal hematomas occur more commonly in association with forceps rotation of a fetus in an occipitoposterior (OP) position. They are often found on the same side as the occiput, perhaps because of long-continued pressure of the fetal head in one posterior quadrant of the vagina. Many vaginal hematomas occur beneath the mucosa opposite the ischial spines in the plane of the midpelvis. Therefore the physician will palpate the vaginal walls to detect a hematoma. During the postdelivery period, if the woman complains of persistent perineal pain or a feeling of fullness in the vagina, a careful inspection of the vulva is made. Once the hematoma is diagnosed, treatment is initiated. The woman is returned to the delivery unit, where (after a suitable anesthetic has been administered) the hematoma is incised and evacuated and deep sutures are placed for control of the bleeding.

Retained Placenta: Nonadherent

The obstetrician must recognize the normal completion of the third stage of labor, or complications may result. If the operator is hasty, for example, the placenta may not have an adequate opportunity to separate. If one waits too long, needless loss of blood may occur.

After birth of the baby but before recovery of the placenta, some women may have only slight bleeding, but others may have considerable blood loss. If no significant bleeding occurs and with proper management, the normally implanted placenta separates with the first or second strong uterine contraction after delivery of the infant. Placental separation occurs within 15 minutes in about 90% of women. If the placenta is not delivered within 30 minutes, most physicians will attempt to remove it manually. Oxytocin may be administered intravenously to hasten placental separation.

Some obstetricians practice elective manual separation and extraction of the placenta to expedite the delivery sequence or to avoid abnormal bleeding, for example, after twin delivery.

Retained Placenta: Adherent

Abnormal adherence of the placenta occurs for reasons unknown, but it is thought to be the result of zygote implantation in a zone of defective endometrium. ***There is no zone of separation*** between the placenta and the decidua. Abnormal adherence of the placenta is diagnosed in only about 1 of every 12,000 deliveries. Approximately 90% of the mothers are multiparous, and many of them have also had abortions. The mother with an abnormally attached placenta is jeopardized mainly by postdelivery hemorrhage leading to hypovolemic shock. There are no sure signs of an abnormally adherent placenta during pregnancy.

Unusual placental adherence may be partial or complete, and the following degrees of attachment are recognized.

- ***Placenta accreta*** (vera): slight penetration of myometrium by placental trophoblast (unusual)
- ***Placenta increta:*** deep penetration by placenta (rare)
- ***Placenta percreta*** (destruans): perforation of uterus by placenta (exceptional)

More cases of partial than complete placenta accreta occur. At least 15% of cases of abnormally adherent placenta (all types) are associated with placenta previa.

Bleeding with complete or total placenta accreta does not occur unless separation of the placenta is attempted. When manual removal of a placenta accreta is attempted, damage to placental tissue and decidua, both rich in thromboplastin, occurs. When this substance is released in quantity into the circulation, DIC may develop.

At vaginal delivery the diagnosis of an abnormally adherent placenta generally is made when manual separation of a retained placenta is attempted. If the placenta will not separate readily (even a portion), immediate abdominal hysterectomy may be indicated.

Inversion of the Uterus

Inversion of the uterus (turning inside out) after delivery is a critical obstetric complication. The inversion may be complete or partial. Fundal pressure, especially when the uterus is flaccid, may result in inversion. Traction on the cord before the placenta has separated can cause inversion.

Prevention—always the easiest, cheapest, and most effective therapy—is especially appropriate in the avoidance of puerperal uterine inversion. ***One must not pull on the umbilical cord unless the placenta has definitely separated.***

Profound shock follows complete inversion; postdelivery hemorrhage accompanies partial uterine inversion. Prompt assistance is imperative because maternal mortality may reach 30%, without immediate corrective therapy. Successful, prompt vaginal replacement is likely in about 75% of women. Uterine inversion may occasionally recur in a subsequent delivery.

Hemorrhagic Shock

Hemorrhage is a major threat to the mother during the childbearing cycle. Shock may result (see danger signs box, p. 431). Shock is an emergency situation in which the perfusion of body organs may become severely compromised and death may ensue. Vigorous treatment of **hemorrhagic shock** is necessary to prevent adverse sequelae (e.g., cellular death, fluid overload, shock lung, and oxygen toxicity). A brief explanation of the physiologic mechanisms is provided to assist the nurse in implementing appropriate actions.

Physiologic Mechanisms. Physiologic compensatory mechanisms are activated in response to hemorrhage (or other trauma such as cardiac arrest). The adrenals release catecholamines, causing arterioles and venules in the skin, lungs, gastrointestinal tract, liver, and kidneys to constrict. The available blood flow is diverted to the brain and heart and away from other organs, including the uterus. If shock is prolonged, the continued reduction in cellular oxygenation results in an accumulation of lactic acid and acidosis (from anaerobic glucose metabolism). Acidosis (lowered serum pH) causes arteriole vasodilatation; venule vasoconstriction persists. A circular pattern is established:

decreased perfusion, increased tissue anoxia and acidosis, edema formation, and pooling of blood further decrease the perfusion. Cellular death occurs.

Nursing Management. Hemorrhagic shock often occurs rapidly. As soon as a woman exhibits the signs and symptoms of shock, the nurse stays with her and summons assistance and equipment. Nurses should have standing orders to start IV fluids and know the type of infusion to use and laboratory tests to order. While waiting for the physician, the nurse should insert an airway to facilitate oxygen administration and suction (not all people in shock require an airway). The nurse can elevate the right hip (if woman cannot be in left sidelying position) to avoid supine hypotensive syndrome. *Trendelenburg's position* (with head down and feet elevated) *is not advised.* This position may interfere with cardiac function. This position should be used on physician request only.

The nurse continues to monitor, assess, and record respirations, pulse, blood pressure, skin condition, urinary output, level of consciousness (LOC), and CVP (see Fig. 23-12) to evaluate effectiveness of management (Royce, 1973):

a. ***Respirations.*** The body rids itself of excess acids by increasing the respiratory rate. Ventilatory assistance with oxygen or respirator or both may be needed.
b. ***Pulse.*** The pulse rate increases and becomes irregular as shock progresses in severity.
c. ***Blood pressure.*** In later stages of shock the systolic pressure decreases.
d. ***Skin.*** Perfusion of the skin is sacrificed in the body's attempt to maintain blood flow to the heart and brain. Therefore the condition of the skin is a valuable index to the severity of shock. The nurse assesses the degree of ischemia or cyanosis of the nail beds, eyelids, and skin inside the mouth (buccal mucosa, gums, tongue). The nurse notes the degree of coolness and clamminess.
e. ***Urinary output.*** The nurse measures hourly output. Poor urinary output (less than 50 ml/hr) may indicate worsening of shock or inadequate fluid therapy; an increased output indicates improvement in the woman's condition.
f. ***Level of consciousness.*** The adequacy of cerebral perfusion may be estimated by an evaluation of the woman's LOC. In early stages of decreased blood flow the woman may complain of "seeing stars," feeling dizzy, or feeling nauseous. She may become restless and orthopneic. As cerebral hypoxia increases, she may become confused and react slowly or not at all to stimuli. An improved sensorium is an indicator of improvement.
g. ***Heart function. CVP***: CVP readings measure the function (e.g., blood pressure) of the right side of the heart. Normal values range between 6 and 12 cm H_2O. A low or falling value indicates inadequate blood volume or hypovolemia. A high or rising value indicates impaired contractility of the heart. ***PA catheter***: A multiple-lumen pulmonary artery (PA) catheter is used to measure both right- and left-side heart functions. ***PAWP***: A PA catheter, when properly placed and when its flexible latex balloon is inflated, is used to measure the pulmonary artery wedge pressure (PAWP), an indicator of left-side heart function.
h. ***Response to shock therapy (fluids, oxygen).*** Hazards of shock therapy include fluid overload, shock lung, and oxygen toxicity (Table 23-4).

Anxiety is contagious. The nurse's calm, confident manner, coupled with brief, simple explanations, is an important adjunct to the interventions just discussed.

A general nursing care plan for hemorrhagic disorders of pregnancy follows on p. 686.

Table 23-4 **Hazards of Shock Therapy**

Hazard	Nursing Action
Fluid overload: moist respirations, stridor, or dyspnea	Alert physician, decrease the drip rate
Shock lung: tachypnea, dyspnea, anxiety, a rise in blood pressure, cyanosis, and harsh loud breaths	Alert physician, maintain ventilator between 50 and 70 mm Hg
Oxygen toxicity: muscular twitching about the face, followed by convulsions resembling grand mal seizures.	Alert physician; take convulsion precautions

General Nursing Care Plan

HEMORRHAGIC DISORDERS OF PREGNANCY

ASSESSMENT	NURSING DIAGNOSIS (ND), PLAN/GOAL (P/G)	RATIONALE/ IMPLEMENTATION	EVALUATION
Vital signs and blood pressure. Affect/LOC. Tenderness. Integument. Time in child-bearing cycle: Prenatal: duration since LMP. Postnatal: duration since delivery. Events preceding symptoms (falls, vaginal examination, coitus, childbirth). Previous obstetric history. Amount of bleeding, presence and size of clots. Associated discomfort: amount and location. Passage of tissue. Blood: Rh and blood group, type and cross-match as necessary; Hgb, Hct; CBC: WBC, platelets. Urine: UTI; chest x-ray study if extrapelvic infection is suspected or if surgery is anticipated.	ND: Decreased cardiac output related to hemorrhage. ND: Fluid volume deficit related to hemorrhage. ND: Impaired gas exchange related to hemorrhage or its therapy. ND: Altered cardiopulmonary tissue perfusion related to hemorrhage. ND: Fluid volume excess related to blood or fluid replacement. ND: Potential for injury related to infection or excessive volume loss. ND: Pain related to procedures and/or complications. P/G: The client will remain physiologically safe as indicated by: a. Vital signs stabilized within normal limits. b. Hemodynamic stability. c. Absence of infection. d. Absence of pain.	*Prompt identification and treatment of hemorrhage will decrease complications:* Report and record findings promptly. Monitor vital signs, blood pressure, LOC, CVP, integument. Save all peripads, linens soaked with blood, clots, and tissue. Start IV infusion. Hang appropriate blood product. Administer medications as ordered. Obtain specimen collection, (blood, urine, culture). Insert retention urine catheter. Provide preoperative and postoperative care as needed. Give Rh_o (D) immune globulin, if indicated.	Woman's blood loss is minimized. Vital signs are stabilized within normal limits. Complications of blood, fluid, and electrolyte replacement are averted. Fluid and electrolyte balance is maintained. Woman's reproductive capability is maintained. Surgical intervention is successful with no adverse sequelae. Comfort is maximized. Client remains free from infection. Fetus/newborn suffers no sequelae related to maternal condition.
Assess woman's learning needs in regard to hemorrhage, its management, and complications.	ND: Knowledge deficit related to identification of and care during a hemorrhagic disorder. P/G: Woman will verbalize understanding of her condition and its management. P/G: Woman will verbalize the danger signals of hemorrhage. P/G: Woman will verbalize the signs and symptoms of infection.	*Knowledge of health problems allows woman and family to be active participants:* Carefully explain known causes, management, and expected outcomes. Assist in identifying questions for the physician. Teach woman about danger signs and symptoms and whom to call should they occur. Counsel regarding antibiotic therapy. Counsel regarding nutrition to prevent anemia. Provide information regarding contraceptives as appropriate. Refer to social services	Woman and family verbalize understanding of the condition and its management. Woman identifies danger signals and whom to notify.

General Nursing Care Plan—cont'd

ASSESSMENT	NURSING DIAGNOSIS (ND), PLAN/GOAL (P/G)	RATIONALE/ IMPLEMENTATION	EVALUATION
Assess for previous experience with loss and positive coping mechanisms utilized. Assess support system. Assess current emotional status of woman. Identify spiritual needs.	ND: Anxiety related to actual or potential loss. ND: Body image disturbance, personal identity disturbance, situational low self-esteem, altered role performance. ND: Ineffective individual or family coping related to loss and grief. ND: Powerlessness related to loss or grief. ND: Spiritual distress related to loss or guilt. P/G: Woman and family will accept a loss in a positive manner (Chapter 29). P/G: Guilt or blame will be averted. P/G: Self-concept will not be disturbed. P/G: Spiritual distress will be averted. P/G: Sense of power will be retained (participates in own care).	*Grief reactions are individualized for each family member:* Explain procedures, sensations, expected outcomes; answer questions. Involve family in planning and care. Encourage verbalization of concerns and feelings. Assist woman and family with emotional reactions. Explain the grief process. Give couples experiencing perinatal loss the opportunity to see fetus or inform them of sex. Baptize products of conception or newborn, or summon clergy if requested. Offer pictures, lock of hair, or footprints as memories for woman and family.	Woman verbalizes understanding of condition and its management. Woman identifies support system. Woman initiates grief process.
Disseminated intravascular coagulation (DIC). Predisposing factors: Retained dead fetus. Infection. PIH. Abruptio placentae. Amniotic fluid embolism. Signs: Spontaneous bleeding (e.g., from gums, nose). Excessive bleeding from site of slight trauma. Reduced laboratory values for platelets, fibrinogen, proaccelerin, antihemophilic factor, and prothrombin. Ecchymoses. Occurrence of sequelae: Acute renal failure. Pituitary insufficiency.	ND: Anxiety, fear, pain, ineffective individual coping related to signs and symptoms of DIC. ND: Knowledge deficit related to DIC, its causes and management. ND: Fluid volume deficit or excess related to DIC or its management. ND: Altered cardiopulmonary tissue perfusion and injury related to DIC. P/G: Mother will demonstrate no serious sequelae to hemorrhage or treatment. P/G: Newborn will demonstrate no evidence of hypoxia.	*Prompt identification and treatment of complications protect mother and fetus:* Assist physician with treatment or removal of predisposing factors: a. Deliver dead fetus. b. Treat existing infection or PIH. c. Deliver fetus and abrupted placenta. Replace clotting factors. Assist with treatment of sequelae.	The woman survives the disease with minimum or no damage to body organs or systems. The woman's blood-clotting mechanism returns to normal. The woman and her family understand the disease process and its management. The newborn survives with no adverse sequelae.

KEY CONCEPTS

- Preeclampsia is characterized by hypertension and proteinuria often accompanied by edema occurring after the twentieth week of pregnancy or during the early postpartum.
- The anticonvulsive drug of choice, magnesium sulfate, requires careful monitoring of respirations, reflexes, and urinary output.
- Management of an eclamptic convulsion directs the caregivers to act to prevent self-injury, to ensure adequate oxygenation, to reduce risk of aspiration, to establish control with magnesium sulfate, and to correct maternal acidemia.
- Pregnancy confers no immunity against infection and both mother and fetus must be considered when the pregnant woman contracts an infection.
- Young sexually active females and males who have multiple sex partners and do not practice safe sex are at greatest risk for STDs.
- Since medical history and examination cannot reliably identify all people with HIV or other bloodborne pathogens, blood and body-fluid precautions should be consistently implemented.
- STDs and genital and perigenital infections are biologic events, for which people have a right to expect objective, compassionate, and effective health care.
- Many spontaneous abortions occur for unknown reasons, but fetoplacental maldevelopment and maternal factors can account for others.
- Ectopic pregnancy is a significant cause of maternal morbidity and mortality even in developed countries.
- Abruptio placentae and placenta previa are differentiated by type of bleeding, uterine tonicity, and presence or absence of pain.
- Postdelivery hemorrhage is the most common and most serious type of excessive obstetric blood loss.
- Hemorrhagic (hypovolemic) shock is an emergency situation in which the perfusion of body organs may become severely compromised and death may ensue.

SUMMARY

Hypertensive disease, infection, and hemorrhage are three distinct pathologic conditions that can lead to inevitable harm to the mother and newborn if not appropriately identified and emergency measures instituted. These complications usually begin in the antepartum period, so the well-being of and optimum outcomes for mother and newborn must be considered. In some instances all three complications may occur simultaneously. The nurse plays a major role in identifying these complications, initiating appropriate nursing and medical treatments, monitoring the response to treatment, and providing appropriate verbal and written communication to other health care workers. Universal precautions are initiated to ensure both client safety and prevention of spread of infection to health care workers. Although all possible medical and nursing interventions are attempted, there still may be maternal or neonatal loss. The nurse also provides emotional support to the family during this period of loss and grief.

LEARNING ACTIVITIES

1. Develop a plan of care, utilizing nursing diagnoses, for a client with preeclampsia. Be certain to include potential problems.
2. Divide students into four groups. Have each group take one STD or TORCH infection and develop a complete nursing care plan for a 22-year-old who is 10 weeks pregnant. (Woman is married.) When finished, compare and contrast the nursing care plans, noting the similarities and differences.
3. Discuss a general nursing care plan for a young mother who has been diagnosed with AIDS. She is being discharged home with her baby. You are to make a home visit and teach her and the family members about her care and infection control.
4. Role-play a nurse caring for each of the following clients:
   a. A 22-year-old unmarried woman threatened with the loss of her first pregnancy at 14 weeks.
   b. A 35-year-old mother of twins who lost 1500 ml of blood at the time of delivery.
   c. A 28-year-old woman whose second pregnancy is complicated by a suspected placenta previa. Following cesarean delivery, she develops DIC.
   d. A 28 year-old G3, P2 at 35 weeks gestation with an abruptio placentae. She admits to IV cocaine use last night.

References

Hypertensive States

Anderson GD: A systematic approach to eclamptic convulsion, Contemp OB/GYN 29(3):65, 1987.

Brazie JE, Gumm JK, and Little VA: Neonatal manifestations of severe maternal hypertension occurring before the thirty-sixth week of pregnancy, J Pediatr 100:265, 1982.

Cunningham FG, MacDonald PC, and Gant NF: Williams obstetrics, ed 18, Norwalk, Conn, 1989, Appleton & Lange.

Egley CC, Gutliph J, and Bowes WA: Severe hypoglycemia associated with HELLP syndrome, Am J Obstet Gynecol 152:576, 1985.

Iams JD and Zuspan FP: Zuspan and Quilligan's manual of obstetrics and gynecology, ed 2, St Louis, 1990, The CV Mosby Co.

Knuppel RA and Drukker JE: High-risk pregnancy: a team approach, Philadelphia, 1986, WB Saunders Co.

Kozier B and Erb G: Fundamentals of nursing, ed 2, Menlo Park, Calif, 1987, Addison-Wesley Publishing Co, Inc.

O'Brien WF: Predicting preeclampsia, Obstet Gynecol 75(3):445, 1990.

Reiss RE et al: The blood pressure source in primiparous pregnancy: a prospective study of 383 women, J Reprod Med 32:523, 1987.

Sachs BP et al: Maternal mortality in Massachusetts: trends and prevention, N Engl J Med 316(11):667, 1987.

Scott JR et al: Danforth's obstetrics and gynecology, ed 6, Philadelphia, 1990, JB Lippincott Co.

Sibai BM: Seeking the best use for magnesium sulfate in preeclampsia–eclampsia, Contemp OB/GYN 29(1):155, 1987.

Weinstein L: The HELLP syndrome: a severe consequence of hypertension in pregnancy, J Perinat 6(4):316, 1986.

Infection

Berkley SF et al: The relationship of tampon characteristics to menstrual toxic shock syndrome, JAMA 258(7):908, 1987.

Bernstein I and Capeless E: Elevated maternal serum alphafetoprotein and hydrops fetalis in association with fetal parvovirus B19, Obstet Gynecol 74(3):456, 1989.

Cates W and Lloyd-Schulz S: Epidemiology of HIV in women, Contemp OB/GYN 30(9):94, 1988.

Centers for Disease Control: Hepatitis B virus and vaccine, Hepatitis Branch, Center for Prevention Services, CDC, Atlanta, Ga, 1986.

Centers for Disease Control: Risks associated with human parvovirus B19 infection, MMWR 38(6):81, 1989.

Chorba R and Anderson L: Erythema infectiosum (fifth disease) Clin Dermatol 7(1):65, 1989.

Corbett M and Meyer JH: The adolescent and pregnancy, Boston, 1987, Blackwell Scientific Publications, Inc.

Ferenczy A, moderator: Symposium: treating condylomata, Contemp OB/GYN 30(3):158, 1987.

Foster SD: Education, the best defense against AIDS: MCN focus on patient teaching, MCN 12(5):311, 1987.

Francis DP and Chin J: The prevention of acquired immunodeficiency syndrome in the United States, JAMA 257(10):1357, 1987.

Friedland GH and Klein RS: Transmission of the human immunodeficiency virus, 317(18):1125, 1987.

Gershon A: Chickenpox: how dangerous is it? Contemp OB/GYN 31(3):41, 1988.

Gotoff S: Prophylaxis for early-onset group B strep, Contemp OB/GYN 30(11):25, 1988.

Guinan ME: Treatment of primary and secondary syphilis: defining failure of three- and six- month follow-up, JAMA 257:359, 1987.

Hecht F: Counseling the HIV-positive woman regarding pregnancy, JAMA 257(24):3361, 1987.

Helstrom KK: Fifth disease and pregnancy: what the childbirth educator should know, Int Childbirth Educ 5(1):Feb 1990.

Huffman DG and Blanco JD: Multiple genital papillomatosis: an indication for cesarean section? JAMA 258(22):3309, 1987.

Keeling RP: AIDS education: a mandate for schools of nursing, Dean's Notes 9(2):1, 1987.

Klug RM: AIDS beyond the hospital: children with AIDS, Am J Nurs 86(10):1126, 1986.

Landesman S et al: Serosurvey of human immunodeficiency virus infection in parturients, JAMA 258(19):2701, 1987.

Markowitz LE et al: Lyme disease during pregnancy, JAMA 255:3394, 1986.

Marvin C and Slevin A: Chlamydia—cause, prevention, and cure, MCN 12(5):318, 1987.

Mead P: Parvovirus B19 infection and pregnancy, Contemp OB/GYN 34(3):56, 1989.

Minkoff HL: Pregnant women with HIV, JAMA 258(19):2714, 1987a.

Minkoff HL et al: Pregnancies resulting in infants with acquired immunodeficiency syndrome: description of the antepartum, intrapartum, and postpartum course, Obstet Gynecol 69:285, 1987b.

Minkoff HL et al: Follow-up of mothers of children with AIDS, Obstet Gynecol 87:288, 1987c.

MMWR: Penicillinase-producing *Neisseria gonorrhoeae*—United States, 1986, JAMA 257(12):1579, 1987.

Rhoads JL et al: Chronic vaginal candidiasis in women with human immunodeficiency virus infection, JAMA 257(22):3105, 1987.

Samra J, Obhrai M, and Constantine G: Parvovirus infection in pregnancy, Obstet-Gynecol 73(5 Pt 2):832, 1989.

Schachter J et al: Erythromycin in the routine treatment of chlamydial infections in pregnancy, N Engl J Med 314:276, Jan 30, 1986.

Shaw NS: Serving your patients in the age of AIDS, Contemp OB/GYN 28(4):141, 1986.

Thurn J: Human parvovirus B19: historical and clinical review, Rev Infect Dis 10(5):1005, 1011.

Towers C and Keegan K: The many forms of viral hepatitis, Contemp OB/GYN 29(8):39, 1987.

Tramont EC: Syphilis in the AIDS era, N Engl J Med 316(25):1600, 1987.

Update: human immunodeficiency virus infection in health care workers exposed to blood of infected patients, MMWR 36:285, 1987.

Washington AE, Browner WS, and Korenbrot CC: Cost-effectiveness of combined treatment for endocervical gonorrhea considering co-infection with *Chlamydia trachomatis*, JAMA 257(15):2056, 1987a.

Washington MD, Johnson RE, and Sanders LL: *Chlamydia trachomatis* infections in the United States, JAMA 257(15):2070, 1987b.

Williams C and Strobino BA: Lyme disease transmission during pregnancy, Contemp OB/GYN 35(6):48, 1990.

Wolf PH et al: Toxic shock syndrome, JAMA 258(7):908, 1987.

Hemorrhage

Athey PA, and Hadlock, FP: Ultrasound in obstetrics and gynecology, ed 2, St Louis, 1985, The CV Mosby Co.

Cocaine use linked to infant defects, San Francisco Chronicle, Jan 19, 1987.

Cole HM, editor: Cardiovascular effects of cocaine, JAMA 257(7):979, 1987.

de Crespigny LC: The value of ultrasound in ectopic pregnancy, Clin Obstet Gynecol 30(1):136, 1987.

Diamond MP and DeCherney AH: Surgical techniques in the management of ectopic pregnancy, Clin Obstet Gynecol 30(1):200, 1987.

Rigby PG: Bleeding: symposium on bleeding disorders in pregnancy, Am J Obstet Gynecol 156(6):1422, 1987.

Royce JA: Shock emergency nursing implications, Nurs Clin North Am 8:377, 1973.

Scott JR et al: Danforth's obstetrics and gynecology, ed 6, Philadelphia, 1990, JB Lippincott Co.

Woods JR, Plessinger MA, and Clark KE: Effect of cocaine on uterine blood flow and fetal oxygenation, JAMA 257(7):957, 1987.

Bibliography

The American National Red Cross: The American Red Cross AIDS prevention program for youth, Washington DC, 1987, The Association.

Becker L and Lagomarsino W: Isolation guidelines for perinatal patients: creating a new protocol, MCN 12(6):400, 1987.

Bennett J: Aids: what precautions do you take in the hospital? Am J Nurs 86(8):952, 1986.

Bennett J: Nurses talk about the challenge of AIDS, Am J Nurs 87(9):1150, 1987.

Birdsall C and Ruggio J: Clinical savvy: mouth-to-mouth resuscitation—is there a safe, effective alternative? Am J Nurs 87(8):1019, 1987.

Brengman SL and Burns MK: Hypertensive crisis in L & D, Am J Nurs 88(3):325, 1988.

Celeste SM and Smith MD: Gestational trophoblastic neoplasms, JOGN Nurs 15:11, Jan/Feb, 1986.

Centers for Disease Control: CDC reports caution obstetric personnel, patients about AIDS virus, NAACOG Newsletter 13(6):1, 1986.

Centers for Disease Control: 1989 sexually transmitted diseases treatment guidelines, MMWR 38(S-B):5, 1989.

Clark SL: Severe preeclampsia: the role of invasive hemodynamic monitoring, The Female Patient 14(12):52, 1989.

Conti MT and Eutropius L: Preventing UTIs: what works? Am J Nurs 87(3):307, 1987.

DeBrow ME: Safer sex, NSNA/IMPRINT ISSUES, p 33, Feb/Mar, 1988.

DeVore N and Baldwin K: Ectopic pregnancy on the rise, Am J Nurs 86(6):674, 1986.

Few BJ: Prostaglandin F_2 for treating severe postpartum hemorrhage, MCN 12(3):169, 1987.

Flint C: Postpartum hemorrhage at home, Nurs Times, 84(3):47, 1988.

Fogel CI et al: Gonorrhea in women: a serious health problem, Health Care Women Int 8(1):75, 1987.

Gillespie L: When cystitis is suspected, what's the next step? NAACOG Newsletter 14(10):1, 1987.

Hodges LC and Poteet GW: The tragedy of AIDS: a new trial for nursing education, Nurs Health Care 8(10):656, 1987.

Jackson MM et al: Clinical savvy: why not treat all body substances as infectious? Am J Nurs 87(9):1137, 1987.

Johnstone HA and Marcinak JF: Candidiasis in the breastfeeding mother and infant, JOGN Nurs 19(2):171, 1990.

Karnes N: Don't let ARDS catch you off guard, Nurs '87 17(5):34, 1987.

Kennedy M: AIDS: coping with the fear, Nurs '87 17(4):44, 1987.

King J: Vaginitis, JOGN Nurs 13:41s, 1984.

Knor ER: Decision making in obstetrical nursing, 1987, BC Decker, Inc.

Kuczynski JJ: Support for the women with an ectopic pregnancy, JOGN Nurs 15(4):306, 1986.

Larson E: Chlamydia: the most prevalent cause of sexually transmitted disease, Health Care Women Int 8(1):19, 1987.

Lewis HR and Lewis ME: What you and your patients need to know about safer sex, RN 53, Sept, 1987.

Loos C and Julius L: The client's view of hospitalization during pregnancy, JOGN Nurs 1(18):52, 1989.

Mims BC: The risks of oxygen therapy, RN, p 20, July, 1987.

Nadal D, Hunziker UA, and Bucher HU: Infants born to mothers with antibodies against *Borrelia burgdorferi* at delivery, Eur J Pediatr 148:426, 1989.

Nze R: Supporting the mother and infant at risk for A.I.D.S., Nurs '87 17(11):44, 1987.

Osguthorpe NC: Ectopic pregnancy, JOGN Nurs 16(1):36, 1987.

O'Sullivan M and Ricci J: Uterine rupture: management alternative, Contemp OB/GYN (special edition): p 83, 1988.

Peck NL: Action stat! Blood transfusion reaction, Nurs '87 17(1):33, 1987.

Reckling JB and Neuberger GB: Understanding immune system dysfunction, Nurs '87 17(9):34, 1987.

Shannon DM: HELLP syndrome: a severe consequence of pregnancy-induced hypertension, JOGN Nurs 16(6):395, 1987.

Sibai B and Moretti M: PIH: still common and still dangerous, Contemp OB/GYN 2(31):57, 1988.

Sumner SM: Action stat! Septic shock, Nurs '87 17(2):33, 1987.

Tcheng D: When pregnancy threatens mother and child (preeclampsia), RN p 46, Dec, 1986.

USPHS AIDS information hotline: 800/342-AIDS

Williams CL, et al: Lyme disease during pregnancy: a cord-blood serosurvey, Ann NY Acad Sci 539:504, 1988.

CHAPTER

24 Endocrine, Cardiovascular, Medical, and Surgical Problems

Irene M. Bobak and Fannie M. Rankin-Hirschhaut

Learning Objectives

Correctly define the key terms listed.

Differentiate diabetes mellitus types I, II, III, and IV and their respective factors in pregnancy.

Discuss each step of the nursing process when the pregnancy is complicated by diabetes mellitus.

Explain effects of selected disorders on pregnancy.

Review the management of pregnant women with cardiovascular disorders.

Discuss anemia during pregnancy.

Relate the care of women whose pregnancies are complicated with autoimmune disorders.

Discuss cancer and pregnancy.

Key Terms

adult respiratory distress syndrome (ARDS)
autoimmune disorders
benign
carcinoma
cardiac decompensation
chemotherapy
diabetes mellitus
diethylstilbestrol (DES)
euglycemia (normoglycemia)
gestational diabetes
gestational trophoblastic neoplasia
glucose tolerance test (GTT)
glycohemoglobin (HbA_{1c})
hyperemesis gravidarum
hyperglycemia
hypoglycemia
hydramnios
insulin
large-for-gestational age (LGA)
macrosomia
malignant
maternal phenylketonuria (PKU)
metastasis
mitral valve prolapse (MVP)
neoplasm
peripartum cardiomyopathy
physiologic anemia of pregnancy
reflex bradycardia
sickle cell hemoglobinopathy
systemic lupus erythematosus
trauma care

It is not uncommon for women with preexisting medical problems to become pregnant. Nor does pregnancy protect women from developing medical problems or sustaining injuries. The maternity nurse is challenged to provide sound care that meets the unique maternal and fetal needs presented by these conditions. The primary objective must be to guide and support the woman and her family in achieving optimum health for the woman and her fetus. The nurse serves as teacher, counselor, and support person to help the woman and family achieve the best possible outcome and deal with the problems and disappointments that may arise.

Endocrine Disorders

Endocrine disorders complicate many pregnancies. Of these disorders, diabetes mellitus is the most common. Hyperemesis gravidarum and disorders of the thyroid, although encountered less often, also require careful planning for care. Phenylketonuria, an inborn error of metabolism, is a relatively new disorder of women of reproductive age (see p. 706). The first portion of this chapter addresses the special needs of women whose pregnancies are complicated by endocrine disorders.

DIABETES MELLITUS

Preexisting **diabetes mellitus** as a complication of pregnancy was a rare occurrence before the discovery of **insulin.** Before insulin therapy was available, most diabetic girls died before or during puberty; many were amenorrheic and therefore infertile or sterile. When pregnancy did occur, the maternal mortality was 25%; fetal-neonatal loss was 50%. Today, techniques such as home glucose monitoring, multiple doses or constant infusion of insulin, and dietary counseling (American Diabetes Association, 1987) are being used to create a normal intrauterine environment for fetal growth and maturation. These therapeutic modalities most often result in the delivery of an infant who is structurally and physiologically normal (Gabbe, 1985). Such measures have also proved a significant benefit to the mother, providing her with techniques that enable her to be an active participant in her care and remain outside the hospital. If she continues to follow this regimen after she has delivered her child, she may reduce long-term morbidity from diabetes mellitus.

Classification

Following is the 1979 classification of diabetes mellitus issued by the National Diabetes Data Group.

type I diabetes mellitus Formerly called juvenile-onset diabetes or insulin-dependent diabetes; onset in people 40 years or *younger;* etiology: genetic, immunologic, viral. Prone to ketosis.

type II diabetes mellitus Formerly called maturity-onset diabetes or non-insulin-dependent diabetes; occurs in all ages, but more usual in the older, overweight person; etiology: primarily genetic. Resistant to ketosis. In pregnancy, insulin is required to control maternal plasma glucose levels (Hollingsworth, 1985).

type III diabetes mellitus Formerly called **gestational diabetes;** intolerance to glucose with onset during pregnancy with return to normal glucose tolerance after delivery.

type IV diabetes mellitus Formerly called secondary diabetes; refers to abnormalities in glucose tolerance following pancreatic disease, endocrine disorders (Cushing's syndrome), drug ingestion (oral contraceptives), cirrhosis, and the like.

hyperglycemia Blood levels of glucose that exceed normal values.

White's classification of pregnant diabetic women (1978) considers age at onset, duration, and vascular or renal changes, if any. White's classification includes glucose intolerance of pregnancy; A (the mildest form), B, C, D, F, H, and R. Although even mild forms of diabetes pose a threat to mother and infant, the incidence of perinatal death increases with the presence and degree of vascular or renal pathologic changes (classes D, F, H and R).

Incidence. Diabetes mellitus is a complication in about 1% to 2% of pregnant women. It has been found that one in four families has a history of diabetes. The incidence of diabetes mellitus increases with age. About 3.8 in every 100 women will become diabetic. Many of these cases will be diagnosed during pregnancy. A significant number of women who exhibit gestational diabetes will show further deterioration of carbohydrate metabolism during the next 15 years of life (Scott et al, 1990).

Pathogenesis. Diabetes mellitus (types I, II and III) is regarded primarily as a genetically determined syndrome. It is usually inherited as a recessive trait but occurs as a dominant trait in some families. If the β-cells of the islets of Langerhans (pancreas) are deficient either in number or in function, the production of endogenous insulin falls short of the need. As a result, glucose is poorly used, and abnormalities of carbohydrate, protein, and fat metabolism appear. The cardinal signs and symptoms of diabetes mellitus are polyuria (excretion of large amounts of urine), and polydipsia (excessive thirst). The body compensates for its inability to convert carbohydrate into energy by burning proteins (muscle) and fats. Unfortunately the end products of this metabolism are ketones and fatty acids, which in excess quantity produce acidosis and acetonuria. Weight loss occurs in the presence of excessive hunger (polyphagia).

Inheritance of the genetic trait (genotype) for diabetes mellitus does not necessarily mean that the individual will demonstrate diabetic glucose intolerance (phenotype). Many people with the genotype do not show any evidence of diabetes until they experience one or more of a variety of precipitating factors. Examples of such stressors include an increase in age, normal developmental periods of rapid hormonal change (menarche, pregnancy, and menopause), obesity, infection, surgery, emotional factors, and tumor or infection of the pancreas (may damage the β-cells so that diabetes occurs as a result of the trauma).

Effects of Pregnancy on Insulin Requirements

During the first trimester the developing embryo-fetus siphons (moves by active transport) glucose across the placenta from the mother. This gestational period

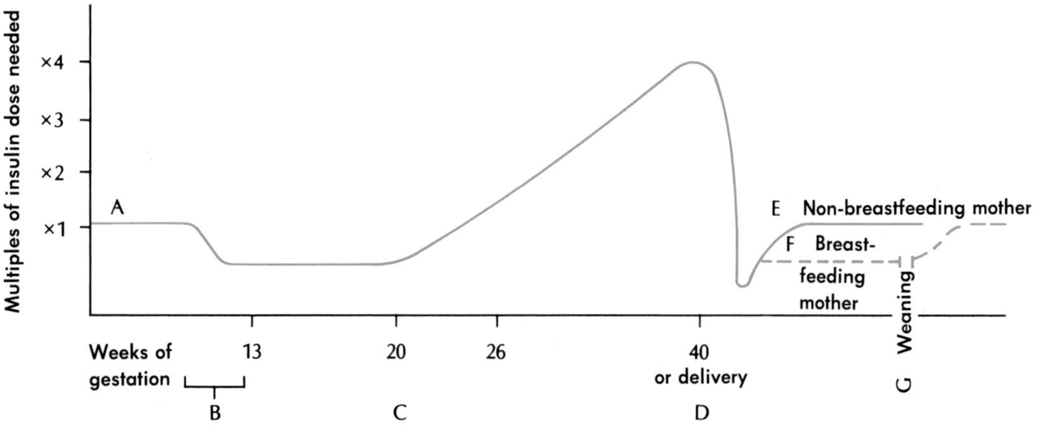

Fig. 24-1 Changing insulin needs during pregnancy caused by properties of placental hormones and enzyme (insulinase) and cortisol.

is characterized by nausea, vomiting, and often, decreased food intake by the mother while glucose use by the embryo-fetus increases. As maternal glucose is used by the fetus, the maternal glucose level drops, thereby decreasing the need for insulin (Fig. 24-1, *A* to *B*). ***Maternal insulin does not cross the placenta.*** By the eighth week of gestation the conceptus secretes her or his own insulin at levels adequate to use the glucose obtained from the mother.

During the second and third trimesters, the development of maternal resistance to insulin keeps pace with the increasing levels of placental hormones (especially hPL), insulinase, and cortisol. Insulin resistance is a glucose-sparing mechanism that assures an abundant supply of glucose to the fetus. The mother's need for insulin increases beginning in the second trimester. Insulin requirements may double or quadruple by term gestation (Fig. 24-1, *C* to *D*).

Delivery of the placenta brings about an abrupt drop in levels of circulating placental hormones, insulinase, and cortisol. Maternal tissues quickly regain their prepregnancy sensitivity to insulin. For the nonbreastfeeding mother, prepregnancy insulin-carbohydrate balance usually returns in about 7 to 10 days (Fig. 24-1, *E*). Lactation utilizes maternal glucose, so that the breastfeeding mother's insulin requirements will remain low for up to 6 to 9 months (Fig. 24-1, *F*). On completion of weaning, prepregnancy insulin requirements are reestablished (Fig. 24-1, *G*).

Effects of Pregnancy on Diabetes Mellitus

Diabetic control is affected by the pregnancy-induced changes in insulin requirements. The insulin doses and food required to control diabetes during the pregnancy may change often. Fatigue and increased stress may reduce exercise and activities and cause higher blood glucose levels. The quality of maternal blood glucose control throughout pregnancy is an important consideration. Ketoacidosis and associated intrauterine death are most common in women with poor blood glucose control.

Whether or not pregnancy worsens diabetes-related macrovascular and microvascular disease depends on the extent of this complication before the pregnancy. The greater the degree of *vasculopathy,* the greater the likelihood of poor outcome for mother and child. Pregnancy can contribute to a worsening of retinal disease in women with a background of proliferative *retinopathy,* especially in the presence of hypertension. Women with active proliferative retinopathy are at greatest risk for loss of visual acuity. Maternal deaths have been reported in women with coronary artery disease.

If kidney function is seriously affected by the diabetes before the pregnancy, with an actual reduction in filtering capacity, kidney function may become worse during the pregnancy. Neuropathy may worsen during the pregnancy, perhaps causing some foot and leg numbness, tingling, or discomfort (American Diabetes Association, 1988). Programs instituting care *before* pregnancy, as well as supervision throughout pregnancy, are associated with the best outcome for the woman and the fetus (Cunningham, MacDonald, and Gant, 1989; Scott et al, 1990).

Effects of Diabetes Mellitus on Pregnancy

Conditions associated with diabetes increase maternal morbidity and mortality. Associated conditions vary slightly with the class of diabetes. In the presence of mild diabetes (classes A to C and glucose intolerance of pregnancy), in which there *is no* associated vascular disease, there is a greater incidence of intensification of preexisting diabetic condition, pregnancy-induced hypertension (PIH), preeclampsia, hydramnios, intranatal fetal death, macrosomia (**large-for-gestational age [LGA]**), and large placenta.

In the presence of more advanced diabetes (classes D to R), in which there *is associated vascular disease,* there is a greater incidence of spontaneous abortions, intrauterine growth retardation (IUGR) (small-for-gestational age [SGA]), and intrauterine fetal deaths and neonatal deaths. Complications associated with mild diabetes occur less commonly.

Infections are much more common and serious in diabetic women who are pregnant (e.g., pyelonephritis, monilial vaginitis). Disorders in carbohydrate metabolism alter the body's normal resistance to infection. The inflammatory response, leukocyte function, and vaginal pH are all affected. The changes of pregnancy predispose any woman to urinary tract infection (UTI). Infection results in increased insulin resistance and ketoacidosis. Unless recognized and treated promptly, ketoacidosis adversely affects the fetus. Ketoacidosis is poorly tolerated by the fetus. Fetal death may occur.

The severity of preeclampsia (occurring in 10% to 20% of pregnant diabetic women) is associated directly with the degree of renal *vascular involvement.* Severe vascular involvement results in deterioration of the placenta and IUGR or death, the need to deliver the baby prematurely because of the risk to the mother in continuing the pregnancy, and possible abruptio placentae (premature separation of the normally implanted placenta, Chapter 23).

Effects of Diabetes Mellitus on Labor and Delivery

Hydramnios (polyhydramnios) occurs about 10 times as often in pregnancies of diabetic women as in pregnancies of nondiabetic women. Hydramnios (amniotic fluid in excess of 2000 ml) increases the possibility of compression of abdominal blood vessels (vena cava and aorta), causing supine hypotension. Hydramnios also causes maternal dyspnea because of upward pressure on the diaphragm. Hydramnios is associated with preterm labor, perhaps because of overstretching of the uterus, and with dystocia (difficult labor and delivery).

There is a greater likelihood of large fetuses (**macrosomia**). Large fetuses are associated with dystocia (Chapter 26), often resulting in operative vaginal delivery (episiotomy and forceps), trauma to the mother's soft tissues or to the baby, and cesarean delivery.

The outcome for both the mother and her child from the embryo stage through birth is determined in large measure by the degree to which diabetes is controlled. If there are no complications of pregnancy, and diabetes is well controlled, mortality for the woman with diabetes is about the same as that for any other woman. The infant from a pregnancy complicated by diabetes mellitus is discussed in Chapter 28.

Perinatal mortality increases threefold to fourfold for the diabetic woman who experiences any of the following conditions: pyelonephritis, severe acidosis, PIH, or poor diabetic control (sometimes because of poor compliance by the woman). Perinatal mortality of 50% follows an acute onset of hydramnios or a rapid drop in insulin requirements.

In the woman who experiences glucose intolerance of pregnancy, the glucose tolerance test (GTT) results typically return to within normal range 3 to 5 weeks after delivery.

Assessment

History and Interview. Early identification of glucose intolerance in a woman is essential so that prompt appropriate therapy can be initiated. Factors in a woman's *history* that are associated with the risk of glucose intolerance of pregnancy include: family history of diabetes (first-degree relatives only [i.e., parents, siblings]); poor obstetric history (e.g., spontaneous abortion, unexplained stillbirth, hydramnois, unexplained prematurity or low birth weight); previous birth of a newborn weighing 4000 g (8 lb 13½ oz) or more; previous birth of a newborn with major congenital anomalies; and high parity (5 or more).

Since emotional stress is a precipitating factor, family and socioeconomic events are reviewed. Certain cultural considerations may present conflict for the pregnant woman (e.g., large infants expected, high food intake encouraged) and should be addressed.

Physical Examination. Findings in the current pregnancy that alert the health care team to the possibility of diabetes (in the absence of a previous diagnosis of the condition) include maternal age of 25 years or older, obesity (weight of 90.7 kg [200 lb] or more), recurrent monilial (*Candida albicans* or "yeast") vaginitis that is not responding to therapy, and glycosuria.

Hydramnios and a large fetus palpated during Leopold's maneuvers warrant further assessment. Women with PIH (Chapter 23) should be assessed for diabetes mellitus. A retinal examination should be done routinely for all gravidas for retinopathy of diabetes and also for changes that may occur with PIH.

If the pregnant woman is insulin dependent, an assessment of her vascular status should include ophthalmologic examination, electrocardiogram (ECG), 24-hour urine for protein, creatinine clearance, and assessment of all peripheral pulses; capillary filling time; lower extremeties; and skin integrity, especially at injection sites, to determine damage or absorption alterations.

Fetal Surveillance. Diagnostic techniques for fetal surveillance (Chapter 22) are often ordered for the woman whose pregnancy is complicated by diabetes mellitus (see box below). Ultrasonography reveals progress of growth and presence of congenital malformations (e.g., caudal regression syndrome). Maternal blood and urine estriol measurement by radioimmunoassay (RIA) reflects the combined function of the placenta and fetus, as well as the clearance of estriol conjugates by the maternal system. Difficulties with this test plus other technologic developments in diagnosis and management have led many physicians to abandon estriol monitoring (Cunningham, MacDonald and Gant, 1989; Scott et al, 1990).

Biochemical analysis of amniotic fluid is done to ascertain fetal lung maturity and congenital malformations (Chapter 22). Since the frequency of neural tube defects in infants of diabetic mothers is more than 10 times that of the general population (Milunsky, et al, 1982), all gravidas with overt diabetes should be offered serum α-fetoprotein (AFP) testing (Cunningham, MacDonald, and Gant, 1989). Another diabetes-associated anomaly, renal agenesis, may result in elevated maternal serum AFP.

Biophysical monitoring is also employed (Chapter 22). Nonstress test (NST), contraction stress test (CST), daily fetal movement count, and biophysical profile are used to expand the data base for assessment. Cardiac anomalies may be reasonably assessed by routine fetal echocardiography (ECHO) (Kleinman, 1982).

Data from all these tests discern some fetuses in jeopardy in pregnancies complicated by diabetes. The specific value of any one test is more difficult to discern. Evidence supports **euglycemia** (**normoglycemia**) as the key to improved perinatal survival.

Determination of Delivery Date. In the past, preterm delivery was often elected to avoid the risk of intrauterine fetal death. Today, delivery can be safely delayed until term gestation in most pregnancies complicated by type I or type III (gestational) diabetes as long as gravidas maintain excellent glycemic control and all parameters of antepartum fetal surveillance have remained normal. In women who have vasculopathy or poor control, who have not adhered to the program of care, or who have had a previous stillbirth, elective delivery to prevent late fetal death may be planned at 38 weeks provided that fetal pulmonary maturation has been confirmed by the analysis of amniotic fluid. (For the pregnancy complicated by diabetes mellitus, fetal lung maturation is better predicted by the amniotic fluid ***phosphatidylglycerol [PG]*** content than by the lecithin/sphingomyelin (L/S) ratio [Scott et al, 1990].) If the fetal lungs are still immature at 38 weeks, delivery should be postponed as long as the results of fetal assessment remain reassuring. Amniocentesis may be repeated to monitor lung maturation. Delivery despite fetal lung immaturity may be essential when testing suggests fetal compromise or if the gravida develops preeclampsia, rapidly worsening retinopathy, or renal failure.

Laboratory Tests. Glycosuria can be diagnosed with Tes-Tape, Clinitest, Diastix, or Chemstrip UG. All of these depend on enzyme reactions *specific for glucose,* not to be confused with fructosuria and lactosuria.

Laboratory tests are required to establish the diagnosis of diabetes mellitus. Two types of laboratory tests are available: tests to identify levels of glucose in blood or plasma and a test to determine the percent of normal adult hemoglobin (HbA) that is glycosylated (**glycohemoglobin** [**HbA_{1c}**]). Some physicians suggest that *all* pregnant women should be screened for plasma glucose using the 50 g, 1-hour glucose screen during the first prenatal visit. Coustan and Carpenter (1985) believe the most efficient time to perform this test is at 24 to 26 weeks of gestation. Most clinical laboratories are now measuring glucose in plasma by more specific glucose oxidase techniques.

The 1-hour glucose screening test can be performed in a clinic or office setting on a woman who has been fasting or nonfasting. A fasting plasma glucose level above 105 mg/dl or a plasma glucose level of 150 mg/dl or greater 1 hour later is considered an indication for diagnostic testing using the 3-hour **glucose tolerance test** (GTT) (Coustan and Carpenter, 1985).

After a 100 g glucose load, the 3-hour GTT is ab-

FETAL SURVEILLANCE

MIDPREGNANCY(16-20 wk): to detect fetal anomalies

Maternal serum α-fetoprotein
Ultrasonography
Fetal echocardiography

LATE PREGNANCY(28 wk to delivery): to assess fetal well-being

Maternal assessment of fetal activity
Nonstress test
Contraction stress test
Fetal biophysical profile
Ultrasonography
Lecithin/sphingomyelin (L/S) ratio and presence of phosphatidylglycerol, lung profile

normal if two or more of the following values are found:

	Plasma (mg/dl)	Venous Whole Blood (mg/dl)	Plasma (Glucose Oxidase) (mg/dl)
Fasting	≥105	≥90	≥95
1 hour	≥190	≥165	≥180
2 hours	≥165	≥145	≥155
3 hours	≥145	≥125	≥140

The above criteria are the same regardless of age, duration of pregnancy, or obesity.

With prolonged hyperglycemia, some of the hemoglobin remains saturated with glucose for the life of the red cell. Therefore a test for HbA_{1c} is a reflection of serum glucose levels during the preceding 4 to 6 weeks (Scott et al, 1990). HbA_{1c} is useful for assessing overall control in type I (insulin-dependent) diabetes. It has not proved useful in screening for glucose intolerance of pregnancy. Glycosylated hemoglobin measures three components of HbA: A_{1a}, A_{1b}, and A_{1c}. Values are as follows (Corbett, 1987):

≤7.5%	Good diabetic control
7.6% to 8.9%	Fair diabetic control
≥9%	Poor diabetic control

Values for the measurement of HbA_{1c} *only* are as follows (Corbett, 1987):

2.2% to 4.8%	Nondiabetic adult
2.5% to 5.9%	Good diabetic control
6% to 8%	Fair diabetic control
≥8%	Poor diabetic control

A decreased incidence of congenital anomalies is associated with HbA_{1c} values that are within normal limits. However, normal HbA_{1c} levels do not guarantee the absence of diabetes-associated anomalies (Mills et al, 1988).

Nursing Diagnoses

Each woman's experience with the serious diagnosis of diabetes mellitus is unique to her and her family. Nursing diagnoses must be carefully formulated to reflect the actual or potential altered health-related responses that can be influenced, improved, or alleviated by nursing interventions. Examples of possible nursing diagnoses follow:

Anxiety (or fear) related to
- The diagnosis

Knowledge deficit related to
- The disorder, its management, and prognosis for self and baby

Potential for injury to self and fetus related to
- Poor control of diabetes

Noncompliance related to
- Insufficient funds or lack of transportation to grocery store
- Insufficient funds to purchase blood glucose or urine testing materials

Altered nutrition: less or more than body requirements

Powerlessness related to
- Unexpected diagnosis that disrupts expectations of "normal" pregnancy

Body image disturbance

Situational low self-esteem

Spiritual distress

Altered family processes

Decisional conflict related to
- Potential job performance change
- When to stop working

Planning

Planning care for women and their families is given direction from identified nursing diagnoses and the medical management of this complication. The plan is individualized, relating specifically to needs identified by the caregivers and to those mutually identified by the woman and caregivers. The information in this chapter is general in nature; not all women experience all problems discussed nor require all facets of care described. See the nursing care plans and client teaching in this chapter.

The ***goals*** of management include:

1. The mother's risk is minimized
2. The woman's need for antepartum hospitalization to maintain or restore diabetic control is minimized
3. The woman and her family learn about diabetes mellitus and its control
4. The woman does not experience perinatal morbidity and mortality
5. The mother maintains her self-esteem
6. The family experiences mutuality and support among its members
7. The family receives health care team support

Implementation

Assisting the woman with stress reduction is central to the care needed by women whose pregnancies are complicated by diabetes mellitus. Stress reduction and relaxation, discussed in Chapter 10, are taught as needed. Space, privacy, and time are provided for the woman and her family to voice their feelings and questions, as well as to problem-solve among themselves. It takes time to adjust to any change in self-concept and expectations. In addition to the support needed in light of this complication, nursing interventions to meet the care needs of any gravida and her family are provided.

Fetal surveillance techniques may identify a congenital malformation incompatible with survival. Parents need supportive care as they consider the option of early pregnancy termination (Van Putte, 1988). The early detection of serious fetal malformations allows for exploration of various options in planning delivery and immediate care of the newborn. The parents may also benefit from the time to prepare for the birth of a child with a congenital abnormality. Even though the testing methods are noninvasive, the investigation of a pregnancy for fetal malformations should be conducted under conditions that are both voluntary and informed (see Informed Consent, Chapter 3). The risks, accuracy, and limitations of the tests should be discussed. The benefits of diagnosis and the options available when a positive diagnosis is obtained should be discussed in advance.

Engaging the woman as an active participant in the health care team maintains or enhances her self-esteem and develops her self-confidence that she will be able to care for herself and her baby. The responsive, reliable, self-assured woman, who has learned to assess her own blood glucose and maintain euglycemia and who communicates openly and frequently with the physician and nurse, often can be seen at the clinic or the office on the same schedule as the nondiabetic gravida. Open communication is encouraged to facilitate client participation in self-care. The need for hospitalization during pregnancy to control diabetes and the need for early delivery are minimized. With this approach to care the nurse-clinician or nurse-practitioner is the primary educator for the woman and her family.

Pregnancy

Dietary or insulin management must be based on blood glucose (not urinary glucose) values. The diet is individualized to allow for increased maternal and fetal metabolic requirements: calories, 35 to 40 kcal/kg of ideal body weight*; protein, 1 g/kg of ideal body weight; complex carbohydrates, 50% to 55% of total calories; body weight; fat, less than 30% of total calories. During pregnancy, sufficient calories, minerals, and vitamins must be provided. Supplements are often recommended. Based on some control trials, the caloric distribution of complex carbohydrates may need to be less as a result of individualized responses to carbohydrate metabolism (Hauenstein and Patterson, 1989).

Regardless of the woman's eating pattern before pregnancy, some changes will be necessary as the pregnancy progresses. Total calories may be distributed among three meals and one evening snack or, more commonly now, three meals and at least two snacks.

The dietary goal is to provide weight gain consistent with a normal pregnancy, to prevent ketoacidosis, and to minimize widely fluctuating blood glucose levels. Women with insulin-dependent diabetes may experience some insulin resistence as the pregnancy progresses and blood glucose levels will vary with foods that previously did not elevate values.

Exercise must be regular to maintain a consistent use of glucose. The woman must be capable of making necessary adjustments to diet and insulin intake if the exercise patterns alter. Some women may need to initiate an exercise pattern.

During the first trimester, *insulin requirements* may be slightly less in the woman with type I diabetes. Hypoglycemic episodes may occur because of fetal drain of glucose and low levels of hormone antagonists to insulin, as well as because of lessened intake as a result of morning sickness. During the second trimester, insulin requirements begin to increase. Insulin adjustments vary from person to person, but for many the ratio between regular and intermediate action insulins change. Often, toward the last few weeks of pregnancy, the amount of insulin needed begins to decline.

Monitoring Blood Glucose. Blood glucose testing at home is now the commonly accepted method for monitoring blood glucose levels. The woman and her family require instructions and rationale for testing and reporting results (Fig. 24-2). Blood glucose levels are monitored by fasting blood sugar and 1½- to 2-hour postprandial tests.

Using a color graph machine (glucose reflectance meter) reduces or eliminates the necessity of obtaining venous blood samples and thereby "saves" accessible veins. Using an automatic pricking device, the woman obtains a blood sample from the side of a finger (all the fingers are used in rotation) (Fig. 24-2). The drop of blood is placed on a glucose reagent strip. After a predetermined number of seconds, the blood is wiped or blotted from the strip and placed in the machine, the color graph is read electronically. The results are recorded and reported to the physician. If blood glucose levels measure less than 100 mg/dl, as a rule the infant is normosomic and has few hypoglycemic problems after delivery.

The advent of home glucose monitoring has been credited with increasing the woman's feeling of control over self, and with decreasing or eliminating hospitalizations and therefore separation from family. It presents the most accurate method to document the degree of control in an out-of-hospital setting. It enables the woman to adjust her insulin dosage on a 24-hour basis.

*The actual number of kilocalories the individual woman should receive varies. The woman needs sufficient kilocalories to achieve optimum weight gain and to prevent acidosis.

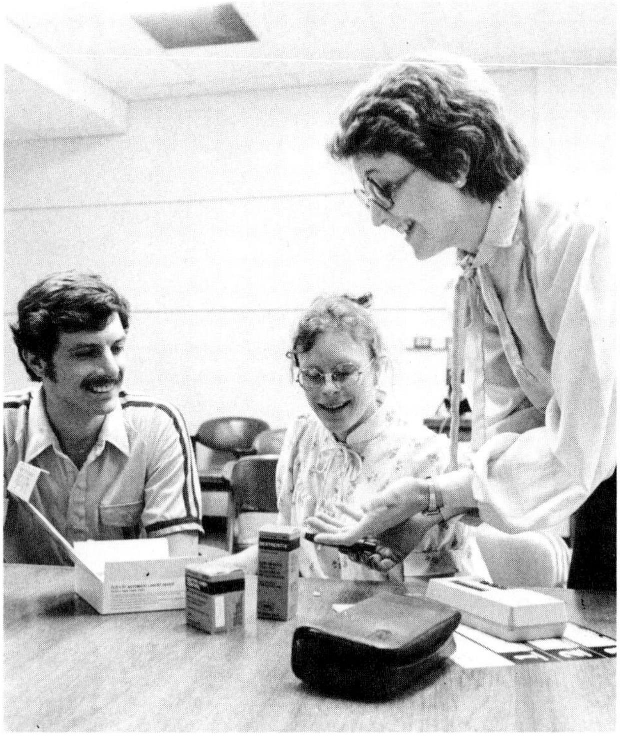

Fig. 24-2 Nurse is teaching family home monitoring of blood glucose. After return demonstration, nurse reviewed with woman how to balance insulin doses with findings. (Courtesy Stanford University Medical Center, Stanford, California.)

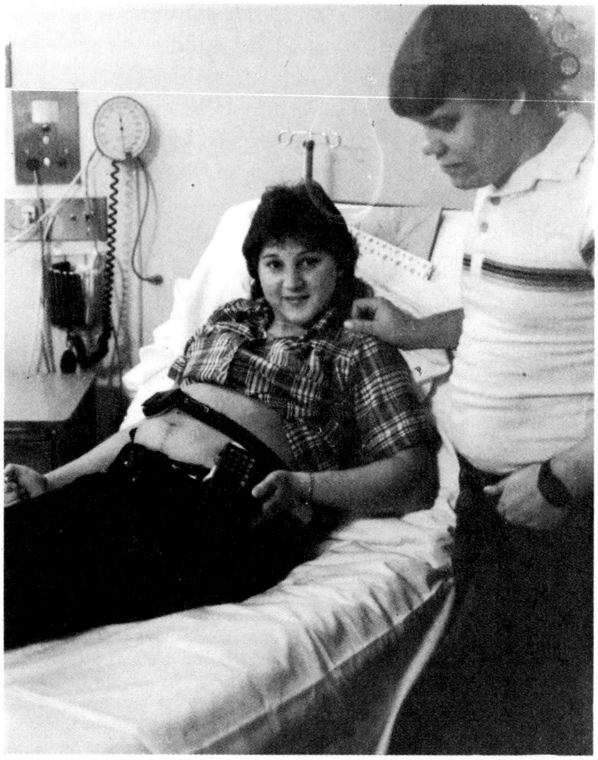

Fig. 24-3 Continuous insulin infusion regulated closely with home monitoring of glucose makes tighter control of diabetes mellitus possible.

Early detection of hypoglycemia is possible even during sleep (Landon and Gabbe, 1985). If used before conception and early in pregnancy, home glucose monitoring may safeguard the conceptus during organogenesis.

Continuous subcutaneous insulin infusion systems (Fig. 24-3) simplify insulin administration for women who need multiple injections per day (Nursing 87). The system infuses insulin at a set basal rate with a bolus dose to cover meals. The infusion tubing from this portable, battery-operated pump can be left in place for several weeks without local complications. Several biochemicals in addition to glucose are also maintained within normal limits, thus decreasing the risk of developing diabetes-related complications. The pump's effects on pregnancy have yet to be determined (Leveno et al, 1988).

If there is a question about the woman's ability to maintain euglycemia, visits are scheduled a minimum of every 2 weeks for the first 32 weeks and then weekly until delivery. A urine sample is checked at each visit throughout pregnancy for blood, glucose, ketones, protein, bilirubin, and pH. Microscopic examination may reveal asymptomatic UTIs, which are frequent and can cause fetal demise. Women having poor control need to be carefully assessed for infection; for example, asymptomatic UTIs may significantly change a woman's insulin requirements. Mycotic (yeast) vaginitis in the diabetic pregnant woman is more common and difficult to control. Women having poor control may be hospitalized from week 34 until delivery (Cunningham, MacDonald, and Gant, 1989).

Fetal well-being is monitored closely (Chapters 14 and 22). The stress of frequent monitoring can be relieved somewhat by meeting the woman's knowledge needs, by referring the woman to social service agencies for assistance with child care and transportation, and by providing a private time and space to discuss concerns.

The diabetic pregnant woman is provided with written instructions as to the need for prompt reporting of ***nausea, vomiting,*** and ***infections*** (see general nursing care plan, pp. 701–705).

Despite the advances in home glucose monitoring some women may require hospitalization for regulation of insulin. Before pregnancy a woman may have been taking an oral hypoglycemic agent, but during pregnancy she may have to change to regular insulin. She may have poor control ("brittle diabetes") so that daily evaluation is necessary. If she develops an infection, intravenous (IV) antibiotic therapy may be indicated. Close monitoring of fetal health may be required as a basis for early termination of the pregnancy.

Labor and Delivery

Most women utilize large amounts of energy (calories) to accomplish the work and manage the stress of labor and delivery. However, each woman expends different amounts of calories. Blood sugar levels and hydration must be controlled carefully during labor. To accomplish this, an IV line is inserted for infusion of glucose and regular insulin by calibrated pump. It is important to reduce considerably or delete the dose of long-acting insulin given on the day of delivery. Regular insulin is used, since insulin requirements drop markedly after delivery (Cunningham, MacDonald, and Gant, 1989). Hourly determinations of blood glucose are made. Insulin and glucose are titrated to maintain blood glucose levels of 70 to 100 mg/dl (Robertson, 1987).

Intranatal insulin requirements involve a prescribed dose of insulin added to 100 ml of 10% dextrose in water for IV solution. NOTE: insulin, a protein, is attracted chemically to the plastic in the IV tubing. It leaves the solution and adheres to the lining of the tubing. Adherence to the tubing can be prevented by flushing the line first with 100 ml of normal saline and 10 units of insulin, which will completely coat the lining. Then the prescribed solution of insulin is begun and will remain stable. (A protein [albumin] may be added to the solution instead; however, it is more expensive.)

The mother should assume a side-lying position during bed rest in labor to prevent supine hypotension because of a large fetus or polyhydramnios. If strong labor and good progress do not ensue within 6 to 8 hours, cesarean delivery may be considered. Poorly controlled diabetes or obstetric indications such as fetopelvic disproportion, positive oxytocin challenge test (OCT), change in estriol levels, or preeclampsia–eclampsia is also an indication for a cesarean delivery. The woman is observed and treated for diabetic complications such as hyperglycemia, ketosis, ketoacidosis, and glycosuria (Table 24-1). A pediatrician should be present at delivery to initiate proper neonatal care.

Postpartum Period

The woman must be closely monitored after delivery. The urine, or preferably the plasma, should be tested for ketones (Cunningham, MacDonald, and Gant, 1989). The woman may require no insulin or only one half to two thirds of her prenatal dosage on the first postpartum day if she is eating a full diet (Scott et al, 1990). Insulin requirements may fluctuate markedly during the next few days. It takes several days after delivery to reestablish carbohydrate homeostasis (see Fig. 24-1). The insulin-dependent woman must realize that *she must eat on time*. This is true even if the baby needs feeding or other pressing demands exist.

Possible *complications* include preeclampsia–eclampsia, hemorrhage, and infection. *Preeclampsia* occurs in one fourth of all diabetic new mothers and in one third of all diabetic new mothers, class C or D. *Hemorrhage* is a possibility if the mother's uterus had been overdistended (hydramnios, macrosomic fetus) or overstimulated (oxytocin induction). Monilial *infection* of the vagina or nipples or other infections are more likely to occur in a woman suffering from diabetes.

Breastfeeding is encouraged. Besides the advantages of maternal satisfaction and pleasure, breastfeeding also has an antidiabetogenic effect. Breastfeeding decreases the dosage for insulin-dependent women. The insulin dosage must be readjusted at the time of weaning (see Fig 24-1, *F* to *G*).

The new mother needs information for *family planning* and *contraception*. To assist in their decision making, couples need to be informed that if the mother has type I diabetes, the offspring have a 22% chance of developing diabetes; if she has type II diabetes, the offspring have a 4% chance. Nearly 100% of offspring of parents who both have noninsulin-dependent diabetes develop that type of diabetes. Only 45% to 60% of the offspring of both parents who have insulin-dependent diabetes will develop the syndrome.* The risk of diabetes doubles with every 20% of excess weight, and this figure applies to the young, as well as to the older, diabetic person. Diabetes is now the sixth leading cause of death by disease in adults and the first leading cause of new cases of blindness between the ages of 20 and 75. If contraception is chosen, the woman may be advised to use the *diaphragm with spermicide*. The use of oral hormonal contraceptives is questioned because of their effect on carbohydrate metabolism. However, much more serious is the possibility of increased risk of ischemic heart disease and cerebrovascular accidents (Steele, 1985). The use of triphasic pills may carry less risk.

Intrauterine devices (IUDs) may be associated with an increased risk of infection for some women. In the presence of severe renal disease and proliferative retinopathy, sterilization may be advised (Steele, 1985).

Evaluation

Evaluation is a continuous process. The woman's responses to the disorder are assessed constantly. Adjustments in the care plan are made in regard to measureable outcome criteria or goals. Clinical findings that represent expected responses are presented under "Evaluation," in the nursing care plan on pp. 701-705.

*Prediction of risk varies from author to author (Steele, 1985).

Table 24-1 Differentiation of Hypoglycemia, Ketoacidosis, and Hyperglycemic Hyperosmolar Nonketotic Coma (HHNK)

Hypoglycemia (Insulin Reaction)	Ketoacidosis (Diabetic Coma)	HHNK
CAUSES		
Too much insulin Not enough food (delayed or missed meals) Excessive exercise or work Indigestion, diarrhea, vomiting	Too little insulin Too much or wrong kind of food Infection, injuries, illness Insufficient exercise	Abnormally high glucose levels without ketoacidosis in mild or suspected diabetic—pancreatic disorders that lower production of insulin Complication of extensive burns, excess steroids (i.e., with steroid therapy), acute stress, TPN,* hemodialysis, peritoneal dialysis
ONSET		
Sudden (regular insulin) Gradual (modified insulin or oral agents)	Slow (days)	Rapid if woman dehydrated
SYMPTOMATOLOGY		
Hunger Sweating Nervousness Weakness Fatigue Blurred or double vision Dizziness Headache (especially with NPH insulin† or PZI) Pallor, clammy skin Shallow respirations Normal pulse Laboratory values Urine: negative for sugar and acetone Blood glucose: 60 mg/dl or less	Thirst Nausea or vomiting Abdominal pain Constipation Drowsiness Dim vision Increased urination Headache Flushed, dry skin Rapid breathing Weak, rapid pulse Acetone (fruity) breath odor Laboratory values Urine: positive for sugar and acetone Blood glucose: 250 mg/dl	Polyuria Thirst (intracellular dehydration) Hypovolemia Blood serum levels Fasting blood sugar (FBS): 600-3000 mg/dl Acetone level: normal or slightly elevated Dry skin Coma, death
NURSING ACTIONS		
Notify physician Give low-fat milk If orange juice is given for a fast supply of sugar, follow it later with milk Obtain blood and urine specimens for laboratory testing	Notify physician Keep woman flat in bed and warm Record intake and output Check and record vital signs	Administer insulin in line with blood glucose levels Monitor IV therapy (sodium and water deficits corrected without extreme shift of fluid into intracellular compartment with no reduction of hyperosmolarity of blood) Monitor woman for dehydration; record intake and output Check and record vital signs Notify physician of changes in symptomatology

Modified from form used at Santa Clara Valley Medical Center, San Jose, Calif.
*TPN (total parenteral nutrition) replaces the term *hyperalimentation*.
†NPH: neutral protamine Hagedorn; PZI: protamine zinc insulin.

General Nursing Care Plan

DIABETES MELLITUS

ASSESSMENT	NURSING DIAGNOSIS (ND), PLAN/GOAL (P/G)	RATIONALE/ IMPLEMENTATION	EVALUATION
PRENATAL CARE			
How long has woman had diabetes mellitus? Has woman administered insulin? Knowledge about diabetes. Knowledge about care needed during pregnancy to prevent sequelae for the mother and fetus.	ND: Knowledge deficit related to diabetes mellitus, its management, and potential effects on the pregnant woman and fetus. ND: Ineffective individual coping related to woman's responsibility in managing her diabetes mellitus during pregnancy. P/G: Woman will learn about diabetes mellitus, its management, and potential sequelae during pregnancy. P/G: Woman will demonstrate technique of home monitoring tests and verbalize understanding of the results she should report.	*Woman needs to understand about diabetes mellitus, its management, and effects on pregnancy to effectively control the disorder:* Review pathophysiology of the disease. Assist woman in formulating questions for the physician. Clarify misconceptions. Teach home monitoring tests, demonstrate techniques, interpretation, and recording of results. Review the effects of diabetes on the pregnant woman and fetus. Teach (written and oral) the danger signs of diabetes and whom to notify. Stress importance of weekly prenatal visits during second half of pregnancy. Refer woman to community diabetic support group.	Woman verbalizes understanding of instruction. Woman accurately demonstrates how to perform home monitoring tests. Woman keeps all scheduled appointments. Woman notifies caregiver if danger signs appear. Woman joins and participates in community diabetic support group.
Assess verbal and nonverbal reactions regarding diabetes and pregnancy. Assess woman's support system. Note previous successful coping mechanisms. Note plans for family/work relationships.	ND: Anxiety, fear, ineffective individual coping, dysfunctional grieving, powerlessness, body image disturbance, self-esteem disturbance, altered role performance, personal identity disturbance, spiritual distress, and altered family processes related to diabetes and its potential sequelae on the pregnant woman and fetus. P/G: Woman will verbalize concerns and feelings regarding diabetes and its potential sequelae on herself and fetus. P/G: Woman will identify her support system. P/G: Woman will identify previous successful coping mechanisms.	*Verbalizing concerns and adjusting to the strict management of her disease will increase woman's ability to cope:* Provide private area for conversation. Discuss issues in an unhurried manner. Provide consistency in caregivers. Encourage verbalization of concerns and feelings. Answer questions honestly. Assist woman in formulating questions for physician. Offer woman choices when possible. Compliment woman on successful learning, problem solving, and coping.	Woman verbalizes her concerns and feelings. Woman participates in her plan of care. Woman identifies her support system. Woman identifies previous successful coping mechanisms.

Continued.

General Nursing Care Plan—cont'd

ASSESSMENT	NURSING DIAGNOSIS (ND), PLAN/GOAL (P/G)	RATIONALE/ IMPLEMENTATION	EVALUATION
		Identify previous successful learning, problem solving, and coping. Identify with woman her support system. Involve significant others in plan of care. Refer to community diabetes support group. Refer to psychologist, clergy, social worker, etc.	
Assess knowledge regarding insulin and its administration. Note any possible objections to animal source or human source insulins.	ND: Knowledge deficit related to insulin effects and its administration. ND: Potential for injury related to improper insulin administration. P/G: Woman will learn the purpose and effects of insulin in the body. P/G: Woman will administer insulin to herself correctly.	*Learning about insulin, its effects on the body, and proper administration takes time and effort:* Explain insulin's effect on the body. Review peak action of insulin and signs of hypoglycemia. Stress importance of administration of correct dose with correct syringe. Demonstrate correct withdrawal and administration of insulin. Explain importance of site rotation and identify the sites that can be used. Teach proper techniques of insulin storage. Monitor woman's self-administration of insulin until techniques are learned and understood. Explain why insulin needs will be higher during the third trimester.	Woman learns the purpose and effect of insulin. Woman administers her own insulin properly. Woman understands changing insulin needs during pregnancy.
Assess knowledge of **hyperglycemia.**	ND: Knowledge deficit related to hyperglycemia or hypoglycemia. ND: Potential for injury related to hyperglycemia or hypoglycemia to the pregnant woman and fetus. P/G: Woman will verbalize the signs and symptoms of hyperglycemia or hypoglycemia. P/G: Woman will seek medical attention when danger signs and symptoms occur.	*Hyperglycemia compromises the woman's and fetus's well-being and must be prevented:* Explain that illness, infection, vomiting, and diarrhea can precipitate ketoacidosis. Encourage woman to call physician when illness occurs and continue to administer insulin. Teach danger signs of ketoacidosis.	Woman learns the signs and symptoms of hyperglycemia. Woman verbalizes danger signs and whom to notify if they occur. Woman notifies caregiver promptly if danger signs appear. Woman experiences no episodes of hyperglycemia.

General Nursing Care Plan—cont'd

ASSESSMENT	NURSING DIAGNOSIS (ND), PLAN/GOAL (P/G)	RATIONALE/ IMPLEMENTATION	EVALUATION
	P/G: Woman will use preventive measures to avoid hyperglycemia and hypoglycemia.		
Assess knowledge of **hypoglycemia,** its signs and symptoms, and its treatment. Assess knowledge of preventive measures for hypoglycemia.		*Hypoglycemia compromises the gravida's and fetus's well-being and must be prevented:* Teach signs and symptoms of hypoglycemia. Review causes and dangers of insulin reaction. Stress importance of carrying fast-acting sugar when traveling and of having milk on hand at home. Review relationship of exercise and diet. Explain importance of seeking medical attention for hypoglycemia. Give Medic-Alert information and encourage woman to wear bracelet or necklace. Review with significant others the signs of hypoglycemia and hyperglycemia and whom to notify when danger signs occur.	Woman verbalizes signs and symptoms of hypoglycemia. Woman carries supply of fast-acting sugar and verbalizes having milk on hand at home. Woman wears Medic-Alert bracelet at all times. Woman experiences no episodes of hypoglycemia. Family verbalizes knowledge of signs of hypoglycemia and its treatment.
Review knowledge of diabetic diet. Assess cultural and financial influences on food served. Who prepares the meals? Who buys the food? Woman's likes/dislikes.	ND: Knowledge deficit related to the diabetic diet and its importance to a woman with diabetes during pregnancy. ND: Altered nutrition: less or more than body requirements, related to diabetes and pregnancy. P/G: Woman will learn about the diabetic diet and verbalize the importance of adhering to its protocol during pregnancy.	*Compliance with diabetes diet management during pregnancy is essential for the gravida's and fetus's well-being:* Consider cultural and financial implications when planning teaching. Ascertain type of diet woman is to follow at home. Refer to registered dietitician (RD). Explain importance of a balanced diet. Encourage woman to design sample menus. Stress importance to maintain or achieve appropriate weight and pattern of weight gain during pregnancy. Stress importance of preplanning food intake during holidays or celebrations.	Woman verbalizes understanding of instruction. Woman gains weight according to protocol for the pregnant woman with diabetes. Woman implements diet prescribed by and developed with caregiver.

Continued.

General Nursing Care Plan—cont'd

ASSESSMENT	NURSING DIAGNOSIS (ND), PLAN/GOAL (P/G)	RATIONALE/ IMPLEMENTATION	EVALUATION
INTRAPARTUM CARE			
Perform assessments for normal laboring woman. Assess for signs of hypoglycemia. Assess for signs of preeclampsia. Assess fetal monitor strip. Assess anxiety level. Assess for excessive uterine size associated with hydramnios and fetal macrosomia. Assess for dyspnea and supine hypotension related to excessive uterine size.	ND: Potential for injury related to hypoglycemia. ND: Potential for injury related to preeclampsia. ND: Anxiety related to labor. ND: Altered cardiopulmonary tissue perfusion related to supine hypotension. P/G: Woman will be monitored closely and treated for signs of hypoglycemia, preeclampsia, and supine hypotension. P/G: Fetus will be monitored closely for signs of distress.	*Maternal and fetal complications occur more often when pregnancy is complicated by diabetes mellitus:* Monitor vital signs, especially blood pressure, frequently. Monitor and report signs and symptoms of preeclampsia and hypoglycemia. Evaluate and record labor pattern. Continuously monitor fetal heart rate (FHR) and report fetal distress. Monitor IV fluids of 10% dextrose in water and insulin as ordered; titrate infusion to frequent blood glucose determinations to maintain euglycemia. Monitor the administration of oxytocin for induction as ordered. Provide supportive labor nursing, which is especially important to prevent hypoglycemia secondary to anxiety. Prepare for induction or cesarean delivery (fetal distress, fetopelvic disproportion, lack of labor progression). Alert pediatrician and nursery personnel.	Woman is monitored and treated promptly for preeclampsia and hypoglycemia. Supine hypotension is avoided. Euglycemia is maintained. Woman remains free of undue anxiety. Woman experiences no adverse sequelae to fluid therapy and oxytocin induction or augmentation of labor. Fetus remains free from distress as indicated by FHR.
POSTDELIVERY CARE			
Perform normal postpartum assessment. Note frequent blood and urine glucose levels. Note signs and symptoms of hypoglycemia or hyperglycemia. Assess signs and symptoms of hemorrhage and infection. See postpartum general care plan (Chapter 21).	ND: Potential for injury related to fluctuating blood glucose levels after delivery. ND: Potential for injury related to complications of involution (hemorrhage, infection), or postpartum appearance of preeclampsia. P/G: Woman's blood glucose level will be monitored closely for initial 24-48 hours postdelivery and remain within normal limits.	*Fluctuating glucose levels occur in the postpartum period and require careful management:* Perform frequent fractional urine tests. Obtain blood for glucose level as ordered. Monitor foods and fluids taken. Evaluate for signs and symptoms of hypoglycemia or hyperglycemia. Adjust insulin intake according to protocol ordered.	Woman's blood glucose stabilizes within normal limits; woman experiences minimum or no sequelae from hypoglycemia or hyperglycemia. Woman remains free of hemorrhage, infection, or preeclampsia. Woman verbalizes understanding of instruction. Woman progresses through involution without complication.

General Nursing Care Plan—cont'd

ASSESSMENT	NURSING DIAGNOSIS (ND), PLAN/GOAL (P/G)	RATIONALE/ IMPLEMENTATION	EVALUATION
	P/G: Woman will progress through normal involution without complication.	Explain the need to increase caloric intake by approximately 300-500 calories and decrease insulin by one half to successfully produce breast milk. If mother develops acetonuria, discard her breast milk until resolved. Explain that hypoglycemia decreases milk production. Counsel woman to eat every meal on time, even if it means others (including infant) must wait.	

HYPEREMESIS GRAVIDARUM

Hyperemesis gravidarum is defined as excessive or pernicious vomiting during pregnancy, leading to dehydration and starvation. Many pregnant women suffer nausea and vomiting at some time during early gestation. The indisposition is mild in most cases, but in about 1 of every 1000 pregnant women, severe intractable emesis will require hospitalization and perhaps even therapeutic abortion.

The cause of hyperemesis during pregnancy is still debated. Psychologically unstable women whose established reaction patterns to stress involve gastrointestinal disturbances often are affected. In some women, however, psychologic causes cannot be elicited. Other causes could be multifetal pregnancy, hormonal abnormalities (elevated thyroxine [T_4]), or trophoblastic disease (hydatidiform mole).

In extreme cases ***dehydration*** leads to fluid-electrolyte complications, particularly acidosis. Rarely does vomitus contain only gastric acid fluids. Most vomiting involves loss of contents (alkali) from deeper within the gastrointestinal tract. This leads to the development of ***metabolic acidosis. Starvation*** causes hypoproteinemia and hypovitaminosis. Degenerative changes produce characteristic symptomatology. Jaundice and hemorrhage as a result of vitamin C and B-complex deficiency and hypothrombinemia lead to bleeding from mucosal surfaces. The embryo or fetus may die, and the mother may die from irreversible metabolic alterations. In most cases hyperemesis gravidarum will respond to therapy; hence the prognosis is good. The woman is discharged home when fluid and electrolyte balance is restored and weight gain begins.

DISORDERS OF THE THYROID GLAND

Hyperthyroidism, which affects about 1 of every 1500 pregnant women, may seriously complicate gestation or endanger the fetus. Hyperthyroidism may be responsible for anovulation and amenorrhea, but the disease is not a cause of abortion or fetal anomaly. Hyperthyroidism is associated with an increased incidence of preterm labor and delivery. Symptoms include weakness, sweating, weight loss (or poor gain), nervousness, loose stools, and heat intolerance. Warm, soft, moist skin, tachycardia, exophthalmos, tremor, and goiter (enlarged gland) with a bruit are characteristic. Enlargement of the thyroid gland is symmetric. Laboratory findings, particularly the basal metabolic rate and the free T_4 index, will be elevated.

Any maternal therapy for thyroid dysfunction may induce fetal thyroid insult. Determination of free T_4 index in cord blood of such a newborn is necessary.

Hypothyroidism may be responsible for anovulation in the woman with impaired fertility. Moreover, thyroid deficiency may cause spontaneous abortion, fetal maldevelopment, or fetal goiter. The metabolic clearance of insulin, like that of most substances, is influenced by the metabolic status. Thus the woman with type I insulin-dependent diabetes may have an alteration in the insulin requirement with the development of hyperthyroidism or hypothyroidism. Since there may be an increased incidence of either hyperthyroidism or hypothyroidism in type I diabetes, this alteration in insulin requirement will be of primary concern when insulin adjustments are made in the pregnant diabetic. The combination of uncontrolled hyperthyroidism and insulin-dependent diabetes may be a considerable clinical challenge. Careful surveillance of the thyroid status and treatment in the pregnant diabetic are essential to maternal and fetal well-being (DeGroot et al, 1984).

MATERNAL PHENYLKETONURIA

Phenylketonuria (PKU) is an inborn error of metabolism caused by an autosomal recessive trait that creates a deficiency in the enzyme phenylalanine hydroxylase. Absence of this enzyme results in the inability to metabolize phenylalanine to tyrosine. Prompt diagnosis of this disorder in the newborn and subsequent dietary intervention have made it possible for individuals to live a productive life with the exception of reproduction. **Maternal phenylketonuria** (PKU) is a relatively new disorder of women of reproductive age, resulting from the improved newborn prognosis. Homozygosity for this disorder in a woman whose fetus is heterozygous produces disastrous fetal results.

Elevated maternal blood phenylalanine levels during pregnancy result in fetal hyperphenylalaninemia. Maternal risk in this disorder is not a factor; however, for the fetus, high frequency of spontaneous abortion, microcephaly, and intrauterine and postnatal growth retardation, including mental retardation, are almost universal. About one fourth of fetuses are malformed. Apparently, a maternal diet low in phenylalanine has questionable preventive value unless followed *before conception* (Cunningham, MacDonald, and Gant, 1989; Scott et al, 1990). A simple urine test (Phenostix) is available and is applied routinely to every woman in early pregnancy.

Cardiovascular Disorders

Every pregnancy taxes the cardiovascular system (Chapter 8). The strain is present during pregnancy and is maintained for a few weeks after delivery. An increase in blood volume begins by the tenth or twelfth week of gestation, reaches a maximum increase of 30% to 50% at 20 to 26 weeks, and levels off after the thirtieth week. Blood volume returns to nonpregnant levels within the first 2 to 3 weeks after delivery. The increase in blood volume is correlated with total birth weight and thus tends to be greater in multigravidas and women with multifetal pregnancies. The relaxation of the great veins causes a decrease in systemic vascular resistance, a decrease in blood pressure and pulse pressure, and an increase in cardiac output. The cardiac output and stroke volume at rest reflect the increase in the blood volume but return to normal by 6 weeks after delivery. The heart rate is accelerated by a maximum of 15 to 20 beats per minute (bpm) in the last trimester. The point of maximum intensity (PMI) is laterally displaced (see Fig. 8-8). A split develops in the first heart sound because of increased venous return to the heart. As many as 90% of women may develop a systolic ejection murmur. With delivery of the placenta and closure of the placental vascular shunt, venous hypertension occurs during the first 24 hours after childbirth.

The normal heart can compensate for these and associated burdens so that pregnancy and delivery are generally well tolerated. If myocardial or valvular disease develops, or if a congenital heart defect is large, cardiac decompensation is likely.

Heart disease is the leading cause of *non*obstetric maternal mortality. A maternal mortality of 1% to 3% is likely with severe heart disease. It ranks fourth overall as a cause of maternal death. A perinatal mortality of up to 50% must be expected with persistent cardiac decompensation. Some degree of cardiac impairment affects 0.5% to 2% of pregnant women (Roberts and Chestnut, 1987).

Congenital heart disease may result from genetic abnormalities, maternal condition, drug ingestion, infection, or a combination of these (Ramin, Maberry, and Gilstrap, 1989). Maternal diabetes, lupus erythematosus, rubella, and ingestion of lithium or alcohol are implicated. Cocaine use is associated with various cardiac complications (p. 742) and vascular phenomena (e.g., abruptio placentae).

The effects of pregnancy on heart disease result from the maternal adaptations during pregnancy. The stress these place on a heart whose function is already taxed can cause cardiac decompensation. Cardiac failure can develop during the last few weeks of pregnancy, during labor, and during the postdelivery period (Cunningham, MacDonald, and Gant, 1989).

Spontaneous abortion is increased, and preterm labor and delivery are more prevalent in the pregnant woman with cardiac problems. Probably because of the low Po_2 level, fetal growth retardation commonly occurs.

Little information is available regarding fetal risk for the majority of cardiac medications. Generally, the disease process carries more risk to the mother and fetus than the medications (Little and Gilstrap, 1989).

The differential diagnosis of heart disease involves ruling out respiratory problems and arrhythmias. The diagnosis of heart disease depends on the history, physical examination, x-ray films, and ultrasonograms when required.

Classification. The degree of dysfunction (disability) of the woman with cardiac disease often is more important in the treatment and prognosis of cardiac disease complicating pregnancy than the diagnosis of the valvular lesion per se. The New York Heart Association's functional classification of organic heart disease, a widely accepted standard, is as follows:

Class I: asymptomatic at normal levels of activity
Class II: symptomatic with increased activity
Class III: symptomatic with ordinary activity
Class IV: symptomatic at rest

No classification of heart disease can be considered rigid or absolute, but this one offers a basic practical guide for treatment, assuming frequent prenatal visits, good client cooperation, and proper obstetric care. Medical therapy is conducted as a team approach with a cardiologist. The functional class of the disease is determined at 3 months and again at 7 or 8 months.

DANGER SIGNS

Cardiac Decompensation

Gravida: Subjective Symptoms

1. Increasing fatigue or difficulty breathing or both with her usual activities
2. Feeling of smothering
3. Need to cough frequently
4. Rapid pulse; feeling that her heart is "racing"
5. Swelling of feet, legs, fingers (rings do not fit anymore), or face

Nurse: Objective Signs

1. Irregular rapid pulse (≥100 bpm)
2. Progressive, generalized edema
3. Crackles (rales) at base of lungs that persist after two deep inspirations
4. Orthopnea; increasing dyspnea
5. Rapid respirations (≥25 per minute)
6. Frequent cough
7. Increasing fatigue

Assessment

During the *prenatal period* the woman is assessed at weekly intervals at home or on a continuous basis if hospitalized. The nurse assesses for factors that would increase stress on the heart, such as anemia, infection, or a home situation that includes responsibility for the house, other children, or extended family members. The woman is observed for signs of **cardiac decompensation,** that is, progressive generalized edema, crackles (rales) at the base of the lungs that persist after one or two deep inspirations, or pulse irregularity (see box above, right). Symptoms of cardiac decompensation may appear abruptly or gradually. Medical intervention must be instituted immediately to correct cardiac status. Unfortunately dyspnea, chest pain, palpitations, and syncope occur commonly in pregnant women and can mask the symptoms of a developing or worsening cardiovascular disorder.

The routine assessment continues for the prenatal period, including monitoring weight gain and pattern of weight gain, edema, vital signs, discomforts of pregnancy, urinalysis, and blood work. The nurse keeps careful check of the side effects and interactions of all medications—including supplemental iron—that the woman is taking and reports them to the physician. Their use also is documented on the client's record.

During the *intrapartum period* assessment includes the routine assessments for all laboring women as well as assessments for cardiac decompensation. The latter include measurements of the pulse and respiratory rate at least 4 times every hour during the first stage of labor and every 10 minutes during the second stage (Cunningham, MacDonald, and Gant, 1989). ***The physician is alerted if the pulse rate is 100 bpm or greater or if respirations are 25 per minute or greater. Respiratory status*** is checked constantly for developing dyspnea, coughing, or crackles (rales) at the base of the lungs. The color and temperature of the skin are noted. Pallor, cooling, and sweating may indicate cardiac shock. The woman is carefully watched for symptoms of emotional stress.

The *immediate postdelivery period* is hazardous for a woman with a compromised heart. Cardiac output remains elevated for at least 48 hours after delivery. Venous return is increased as extravascular fluid is remobilized into the vascular compartment and pressure on the inferior vena cava is reduced. Stroke volume is increased and **reflex bradycardia** occurs. Some physicians favor the application of the abdominal binder or alternating tourniquets on the extremities to minimize the effects of this rapid change in the early puerperium. By 2 to 3 weeks postpartum, these changes have returned to nonpregnant levels.

Cardiac monitoring for decompensation continues through the first weeks after delivery because it has been known to occur as late as the sixth postpartum day. Routine assessment as for any newly delivered woman is instituted; for example, vital signs, bleeding, uterine contractility, urinary output, pain, rest, diet, and daily weight. Laboratory (e.g., hemoglobin, hematocrit, and urinalysis) results are noted and reported if indicated to the physician. It is important to assess the woman's support systems, since activity will be curtailed until the cardiac system is recovered. The family response to the birth and infant needs to be observed because the mother may not be directly involved in the infant's care for a period of time (e.g., prematurity of infant, health of mother).

Nursing Diagnoses

Following are examples of nursing diagnoses that may be formulated. As always, individualization of diagnoses is vital.

Prenatal

Potential altered tissue perfusion related to
- Hypotensive syndrome

Impaired home maintenance management related to
- Mother's confinement to bed

Intrapartum

Anxiety related to
- Fear for neonate's safety

Fear of dying related to
- Perceived physiologic inability to cope with the stress of labor

Postpartum

Self-care deficit related to
- Need for bed rest

Situational low self-esteem related to
- Restriction placed on involvement in care of newborn

Planning

The nursing diagnoses derived from analyses of clinical findings act as guides to develop a plan of care (see general nursing care plan, p. 711). The mother who has cardiovascular problems faces curtailment of her activities. These restrictions can have physical and emotional implications. The community health nurse, social worker, and pediatrician are some of the resource people whose services may need to be incorporated into the plan of care. Goals such as the following might be appropriate.

General ***goals*** for care include the following:

1. Woman and family understand the disorder, management, and probable outcome.
2. Woman and family understand their role in management, including when and how to take medication, diet, and preparation for and participation in treatment.
3. Woman and family cope with emotional reactions to pregnancy and newborn at risk.

Implementation

Therapy is focused on minimizing stress on the heart. Factors that increase the risk of cardiac decompensation are treated. The work load on the cardiovascular system is reduced by appropriate treatment of any coexisting emotional stress, hypertension, anemia, hyperthyroidism, or obesity. Infections are treated promptly since respiratory, urinary, or gastrointestinal tract infections can complicate the condition by accelerating heart rate and by direct spreading of organisms (e.g., *Streptococcus*) to the heart structure. Sodium intake is restricted and accompanied by careful monitoring for hyponatremia. The woman's intake of potassium is monitored to prevent hypokalemia. Hypokalemia is associated with heart and other muscular weakness and dysfunction. Anticoagulant therapy, if used, is monitored. Tests for fetal maturity and well-being, and placental sufficiency may be necessary. Other therapy is directly related to the functional classification of heart disease.

Class I. The pregnant woman with class I heart disease should limit stress to protect against cardiac decompensation. Frequent evaluations, and the early and effective treatment of respiratory and other infections should be stressed. Vaccines against pneumococcal and influenza infections are recommended. Therapeutic abortion is never medically warranted. If there are no obstetric problems, vaginal delivery is recommended. This is accomplished using epidural or pudendal block anesthesia with forceps for shortening of the second stage of labor.

Class II. A program similar to that for class I should be followed for the pregnant woman with class II heart disease. However, the woman should be admitted to the hospital near term (if signs of cardiac overload or arrhythmia develop) for evaluation and treatment.

Penicillin prophylaxis of nonsensitized pregnant women against bacterial endocarditis in labor and during the early puerperium may be ordered. Mask oxygen and pudendal block anesthesia are important. Ergot products should not be used because they tend to increase blood pressure. Dilute intravenous oxytocin immediately after delivery may be employed to prevent postdelivery hemorrhage. Tubal sterilization may be performed, but surgery is delayed several days at least to ensure homeostasis. If sterilization is not achieved, effective contraception without the use of estrogen and progesterone must be provided.

Class III. Bed rest for much of each day is necessary

for pregnant women with class III cardiac disease. About 30% of these women experience cardiac decompensation during pregnancy. With this possibility the woman may be hospitalized for the remainder of pregnancy and the early puerperium. Early therapeutic abortion may be suggested, particularly if the woman experienced a previous episode of cardiac failure. Breastfeeding is contraindicated. Sterilization should be postponed until a later date, but explicit contraceptive advice must be given.

Class IV. Because persons with class IV cardiac disease have decompensation even at rest, a major initial effort must be made to improve the cardiac status of pregnant women in this category. Early therapeutic abortion, although not without risk, may be feasible with regional anesthesia in some cases. Prophylactic antibiotic therapy may be ordered with the procedure. Vaginal delivery of women with class IV lesions is the safest approach if abortion is not done. Maternal mortality approaches 50% in class IV heart disease; the perinatal mortality is even higher.

Heart Surgery During Pregnancy. Operations for the correction of congenital or acquired heart disease should be done before pregnancy if possible. However, valve replacement and mitral valvotomy are surprisingly well-tolerated during pregnancy. Closed cardiac surgery, such as release of a stenotic mitral orifice, can be accomplished with little risk to mother or fetus. Open heart surgery requires extracorporeal circulation, and under these circumstances, fetal hypoxia may develop. With current surgical and anesthetic techniques, the theoretical risk to the fetus is decreased.

If anticoagulant therapy is required during pregnancy, ***heparin*** should be used because this large-molecule drug does not cross the placenta (Cunningham, MacDonald, and Gant, 1989; Anticoagulants, 1990; Scott et al, 1990). Even though heparin is the anticoagulant of choice during pregnancy, it is not without risk. Heparin use can result in maternal hemorrhage, preterm birth, and stillbirth. Oral anticoagulants, such as warfarin (Coumadin) compounds, cross to the fetus and may cause anomalies or hemorrhage in the infant (Anticoagulants, 1990).

Prenatal Period

Signs and symptoms of cardiac decompensation are reviewed with the gravida and her family. The woman requires *adequate rest.* She should sleep 8 to 10 hours every day and 30 minutes after meals. Her activities are restricted; for example, if the woman is at home, she needs to limit housework, shopping, walking, and laundry to the amount allowed for her functional classification of heart disease. *Nutrition* counseling is necessary for her in the presence of her family. Adequate nutrition may be difficult to achieve especially when someone else shops and cooks for her. The woman needs a diet high in iron and protein and adequate enough in kilocalories to gain 10.8 kg (24 lb) during pregnancy. To prevent pyrosis (heartburn) the woman is advised to assume a semi- or low-Fowler's position after eating.

The woman may need to learn to self-administer heparin. She is cautioned to avoid foods high in vitamin K, such as raw, deep green, leafy vegetables, which counteract the effects of the heparin. Therefore she will require a substitute source of folic acid in her diet (Chapter 11).

Infection adds considerable stress to cardiac function. The woman should notify her physician at the first sign of infection or when she is exposed to infection. Hospitalization may be required until the infection is cured.

The nurse may need to reinforce the physician's explanation for the need for close medical supervision. Information about management of the woman's labor and her early postdelivery period is reviewed. The woman and her family will need time to plan for the necessary extra care the mother will require.

Labor and Delivery

Nursing care during labor and delivery focuses on the promotion of cardiac function. *Anxiety is alleviated* through maintaining a calm atmosphere and keeping the woman and her family informed. *Uterine perfusion* is facilitated by placing the woman in a side-lying position. *Cardiac function* is supported by keeping her head and shoulders elevated and body parts resting on pillows. Bearing down (Valsalva maneuver) must be avoided, since this reduces diastolic ventricular filling and obstructs left ventricular outflow (Scott et al, 1990). Since pain can contribute to cardiovascular stress, discomfort is relieved with medication and supportive care. For delivery the nurse will assist in the administration of pharmacologic relief of discomfort. Epidural regional anesthesia provides better pain relief than narcotics and fewer alterations in hemodynamics (Gilbert and Harmon, 1986; Cunningham, MacDonald, and Gant, 1989). ***Hypotension must be avoided.***

Vaginal delivery is accomplished with the woman in the left side-lying position, or if placed in the supine position, a pad is positioned under the right hip to minimize the danger of supine hypotension. The knees are flexed, and the feet are flat on the bed. Stirrups are not used to prevent compression of popliteal veins and an increase in blood volume in the chest and trunk as a result of the effects of gravity. An episiotomy and the use of outlet forceps also decrease the work of the heart.

β-*adrenergic agents* (i.e., ritodrine and terbutaline) should not be used for tocolysis. These agents are associated with myocardial ischemia. *Syntocinon,* a synthetic oxytocin, can be used for induction of labor (Chapter 26). This drug does not appear to cause significant coronary artery constriction in doses prescribed for labor induction or control of postpartum uterine atony.

Postpartum Period

Care in the postpartum period is tailored to the woman's functional capacity. The woman must be protected from infection. A private room is one method to restrict traffic into her room. Positioning in bed is the same as that for the labor; that is, the head of the bed is elevated and the woman is encouraged to lie on her side. Bed rest may be ordered with or without bathroom privileges. The nurse may need to help the woman meet her grooming and hygiene needs and even help her with turning in bed, eating, and other activities. Boredom and respiratory and circulatory sequelae to immobility must be addressed. Progressive ambulation may be permitted as tolerated. The nurse assesses the woman's pulse, skin, and affect before and after walking.

Bowel and bladder elimination require special attention. Bowel movements without stress or strain are promoted with stool softeners, diet, and fluids, plus mild analgesia and local anesthetic spray. Overdistension of the bladder is prevented, because a distended bladder can result in an atonic uterus and hemorrhage. Anemia may result, adding additional stress to cardiac function. Rapid emptying of the bladder is avoided however. Rapid decompression of the bladder results in a precipitous drop in intraabdominal pressure, leading to ***splanchnic engorgement*** and generalized hypotension.

Mother-child interactions receive special planning. The interactions should not stress the mother. The mother may direct care of the infant by a designated family member. Women in classes I and II (where there was no evidence of cardiac embarrassment) may breastfeed. Those mothers whose functional capacity is classified as class III or IV are advised against breastfeeding. The fed baby can be brought regularly to the mother, held at her eye level and by her lips, and brought to her fingers so that she can establish an emotional bond with her baby with a low expenditure of her energy. At the same time, involving the mother passively in her infant's care helps the mother feel vitally important—as she is—to the infant's well-being (e.g., "You can do something no one else can: provide your baby with your sounds, touch, and rhythms that are so comforting"). Perhaps the mother can be encouraged to make a tape recording of her talking, singing, or whispering, to be played for the baby in the nursery, to help the infant feel her presence and be in contact with her voice.

Before discharge the nurse assesses the home support for the woman and infant. Preparation for discharge is carefully planned with the woman and family. Provision of help in the home for the mother by relatives, friends, and others must be addressed. If necessary, the nurse refers the family to community resources (e.g., for homemaking services). Rest and sleep periods, activity, and diet must be planned. The couple will want information about reestablishing sexual relations, contraception, sterilization of the man or the woman (especially if the woman is classified as classes II, III, or IV), and medical supervision.

A general nursing care plan for a childbearing woman with heart disease is shown on pp. 711-713.

Evaluation

The nurse uses the following criteria as *overall indications* for the success of therapy:

1. The woman is able to tolerate the stresses imposed by pregnancy. These include increase in cardiac output by more than one third, increase in pulse rate by 10 bpm, expansion of blood volume by 25%, and psychologic stress common to pregnancy and related to the heart condition.
2. Congestive heart failure, the primary cause of maternal mortality in women with cardiac disease, is prevented.
3. The home situation is controlled, with assistance provided as necessary.
4. The mother and family accept the limitations imposed on the woman by the presence of heart disease.
5. The parent-child relationship is fostered by the family.

❑ CARDIOVASCULAR CONDITIONS

Mitral valve prolapse (**MVP**) is a common condition occurring in nearly 10% of women of reproductive age (Cunningham, MacDonald, and Gant, 1989). The mitral valve leaflets prolapse into the left atrium during ventricular systole, allowing some backflow of blood. Midsystolic *click* and late systolic *murmur* are hallmarks of this syndrome. Most women are asymptomatic. A few women have a peculiar chest pain or palpitations, which usually respond to β-blockers such as propranolol (Inderal). Pregnancy is usually well tolerated unless bacterial endocarditis occurs.

Marfan's syndrome, an autosomal dominant disorder, is characterized by a generalized weakness of connective tissue. About 90% of individuals with this

General Nursing Care Plan

HEART DISEASE AND CHILDBEARING

ASSESSMENT	NURSING DIAGNOSIS (ND), PLAN/GOAL (P/G)	RATIONALE/ IMPLEMENTATION	EVALUATION
PRENATAL CARE			
Assess for factors that increase stress on the heart (anemia, infection, household activities). Assess for signs of cardiac decompensation: generalized edema, rales at the base of lungs, pulse irregularity. Patterns of weight gain. Vital signs. Edema. Discomforts of pregnancy. Urinalysis (protein, blood, acetone, glucose). Blood work (Hgb, Hct, WBC, platelets). Check for side effects and interactions of medications. Assess dietary patterns.	ND: Altered tissue perfusion related to hypotensive syndrome. ND: Increased cardiac output related to pregnancy. ND: Impaired home maintenance management related to mother's restricted household activities or confinement to bed. P/G: Woman will maintain adequate perfusion as exhibited by stable blood pressure, clear lung fields, no edema, and regular pulse. P/G: Woman will attend scheduled appointments. P/G: Woman will avoid restricted activities and achieve adequate rest. P/G: Woman will self-administer heparin as ordered.	*A gravida with heart disease is at risk for cardiac decompression and embolism:* Reinforce physician's explanation for need of close medical supervision. Schedule weekly appointments and evaluate problems pertaining to missed appointments. Review symptoms of cardiac decompensation. Monitor weight and dietary patterns. Monitor vital sign patterns. Note and report edema ("Are your shoes getting tight?") Obtain urine and blood specimens, and evaluate and report results. Monitor for side effects and interactions of medications. Encourage adequate rest. Review rest and activities. Refer to child care and home health agencies. Teach woman how to self-administer heparin as ordered.	Woman remains free from cardiac decompensation. Woman attends weekly health care appointments. Woman obtains adequate rest and avoids restricted activities. The home situation is controlled with community assistance provided as necessary. Woman self-administers heparin as ordered by a physician.
Assess woman's baseline knowledge of her heart disease. Assess woman's knowledge of how pregnancy will affect her heart disease.	ND: Knowledge deficit related to care required by a woman with heart disease during pregnancy. ND: Fear related to increased peripartum risk. P/G: Woman and family will learn how to monitor and care for her heart disease during pregnancy. P/G: Woman and family will learn the risks of pregnancy on her heart disease.	*Knowledge of heart disease enables the woman to care for herself during pregnancy:* Review effects pregnancy will have on her health. Help woman formulate questions for the physician. Evaluate woman's desire to continue with the pregnancy given all the peripartum risks and review her option for termination of the pregnancy. Teach symptoms of cardiac decompensation (verbal and written). Review restricted activities and need for rest. Teach nutrition and the need for a high iron, high protein, and adequate caloric diet to gain	Woman and family verbalize an understanding of the risks of pregnancy on woman's health. Woman learns how to care for herself during pregnancy and knows whom to contact should danger signs present. Woman and family utilize community resources and support. Woman and family follow prescribed diet and treatment regimen.

Continued.

ASSESSMENT	NURSING DIAGNOSIS (ND), PLAN/GOAL (P/G)	RATIONALE/ IMPLEMENTATION	EVALUATION
		about (10.8 kg) 24 lb during pregnancy. Tell woman to avoid foods high in Vitamin K if she is receiving heparin therapy. Teach woman regarding danger of infection, its signs, and symptoms. Review information pertaining to management of labor and the early postdelivery period.	
INTRAPARTUM CARE			
Routine assessments for a laboring woman. Vital signs every 10 to 15 minutes. Alert physician to heart rate ≥100 or ≥25 respirations per minute. Assess respiratory status frequently for dyspnea, coughing, or rales at base of lungs. Note and record color and skin temperature. Assess for signs of cardiac shock. Assess for suspicious FHR deceleration patterns (Chapter 14).	ND: Increased cardiac output related to the stress of labor and delivery. ND: Altered cardiopulmonary tissue perfusion related to hypotension (maternal or fetal). P/G: Woman will maintain adequate perfusion, exhibited by stable blood pressure, regular pulse, warm pink extremities, and clear lung field. P/G: Woman will maintain adequate perfusion to the placenta as exhibited by a stable FHR during labor.	*Adequate perfusion assists in alleviating cardiac stress:* Promote cardiac function by: Alleviating anxiety. Placing woman in side-lying position. Medicating or sedating for discomfort. Preventing, recognizing, reporting, and treating hypotension, which may follow anesthesia. For delivery, place on left side or supine with right hip elevated. Administer medications and report signs of cardiac decompensation. Monitor contractions and FHR response.	Woman maintains adequate perfusion during labor and delivery. Fetus will remain adequately perfused in utero as demonstrated by acceptable FHR patterns.
Watch for symptoms of emotional stress.	ND: Anxiety related to fear for infant's safety. ND: Fear of dying related to perceived inability to control stress of labor. P/G: Woman will be comforted and anxiety relieved by stress reduction techniques.	*Control reduces workload:* Answer any questions of concern the woman might have about labor and delivery. Help woman formulate questions for the physician. Correct misconceptions. Explain upcoming procedures, feelings, or sensations she might experience. Encourage support person to provide comfort techniques (back rub, pressure to lumbar spine, etc.). Encourage support person to remain at bed side with the woman as a comfort measure. Administer medications for discomfort or sedation as ordered.	Woman reports comfort or demonstrates reduced anxiety by measures instituted.

General Nursing Care Plan—cont'd

ASSESSMENT	NURSING DIAGNOSIS (ND), PLAN/GOAL (P/G)	RATIONALE/ IMPLEMENTATION	EVALUATION
POSTDELIVERY CARE			
Close assessment for cardiac decompensation. Routine postpartum assessments. Assess for signs and symptoms of infection and hemorrhage. Monitor intake/output closely.	ND: Decreased cardiac output related to fluid shifts after delivery. ND: Altered cardiopulmonary tissue perfusion related to rapid fluid shifts on a compromised cardiovascular system. ND: Potential for injury related to hemorrhage or infection. ND: Knowledge deficit regarding methods to reduce stress on cardiac system. P/G: Woman will not demonstrate signs of cardiac decompensation after delivery.	*A parturient with heart disease is at risk for cardiac decompression:* Evaluate for cardiac decompensation up to 7 days after delivery. Apply abdominal binder or tourniquets as ordered by physician after delivery. Administer medications as ordered (oxygen, digitalization therapy, etc.) Elevate head of bed and encourage side-lying. Teach regarding stool softeners, fluids and diet to reduce strain of bowel movements. Prevent overdistended bladder after delivery. Isolate from sources of infection. Prevent or promptly treat hemorrhage or infection. Facilitate mother-infant interactions that do not stress the mother.	Woman remains free from signs and symptoms of cardiac decompensation. Woman remains free from hemorrhage and infection. Woman verbalizes understanding of instructions. Woman experiences normal involution.
Assess woman's support system. Assess family's response to the birth and infant. Assess the need for outside resources (home care, child care).	ND: Ineffective family coping: compromised, related to added child care and household tasks. ND: Altered family processes related to assuming woman's responsibilities after delivery. ND: Self-care deficit related to need for bed rest. ND: Situational low self-esteem related to restriction placed on involvement in care of infant. P/G: Woman will rest and recuperate after delivery. P/G: Woman will not be stressed by child care or household activities after delivery.	*Rest promotes recuperation; the nurse will:* Identify with the woman her support systems. Observe the family's response to the infant and child care activities. Examine the family's time and resources to assist the woman with child care and household tasks. Notify outside resources to assist with the care of the woman, house, and child (homemaker, child care, home health care). Encourage woman to spend "quiet moments" with her child but to allow family to provide most of the child care activities. Remind woman that she can assume all child care activities once she allows her body to recuperate from childbirth.	Woman achieves the needed rest to recuperate. The mother and family accept the limitations imposed on the woman by the presence of heart disease. Woman's family or outside services assumes responsibility of children and household tasks until woman recuperates. The parent-child relationship is fostered by the family.

symptom have mitral valve prolapse, and 25% have aortic insufficiency. There is an increased risk of *aortic dissection* and rupture during pregnancy, and maternal mortality is reported at 25% to 50% (Scott et al, 1990). Management during pregnancy is by restricted activity and propranolol therapy.

Cardiovascular accidents (CVAs) can occur. Uncontrolled hypertension can result in cerebral hemorrhage (Chapter 23) (Cunningham, MacDonald, and Gant, 1989). CVAs have been reported with cocaine use (Cregler and Mark, 1986).

Infective endocarditis is an uncommon condition during pregnancy (Cox and Levano, 1989). However, at some hospitals the incidence in recent years has been 1:16,000 deliveries (Cox et al, 1988). It is seen commonly in women taking illicit drugs intravenously. Bacterial endocarditis, leading to incompetence of heart valves and cerebral emboli, can result in death. Seaworth and Durack (1986) report a 33% maternal mortality rate.

Rheumatic Heart Disease

The woman who has rheumatic heart disease as a result of rheumatic fever may experience ***chorea gravidarum*** (Sydenham's chorea). This condition is characterized by involuntary purposeless contractions of the muscles of the trunk and extremities, anxiety, and impairment of memory. Recovery occurs within 6 to 10 weeks of delivery. Treatment consists of rest for the body and mind.

Mitral valve stenosis, the most common lesion of rheumatic heart disease, is the most important hemodynamically (Brady and Duff, 1989). A tight stenosis plus the increased preload and cardiac output of normal pregnancy (Chapter 8) may cause ventricular failure and pulmonary edema; hemoptysis may occur. Atrial fibrillation is common. Cardiac failure occurs during pregnancy for the first time in 25% of women with mitral valve stenosis. Digoxin prophylaxis may be warranted. Atrial fibrillation also predisposes the woman to thromboembolism, especially in cerebral vessels (Brady and Duff, 1989). Mitral valvotomy often brings dramatic relief of heart failure. Epidural anesthesia for labor and *avoidance* of intravenous fluid overload are appropriate (Cunningham, MacDonald, and Gant, 1989). Prophylaxis for intrapartum endocarditis and pulmonary infections is usually provided.

Surgically Corrected Heart Disease: Valve Replacement

Some women who are asymptomatic after cardiac surgery undergo frightening deterioration of their condition during pregnancy. This is especially true of women with prosthetic heart valves (Metcalfe, McAnulty, and Ueland, 1986). The hemodynamic demands of pregnancy compromise their cardiac status. Should such a woman become pregnant, abortion before the hemodynamic demands are fully manifest is the most therapeutic course if it is acceptable to the woman and her family. Most women opt for careful contraception to avoid pregnancy rather than for therapeutic interruption.

Women with prosthetic heart valves or valvular heart disease continue to require anticoagulants to prevent or treat systemic embolism (Cunningham, MacDonald, and Gant, 1989; Anticoagulants, 1990) (p. 709). Valvuloplasty clients should receive penicillin or other antibiotic prophylaxis against bacterial endocarditis during gestation. The incidence of pregnancy wastage is greater than in the unaffected population. There is an increased incidence of spontaneous abortion, stillborns, low-birth-weight infants, and malformed fetuses.

Peripartum Heart Failure

Peripartum heart failure can result from an underlying chronic hypertension, previously unrecognized mitral valve stenosis, obesity, viral myocarditis, or idiopathic **peripartum cardiomyopathy** (Cunningham, MacDonald, Gant, 1989). Anemia and infection are two factors that contribute to congestive heart failure. Both force the heart to work harder, since both conditions require an increase in cardiac output. Cardiac output must be increased in anemia because of decreased oxygen per volume of blood; and, in infection with fever, because oxygen utilization is greatly increased. Peripartum heart failure from an explainable cause such as an underlying heart disease usually responds well to therapy. The typical response is rapid reversal of heart failure with furosemide (Lasix) diuresis and correction of associated obstetric complications (Cunningham, MacDonald, Gant, 1989). Within days the heart size of these women returns to normal; their long-term prognosis depends on the underlying heart disease condition (e.g., hypertrophic cardiomyopathy).

Peripartum Cardiomyopathy: Hypertrophic Cardiomyopathy. Most clients with hypertrophic cardiomyopathy (HCM) are asymptomatic until late adolescence or early adulthood (childbearing years) or more rarely middle age. Symptoms include angina pectoris, exertional dyspnea, supraventricular and ventricular arrhythmias, dizziness, and syncope. Most deaths associated with HCM are sudden, unexpected, and unrelated to functional status. HCM may be precipitated by physical or emotional stress, and the myocardial ischemia resulting from stress may promote ventricular fibrillation (Veille, 1984). Propranolol is given if symp-

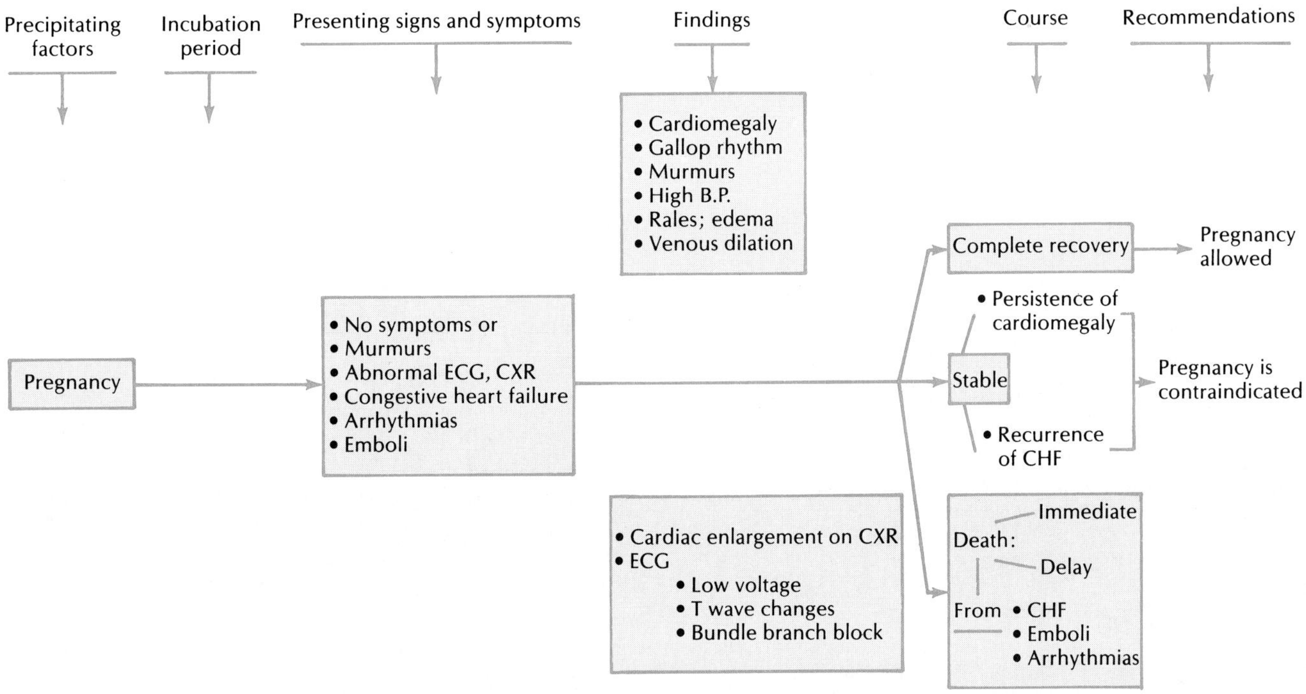

Fig. 24-4 Summary of course of peripartum cardiomyopathy. (From Veille JC: Am J Obstet Gynecol 148:805, 1984.)

toms develop (Cunningham, MacDonald, and Gant, 1989).

The incidence of peripartum cardiomyopathies has been reported as 1 in 3000 to 4000 pregnancies. It occurs more often in the multiparous woman. The maternal mortality has been estimated in the range of 30% to 60%, the infant mortality approximately 10%. *Clinical findings* are those of congestive heart failure (left ventricular failure). Findings include breathlessness, tachyarrhythmias, and edema (Fig. 24-4) with radiologic findings of cardiomegaly. The *prognosis* is good if cardiomegaly is not persistent after 6 months. The prognosis for women whose hearts remain enlarged is not as favorable. *Future pregnancies* usually result in some cardiac failure (50% to 88%). Mortality has been estimated as high as 60%.

Idiopathic Cardiomyopathy. Idiopathic peripartum cardiomyopathies comprise a syndrome of heart failure (1) occurring during the peripartum period, (2) with no previous history of heart disease, and (3) with no specific etiologic factors (Demakis and Rahimtoola, 1971). Autoimmune factors may be implicated (Sanderson et al, 1985; Lee and Cotton, 1989). Idiopathic cardiomyopathy in nonpregnant people results in death in over 75% from unrelenting cardiomegaly (enlarged heart) and heart failure (Homans, 1985).

Medical Management. Bed rest for the pregnant woman is advocated up to 7 months, with some women requiring 20 to 22 months after diagnosis. The rationale for instituting bed rest is to decrease the heart rate, stroke volume, and arterial pressure.

Low sodium intake (1.5 to 2 g per day) is ordered for women with severe congestive failure. The use of diuretics (e.g., furosemide), digitalis, and anticoagulants require close medical supervision to detect toxicity. Suppression of lactation is often recommended with no particular rationale other than to minimize stress. (All women experience some rise in blood pressure at the onset of lactation.)

Nursing Care. The nursing care of clients with peripartum cardiomyopathies is essentially the same as for those with other types of cardiac problems. The use of Trendelenburg's position for relief of syncope has been demonstrated. The necessity for prolonged bed rest can pose social and economic hardships for a family; therefore referral to community resources for assistance may be necessary. Because sudden death is a feature of this condition, the family needs to be trained in cardiopulmonary resuscitation. Clients need to have ready access to emergency care. (Some hospitals provide special numbers to dial for immediate dispatch of a medically staffed ambulance.)

Cardiopulmonary Resuscitation of the Pregnant Woman

Trauma, pulmonary embolism, anesthesia complications, drug overdose, or hypovolemia or septic shock

EMERGENCY PROCEDURE

CARDIOPULMONARY RESUSCITATION (CPR) FOR PREGNANT WOMAN

DEFINITION

A basic emergency procedure for life support.

PURPOSE

To restore cardiac and/or respiratory function.

EQUIPMENT

Resuscitation equipment should be readily available in areas in which respiratory arrest might take place, and the status of this equipment should be checked regularly, at least once a day.

NURSING ACTIONS	RATIONALE
Wash hands before and after touching woman and equipment. Glove if possible.	Prevents nosocomial infection and implements universal precautions.
CPR	
Position woman on a flat firm surface with the uterus displaced laterally (manually or with a wedge or rolled towel under her right hip).	Prevents supine hypotension.
HEIMLICH MANEUVER (Fig. 24-5)	
Provide external *chest* compressions (NOT subdiaphragmatic thrusts) at a rate of 80 to 100/min.	Prevents injury to fetus.

may result in cardiopulmonary arrest. Preexisting disorders, such as heart or pulmonary disease, hypertension, or autoimmune collagen vascular disease, increase this risk (Newkirk and Fry, 1985; Songster and Clark, 1985; Troiano, 1989). Some modifications of the procedure for cardiopulmonary resuscitation (CPR) and the Heimlich maneuver are needed (see emergency procedure, above, and Fig. 24-5).

Complications may be associated with CPR of a gravid woman. These complications may include laceration of the liver, rupture of the uterus, hemothorax, or hemoperitoneum (Troiano, 1989). Fetal complications may also occur. These include cardiac arrhythmia or asystole related to maternal defibrillation and medications; central nervous system (CNS) depression related to antiarrhythmic drugs and inadequate uteroplacental perfusion; and, onset of preterm labor (Lee et al, 1986).

After successful resuscitation, the gravida and her fetus must be carefully monitored. The gravida remains at increased risk for recurrent pulmonary arrest and arrhythmias (ventricular tachycardia, supraventricular tachycardia, bradycardia). Therefore the gravida's cardiovascular, pulmonary, and neurologic status should be assessed continuously. Uterine activity and resting tone must be monitored. Fetal status and gestational age should be determined. All assessment data influence both the medical and nursing plans of care.

Medical Disorders During Pregnancy

Medical conditions may complicate pregnancy. The most common of these is anemia, especially anemia caused by iron or folic acid deficiency, sickle cell trait or disease, and thalassemia. Pulmonary, gastrointestinal, integumentary, neurologic, autoimmune, and neoplastic disorders also may be encountered. Pregnancy-related aspects of these conditions are addressed in the following sections.

❑ ANEMIA

Anemia, the most common medical disorder of pregnancy, affects at least 20% of pregnant women. Anemia, either chronic from iron deficiency or acute after hemorrhage, stresses ventricular function. Therefore anemia, working in concert with any other complication (e.g., preeclampsia) may result in congestive heart failure. Anemia increases the woman's vulnerability to other puerperal complications such as infection.

Anemia results in reduction of the oxygen-carrying capacity of the blood. An indirect index of the oxygen-carrying capacity is the packed red blood cell volume (PCV), or hematocrit level. The normal hematocrit range in nonpregnant women is 38% to 45%. How-

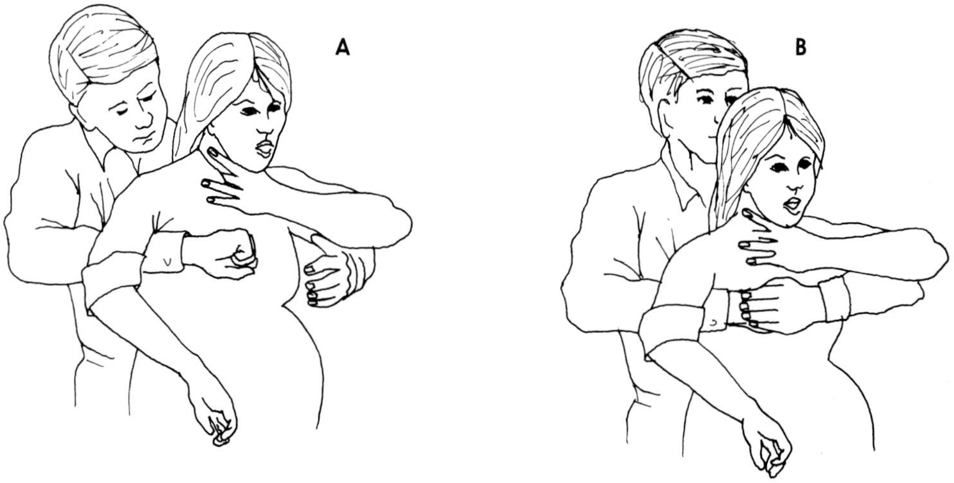

Fig. 24-5 Clearing an airway obstruction and performing chest compressions. **A,** Place top of clenched fist against middle of sternum; place other hand on top of clenched fist. Perform chest thrusts until the obstruction is expelled or woman loses consciousness. **B,** If woman is unconscious, give chest compressions as for woman without a pulse.

ever, normal values for pregnant women with adequate iron stores may be as low as 34%. This has been explained by hydremia (dilution of blood), or the **physiologic anemia of pregnancy.**

About 90% of cases of anemia in pregnancy are of the iron-deficiency type. The remaining 10% of cases embrace a considerable variety of acquired and hereditary anemias, including folic acid deficiency and hemoglobinopathies.

Normal and abnormal changes confuse the hematologic profile during pregnancy. The blood values of pregnant women differ significantly from those of nonpregnant women. All the constituents of blood normally increase during pregnancy: plasma volume, by 30% to 35%; red cell volume, by 20% to 30%; and hemoglobin mass, by 12% to 15%. The dilution of red blood cells and hemoglobin resulting from the relatively greater increase in plasma volume does not significantly change cell indices such as the mean corpuscular volume (MCV). However, this dilution does affect red blood cell count (RBC), hemoglobin, and hematocrit values. Laboratory values drop progressively to a low between the thirtieth and thirty-fourth weeks of pregnancy.

At or near sea level, during the *first* trimester, the pregnant woman is anemic when her hemoglobin level is less than 11 g/dl or her hematocrit level falls below 37%. She is anemic in the *second* trimester when the hemoglobin level is less than 10.5 g/dl or the hematocrit level falls below 35%; and she is anemic in the *third* trimester when the hemoglobin level is less than 10 g/dl or the hematocrit level is less than 33%. Much higher values are indicative of anemia in areas of high altitude; for example, at 1500 m (5000 ft) above sea level, a hemoglobin level less than 14 g/dl indicates anemia.

Iron Deficiency Anemia

Without iron therapy even pregnant women who enjoy excellent nutrition will conclude pregnancy with an iron deficit. Diet alone cannot replace gestational iron losses. Inadequate nutrition without therapy will certainly mean iron deficiency anemia during late pregnancy and the puerperium.

Successful iron therapy during pregnancy can be carried out in the vast majority of cases with oral iron supplements (e.g., ferrous sulfate, 0.3 g 3 times a day). Some pregnant women cannot tolerate or fail to take the prescribed oral iron. In such cases the woman should receive parenteral iron such as the iron-dextran complex (Imferon).

Folic Acid Deficiency Anemia

Folic acid deficiency anemia occurs in at least 2% of pregnant women in North America, an incidence much higher than that suspected even 5 years ago. Anemia compromises the women's defenses, making her more vulnerable to urinary tract infections and hemorrhage.

Poor diet, cooking with large volumes of water, or canning of food may lead to folate deficiency. Also, malabsorption or increased folate use may play a part in the development of anemia caused by a lack of folic acid.

During pregnancy the recommended daily intake is 150 μg of folic acid. In folate deficiency a dosage of about 5 mg per day orally for several weeks should ensure a remission. A generous maintenance dose each day should prevent a relapse. Because iron deficiency anemia may also accompany folate deficiency, augmented iron intake should also be provided.

Sickle Cell Hemoglobinopathy

Sickle cell trait (SA hemoglobin pattern) is sickling of the red blood cells but with a normal red blood cell life span. Pregnant women with sickle cell trait (**sickle cell hemoglobinopathy**) are susceptible to urinary tract infection. Hematuria is common.

Sickle cell anemia (sickle cell disease) is a recessive, hereditary, familial hemolytic anemia peculiar to those of black or Mediterranean ancestry. These individuals usually have abnormal hemoglobin types (SS or SC). Persons with sickle cell anemia have recurrent attacks (crises) of fever and pain in the abdomen or extremities beginning in childhood. These attacks are attributed to vascular occlusion (from abnormal cells), tissue hypoxia, edema, and red blood cell destruction. Crisis may be caused by hypotension, acidosis, dehydration, exertion, sudden cooling, and low-grade fever. Crises are associated with normochromic anemia, jaundice, reticulocytosis, positive sickle cell test, and the demonstration of abnormal hemoglobin (usually SS or SC).

Almost 10% of blacks in North America have the sickle cell trait, but less than 1% have sickle cell anemia. The anemia is often complicated by iron and folic acid deficiency.

Pregnancy usually results in a worsening of most aspects of the disease (Scott et al, 1990). Pregnant women with sickle cell anemia are prone to pneumonia, pyelonephritis, leg ulcers, bone infarction, congestive heart failure, and preeclampsia. Assessments for asymptomatic bacteriuria and determinations of hemoglobin and hematocrit are done frequently. An aplastic crisis may follow serious infection. Medical therapy, including transfusions to maintain the hematocrit level at 30% at least is essential. Crises are treated with analgesics, oxygen, and vigorous hydration. Cesarean delivery is warranted only on obstetric indications. Postpartum hemorrhage may be the result of heparin therapy. Oxytocin or protamine may be ordered.

Pregnancy may impose critical complications in sickle cell disease. Maternal mortality often ranges between 5% and 10%. The perinatal mortality may reach 30%. Therapeutic abortion is not medically indicated.

Thalassemia

Thalassemia (Mediterranean or Cooley's anemia) is a relatively common anemia in which an insufficient amount of globin is produced to fill the red blood cells. Thalassemia is a hereditary disorder that involves the abnormal synthesis of the α- or β-chains of globin. β-Thalassemia is the more common variety in the United States and is often diagnosed in individuals of Italian, Greek, or southern Chinese descent. The unbalanced synthesis of globin leads to premature red blood cell death resulting in severe anemia. Thalassemia major is the homozygous form of the disorder; thalassemia minor is the heterozygous form.

Thalassemia major may complicate pregnancy. Preeclampsia is more common in women with thalassemia major. Thalassemia major may be associated with low-birth-weight infants and increased fetal wastage. Placental weight often is increased, perhaps as a result of maternal anemia. The frequency of fetal distress from hypoxia is greater than in control women. Therefore pregnant women with thalassemia major should be monitored more closely than normal pregnant women.

Regular transfusion may be necessary. Folic acid should be given to avoid folate deficiency. Partial exchange transfusion may be warranted in severe thalassemia. Splenectomy may be necessary if enlargement and pain occur. Women with thalassemia major may die of chronic infection or progressive hepatic or cardiac failure, the result of excessive iron deposition.

Persons with *thalassemia minor* have a mild persistent anemia, but the RBC may be normal or even elevated. However, no systemic problems are caused by the anemia that is a part of the minor form of the disease. Thalassemia minor must be distinguished principally from iron deficiency anemia.

Pregnancy will neither worsen thalassemia minor nor will it be compromised by the disease. The anemia will not respond to iron therapy. Prolonged parenteral iron can lead to harmful, excessive iron storage. Infants born to parents with thalassemia will inherit the disorder. Persons with thalassemia minor should have a normal life span despite a moderately reduced hemoglobin level.

❑ PULMONARY DISORDERS

Bronchial Asthma

Bronchial asthma occurs in less than 1% of pregnant women. The effect of pregnancy on asthma is unpredictable. Psychologic alterations induced by pregnancy do not make the pregnant woman more prone to asthmatic attacks. Asthma increases the incidence of abortion and preterm labor, but the fetus per se is unaffected. In severe cases, asthma may be life threatening for the gravida. The prognosis for both mother and fetus will be good in most cases.

Therapy for bronchial asthma has two objectives: (1) relief of the acute attack and (2) prevention or limitation of later attacks. In all asthmatics, known allergens should be eliminated and a comfortable home temperature maintained. Respiratory infections should be treated and mist or steam inhalation employed to aid expectoration of mucus. Bronchial asthma therapy is initiated. Acute episodes may require steroids, aminophylline, oxygen, and correction of fluid-electrolyte imbalance. See medical-surgical texts for general care.

Adult Respiratory Distress Syndrome

Adult respiratory distress syndrome (**ARDS,** shock lung) occurs when the lungs are unable to maintain levels of oxygen and carbon dioxide within normal limits. Marked tachycardia, dyspnea, and cyanosis that does not respond to nasal oxygen or intermittent positive pressure breathing are the most noted signs. ARDS is not a condition specific to pregnancy; it can also result from chest trauma, drug ingestion, severe acute hemorrhage, or pneumonia. When ARDS is associated with pregnancy, pulmonary embolism, disseminated intravascular coagulation (DIC) (Chapter 23), and aspiration pneumonia are the precipitators. The postpartum incidence of ARDS is not affected by the means of delivery, but by the amount of trauma experienced during pregnancy and delivery. It also may occur after spontaneous or medically induced abortion.

Laboratory reports are important in identifying the origin of acute pulmonary problems. The important observations for the nurse to note are vital signs, signs of thrombophlebitis, and hemorrhage.

Temperature elevation may indicate the development of thrombophlebitis. The *pulse rate* increases to compensate for respiratory insufficiency of any origin. The pulse rate rises as the severity of the pulmonary problem increases. An initial rise in blood pressure occurs as cardiac output increases to try to supply the bloody tissue with oxygen. When lung damage is severe, the *blood pressure* drops. Respiratory changes are the most important indicators of ARDS. The rate, depth, respiratory pattern, symmetry of chest movement, and use of accessory muscles should be noted; therefore observation of respiratory characteristics after activity is important. If there is any indication of abnormality, respirations are counted for a full minute; an error of plus or minus four may be highly significant. During the postdelivery period, apprehension, distended neck veins, cyanosis, diaphoresis, and pallor may be clues to watch for. Also mental confusion or disorientation may be noted. On auscultation of the lungs, crackles (rales), rhonchi, wheezes, or a pleural friction rub need to be reported, especially when they have occurred since an earlier normal assessment. The pregnant woman should be positioned for breathing comfort. Oxygen and emergency equipment should be available while the physician is notified. The woman should be reassured so that her anxiety is lessened.

The lower extremities need to be checked for swelling, pain, inflammation, venous distension, and Homan's sign. If *thrombophlebitis* is suspected, the woman should be kept on bed rest until the physician can be notified. Sudden movement or straining can dislodge a clot and lead to pulmonary embolism. Thrombophlebitis can result in ARDS (emboli from thromboembolism cause obstruction in the pulmonary circulation).

Food eaten as long as 24 to 48 hours before labor can be vomited and then aspirated. Aspiration of solid foods and liquids may cause bronchial obstruction leading to bronchoconstriction, which in turn can result in ARDS. Large particles can be removed by coughing, suctioning, or bronchoscopy, but liquids are harder to remove. The hydrochloric acid in the aspirated stomach contents may cause an asthmatic-like syndrome with necrotizing bronchitis. For this reason an antacid is given preoperatively as a prophylactic measure.

The syndrome carries a high rate of mortality. The prognosis is good if the woman is otherwise healthy and if ventilatory support can be maintained until the underlying disease can be treated (Cunningham, MacDonald, and Gant, 1989).

Cystic Fibrosis

Improvements in diagnosis and treatment of cystic fibrosis have allowed an increasing number of females to survive to adulthood. Most are infertile; however, pregnancy is not uncommon. The pregnancy is often complicated by chronic hypoxia and frequent pulmonary infections. Increased maternal and perinatal mortality is related to severe pulmonary infection.

❑ GASTROINTESTINAL DISORDERS

Compromise of gastrointestinal function during pregnancy is apparent to all concerned. There are psychogenic overtones generally admitted in nausea and vomiting of pregnancy. However, a capricious food choice is observed in many women during pregnancy. In addition, obvious physiologic alterations, such as the greatly enlarged uterus, and less apparent changes, such as hypochlorhydria, require understanding for proper diagnosis and treatment.

Peptic Ulcer

Peptic ulcer is less common in women than in men, and this problem is even more uncommon during pregnancy. Moreover, women with a diagnosed peptic ulcer generally improve during gestation. Therefore hemorrhage and perforation are unlikely. Fortunately emergency surgery for peptic ulcer complications rarely jeopardizes the pregnancy. Postdelivery reactivation of the ulcer may occur. Medical therapy is similar to that recommended for nonpregnant individuals.

Cholelithiasis and Cholecystitis

Maternal adaptation significantly alters gallbladder function (Scott et al, 1990). Gallbladder emptying time is delayed and volume is increased. Sluggish function (cholestasis) and increased biliary cholesterol make the gravida more vulnerable to cholelithiasis (gallstones). Cholecystitis does not commonly occur during pregnancy.

Generally, gallbladder surgery should be postponed until the puerperium. Impaction of a stone in the cystic or common duct during pregnancy may require immediate cholelithotomy or cholecystectomy. Meperidine (Demerol), morphine, or atropine alleviates ductal spasm and pain.

Ulcerative Colitis

The cause of ulcerative colitis is unknown. Its effect on pregnancy is minimal unless there is marked debilitation, whereupon spontaneous abortion, fetal death, or preterm delivery may occur. In general, when pregnancy coincides with active ulcerative colitis, the great majority of women will experience a severe exacerbation of the disease. When pregnancy occurs during a period of inactivity of the disorder, a flare-up is unlikely. There is no specific therapy for ulcerative colitis, but adrenocorticosteroids and antibiotics may be beneficial.

❏ INTEGUMENTARY DISORDERS

Dermatologic disorders induced by pregnancy (see Table 10-13 and p. 200) include melasma (chloasma), herpes gestationis, noninflammatory pruritus of pregnancy, vascular spiders, palmar erythema, and pregnancy granulomas (including epulides). Skin problems generally aggravated by pregnancy are acne vulgaris (in the first trimester),* erythema multiforme, herpetiform dermatitis, granuloma inguinale, condylomata acuminata, neurofibromatosis, and pemphigus. Dermatologic disorders usually improved by pregnancy include acne vulgaris (in the third trimester), seborrhea dermatitis, and psoriasis. An unpredictable course during pregnancy may be expected in atopic dermatitis, lupus erythematosus, and herpes simplex.

Therapeutic abortion or early delivery may be justified for some dermatologic conditions. These conditions include herpes gestationis, disseminated lupus erythematosus, and neurofibromatosis (von Recklinghausen's disease).

Explanation, reassurance, and common sense measures should suffice for normal skin changes (see Table 10-13 and p. 200). In contrast, disease processes during and soon after pregnancy may be extremely difficult to diagnose and treat.

❏ NEUROLOGIC DISORDERS

Epilepsy

Epilepsy may result from developmental abnormalities or injury. Epilepsy seriously complicates about 1 of every 1000 gestations. Convulsive seizures may be more frequent or severe during complications of pregnancy, such as edema, alkylosis, fluid-electrolyte imbalance, cerebral hypoxia, hypoglycemia, and hypocalcemia. Seizures must be prevented, since they can result in fetal hypoxia and acidosis. On the other hand, the effects of pregnancy on epilepsy are unpredictable. Pregnancy usually alters pharmokinetics. In addition, nausea and vomiting may interfere with ingestion and absorption of medication.

The differential diagnosis of epilepsy vs. eclampsia poses a problem. Epilepsy and eclampsia can coexist. However, a past history of seizures, the absence of hypertension, generalized edema, or proteinuria, and a normal plasma uric acid level point to epilepsy. Electroencephalography (EEG) rarely is diagnostic.

Grand mal seizures can be controlled by intravenous sodium amobarbital or magnesium sulfate. Phenytoin (Dilantin) and its analogs may be fetotoxic (Chapter 28, fetal hydantoin syndrome). Diazepam (Valium) does cross the placenta and accumulates in fetal circulation. Cleft lip or cleft palate or other malformations may be associated with its use (Mattison et al, 1989). Epilepsy is not an indication for therapeutic abortion or cesarean delivery. Diazepam and chlordiazepoxide may cause respiratory depression in the newly delivered infant.

Multiple Sclerosis

Multiple sclerosis, a patchy demyelinization of the spinal cord and CNS, may be a viral disorder. Multiple sclerosis is more common during the childbearing

*ALERT: Isotretinoin (Accutane), commonly prescribed for cystic acne, is highly teratogenic. There is a 26-fold risk for craniofacial, cardiac, and CNS malformations in exposed fetuses (Lammer et al, 1985).

years. Multiple sclerosis may occasionally complicate pregnancy, but exacerbations and remissions are unrelated to the pregnant state. There seems to be no medical reason for elective abortion. The burden of pregnancy and subsequent care of the child may warrant early interruption of pregnancy and sterilization in extreme cases. The incidence of multiple sclerosis in the offspring is about 3% (Frith and McLeod, 1988). Women with multiple sclerosis occasionally may have an almost painless labor. The character of uterine contractions is unaffected by the disease, however.

Myasthenia Gravis

Myasthenia gravis, an autoimmune motor (muscle) end plate disorder that involves acetylcholine use, affects the motor function at the myoneural junction. Muscle weakness, particularly of the eyes, face, tongue, neck, limbs, and respiratory muscles results. The peak prevalence of myasthenia gravis is about 25 years of age. Pregnancy may complicate the disorder, although some women experience a remission during gestation. Pregnancies in women with this disease can be carried to safe delivery if certain precautions are taken. Moreover, congenital myasthenia gravis is rare. Therefore the disorder is not an indication for therapeutic abortion.

The nurse and physician should be alert to symptomatology, which includes easy fatigue, intermittent double vision, upper eyelid drooping, and facial muscle weakness. In more serious cases, upper arm weakness and breathing difficulty are seen. Infections may precipitate the onset or relapse and must be treated aggressively during pregnancy.

Women with myasthenia gravis usually tolerate labor well, because they already have some degree of muscle relaxation. During the second stage, some women may show impairment of voluntary expulsive efforts. Meperidine is the obstetric analgesic of choice. Local anesthesia is preferred. Oxytocin may be given, but scopolamine and muscle relaxants (e.g., magnesium sulfate) are contraindicated. After delivery, women must be carefully supervised, because relapses often occur during the puerperium.

Occasionally an infant born to a mother with severe myasthenia gravis also shows myasthenic signs sufficient to require neostigmine treatment for 1 to 2 months. Complete recovery of the infant is the rule. However, infants born with the disorder do not have as good a prognosis as do infants born without the disorder.

Bell's Palsy

An association between idiopathic facial paralysis and pregnancy was first cited by Bell in 1830, but it was not until 1975 that Hilsinger and colleagues proved this association. Not all neurologists agree with this association, however (Aminoff, 1978). There does not seem to be any causative relationship between the appearance of Bell's palsy and any of the complications of pregnancy.

No effects of maternal Bell's palsy have been observed in infants. Maternal outcome is generally good. Electromyography and nerve conduction velocity studies are useful in predicting the outcome. Evidence of a complete block in conduction carries a worse prognosis. Loss of taste also carries a less favorable prognosis. Steroids are sometimes prescribed for the condition, but they do not hasten recovery (McGregor, Guberman, and Goodlin, 1987). In most affected women, 90% or more return of facial function can be expected (Cunningham, MacDonald, and Gant, 1989). Supportive care includes prevention of injury to the exposed cornea, facial muscle massage, careful chewing and manual removal of food from inside the affected cheek, and reassurance that return of total neurologic function is likely.

Spinal Cord Injured Women

Debra I. Craig

In 1982 it was estimated that approximately 10,000 people would suffer spinal cord injuries. Of these 10,000, approximately 1000 of the injuries would occur in women aged 15 to 25. It was also predicted that this number would increase each year (Axel, 1982). Role function is influenced by one's self-expectation and the expectations held by others (Sarbin and Allen, 1968). It is an accepted role function of women to bear children, and one's feminine identity may be tied to the ability to give birth. As spinal cord injured (SCI) women enter the childbearing process, it is essential that nurses be prepared to assist these women in the development of a positive experience throughout the perinatal period. Axel (1982) states that there is a correlation between a positive self-image and role definition and the ability to achieve pregnancy in SCI women.

There is no physiologic reason for SCI women to believe that they cannot achieve a normal pregnancy. Fertility is not impaired by their injury and there is no greater incidence of spontaneous abortion or fetal abnormalities among this population (Goller and Paeslack, 1971, 1972; Ohry et al, 1978; Young, Kutz, and Klein, 1983). However, the SCI woman must deal with her own expectations regarding parenting, the expectations of her significant others, and the perceived expectations of both the medical profession and society. Women with spinal cord injuries experience reactions similar to other women when their pregnancies are confirmed: shock, elation, disbelief, relief, and joy. The reactions of significant others range from shock and joy to concern regarding the effect of the pregnancy on the woman. SCI women receive a variety of responses to their impending or confirmed pregnancy from the medical profession. Some have been counseled to seek psychologic help, others to avoid becoming pregnant because it may be too dangerous, or to consider abortion. SCI women have had to search for physicians willing to take them as clients, although some have found supportive physicians from the onset of their pregnancies.

These women encounter a variety of responses within the hospital environment. They perceive the staff to be ill-at-ease in caring for them. "Perhaps the nurses were unsure about our needs and what to expect from us during labor," was a comment made by one paraplegic mother. Another quadriplegic woman stated she felt like she had been "raped" by the system because no one seemed to listen to her requests and desires. SCI women tend to be more in touch with their bodies and its responses because of their injuries and are more directive in their care. They find that hospitals are not designed to accommodate people who spend their lives in wheelchairs. Most of the rooms are too small, as are the showers and bathrooms. The quadriplegic woman may need a specialized call light to obtain help. Commonly, these lights are not readily available to them.

The SCI woman also needs additional help in providing care to her newborn. Her concerns regarding her ability to care for the newborn are often verbalized during pregnancy, but not readily considered by hospital staff. SCI mothers express appreciation for those nurses who take extra time to help problem-solve infant care needs. SCI women have been very imaginative in developing adaptive equipment for the safety and care of their children. Some of the adaptations include redesigning the crib so that the side can be raised and the baby moved directly onto the mother's lap. Mothers have also designed special equipment to pick a baby up from a play pen or the floor. In addition to worrying about the physical care of their children, the mothers worry about how their children will adapt to their disabilities. The children of an SCI parent are usually accepting of their parent's disability and commonly educate their classmates regarding the functional ability of their parent.

Physiologic Problems. Physiologically the SCI woman encounters many of the same problems that pregnant women in general experience. All woman suffer from urinary frequency during their pregnancy. This is more of a problem for the SCI women because of their alteration in voiding methods. Some SCI women use an indwelling catheter, some catheterize themselves at specific intervals, and others créde themselves to empty their bladder. Generally the increased urine production of pregnancy forces the women to increase the number of times they void daily, which increases the number of times they must transfer and undress themselves. Pressure on the bladder by the enlarging uterus increases the incidence of incontinence. Most SCI women find that a padding system is needed, especially during the third trimester. The most common materials used for padding are disposable diapers, either infant or adult size, and sanitary napkins. Many SCI women are unable to return to their prepregnant level of bladder functioning and must continue to wear padding after the birth of the baby.

The alteration in bladder functioning increases the SCI woman's susceptibility to bladder and kidney infections. UTIs affect about 10% of the pregnant nonspinal cord injured population and the majority of pregnant SCI women. SCI women generally experience an increase in the number and frequency of UTIs beginning in the second trimester and continuing through delivery. The SCI woman must work closely with her urologist and obstetrician to treat the infection without hurting the fetus.

Constipation is another problem that plagues the pregnant woman. The SCI woman has developed a bowel program as part of her routine of daily living. This usually includes either stool softeners or bulk-producing medication. During pregnancy this program must be altered to accommodate both the hormonal effect, slowing of the gastrointestinal tract, and pressure from the enlarging uterus on the intestinal tract. Adaptations used during pregnancy to combat constipation include increasing the frequency and amount of stool softeners or bulk producers, increasing the frequency of bowel movements, adding more roughage to the diet, and maintaining a high fluid intake.

Having to use the bathroom more frequently is just one of the mobility problems that the SCI woman encounters. SCI women use the prone position to sleep to relieve pressure on the ischial spines and gluteal muscle and to straighten joints. As a pregnancy progresses it becomes impossible for the SCI woman to lie prone. This necessitates more frequent repositioning during the night and often involves the significant other more dramatically in the caregiving. Transfers to and from the wheelchair, bathroom, bed, and car become more difficult as the pregnancy progresses. This difficulty in transfering threatens to hinder the woman's independence. Mobility is also a question that must be faced when the SCI woman visits the obstetrician. Is there room for her to undress? How does she get on and off of the examining table? Does the office staff know how to assist her with her needs?

A decrease in mobility correlates with the increased risk of developing pressure areas. Young, Kutz, and Klein (1983) list the development of decubiti as a major complication of SCI women. A recent unpublished study indicates that only a small proportion of SCI women develop decubiti (Craig, 1985). SCI women are aware of the possibility of developing pressure areas and take proactive measures to prevent their development.

Labor and Delivery. It has been assumed that since SCI women have impaired sensation they will not be able to tell when they are in labor. This has not proven to be true. They may not experience labor in the same manner as other women, but because they are in tune with their bodies they know that something is happening. Some sense their abdomen tightening, others suffer increased spasms, others have a rhythmic need to void or defecate, and still others who had sparing (incomplete cord damage with occasional areas of remaining sensation) experience menstrual-like cramps or actual labor. Women who are injured at the level of T5 or above may correlate increasing symptoms of autonomic dysreflexia with labor.

Autonomic dysreflexia results from hyperstimulation of the splanchnic (abdominal) nerves and loss of central control over sympathetic spinal reflexes. Hyperstimulation may result from distension of pelvic viscera, uterine contractions, muscle spasms, bladder or bowel distension, or chest pressure. Autonomic dysreflexia may be manifested by sweating, facial flushing, a pounding headache, pilomotor erection, and severe hypertension (Tabsh, Brinkman, and Reff, 1982; Young, Kuntz, and Klein, 1983). The symptoms of dysreflexia are more prevalent during the end of the first stage of labor and all of the second stage as perineal pressure and distension occur. These symptoms, a pounding headache and an increased blood pressure, must not be confused with pregnancy-induced hypertension. The most common treatment for dysreflexia is epidural anesthesia and/or the delivery of the baby.

Delivery of the infant is usually accomplished vaginally. The SCI woman experiences no higher incidence of cesarean birth than a noninjured woman. There is no reduction in the power of the uterine contractions and spontaneous labor. Adequate contractions can and do occur even when the cord transection is above the motor nerve supply of the uterus. The SCI woman has no difficulty with a vaginal delivery even though she has no ability to push. Uterine contractions plus a relaxed perineum facilitate a vaginal delivery. The indications for a cesarean delivery are the same for a SCI woman as for any other woman.

After the delivery of the baby the SCI woman is confronted with the problem of maintaining the integrity of the episiotomy. Ohry et al (1978) state that the use of nonabsorbable sutures to repair episiotomies reduces infections, abcesses, and the probability of dehiscence in the SCI woman. The SCI woman must be assisted in checking her episiotomy at least twice a day for healing, especially since the SCI woman experiences decreased or absent perineal sensation. Sitz baths cannot be used because of the woman's inability to transfer into or onto one. Heat lamps must be used with extreme caution since the SCI woman has little or no sensation and might suffer a burn. The long sanitary napkins used in maternity are ideal for the SCI woman since they decrease the possibility of the pad causing a pressure area. Pressure areas may also result from the use of sanitary belts, and the woman should be cautioned against their use.

During pregnancy both the SCI and the noninjured woman must adapt to physiologic and psychologic changes. The SCI woman has already made major adaptations in her life-style. With pregnancy she must make additional adaptations, but she has a background in successful problem solving to assist her. Through education and timely interventions, nurses can assist with these adaptations and facilitate a positive perinatal experience.

❑ AUTOIMMUNE DISORDERS

Autoimmune disorders have a predilection for women in their reproductive years; therefore associations with pregnancy are not uncommon (Scott et al, 1990). Pregnancy may affect the disease process. Some disorders adversely affect the course of pregnancy or are detrimental to the fetus. Autoimmune connective tissue or collagen vascular disorders include rheumatoid arthritis, systemic lupus erythematosus, hyperthyroidism, myasthenia gravis (p. 721), and immunologic thrombocytopenic purpura (Chapter 23). Autoantibodies from rheumatoid arthritis do *not* cross the placenta; those of the other disorders do. The woman with immunologic thrombocytopenic purpura may deliver a child who demonstrates thrombocytopenia. Petechiae and bleeding into the gastrointestinal and genitourinary tracts and into the brain may be evident. If the mother has myasthenia gravis, the newborn may exhibit a weak cry, sucking mechanism, and facial muscles and may have respiratory problems. Thyrotoxicosis is probable in the newborn of the mother with hyperthyroidism.

Rheumatoid Arthritis

Approximately three of every four women with rheumatoid arthritis (RA) find that the severity of symptoms decreases during pregnancy (Cecere and Persellin, 1981). For this reason many affected women attempt to become pregnant as often as possible; however, many are subfertile because of the RA. During normal pregnancy an increase in α_2-glycoprotein surpasses 40 mg/dl in about 75% of women (Cecere and Persellin, 1981). In addition, total plasma and free cortisol (especially estrogens and progesterones) show an increase (Nolten and Reuckert, 1981). This combination apparently leads to depressed cellular immunity (Persellin, 1981). Women in whom the rheumatoid factor (autoantibodies found in the synovial fluid) decreases during pregnancy report improvement in their symptoms. Researchers are now investigating the possibility of a positive effect on RA associated with the use of oral contraceptives.

The woman with RA needs to be informed of the positive and negative aspects that accompany pregnancy. She must be cautioned that although symptoms may subside during pregnancy, she should anticipate a return of her symptoms after delivery. Exacerbations often recur about a month after delivery. "In short, she will be trading off a 75% chance that she will feel better against the strong possibility that she could 'crash' when the infant is about a month old" (Baum, 1984).

Management of rheumatoid arthritis during pregnancy includes an appropriate balance of rest and exercise, heat and physical therapy, and salicylates. Aspirin probably remains the safest and most useful antiinflammatory drug in these women. Mild hemostatic changes in the newborn, an increase in the average length of gestation, and possibly premature closure of the ductus arteriosus are attributed to maternal ingestion of large doses of aspirin, however (Cunningham, MacDonald, and Gant, 1989).

Systemic Lupus Erythematosus

One of the most common serious disorders of childbearing age, **systemic lupus erythematosus** (SLE), is a chronic multisystem inflammatory disease. The condition is not rare; more than 250,000 persons are known to have SLE, with an estimated 50,000 new cases per year. Although the antibody may be formed in response to a virus, a familial tendency seems to be involved. The vague early symptoms, such as fatigue, may be overlooked. Eventually all organs become involved. The condition is characterized by a series of exacerbations and remissions.

If the diagnosis has been established and the woman desires a child, she is advised to wait for 2 years. At that time, if the disease has been controlled well on low doses of corticosteroids, pregnancy may be reasonably considered (Scott et al, 1990). Oral contraceptives are contraindicated. Diaphragms and condoms are the preferred methods of fertility management if pregnancy is desired in the future. Sterilization is suggested if no more children are desired. The outlook for persons with SLE has improved markedly in the past few years. The survival rate is now more than 90% for 5 years and more than 80% for those who survive for 10 years after diagnosis.

The effect of pregnancy on SLE seems inconsistent. The rate of spontaneous abortion is high. Maternal complications correlate with the degree of cardiac or renal involvement (Scott et al, 1990). Renal failure, hypertension, and death are associated with diffuse proliferative lupus glomerulonephritis. When the kidneys are involved, gravidas are subject to superimposed preeclampsia, stillbirths, preterm delivery, and low-birth-weight infants. However, if the disease is stable during pregnancy, the risk that the disease will worsen with gestation is only slight.

Obstetric management includes surveillance of the woman's renal and cardiovascular status and determination of fetal status. Corticosteroid (prednisone) therapy is maintained throughout pregnancy; hydrocortisone is administered intravenously during labor and delivery. Corticosteroid therapy is continued for about 2 months after delivery.

The relationship with immunosuppresive drugs (such as corticosteroids) and infection must be appreciated. Infection is now a leading cause of death among people with SLE. Nursing care is directed by nursing diagnoses, which often include pain, activity intolerance, altered nutrition, impaired skin integrity, personal identity disturbance, and altered parenting.

Although the antibodies cross the placenta, their amount varies so that the effect on the fetus also varies. The most severely affected newborns suffer from discoid lupus, anemia, neutropenia, thrombocytopenia, and congenital complete heart block. Great strides in diagnosis, drug therapy, and knowledge about the immune system provide hope for the future.

❑ CANCER AND PREGNANCY

Fortunately the peak incidence for most malignant diseases does not occur during the reproductive years (DiSaia and Creasman, 1989). However, an estimated 1 in 1000 women will be afflicted by cancer during pregnancy (Donegan, 1983). The most common cancers reported during pregnancy in order of frequency are breast cancer, Hodgkin's disease, melanoma, and various gynecologic cancers.

Cancer of the Breast

Approximately 1% to 2% of women are pregnant or lactating at the time of diagnosis of cancer of the breast (DiSaia and Creasman, 1989). Breast cancer complicates about 1 in 3000 to 1 in 10,000 pregnancies (Parente et al, 1988). Diagnosis is often delayed because the normal changes in the breast obscure the disease. Pregnancy does not appear to influence the course of mammary cancer and therapeutic abortion does not improve its prognosis (Cunningham, MacDonald, and Gant, 1989). Pregnancy or lactation is not a contraindication to surgery. Treatment is the same as for the nonpregnant woman. For advanced disease in the second or third trimester, alkylating agents, 5-fluorouracil, and vincristine are relatively safe for the fetus (DiSaia and Creasman, 1989). Chemotherapy may significantly improve the survival of these women.

After diagnosis, breastfeeding is contraindicated on two counts: (1) if one of the oncogens for breast cancer is a virus, as many have postulated, then the remaining breast may be contaminated and the virus may be passed to the newborn and may act as a latent inducer of breast carcinoma, and (2) lactation increases vascularity in the remaining breast, which may contain a neoplasm.

The question of subsequent pregnancies depends on the disease-free interval and the status of the lymph nodes (Morrow and Townsend, 1987). A disease-free interval of 2 years, no evidence of metastatic disease, and negative nodes are good prognostic signs. That is, prognosis is not adversely affected by a subsequent pregnancy (Harvey et al, 1981; Morrow and Townsend, 1987).

A 70% 5-year survival rate is anticipated after therapy when the neoplasm is confined to the breast. If axillary metastases are present, the 5-year survival rate after therapy is 30% to 40%. Earlier diagnosis in pregnant women and improved therapy underlie the improvement in the overall survival rate.

Hodgkin's Disease (Lymphoreticuloma)

Hodgkin's disease is a malignant lymphoma that affects many younger people and complicates about 1 in 6000 pregnancies. Younger women (under 40) have a better prognosis.

Although pregnancy in the early stages does not appear to affect the course of the disease adversely, aggressive radiotherapy and chemotherapy has improved overall survival considerably. However, both of these therapies increase susceptibility to infection and sepsis. Unless gestation is well into the third trimester, delay in initiating therapy should be minimal. Radiotherapy to diseased areas above the diaphragm can be initiated during the third trimester with proper shielding of the fetus. Chemotherapy is strongly contraindicated during the first trimester and is relatively contraindicated in the second and third trimesters.

If the gravida and her family refuse any therapy until pregnancy terminates naturally, the physician respects their choice. However, termination of the pregnancy before initiating radiotherapy or chemotherapy is most desirable (DiSaia and Creasman, 1989).

Melanoma

Malignant melanoma was previously thought to be adversely affected by pregnancy. Adverse effects on survival have not been found regardless of whether melanoma developed before or during pregnancy (Holly, 1986). Diagnosis is established by biopsy. Therapy consists of radical local excision.

For most other malignancies, the placenta is unexplainably resistant to invasion by maternal cancer. Though melanoma accounts for few cases of malignant disease during pregnancy, almost 50% of the *placental metastases* and nearly 90% of fetal metastases occur from maternal melanoma (DiSaia and Creasman, 1989).

Despite this, most authorities recommend that women who have histories of malignant melanomas avoid pregnancy for approximately 3 years after complete surgical excision, because this is the period of highest risk of relapse (DiSaia and Creasman, 1989).

Pelvic Malignancies

Cancer of the Vulva. The diagnosis of preinvasive (vulvular intraepithelial neoplasia [VIN]) disease during pregnancy is not uncommon. Therapy is postponed until the postpartum period. If invasive disease is diagnosed during the first trimester, vulvectomy with bilateral groin dissection may be done after the fourteenth week. When it is diagnosed in the third trimester, local wide excision is done deferring definitive surgery until after delivery. Pregnancy does not alter the course of the disease.

Cancer of the Vagina. Except for clear-cell adenocarcinoma of **diethylstilbestrol** (DES)-exposed women, cancer of the vagina is not common. If clear-cell adenocarcinoma of the cervix and vagina or sarcoma is found in the upper vagina, the preferred surgery is radical hysterectomy, upper vaginectomy, and bilateral pelvic lymphadenectomy, followed by chemotherapy. If disease is advanced, the preferred treatment is to empty the uterus and begin radiotherapy.

Cancer of the Cervix. Rarely an invasive **carcinoma** (a malignant tumor made up of connective tissue enclosing epithelial cells; tends to become progressively worse and to result in death) of the cervix is discovered during pregnancy. The major risk to the woman of delivery through a cervix containing invasive carcinoma is the risk of hemorrhage as a result of tearing of the tumor during cervical dilatation and delivery. Therefore abdominal surgical delivery is preferred (Droegemueller et al, 1987).

The cancer itself does not harm the pregnancy: stage for stage, the outcome for the gravida with cervical cancer is roughly the same as for the nonpregnant woman (Droegemueller et al, 1987; DiSaia and Creasman, 1989). Carcinoma of the cervix is curable if diagnosed and treated in its early stages. Diagnosis and therapy is the same regardless of whether the woman is pregnant. The beliefs and desires of the woman and her family are important in terms of initiating therapy that can interrupt the pregnancy as opposed to postponing the therapy until fetal viability is achieved.

Cancer of the uterus, uterine tube, or ovary is an infrequent complication during pregnancy. Malignancy of the ovary occurs approximately once in 8000 to 20,000 deliveries. The pregnancy does not alter the woman's prognosis if an aggressive therapeutic approach is taken. Fortunately, ovarian germ cell neoplasms occurring in pregnancy are usually **benign** (not recurrent or not tending to progress) (DiSaia and Creasman, 1989).

Therapy During Pregnancy

Chemotherapy. Many cytotoxic agents are teratogenic early in pregnancy and would result in either spontaneous abortion or fetal abnormality if administered. In addition, these drugs theoretically are mutogenic, abortifactants, and lethal to the fetus at any time. Nothing is known about the long-term effects of in utero exposure should the child survive. Chemotherapy with some drugs (aminopterin and methotrexate) in the second and third trimesters may not cause observable harm to the fetus.

Radiotherapy. During embryonic development, tissues are extremely radiosensitive. If cells are genetically altered or killed during this time, the child either will fail to survive or will be deformed. From a radiologic stance there are three significant periods in embryonic development:

1. *Preimplantation:* If irradiation does not destroy the fertilized egg, it probably does not affect it significantly.
2. *Critical period of organogenesis:* During this period, especially between days 18 and 38, the organism is most vulnerable; microcephaly, anencephaly, eye damage, growth retardation, spina bifida and foot damage may occur.
3. *After day 40:* Large doses may still cause observable malformation and damage to the CNS.

Irradiation of gonads involves genetic damage—gene mutation and chromosome breakage—even at relatively low doses. Most mutations are recessive so that mutant effects may not surface for many generations.

Gestational Trophoblastic Neoplasm

Gestational trophoblastic neoplasia follows a hydatidiform mole in 50% of cases, an abortion in 25% of cases, or a normal pregnancy in 25% of cases. Nearly 20% of complete (classic) moles (p. 675 and Fig. 23-7) progress to gestational trophoblastic neoplasia (Cunningham, MacDonald, and Gant, 1989). Gestational trophoblastic neoplasia can be nonmetastatic or metastatic; the latter cases are further divided into those women with good and those with poor prognoses (Cunningham, MacDonald, and Gant, 1989). A *good* prognosis can be expected if metastatic disease is present less than 4 months, human chorionic gonadotropin (hCG) is $\leq$40,000 U/ml, and there has been no prior chemotherapy. A *poor* prognosis can be expected if any of the following is present: disease persists more than 4 months, hCG is $\geq$40,000 U/ml, brain or liver **metastasis** is seen, prior chemotherapy failed, or disease follows a term pregnancy.

In a sizeable proportion of women, gestational trophoblastic disease regresses spontaneously or is cured by surgical procedures (e.g., curettages, hysterectomy). In a few cases the disorder progresses to choriocarcinoma or invasive mole. An extremely **malignant** form of trophoblastic neoplasia is ***choriocarcinoma.*** In choriocarcinoma, the villi are absent and the **neoplasm** is composed of sheets of malignant trophoblast. Hemorrhage and necrosis, common in choriocarcinoma, result from the lack of vascular supply. Metastases develop early and are blood-borne. Of affected women, 75% show metastases to the lungs; 50% to the vagina (Cunningham, MacDonald, and Gant, 1989). Metastases are found in many cases in the vulva, kidneys, liver, ovaries, brain and bowel.

An ***invasive mole*** is locally invasive with little tendency to widespread metastasis. Excessive trophoblastic growth and extensive penetration by trophoblastic elements, including whole villi, occur deep in the myometrium. Sometimes the peritoneum, adjacent parametrium, or vaginal vault is affected.

The clinical history reveals a recent normal pregnancy or one complicated by hydatidiform mole, abortion, or ectopic implantation. A common sign is irregular bleeding in the immediate puerperium in association with uterine subinvolution. The bleeding may be intermittent, constant, or sudden, with sometimes massive hemorrhage. If the uterus is perforated, extension into the parametrium or intraperitoneal hemorrhage causes pain and other symptoms of pelvic inflammatory disease. Metastatic lesions cause symptoms. Cough and bloody sputum accompany pulmonary lesions. Tumors of the vagina or vulva may be found.

Diagnosis is confirmed by examination of tissue obtained by curettage when investigating postpregnancy or postabortal bleeding. Radioimmunoassay based on the β-subunit of hCG permits detection of a very low level of this hormone. Persistent or rising hCG titers in the absence of pregnancy are indicative of trophoblastic neoplasia (Cunningham, MacDonald, and Gant, 1989). A chest x-ray study reveals metastatic lesions. Computed tomography (CT scan) or magnetic resonance imaging (MRI) is used to evaluate the brain, lungs, liver, and pelvis for metastatic lesions.

Before 1956, metastatic gestational trophoblastic disease had a short clinical course and was fatal. In 1956, complete remission with methotrexate in some women was reported (Li, Hertz, and Spencer). In 1960, actinomycin D (dactinomycin), when given sequentially with methotrexate, improved the remission rate from 50% to approximately 75%. Current treatment for gestational trophoblastic neoplasia is much more successful than that used in the past (Cunningham, MacDonald, and Gant, 1989). The overall cure rate has been about 90% (Lewis, 1980). Almost 100% of women at low risk with good prognoses have been cured. For these women, single-agent chemotherapy is used (i.e., either methotrexate or actinomycin D). Others require a combination of these drugs to affect a cure. For women at high risk, cure has been achieved by combining chemotherapy (methotrexate, actinomycin-D, and cyclophosphamide) with irradiation of metastatic lesions.

Women who have experienced gestational trophoblastic disease are at increased risk for recurrence in a subsequent pregnancy. However, women who have received chemotherapy are not at increased risk for fetal anomalies in subsequent pregnancies (Song et al, 1988; Rustin et al, 1989).

Surgery During Pregnancy

The need for immediate abdominal surgery occurs as frequently among pregnant women as among nonpregnant women of comparable age. Diagnosis is more difficult in the pregnant woman, however. An enlarged uterus and displaced internal organs may prevent adequate palpation and alter the position of the surgical procedure.

Differential diagnosis includes consideration of obstetric complications (e.g., ectopic pregnancy and premature separation of the placenta) and the onset of labor. Mild leukocytosis and increased serum values of alkaline phosphatase and amylase are characteristic of pregnancy, as well as surgical intraperitoneal processes. Rising or abnormally high laboratory values are suspect, however. X-ray evaluation, a valuable adjunct to diagnosis, is contraindicated, particularly in the first trimester, except in extreme cases. The surgeon is confronted with both a surgical and an obstetric problem.

Laparotomy or laparoscopy may be required. Hazards of these procedures include abortion and preterm labor. But surgical or anesthetic intervention does not affect the incidence of congenital malformations.

Assessment

Fetal vital signs and activity and uterine contractility (labor may have begun) are monitored, and constant vigilance for symptoms of impending obstetric complications is maintained. The woman and her family may have heightened concerns regarding effects of the procedure and medication on fetal well-being and the course of pregnancy.

The extent of presurgery assessment of the mother is determined by the immediacy of surgical intervention and the specific condition that requires surgery (Phipps, Long, and Woods, 1991).

Nursing Diagnoses

Nursing diagnoses also vary with the surgical condition and the immediacy of surgical intervention. Nursing diagnoses may include the following:

Knowledge deficit related to
- The surgical condition
- The surgical procedure
- Recovery
- Potential sequelae for self and infant

Potential for injury related to
- Effects of postoperative immobility

Spiritual distress related to
- High-risk status

Planning

The preoperative and postoperative plans for care incorporate consideration for the family's and woman's concern for the newborn as well as for the woman.

Goals for care vary with each individual client. However, general goals apply in all situations. These general goals include:

1. Woman and family meet their spiritual care needs
2. Woman and family understand the condition, rationale for surgical intervention, expected outcome, and postoperative course and management

3. Well-being of maternal-fetal-placental unit is maintained
4. Mother and fetus-neonate suffer no adverse sequelae
5. Mother complies with scheduled postoperative follow-up care

Implementation

Preoperative Period

Preoperative care for a pregnant woman differs from that for a nonpregnant woman in one significant aspect: the presence of at least one other person, the fetus. Procedures such as preparation of the operative site and the time of insertion of IV lines and urinary retention catheters vary with the physician and the facility. However, in every instance there is a total restriction of solid foods and liquids or a clear specification of the type, amount, and time at which clear liquids may be taken before surgery. Food by mouth is restricted for several hours before a scheduled procedure. Even if she has had nothing by mouth, but, more important, if surgery is unexpected, the woman is in danger of vomiting and aspirating, and special precautions are taken before anesthesia is administered (Chapter 13).

General preoperative observations and ongoing care are the same as for any surgery (Phipps, Long, Woods, 1991), with the addition of fetal surveillance. A notation of FHR, fetal status, and uterine activity is important.

Postoperative Period

Most recovery rooms have special forms used as checklists for assessing the client's postoperative status and progress. General observations and ongoing care pertinent to postoperative recovery are initiated. This includes maintaining fluid and electrolyte balance by diligent attention to intake and output. The nurse promotes physical and emotional rest through the appropriate use of nurse-ordered comfort measures and physician-ordered medications and procedures. If intrauterine pregnancy continues, fetal monitoring and monitoring of uterine activity are continued (Chapter 14).

Client safety remains an important component of care. The family is called on to assist in maintaining client safety through orientation of the woman (and her family and friends) to the need to use side rails, to call for assistance when getting out of bed, to protect the IV infusion and incision sites, and to cleanse the perineum.

Some causes of vital sign changes early in the postoperative phase are listed in Table 24-2.

Table 24-2 Some Causes of Vital Sign Changes in Early Postoperative Phase

Increase	Decrease
TEMPERATURE	
Stress reaction (low-grade fever)	Cold operating room and recovery room
PULSE RATE	
Jarring during transfer Shock, hemorrhage Hypoventilation Acute gastric dilatation Pain Anxiety Cardiac arrhythmias	Digitalis overdose Cardiac arrhythmias
RESPIRATORY RATE	
Hypoventilation: poor positioning, right chest or upper abdominal dressing, obesity, gastric dilatation	Drugs: anesthetics, narcotics, sedatives
BLOOD PRESSURE	
Anxiety (↑ systolic) Pain	Jarring during transfer Severe pain Cardiac arrhythmias Shock: fluid loss, hemorrhage, acute gastric dilatation

From Phipps WJ, Long BC, and Woods NF: Medical-surgical nursing: concepts and clinical practice, ed 4, St Louis, 1991, The CV Mosby Co.

Discharge Planning

Planning for discharge begins when the gravida first enters the health care delivery system. The extent to which the goals of care can be met before surgery is reviewed, and adjustments are made accordingly. For example, if the surgery was an emergency, such as for appendicitis, there is little time for preoperative preparation. After the woman has recovered from the effects of the surgery, the nurse needs to take time to encourage her to voice her fears, concerns, and questions. She may have questions regarding the effect of the surgery and anesthesia on the fetus. If she is unable to express these concerns to the physician, the nurse acts as client-advocate and informs the physician.

The participation of the woman and her family in discharge planning is necessary to individualize the care to fit with the available family support systems, the home situation, and the facilities. If the woman is to perform some type of treatment or exercises at home, the family member or friend who will be caring for her is included when she is taught these activities, and her mastery is evaluated. The woman may be demonstrating symptoms of grief and loss, and her participation in discharge planning may be minimal. She may need assistance coping with these feelings (Chapter 29).

The woman may need referral service to various community agencies for evaluation of the home situation, child care, home health care, and financial or other assistance. All arrangements for her return home and for convalescent care should be completed as early as possible before the expected date of discharge. Topics covered vary but may include the following:

1. Care of incision site.
2. Return of gastrointestinal function: diet, elimination.
3. Signs and symptoms of developing complications: wound infection, thrombophlebitis, pneumonia. These should be given to the woman in printed form as well.*
4. If the woman is expected to assess her temperature, she will need a thermometer and must know how to use it.
5. Resumption of activities of daily living. For example, the woman should not lift heavy objects and usually should not resume driving for 2 to 4 weeks or longer.
6. Treatments and medications ordered.
7. List of resource people and phone numbers that can be used for different services.
8. Schedule of follow-up visit.

The follow-up examination at the physician's office is scheduled usually 1 to 2 weeks after discharge. The nurse plays a vital role in helping clients understand the importance of follow-up care.

Evaluation

The nurse can be reasonably assured that care has been effective if the goals of care have been achieved.

Appendicitis

Acute suppurative appendicitis complicates about 1 in every 1000 pregnancies. This disorder poses the following special problems during gestation:

1. Appendicitis is more difficult to diagnose during pregnancy. The appendix is carried high and to the right, away from McBurney's point, by the enlarged uterus.
2. Appendiceal rupture and peritonitis occur 2 to 3 times more often in pregnant women than in nonpregnant women.
3. Maternal and perinatal morbidity and mortality are greatly increased when appendicitis occurs during pregnancy.

Most cases of acute appendicitis occur during the first 6 months of gestation, with decreasing frequency through the third trimester, labor, and puerperium. The differential diagnosis of appendicitis during pregnancy is also difficult because of gastrointestinal or genitourinary problems that may be confused with appendicitis. A high level of suspicion is important in the diagnosis of appendicitis.

Appendectomy before rupture is extremely important. Antibiotic therapy before rupture is of questionable value; after rupture it may be lifesaving. Therapeutic abortion is never indicated in appendicitis. Cesarean delivery at or near term may be justified in association with appendectomy.

Maternal mortality increases to about 10% in the third trimester and is about 15% when appendicitis develops during labor. Perinatal mortality is approximately 10% with unruptured appendicitis but is at least 35% with peritonitis.

Intestinal Obstruction

Although intestinal obstruction (dynamic ileus) is not common during pregnancy, any woman with a laparotomy scar or a history of pelvic inflammatory disease (PID) is more likely to suffer intestinal obstruction during gestation. Adhesions as a result of previous surgery or PID, an enlarging uterus, and displacement of the intestines are etiologic factors.

Persistent abdominal, cramplike pain; vomiting; auscultatory rushes within the abdomen; and "laddering" of the intestinal shadows on x-ray films aid in the diagnosis of intestinal obstruction. Immediate surgical intervention is required for release of the obstruction. Pregnancy is rarely affected by the surgery, assuming the absence of complications such as peritonitis. Cesarean delivery is not indicated in intestinal obstruction.

Abdominal Hernias

The incidence of abdominal hernias and related incarceration of the bowel is reduced during pregnancy despite permanent enlargement of umbilical or incisional hernial rings. Displacement of a nonadherent bowel by the enlarging uterus and its shielding of so-called weak areas of the abdominal wall are responsible. In fact, temporary spontaneous reduction of some abdominal wall hernias occurs during gestation. In contrast, however, the uncommon irreducible or adherent hernias may become incarcerated as pregnancy progresses.

Straining or bearing down during the second stage

*The client's ability to read, comprehend, and comply with the printed instructions must be assessed as well.

of labor may be contraindicated for women with hernias. Therefore low forceps delivery may be planned. Abdominal hernia is not an indication for cesarean delivery; herniorrhaphy should be done between pregnancies.

Gynecologic Problems

Ovarian cysts and twisting of ovarian cysts or adnexal tissues may occur. Pregnancy predisposes a woman to ovarian problems, especially during the first trimester. Conditions include retained or enlarged cystic corpus luteum of pregnancy, ovarian cyst, and bacterial invasion of reproductive or other intraperitoneal organs. Laparotomy or laparoscopy is required to discriminate between ovarian problems and early ectopic pregnancy, appendicitis, or other infectious processes.

Injuries During Pregnancy

Minor injury during pregnancy is a common occurrence; most trauma (more than 50%) occurs during the third trimester. Maternal adaptations to pregnancy are responsible for syncope, loss of balance, and general clumsiness. Discomfort such as a contracting uterus or vigorous fetal movement may be distracting while the woman is driving or working; an estimated 7% of pregnant women sustain accidental injury (Smith and Payne, 1984). The leading cause of death in women of reproductive age is trauma and not neoplasms or obstetric complications (Bremer and Cassata, 1986; Daddario, 1989).

Assessment

The woman's condition is the initial concern. The injury sustained determines the type and extent of assessment conducted. Attention is focused first on the basic ABCs: **a**irway, **b**reathing, and **c**irculation (Fig. 24-6). The woman's abdomen is assessed for ruptured uterus and uterine activity. As indicated, health assessment is performed. When available, the woman's prenatal record is reviewed.

Physical Examination

Findings from the injury must not be confused with the normal physiologic changes during pregnancy:

1. Usual signs of organ rupture (i.e., guarding, rebound tenderness, and rigidity) may only be responses to stretching of the abdominal wall.
2. Examination of the woman in a supine position results in hypotension and a systolic value as low as 80; changing her position to left lateral or simply moving the fetus raises the systolic value to more than 100.
3. A "silent" abdomen, a sign of bowel trauma, may be a normal finding because of the decreased motility found during pregnancy.
4. Delayed emptying time of the stomach during pregnancy poses a threat of vomiting and possible aspiration if the woman has eaten within the last several hours.
5. During pregnancy, the woman may sustain a significant blood loss (about 30% reduction in circulating blood volume) without the usual signs and symptoms of hypovolemia. Pelvic blood vessels (retroperitoneal and parametrial arteries) enlarge greatly during pregnancy so that they are damaged and perhaps rupture more easily as a result.
6. The large uterus can compartmentalize and hide hemorrhage originating in the liver and spleen.
7. A rapid pulse may reflect only the usual increase of 10 to 15 bpm, or it may be a sign of hypovolemia.

Laboratory Tests

The type of test is determined by the type of injury. Appropriate blood studies include tests for serum amylase and blood gases; baseline bleeding profile; and complete blood count, typing and cross-matching. In normal pregnancies a white blood count of 18,000/mm^3 in the last trimester and 25,000/mm^3 during labor is usual; these same values are also indicative of intraabdominal hemorrhage. DIC can complicate severe trauma, placental abruption, and sepsis.

An indwelling urinary bladder catheter for drainage facilitates management of fluid therapy and aids diagnosis; for example, difficulty in passing the catheter suggests urethral disruption, and hematuria suggests a ruptured bladder. The catheter also provides access for retrograde cystogram x-ray examination.

Intraperitoneal hemorrhage must be detected. Radiology, realtime ultrasound, and CT scan are useful diagnostic modalities. The physician places a peritoneal lavage catheter for detecting intraperitoneal hemorrhage. The procedure is performed with the woman under local anesthesia through a small incision into the peritoneum. The test is positive for bleeding if the aspirate exceeds 10 ml of nonclotting blood or if, after instillation of 1 L of lactated Ringer's solution, bloody fluid is recovered. Radiographic studies may be necessary to guide management.

Posttraumatic Uterine and Fetal Surveillance

When the mother has been stabilized, attention is turned toward monitoring the fetus and monitoring for

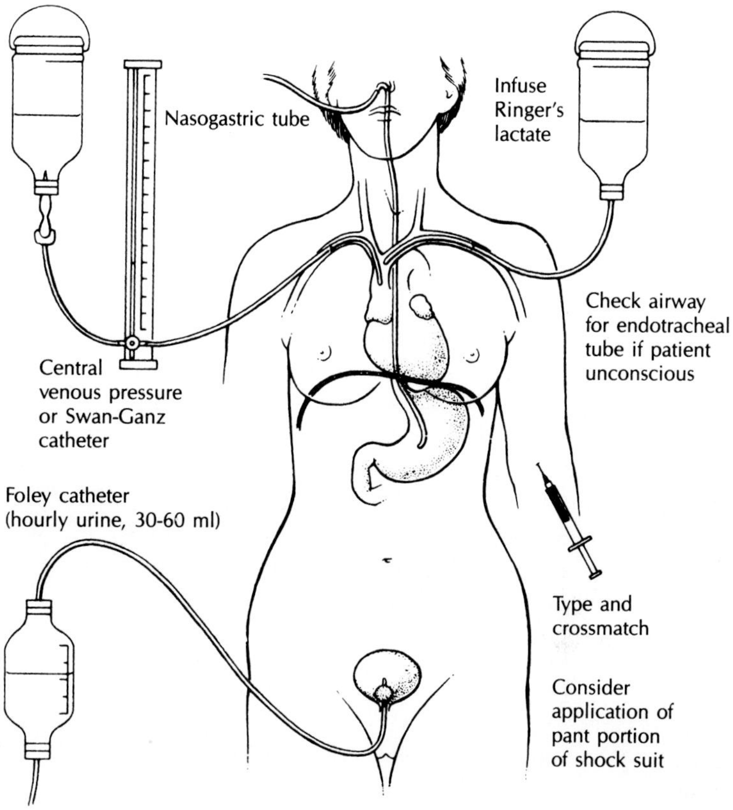

Fig. 24-6 Summary of technique used for resuscitation. Trauma care should begin in field where injury occurred, always with attention to basic ABCs: airway, breathing, and circulation. (From Higgins SD: Contemp Obstet Gynecol 21(3):32, 1983.)

preterm labor and placental abruption. Usually, if these complications occur, they happen within 24 to 48 hours after the accident.

In the case of minor trauma, the woman is hospitalized and evaluated for the following: vaginal bleeding, uterine irritability, abdominal tenderness, abdominal pain or cramps, evidence of hypovolemia, a change in or absence of fetal heart tones, and leakage of amniotic fluid (Rothenberger, 1978).

After injury, if ***placental abruption*** (abruptio placentae) is to occur, it usually manifests itself within 48 hours. ***Uterine rupture*** can occur at the site of a previous scar or over the site of implantation, which is weakened by increased vascularity at the site. Expulsion of the uterine contents into the abdominal cavity may occur and is usually followed by massive hemorrhage.

Nursing Diagnoses

The nursing diagnoses are formulated from assessment findings. Examples of possible nursing diagnoses include the following:

Anxiety, fear related to
- Uncertainty of outcome for the gravida and fetus

Knowledge deficit related to
- Inadequate pretreatment preparation time

Potential for injury related to
- Recent food intake before need for anesthesia

Planning

Planning with the gravida may not be possible in all situations. The gravida and family are included in planning at the earliest possible time.

Goals are derived from the injury, its management and course, and based on the gravida's and family's individual needs. ***Goals*** include the following:

1. The woman's injuries resulting from accidents are diagnosed and treated accurately and rapidly
2. Woman and fetus sustain no permanent adverse sequelae
3. Woman and family grieve appropriately
4. Injuries are prevented through prenatal education on safety in view of normal maternal adaptations to pregnancy (e.g., balance).

Implementation

Intervention begins with *prevention*. The woman is counseled to discontinue activities requiring balance and coordination, to use seat belts appropriately, to recognize early adverse symptoms, and to seek therapy immediately. If the woman is hospitalized only for observation, she is involved in assessment for signs and symptoms of complications.

Immediate **trauma care** consists of attention to the ABCs. While hypoxia and hypovolemia are being corrected, the woman should be transferred to a trauma center with obstetric and neonatal backup, if possible. During transfer, attendants must remember the aortocaval (supine hypotensive) syndrome. The woman should be positioned on her side or the uterus displaced laterally by a uterine displacer or by a pillow placed under her right hip. Hypotension must be avoided to prevent compromise of cardiac output followed by a decrease of blood flow to the uterus.

A nasogastric tube is inserted, if indicated, because delayed gastric emptying time and increased intestinal transit time increase the risk of vomiting and aspiration (see Fig. 24-6). Mouth care and reassurance are used to counter the annoyance the woman may feel because of the presence of the tube. Fluid and electrolyte replacement is instituted and monitored. Oxygen needs are met.

Penetrating abdominal wounds, internal hemorrhage, and ruptured uterus are all indications for immediate *surgical intervention.* Wounds high in the abdomen have most likely penetrated a vital structure because organs such as the bowel, liver, and spleen have been displaced upward by the enlarging uterus.

Cesarean Delivery

Indications for immediate cesarean delivery (Chapter 26) include fetal distress and maternal infection, ruptured diaphragm, unstable spinal fractures, and complicated pelvic fractures. The enlarged uterus can hamper control of hemorrhage and repair of vital structures. A ruptured diaphragm must be repaired immediately, but the family must be informed that even in nonpregnant persons, the morbidity and mortality are high. During pregnancy, increased intraabdominal pressure generated by the uterus and bearing-down efforts during labor increase the risk. Unstable spinal fractures cannot be tolerated by the pregnant woman because of inability to remain in the supine position and of the stress of vaginal delivery. A pelvis distorted by extensive fracture in itself is incompatible with vaginal delivery, but vaginal delivery may also cause extensive damage to the urethra and bladder that do not have the protection of an intact and well-formed pelvis.

Fetal outcome of the uninjured fetus is likely to be good if the interval is less than 10 but no more than 20 minutes since the mother's death. The family will need supportive care to deal with the grief of losing a loved one (Chapter 29).

Evaluation

The nurse can be assured that care has been effective if the goals of care have been achieved.

SUMMARY

Pathophysiology, medical treatment, and nursing care of several disorders are presented in this chapter. These disorders have immediate and long-term consequences for the mother and her fetus or newborn. This chapter discusses the knowledge base for understanding how to implement the nursing process with problems that occur during pregnancy. As always, sensitivity to the woman and her family during the childbearing experience that is complicated by a physical disorder is as important as expert technologic assistance. Nursing care of the pregnant woman with a medical or surgical complication presents a challenge that offers the potential of fulfillment on both a professional and personal level.

LEARNING ACTIVITIES

1. Develop a teaching plan for a non-English-speaking pregnant diabetic woman. Incorporate materials, both written and illustrated, and audiovisual aids as available.
2. Participate in the assessment and implementation of a teaching plan for a newly diagnosed gestational diabetic, either in a clinic or physician's office. Discuss the experience in postclinical conference.
3. Develop plans of care for a woman with hyperemesis gravidarum, including psychologic considerations.
4. Develop a care plan for a woman who does not follow her prescribed treatment. Role play one part of the care plan in front of a group. Explore the feelings, beliefs, and values that emerge in the group discussion that follows.
5. Discover resources in your community that offer financial, counseling, or educational services to pregnant clients with heart disease. What criteria must the client meet to be eligible for service? Interview a staff member and report your findings back to your group.
6. Follow a pregnant client through the perioperative phase. Discuss what considerations were given to the client's obstetric needs and what measures were taken to protect the fetus.

KEY CONCEPTS

- Alteration in the maternal metabolic milieu characteristic of diabetic mellitus may be responsible for congenital malformations that occur sometime before the fourth to the seventh week of gestation.
- Maternal insulin does not cross the placenta; the fetus begins to secrete its own insulin at the tenth gestational week.
- After the tenth week of gestation, fetal hyperinsulinism results from maternal hyperglycemia (fetal hyperinsulinism is responsible for fetal disorders, discussed in Chapter 28).
- Poor control of diabetes mellitus during pregnancy is responsible for dystotic labor from hydramnios and macrosomia, infections, vascular damage, and an increased risk for PIH.
- Home monitoring for glucose, multiple doses or constant infusion of insulin, and dietary counseling are being used to create a normal intrauterine environment for fetal growth and maturation in the pregnancy complicated by diabetes mellitus.
- Abnormalities in thyroid function may adversely affect control of diabetes mellitus during pregnancy as a result of changes in the metabolism of insulin.
- The woman who is being treated for hyperemesis gravidarum is discharged home when fluid and electrolyte balance is restored and weight gain begins.
- The stress of normal maternal adaptations to pregnancy on a heart whose function is already taxed may cause cardiac decompensation.
- Anemia, the most common medical disorder of pregnancy, affects at least 20% of pregnant women.
- The chance of developing adult respiratory distress syndrome (ARDS) increases with the amount of trauma experienced during pregnancy or delivery.
- Autoimmune disorders (e.g., systemic lupus erythematosus, myasthenia gravis) have a predilection for women in their reproductive years, therefore associations with pregnancy are not uncommon.
- In the gravida, an enlarged uterus, displaced internal organs, and altered laboratory values may confound differential diagnosis when the need for immediate abdominal surgery occurs.
- Preoperative care for a pregnant woman differs from that for a nonpregnant woman in one significant aspect: the presence of at least one other person, the fetus.
- Cancer and its therapy are emotionally and physically draining on the woman, her family, and the caregiver.

References

Endocrine Disorders

American Diabetes Association: Physician's guide to insulin-dependent (type I) diabetes: diagnosis and treatment, Alexandria, Vir, 1988, American Diabetes Association.

American Diabetes Association: Position statement: Nutritional recommendations and principles for individuals with diabetes mellitus: 1986, Diabetes Care 10:126, 1987.

Corbett JV: Laboratory tests and diagnostic procedures with nursing diagnoses, ed 2, Norwalk, Conn, 1987, Appleton & Lange.

Coustan DR and Carpenter MW: Detection and treatment of gestational diabetes, Clin Obstet Gynecol 28(23):507, 1985.

Cunningham FG, MacDonald PC, and Gant, NF: Williams obstetrics, ed 18, Norwalk, Conn, 1989, Appleton & Lange.

DeGroot LJ et al: The thyroid and its diseases, New York, 1984, John Wiley & Sons.

Gabbe SG: Diabetes in pregnancy, Clin Obstet Gynecol 28(3):455, 1985.

Hauenstein D and Patterson AM: Redefining "gestational" diabetes: a case report, Diabetes Professional: The publication for health professionals, p 17, Spring, 1989.

Hill CS, Jr, et al: Effect of pregnancy after thyroid carcinoma, Surg Gynecol Obstet 122:1219, 1966.

Hollingsworth DR: Maternal metabolism in normal pregnancy and pregnancy complicated by diabetes mellitus, Clin Obstet Gynecol 28(3):457, 1985.

Kleinman CS: Fetal echocardiography. In Sanders R, editor: Ultrasound annual, New York, 1982, Raven Press.

Landon MG and Gabbe SG: Glucose monitoring and insulin administration in the pregnant diabetic patient, Clin Obstet Gynecol 28(3):496, 1985.

Leveno KG et al: Continuous subcutaneous insulin infusion during pregnancy, Diabetes Res Clin Pract 4:257, 1988.

Mills JL et al: Lack of relation of increased malformation rates in infants of diabetic mothers to glycemic control during organogenesis, N Engl J Med 318:671, 1988.

Milunsky A et al: Prenatal diagnosis of neural tube defects. VIII. The importance of serum alpha-fetoprotein screening in diabetic pregnant women, Am J Obstet Gynecol 142:1030, 1982.

Nursing 87 Books: 1987 Nursing photobook annual, Springhouse, Penn, 1987, Springhouse Corp.

Robertson C: When your pregnant patient has diabetes, RN, p 18, Nov, 1987.

Scott JR et al: Danforth's obstetrics and gynecology, ed 6, Philadelphia, 1990, JB Lippincott Co.

Steele JM: Prepregnancy counseling and contraception in the insulin-dependent diabetic patient, Clin Obstet Gynecol 28(3):553, 1985.

VanPutte AW: Perinatal bereavement crisis: coping with negative outcomes from prenatal diagnosis, J Perinat Neonat Nurs 2(2):12, 1988.

White P: Classification of obstetric diabetes, Am J Obstet Gynecol 130:228, 1978.

Cardiovascular Disorders

Anticoagulants: how safe are they during pregnancy? Contemp OB/GYN 35(1):182, 1990.

Brady K and Duff P: Rheumatic heart disease in pregnancy, Clin Obstet Gynecol, 31(1):21, 1989.

Cox SM et al: Bacterial endocarditis: a serious pregnancy complication, J Reprod Med 33:671, 1988.

Cox SM and Leveno KJ: Pregnancy complicated by bacterial endocarditis, Clin Obstet Gynecol 31(1):48, 1989.

Cregler LL and Mark H: Cardiovascular dangers of cocaine abuse, Am J Cardio 57:1185, May, 1986.

Cunningham FG, MacDonald PC, and Gant NF: Williams obstetrics, ed 18, Norwalk, Conn, 1989, Appleton & Lange.

Demakis JG and Rahimtoola SH: Peripartum cardiomyopathy, Circulation 44:964, 1971.

Gilbert ES and Harmon JS: High risk pregnancy and delivery, St Louis, 1986, The CV Mosby Co.

Homans DC: Peripartum cardiomyopathy, N Engl J Med 312:1432, 1985.

Lee RV et al: Cardiopulmonary resuscitation of pregnant women, Am J Med 81:311, 1986.

Lee W and Cotton DB: Peripartum cardiomyopathy: current concepts and clinical management, Clin Obstet Gynecol 31(1):54, 1989.

Little BB and Gilstrap LC: Cardiovascular drugs during pregnancy, Clin Obstet Gynecol 31(1):13, 1989.

Metcalf J, McAnulty JH, and Ueland K: Burwell and Metcalfe's heart disease and pregnancy: physiology and management, ed 2, Boston, 1986, Little, Brown & Co, Inc.

Newkirk EJ and Fry ME: Trauma during pregnancy, Focus Crit Care 12(6):30, 1985.

Ramin SM, Maberry MC, and Gilstrap LC: Congenital heart disease, Clin Obstet Gynecol 31(1):41, 1989.

Roberts SL and Chestnut DH: Anesthesia for the obstetric patient with cardiac disease, Clin Obstet Gynecol 30(3):601, 1987.

Sanderson JE, Olsen EGJ, and Gatei D: Peripartum heart disease: an endomyocardial biopsy study, Br Heart J 56:285, 1986.

Scott JR et al: Danforth's obstetrics and gynecology, ed 6, Philadelphia, 1990, JB Lippincott Co.

Seaworth BJ and Durack DT: Infective endocarditis in obstetric and gynecologic practice, Am J Obstet Gynecol 154:180, 1986.

Songster GS and Clark SL: Cardiac arrest in pregnancy—what to do, Contemp OB/GYN 26:141, 1985.

Troiano NH: Cardiopulmonary resuscitation of the pregnant woman, J Perinat Neonat Nurs 3(2):1, 1989.

Veille JC: Peripartum cardiomyopathies: a review, Am J Obstet Gynecol 148:805, 1984.

Medical Disorders

Aminoff MJ: Neurological disorders and pregnancy, Am J Obstet Gynecol 132:325, 1978.

Axel SJ: Spinal cord injured women's concerns: menstruation and pregnancy, Rehab Nurs 7(5):10, 1982.

Baum J: Arthritis and pregnancy, Contemp OB/GYN 23(3):97, 1984.

Cecere FA and Persellin RH: The interaction of pregnancy and the rheumatic diseases, Clin Rheum Dis 7:747, 1981.

Craig DI: Adaptation to pregnancy by spinal cord injured women. Unpublished research for MSN degree requirement, University of San Diego, 1985.

Cunningham FG, MacDonald PC, and Gant NF: Williams obstetrics, ed 18, Norwalk, Conn, 1989, Appleton & Lange.

DiSaia PJ and Creasman WT: Clinical gynecologic oncology, ed 4, St Louis, 1989, The CV Mosby Co.

Donegan WL: Cancer and pregnancy, CA 33:194, 1983.

Droegemueller W et al: Comprehensive gynecology, St Louis, 1987, The CV Mosby Co.

Frith JA and McLeod JG: Pregnancy and multiple sclerosis, J Neurol Neurosurg Psychiatry 51:495, 1988.

Goller H and Paeslack V: Our experiences about pregnancy and delivery of the paraplegic woman, Paraplegia 8:161, 1971.

Goller H and Paeslack V: Pregnancy damage and birth complications of paraplegic women, Paraplegia 10:213, 1972.

Harvey JC et al: The effect of pregnancy on the prognosis of carcinoma of the breast following radical mastectomy, Surg Gynecol Obstet 153:723, 1981.

Holly EA: Melanoma and pregnancy, Recent Results Cancer Res 102:118, 1986.

Lammer EJ et al: Retinoic acid embryopathy, N Engl J Med 313:837, 1985.

Lewis JL, Jr: Treatment of metastatic gestational trophoblastic neoplasms, Am J Obstet Gynecol 136:163, 1980.

Li M, Hertz R, and Spencer DB: Effects of methotrexate therapy upon choriocarcinoma and chorioadenoma, Proc Soc Exp Biol Med 93:361, 1956.

Mattison DR et al: Pharmacology: effects of drugs and chemicals on the fetus, Contemp OB/GYN 33(4):97, 1989.

McGregor JA, Guberman A, and Goodlin R: Idiopathic facial nerve paralysis (Bell's palsy) in late pregnancy and the early puerperium, Obstet Gynecol 69:435, 1987.

Morrow CP and Townsend DE: Synopsis of gynecologic oncology, ed 3, New York, 1987, John Wiley & Sons.

Nolten WE and Rueckert PA: Elevated free cortisol index in pregnancy: possible regulatory mechanism, Am J Obstet Gynecol 139:492, 1981.

Ohry A et al: Sexual function, pregnancy and delivery in spinal cord injured women, Gyn Obstet Invest 9(6):281, 1978.

Parente JT et al: Breast cancer associated with pregnancy, Obstet Gynecol 71:861, 1988.

Persellin RH: Inhibitors of inflammatory and immune responses in pregnancy serum, Clin Rheum Dis 7:769, 1981.

Rustin GJ et al: Pregnancy after cytotoxic chemotherapy for gestational trophoblastic tumours, Br Med J 288:103, 1984.

Sarbin TR and Allen VL: Role theory. In Lindzey G and Aronson E, editors: The handbook of social psychology, vol 1, ed 2, Reading, Mass, 1968, Addison-Wesley Publishing Co, Inc.

Scott JR et al: Danforth's obstetrics and gynecology, ed 6, Philadelphia, 1990, JB Lippincott Co.

Song HZ, et al: Pregnancy outcomes after successful chemotherapy for choriocarcinoma and invasive mole: long-term follow-up, Am J Obstet Gynecol 158:538, 1988.

Tabsh KMA, Brinkman CR, III, and Reff RA: Autonomic dysreflexia in pregnancy, Obstet Gynecol 60(1):119, 1982.

Young BK, Kutz M, and Klein SA: Pregnancy after spinal cord injury: altered maternal and fetal responses to labor, Obstet Gynecol 62(1):59, 1983.

Surgery During Pregnancy

Phipps WJ, Long BC, and Woods NF: Medical-surgical nursing: concepts and clinical practice ed 4, St Louis, 1991, The CV Mosby Co.

Injuries During Pregnancy

Bremer C and Cassata L: Trauma in pregnancy, Nurs Clin North Am 21:705, 1986.
Daddario JB: Trauma in pregnancy, J Perinat Neonat Nurs 3(2):14, 1989.
Rothenberger D: Blunt maternal trauma: a review of 103 cases, J Trauma 18:173, 1978.
Smith LG and Payne T: Pregnant trauma victims, Am J Nurs 84:14, 1984.

Bibliography

Endocrine Disorders

American Diabetes Association and The American Dietetic Association: A guide for professionals: diabetes nutrition and meal planning, Alexandria, Vir, 1988, American Diabetes Association.
Franz MJ: Nutrition recommendations for the eighties, Practical Diabetology 7(4):1, 1988.
Hollander P: Gestational diabetes: the diabetes of pregnancy, Practical Diabetology 7(2):14, 1988.
Jovanovic L: Insulin on the go, Practical Diabetology 7(2):10, 1988.
Ney DM: Nutritional management of diabetes during pregnancy, Practical Diabetology, 7(2):1, 1988.
Robertson C: When your pregnant patient has diabetes, RN, p 18, Nov, 1987.

Cardiovascular Disorders

Brown CE and Wendel GD: Cardiac arrhythmias during pregnancy, Clin Obstet Gynecol 31(1):89, 1989.
Gardezi N: Cardiovascular effects of cocaine, JAMA 257(7):979, 1987.
McColgin SW, Martin JN, and Morrison JC: Pregnant women with prosthetic heart valves, Clin Obstet Gynecol 31(1):76, 1989.
McKeon VA and Perrin KO: The pregnant woman with myocardial infarction: nursing diagnosis, Dimensions of Crit Care Nurs 8(2):92, 1989.
Nolan TE and Hankins GD: Myocardial infarction in pregnancy, Clin Obstet Gynecol 31(1):68, 1989.
Schmidt J, Boilanger M, and Abbot S: Peripartum cardiomyopathy, JOGN Nurs (6):465, Nov-Dec, 1989.
Woods JR, Plessinger MA, and Clark KE: Effect of cocaine on uterine blood flow and fetal oxygenation, JAMA 257(7):957, 1987.
Yeomans ER and Hankins GD: Cardiovascular physiology and invasive cardiac monitoring, Clin Obstet Gynecol 31(1):2, 1989.

Medical Disorders

Anderson J: Facing up to mastectomy, Nurs Times, 84(3):36, 1988.
Birk KA and Rudick RA: Caring for the OB patient who has multiple sclerosis, Contemp OB/GYN 34(1):58, 1989.
Birk K et al: The clinical course of multiple sclerosis during pregnancy and the puerperium, Arch Neurol 47:738, 1990.
Conley NJ and Olshanski E: Current controversies in pregnancy and epilepsy: a unique challenge to nursing, JOGN Nurs 16(5):321, 1987.
Drachman DB: Present and future treatment of myasthenia gravis, N Engl J Med 316(12):743, 1987.
Goldstein J and Kappy KA: Pharmacology: nonrheumatoid arthritis during pregnancy, Contemp OB/GYN 34(1):89, 1989.
Hilgers RD: Improving the outcome of high-risk gestational trophoblastic neoplasia, Contemp OB/GYN 29(5):73, 1987.
Karacic B: Antepartal nursing management of Graves' disease, JOGN Nurs 15(3):214, 1986.
MacMullen NJ and Brucker MC: Pregnancy made possible for women with cystic fibrosis, MCN 14(3):196, 1989.
McGee IE: Management of cervical dysplasia in pregnancy, Nurse Pract 12:34, March, 1987.
Nass T: Helping the patient who has lupus, RN, 69, Oct, 1987.
Petri M: Outcomes encouraging in mothers with lupus, Contemp OB/GYN 31(3):103, 1988.
Thornton NG and Dewis M: Multiple sclerosis and female sexuality, Can Nurse, p 16, April, 1989.
Twiggs LB and Savage JE: Nonmetastatic GTD: a curable disease, Contemp OB/GYN 29(5):61, 1987.

Surgery and Injuries During Pregnancy

Boyanowski C, Hill K, and Martin D: Assessment of the pregnant trauma patient, Dimensions Crit Care Nurs 7(6):356, 1988.
Buchsbaum HJ: Trauma in pregnancy, ACOG Update 12(4):1, 1986.
Clinical News: Pregnant trauma victims, Am J Nurs 84(1):14, 1984.
Droegemueller W et al: Comprehensive gynecology, St Louis, 1987, The CV Mosby Co.
Foster CA: The pregnant trauma patient, RN 14(11):58, 1984.
Higgins SD: Perinatal protocol: trauma in pregnancy, J Perinatol 8:288, 1988.
Reveille JD: Systemic lupus erythematosus. I. A clinical and diagnostic challenge, The Female Patient 15(4):78, 1990.
Reveille JD: Systemic lupus erythematosus. II. Issues in long-term management and pregnancy, The Female Patient 15(5):21, 1990.

CHAPTER

25 Psychosocial Conditions Complicating Pregnancy

Dorothy K. Fischer

Learning Objectives

Correctly define the key terms listed.

Assess the effects of poverty on the childbearing cycle.

Review the care of women experiencing emotional complications during the childbearing cycle.

Explain the care of women who use, abuse, or are dependent on drugs such as alcohol, opioids, and cocaine.

Identify the myths about abuse and battering and how they might influence nursing care.

Explain the cycle of violence and the nursing process for each phase.

Describe alleged rape, rape, and the rape trauma syndrome.

Key Terms

absence of consent
abuse
affective disorders
alleged rape
battered women
cycle of violence
depressive reactions
domestic violence
incest
postpartum psychosis
psychoactive drugs
rape
rape trauma syndrome
schizophrenia
sexual assault
Stockholm syndrome
toxicology screen
trauma care
withdrawal

Psychosocial conditions have implications for the health of the mother and newborn. These conditions can interfere with family integration and restrict attachment to the newborn. Some may threaten the safety and well-being of the mother and newborn. This chapter explores poverty, emotional disorders, psychoactive substance use (drug dependency), and abuse and violence toward women. The nursing process with affected women and their families is emphasized.

❑ POVERTY

The very poor, the social class of people who consistently live at or below the poverty level, are in a perpetual state of despair. Their limited skills give them no bargaining power in the job market. Education needed to improve their status is beyond them. The poor desire a better life for their children but are trapped in a circular pattern that perpetuates their condition. Their powerlessness to control their fate or condition is a source of fatalism and resignation that is characteristic of the group in general. This fatalistic attitude is a significant impediment to occupational and educational aspirations and to seeking health care (Whaley and Wong, 1991).

The term *poverty* implies both visible and invisible impoverishment. *Visible poverty* refers to lack of money or material resources, which includes insufficient clothing, poor sanitation, and deteriorating housing. *Invisible poverty* refers to social and cultural deprivation such as limited employment opportunities, inferior educational opportunities, lack of or inferior medical services and health-care facilities, and an absence of public services (Spector, 1979).

Factors Related to Poverty. One factor that notably affects women is employment and wage discrimination. Poverty and undue stress occur in response to the discrimination and exploitation that women experience in paid employment. Most seriously affected are the swelling numbers of single-parent families headed by women (Griffith-Kenney, 1986). There are also increasing numbers of women with young children who are now being counted among the homeless.

Certain ethnic or racial groups are overrepresented in the impoverished population. The most obvious of these are the blacks, Hispanics, and Native Americans.

Migrant Families. One of the most disadvantaged groups is migrant farm workers and their families. The low position of these families on the economic scale and their rootless, mobile existence subject them to inadequate sanitation, substandard housing, social isolation, and lack of educational opportunities and medical services. This is especially deleterious to the mothers and children. Health care is generally inadequate. Families are apt to live in a number of localities in the course of a year with no continuity in what health care is available. Pesticides and herbicides have been identified as mutagenic and teratogenic. Since both parents usually work in the fields, both are exposed to potential mutagens: the women may be exposed to teratogens during pregnancy. Accident rates are high and meals may be erratic.

Some migrants have a home base to which they return at the end of a growing season; others travel continuously, migrating north in summer and south in winter. With most there is little if any integration into the dominant culture; therefore migrant groups suffer social isolation. Groups who travel together, especially those with the same ethnic background, develop a cohesiveness and form their own set of values and customs. Sometimes a migrant family will leave the migration stream and become a part of a permanent community. However, this involves adaptation to a new environment and life-style that can be stress provoking to these families (Whaley and Wong, 1991).

Preventive Health Care. The vulnerability of economically and socially deprived persons in our society to health problems is apparent across the spectrum of health care from prevention to rehabilitation. Preventive health is more than the prevention of disease states. It involves those factors in an individual's life that protect the individual and allow for growth and development of potential. Adequate clothing and shelter, proper nutrition, education, a safe environment, all taken for granted by the economically advantaged, are noticeably lacking in the health experience of many low-income groups.

The concept of preventive health is often missing. The development of a concept of preventive health begins in childhood as the child is directed and encouraged to "eat your dinner and grow up to be a strong boy," "brush your teeth," "go to the doctor for a checkup," and "get enough sleep." These repeated admonitions eventually result in a concept of health care that includes prevention as well as cure. For women who have experienced this indoctrination, acceptance of the necessity for prenatal care comes more readily. For those women who have only gone to a physician when they were very ill, the relative health of the pregnant state precludes full use of care available. For some low-income women a choice between prenatal care (preparation for birth) and providing their families with necessities results in their foregoing prenatal care.

In some communities clinics have been established specifically for high-risk mothers and their infants. Adolescent mothers and preterm infants make up a large part of the client population at these clinics. Although prevention of the problem is probably the best approach, follow-up care is of great importance. Helping mothers develop parenting skills will do much to promote the optimum growth and development of these disadvantaged children. Nursing and nurse-researchers are in the forefront of efforts to provide care for childbearing families.

Reproductive Experience

Low-income women tend to begin reproducing at an earlier age and to end at a later age than other women. In addition, they have many pregnancies, and these are adversely affected by the close spacing of the gestations. Birch and Gussons (1970) describes this phenomenon as "too young, too old, and too often." This has not changed in recent years. Maternal age and parity are implicated in perinatal mortality. There is increased risk to the fetus, infant, and mother when the mother is at either extreme of age or parity. Preterm delivery, low birth weight, and their complications remain the chief causes in perinatal mortality. Low-income mothers are more likely to give birth to preterm infants than are mothers in the population at large.

Pregnancy Outcomes. The differences in pregnancy outcomes related to socioeconomic class have been well documented for over half a century. Studies have consistently demonstrated a relationship between economic class and maternal and infant morbidity and mortality. These discrepancies have been of major concern to nursing groups as they have attempted to improve the health and well-being of all individuals in society. Researchers have repeatedly identified two recurrent factors that predispose low-income women to poor pregnancy outcomes (Osofsky and Kendall, 1973). The first relates to reproductive experience of the women and the second to the specific obstetric and neonatal complications involved.

Complications. Low-income mothers are more predisposed to intercurrent illness and obstetric complications during pregnancy. Obstetric complications such as placenta previa, abruptio placentae, and placental insufficiency often result in preterm births, low birth weight, or small-for-gestational-age newborns and subsequent infant difficulties. Many obstetric complications have life-threatening consequences for the mother as well as for the infant. Examples of complications include hemorrhage, cardiac disease, or uncontrolled infection.

The problems faced by low-income mothers have direct implication for nursing service. Much of our current knowledge could be used to ameliorate or prevent the occurrence of the problems. One of the prerequisites to providing assistance to the low-income mother is to find better and more effective ways to deliver safe and meaningful care to her.

EMOTIONAL COMPLICATIONS

Mental health problems can complicate pregnancy, childbirth, and the puerperium. Developmental and personality disorders generally have an onset in childhood or adolescence. They usually persist in a stable form into adulthood (Stuart and Sundeen, 1991). Mental retardation, autism, and disruptive behavior disorders are examples.

Mental health disorders generally predate pregnancy. Sleep and arousal disorders, schizophrenic disorders, delusional (paranoid) disorders, and anxiety disorders are a few behavioral categories.

Pregnancy per se is not a cause of psychiatric illness. The psychologic and physical stresses relating to pregnancy or to the new obligations of motherhood may, however, bring on an emotional crisis (Affonso, 1984). The principal emotional disturbances complicating gestation are mood (affective) disorders and schizophrenia. Organic mental syndromes and disorders (non-substance-induced) may also be seen. The mood disturbances include depression or depression with manic episodes (bipolar disorders). Paranoia or other disorganizational problems may characterize schizophrenic disorders. Toxic delirium associated with substance abuse, excessive analgesia, or serious metabolic disorders is not common. Rarely, psychosis secondary to alcoholism or syphilis may complicate both prenatal and postdelivery progress. Psychoactive substance-induced organic mental disorders are seen more often today. They are discussed later in this chapter.

No one single factor has been isolated as responsible for precipitating postpartum mental illness. Predisposing factors have been categorized by Herzog and Detre (1976) as follows: (1) genetic-constitutional, (2) social-environmental, and (3) physiologic-endocrine.

Emotional illnesses arising during the puerperium are diagnosed by their initial features: affective, schizophrenic, or organic. Those illnesses that do not meet the criteria for any of these disorders are designated "postpartum psychoses" (American Psychiatric Association, 1980).

Mood (Affective) Disorders

Although the cause of **affective disorders** is unknown, the family history may record one or more adults who have had this problem. Moreover, women who have psychiatric complications during the course of pregnancy often have had similar crises previously. Over 50% of pregnancy-related mental illnesses are affective reactions. Of these, about 10% are predelivery manic or depressive states; the remainder disturb the postdelivery period. Younger women seem more prone to manic reactions, but depression is the more common problem for most women.

Rejection of the infant, often caused by abnormal jealousy, is a prominent feature of affective disorders. The mother may be obsessed by the notion that the offspring may take her place in her husband's affections. In other instances, guilt regarding aversion to pregnancy, attempted abortion, or other personal conflicts may be the basic problem.

Depressive reactions, far more common than manic reactions, may begin as a mild feeling of discouragement during the first week after delivery. However, anxiety, anorexia, and exaggerated fatigue soon color the despondency. The woman seems helpless; she is self-accusatory and often expresses strange or inappropriate thoughts or feelings. Occasionally a severely disconsolate mother may kill her infant and/or herself.

Depression may continue for weeks or months. Amphetamines are not helpful and may add to agitation. However, a tranquilizer with a prominent stimulatory effect, such as trifluoperazine (Stelazine), may be beneficial. Psychotherapy must be intensive and often prolonged. Meanwhile, separation of mother and infant is necessary. If the depression lifts within several weeks, the prognosis is good. However, women who have been depressed previously, especially those who have had even longer depressions, have a poor prognosis.

Manic reactions often occur during the first or second week of the puerperium, perhaps after a brief depression. Agitation, excitement, and volubility, often with rhyming or punning, develop. The woman becomes disinterested in personal care and food. Because dehydration or exhaustion may occur, prompt and effective supportive treatment is essential.

Psychiatric therapy may include a tranquilizer with a prominent sedative effect, for example, promethazine

(Phenergan). Lithium may be given later for more prolonged control. Psychotherapy is essential. The usual duration of the manic state is 1 to 3 weeks. The prognosis for mother and infant is good after initial separation and gradual reunion.

Schizophrenia

Schizophrenic reactions, now suspected of being a disorder of cerebral metabolism, affect adolescents and younger adults rather than older persons. Abnormal personality features are common. Unusually shy, retiring, hypersensitive, or overly suspicious women are prone to **schizophrenia.** A sudden onset of delusions or hallucinations may alter a seemingly well-accepted normal pregnancy. The symptoms indicate the woman's inability to adjust to and cope with her new obligations as a mother.

The husband and infant are totally rejected. Hostility toward the spouse and the medical staff is obvious. The woman abandons reality and retreats completely into her own world of unreality. The mother totally neglects her infant. Suicide is unlikely. A phenothiazine type of tranquilizer, for example, chlorpromazine (Thorazine), will be useful. Transfer of the woman to a psychiatric hospital usually is necessary. A good prognosis is likely with the first psychotic episode, especially if it occurs unexpectedly during the puerperium.

Postpartum Mental Illness

Postpartum mental illness may be acute or chronic and appears cross-culturally. It ranges from a transitory depression to severe postpartum emotional disturbances. The transitory depression, "maternity blues" or "baby blues," may occur in 30% to 80% of all childbirths (Ketai and Marvin, 1979) (Chapter 21). Transitory depression begins the second or third day after birth. The symptoms include anxiety, poor concentration, tearfulness, and despondency. The symptoms usually subside within the first week. No hospitalization is required.

However, approximately 40% of women with mild depression have symptoms that persist as long as 1 year (Tentoni and High, 1980). Illnesses of intermediate severity occur in 11% of all childbirths (Hayworth et al, 1980). Severe postpartum emotional disturbance is noted in only 1% to 2% of all normal childbirths. However, 2% to 9% of women admitted to mental hospitals are admitted for conditions related to childbearing (Ketai and Marvin, 1979; Weiner, 1982).

The onset of **postpartum psychosis** is usually abrupt and occurs within days of delivery. The symptoms center around the mother's relationship with the baby. The mother's response may be of an overprotective or of a rejecting nature (Hurt and Ray, 1985). The mother may be convinced that someone is trying to take her baby from her and will clutch it protectively. Or she may believe that the baby is dead or defective or that God is caring for it and so the baby does not need care.

The presenting symptoms form the basis for management (American Psychiatric Association, 1980; Hurt and Ray, 1985). Schizophrenia-like symptoms are treated with psychotropic medications. Lithium may be prescribed with or without psychotropic medications for bipolar affective disorders. Depression may be treated with electroconvulsive therapy (ECT) if suicidal or infanticidal thoughts are identified. Women may need assistance for alterations in patterns of sleep-rest, self-care (basic hygiene), nutrition and fluid balance, elimination, self-esteem, and family coping and processes. Discharge planning focuses on preparation for meeting the demands of an infant while the mother is still integrating her experience with psychosis, supporting the husband, and exploring the effects of the illness on their family (Hurt and Ray, 1985).

Assessment

The nursing care plan must reflect the expected behavioral responses of the particular disorder. Characteristics of the woman and her specific circumstances are utilized to individualize the plan.

Nursing Diagnoses

Nursing diagnoses relevant to any emotional illness that complicates pregnancy may include the following:

Potential for injury to fetus related to
- Psychotropic medication
- Maternal suicide

Potential for injury to newborn related to
- Unmet needs (e.g., hygiene, nutrition) and safety precautions
- Mother's poor impulse control

Ineffective family coping related to
- Increased care needs of mother-fetus-newborn

Impaired home maintenance management related to
- Increased care needs of mother-fetus-newborn

Potential altered parenting related to
- Lack of supervised opportunities for attachment to infant

Potential altered growth and development of infant related to
- Lack of intellectual stimulation

Planning

Planning focuses on the mother's dependency needs, attachment to the infant, family integration, parenting skills and care of the infant, and home maintenance management. Supervision of the mother and family in the home is a prime concern.

Goals of care may include the following:

1. The mother and newborn maintain physical well-being
2. Effective individual and family coping are established.
3. Each family member continues healthy growth and development.

Implementation

Community resources such as the community health nurse, homemaker service, or foster care are utilized as necessary. Discharge planning carefully developed with the family in collaboration with a hospital-community health care team is vital.

Evaluation

Evaluation of interventions occurs over a varying period. "Postpartum psychoses" may resolve in a period of weeks. Other disorders, including mental retardation, extend indefinitely.

❑ PSYCHOACTIVE SUBSTANCE USE

The use of **psychoactive drugs** is pandemic. In this discussion, substance abuse is defined as the use of any mind-altering agent to such an extent that it interferes with the individual's biologic, psychologic, or sociocultural integrity (Stuart and Sundeen, 1991). Interference with biologic integrity might be exemplified (during pregnancy) in poor nutrition leading to poor weight gain, anemia, and a predisposition to infection and pregnancy-induced hypertension (PIH). Some drugs (morphine, heroin, diazepam, and others) induce platelet disorders that predispose the woman to hemorrhage (Scott et al, 1990). Psychologic consequences may include acute psychosis in a pregnant teenager who has been taking PCP or the inability of a new mother to "bond" with her infant (see discussion of emotional disturbances). Expectant and new mothers using psychoactive drugs receive negative feedback from society, as well as from health care providers who condemn them for endangering the unborn and the newborn infant and who may withhold support. Pregnant women who are drug dependent often do not seek prenatal care until labor begins. They will take the drug just before seeking admission; therefore **withdrawal** symptoms can be delayed until 6 to 12 hours after delivery. The care of the substance-dependent pregnant woman is based on historical data, symptoms, physical findings, and laboratory results. As a result of the woman's defensiveness and frequent denial, history taking has to be done in a sensitive and competent manner.

The woman dependent on a drug tends to exhibit a passive response to life and its responsibilities. She may show a high degree of depression. Drug use has meant a way for her to relieve psychologic distress, to encourage social interaction, and to blunt the feelings of loneliness and emptiness that are part of depression. Pregnancy is not planned. It occurs as an "accidental" phenomenon. It may serve as a positive event, confirming her worth as a woman.

After birth, however, the woman is faced with the parental tasks of caring for and nurturing a completely dependent infant and of forming a warm, close, intimate relationship with the child. Care of the woman addicted to a drug offers a tremendous challenge to nursing.

Realization of the difficulty of the nursing challenge becomes apparent. The demands of motherhood are being made of a person who is herself dependent and arrested at the stage of taking and receiving rather than giving. Most substance-dependent people are unable to establish positive intimate relationships and lack a meaningful support system. The mother's ability to care for her infant after discharge from the hospital should be assessed by frequent observations, including some in the home setting.

This discussion focuses on the use and abuse of alcohol, heroin, cocaine, and methamphetamine. Many other substances are abused. The care needed by the individual varies with the particular circumstances of that individual and the substance abused. However, the nursing process is similar for all.

Alcohol

Identification of the woman with an alcohol problem may be difficult. Denial of the problem or its consequences is seen commonly. A concerned, nonjudgmental, matter-of-fact approach is used in the hope that the woman admits a problem if it exists. Inability to form positive relationships is often secondary to manipulative behavior. A low tolerance for frustration or anxiety and expressions of guilt related to alcoholic behavior patterns may be evident. Physical signs and symptoms may also be present (Table 25-1). During withdrawal, central nervous system (CNS) agitation is expressed as fatigue, insomnia, agitation, restlessness,

Table 25-1 Psychoactive Substance Effects

Drug	Psychologic Signs	Physiologic Signs
ALCOHOL		
Intoxication	Mood lability or change Impaired attention or memory Irritability Talkativeness	Slurred speech Flushed face Incoordination, unsteady gait Nystagmus
Withdrawal	Anxiety Depressed mood or irritability Maladaptive behavior	Nausea and vomiting Malaise or weakness Hyperactivity Coarse tremor of hands, tongue, eyelids Orthostatic hypotension
HEROIN		
Intoxication	Euphoria, dysphoria Psychomotor retardation Apathy Maladaptive behavior Impaired attention or memory	Pupillary constriction Drowsiness Slurred speech
Withdrawal	Insomnia	Lacrimation, rhinorrhea Pupillary dilatation Sweating Diarrhea Yawning Mild hypertension Tachycardia Fever
COCAINE "CRACK"		
Intoxication	Psychomotor agitation Elation Grandiosity; talkativeness Hypervigilance Maladaptive behaviors	Tachycardia Pupillary dilatation Hypertension Perspiration; chills Nausea; vomiting
Withdrawal	Depressed mood Disturbed sleep Increased dreaming	Fatigue
METHAMPHETAMINE "ICE"		
Intoxication	Hyperactivity Insomnia Restlessness Irritability Aggressiveness	Tachycardia, palpitations Tachypnea Nausea, vomiting Constipation Impotence
Withdrawal	Depression Increased sleeping Lethargy	Headache Nausea, vomiting Muscle pain Weakness

and belligerence. Bruises, rashes, and other injuries may be found on observation. Poor physical hygiene and malnutrition are potential problems, especially in the chronic alcoholic. Assessment for maternal and fetal well-being follows the protocols discussed for other clients.

Cocaine

The cocaine abuser often has a constellation of cocaine-related problems: family problems, employment difficulties, various health issues, psychologic stress, guilt, and anger (Landry and Smith, 1987). Coexisting psychiatric disorders cloud differential diagnosis. Decreased amounts of ***norepinephrine*** and ***serotonin*** have been implicated in people with biologically based depression. Dysfunction of serotonin metabolism is seen in disorders such as violence, rage, and maladaptive behavior. Cocaine raises norepinephrine and serotonin levels rapidly and then depletes them precipitously. Schizophrenics display excessive dopamine levels in some areas of the brain. The biochemical systems of norepinephrine, serotonin, and dopamine play a vital role in mood regulation and mental health; all three systems are affected by cocaine.

The increase in the use of cocaine and the even more addictive "crack" among childbearing women has been phenomenal in the past few years (Tracy, 1988). Crack is cocaine mixed with baking soda and heated until it reaches its purest form. It is sold in the form of "rocks," which are smoked in pipes. Whereas its use may cross all cultural groups, its inexpensiveness and availability are making it the drug of choice among many of the country's poorer populations. Since crack is highly addictive, it poses new problems to health care providers who may first see the pregnant addict in the labor and delivery area. The effects of crack on newborns is covered in Chapter 28.

Diagnostic protocol to distinguish between drug use and drug addiction requires considerable knowledge and is beyond the scope of this text. An appropriate plan of care is designed depending on the diagnosis (i.e., substance use problems or addiction disease) (Landry and Smith, 1987). The focus of this section is the identification of the pregnant cocaine-user and the effects of cocaine on the pregnancy. The care of the cocaine-affected newborn is addressed in Chapter 28.

The nurse or physician takes a history of the drug abuse (95% are also addicted to heroin or methadone), type of drug and mode of administration, and participation (if any) in drug programs; assesses the woman's feelings and plans for this pregnancy (infant); and determines the expected date of delivery (EDD). The social worker or psychiatric social worker is brought in to evaluate the woman's social, economic, home, and ethnic problems; welfare requirements; and educational or vocational status and needs.

Medical Complications. Pregnancy is compromised by cocaine-related medical complications that are encountered by the infrequent, as well as frequent, high-dose user. A variety of less serious medical problems is seen, including lack of energy, insomnia, nasal sinus problems, nose-bleeds, sore throat, and decreased libido. More serious problems develop as general health deteriorates. The nasal septum perforates. Cardiovascular stress increases, tachycardia, systemic hypertension, ventricular arrhythmias, sudden coronary artery spasm, and myocardial infarction develop. Cocaine-associated complications also include liver damage, intestinal ischemia, seizures, hemorrhagic bronchitis, headache, and death. Needle-borne diseases such as hepatitis B and acquired immunodeficiency syndrome (AIDS) are common: "Tracks," septic phlebitis, cellulitis, and superficial abscesses are seen in intravenous drug users. Many users are poorly nourished and commonly have sexually transmitted diseases (STDs). Pulmonary disease with acute pulmonary edema is a commonly encountered complication. A **toxicology** (urine) **screen** or other laboratory tests for liver damage and anemia may be ordered when drug use is suspected. An assessment of the woman's support system adds valuable data for developing a plan of care. The presence of any of the medical complications, results of laboratory tests, or signs and symptoms of intoxication or withdrawal (Table 25-1) assist in the identification of substance use problems and addictive disease.

Cocaine users typically mediate the side effects of cocaine by a CNS depressant such as alcohol (Landry and Smith, 1987). Thus the woman and her fetus are exposed to the risks of cocaine and alcohol. In some areas of the United States it is estimated that 10% of pregnant women use cocaine (Chasnoff et al, 1985).

Cocaine produces tachycardia and a rise in blood pressure by increasing the levels of catecholamines (Woods, Plessinger, and Clark, 1987). During pregnancy, uterine blood vessels are maximally dilated, but they vasoconstrict readily in the presence of catecholamines. Separation of the placenta (abruption) or acute onset of labor following intravenous cocaine administration is probably secondary to acute spasm of uterine blood vessels (Woods, Plessinger, and Clark, 1987). Use of the drug during pregnancy can lead to small-for-gestational-age neonates and fetal death (Woods, Plessinger, and Clark, 1987). Neonate addiction is discussed in Chapter 28.

Heroin

Assessment of heroin use is similar to that for alcohol and cocaine use. Interview and open discussion may disclose the problem and its extent (e.g., length of addiction, amount needed in cost per day). Physical examination reveals intravenous tracks, cellulitis, and surface abscesses at the administration sites. Further assessment of the peripheral vascular system may reveal burning paresthesia or decreased or absent peripheral pulses (or both) in the extremity used for self-injection. Signs of STDs and urinary tract infections (UTIs) are often present.

Laboratory tests are ordered for toxicology, STDs, hepatitis B, and AIDS antibody. Blood urea nitrogen (BUN), serum creatinine, total protein levels, albumin-to-globulin ratio, total iron-binding capacity, hemoglobin, and hematocrit values are obtained. Chest x-ray study may be ordered for pulmonary disease. Hilar lymphadenopathy in 95% of addicts, pulmonary edema, bacterial pneumonia, and foreign body emboli (from the substances used to "cut" street drugs) may be revealed.

Initial and serial ultrasound studies are used to determine gestational age because amenorrhea, common among drug users, precludes dating by history of last menstrual period (LMP). However, nonstress and stress testing are not too helpful in assessing fetal well-being. The addicted fetus is nonreactive. Estriol measurements are inaccurate. The heroin-addicted woman is more likely to experience premature rupture of membranes (PROM) and preterm labor.

Methamphetamine

The active metabolite of methamphetamine is amphetamine, a CNS stimulant. Powdered methamphetamine is known as "speed" and "meth." Methamphetamine-exposed gravidas have higher rates of preterm deliveries and intrauterine-growth-retarded fetuses with smaller head circumferences than found in gravidas in a drug-free comparison group (Oro and Dixon, 1987). Neonatal behavioral patterns are altered. They are characterized by abnormal sleep patterns, poor feeding, tremors, and hypertonia. These behaviors are seen if the fetus was exposed to cocaine, methamphetamine, or their combination (Oro and Dixon, 1987). The addition of cocaine significantly increases the rate of placental hemorrhage and stillbirth. Other neonatal behaviors include state disorganization and decreased sleep. Feeding may be prolonged and accompanied by disorganized rooting and sucking. Tube feeding may be required. Withdrawal symptoms may be treated with phenobarbital or opium tincture (Paregoric).

Ice. The crystalline form of methamphetamine is known as "ice." This smokable form is odorless. It gives users a very long steady high, is more addictive than heroin, and is more potent than "crack" cocaine ("Ice," 1989). Ice enables a person to go without rest or food for 24 hours, only to "crash" for the next 24 hours. Common signs include tachycardia, tachypnea, paranoid illusions, and violent behavior. Symptoms of amphetamine abuse appear after 2 years of use: paranoia, and delusional, irrational, and illogical behavior. Convulsions, coma, and death follow overdose (New drug, 1989).

The drug is very popular with young women who want to lose weight rapidly and with teenagers who want to stay up all night. Drug dependency has serious consequences for the woman who is pregnant. The drug causes convulsions in the mother and the newborn. Other effects on the fetus/newborn are thought to be similar to those experienced by the fetus/newborn exposed to powdered methamphetamine.

Assessment

Each client is assessed for signs and symptoms of psychoactive substance use. Psychologic and physiologic symptomatology is described and reported.

Nursing Diagnoses

The following are examples of nursing diagnoses formulated from the assessment data:

Potential fluid volume deficit and altered nutrition: less than body requirements, related to
- Effects of excessive use of psychoactive drugs

Potential for injury to self, fetus, or newborn related to
- Sensory effects of drug

Potential for infection related to
- Life-style
- Dehydration and malnutrition
- Method of administration of drug or effects of drug

Self-care deficit, bathing/hygiene related to
- Effects of drug

Knowledge deficit related to
- Effects of psychoactive drug on developing fetus and pregnancy

Ineffective individual coping related to
- Lack of support system
- Low self-esteem
- Lack of healthy mechanisms for recognition and release of anger

Planning

Planning for care must be accomplished with recognition of the woman's life-style and habits. The ideal long-term goal would be total abstinence. However, the woman may be unable to face that level of commitment at this time. The thought of relinquishing the substance forever is anxiety provoking. It is rare for a substance-dependent person to stop use of that substance suddenly. Short-term goals are necessary. The woman must participate in the decision-making process in formulating the goals. It is particularly important that the goals be phrased so that it is clear that the woman has responsibility for her behavior. The goals are written into a contract signed by the woman and the nurse (or physician). One copy is kept by the woman.

Short-term Goals:

1. Woman's physiologic status is stabilized
2. Woman keeps appointments for prenatal and postpartum care for herself and her infant
3. Fetal effects are minimized; baby remains safe and receives care

Long-term Goal:

1. Woman voluntarily becomes involved in long-term medical, social, psychiatric, and vocational rehabilitation.

Implementation

A multidisciplinary approach is needed to plan for the care of the expectant mother. In increasing numbers, pregnant psychoactive drug users are seen on maternity units. Their presence and needs present special challenges to nurses. A "standardized" nursing care plan may be best developed by the total team of nurses on the maternity unit. A starting point in the development of a care plan may need to be a values clarification experience. It is not uncommon for nurses to harbor negative feelings for psychoactive drug users' behaviors. Collaboration with psychiatric nurses may be necessary to augment the maternity nurse's therapeutic potential with these clients. Comprehensive care involves many organizations, child protective services, human resource agencies, and the community health department (Mondanaro, 1987).

The need for biologic support may be related to overdose, withdrawal, allergy, or toxicity. Physical deterioration results from the deleterious effects of drugs, including conditions such as malnutrition, dehydration, and various infections. The acute physical condition takes priority over the woman's other health needs.

Interactive interventions are initiated as soon as they are appropriate. The type of interactive intervention is directed toward alleviating the stressors that apply to each individual and is identified in the nursing diagnoses. Examples of interactive intervention include group support, client education, or individual counseling. Psychiatric nurses are skilled in intervening in denial, dependency, manipulation, and anger. Other required skills include establishing behavioral contracts and increasing self-esteem. The primary focus of care is the woman. Usually she is already acutely aware of the dangers to the fetus resulting from her behavior. Emphasis on the fetus's well-being instead of on her own may add to her guilt, frustration, and low self-esteem.

Social support systems are mobilized. Family counseling, self-help groups, transitional living programs, and community treatment programs are involved. Employee assistance programs are now available in many industries, including hospitals (Clemmer, 1987).

Labor room nurses also need to work out a "standardized" plan for care. Typically the woman displays poor control over her behavior and a low threshold for pain, which is especially noticeable when she is in labor. Increased dependency needs are apparent. Intoxication or withdrawal signs and symptoms of the mother and fetus (see Table 25-1) may challenge the staff. Staffing should be sufficient to ensure strict surveillance of visitors to prevent unsupervised drug administration.

Advice regarding ***breastfeeding*** is individualized. Small amounts of some drugs (e.g., heroin) appear in breast milk and the baby's eating and safety needs must of course be considered. Breastfeeding necessitates a closeness between the mother and child, and the baby may be more irritable and difficult to console. These women, who are already in a fragile state with depleted energy reserves and coping capability, commonly experience severe emotional decompensation. This can be aggravated by breastfeeding and care of the infant, which are exhausting under ideal circumstances. For some women the need to breastfeed and care for the infant provides the impetus they need to break the drug dependency habit. Community health agencies may be mobilized for home supervision or guidance in antepartum and infant care or for putting the infant up for adoption. Day/night-center care programs or halfway houses may be indicated.

Discharge planning should begin with the first contact with the woman. If the woman is to be discharged to the care of her parents, several nursing actions may be employed. The client is involved in decision making whenever possible. The mother is involved with the care of her infant when she is willing. Mother-child attachment is promoted. Angry, argumentative encounters between the mother and nurse are avoided; the nurse needs to respond with patience, sympathy, consistency, and at times, with firmness. The mother's positive maternal responses and feelings are supported even if she is relinquishing her infant for adoption.

Evaluation

Evaluation is difficult because the long-range effects cannot be projected. Short-term positive achievements are indicators of success (e.g., if the mother keeps her appointments or improves her nutrition and personal hygiene or learns to diaper the baby). It is not reasonable to expect to see evidence of significant strides, such as complete abstinence from drugs and assumption of adult maturity behaviors within a short period.

❑ ABUSE AND VIOLENCE

Hazards to women's health cover a wide spectrum. Battering, sexual assault, incest and rape are significant problems with each carrying the potential for serious physical, psychologic, and emotional injury or impairment.

Battered women are victims of assault, a violent physical attack. Clinical findings include bruises, lacerations, burns, hematomas, and fractures. A **sexual assault** is any aggressive or violent act involving sexual intimacy performed by one person on another *without that person's consent.* **Abuse** of women is defined as physical, emotional, or sexual mistreatment: aggressive behavior, including acts of a sexual or physical nature, verbal belittling, or intimidation. Battery, abuse, and assault are often used interchangeably.

Accurate statistics are not available as the following estimates demonstrate. It has been estimated that in the United States, 1 woman is beaten every 18 seconds (Battered, 1987). Delgaty (1985) reports that 1 in 10 married Canadian women is physically abused each year. These numbers are impressive since assault within families is the most underreported of all crimes (Klaus and Rand, 1984; Hillard, 1986). Pregnancy is a time of increased battering episodes (Hillard, 1985).

Every 3½ minutes (Battered, 1987) to every 6 minutes (Riesenberg, 1987) a woman is a victim of rape or attempted rape. About 80% of rapes go unreported, and many of the victims do not seek health care (Hicks, 1981).

An estimated 100,000 cases or more of incest occur per year; 12% to 24% of the female victims become pregnant (Zdanuk, Harris, and Wisian, 1987).

The overwhelming physical evidence of the prevalence of these serious crimes precludes the need to identify them as major issues in current society.

Although both women and men may take on either role or both roles—abuser and/or victim—this chapter focuses only on women (from adolescence through adulthood) as victims of violence. The vast areas of child abuse and molestation and of men as victims of spouse battering and rape are beyond the scope of this text.

Nurses will see victims in all age groups and in every area of their practice. Because of the magnitude of the problems of violence against women, maternity nurses cannot ignore this reality of client care. There is a need to focus on prevention, effective nursing actions, and long-term counseling of victims.

Battered Women

Women should have the right to move about within the confines of their homes among those persons with whom they share the most intimate, interpersonal relationships without fearing for their safety and well-being, or for life itself. In general, women accept and expect that right as a given (Drake, 1982). Battering is a criminal act; in a marriage, it is a fundamental betrayal of trust (Delgaty, 1985).

The abuse of spouses occurs at all socioeconomic levels, as well as all educational levels. The myth that only persons in the low socioeconomic classes or that those with little education are the primary perpetrators of wife abuse has been refuted. Wives are more likely to be abused than are husbands, although it is not entirely unknown for a man to report physical or emotional abuse by his spouse.

The problem of wife abuse is particularly significant because 90% of homicides in families are preceded by family violence. Battering precipitates one in every four suicides by all women and half of all suicides by black women in the United States.

It is estimated that 50% of all women will be battered at some time. Since nurses come from the general population, how many have themselves been abused (or have been abusers)? What effect has the experience had on their ability to cope with the crisis state presented by victims who have come for medical care?

Wife battering, spouse abuse, and domestic (family) violence are all terms applied to physical trauma inflicted by the male partner on the female partner in a marriage or marital-like relationship. An extraordinary variety of other definitions have been formulated for this behavior. Some common elements in these definitions are repetition of episodes, some demonstrable injury or injuries resulting from the violence, and violence that is deliberate and severe.

These elements preclude the occasional physical acts of shoving, shaking, or restraining that occur in some marriages. At present, family violence generally is considered a part of family life by both the law and large numbers of women. Some people are socialized to believe that **domestic violence** is an acceptable way of dealing with the stresses of family life (Mandel, 1986;

Battered, 1987; Stuart and Sundeen, 1991); for example, women have reported that they believe it is acceptable for a husband to beat his wife "every once in a while."

Characteristics of Victims and Abusers. Every socioeconomic group is represented among abused wives. As noted earlier in this chapter, race, religion, social background, age, and educational level are not significant factors in differentiating women at risk.

Battered wives may feel they are to blame for their situation because they are "not good-enough wives." They fear societal rejection if they discuss their problem openly. This fear is justified in many cases because society has stereotyped these women as masochistic. It is impossible for many people to comprehend why a woman would remain in a situation where she is repeatedly beaten and injured.

One explanation may be the tendency for some victims to form a symbiotic relationship, sometimes called the victim-victimizer bond or the **Stockholm syndrome.** This type of relationship is named after a female bank teller in Stockholm who was abducted and became romantically involved with her captor. After being released, a hostage suffering from this bond exhibits the negative effects of the syndrome: nightmares, tremors, sweating, substance (drug, food) abuse, various phobias, and stress reactions such as ulcers, hypertension, allergies, and depression. These psychosomatic responses are attributed to a growing realization of the humiliation and demoralization suffered during the experience.

Women who were victims of incest or whose mothers were victims of domestic violence are at significant risk for battering. Similarly, men who, as children, observed their fathers abuse their mothers or sisters are more likely to abuse their wives. It appears that some women are not "innocent victims," nor do they consciously precipitate violence, but, rather, they unconsciously or subconsciously collaborate with their mates to initiate violent episodes. Such a woman may seek a particular type of mate with whom she will reenact her own childhood family experience. In one study Parker and Schumacher (1977) found that battered wives come from families that exhibited one of three types of interaction patterns: families in which mothers used subtle methods of control and fathers were merely figureheads; families in which mothers were submissive and fathers were dominant; and families consisting of disturbed mothers and multiple "fathers."

Myths About Battered Women. Health professionals often become frustrated by women who remain in battering relationships. As with other human dynamics that are not easily explained, a number of myths have emerged to account for this perceived self-destructive behavior (Griffith-Kenney, 1986; Collier, 1987). Some myths about abuse and battering include the following:

Battering occurs only in lower-class families.

Battered women like to be beaten and deliberately provoke the attack. They are masochistic.

Batterers are uneducated men who are unable to cope with the world.

Alcohol and drug abuse causes battering.

Batterers and battered women cannot change.

Cycle of Violence. When the woman is asked why she remains with a battering mate, she may say that there are times when their relationship is fine. A cyclic pattern to the battering behavior has been described as a period of increasing tension leading to the battery, followed by an aftermath characterized by kind, loving behavior and a plea for forgiveness by the husband (Hillard, 1986). Reconciliation is characterized by loving behavior and promises never to do it again. The batterer believes that he has taught the woman a lesson and will not have to repeat the experience. The victim wants to believe that the man loves her and is serious about not hurting her again.

Women in chronic battering situations may also stay with the batterer because they have no job skills, are economically dependent, are afraid of being alone, or are even fearful of retaliation if they leave. Gelles (1979) reported that the less power and resources the woman has the more likely she is to stay in the situation. Pfouts (1978) described a "cost-benefit analysis" employed by abused women as they choose a method for coping with the abuse. This analysis involves a decision-making process wherein the woman weighs the benefits of remaining in the relationship against the costs.

The **cycle of violence** often begins in the first year of marriage (Lichtenstein, 1981). Many victims remain in the abusive situation for an average of 6 to 7 years, especially when there are small children involved.

Many women report that they were first beaten when their husbands learned of their pregnancy. The blows are often directed toward the breasts, abdomen, and genitals. It has been hypothesized that jealousy of the baby's intrusion on the couple's relationship and the increased strain on the marriage either triggers or exacerbates abuse.

The battered pregnant woman should be treated as a high-risk obstetric client because she often has more medical, social, or psychologic needs (Mercer, 1977) that require special attention. She is at additional risk for repeated physical trauma and for psychologic trauma because of a deficient support system.

Pregnancy is a time of increased battering episodes for a variety of reasons: (1) The biopsychosocial stresses of pregnancy may strain the relationship beyond the couple's ability to cope; frustration is followed by violence. (2) The man may be jealous of the fetus, resenting its intrusion into the couple's relationship. As one expectant father succinctly stated, "I don't get the TLC I got before that thing came along." (3) The beating may be the man's conscious or subconscious attempt to end the pregnancy. After delivery the mother may be so physically and emotionally drained that she may have difficulty bonding with her infant. She is considered at risk of becoming an abusive mother whether she chooses to stay in the abusive relationship or not. If she remains with her husband, the chances are 1 in 3 or 4 that he will batter the child as well.

Battered women are reluctant to seek help for various reasons: the need to avoid the stigma associated with the nature of the family violence, the fear that they will not be believed, the fear of reprisal from their husbands, and in some states in which battering is a reportable crime, the wish to avoid involvement with police. A study by Bowker and Maurer (1986) reports that women's groups are more effective than traditional forms of counseling utilized by battered wives.

Exactly what drives a woman to seek assistance is not clear, but apparently it may be the result of a behavioral change in the woman. The women who display any of the following three characteristics are more likely to seek assistance:

1. Women who are beaten frequently and severely
2. Women who have not experienced or witnessed family violence in their family of origin
3. Women who see an alternative to life in their marriages—specifically, women with jobs

Assessment

Careful assessment of all clients, pregnant or not, may reveal findings that alert the nurse or physician to the possibility of battering. The diagnosis is missed in a significant number of cases. The *history* may contain data with a high index of suspicion for battering: drug or child abuse; repeated injury to the head, face, neck, chest, abdomen, and upper extremities; a time delay between the injury and seeking treatment; previous abuse; and chronic depression. Women who wear sunglasses should be asked to remove them for an assessment for bruises around the eyes. The presenting problem may be broken bones, serious bleeding injuries (nosebleed, lacerations), and/or burns from a variety of sources. Women may be vague or evasive in their account of the cause of the injuries.

If the woman is seen during the tension-building period of the battering cycle, her symptoms usually contain an emotional element (e.g., chest pain, hyperventilation, gastrointestinal disorders, and headache).

Interviewing skills are essential. The validating interview should take place in a quiet, private area. In a nonjudgmental, caring manner, the interviewer may comment that the woman's signs and symptoms do not fit with the description of the accident but that they are consistent with injury inflicted by another person. The nurse may then comment that it is not uncommon to find such injuries when wives are hurt by their husbands. Finally, the nurse can ask the woman if, indeed, she was hurt by her husband (Finley, 1981). Types of questions that could be asked include: Do you and your partner fight? Does the fighting ever become physical? Is there a history of abuse in your partner's family? How did this happen? Did someone do this to you?

As stated earlier, pregnancy increases the likelihood of domestic abuse. Therefore a clustering of the following situations may indicate a battering situation: incidence of abortion, miscarriage, or preterm delivery; injuries or bruises acquired during pregnancy; sexual dysfunction during pregnancy; divorce or separation during pregnancy; persistent gynecologic complaints (especially abdominal pain or dyspareunia); attempted suicide; and repeated missed office visits and/or alcohol or other substance abuse (Chez, 1987).

Nursing Diagnoses

Nursing diagnoses are individualized for each woman. Following are examples of potential nursing diagnoses for battered women.

Actual injury related to
- Battering episode

Personal identity/self-esteem disturbance related to
- Continuing victim-abuser relationship

Ineffective individual and family coping related to
- Persistence of victim-abuser relationship

Knowledge deficit related to
- The phenomenon of battering
- Cycle of violence
- Community resources for protection and support

Spiritual distress related to
- Continuing victim-abuser relationship

Planning

To develop an effective plan, the caregiver must be comfortable working with the victim and her family. In addition, the caregiver must have a broad knowledge base of this phenomenon, excellent communication skills, and access to appropriate community resources. If possible, continuity of care is planned with the health care provider(s) with whom the woman develops a relationship of trust.

Goals are formulated in client-centered terms. Following are examples of goals for care.

1. The battered woman is identified
2. The woman's physical injuries are treated promptly
3. The woman increases her knowledge of the following:
   a. Alternatives, options, and choices
   b. Community resources (shelters, financial aid, child care, education, etc.)
   c. Roles of members of the health care team
4. If the woman is pregnant or has children, the fetus and children are protected from abuse.
5. The woman is protected from further abuse
6. The woman perceives herself as deserving of respect and not as "deserving" to be victimized
7. The woman reestablishes a feeling of control
8. The woman identifies her areas of strength and develops goals for herself

Implementation

A support network is developed with the other maternity nurses who will be involved in the pregnant woman's care during the peripartum period. Each nurse can plan care that will point out the woman's strengths and raise her self-esteem. The husband is welcomed to attend prenatal visits and classes and is included in other ways if the woman choses to stay with him. Counseling services are offered to both spouses. The first days after delivery are particularly crucial—the mother is physically and emotionally vulnerable and usually tired, and the baby's crying may be intolerable to both the father and the mother. The danger of abuse to mother and child is acute during this time. A support network of maternity and pediatric staff, community health nurses, and parental crisis center personnel is needed to coordinate efforts to provide support during this crucial period.

The nurse does do the following:

1. Treat the woman with dignity and concern to help her reduce her feelings of isolation, embarrassment, shame, and guilt.
2. Encourage the woman to refer to herself specifically, using statements such as "I am" rather than referring to herself in general terms (Finley, 1981).
3. Indicate sensitivity to and acceptance of the woman's state of confusion.
4. Indicate that hope exists. As the woman develops a sense of hope, her ability to formulate realistic goals increases.
5. Help the woman identify and explore her options; for example, remaining in the relationship is one option among several. The woman's feeling of being controlled by the situation may be reduced as she considers her choices.
6. Offer family planning counseling, since unplanned or unwanted pregnancy is a precipitating factor in wife abuse.
7. Offer referrals for treating substance abuse and for learning problem-solving behaviors and techniques for "fighting fair" to replace violence.

The nurse does not do the following:

1. Berate the woman's husband. The woman may be very protective of him, and negative input from the nurse may force her to sever therapeutic ties.
2. Urge or encourage the woman to leave home. She alone must make this decision. Leaving before a commitment to a different way of life is firm can bring the woman back into the situation. Studies indicate that this is a high-risk time for homicide (Elbow, 1977).

A woman indicates her readiness to leave the relationship when she indicates she is capable of planning for herself, investing in herself as a person, recognizing that the abuse is part of a continuing pattern, and is able to express the desire to leave when no abuse is occurring at the moment.

Many nurses become frustrated when women return time after time with injuries. As client advocates, nurses must be sensitive to the battered woman's problems and be able to tolerate their own empathic feelings of fear and terror (Griffith-Kenney, 1986). This is particularly true for the nurse who is herself a battered woman (Collier, 1987). A nursing care plan for the battered postpartum mother appears on pp. 749-750.

Evaluation

Evaluation may be somewhat difficult because some changes are hard to evaluate objectively or because the woman (family) may not return for care. Intervention can be considered effective if the woman (couple) has developed self-esteem and a sense of self-worth, no longer views herself as a deserving victim, affirms her own individuality, has developed problem-solving behaviors, and is comfortable with her choices, and when no further battering or abusive episodes occur.

Rape, Sexual Assault, and Incest

Forcible rape is a crime that women may fear more than any other. **Rape**, a legal, not a medical entity, is defined differently from state to state. In many jurisdic-

Specific Nursing Care Plan

BATTERED POSTPARTUM WOMAN

Rosemary has just been admitted to the postpartum floor. As the nurse is helping her into the bed she notices bruises, scars, and scratches covering parts of Rosemary's body. When the nurse questions Rosemary she replies, "I fell down the steps." Rosemary appears withdrawn and does not make eye contact with the nurse when speaking to her. Staff recognize some difficulty with bonding. Twelve hours postdelivery Rosemary is still requesting that her baby stay in the nursery. Her husband has not visited, but a dozen roses were delivered to her from him. The nurse manager calls the physician, who asks the social service department to visit Rosemary. When Marge, the social worker, comes to see Rosemary, the husband is in the room. When he finds out who she is he becomes angry, ejecting Marge from the room and throwing the water pitcher at the door after her. As Marge is leaving the room she notices Rosemary cowering and sobbing in bed.

ASSESSMENT	NURSING DIAGNOSIS (ND), PLAN/GOAL (P/G)	RATIONALE/ IMPLEMENTATION	EVALUATION
Physical and emotional fatigue.	ND: Activity intolerance related to potential physical abuse, labor, and delivery of infant. P/G: Rosemary is able to rest to regain physical strength.	*Rest increases energy reserves:* Provide a quiet nonthreatening environment. Assist with activities of daily living (ADL). Limit visitors with Rosemary's permission. Reassure Rosemary she can call the nurse at any time for any thing she may want or need.	Rosemary sleeps. Rosemary begins to ambulate and take responsibility for own ADL. Rosemary calls on nurses for assistance, to converse, and to share information.
Rosemary not bonding with infant.	ND: Altered parenting related to lack of attachment behaviors. P/G: Rosemary begins to show attachment behaviors.	*A safe environment promotes attachment to newborn:* Bring infant to mother when she is well rested. Sit and feed infant while mother observes or touches infant. Allow infant to sleep in room beside mother's bed. Allow time for questions. Have mother observe baby care if she is too tired to do it herself.	Mother begins to touch, stroke, and kiss infant. Mother asks questions about infant care. Mother begins to feed and care for infant without prompting from nurses.
Avoiding making eye contact with person speaking to her.	ND: Self-esteem disturbance related to feelings of worthlessness. P/G: Rosemary starts to feel good about herself.	*A caring environment helps bolster self-esteem:* Praise Rosemary's accomplishments. Ask Rosemary's opinion about care of herself and her infant.	Rosemary starts making eye contact. Rosemary smiles.
Stays to self, doesn't socialize with roommate.	ND: Social isolation related to fear and low self-esteem. P/G: Rosemary begins to converse with roommate and staff.	Be sincere in behavior. Provide choices. Respect Rosemary's right to privacy. Speak to roommate—tell her it is nothing personal with her. Let Rosemary make the first move.	Rosemary initiates conversation with nurse. This may not resolve itself in the 2 to 3 days Rosemary is in the hospital. However, even a "good morning" to the roommate is a step forward.

Continued.

Specific Nursing Care Plan—cont'd

ASSESSMENT	NURSING DIAGNOSIS (ND), PLAN/GOAL (P/G)	RATIONALE/ IMPLEMENTATION	EVALUATION
Anxious and fearful. Husband-wife relationship strained.	ND: Anxiety, moderate, related to potential or real family relationship problems. ND: Ineffective individual and family coping related to problems with husband-wife relationship. P/G: Rosemary appears to be and verbalizes that she feels "better" P/G: Rosemary accepts assistance.	*Reduction of anxiety promotes positive coping:* Provide support. Provide reassurance. Inquire about support systems in the family. Assist Rosemary with obtaining community support. Do not take sides. Keep a sense of humor. Keep a sense of reality.	Rosemary's verbal and nonverbal cues are less anxious. Rosemary accepts assistance and speaks to social worker about networking for support and assistance.
Bruises and cuts on body. Episiotomy.	ND: Pain related to bruises, wounds, and episiotomy. P/G: Rosemary states she is more comfortable.	*Comfort increases ability to cope:* Provide comfort measures. Provide medication as ordered.	Rosemary verbalizes increased comfort.
	ND: Impairment of skin integrity related to cuts on body and episiotomy. P/G: Infection does not occur.	*Absence of infection promotes healing:* Teach Rosemary how to keep areas clean. Give antibiotics as ordered. Promote good nutrition.	Rosemary does not develop infection.
Suspected victim of abuse. Possible perpetuation of violence.	ND: Potential for violence related to being abused. P/G: Violence in the family is prevented.	*The newborn can become a victim of family violence:* Discuss this openly with Rosemary in a nonaccusatory manner. Contact social service department with physician's order. Consult a psychiatrist or psychologist to speak to Rosemary. Refer to appropriate community agencies (Appendix I).	Rosemary speaks freely with nurse. Rosemary agrees to seek help. Representative of community agency visits with Rosemary (and her husband if he wishes to be present).

tions, rape, in its strictest sense, is the penile penetration of the female sex organ, or labia in some states, without her consent. Penetration by any other male appendage or other object or penile penetration of any other orifice constitutes ***sexual assault,*** another legal term. Hymenal penetration or ejaculation does not have to occur. The key feature to establish rape is the **absence of consent**; threat or coercion implies the lack of consent. The victim who is mentally retarded, is unconscious or otherwise physically unable to move, has been drugged without her knowledge, or is a minor (statutory rape) is not capable of giving consent. It is up to the court to prove absence of consent; hence the term **alleged rape** or *alleged sexual assault* is used in medical records.

Incest has been defined by Warner (1980) as "inappropriate sexual behavior among surrogate family members." This includes sexual contact from an adult to a child (such as rape), genital fondling, or oral-genital contact. In addition, sexual contact between nuclear or extended family members (either biologic or step relations) is included in the definition of incest.

Although incest is a universal taboo, an estimated 100,000 cases or more of incest occur each year in the United States. Pregnancy occurs in 12% to 24% of the female victims. Simens (1982) reports that 20% to 35% of all adult women surveyed were sexually molested as children. Nurses who work in schools, public health, pediatrics, obstetrics, and emergency rooms are in an excellent position to identify victims and strategically intervene (Zdanuk, Harris, and Wisian, 1987).

Several states have laws defining rape in terms of a *perceived threat* to the victim's well-being. Sometimes the threat is simple to describe. If the rapist uses a weapon such as a gun or knife, the threat is obvious; if he first engages the intended victim in conversation or is admitted by her into her home and then rapes her without a weapon, the threat she perceives may be more difficult to prove. Cases are brought to court only to be dismissed because the victims cannot prove the presence of a threat. Defense attorneys have used the argument that the woman gave implicit consent for intercourse by the fact that she let the rapist into her apartment, engaged in conversation with him in a bar, or made no attempt to get help during the attack.

Some couples willingly engage in violent sexual acts, considered perverse by many; legal defense could focus on showing that the victim gave consent to enter into sexual behaviors in spite of the potential for injury.

Rape is a violent crime on the increase. Since there are many reasons that deter a woman from reporting the crime, accurate statistics concerning psychosocial and demographic variables relating to rape are not available. Women do not report rape because of the associated stigma or out of embarrassment, guilt that in some way they provoked the assault, fear of retribution from the rapist or his friends, dread of being humiliated and figuratively "raped" again by the police or the court, and discouragement generated by the dismally small number of convictions, to name a few reasons. Victims often fear the reactions of husbands, lovers, friends, family, and children and prefer to suffer alone.

The true incidence will not be known until women feel free to report the crime.

Violent Nature of Rape. *Myths* about rape continue to exist; for example, "there is no such thing as a *real* rape," "women *want* to be taken by force," women "ask for it" by dressing and acting in sexually provocative ways, and, the most dangerous of the myths, "it can't happen to me."

Rape is not an act of lust, nor is it an overzealous release of passion. *Rape is a violent, aggressive assault on the body and integrity of the victim.* As one victim said: "No matter how terrible people think rape is, it's worse than they know. It's like a bomb going off at the center of your soul."

The rapist has no regard for his victim's age, race, sexual attraction, or physical condition—10-day-old infants, as well as handicapped elderly women confined to wheelchairs, have been raped. Most rapes occur *intra*racially rather than *inter*racially. The attacker may be a complete stranger to the victim, or she may know the attacker as a casual acquaintance or a friend of long standing. This is termed *acquaintance rape,* and is more prevalent than previously acknowledged.

Socialization into violence may be a key. In 1935 Margaret Mead (a sociologist) noted that in cultures where males are socialized to be nurturant, not aggressive, rape is unknown.

Nichaus (1986) describes five categories of rape:

Blitz rape: victim and assailant are strangers. A woman pulled into an alley is blitz raped.

Confidence rape: deceit is the major characteristic of confidence rape; for example, the date who uses coercion to obtain sex when the partner is a reluctant, unconsenting acquaintance. This kind of rape is common and seldom reported because the woman is afraid of being considered an accomplice to the rape.

Power rape: the man's victims are usually strangers attacked in a blitz rape. By dominating his victim, the man places the woman in the powerless position he experiences and despises. He fantasizes sexual conquest as a demonstration of his strength and potency. He believes that the woman enjoys the experience.

Anger rape: this is a revenge rape. The assailant uses rape to symbolically punish a significant woman in his life. These are impulse rapes characterized by considerable brutality and trauma.

Sadistic rape: sadism usually characterizes all of the sadistic rapist's relationships. They eroticize their aggression. They abuse and torture the woman until they are completely out of control. In a frenzy, he may commit a "lust murder."

Rape Trauma Syndrome. Regardless of the absence or severity of physiologic trauma present, rape is a serious psychologic emergency; priority consideration in the emergency department is imperative. The degree of support the woman receives in the immediate post-trauma period may have long-range consequences.

Burgess and Holmstrom (1975) described the progressive manifestations of **rape trauma syndrome.** *Disorganization characterizes the acute phase.* Initially, women react in one of two styles of response; *expressed,* evidenced in behaviors such as crying or restlessness; and *controlled,* reflected in a calm, composed, or subdued affect. Somatic reactions include physical discomfort, skeletal muscle tension, gastrointestinal irritability, and genitourinary disturbance (itching or burning on urination). Emotional reactions include fear, humiliation, degradation, and embarrassment; anger, need for revenge, and self-blame; and not uncommonly, mood swings.

The long-term process of reorganization involves increased motor activity such as changing residence and/or phone number. Nightmares and trauma phobia are common. The woman may express fear of indoors or outdoors (depending on site of rape), of being alone, of crowds, or of people walking or standing behind the woman. Sexual fears are common.

Burgess and Holmstrom (1974a,b) have been instrumental in educating professional and lay people about the victim, the physical and psychologic effects of rape, and therapeutic management of rape victims. The victim's crisis response after a rape develops in four stages (Foley and Davies, 1983):

1. Tension rises as the victim tries her habitual problem-solving techniques
2. The woman's stress and discomfort increase because she cannot cope and cannot restore homeostasis
3. The additional stress acts as an internal stimuli to mobilize the woman's internal and external resources to solve her problem, and
4. If disequilibrium continues and cannot be resolved or avoided, tension increases and major disorganization and/or disintegration of personality occurs.

In the therapeutic management, Foley and Davies (1983) emphasize crisis intervention to protect the victim from further psychologic trauma.

Welch (1977) describes rape as a psychologic emergency, after which recovery follows a devious course. Each of three identified phases can last days, months, or years. In the first phase the victim's *acute reaction* is manifested by shock, dismay, generalized anxiety, fear, and immobilization. To the casual observer the victim in the second phase appears outwardly to have *adjusted;* for example, she indicates that she has no further need of help. Now she just wants to forget the incident and return to her previous activities at work and in the home. During the third phase, *ultimate integration and resolution,* the woman who is unfamiliar with symptoms of this phase of recovery may be surprised by the onset of depression and disrupted eating and sleep patterns and by a renewed need to talk about the experience. Surprises can be ego weakening, whereas prior preparation for this eventuality can be ego strengthening. Hilberman (1976) discusses the often-overwhelming feelings of powerlessness and helplessness described by rape victims.

Rape affects everyone who comes in contact with the victim. The family of the rape victim also experiences the two phases of response: an acute reaction and a long-term reorganization process (Burgess and Holmstrom, 1974a).

Assessment

Sexual assault treatment centers usually have a standard form for obtaining and recording pertinent data (Shepard, 1983).

Consent forms must be signed before evidence can be collected and released to the police and before photographs can be taken. If the victim is under 16 years of age, a pediatrician is notified. A parent or guardian is required to sign the consent forms. The children's protective service may need to be called to facilitate consent.

History. The history includes the client's age, allergies, and *menstrual* history, including the age of menarche, date of LMP, and menstrual pattern. If LMP was not normal, the woman is asked to describe it. Her *obstetric* history is determined: gravidity, parity, date of termination of last pregnancy, and, if she thinks she may be pregnant now, symptoms she is experiencing. She is asked to describe her *sexual* history: the date and time of the most recent coitus before the alleged assault and whether a condom was used, her current mode of contraception, whether she was a virgin before the assault, whether she uses tampons, whether she uses douches, and the date of the last douche.

The woman is asked to describe the *assault* (she may need support and assistance in verbalizing the offender's acts): Did the penis enter the vagina? Did he have an orgasm? Was there oral or anal penetration? Did he wear a condom? She is asked to recount her *activity since the assault;* Did she douche, bathe or shower, or defecate or urinate? How, when, and from whom did she seek assistance afterward?

Physical Examination and Laboratory Tests. The physical examination is conducted after the procedure is explained to the woman. She remains clothed* while her vital signs and blood pressure are determined, and her clothing is inspected for stains, tears, and foreign material. She is assisted to undress and is draped; a female attendant, rape counselor, or other person of her choice may remain with her during the examination. The physician informs her of every step of the procedure. Her body is inspected for bruises, swelling, scratches, lacerations, stab wounds, and body lice. A head-to-toe examination is performed. Special attention is given to the area assaulted (e.g., pelvic structures and genitals).

*An ultraviolet light (Wood's lamp) will cause semen to fluoresce even if the man has had a vasectomy. The fluorescent areas of the body and clothing can then be identified for further examination and for sources of specimens for acid phosphatase determination. Specimens can be aspirated or scraped off, appropriately packaged, and labeled.

External genitals, thighs, buttocks, and lower abdomen are assessed, and if there are injuries, photographs may be taken or drawings made. A new test, not yet acceptable to the courts, is toluidine blue staining; a positive toluidine blue staining of the vulva occurs in a significant percentage of rape victims but rarely in women who have coitus with consent (Lauber and Souma, 1982; Shepard, 1983).

A speculum examination (no lubricant is used) is performed gently to detect tears or bruises and to collect appropriate specimens. The cervix is scraped for *Neisseria gonorrhoeae* culturing, and vaginal fluid is obtained for analysis. One slide is fixed and dried to be stained and examined for sperm, a swab of fluid is placed in saline solution for potential sperm serovaring and a sample is assayed for acid phosphatase.*

A bimanual pelvic examination is performed carefully to determine the size and position of the uterus and adnexa. If a pelvic mass is palpated, it may be caused by bleeding into the broad ligament. If pregnancy is a possibility, a pregnancy test is done. Internal pelvic assessment is ended with a rectovaginal examination.

Blood is drawn for a Venereal Disease Research Laboratory (VDRL) test. Any x-ray films or photographs that were taken are noted at this time.

Additional specimens are obtained for evidence to document the identity of the offender. *Swabs* are taken from all orifices if the woman is unconscious, or as deemed appropriate from the woman's history. Slides are prepared from the material on the swabs and allowed to air-dry. The slides are placed into mailers; the swabs are put into one test tube. *Contents of the vaginal vault* are aspirated and put into another test tube. The woman's *pubic hair* is combed; the comb and adhering hair are placed into an envelope, sealed, and labeled "combings." At least 12 of her pubic hairs are pulled out by the roots (or hair is clipped very close to the skin), placed into an envelope, and labeled "pubic hair samples." *Fingernail scrapings* are placed into a separate envelope and labeled.

All slides, envelopes, test tubes, and slide mailers must be labeled personally by the examining physician with a Carborundum pencil, with the woman's name, the date and time, and the site from which the specimen was taken. Her clothes are put into a paper bag, sealed, and labeled. All transactions—obtaining her specimens, packaging them, labeling them, and giving them over to either the police or a laboratory technician—are witnessed and signed by both the giver and the receiver; the time and date are also noted.

*Acid phosphatase is an enzyme found in high concentrations in seminal fluid.

During the examination the woman's *emotional status* is assessed and findings are recorded; which impact reactions she is exhibiting, her orientation to time and place, and her attention span, affect, and verbal description and feelings about the assault. The availability of family or peer support systems is assessed. She is asked about her plans to report or not report the crime to the police.

Nursing Diagnoses

Following are nursing diagnoses for the immediate and later posttrauma periods.

Immediate posttrauma period

Anxiety/fear related to
- The experience itself
- The interactions with police, caregivers
- The physical examination to assess injury and collect evidence
- The possibility of pregnancy and/or infection.

Pain related to
- The experience itself
- The examination

Rape trauma syndrome: silent or compound reaction, related to
- The experience

Injury related to
- The experience

Self-esteem disturbance related to
- Posttrauma syndrome

Later posttrauma period

Posttrauma phobias related to
- Posttrauma syndrome

Potential for infection with STDs related to
- The experience

Potential alterations in ability to form meaningful relationships related to
- Rape trauma syndrome

Planning

Planning for care for victims of rape, sexual assault, or incest requires the same sensitivity, understanding, and knowledge as that needed for the care of the battered woman.

Priorities of personnel who provide care to victims of rape or sexual assault in hospital-based sexual assault centers or in community-based rape crisis centers should include the following (Klingbeil et al, 1976):

1. An emotional support system for the family, friends, and parents, as well as for the victim
2. A sensitive health care system to provide optimum care and to document objective data

3. Presentation of information and education sessions to health care providers, educators, students, members of criminal justice systems, and community groups
4. Interaction and effective communication with the criminal justice system at all levels
5. Involvement with community interest groups concerned with the problems of sexual assault

Goals for the victim of rape include:

1. The woman receives care that is provided in a nonjudgmental, caring, and unhurried manner
2. All evidence is collected during the examination, and all laboratory specimens are individually packaged and carefully labeled, dated, and sealed; receipts are obtained from the laboratory technicians and police
3. The woman does not perceive herself to be victimized by the health care providers
4. The woman does not develop an infection
5. The woman does not become pregnant; if pregnancy results, the woman is able to make an informed decision about its management
6. The woman's physical injuries heal without disfigurement or loss of function
7. The woman participates in scheduled follow-up care
8. The woman understands the phases of the rape trauma syndrome
9. The woman successfully passes through all the stages in the rape trauma syndrome
10. Family bonds are strengthened; family members are supportive of each other

Implementation

Medical management includes (1) treating the physical injuries, (2) providing prophylaxis for infection (e.g., gonorrhea, tetanus) and (3) providing prophylaxis for pregnancy if the woman is not pregnant already. If physical trauma is life-threatening, appropriate intervention takes precedence over collecting evidence.

Immediate Care. If the victim is menarchal, is using no contraception, and is at a time of high risk for pregnancy in her cycle, hormonal therapy may be prescribed for her. Hormonal therapy such as ethinyl estradiol (Estinyl) is prescribed for 5 days to prevent pregnancy if the assault occurred within the previous 48 hours. She is told that the drug can cause nausea and that she should expect withdrawal bleeding shortly after finishing the therapy. Antinauseant therapy in the form of a prochlorperazine preparation (Compazine) is also prescribed to counter the side effects of high doses of estrogens. She is apprised of the availability of abortion or menstrual extraction as a backup measure. If she misses a menstrual period in spite of therapy or if she fails to have withdrawal bleeding from the estrogens, she is assessed for the β-subunit of human chorionic gonadotropin in 2 to 3 weeks (a highly accurate test for pregnancy). She has the option of continuing a pregnancy if pregnancy does occur but is warned about the teratogenic effects of estrogen in these doses.

If the woman is pregnant at the time of the assault, she should be observed for several hours for uterine contractility.

Psychologic support is provided by the manner in which the woman is signed into the emergency room, the respect she is shown, the privacy that is provided for the examination and consultation, and the manner in which the examination is carried out. Access to supplies (including mouth wash) and facilities in which to clean up, clothes to wear home, money as needed, and transportation to wherever she is staying (an alternate place may need to be found for her) add to the woman's comfort and perception of being in control.

In some facilities the social worker is notified the moment a victim is admitted; other facilities contact local rape crisis centers, usually staffed by specially trained volunteers on 24-hour call for just these types of emergencies. The victim needs to be informed of all the steps involved in the rape examination and follow-up. Rape counselors provide ongoing support in a variety of ways. In addition to providing emotional support, transportation, etc., the counselor helps her interact with her family, friends, and various authorities, informs her of the rape trauma syndrome, and finds other resources for her as needed. Male volunteers help counsel male members of the victim's family and peers.

Discharge. The woman is discharged with medications and printed instructions about their use, printed instructions for self-care, and names and phone numbers of resource people should she require assistance. Medical follow-up in the gynecology or pediatric clinic is scheduled for 1 week for a repeat culture for gonorrhea, at 6 weeks for assessment of healing of injuries, and at 8 weeks for a repeat VDRL test and test for AIDS antibodies. Repeat tests are rescheduled as necessary. The woman and her counselor determine whether there is a need for additional medical or psychologic follow-up between the scheduled visits. The woman has a choice of site for follow-up—some women choose to continue with the physician who first performed the examination, others prefer their private physician, and still others need referral to a clinic in the area (city, state) to which they have moved.

Because of the phases of recovery, follow-up telephone contact is continued until the woman has no further need of such help.

A bill for laboratory work and treatment, if sent to the victim, adds insult to injury. Not only can the bill impose a financial burden, but it is a tangible reminder of the assault and adds the indignity of having to pay a financial penalty for being a victim. Today, many municipalities are assuming the cost of examination and treatment for rape.

Evaluation

The nurse can be reasonably assured that care was effective when goals of care (p. 753) have been met. The woman receives care that is nonjudgmental and caring. The examination is accomplished in a nonhurried manner and meets all legal specifications. The woman does not perceive herself as a victim; she receives anticipatory guidance regarding delayed reactions; STDs and pregnancy are prevented; and family bonds are supported and strengthened. Later the woman has no adverse physical, psychologic, or emotional sequelae.

SUMMARY

This chapter discusses the knowledge base needed to assist the nurse in understanding the impact that poverty and psychosocial issues have on pregnant women and their families. Drug dependence and addiction by women, the provision of mental health services, and violence against women are major social problems. Society and health professionals need to move beyond only recognizing these problems to understanding the dynamics of these social ills. Nurses need to be advocates for the women and families in the areas of homelessness, social support programs, community agency involvement, and government assistance for various programs. As always, sensitivity to a woman and her family during a childbearing experience complicated by a psychosocial disorder is as important as expert technologic assistance.

LEARNING ACTIVITIES

1. Visit a high-risk or free prenatal clinic. Assess the risk factors for the clients. What nursing actions may alleviate potential complications for the low-income client? What is the reproductive history of the low-income client?
2. It is difficult to remain objective with substance abuse clients, especially when fetal damage occurs. Activities to raise the awareness might include inviting a speaker from a community agency or half-way house, attending a self-help group meeting, or role-playing two situations:
   a. A nurse caring for a drug-dependent mother who has given birth to an addicted infant.
   b. The same nurse expressing her feelings to a peer. Have the group discuss the implications for effective nursing care.
3. Visit or volunteer time at a battered women's shelter or a victims' hotline.
4. Set up and conduct the following role-playing situations in class:
   a. A nursing student raped in the dorm.
   b. A woman brought to the emergency room with black eyes, a broken leg, and multiple cuts and bruises.
5. Visit a rape crisis center. Describe the supportive role of the nurse. What procedures are carried out in collection of evidence? Obtain the "rape kit" used and review the use and purpose of the contents. Describe your feelings regarding the victim.

KEY CONCEPTS

- Low-income mothers are more predisposed to intercurrent illness and obstetric complications during the childbearing cycle.
- Psychosocial conditions that may complicate childbearing can interfere with family integration and restrict bonding with the infant.
- Developing a nursing care plan for women who are dependent on psychoactive substances may be most therapeutic if it is a collaborative effort of the total health delivery team following a values clarification experience.
- It has been estimated that one out of every six U.S. couples engage in family violence at least once a year.
- Pregnancy is a time of increased battering episodes.
- The abuse of spouses occurs at all socioeconomic levels, as well as at all educational levels.
- Battered women may feel that they are to blame for their situation.
- To develop an effective plan, the caregiver must be comfortable working with the victim (of rape, incest, or battering) and her family.
- Although incest is a universal taboo, an estimated 100,000 cases or more of incest occur each year in the United States.
- The true incidence of rape will not be known until women feel free to report the crime.
- The rapist has no regard for his victim's age, race, sexual attraction, or physical condition.
- Rape is not just a woman's problem; it is a community problem.

References

Poverty

Birch HG and Gussons JD: Disadvantaged children: health, nutrition, and failure, New York, 1970, Harcourt Brace & World.

Griffith-Kenney J: Contemporary women's health: a nursing advocacy approach, Menlo Park, Calif, 1986, Addison-Wesley Publishing Co, Inc.

Osofsky HJ and Kendall N: Poverty as a criterion of risk, Clin Obstet Gynecol 16:103, 1973.

Spector RE: Cultural diversity in health and illness, New York, 1979, Appleton-Century-Crofts.

Whaley LF and Wong DL: Nursing of infants and children, ed 4, St Louis, 1991, The CV Mosby Co.

Emotional Complications

Affonso D: Postpartum depression. In Fields P, editor: Recent advances in perinatal nursing, New York, 1984, Churchill Livingstone, Inc.

American Psychiatric Association: Diagnostic and statistical manual of mental disorders, ed 3, Washington, DC, 1980, The Association.

American Psychiatric Association: Draft of the DSM-III-R in Development (subject to change), as proposed by the Work Group to Revise DSM-III. American Psychiatric Association, October, 1985.

Hayworth J et al: A predictive study of postpartum depression: some predisposing characteristics, Br J Med Psychol 53:161, 1980.

Herzog A and Detre T: Psychotic reactions associated with childbirth, Dis Nerv Sys 37:229, 1976.

Hurt LD and Ray CP: Postpartum disorders: mother-infant bonding on a psychiatric unit, J Psychosoc Nurs 23(2):15, 1985.

Ketai RM and Marvin AB: Childbirth-related psychosis and familial symbiotic conflict, Am J Psychiatry 136:190, 1979.

Spielvogel A and Wile J: Treatment of the psychotic pregnant patient, Psychosomatics 27(7):487, 1986.

Stuart GW and Sundeen SJ: Principles and practice of psychiatric nursing, ed 4, St Louis, 1991, The CV Mosby Co.

Tentoni S and High K: Culturally induced postpartum depression, JOGN Nurs 9:246, July/Aug, 1980.

Weiner A: Childbirth related psychiatric illness, Compr Psychiatry 25:143, 1982.

Psychoactive Substance Use

Chasnoff I et al: Cocaine use in pregnancy, N Engl J Med 313(11):666, 1985.

Clemmer J: When an addicted nurse comes back to work, RN, p 62, Oct 1987.

Finnegan LP and Macnew BA: Nursing care of the addicted infant, Am J Nurs 74:685, 1974.

"Ice" drug now used at work, officials say, San Francisco Chronicle, Wednesday, Oct 25, 1989.

Landry M and Smith DE: Crack: anatomy of an addiction, part 2, Calif Nurs Rev 9(3):28, 1987.

Mondanaro J: Strategies for AIDS prevention: motivating health behavior in drug dependent women, J Psychoactive Drugs 19(2):143, 1987.

New drug "Ice" called worse peril than crack, San Francisco Chronicle, Thursday, Aug 31, 1989.

Oro AS and Dixon SD: Perinatal cocaine and methamphetamine exposure: maternal and neonatal correlates, J Pediatr 111(4):571, 1987.

Scott JR et al: Obstetrics and gynecology, ed 6, Philadelphia, JB Lippincott Co.

Stuart GW and Sundeen SJ: Principles and practice of psychiatric nursing, ed 4, St Louis, 1991, The CV Mosby Co.

Tracy CE: Women suffer most from drugs, The Philadelphia Inquirer, p 7E, November 27, 1988.

Woods JR, Plessinger MA, and Clark KE: Effect of cocaine on uterine blood flow and fetal oxygenation, JAMA 257:957, 1987.

Abuse and Violence

Battered wives testify—'no legal recourse,' San Francisco Chronicle, p A18, Sept 17, 1987.

Bowker L and Maurer L: The effectiveness of counseling services utilized by battered women, Women and Therapy 5(4):65, 1986.

Burgess AW and Holmstrom LL: Crisis and counseling requests of rape victims, Nurs Res 23:196, 1974.

Burgess AW and Holmstrom LL: Rape: victims of crisis, Bowie, Md, 1974b, Robert J Brady Co

Burgess, AW and Holmstrom LL: Rape trauma syndrome: coping behavior of the rape victim, Nurs Dig 3:17, May/June, 1975.

Chez RA, moderator: If you suspect a patient is a victim of abuse, Contemp OB/GYN 29(6):132, 1987.

Collier JA: When you suspect your patient is a battered wife, RN, p 33, May, 1987.

Delgaty K: Battered women: the issues for nursing, NAACOG Newsletter, 12(10):9, 1985.

Drake VK: Battered women: a health care problem in disguise, Image 14:40, June, 1982.

Elbow M: Theoretical considerations of violent marriages, Social Casework, p 515, Nov, 1977.

Finley B: Nursing process with the battered woman, Nurse Pract 6(4):11, 1981.

Foley TS and Davies MA: Rape: nursing care of victims, St Louis, 1983, The CV Mosby Co.

Gelles RJ: Abused wives: why do they stay, J Marriage Fam, Nov, 1976.

Gelles RJ: The myths of battered husbands, Ms 8(4):65, 1979.

Griffith-Kenney J: Contemporary women's health: a nursing advocacy approach, Menlo Park, Calif, 1986, Addison-Wesley Publishing Co, Inc.

Hicks DJ: Sexual battery: management of the rape victim. In Sciarra JJ, editor: Obstetrics and gynecology, New York, 1981, Harper & Row, Publishers, Inc.

Hilberman E: The rape victim, New York, 1976, Basic Books Inc, Publishers.

Hillard PJ: Physical abuse in pregnancy, Obstet Gynecol 66:185, 1985.

Hillard PJ: Physical abuse and pregnancy, Fam Pract Recertification 8(9):89, 1986.

Klaus PA and Rand MR: Family violence, Bureau of Justice Statistics (special report), Washington, DC, 1984.

Klingbeil KS et al: Multidisciplinary care for sexual assault victims, Nurs Pract 1(6):21, 1976.

Lauber AA and Souma ML: Use of toluidine blue for documentation of traumatic intercourse, Obstet Gynecol 60:644, 1982.

Lichtenstein VR: The battered woman: guideline for effective nursing intervention, Issues Ment Health Nurs 3:237, 1981.

Mandel B: Woman victimized twice—by her ex-lover and the system, San Francisco Examiner, Nov 2, 1986.

Mercer RT: Nursing care for parents at risk, Thorofare, NJ, 1977, Charles B Slack, Inc.
Nichaus MA: Rape. In Griffith-Kenney J: Contemporary women's health: a nursing advocacy approach, Menlo Park, Calif, 1986, Addison-Wesley Publishing Co, Inc.
Parker B and Schumacher DN: The battered wife syndrome and violence in the nuclear family of origin: a controlled pilot study, Am J Public Health 67:760, 1977.
Pfouts JH: Violent families: coping responses of abused wives, Child Welfare 57:101, 1978.
Riesenberg D: Treating a societal malignancy—rape, JAMA 257(6):726, 1987.
Shepard M: Guide to managing the victim of rape, Contemp OB/GYN 22(3):253, 1983.
Simens S and Brandzel RC: Sexuality: nursing assessment and intervention, Philadelphia, 1982, JB Lippincott Co.
Straus MA et al: Behind closed doors: violence in the American family, Garden City, NY, 1980, Anchor Books.
Stuart GW and Sundeen SJ: Principles and practice of psychiatric nursing, ed 4, St Louis, 1991, The CV Mosby Co.
Warner CG: Rape and sexual assault, Germantown, Penn, 1980, Aspen Publishers, Inc.
Welch MS: Rape and the trauma of inadequate care, Nurs Dig 5:50, Spring, 1977.
White EC: Chain, chain, change: for black women dealing with physical and emotional abuse, Seattle, 1985, Seal Press, New Leaf Series.
Witkin-Lanoil G: Too close to home, Health, p 6, Jan, 1987.
Zdanuk JM, Harris CC, and Wisian NL: Adolescent pregnancy and incest: the nurse's role as counselor, JOGN Nurs 16(2):99, 1987.

Bibliography

Poverty

Carter ER: Quality maternity care for the medically indigent, MCN 11(2):85, 1986.
Damrosch SP et al: On behalf of homeless families, MCN 13(4):259, 1988.
Johnson SH: Nursing assessment and strategies for the family at risk: high-risk parenting, ed 2, Philadelphia, 1986, JB Lippincott Co.
Moleti CA: Caring for socially high-risk pregnant women, MCN 13(1):24, 1988.
Thompson P: Health promotion with immigrant women: a model for success, Can Nurse, p 20. Dec, 1987.

Emotional Complications

Carmack BJ and Corwin TA: Nursing care of the schizophrenic maternity patient during labor, MCN 5:107, 1980.
Fisher LY: Nursing management of the pregnant psychotic patient during labor and delivery, JOGN Nurs 17(1):25, 1988.
Hans A: Postpartum assessment: the psychological component JOGN Nurs 15(1):49, 1986.
Lagerlof JM: Maternal fetal "conflict": balancing our values, Calif Nurs Rev p 34, Jan/Feb, 1988.
Petrick J: Postpartum depression: identification of high-risk mothers, JOGN Nurs 13(1):37, 1984.

Psychoactive Substance Use

Bingue N et al: Teratogenicity of cocaine in humans, J Pediatr 110:93, 1987.
Chasnoff IJ et al: Perinatal cerebral infarction and maternal cocaine use, J Pediatr 108:456, 1986.
Drug abuse and pregnancy, ACOG Technical Bulletin 96:Sept, 1986.
Drug abuse in adolescents, Child Care Newsletter 6(2):issue, Fall, 1987 (An educational service of Johnson & Johnson, Dept. CCN, PO Box 836, Somerville, NJ 08876).
NAACOG: Pregnancy and alcohol: a hazardous mix, NAACOG Newsletter 15(3):1, 1988.
NAACOG: Caring for cocaine mothers and babies, NAACOG Newsletter, 16(10):1, 1989.
Pitts K and Weinstein L: Cocaine and pregnancy—a lethal combination, J Perinatol 10(2):180, 1990.
Ronkin S et al: Protecting mother and fetus from narcotic abuse, Contemp OB/GYN 31(3):178, 1988.
Silver H et al: Addiction in pregnancy: high risk intrapartum management and outcome, J Perinatol 793:178, 1987.
Smith J: The dangers of prenatal cocaine use, MCN 13(3):174, 1988.

Abuse and Violence

The battered woman, ACOG Technical Bulletin 124:Jan, 1989.
Bullock LF and McFarlane J: The low birth-weight/battering connection, Am J Nurs 89(9):1153, 1989.
Helton AS et al: Battered and pregnant: a presumptive study Am J Public Health 77(10), 1339, 1987.
Moehling K: Battered women and abusive partners: treatment issues and strategies, J Psychosoc Nurs Ment Health Serv 26(9):9, 1988.
Aguilera DC and Messick JM: Crisis intervention: theory and methodology, ed 6, St Louis, 1989, The CV Mosby Co.
Heinrich KT: Effective responses to sexual harassment, Nurs Outlook 35(2):70, 1987.
Helton A: Battering during pregnancy, Am J Nurs 86(8):910, 1986.
Helton AS and Snodgrass FG: Battering during pregnancy: intervention strategies, BIRTH 14(3):142, 1987.
Matteson PS: Pregnant and battered, Childbirth Educator 5(2):46, 1985-86.
Moleti CA: Caring for socially high-risk pregnant women, MCN 13(1):24, 1988.
Payne JS, Downs S, and Newman K: Helping the abused woman, Nurs '86 16(9):52, 1986.
Reedy NJ: Trauma in pregnancy, NAACOG update series, lesson 23, vol 1, 1984.
Snodgrass F: Where do women turn? Am J Nurs 86(8):912.

CHAPTER

26 Dystocia and Preterm and Postterm Labor and Birth

Deitra Leonard Lowdermilk

Learning Objectives

Correctly define the key terms listed.

Discuss assessment for different types of dystocia.

Formulate nursing diagnoses based on assessment of dystocia.

Describe interventions for different types of dystocia.

Discuss criteria for evaluating nursing care of clients experiencing dystocia.

Identify nursing assessments and interventions for clients experiencing induction/augmentation of labor.

Explain management of clients experiencing multifetal pregnancy.

Compare management of preterm labor at home with management in the hospital setting.

Identify needs of clients experiencing cesarean delivery and other operative obstetric procedures.

Describe assessment and management of clients experiencing postterm labor.

Key Terms

amniotomy
augmentation of labor
breech presentation
cesarean delivery
dysfunctional labor
dystocia
episiotomy
external cephalic version
Ferguson's reflex
fetal lung maturity
fetopelvic disproportion
forceps delivery
induction of labor
magnesium sulfate
multifetal pregnancy
oxytocin
pelvic dystocia
postterm birth
precipitous labor
preterm birth
prolonged labor
prostaglandin
ritodrine
soft tissue dystocia
terbutaline
trial of labor
vacuum extraction
vaginal birth after cesarean (VBAC)

When there are complications during labor and delivery, perinatal morbidity and mortality increase. Some complications are anticipated, especially if the mother is identified as high risk during the antepartum period; others are unexpected or unforeseen. It is crucial for nurses to have an understanding of the normal birth process to prevent and detect deviations from normal and to implement nursing measures when complications arise. Optimum care of the laboring woman, fetus, and family experiencing complications is possible only when the nurse and other members of the obstetric team use their knowledge and skills in a concerted effort for the provision of care.

Dystocia

Dystocia is defined as difficult birth as opposed to easy (normal) birth, or eutocia. Dystocia results from differences in the normal relationships between any of the five essential factors of labor (Chapter 12). The five factors are as follows:

1. Powers
   a. Primary powers: intensity, duration, and frequency of uterine contractions
   b. Secondary powers: bearing-down efforts
2. Passageway

a. Configuration and diameters of the maternal pelvis
b. Distensibility of the lower uterine segment, cervical dilatation, and capacity for distension of the vaginal canal and introitus

3. Passenger
   a. Fetus: gestational age, size, attitude, presentation, and position of the fetus; number of fetuses
   b. Placenta: type, sufficiency of, and site of insertion
4. Position of the mother: standing, walking, side-lying, squatting, hands and knees
5. Psychologic response: previous experiences, emotional readiness, preparation, cultural-ethnic heritage, support systems, and environment

These five factors are interdependent. Interactions among the factors and how they influence labor progress must be considered in assessing the woman for an abnormal labor pattern. Dystocia is suspected when there is a lack of progress in the rate of cervical dilatation, a lack of progress in fetal descent and expulsion, or an alteration in the characteristics of uterine contractions.

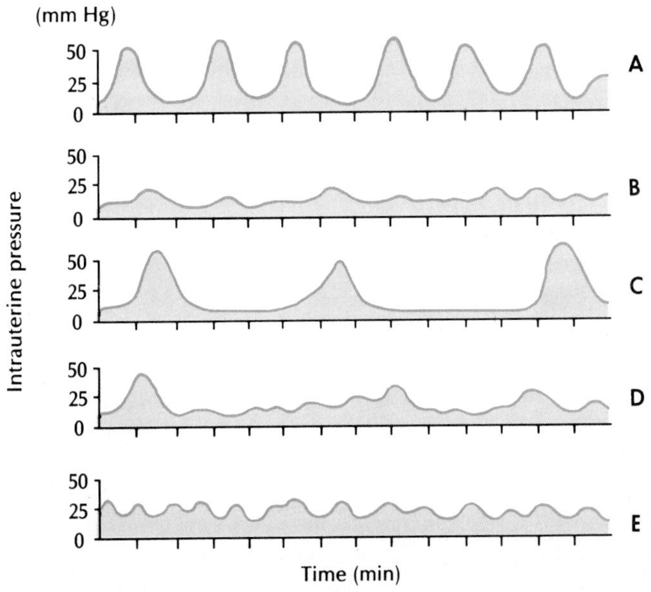

Fig. 26-1 Uterine contractility patterns in labor. **A,** Typical normal labor. **B,** Subnormal intensity, with frequency greater than needed for optimum performance. **C,** Normal contractions, but too infrequent for efficient labor. **D,** Incoordinate activity. **E,** Hypercontractility.

❑ POWERS: DYSFUNCTIONAL LABOR

Dysfunctional labor is described as abnormal uterine contractions that prevent normal progress of cervical dilatation, effacement (primary powers), and/or descent (secondary powers). Figs. 26-1 and 26-2 compare the typical normal labor pattern with uterine patterns that are dysfunctional.

Primary Powers

Dysfunction of uterine contractions can be further described as primary or secondary. The woman who is experiencing *primary dysfunctional labor,* or *hypertonic uterine dysfunction,* is often an anxious nullipara who is having painful contractions that are out of proportion to their intensity and that do not cause cervical

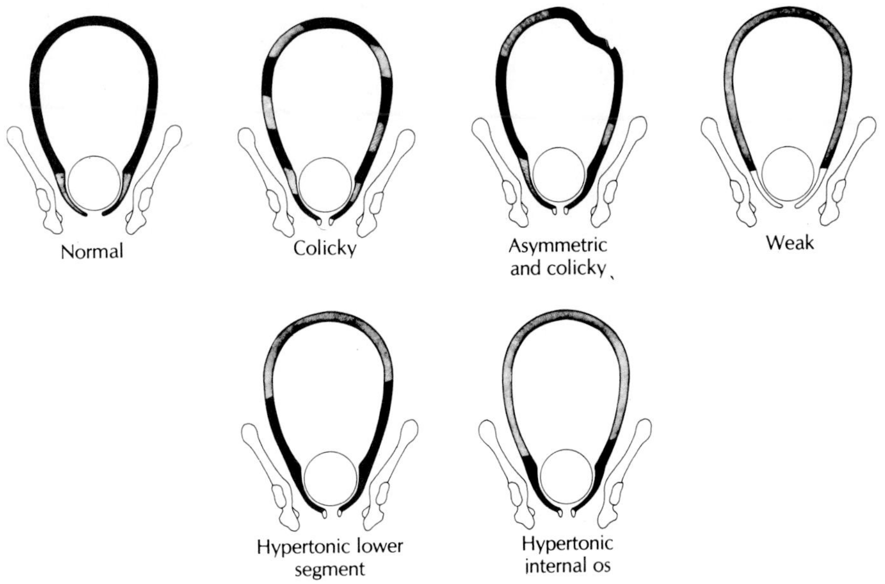

Fig. 26-2 Normal and dysfunctional uterine contraction types. *Darker area,* strong contraction; *grey area,* slight contraction; *white area,* atonic areas.

dilatation or effacement. These contractions usually occur in the latent stage (cervical dilatation <4 cm) and are usually uncoordinated and frequent. The force of the contraction may be in the midsection of the uterus rather than in the fundus, and the uterus may not completely relax between contractions.

Women experiencing hypertonic uterine dysfunction may be exhausted and express concern about loss of control because of the intense pain and lack of progress. Management of primary uterine dysfunction is therapeutic rest, which is achieved through the administration of effective analgesics such as morphine or meperidine to reduce the pain and encourage sleep. Often these women will awaken with normal uterine activity.

The second and more common type of uterine dysfunction is *secondary uterine inertia,* or *hypotonic uterine dysfunction.* The woman, who may be a nullipara or multipara, initially makes normal progress into the active stage of labor; then the contractions become weak and inefficient or stop altogether. The uterus is easily indentable even at the peak of contractions. Fetopelvic disproportion and malpositions are common causes.

Women experiencing hypotonic uterine dysfunction may become exhausted and are at risk for infection. Medical management usually includes ruling out fetopelvic disproportion, followed by augmentation of dysfunctional labor with oxytocin (p. 767).

Secondary Powers

Bearing down efforts are compromised by large amounts of analgesic. Anesthesia may block the bearing-down reflex and alter the effectiveness of voluntary efforts. Exhaustion from lack of sleep or long labor and fatigue from inadequate hydration and food affect the woman's voluntary efforts. Maternal position can work against the forces of gravity, as well as decrease the contraction's strength and efficiency. Gravity adds 10 to 35 mm Hg to the pressure exerted by the presenting part (Fenwick and Simkin, 1987). Table 26-1 summarizes dysfunctional labor.

Precipitous labor is defined as labor that lasts less than 3 hours from onset of contractions. Hypertonic uterine contractions may result in precipitous labor, characterized by tetanic-like contractions. Since labor is rapid, maternal and fetal complications can occur. Maternal complications include uterine rupture, lacerations of the birth canal, amniotic fluid embolism, and postpartum hemorrhage. Fetal complications include hypoxia caused by decreased periods of uterine relaxation between contractions and intracranial hemorrhage related to rapid delivery.

❑ PASSAGEWAY

Pelvic Dystocia

Pelvic dystocia can occur with contractures of the pelvic diameters that reduce the capacity of the bony pelvis, including the inlet, midpelvis, outlet, or any combination of these planes. Pelvic contractures may be caused by congenital abnormalities, maternal malnutrition, neoplasms, and lower spinal disorders. Immature pelvic size predisposes some adolescent gravidas to pelvic dystocia. Pelvic deformities may be the result of automobile or other accidents.

Inlet contracture occurs in 1% to 2% of term deliveries and is diagnosed when the diagonal conjugate is less than 11.5 cm. The incidence of face and shoulder presentation increases. These presentations prevent engagement and fetal descent, thereby increasing the risk of prolapse of the umbilical cord. Inlet contracture is associated with maternal rickets and a flat pelvis.

Midplane contracture, the most common cause of pelvic dystocia, is diagnosed when the sum of the interischial spinous and posterior sagittal diameters of the midpelvis is 13.5 cm or less. Fetal descent is arrested (transverse arrest of the fetal head), since the head cannot rotate internally. Cesarean delivery is the usual management, but vacuum extraction has been used safely if the cervix is fully dilated. Midforceps delivery is usually avoided because of increased perinatal mobidity associated with this intervention.

Outlet contracture exists when the interischial diameter is 8 cm or less. It rarely occurs without midplane contracture. Outlet contracture is associated with a long narrow pubic arch and an android pelvis (see Fig. 12-13). Fetal descent is arrested. Maternal complications include extensive perineal lacerations during vaginal delivery because the fetal head is pushed posteriorly.

Soft Tissue Dystocia

Soft tissue dystocia results from obstruction of the birth passage by an anatomic abnormality other than that of the bony pelvis. The obstruction may result from placenta previa (low-lying placenta) that partially or completely obstructs the internal os of the cervix. Care relative to placenta previa is discussed in Chapter 23. Other causes, such as leiomyomas (uterine fibroids) in the lower uterine segment, ovarian tumors, and a full bladder or rectum, may prevent the fetus from entering the pelvis. Occasionally, *cervical edema* occurs in labor when the cervix is caught between the presenting part and the symphysis, preventing complete dilatation.

Bandl's ring, a pathologic retraction ring (see Fig. 12-14), may cause second-stage dystocia.

Table 26-1 **Dysfunctional Labor: Primary and Secondary Powers**

Hypotonic Uterine Dysfunction	Hypertonic Uterine Dysfunction	Inadequate Voluntary Expulsive Forces
DESCRIPTION		
Cause may be contracture and fetal malposition, overdistension of uterus (twins), or unknown (primary powers) (Figs. 26-1 and 26-2)	Usually occurs before 4 cm dilatation; cause not yet known, may be related to fear and tension (primary powers) (Figs. 26-1 and 26-2)	Involves abdominal and levator ani muscles Occurs in second stage of labor; cause may be related to conduction anesthesia, heavy analgesia, paralysis or intense pain with contractions (secondary powers)
CHANGE IN PATTERN OF PROGRESS		
Contractions decrease in frequency and intensity Uterus easily indentable even at peak of contraction Uterus relaxed between contractions (normal)	Pain out of proportion to intensity of contraction Pain out of proportion to effectiveness of contraction in effacing and dilating the cervix Contractions increase in frequency Contractions uncoordinated Uterus is contracted between contraction (basal hypertonus), cannot be indented.	No voluntary urge to push or bear down
POTENTIAL MATERNAL EFFECTS		
Infection Exhaustion Psychologic trauma	Loss of control related to intensity of pain and lack of progress Exhaustion	Spontaneous vaginal delivery prevented
POTENTIAL FETAL EFFECTS		
Fetal infection Fetal and neonatal death	Fetal asphyxia with meconium aspiration	Fetal asphyxia
MEDICAL MANAGEMENT		
Oxytocic stimulation of labor (p. 767) **Prostaglandin** stimulation of labor (p. 766)	Analgesic (morphine, meperidine) if membranes not ruptured or fetopelvic disproportion not present Relief of pain permits mother to rest; when she awakens, normal uterine activity may begin	Coach mother in bearing down with contractions Analgesia to counteract pain Cesarean delivery only if fetal distress

❏ PASSENGER: DYSTOCIA OF FETAL ORIGIN

Dystocia may be caused by fetal anomalies, excessive size, or malpresentation or malposition of the fetus. Although these conditions are uncommon, they constitute obstetric emergencies.

Fetal dystocia may be classified according to the cause of the abnormality.

Fetal Anomalies

Gross ascites, abnormal tumors, myelomeningocele, and hydrocephalus are fetal anomalies that can cause dystocia.

Fetopelvic Disproportion

Excessive *fetal size* is arbitrarily 4000 g (8 lb 13½ oz) or more in North America. Shoulder dystocia can be anticipated in large fetuses (Lee, 1987). **Fetopelvic disproportion** represents about 5% of term births. Commonly excessive fetal size is a result of diabetes mellitus, obesity, maternal multiparity, or the large size of one or both parents.

Fetal Malposition

The most common fetal malposition is persistent occipitoposterior position (right occipitoposterior [ROP]

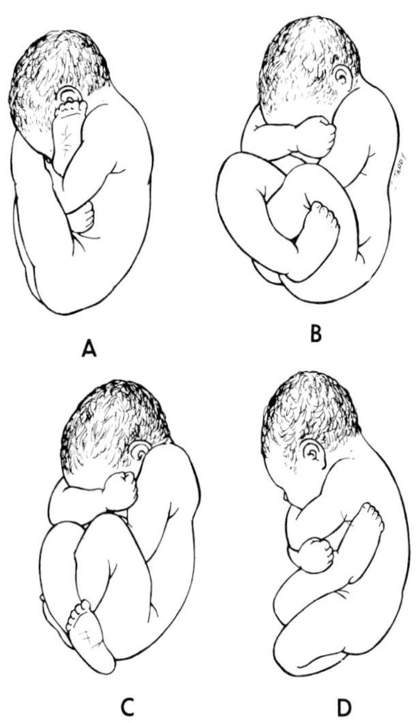

Fig. 26-3 Types of breech presentation. **A**, Frank breech: thighs are flexed on hips; knees are extended. **B**, Complete breech: thighs and knees are flexed. **C**, Incomplete breech: foot extends below buttocks. **D**, Incomplete breech: knee extends below buttocks.

or left occipitoposterior [LOP]; see Fig. 12-4), occurring in about 25% of all labors. Labor is prolonged, especially the second stage; the mother complains of severe back pain from the pressure of the fetal head against her sacrum. Counterpressure to the sacral area and frequent position changes may decrease the pain. The hands and knees or lateral position has been used to facilitate rotation of the fetus from a posterior to an anterior position (Lehrman, 1985; Fenwick and Simkin, 1987). Whereas the fetus will usually rotate spontaneously, delivery may be accomplished by use of low forceps or manual rotation.

Fetal Malpresentation

Breech presentation is the most common example of malpresentation, occurring in 3% to 4% of all deliveries and up to 25% of preterm deliveries. There are four main types of breech presentation: frank breech (thighs flexed, knees extended), complete breech (thighs and knees flexed), incomplete breech (foot extends below buttocks), and incomplete breech (knee extends below buttocks) (Fig. 26-3). Breech presentations are associated with multiple gestation, fetal and maternal anomalies, hydramnios, and oligohydramnios. Diagnosis is made by abdominal palpation and vaginal examination, and is confirmed by ultrasound or x-ray studies.

During labor, fetal descent may be slow because the breech is not as good a dilating wedge as the fetal

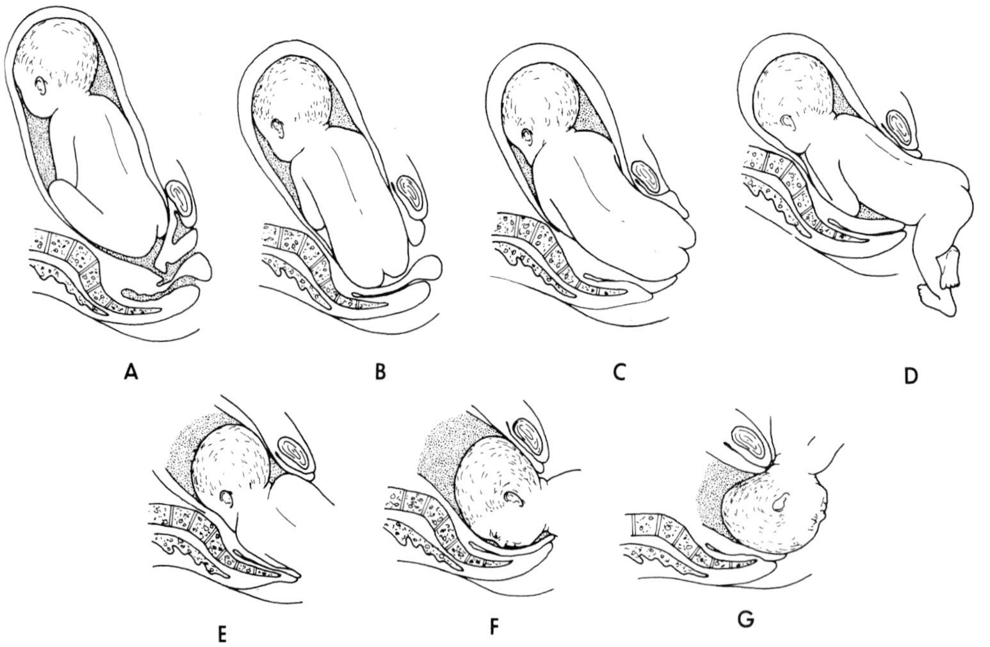

Fig. 26-4 Mechanism of labor in breech position. **A**, Breech before onset of labor. **B**, Engagement and internal rotation. **C**, Lateral flexion. **D**, External rotation or restitution. **E**, Internal rotation of shoulders and head. **F**, Face rotates to sacrum when occiput is anterior. **G**, Head is delivered by gradual flexion during elevation of fetal body.

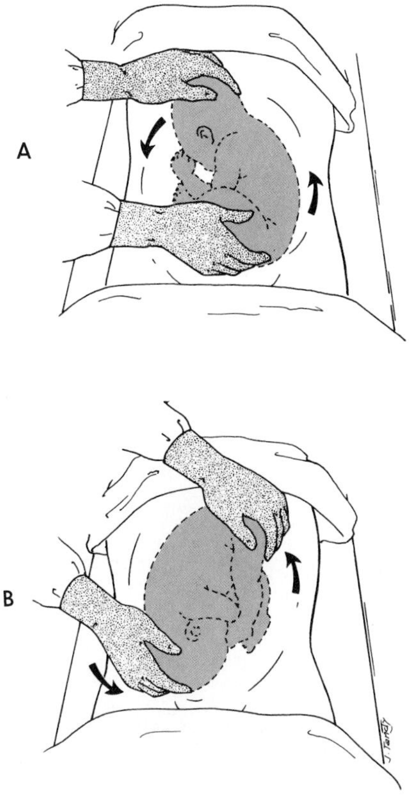

Fig. 26-5 External version of fetus from breech to vertex presentation. This must be achieved without force. **A,** Breech is pushed up out of pelvic inlet while head is pulled toward inlet. **B,** Head is pushed toward inlet while breech is pulled upward.

head, but labor is usually not prolonged. There is a risk of prolapsed cord if membranes rupture in early labor. Presence of meconium in amniotic fluid is not necessarily a sign of fetal distress, since it is caused by pressure on the fetal abdominal wall as it traverses the birth canal. Fetal heart tones are best heard at or above the umbilicus. Vaginal delivery is accomplished by mechanisms related to birth of the buttocks and lower extremities (Fig. 26-4). Piper's forceps are sometimes used to deliver the head (see Fig. 26-9).

Alternatives to vaginal delivery of the breech are external cephalic version and cesarean delivery. **External cephalic version** may be attempted in a labor and delivery setting after 37 weeks of gestation, and is accomplished by gentle, constant pressure accompanied by continuous fetal heart surveillance (Fig. 26-5). A tocolytic agent, such as ritodrine or terbutaline (p. 784) may be given intravenously to relax the uterus and facilitate the maneuver. Ultrasound may be used to identify potential problems such as cord entanglement and placental separation (Englinton, 1988). Cesarean delivery is commonly performed for women with fetuses es-

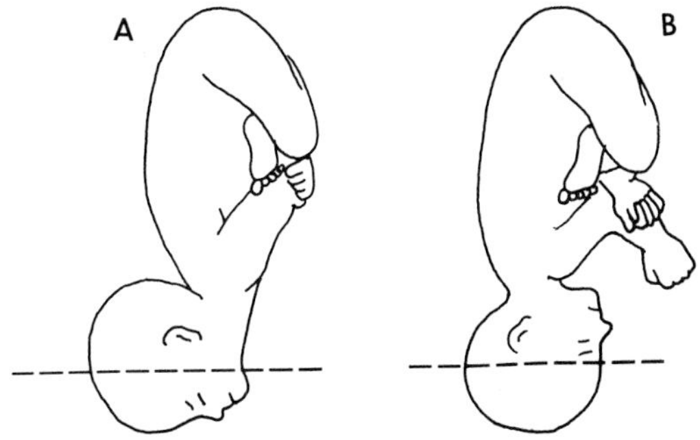

Fig. 26-6 Extension of normally flexed head. **A,** Face, and **B,** brow presentations.

timated to be larger than 3360 g (7¼ lb), if labor is ineffective, or when complications arise.

Face and brow presentations (Fig. 26-6) are uncommon and are associated with fetal anomalies, pelvic contractures, and fetopelvic disproportion. Vaginal delivery is possible if the fetus flexes to a vertex presentation, although forceps are often used. Cesarean delivery is indicated when the presentation persists, if there is fetal distress, or if labor progress stops.

Multifetal Pregnancy

Multifetal pregnancy is the gestation of twins, triplets, quadruplets, or more infants (Chapter 7). Infants of multifetal pregnancies account for 2% to 3% of all viable births and are associated with more complications, including dysfunctional labor, than single births. The high incidence of complications and risk of perinatal mortality are primarily related to low-birth-weight infants resulting from preterm birth and intrauterine growth retardation. In addition, fetal complications such as congenital anomalies and abnormal presentations can cause dystocia and increased incidence of cesarean delivery. For example, only half of all twin pregnancies will have both fetuses presenting in the vertex position, the most favorable for vaginal delivery; one third may present as one twin in vertex and one in breech (Perkins, 1987).

❑ POSITION OF THE MOTHER

The functional relationships between the uterine contractions, the fetus, and the mother's pelvis are altered by maternal positioning. In addition, positioning can provide either a mechanical advantage or disadvantage to the mechanisms of labor by altering the effects of gravity and the relationships among body parts that are significant to labor progress (Fenwick and Simkin, 1987). Discouraging maternal movement or restricting labor to the recumbant or lithotomy position may compromise labor. The positions commonly chosen by laboring women for comfort may also reduce the length of labor, thus reducing the possibility of dystocia (Fenwick and Simkin, 1987). Freedom of movement (e.g., walking, squatting, sitting) offers a greater variety of angles to the presenting part, increasing the chances of a better fit between fetus and pelvis (Chapter 15).

❑ PSYCHOLOGIC RESPONSE

Hormones released in response to stress can cause dystocia. Sources of stress vary for each individual, but pain and the absence of a support person are two accepted factors. Maternal position can decrease the efficiency of labor and increase pain (Caldeyro-Barcia, 1979). Confinement to bed and restriction of maternal movement add a potential psychologic stress to compound the physiologic stress of immobility in the unmedicated parturient. Women who are upright in the second stage of labor produce lower levels of stress-related hormones (β-endorphin, adrenocorticotropic hormone [ACTH], cortisol, and epinephrine) than women who are supine. These women report less tension and anxiety when sitting upright. The labor-inhibiting effects of excessive levels of these hormones are well documented (Simkin, 1986) and may be associated with dystotic labor patterns (Fenwick and Simkin, 1987).

❑ PROLONGED LABOR

Labor extending beyond 24 hours is **prolonged labor** (Ledger, 1987). It may result from various causes previously described as factors associated with dystocia: ineffective uterine contractions, pelvic contractures, fetopelvic disproportion, and abnormalities of fetal presentation and position. In prolonged labor, progress in either the first or second stage of labor is delayed or protracted. Abnormal progress can be recognized when cervical dilatation is plotted on a labor graph and compared with a normal labor curve. Fig. 26-7, *A* is a graphic representation of normal labor progress of a nullipara.

The *latent phase* includes that portion of the first stage between the onset of labor contractions and the acceleration in rate of cervical dilatation. The upswing in the curve denotes the onset of the *active phase* of the first stage of labor, which includes the *acceleration phase*, the *phase of maximum slope*, and the *deceleration phase*. Compare this with Fig. 26-7, *B*, which shows major types of deviation from normal progress of labor. These can be detected by noting the dilatation of the cervix at various intervals after labor begins. If a woman exhibits an abnormal labor pattern as depicted by the broken lines, the physician should be notified immediately (Sheen and Hayashi, 1987.)

1. Cervical dilatation patterns: report to physician
   a. Prolonged latent phase: 20 hours or longer in the nullipara and 14 hours or longer in the parous woman
   b. Protracted active phase: cervical dilatation of less than 1.2 cm/hr in the nullipara and less than 1.5 cm/hr in the parous woman
   c. Arrest of the active phase: no progress in the active phase for more than 2 to 4 hours
   d. Precipitate labor: labor of less than 3 hours
2. Descent patterns: report to physician
   a. Protracted descent pattern in the active phase: rate of descent less than 1 cm/hr in the nullipara and less than 2 cm/hr in the parous woman
   b. Arrest of descent in the active phase: no progress for 1 hour or more in the nullipara and 30 minutes in the parous woman
   c. Failure of descent during deceleration and second stage

Fetal mortality increases sharply after 15 hours of the active first stage of labor. Maternal morbidity and mortality may occur as a result of uterine rupture, infection, serious dehydration, and postpartum hemorrhage. A long difficult labor can have an adverse psychologic effect on the mother, father, and family. A summary of normal and prolonged labor patterns is given in the box below.

LABOR PATTERNS IN NORMAL AND PROLONGED LABOR

NORMAL LABOR

1. Dilatation: continues
   a. Latent phase: <4 cm and low slope
   b. Active phase: >5 cm or high slope
   c. Deceleration phase: ≥ 9 cm
2. Descent: active at ≥ 9 cm dilatation
3. Normal labor progresses rapidly; multiparas faster than nulliparas

PROLONGED LABOR PATTERNS	NULLIPARAS	MULTIPARAS
1. Prolonged latent phase	>20 hr	>14 hr
2. Protracted active-phase dilatation	<1.2 cm/hr	<1.5 cm/hr
3. Secondary arrest: no change for	≥2 hr	≥2 hr
4. Prolonged deceleration phase	>3 hr	>1 hr
5. Protracted descent	<1 cm/hr	<2 cm/hr
6. Arrest of descent	≥1 hr	≥½ hr

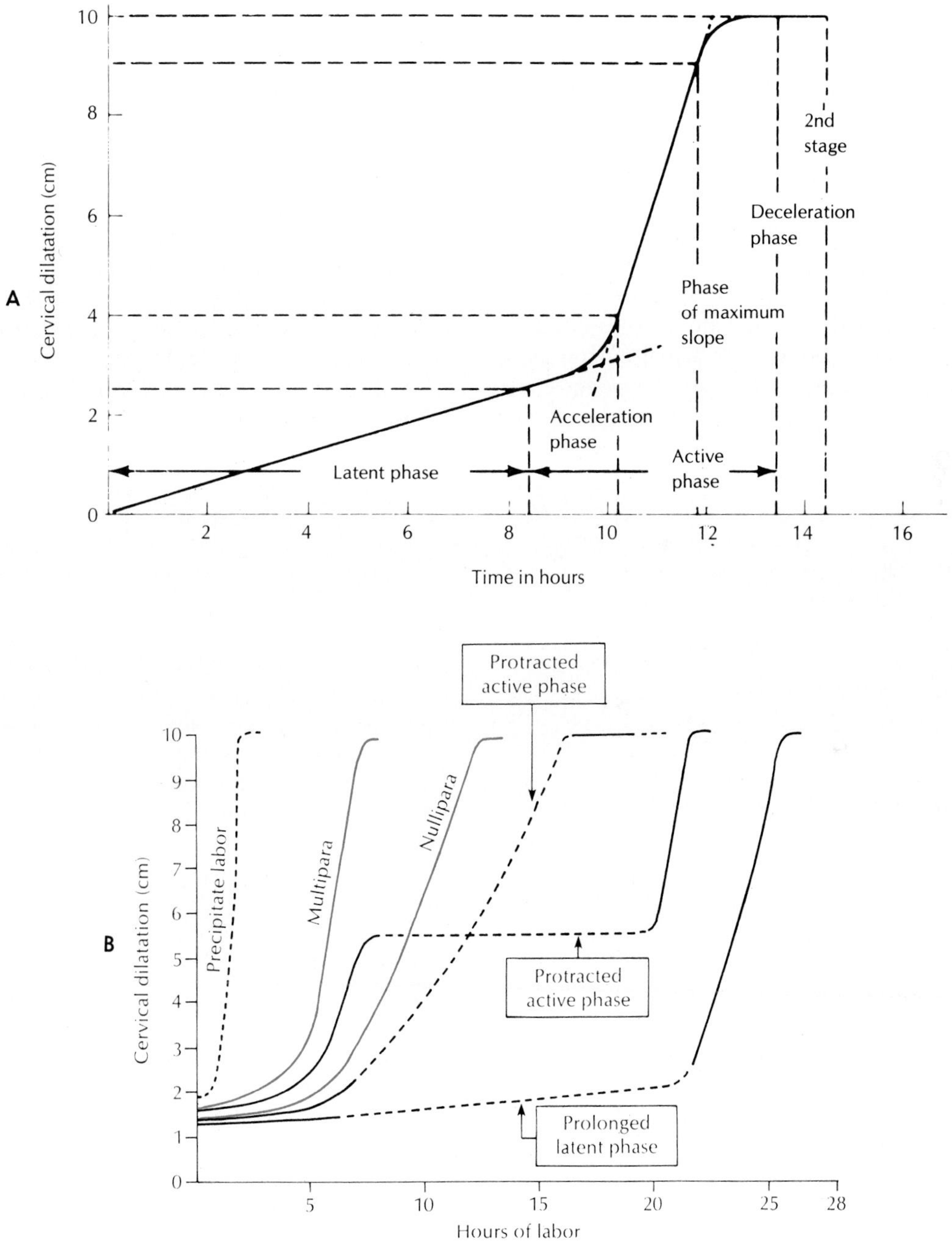

Fig. 26-7 **A,** Partogram of a normal labor. **B,** Major types of deviation from normal progress of labor may be detected by noting dilatation of cervix at various intervals after labor begins. If a woman exhibits an abnormal labor pattern as depicted by broken lines, physician should be notified immediately.

Assessment

Risk assessment is a continuous process. Information from the woman's history, physical examination, laboratory tests, observation of her psychologic response to labor, and maternal-fetal monitoring contribute to accurate identification of potential and actual nursing diagnoses related to dystocia and maternal-fetal compromise.

Nursing Diagnoses

Nursing diagnoses vary with the type of dystocia present as well as with the individual needs of the woman and her family. Potential or actual nursing diagnoses that might be identified for clients experiencing dystocia include:

Anxiety related to
- Slowed labor progress

Pain related to
- Dystocia

Potential for fetal injury: fetal compromise
Potential for maternal injury: infection
Powerlessness related to
- Loss of control

Ineffective individual coping related to
- Disappointment
- Pain
- Fear
- Exhaustion

Knowledge deficit related to
- Procedures, positioning, relaxation techniques, etc.

Situational low self-esteem related to
- Inability to labor and give birth as expected

Fluid volume excess related to
- Intravenous infusion with oxytocin

Fluid volume deficit related to
- NPO status

Planning

Nursing diagnoses provide direction for care. During this important step, goals are set in client-centered terms, and the goals are prioritized. Nursing actions are selected with the client, as appropriate, to meet the goals.

Goals for the woman who is experiencing dystocia may include:

1. Client education about dysfunctional labor
2. Prevention of complications such as hemorrhage and infection
3. Promotion of feelings of self-esteem
4. Provision of physical and psychologic support during labor.

Goals for the fetus may include:

1. Maintenance of a healthy intrauterine environment
2. A safe and healthy adjustment to extrauterine life

The most important goal for the family is the promotion of attachment between parents and the infant.

Implementation

Nurses assume many caregiving roles when labor is complicated. The nurse's roles are both supportive and teacher/counselor/advocate. Knowledge of medical management for each condition is essential to implementation of the nursing process. This knowledge enables the nurse to work collaboratively with the physician and to meet the client's knowledge and emotional needs.

TRIAL OF LABOR

A **trial of labor** (TOL) is a reasonable period (4 to 6 hours) of active labor allowed for assessment of the possibility of a safe vaginal delivery for the mother and infant. TOL may be initiated when the mother has a questionable pelvis (size or shape), when she wishes to have a vaginal delivery after a previous cesarean birth, and for abnormal presentations of the fetus. Fetal sonography and/or maternal pelvimetry are used before a TOL to rule out fetopelvic disproportion. The cervix must be soft and dilatable. During TOL, the woman is evaluated for active labor including adequate contractions, engagement and descent of the presenting part, and effacement and dilatation of the cervix. Induction of labor is seldom implemented.

The nurse assesses the condition of the mother and fetus during this TOL. If maternal or fetal complications are identified, the nurse is responsible for initiating appropriate actions, including notifying the obstetrician, and evaluating and documenting the maternal or fetal response to the interventions.

INDUCTION OF LABOR

Induction of labor is the initiation of uterine contractions before their spontaneous onset for the purpose of bringing about delivery. Induction may be indicated for a variety of medical and obstetric reasons, including pregnancy-induced hypertension, diabetes mellitus and other maternal medical problems, postterm gestation, and suspected fetal compromise (e.g., intrauterine growth retardation). With such conditions, the risk of delivery to the mother or fetus is less than the

Table 26-2 **Bishop's Scale**

	Score			
	0	1	2	3
Dilatation (cm)	0	1-2	3-4	5-6
Effacement (%)	0-30	40-50	60-70	80
Station (cm)	−3	−2	−1	+1
Cervical consistency	Firm	Medium	Soft	
Fetal position	Posterior	Midline	Anterior	

risk of continuing the pregnancy (Marshall, 1985). *Elective induction* may be indicated when there is a risk of a precipitate delivery (≤3 hours of labor) to prevent an uncontrolled out-of-hospital delivery.

Both chemical and mechanical methods are used to induce labor. Intravenous oxytocin and amniotomy are the most common methods used in the United States. Prostaglandin gel and other cervical ripening agents are also used, but have not yet been approved by the U.S. Food and Drug Administration (FDA) (NAACOG, 1988). Less commonly used methods of induction include nipple stimulation, ingestion of castor oil, soapsuds enema, and acupuncture. Continued research is needed to evaluate the effectiveness of these methods.

Success rates for induction of labor are higher when the cervix is favorable, or inducible. A scoring system such as Bishop's scale (Table 26-2) can be used to evaluate inducibility. For example, a score of 9 or more on this scale indicates the cervix is soft, anterior, 50% effaced, and dilated 2 cm or more; the presenting part is engaged. Labor should be successful.

Amniotomy

Amniotomy (artificial rupture of membranes [AROM]) can be used to stimulate labor when the cervix is favorable. Before the procedure, an explanation of what to expect is given to the mother; she is also assured the procedure is painless for her and the fetus. The membranes are ruptured with an amnihook or other sharp instrument; amniotic fluid is allowed to drain slowly. The fluid is assessed for color, odor, and consistency (i.e., absence of meconium or blood). The fetal heart rate (FHR) is assessed before and after the procedure to detect changes that may indicate presence of cord compression or prolapse.

Labor usually begins within 12 hours of the rupture; however, if amniotomy does not stimulate labor, prolonged rupture may lead to infection. For this reason, amniotomy is often used in combination with oxytocin induction.

Oxytocin

Stimulation of labor with **oxytocin** may be used either to induce the labor process or to augment a labor that is progressing slowly because of inadequate uterine contractions. It can also be used to assess fetal response to the stress of labor contractions (oxytocin challenge test [OCT]); see Chapter 14.

The *indications* for oxytocin induction of labor may include, but are not limited to, the following:

1. Slowing of progress of labor
2. Management of abortion, to stimulate the uterus to pass the conceptus
3. Prolonged rupture of membranes
4. Prolonged pregnancy (42 to 43 weeks)
5. Preterm delivery in diabetic mother or mother with severe isoimmunization
6. Severe preeclampsia, abruptio placentae, or fetal death necessitating termination of the pregnancy artificially
7. Multigravidas with a history of precipitate labor who live a long distance from the hospital

The management of stimulation of labor is the same regardless of indication. Because of the potential dangers associated with the use of injectable oxytocin in the prenatal and intranatal periods, the FDA has issued restrictions on its use.

Contraindications to oxytocic stimulation of labor include, but are not limited to, the following:

1. Fetopelvic disproportion
2. Fetal distress
3. Placenta previa
4. Prior classic uterine incision or uterine surgery
5. Active genital herpes infection

Hazards of oxytocin stimulation to both mother and infant include the following:

1. Maternal
   a. Tumultuous labor and tetanic contractions, which may cause premature separation of the placenta, rupture of the uterus, laceration of the cervix, or post-delivery hemorrhage
   b. Sequelae to above complications: infection, disseminated intravascular coagulation (DIC), amniotic fluid embolism
   c. Fear or anxiety: may be compounded if the procedure is not successful (the woman must be aware of this possibility and of what other techniques can be used)
2. Fetal
   a. Fetal asphyxia and neonatal hypoxia from too frequent and prolonged uterine contractions
   b. Physical injury
   c. Prematurity, if the estimated date of delivery (EDD) has been estimated inaccurately

Initiation of induction or augmentation of labor with oxytocin is the responsibility of the physician, although the medication is often administered by a nurse. A written protocol for the preparation and administration of oxytocin should be established by the obstetric department in each institution. Until recently, the aim of induction with oxytocin was to achieve a contraction pattern that simulated the active phase of labor as quickly as possible. Recent research on uterine tolerence to oxytocin has shown that lower doses given at longer intervals are as effective as previous protocols and are less likely to cause uterine hyperstimulation and dysfunctional labor (Seitchik, 1987).

After the woman has been evaluated for induction, the following recommended procedures are to be carried out in a labor and delivery setting (NAACOG, 1988):

1. Use of a primary intravenous infusion of a physiologic electrolytic fluid. Intravenous medications other than oxytocin can be administered through this line.
2. Use of a secondary intravenous infusion containing dilute oxytocin (usually 10 U/1000 ml). This line should be connected close to the primary venipuncture site. No medication except oxytocin should be given through this line.
3. Initial dose of 0.5 to 1 mU/minute, with increases at 30- to 60-minute intervals until the desired contraction pattern is achieved.
4. Once the cervix is dilated 5 to 6 cm and labor is established, the oxytocin dose can be reduced by similar decrements.
5. Usually no more than 20 to 40 mU of oxytocin/minute are needed to achieve progressive cervical dilatation.
6. The FHR, uterine resting tone, and frequency, duration, and intensity of contractions are monitored continuously; maternal blood pressure and pulse are monitored at 30- to 60-minute intervals and/or when doses are changed.
7. ***Oxytocin is discontinued immediately and the physician notified of uterine hyperstimulation or non-reassuring FHR.*** With the latter, other nursing interventions, such as administration of oxygen by face mask and positioning the woman on her left side, are implemented immediately.
8. Documentation of maternal and fetal assessments is necessary in the medical record and on the fetal monitor tracing.

Induction of Labor for Intrauterine Fetal Demise

Labor is often spontaneous within several weeks of intrauterine fetal demise (IUFD). If there are complications, or if the woman and physician decide to terminate the pregnancy after the diagnosis is confirmed, induction of labor may be planned. Oxytocin induction procedures except for monitoring FHR are appropriate.

Prostaglandin E_2 suppositories may also be used to induce delivery safely up to 28 weeks of gestation, and after 28 weeks with careful assessment for hyperstimulation and uterine rupture (ACOG, 1987).

Augmentation of Labor

Augmentation of labor refers to the use of oxytocics or other methods to add or increase the action of the uterine muscle. Augmentation is usually implemented for hypotonic dysfunctional labor. The procedures used are the same as those used for oxytocin induction of labor.

Procedure 26-1 summarizes the nursing responsibilities for induction of labor by amniotomy and oxytocin administration.

❑ FORCEPS DELIVERY

Obstetric forceps are made from two double-curved, spoonlike articulated blades. They are used to assist in the expulsion of the fetal head. The commonly employed forceps have a cephalic curve shaped similarly to that of the fetal head. A pelvic curve of the blades conforms to the pelvic axis. The blades are joined by a pin, screw, or groove arrangement. These locks prevent the forceps from compressing the fetal skull. Indications for **forceps delivery** may be maternal or fetal, and include the following:

1. *Maternal.* To shorten the second stage in dystocia (difficult labor), or when the mother's expulsive efforts are deficient (e.g., she is tired or she has been given spinal anesthesia), or when the woman is endangered (e.g., cardiac decompensation).
2. *Fetal.* To deliver a fetus in distress, in certain abnormal presentations, in arrest of rotation, and to deliver an aftercoming head in a breech presentation.

Prerequisites for Forceps Operations

The following conditions must apply for successful forceps delivery:

1. *Fully dilated cervix.* Severe lacerations and hemorrhage may ensue if a rim of cervical tissue remains.
2. *Head engaged.* The extraction of a mature fetus with a "high" (unengaged) head usually is disastrous.
3. *Vertex presentation or face presentation* (mentum anterior). Other presentations require wider-than-average pelvic diameters.

PROCEDURE 26-1

INDUCTION OF LABOR

DEFINITION

An obstetric procedure in which labor is started or augmented artificially by means of amniotomy or administration of oxytocics.

PURPOSE

To initiate or augment the uterine contractions of labor.

EQUIPMENT

Oxytocin (Pitocin or synthetic oxytocin [Syntocin]) 10 U.
1000 ml 5% dextrose in water or Ringer's lactate or normal saline for piggyback set-up (maintenance IV).
1000 ml 5% dextrose in water, Ringer's lactate, or normal saline for oxytocin solution
Infusion pump (e.g., IVAC) or standard pump (Harvard)
Amnihook or Allis clamp for amniotomy. Also bedpan or fracture pan.

NURSING ACTIONS	RATIONALE
Apply fetal and maternal electronic monitor before beginning induction or augmentation.	Obtains constant, accurate recording of FHR and contractions.
	Obtains baseline reading.
Explain technique, rationale, and reactions to expect:	Promotes cooperation of woman and family.
Route and rate: what "piggyback" is for.	Lessens anxiety over technique.
Reasons for use:	Assures woman and family of careful monitoring.
▪ Induce labor.	Prepares woman and family for chances of success.
▪ Improve (augment) labor.	
Reactions to expect—nature of contractions: "Intensity of contraction increases more rapidly, holds the peak longer, and ends more quickly. The contractions will begin to come regularly and more often."	
Monitoring to anticipate:	
▪ Maternal: blood pressure (BP), pulse (P), uterine contractions, uterine tone.	
▪ Fetal: heart rate, activity.	
Success to expect—a favorable outcome will depend on inducibility of the cervix (Bishop's scale score of 9 or more).	
Position woman in left lateral position.	Maximizes placental perfusion and oxygenation of fetus.
Prepare solutions and administer according to prescribed orders with pump delivery system:	Promotes safety. A piggyback setup permits the induction solution to be stopped while the vein remains open with the second solution.
▪ Infusion pump and solution is set up	
▪ Piggyback solution is connected to IV line	
▪ Solution with oxytocin is flagged with a medication label	
▪ Begin induction at 0.5 to 1 mU/minute.	Ensures that only amount of medication necessary for success is used.
▪ Increase dose by 1 to 2 mU/minute at 30- to 60-minute intervals.	Determines minimum amount of medication necessary for success.
Maintain dose when:	Maintains needed stimulation and avoids overstimulation.
▪ Intensity of contraction results in intrauterine pressures of 50 to 75 mm Hg (by internal monitor).	
▪ Duration of contraction is 40 to 60 seconds.	
▪ Frequency of contractions is 2½ to 4-minute intervals.	
▪ Assess intake and output; limit IV intake to 1000 ml/24 hours; output should be 120 ml or more every 4 hours.	Avoids water intoxication (fluid overload).
▪ Monitor for nausea, vomiting, headache, hypotension	Identifies signs of water intoxication.
Discontinue infusion of oxytocin, keep maintenance line open, and notify physician if ***danger signs*** occur:	Prevents further complication.
▪ ***Contractions:*** excessive intrauterine pressure above 75 mm Hg, duration over 90 seconds, and frequency more than every 2 minutes.	Overstimulation of the uterine muscle can cause tetany and rupture of the uterus.
▪ ***Fetal distress:*** fetal bradycardia, tachycardia, or heart irregularity.	Fetoplacental unit may not be able to withstand the stress of labor.
Keep woman and family informed of progress.	Reduces anxiety.

Continued.

PROCEDURE 26-1— cont'd

NURSING ACTIONS	RATIONALE
For amniotomy:	
Position woman on bedpan or fracture pan.	Catches amniotic fluid when amniotic sac is torn.
Person performing procedure puts on gloves and inserts first two fingers of one hand into cervix until membranes are identified.	Maintains clean environment. Serves as a guide for the amnihook or Allis clamp.
Amnihook or Allis clamp is inserted alongside fingers and membranes are hooked and torn by the instrument.	Allows for release of amniotic fluid.
Assess FHR.	Checks for compression or prolapse of umbilical cord.
Assess color, odor, and consistency of fluid.	Discoloration or foul odor signals meconium passage by fetus or infection.
Charting Medication: kind, amount, time of beginning, increasing dose, maintaining dose, and discontinuing medication in client record and on monitoring strip. Reactions of mother and fetus: ▪ Pattern of labor. ▪ Progress in labor. ▪ FHR. Signs of maternal or fetal stress.	Provides data base against which to compare future findings. Provides data base for implementation. Promotes collaboration with other members of health care team. Documents maternal-fetal surveillance.

4. *Membranes ruptured* to ensure a firm grasp of the forceps on the fetal head.
5. *No cephalopelvic disproportion.* If there is engagement, there must be no outlet contracture or gross sacral deformity.
6. *Empty bladder and bowel* to avoid visceral laceration and fistula formation.

Level of Forceps Application

The station of the head determines the level of forceps application and, generally, the relative difficulty to be expected in forceps operations.

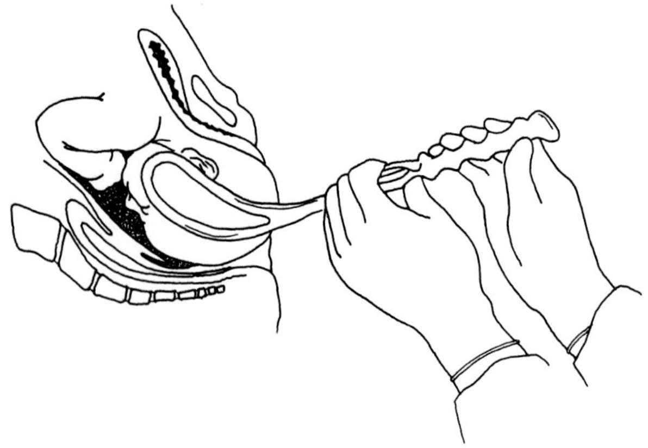

Fig. 26-8 Low forceps extraction of the head.

High Forceps. The biparietal diameter of the vertex is above the ischial spines (not engaged) when the forceps are applied. There is rarely, if ever, justification for their use because of the risk of maternal and fetal morbidity and mortality (Krieger, 1987).

Midforceps. The vertex is at the ischial spines, almost to the ischial tuberosities on application of the forceps. The delivery often is difficult, depending on the size of the vertex, its position, and the pelvic architecture and diameters. The use of midforceps remains controversial (Hayashi, 1985; Friedman, 1987).

Outlet (Low) Forceps. Forceps are applied when the scalp is visible at the introitus without separating the labia. The blades are applied principally to provide control and guidance of the head (Fig. 26-8).

Nursing Care

The nurse obtains forceps designated by the physician (Fig. 26-9). The FHR is checked, reported, and recorded *before* forceps are *applied.* The mother is informed that the forceps blades fit like two tablespoons around an egg. The blades come over the baby's ears. The FHR is rechecked, reported, and recorded *before traction* is applied after application of forceps. Compression of the cord between the fetal head and the forceps would cause a drop in FHR. The physician would then remove and reapply the forceps.

After delivery, the mother is assessed for vaginal and cervical lacerations (bleeding occurs even with a contracted uterus) and urine retention, which may result

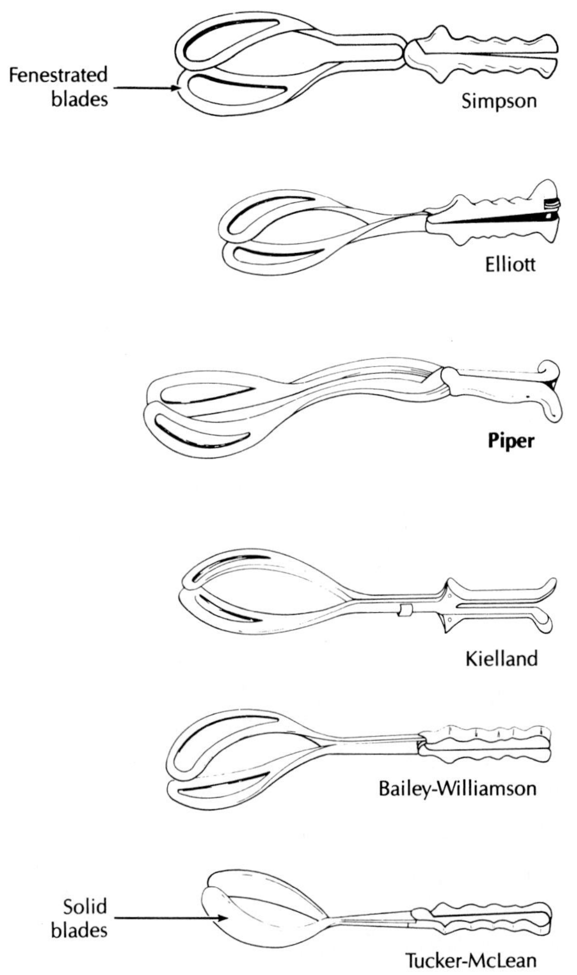

Fig. 26-9 Types of forceps. Piper forceps are used to assist birth of the head in breech delivery.

from bladder injuries. The infant should be assessed for bruising or abrasions at the site of the blade applications, facial palsy resulting from pressure of the blades on the facial nerve, and subdural hematoma.

❑ VACUUM EXTRACTION

Vacuum extraction is a delivery method involving the attachment of a vacuum cup to the fetal head, using negative pressure. It is a popular alternative to forceps delivery in Europe, but is not as popular in the United States. Indications for use are similar to those for outlet forceps, but especially failure to rotate and arrest of second stage of labor (Galvan and Broekhuizen, 1987). Prerequisites for use include a vertex presentation, ruptured membranes, and absence of fetopelvic disproportion.

The woman is prepared for a vaginal delivery in the lithotomy position to allow for sufficient traction. The cup is applied to the fetal head and a caput develops inside the cup as the pressure is initiated (Fig. 26-10, *A*). Traction is then applied to facilitate descent of the fetal head. As the head crowns, an **episiotomy** is performed if necessary, and the vacuum cup is released and removed after delivery of the head (Fig. 26-10, *B*). If vacuum extraction is not successful, a forceps or cesarean delivery will be performed.

Risks to the newborn include cephalhematoma, scalp lacerations, and subdural hematoma. Maternal complications are uncommon but may include perineal, vaginal, and cervical lacerations.

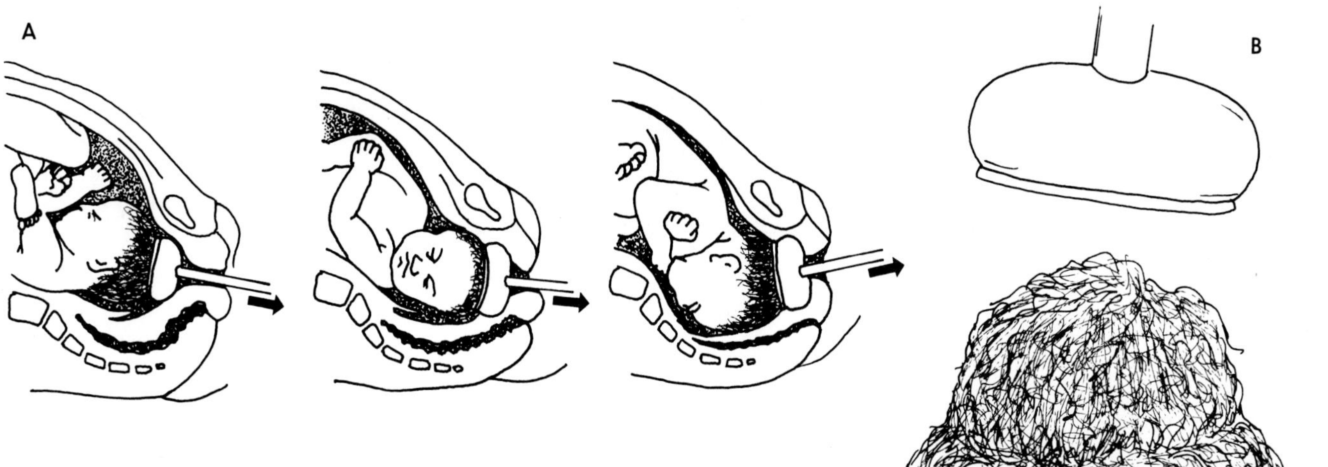

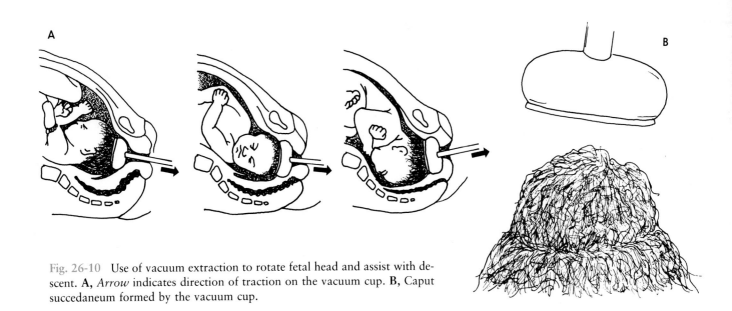

Fig. 26-10 Use of vacuum extraction to rotate fetal head and assist with descent. **A,** *Arrow* indicates direction of traction on the vacuum cup. **B,** Caput succedaneum formed by the vacuum cup.

Nursing Care

The nurse's role for the woman delivering by vacuum extraction is one of support person and educator. The nurse can prepare the woman for the delivery and encourage her to remain active in the birth process by pushing during contractions. After delivery, the newborn should be observed for signs of infection at the application site and cerebral irritation (e.g., poor sucking, listlessness). The parents may need to be reassured that the caput succedaneum will begin to disappear in a few hours.

❑ CESAREAN DELIVERY

Cesarean delivery is the delivery of a fetus through a transabdominal incision of the uterus. Although the myth persists that Julius Caesar was delivered in this manner, the derivation of the term is more likely from the Latin word *caedo* meaning "to cut." Whether cesarean delivery is planned (elective) or unplanned (emergency), the loss of the experience of delivering a child in the traditional manner may have a negative effect on a woman's self-concept. In an effort to maintain the focus on the *birth* of a child rather than the operative procedure, the term *cesarean delivery* or *cesarean birth* has come into common usage. The mother experiences abdominal rather than vaginal birth.

The basic purpose or use of cesarean delivery is to preserve the life or health of the mother and her fetus. The use of cesarean delivery is based on evidence of maternal or fetal stress. Maternal and fetal morbidity and mortality have decreased since the advent of modern surgical methods and care. However, cesarean delivery still poses threats to the health of both mother and infant. The technique of cesarean surgery has changed. Today incisions into the lower uterine segment rather than into the muscular body of the uterus permit a more effective healing.

The incidence of cesarean births has increased dramatically in the last 25 years. From the mid-1960s to the late 1980s, the cesarean delivery rate has increased from less than 5% to more than 24% (NCHS, 1989), or about one fourth, of all births.

Indications. There are few absolute indications for performing a cesarean delivery. Today most are performed primarily for the benefit of the fetus. Four diagnostic categories are responsible for 75% to 90% of the cesarean births: dystocia, repeat cesarean, breech presentation, and fetal distress (Pauerstein, 1987). Other indications for the procedure include active herpes viral infection, prolapsed umbilical cord, medical complications such as pregnancy-induced hypertension, placental abnormalities such as placenta previa and premature separation (abruption), malpresentations such as shoulder presentation, and fetal anomalies such as hydrocephaly.

Surgical Techniques. The two main types of cesarean operation are *classic* and *lower segment* cesarean deliveries. Classic cesarean delivery is rarely performed today. It may be used when rapid delivery is necessary and in some cases of shoulder presentation and placenta previa. The incision is vertical into the upper body of the uterus (Fig. 26-11, *A*). The procedure is associated with a higher incidence of blood loss, infection, and uterine rupture in subsequent pregnancies than lower segment cesarean delivery.

Lower segment cesarean delivery can be performed through a vertical (Krönig) or transverse (Kehr) incision (Fig. 26-11, *B* and *C*). The transverse incision is more popular because it is easier to perform, is associated with less blood loss and fewer postoperative infections, and is less likely to rupture in subsequent pregnancies (Cunningham, MacDonald, and Gant, 1989).

Elective Cesarean Delivery. Women electing to have cesarean delivery have time for psychologic preparation. The psychic response of women in these groups may differ. Those women scheduled for *repeat surgery* may have disturbing memories of the conditions preceding the initial surgical delivery and their experiences in the postoperative recovery period. The added burden of care of an infant while recovering from a surgical operation may be faced with great concern. Some women elect the repeat cesarean birth because they can exert more *control* over events than if a trial of labor fails and an unplanned cesarean delivery is necessary. Other women desire the convenience of a planned birth experience.

Women who face elective cesarean delivery for the *first time* share with other surgical clients the same apprehensions concerning surgery. These anxieties are coupled with the uncertainty of being able to cope with child care after a major operation.

Emergency Cesarean Delivery. Women having emergency cesarean deliveries share with their families abrupt changes in their expectations for birth, postdelivery care, and the care of the new baby at home. This may be an extremely traumatic experience. The woman approaches surgery usually tired and discouraged after a fruitless labor. She is worried about her own and the child's condition. She may be dehydrated, with low glycogen reserves. All preoperative procedures must be done quickly and competently. The time for explanation of procedures and of operation is short. Since maternal and family anxiety levels are high, much of what is said is forgotten or perhaps misconstrued. Postoperatively, time must be spent reviewing the events preceding the operation and the operation itself to ensure that the woman understands what has happened. Fatigue is often noticeable in these women. They need much supportive care.

Many women who experience a cesarean birth speak of the feelings that interfere with their maintain-

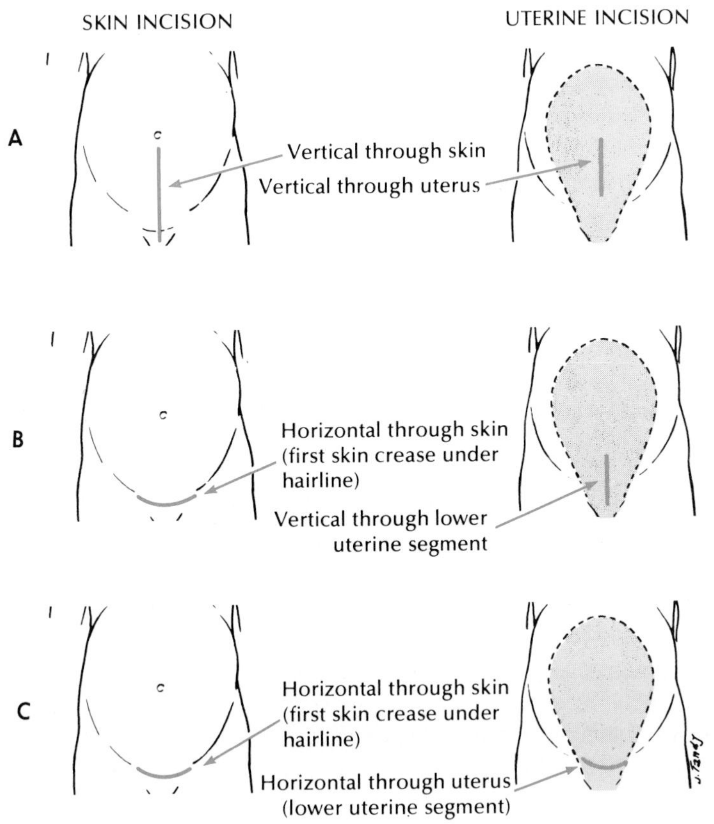

Fig. 26-11 Cesarean delivery: skin and uterine incisions. **A,** Classic: vertical incisions of skin and uterus. **B,** Low cervical: horizontal incision of skin; vertical incision of uterus. **C,** Low cervical: horizontal incisions of skin and uterus.

ing an adequate self-concept. These feelings include fear, disappointment, frustration at losing control, anger (the "why me" syndrome), and loss of self-esteem as their body image is not sustained. Success in mothering activities and in the recovery process can do much to restore these women's self-esteem. Some women see the scar as mutilating, and worries concerning sexual attractiveness may surface. Some men are fearful of resuming intercourse because of the fear of hurting their mates.

Professional staff can expect some anger directed toward them. Parents will wonder if it was absolutely necessary for them to have a cesarean delivery. Such feelings may surface even years later.

Prenatal Preparation for Cesarean Birth

Concerned professional and lay groups in the community have established councils for cesarean birth to meet the needs of these women and their families. Such groups advocate including preparation for cesarean birth in all parenthood preparation classes. No woman can be guaranteed a vaginal delivery, even if she is in good health and there is no indication of danger to the fetus before the onset of labor. Every woman needs to be aware of and prepared for this eventuality. The unknown and unexpected are ego weakening.

Childbirth educators stress the importance of emphasizing the similarities as well as differences between cesarean and vaginal birth. Also, in support of the philosophy of family-centered birth, many hospitals have changed policies to permit fathers to share in these births as they have in vaginal ones. Women undergoing cesarean birth agree that the continued presence and support of their partners have helped them experience a positive response to the whole process.

Client teaching guidelines for preparing the expectant woman and her family for cesarean birth are presented on pp. 774-775.

Care During Cesarean Delivery

The goal for the woman and her family is family-centered care for a cesarean delivery. Facing cesarean delivery relates to the option for father to be present at the birth, availability of regional as well as general an-

Guidelines for Client Teaching

PREPARATION FOR CESAREAN DELIVERY

ASSESSMENT

1. Woman in third trimester of pregnancy.
2. Woman to be prepared for possible cesarean delivery.
3. Woman to have repeat cesarean delivery.

NURSING DIAGNOSES

Knowledge deficit related to cesarean delivery.

Knowledge deficit related to testing for fetal well-being and **fetal lung maturity.**

Anxiety and fear related to possible or actual cesarean delivery.

Self-esteem disturbance related to unsatisfied planned birth experience.

Potential altered parenting.

Personal identity disturbance related to loss of control over decisions and powerlessness.

GOALS

Short-term

Woman (couple) will learn that a cesarean delivery can be a positive birth experience.

Woman (couple) will learn the reasons for the cesarean delivery.

Intermediate

Woman (couple) will learn the rationale for prenatal testing and how the results determine cesarean delivery.

Woman (couple) will learn about medications and forms of anesthesia given for cesarean deliveries.

Long-term

Woman (couple) will take a tour of the operating room/delivery room.

Woman (couple) verbalizes feelings about cesarean delivery.

Woman (couple) will learn immediate preoperative preparation for cesarean delivery.

Woman (couple) understands breastfeeding is still an option.

Woman understands that pain relief will be provided.

REFERENCES AND TEACHING AIDS

Books and pamphlets describing cesarean delivery in a positive way.

Discussion and lecture, use of slides, charts, illustrations.

Films or videos depicting a cesarean birth.

Tour of the hospital's labor and delivery suite, including the operative area and recovery area.

Discussions with parents who have experienced cesarean delivery.

RATIONALE/CONTENT	TEACHING ACTIONS
Knowledge and support provide a basis for making informed choices and minimize feelings of loss of control, fear, and anxiety:	
Explain similarities between vaginal and cesarean births.	Use charts, diagrams, and audiovisual aids to show differences and similarities between vaginal and cesarean births.
Discuss possible prenatal testing and how fetal well-being is illustrated (e.g., nonstress test [NST], contraction stress test [CST], or oxytocin challenge test [OCT], ultrasonography, amniocentesis, foam stability index, and biophysical profile) (Chapter 22).	Use diagrams or audiovisual aids for tests if possible. Discuss rationale for each test. Explain where tests are done and by whom. Explain what information the tests provide about fetal well-being or maturity. Indicate that interpretations of tests will be explained as soon as results are available.
Anticipatory guidance for preoperative and postoperative care assists with individual coping:	
Discuss types of anesthesia that are used for cesarean delivery—general, spinal, epidural	Show a diagram or picture of a woman receiving an epidural or spinal.
Explain preoperative preparation and postoperative assessments that will be implemented.	Explain shaving the abdomen, insertion of an indwelling urinary catheter, and starting intravenous infusion. Explain blood drawing for laboratory tests such as baselines for hemoglobin and hematocrit, and blood type to cross-match for possible transfusion. Explain NPO status. Discuss what will be done in the recovery area after the operation

Guidelines for Client Teaching—cont'd

RATIONALE/CONTENT	TEACHING ACTIONS
	Explain postoperative procedures such as turn, cough, deep breathe (TCDB), fundal and incision checks, and pain relief.
	Reassure woman, if she is up to it, and her newborn is well, she may hold the baby at this time.
	The father may also interact with the newborn.
Discuss alternate positions for breastfeeding so that the incision is not interfered with.	Reassure woman that she may still breastfeed.
Arrange for a tour of the labor and delivery area, include the operating and recovery areas.	Take woman (couple) on a tour. Point out important sights, sounds, and smells at that time. Leave time for questions.

EVALUATION Couple verbalizes understanding of information presented; they ask appropriate questions. Woman (couple) sees cesarean delivery as a positive, alternate method of childbirth, and it is a satisfying experience for them.

esthesia, and receiving support from the health care staff.

The *preparation* of the woman for cesarean birth is the same for either elective or emergency surgery. The obstetrician discusses the need for the cesarean delivery and the prognosis for mother and infant with the woman and her family. The anesthesiologist assesses the woman's cardiopulmonary system and presents the options for anesthesia. Informed consent is obtained for the procedure. Procedure 26-2 contains the nursing care necessary in preparation for surgery.

Once the woman has been taken to surgery her care becomes the responsibility of the obstetric team, surgeon, anesthesiologist, pediatrician, and nursing staff (Fig. 26-12). If possible, the father, gowned appropriately, accompanies the mother to the surgical unit and remains close to her.

If the father is not allowed or chooses not to be present, the nurse can stay in communication with him and give progress reports when possible. If the mother is awake during the delivery, the nurse can tell her what is happening and provide support. The mother may be anxious about the sensations she is experiencing, such as cold solutions used to prep the abdomen and pressure or pulling during the actual delivery of the infant. She may also be apprehensive because of the bright lights, unfamiliar equipment present, and masked and gowned personnel in the room.

Care of the infant is delegated to a pediatrician and a nurse because these infants are considered to be at risk until there is evidence of physiologic stability after delivery.

A crib with resuscitative equipment is readied before surgery. Those responsible for care are expert in resuscitative techniques, as well as in observational skills for detecting normal infant responses. After birth, if the infant's condition permits, she or he is given to the father to hold and to show to the mother (Fig. 26-13). The attachment process can continue uninterrupted. Some mothers are able to breastfeed the infant in the recovery room area. However, many are not ready for this direct participation. They need to be reassured that the parent-child attachment process will not be impaired.

If compromised, the infant is transported immediately to the infant intensive care unit. Personnel keep the family informed of the infant's progress. Father-child contacts are initiated as soon as possible.

If the family-oriented approach is not feasible, the family is directed to the surgical waiting room. The physician reviews with the family members the condition of the mother and child after the birth is completed. Family members may accompany the infant as she or he is transferred to the nursery. This gives the family opportunity to see and admire the infant.

Postpartum Care

The care of the woman after cesarean delivery combines surgical and obstetric nursing. Once surgery is completed, the mother is transferred to the recovery room for intensive care until her condition stabilizes. Then she is moved to the postdelivery unit. See specific nursing care plan on pp. 778-780.

Text continued on p. 781.

PROCEDURE 26-2

PREPARATION FOR CESAREAN DELIVERY

DEFINITION

Delivery of the fetus by an abdominal and uterine incision.

PURPOSE

To complete the preparation for surgery as competently and quickly as possible.

To provide emotional support through a caring attitude, calm manner, and technical competence.

To decrease client anxiety by reassurance.

EQUIPMENT

Skin preparation kit (for shaving); retention (Foley) catheter kit; IV infusions (as ordered); medications (as ordered).

NURSING ACTIONS	RATIONALE
Wash hands before and after touching woman and equipment. Glove, prn.	Prevents nosocomial infection and implements universal precautions.
Explain procedures to be carried out.	Keeps the family informed, decreases anxiety, and elicits cooperation.
Take and record vital signs, blood pressure, FHR.	Establishes baseline data.
Complete preoperative preparation of abdomen. The abdomen is shaved beginning at the level of the xiphoid process and extending to the flank on both sides and down to the pubic area.	Minimizes potential for infection.
Insert a retention catheter (Foley). It is attached to a continuous drainage system. Care must be taken that catheter is placed properly within the bladder and is draining adequately.	Ensures the bladder remains empty during the operation.
Administer preoperative medications as ordered:	
Analgesia.	Promotes relaxation before surgery.
Atropine.	Minimizes amount of secretions in bronchial tree.
Antacid.	Prevents irritative pneumonia if aspiration of gastric juice from stomach occurs.
If spinal or epidural anesthesia is used, an antacid may be the only medication administered.	
Begin IV infusion. 1000 ml Ringer's lactate solution, or 5% dextrose in water or saline.	Maintains hydration. Provides an open line for administration of blood, medications, etc. if needed.
Send specimens to laboratory for analysis:	
Send blood for typing and cross-matching. Two units of matched blood are kept in reserve for 48 hours after surgery.	Replaces blood loss during surgery or postpartum if excessive.
Send urine for routine analysis.	Establishes baseline data.
Send blood for CBC and chemistry.	Establishes baseline data.
Complete preoperative care including removal of dentures, contact lenses, rings, and fingernail polish. Valuables are given to support person or put into safekeeping.	Protects client.
Ready the woman's chart for use in surgery and see whether permission forms for care of the mother and infant are signed. If the woman has received an analgesic or anesthetic, the responsible adult accompanying the woman signs the necessary forms.	Provides data base for future comparison. Provides data base for implementation of the next steps in the nursing process. Promotes collaboration with other members of the health care team.
Provide as much information as possible to the woman and her family while carrying out the necessary care.	Relieves apprehension and promotes understanding.
Notify nursery and pediatrician of impending cesarean birth.	Ensures availability of equipment and personnel for immediate infant care.
Encourage the support person's presence as much as possible during preparation.	Provides continued emotional support.
Assess perceptions about having a cesarean delivery.	Promotes ventilation of feelings and identifies potential for disturbance in self-concept during the postpartum period.

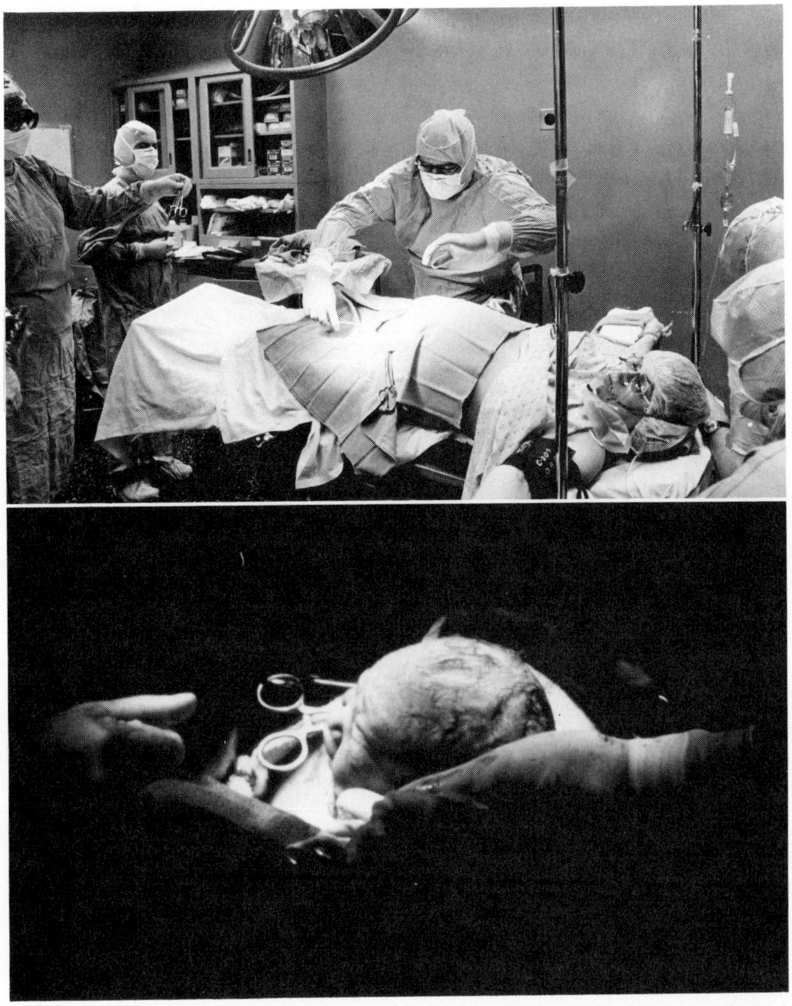

A

B

Fig. 26-12 **A,** Surgical team preparing woman for surgery. **B,** Birth of infant. (**A,** Courtesy Jose Mercado. From News and Publication Service, Stanford University, Stanford, Calif. **B,** Courtesy Marjorie Pyle, RNC Lifecircle, Costa Mesa, Calif.)

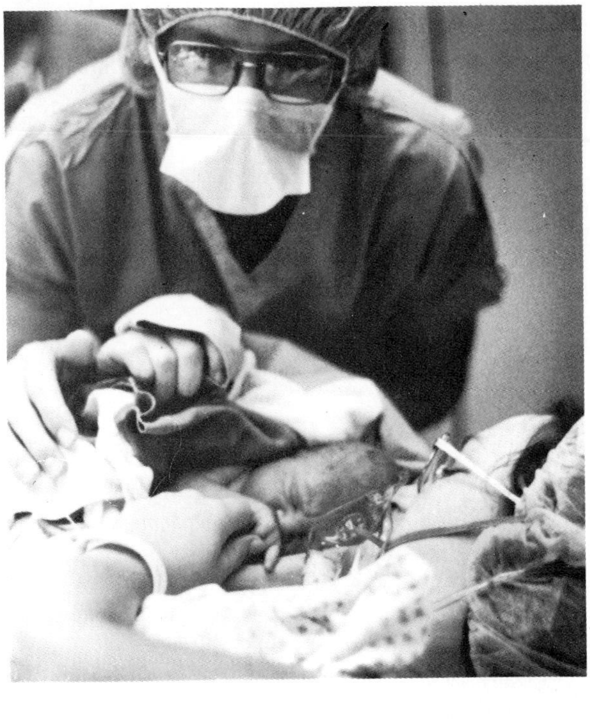

Fig. 26-13 Parents and their newborn. (Courtesy Captain Barbara Kalmen.)

Specific Nursing Care Plan

CARE AFTER CESAREAN DELIVERY

Maggie V., a nullipara, had an unplanned low transverse cesarean delivery for fetopelvic disproportion. Maggie had epidural anesthesia. She and her husband had attended childbirth classes and had anticipated a normal vaginal delivery without anesthesia. Maggie delivered a viable female (Apgar scores 8-9, weight 3800 g), who was admitted to the newborn nursery after being checked by a pediatrician and shown to the parents. Maggie's husband was present during the delivery and recovery period.

After the delivery, Maggie was transferred to the recovery unit. She was awake and moved all extremities when asked. She had an IV of 5% dextrose in Ringer's lactate, with 20 U of oxytocin added, infused at a rate of 125 ml/hour. The indwelling urinary catheter was in place and draining well.

Initial assessment revealed the following:

1. Fundus firm at 2 cm above umbilicus.
2. Small amount of lochia rubra present.
3. Abdominal dressing dry and intact.
4. Blood pressure—120/86.
5. Temperature—37° C (98.6° F); pulse—90 bpm; respirations—16/minute.
6. Complaining of pain at incision site.
7. Wants to rest before seeing daughter.

Standard postoperative (cesarean) orders per hospital policy or physician.

ASSESSMENT	NURSING DIAGNOSIS (ND), PLAN/GOAL (P/G)	RATIONALE/ IMPLEMENTATION	EVALUATION
Experiencing postoperative pain.	ND: Pain related to incision. P/G: Maggie will verbalize decrease in pain after interventions implemented.	*Discomfort can delay healing and attachment and compromise coping:* Assess nature of pain and where it's located. Administer pain medication every q3-4h as ordered and evaluate response. Provide comfort measures (e.g., position changes, support body parts with pillows). Encourage relaxation techniques.	Maggie verbalizes a decrease in pain.
Maggie is very tired after delivery and has not seen daughther except briefly after delivery.	ND: Potential altered parenting related to unplanned cesarean delivery. P/G: Couple will display positive bonding and attachment behaviors.	*Maggie (couple) needs assistance in beginning attachment to her (their) infant:* Model bonding techniques to parents. Encourage frequent visiting between parents and newborn. Encourage participation in infant care as soon as Maggie feels able. If feeding is attempted, the infant can be placed on pillows to relieve pressure on mother's abdomen, or Maggie can use the side-lying position.	Couple states positive feelings toward baby. Maggie (couple) demonstrates positive attachment—eye contact, cuddling, etc.

Specific Nursing Care Plan—cont'd

ASSESSMENT	NURSING DIAGNOSIS (ND), PLAN/GOAL (P/G)	RATIONALE/ IMPLEMENTATION	EVALUATION
Assess for signs of infection at surgical incision site (Fig. 26-14).	ND: Potential for infection related to cesarean birth. P/G: Maggie does not develop infection.	*Postpartum or incisional infection is a potential complication:* Assess vital signs, especially temperature, q4h × 24 hr; then q8h if within normal limits. Assess incisional healing, odor of lochia q8h. Provide good perineal care with each pad change. Change abdominal dressing as needed and/or provide heat lamp to incision as ordered. Maintain nutrition and hydration. Administer postoperative antibiotics as ordered.	Maggie remains afebrile. Maggie does not develop postpartum/ postoperative infection.
Assess for postoperative complications as a result of immobility: respiratory, gastointestinal, neuromuscular, cardiovascular (including coagulopathy), urinary, and emotional.	ND: Potential for injury related to sequelae of immobility. P/G: Maggie will experience no complications as a result of immobility.	*Postoperative sequelae to immobility are possible complications:* Assess heart rate, respirations, breath sounds, bowel sounds, Homans' sign at least q8h. Monitor intake and output at least q8h. Assess affect and emotional responses q8h. Teach and encourage coughing and deep breathing and use of incentive spirometry (if ordered) q2-4h × 24 hr. Encourage and assist with range of motion q2h × 24 hr and ambulation as tolerated. Medicate and provide comfort measures to promote mobility.	Maggie experiences no respiratory, gastrointestinal, neuromuscular, emotional, urinary, or cardiovascular problems as a result of immobility.

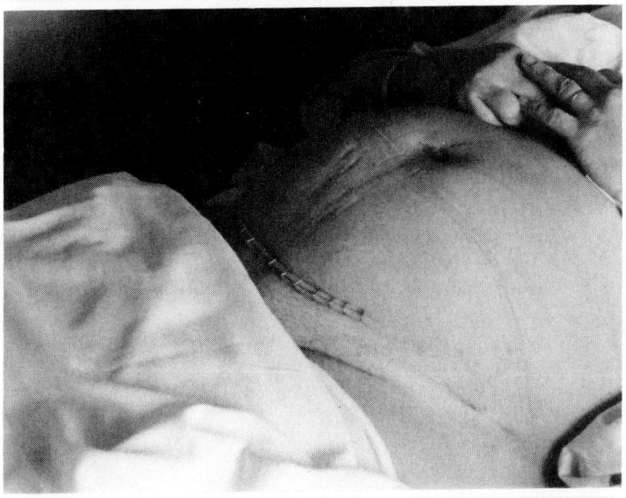

Fig. 26-14 Typical incision for cesarean birth. Note "skin clips" used to suture incision.

Continued.

Specific Nursing Care Plan—cont'd

ASSESSMENT	NURSING DIAGNOSIS (ND), PLAN/GOAL (P/G)	RATIONALE/ IMPLEMENTATION	EVALUATION
Assess for feelings of powerlessness and disappointment with change from birth plans.	ND: Situational low self-esteem related to loss of control and unplanned cesarean delivery. P/G: Maggie (couple) will discuss feelings openly and participate in decision-making process when appropriate; will verbalize acceptance of self and method of delivery.	*Maggie needs assistance in resolving negative feelings and accepting the situation:* Assess Maggie's (couple's) verbal/nonverbal communication. Encourage open discussion. Provide information to assist with interpretation of experience and "fill in gaps" in her labor and delivery process. Provide options for care when appropriate.	Couple verbalizes understanding of information given. Couple states satisfaction with participation in decision-making about care options. Couple verbalizes they feel good about themselves and that the cesarean delivery was necessary for the health and safety of mother and infant.
Assess urinary elimination.	ND: Potential altered patterns of urinary elimination related to epidural anesthesia and immobility. P/G: Normal pattern of urinary function is established.	*Urinary complications should be prevented:* Record intake and output q4-8h × 24 hr. Note whether catheter is draining properly. Note character of drainage. Give fluids intravenously or by mouth as ordered. Assess bladder for distension q8h after catheter is removed and voiding pattern is reestablished.	Urinary complications such as infection or inability to void after catheter is removed do not occur. Normal pattern of urinary function is reestablished.
Assess Maggie's (couple's) need for understanding of care needed after discharge.	ND: Knowledge deficit related to differences in care needed after cesarean delivery. P/G: Maggie (couple) will understand specific needs and will demonstrate self-care.	*Knowledge enables Maggie (couple) to provide care needed:* Encourage assistance at home and rest several times during the day. Exercises can be started after abdominal discomfort has eased or after the postoperative checkup. Nothing heavier than the infant should be lifted for about 2 weeks. Give instructions about breast care, diet, contraception, medications. Instruct Maggie to report the following signs of complications immediately: fever >38.6° C (101.4° F), dysuria, urinary frequency, lochia heavier than a normal period, wound separation, redness, oozing at the incision site, or severe abdominal pain. Give Maggie phone numbers for emergencies and counseling.	Maggie demonstrates knowledge by performing self-care and verbalizes understanding of information given. During postdischarge follow-up, parents express satisfaction with assistance they received to be able to meet demands of early weeks after birth.

❑ VAGINAL DELIVERY AFTER CESAREAN

The incidence of primary cesarean delivery is 17.4% (NCHS, 1989). Indications for primary cesarean delivery, such as dystocia, breech presentation, or fetal distress, are often nonrecurring. Therefore a woman who has had a cesarean delivery may subsequently become pregnant and not have any contraindications to labor and vaginal delivery.

The continued practice of "once a cesarean, always a cesarean" is no longer recommended by most obstetricians. A trial of labor and vaginal birth after cesarean (VBAC) are now recommended as routine procedures by the American College of Obstetricians and Gynecologists for women who have had one previous cesarean delivery by low transverse incision (ACOG, 1988). Studies have shown that such vaginal delivery is relatively safe (Lavin et al, 1982), with only a 0.5% risk of uterine rupture through a lower uterine segment scar (Knuppel and Drukker, 1986). Labor and vaginal delivery are not recommended if contraindications, such as a previous classic cesarean scar or evidence of fetopelvic disproportion, are present.

According to Scott et al (1990), 60% to 75% of women can deliver vaginally after a trial of labor. A trial of labor (p. 766) is recommended for women who meet the requirements for VBAC. This labor should occur in a hospital facility that has the equipment and personnel available within 30 minutes from the time a decision is made for cesarean delivery to the beginning of the procedure. Ideally, the woman is admitted to the labor and delivery unit at the onset of spontaneous labor. Normal activities should be encouraged in the latent phase of labor. FHR and uterine activity are usually monitored electronically. There is no evidence that administration of oxytocin to induce or augment labor or use of epidural anesthesia is contraindicated, although some physicians may not elect these procedures (Flamm et al, 1987, 1988).

Attention should be given to the woman's psychologic, as well as physical, needs during the trial of labor. Anxiety can inhibit release of oxytocin, delaying labor progress, and leading to failure and repeat cesarean delivery. The woman can be encouraged to use breathing and relaxation techniques. The husband or support person can be encouraged to provide comfort measures and emotional support.

Evaluation

The woman with dystotic labor requires frequent assessments to adjust the care plan to meet her changing needs. The goal for the woman is the completion of labor with the least amount of fatigue, some degree of comfort, and no maternal or neonatal complications. When the woman and her family state they are satisfied with the management of the labor, the nurse can feel relatively reassured that emotional and physical supportive goals were met.

Preterm Labor and Birth

Preterm birth is traumatic for both child and parent. The infant is faced with adjustment to extrauterine existence before final readiness for the event. Parents are faced with an unexpected emotional crisis as a result of the natural process of pregnancy and birth being altered. Parents and child often are separated. The separation extends over a period of time. Death or disability of the infant is a possibility that must be faced. The elements that foster parent-child attachment, that is, closeness, positive perception of the self and the child, and infant responsiveness, are radically changed. Child and parents experiencing the crisis of preterm labor and birth need the concerted support of all members of the health care team.

Preterm birth is that which occurs after the twentieth but before the end of the thirty-seventh week of gestation. The overall incidence of preterm birth in the United States ranges from 5% to 11% (Pauerstein, 1987) and has remained stable for the last 20 years.

The *diagnosis* of preterm labor contractions may be difficult to distinguish from painful Braxton Hicks contractions or false labor. True labor is progressive and associated with cervical dilatation, effacement, or both.

Preterm birth is responsible for almost two thirds of infant deaths. The infant born prematurely does not possess the growth and development necessary for uncomplicated adjustment to extrauterine life. Her or his prospects for survival or good health may be severely compromised. Most of these deaths occur in infants born between 20 and 32 weeks of gestation. Infants weighing more than 2500 g (5½ lb) and delivered after 37 weeks have the best prospects of survival. Advances in neonatal care have improved preterm birth survival rates; some tertiary care centers report almost 100% survival of infants delivered after 32 weeks of gestation (Konte et al, 1986).

❑ ETIOLOGY

History of multiple abortions, abdominal surgery, pregnancy-induced hypertension, uterine anomalies, incompetent cervix, or infection (especially nephritis) often contributes to preterm labor. Smoking (>10 cigarettes a day), low socioeconomic status, maternal age under 18 years or over 40 years, single parenthood, poor nutrition, and heavy or stressful work are also implicated as causes of preterm labor.

Multifetal pregnancy, hydramnios, and premature

rupture of membranes are also notable, as are placental complications such as placenta previa or placental separation. Transplacental infections such as rubella, toxoplasmosis, or syphilis may be responsible for preterm labor.

In approximately two thirds of preterm deliveries, no definite cause can be identified. Twenty to thirty percent of preterm labors occur after premature rupture of membranes (Benson, 1986). It is important for nurses to convey this information to parents experiencing preterm labor.

❑ MANAGEMENT OF PRETERM BIRTH

Obstetric management of prematurity involves early detection of preterm labor, suppressing uterine activity, and improving intrapartum care of the fetus destined to be born early.

Many women are unaware of the danger of preterm delivery and need to be informed of how they might reduce the risk. Client education programs have been established by concerned professional groups for the purpose of early detection of preterm labor. If preterm labor can be detected, early preventive therapy can be initiated. Research indicates treatment needs to be started in the early latent phase of labor to be successful (Cunningham, MacDonald, and Gant, 1989).

All pregnant women are screened according to risk factors associated with preterm labor at their initial prenatal visit. They are assessed at 22 to 26 weeks of gestation. Women who are considered at high risk for preterm labor are followed in the preterm labor clinic.

Women in the high-risk group for preterm labor are seen weekly. They receive education in the symptoms of preterm labor (guidelines in Chapter 10—Preterm Labor Recognition), and instruction in palpation and timing and reporting of uterine contactions. Recently an ambulatory tocodynomometer device (Fig. 26-15) was developed to detect excessive uterine contractions before they can be perceived by the woman herself. The data are transmitted twice per day, via the telephone, to the hospital for analysis. Ambulatory home monitoring may represent a new and effective means for accurate and early diagnosis of preterm labor. Data from the tocodynomometer or from frequent assessment of the cervix are analyzed and appropriate therapy instituted if labor is suspected.

Therapy for Prevention

Attempts to arrest labor are justified if the following conditions are present.

1. Labor is diagnosed. There are three or more contractions of moderate intensity and duration per 20 minutes; the cervix is dilated no more than 4 cm or effaced no more than 50%; but the membranes must be intact with no bulging.

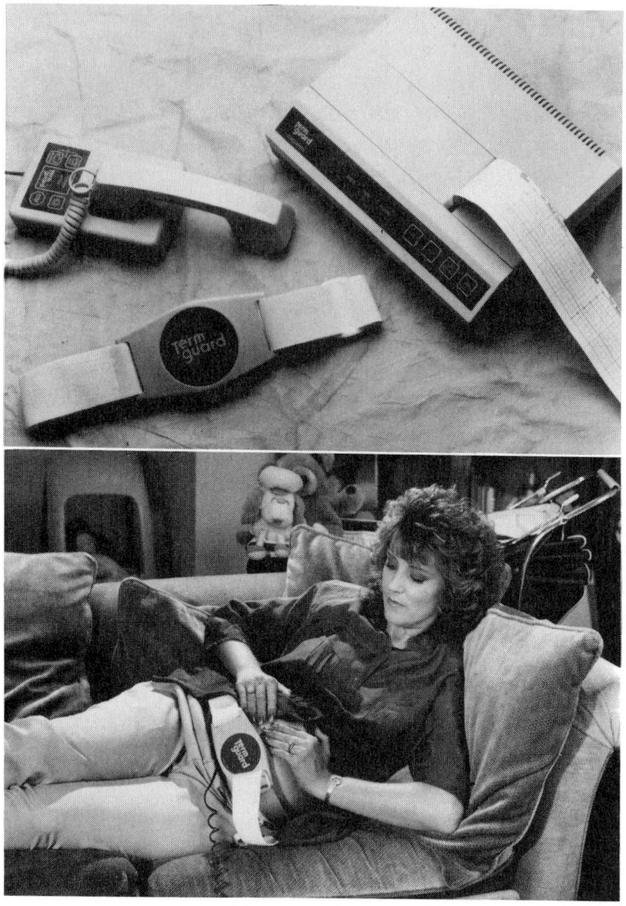

A

B

Fig. 26-15 Home uterine activity monitoring. **A,** Lightweight ambulatory tocodynamometer and recording unit used to transmit data over the phone. **B,** Tocodynamometer in place at center of abdomen below umbilicus.

2. The fetus must be live and viable (some hospitals specify 20 to 36 weeks; others, 27 to 37 weeks' inclusive gestation). Estimation of gestational age by ultrasonography is the preferred technique.
3. There are no signs of fetal distress or disease.
4. There must be no medical or obstetric disorder or clinically significant abnormalities in laboratory findings that are a contraindication to the continuation of pregnancy.
5. The woman is both willing and capable of giving an informed consent. She should be able to comply with the prescribed regimen of medication (on an out-of-hospital basis) and weekly visits until delivery and to return for the 6-week postdelivery examination.

Home Management

Preterm labor may be treated by bed rest in the home. Guidelines for client teaching are provided on pp. 783-784.

Guidelines for Client Teaching
PRETERM LABOR: HOME MANAGEMENT

ASSESSMENT
Gravida 2, 30 weeks' gestation.
First baby born at 34 weeks' gestation.
Preterm labor has been diagnosed and treated; woman is now ready for discharge with medication; or,
Preterm labor is to be treated at home.

NURSING DIAGNOSES
Knowledge deficit related to management of preterm labor.
Potential for injury: maternal and fetal, related to recurrence of preterm labor and delivery.
Anxiety, mild to moderate, related to possible recurrence of preterm labor and delivery.

GOALS
Short-term
Gravida learns home management after preterm labor episode.

Intermediate
Gravida implements home management.

Long-term
Gravida carries pregnancy to or near term and gives birth to healthy mature neonate.

REFERENCES AND TEACHING AIDS
Printed materials available through drug companies, hospitals, and clinics.

RATIONALE/CONTENT	TEACHING ACTIONS
Knowledge provides a basis for decision making re self-care:	
Review guidelines for client teaching: preterm labor recognition, Chapter 10. Teach self-care:	Implement teaching actions as required from guidelines, Chapter 10.
Bed rest Bed rest is intended to keep the pressure of the fetus off the cervix and to enhance uterine perfusion. Kneeling or sitting in bed does not keep the fetus from pressing on the cervix. Physical rest is facilitated by peace of mind. Someone other than the mother must assume care of older children, cooking, and cleaning. Many women are allowed out of bed only for use of the bathroom. Feet may be elevated.	Develop care plan mutually with woman/couple/family. Mobilize assistance for home management. Advise woman to lie on her left side with her head flat or raised on a small pillow.
Medications If the woman is being maintained at home on an *oral* dose of tocolytic medication (ritodrine or terbutaline), woman must know rationale, side effects, and danger signs (boxes, p. 786).	Medications are reviewed and the woman is given written instructions regarding care. Inform woman about the action and side effects of the drug. Instruct her how to take her pulse and report any rate greater than 120 bpm to her physician, and instruct her how to report symptoms, including palpitations, tremors, agitation, and nervousness. Schedule drugs to be taken around the clock.
Some over-the-counter drugs may have deleterious effects. Oral administration may be better tolerated when taken with food.	Caution woman not to use ritodrine with any over-the-counter drugs unless her physician approves.
Sedation is often ordered to facilitate relaxation and rest.	Advise and give written instructions (for woman and her family) regarding the medication. This includes the prescription for sedation, dosage, times for administration, and side effects.
Avoidance of activities that could stimulate labor: Sexual stimulation is contraindicated because (1) prostaglandins in semen can stimulate labor in a susceptible woman and (2) touching the cervix or pressure against the posterior wall of the vagina may stimulate Ferguson's reflex. **Ferguson's reflex** is the increase in myometrial contractility that follows mechanical stretching or touching of the cervix. ***Nipple stimulation*** may induce oxytocin production, which can cause recurrence of uterine activity.	Encourage discussion of this sensitive topic.

Continued.

Guidelines for Client Teaching—cont'd

RATIONALE/CONTENT	TEACHING ACTIONS
Early identification and timely intervention assist with management of preterm labor: Review danger signs, boxes, p. 786. Review danger of infection if membranes are not intact.	Review verbally and provide written instructions regarding: a. What to do and whom to notify in case of onset of labor or rupture of membranes. b. Maintaining personal hygiene if membranes have ruptured earlier. c. Assessing for signs of infection (e.g., odor of vaginal discharge, increase in body temperature).
Home maintenance may be required, therefore the nurse may need to plan with the gravida for community service: Social service consultation may be helpful if the woman has to be transported into a center from an outlying area. Living arrangements, meals, transportation, and financial assistance may be needed for some families.	Refer to appropriate agency after discussion and mutual planning with family.

EVALUATION The nurse can be reasonably assured that teaching was effective if the goals for care are achieved. The woman and her family are able to implement self-care so that preterm labor is stopped, there are no adverse sequelae to medication, and positive family processes are maintained. The woman delivers a healthy infant at or near term.

Inhospital Pharmacologic Management

If uterine contractions persist, or cervical changes occur, tocolytic treatment may be used to stop labor. *Tocolytic* agents are drugs that inhibit uterine contractions. *Toko-* and *toco-* are Greek roots referring to obstetrics; *-lytic* is also Greek, and means "to break down" or stop. The agents used include β-adrenergic drugs such as ritodrine or terbutaline and magnesium sulfate (Scott et al, 1990).

Ritodrine. Ritodrine (Yutopar) was the first, and remains the only, β-sympathomimetic drug approved by the FDA for use in the United States to inhibit preterm labor (Barden et al, 1980; Cunningham, MacDonald, and Gant, 1989). Ritodrine acts on type II β-adrenergic receptors, which cause uterine muscle relaxation, vasodilatation, bronchodilatation, and muscle glycogenolysis. Decrease in serum potassium levels may cause arrhythmias. The initial dose is usually given intravenously, followed by intramuscular and/or oral therapy. The dose is determined by the physician and the woman's response to the medication.

Contraindications for use include maternal diseases such as cardiovascular disease, severe preeclampsia, severe antepartum hemorrhage, chorioamnionitis, and hyperthyroidism. Fetal death and gestational age of less than 20 weeks confirmed by ultrasound are two fetus-related contraindications.

A delay of preterm delivery has potential *beneficial effects* for the fetus. In addition, the tocolytic agents available are usually able to delay delivery long enough for the use of glucocorticoids to effect fetal pulmonary maturation.

Cardiopulmonary complications are possible. Therefore careful assessment and monitoring are essential. Because of the possible cardiopulmonary effects, an electrocardiogram may be ordered before the treatment. A cardiac monitor for the mother may be indicated to maintain continuous assessment for *tachycardia* and *arrhythmia.* See Procedure 26-3 for a summary of the hazardous complications and the care required for a client receiving ritodrine. See box, p. 786, for danger signs for ritodrine and terbutaline toxicity. The danger box for terbutaline is included because this drug is used by some physicians.

Terbutaline. Terbutaline (Brethine) is another β-adrenergic agent often used for preterm labor. Administration and contraindications are similar to those described for ritodrine. The administration of tocolytic drugs must be supervised closely by health professionals qualified to identify and manage complications of drug administration or pregnancy. The box on p. 786 describes the danger signs of ritodrine and terbutaline toxicity.

Magnesium Sulfate. Magnesium sulfate is known to decrease uterine activity. It is being investigated for its use as a tocolytic agent because it is safer than rito-

PROCEDURE 26-3

NURSING CARE OF A WOMAN RECEIVING RITODRINE

DEFINITION

The use of a β-sympathomimetic agent to stop the uterus from contracting, thereby stopping preterm labor.

PURPOSE

Suppression of preterm labor.

EQUIPMENT

Intravenous infusion pump equipment, sphygmomanometer, stethoscope, equipment for cardiopulmonary arrest, fetal monitoring equipment.

HAZARDOUS SYMPTOMS

See danger signs: ritodrine, p. 786.

NURSING ACTIONS	RATIONALE
Identify client and check physician's orders.	Provides the right therapy for the right person.
Wash hands before and after touching client or equipment. Glove, prn.	Prevents nosocomial infection and implements universal precautions.
Assess maternal vital signs and FHR.	Obtains baseline data.
Administer dose as ordered, increasing infusion rate every 10 to 30 minutes depending on uterine response.	Achieves tocolysis.
Do not exceed maximum intravenous rate of 125 ml/hr.	Prevents overhydration.
Monitor uterine activity continuously.	Assesses effectiveness of tocolysis.
Monitor vital signs and blood pressure every 15 minutes until stable and then follow hospital protocol. *Maternal pulse should not exceed 140 bpm.* Note regularity and quality.	Detects complications: cardiac arrhythmias are adverse effects of β-adrenergic therapy, pulmonary edema, and fluid overload.
Prepare mother for use of cardiac monitor and/or fetal monitor during intravenous therapy.	
Note breath sounds when counting respiratory rate.	
Auscultate lungs every 8 to 12 hours.	
Monitor FHR: *should not exceed 180 bpm.* Intermittent evaluation should continue during oral therapy also.	
Observe for any untoward symptoms.	
Ask woman to report symptoms.	Elicits subjective symptoms.
Send blood samples to laboratory for analysis of levels of glucose, potassium, and hematocrit.	Assesses for hypokalemia and hyperglycemia. As glucose moves into cells, potassium shifts from the extracellular space.
Maintain absolute bed rest during intravenous infusion.	Minimizes stress and reduces pressure on cervix.
Prevent hypotension; keep woman in left-lateral position or place wedge under right hip if in supine position.	Maintains placental perfusion.
Apply antiembolism stockings.	Prevents pooling of blood in lower extremities.
Encourage passive leg exercises.	
Maintain adequate hydration, 2000 to 3000 ml total fluid daily.	Maintains cardiac output.
Prevent overhydration:	
Measure intake and output.	Detects overhydration.
Weigh daily.	
Prevent undue stress:	Promotes relaxation through anticipatory guidance.
Prepare woman for potential side effects (i.e., agitation, palpitations, nervousness, tremors, tachycardia).	
Treat for complications:	
Hold medication. If intravenous, keep line open with maintenance solution.	Minimizes effects of medication.
Notify physician and prepare antidote as ordered. β-blocking agents such as propanolol (Inderal) should be available.	Initiates immediate therapy.
Maintain woman in high Fowler's position.	Minimizes effects of possible pulmonary edema.
Administer oxygen.	Maintains sufficient oxygenation.
Initiate CPR for arrest if necessary.	Maintains oxygenation and body functions.

DANGER SIGNS

Ritodrine Toxicity

1. Central nervous system: severe nervousness or anxiety, tremulousness, headache, restlessness.
2. Respirations: dyspnea, hyperventilation.
3. Cardiovascular system: severe palpitations or cardiac irregularities, chest pain; pulmonary edema.
4. Gastrointestinal: severe nausea or vomiting, epigastric distress, diarrhea.

Terbutaline Toxicity

1. Central nervous system: severe dizziness, drowsiness, headache, nervousness, restlessness; clouded sensorium.
2. Blood pressure: severe hypertension.
3. Heart rate: continuous palpitations.
4. Musculoskeletal: severe muscle cramps and weakness.
5. Gastrointestinal: continuous nausea and vomiting.

drine for the woman. It is usually given intravenously, but intramuscular and oral routes may be used (Niebyl et al, 1986). Nursing assessments and interventions are the same as for the woman receiving magnesium sulfate for severe preeclampsia (Chapter 23).

Promotion of Fetal Lung Maturity

Respiratory distress syndrome (RDS) was formerly known as hyaline membrane disease (HMD) of the newborn. RDS is common in small preterm infants who have fetal lung immaturity. The incidence and severity of RDS has been found to be reduced if glucocorticoids (e.g., betamethasone) are administered to the mother at least 24 to 48 hours before the delivery. The fetus must be less than 34 weeks of gestation. The administration must be made at least 24 hours before delivery and no longer than 7 days before delivery (Benson, 1986). Children who have been exposed to the stated levels of glucocorticoids in utero appear to grow and develop normally during the early years of life (Liggins, 1982). Hence some authorities consider that the chance of benefit to the fetus far outweighs the chance of harm.

Care During Irreversible or Acceptable Preterm Labor

The preterm labor is conducted according to the principles that apply to a low-birth-weight (easily compromised) fetus. If vaginal delivery is chosen, the analgesia is limited, and continuous FHR monitoring is applied. Artificial rupture of membranes (AROM) is delayed until the cervix is more than 6 cm dilated and there is sufficient descent of the presenting part to avoid prolapse of the cord.

If augmentation of labor is advisable, a low concentration of oxytocin is infused continuously. Pudendal block anesthesia is desirable. An episiotomy is done to limit the length of the second stage and excessive pressure on the fragile fetal head. Outlet (low) forceps are used for delivery unless easy spontaneous birth is likely. A cesarean delivery may be performed for malpresentation or maternal or fetal distress. A pediatrician and a nurse from the infant intensive care unit are present at the birth so that resuscitative and supportive care for the infant can be initiated immediately if necessary (Chapter 28). The newborn is permitted several breaths before clamping the cord; if resuscitation is required, however, the cord is clamped and cut immediately.

Parental concern for the well-being of the infant is apparent during labor. Parents need to be aware of the interest and support of the staff. However, false assurance of fetal health must be avoided. For some parents the reality of the situation is not appreciated until they see their daughter or son in the intensive care unit. For others who experience fetal or neonatal death, the loss intensifies once the stress of labor and delivery is over (Chapter 29).

During the postpartum period physical care of the mother is similar to that required for any vaginal delivery. However, the family will be very anxious concerning the health and prognosis of their infant (Sammons and Lewis, 1985). Nursing care of the preterm infant involves not only medical and nursing personnel but also the participation of the parents (Chapter 28). The nurse must be aware of the impact that preterm birth may have on family dynamics (Richardson, 1987). Parents must accept that the infant has special needs and learn to meet these needs prior to discharge so that they will have more realistic expectations when they are at home (Sosa, 1982).

Postterm Labor and Birth

Postterm birth is the delivery of an infant beyond the end of the forty-second week of gestation, or 2 weeks beyond the EDD figured from Nägele's rule (see p. 80). The infant whose gestational age is beyond 42 weeks is referred to as "postterm" if healthy and "dysmature" if signs of intrauterine nutritional deprivation are present (Chapter 28).

Maternal risks are related to the delivery of an excessively sized infant. Fetal risks appear to be twofold. The first is related to the possibility of birth trauma and asphyxia through fetopelvic disproportion. The second risk is felt to result from the compromising effects on the fetus of an "aging" placenta. Scott et al (1990) note that placental function decreases after 40 weeks of gestation and amniotic fluid volume declines. If placental insufficiency is present, there is a high incidence of fetal distress during labor. Postterm babies have increased mortality, increased feeding and sleeping problems, more illness, and low developmental and mental scores (Scott et al, 1990).

The management of postterm pregnancy is still controversial. Induction of labor at 42 weeks is suggested by some authorities, while others allow pregnancy to proceed to 43 weeks as long as tests of fetal well-being are performed and results are normal. Antepartum assessments for postterm pregnancy may include daily fetal movement counts (DFMC) (at least 10 in a 12-hour period) and abdominal girth measurements (to detect oligohydramnios). Nonstress and stress tests may be performed weekly, as well as realtime ultrasound scanning (to assess fetal movements, fetal breathing movements, and amniotic fluid volume). Amniocentesis or amnioscopy may be performed to detect meconium in the amniotic fluid (Hendricksen, 1985; Scott et al, 1990) (also see Chapter 22).

Labor of a woman with a postterm fetus should be monitored for signs of fetal distress. The woman should be encouraged to come to the hospital in early labor so the fetus can be monitored electronically for more accurate assessment of the FHR pattern. Fetal scalp pH sampling may be obtained if meconium is present in the amniotic fluid. Accurate assessment of the woman's labor pattern is also important, since dysfunctional labor is common (Hendricksen, 1985).

Emotional support is essential for the postterm woman and her family. A vaginal delivery is anticipated, but the couple should be prepared for a forceps (or vacuum extraction) or cesarean delivery if complications arise.

SUMMARY

Complications during birth have both physical and emotional sequelae. The mother faces hazards to her life. Prolonged and difficult labor can be physically debilitating. The consequent fatigue may interfere with the initial interactions with her newborn. Memories of a difficult birth can resurface years later as a stress factor in subsequent births. The family will be faced with long-term grief reaction if the infant suffers disability. If death of either mother or infant occurs, the family, as it was, no longer exists. Parents, during this time of crisis, need the best possible medical and nursing care that our technically and psychologically knowledgeable society can offer.

KEY CONCEPTS

- Dystocia results from differences in the normal relationships between any of the five essential factors of labor.
- The differences between dystocia and eutocia relate to changes in the pattern of progress in labor.
- The functional relationships between the uterine contractions, the fetus, and the mother's pelvis are altered by maternal positioning.
- Uterine contractility is increased by oxytocin and PGE and is decreased by tocolytics.
- All expectant parents benefit from learning about operative obstetrics (e.g., use of forceps, cesarean delivery) and preterm labor during the prenatal period.
- The basic purpose of cesarean delivery is to preserve the life or health of the mother and her fetus.
- Under certain conditions, vaginal birth is possible after previous cesarean birth.
- The gravida and her family can be taught to treat preterm labor at home with bed rest, tocolytics, and avoidance of activities that stimulate the uterus.
- Inhospital treatment for preterm labor involves the use of tocolytics and pharmacologic stimulation of lung maturity.
- Postterm birth poses a risk to both the mother and the fetus.

LEARNING ACTIVITIES

1. Develop a teaching plan for a client needing:
   a. Self-assessment to identify preterm labor.
   b. Inhospital tocolysis with ritodrine and pharmacologic stimulation of fetal lung maturity.
2. Discuss assessment and management of the following types of dystocia related to:
   a. Breech delivery.
   b. Fetopelvic disproportion.
   c. Prolonged latent stage.
3. Describe nursing considerations when caring for postterm clients.
4. In small groups, develop nursing care plans for the following types of labors; in the total group, compare and contrast the care plans. Select from the following, or from actual cases on your unit:
   a. Woman experiencing preterm labor; previous labor was also preterm and the infant died at 3 days of age.
   b. Woman is having a cesarean delivery scheduled during the prenatal period because of a known obstetric problem.
   c. Woman is having an emergency cesarean delivery.
   d. Woman is having prolonged labor; she is in optimum condition and fetal monitor tracings indicate her twins are responding well to labor.
5. Follow a woman through the perioperative period of a cesarean delivery. What preparation was provided to her? What needs are expressed in the postpartum period that are different from postpartum needs of women who have had a vaginal delivery?

References

American College of Obstetricians and Gynecologists: Technical bulletin number 110: induction and augmentation of labor, Washington, DC, 1987, ACOG.

American College of Obstetricians and Gynecologists: ACOG committee opinion, #64: guidelines for vaginal delivery after a previous cesarean birth, Washington, DC, October, 1988, ACOG.

Barden TP et al: Ritodrine hydrochloride: a betamimetic agent for use in preterm labor, Obstet Gynecol 56:1, 1980.

Benson RC: Preterm labor. in Danforth DN and Scott JR, editors: Obstetrics and gynecology, ed 5, Philadelphia, 1986, JB Lippincott Co.

Brown, ER et al: Reversible induction of surfactant production in fetal lambs treated with glucocorticoids, Pediatr Res 13:491, 1979.

Caldeyro-Barcia R: The influence of maternal position on time of spontaneous rupture of the membranes, progress of labor, and fetal head compression, Birth Fam J 6:7, 1979.

Cunningham FG, MacDonald PC, and Gant NF: Williams obstetrics, ed 18, Norwalk, Conn, 1989, Appleton & Lange.

Englinton GS: External version in modern obstetrics. In Phelan JP and Clark SL, editors: Cesarean delivery, New York, 1988, Elsevier Science Publishing Co, Inc.

Fenwick L and Simkin P: Maternal positioning to prevent or alleviate dystocia in labor, Clin Obstet Gynecol 30(1):83, 1987.

Flamm BL et al: Oxytocin during labor after previous cesarean section: results of a multicenter study, Obstet Gynecol 70(5):709, 1987.

Flamm BL et al: Vaginal birth after cesarean section: results of a multidimensional study, Am J Obstet Gynecol 158(5):1079, 1988.

Friedman EA: Midforceps delivery: no? Clin Obstet Gynecol 30(1):93, 1987.

Galvan BJ and Broekhuizen FF: Obstetric vacuum extraction, JOGN Nurs 16(4):242, 1987.

Hayashi RH: Midforceps delivery: yes? Clin Obstet Gynecol 30(1):90, 1985.

Hendricksen A: Prolonged pregnancy: a literature review, J Nurse Midwife 30(1):33, 1985.

Krieger JA: Operative obstetrics. In Hale RW and Krieger: Obstetrics, New York, 1987, Medical Examination Publishing Co.

Knuppel RA and Drukker JE: High-risk pregnancy: a team approach, Philadelphia, 1986, WB Saunders Co.

Konte JM et al: Short-term neonatal morbidity associated with preterm birth and effect of a preterm birth prevention program on expected incidence of morbidity, Am J Perinatol 3:283, 1986.

Lavin JP et al: Vaginal delivery in patients with a prior cesarean section, Obstet Gynecol 59(2):135, 1982.

Ledger WJ: Dystocia and prolonged labor. In Willson JR and Carrington ER, editors: Obstetrics and gynecology, St Louis, 1987, The CV Mosby Co.

Lee CY: Shoulder dystocia, Clin Obstet Gynecol 30(1):77, 1987.

Lehrman E: Birth in the left lateral position, J Nurse Midwife 30(4):193, 1985.

Liggins GC: Report on children exposed to steroids in utero, Contemp OB/GYN 19:205, 1982.

Marshall C: The art of induction/augmentation of labor, JOGN Nurs 14(1):22, 1985.

Morrison et al: Cesarean section: what's behind the dramatic rise? Perinat Neonat 6:87, 1982.

NAACOG: The nurse's role in the induction/augmentation of labor, OGN Nursing Practice Resource, Jan, 1988 (PO Box 71437, Washington, DC 20024-1437).

NCHS: Vital and health statistics: detailed diagnosis and procedures, National Hospital Discharge Survey, 1987. Series 13, No 100, US Department of Health and Human Services, March, 1989.

Niebyl J et al: Tocolytics: when and how to use them, Contemp OB/GYN 27(6):146, 1986.

Pauerstein CJ: Clinical obstetrics, New York, 1987, John Wiley & Sons, Inc.

Perkins RP: Fetal dystocia, Clin Obstet Gynecol 30(1):56, 1987.

Richardson P: Women's important relationships during pregnancy and the preterm labor event, W J Nurs Res 9(2):203, 1987.

Sammons WA and Lewis JM: Premature babies: a different beginning, St Louis, 1985, The CV Mosby Co.

Scott JR et al: Danforth's obstetrics and gynecology, ed 6, Philadelphia, 1990, JB Lippincott Co.

Seitchik J: The management of functional dystocia in the first stage of labor, Clin Obstet Gynecol 30(1):42, 1987.

Sheen PW and Hayashi RH: Graphic management of labor: alert/action line, Clin Obstet Gynecol 30(1):33, 1987.

Simkin P: Stress, pain and catecholamines in labor. I. A review, Birth 13(8): 1986.

Bibliography

Adamsons K and Wallach RC: Treating preterm labor with diazoxide, Contemp OB/GYN 31(1):161, 1988.

Andrews CM: Changing fetal position through maternal posturing. In Raff BS, editor: Perinatal parental behavior: nursing research and implications for newborn health, White Plains, NY, 1981, March of Dimes Foundation.

Baxi LV and Petrie RH: Pharmacologic effects on labor: effects of drugs on dystocia, labor, and uterine activity, Clin Obstet Gynecol 30(1):19, 1987.

Bell R: The prediction of preterm labour by recording spontaneous uterine activity, Br J Obstet Gynaecol 90:884, 1983.

Carlson JM et al: Maternal positioning during parturition in normal labor, Obstet Gynecol 68:443, 1986.

Cetrulo CL and Cetrulo LG: Medicolegal dystocia, Clin Obstet Gynecol 30(1):106, 1987.

Compton AA: Soft tissue and pelvic dystocia, Clin Obstet Gynecol 30(1):69, 1987.

Cranley M et al: Women's perceptions of vaginal and cesarean deliveries, Nurs Res 32:11, 1983.

Cox B and Smith E: The mother's self-esteem after a cesarean delivery, MCN 7:309, 1982.

Droegemueller W et al: Comprehensive gynecology, St Louis, 1987, The CV Mosby Co.

Fawcett J and Henklein JC: Antenatal education for cesarean birth: extension of a field test, JOGN Nurs 16(1):61, 1987.

Few B: Indomethacin for treatment of premature labor, MCN 13(2):93, 1988.

Filly RA: Twins: sonographic aids to management, UCSF Antepartum and intrapartum management, San Francisco, Calif, June 1987.

Finley BE et al: Emergent cesarean delivery in patients undergoing a trial of labor with a transverse lower-segment scar, Am J Obstet Gynecol 155:936, 1986.

Fitzgerald JG: Preterm labor. II. Management, NAACOG Update Series 1(3):1, 1983.

Flanagan T et al: Management of term breech presentation, Am J Obstet Gynecol 156(6):1492, 1987.

Fortier JC: The relationship of vaginal and cesarean births to father-infant attachment, JOGN Nurs 17(2):128, 1988.

Garfield RE: Cellular and molecular bases for dystocia, Clin Obstet Gynecol 30(1):3, 1987.

Gennaro S: Postpartal anxiety and depression in mothers of term and preterm infants, Nurs Res 37(2):82, 1988.

Gilbert ES and Harmon JS: High-risk pregnancy and delivery: nursing perspectives, St Louis, 1986, The CV Mosby Co.

Gill PJ and Katz M: Early detection of preterm labor: ambulatory home monitoring of uterine activity, JOGN Nurs 15(6):439, 1986.

Glazer G and Hulme MA: Prostaglandin gel for cervical ripening, MCN 12(1):28, 1987.

Grundy HW: Tocolysis: who to treat? When to start? UCSF Antepartum and intrapartum management conference, San Francisco, Calif, June, 1987.

International Medical News Service: Standing, sitting during delivery not dangerous. Report of a presentation by H. Nagai at the 11th World Congress of Gynecology and Obstetrics in Berlin, Obstet Gynecol News 20:10, 1985.

Jacobs MM: Role of prostaglandins in cervical ripening—should you be using it? UCSF Antepartum and intrapartum management conference, San Francisco, June, 1987.

Katz MM: The role of home tocodynamometry in clinical practice, UCSF Antepartum and intrapartum management conference, San Francisco, June, 1987.

Katz M and Gill PJ: Comprehensive preterm birth prevention program, Clin Res 32(2):296A, 1984.

Katz M and Gill PJ: Initial evaluation of an ambulatory system for home monitoring and transmission of uterine activity data, Obstet Gynecol 66(2):273, 1985.

Kemp VH and Page CK: Antenatal education for cesarean birth: extension of a field test, JOGN Nurs 16(3):179, 1987.

Knor ER: Decision making in obstetrical nursing, 1987, BC Decker, Inc.

Kopelman JN: Computed tomographic pelvimetry in the evaluation of breech presentation, Obstet Gynecol 68:455, 1986.

Lam F: Tocolytic infusion at home, UCSF Antepartum and intrapartum management conference, San Francisco, June, 1987.

Laros RK: Twins: current obstetrical management, UCSF Antepartum and intrapartum management conference, San Francisco, June, 1987.

Levine MG et al: Birth trauma: incidence and predisposing factors, Obstet Gynecol 63:792, 1984.

Lupe PJ and Gross TL: Maternal upright posture and mobility in labor: a review, Obstet Gynecol 67:727, 1986.

Main D et al: Can preterm deliveries be prevented? Am J Obstet Gynecol 151:892, 1985.

Miller C and Sutter C: Vaginal birth after cesarean, JOGN Nurs 14(5):383, 1985.

NAACOG: Preterm labor prevention: annotated bibliography, OGN Nursing Practice Resource, 1988 (PO Box 71437, Washington, DC 20024-1437).

Nager CW, Key TC, and Moore TR: Cervical ripening and labor outcome with preinduction intracervical prostaglandin E_2 (Prepidil) gel, J Perinatal 7(3):189, 1987.

Notzon FC et al: Comparisons of national cesarean-section rates, N Engl J Med 316(7):386, 1987.

Odent M: Birth reborn, New York, 1984, Random House, Inc.

Ogburn MD: The mystery of preterm labor, Childbirth Educator, p 20, Summer, 1986.

Petitti E: Recent trends in cesarean delivery rates in California, Birth 12:25, Spring, 1985.

Phelan JP and Clark SL, editors: Cesarean delivery, New York, 1988, Elsevier Science Publishing Co, Inc.

Plosh D and Duhring JL: Management of postdates pregnancy, Am Fam Practitioner 36(2):184, 1987.

Shearer MH and Estes M: A critical review of the recent literature on postterm pregnancy and a look at women's experiences, Birth 12(2):95, 1985.

Stewart DB: The pelvis as a passageway. I. Evolution and adaptions, Br J Obstet Gynecol 91:611, 1984.

Struyk APHB and Treffers PE: Ovarian tumors in pregnancy, Acta Obstet Gynecol Scand 63:421, 1984.

Stubblefield PG: Causes and prevention of preterm birth: an overview. In Fuchs F and Stubblefield PG, editors: Preterm birth: causes, prevention and management, New York, 1984, MacMillan Publishing Co.

Tucker SM et al: Patient care standards: nursing process, diagnosis, and outcome, ed 4, St Louis, 1988, The CV Mosby Co.

Symposium: Alternatives to cesarean section, Contemp OB/GYN 31(1):191, 1988.

Weiss JD: Management of dystocia, UCSF Antepartum and intrapartum management conference, San Francisco, June, 1987.

Young J and Poppe C: Breast pump stimulation to promote labor, MCN 12(2):124, 1987.

CHAPTER 27

Adolescent Pregnancy and Parenthood

Janice M. Spikes and Linda A. Drapp

Learning Objectives

Correctly define the key terms listed.

Discuss dynamics of adolescent sexual development.

Explain the decision tree for adolescent sexual decision making.

Examine the incidence and cost of adolescent pregnancy and parenthood.

Compare and contrast the developmental tasks of adolescence and of pregnancy.

Compare and contrast the nutritional needs of the nonpregnant, pregnant, and lactating adolescent.

Discuss nursing care of the adolescent father.

Key Terms

denial
developmental tasks
infant responsiveness
parenting ability
personal costs
physiologic consequences
public cost
readiness for the task of childbearing
risk-taking behavior
sexual decision-making tree

Adolescent clients present the maternity nurse with a unique challenge. A significant number are sexually active and in need of contraceptive counseling; many become pregnant. The pregnant adolescent, her family, and her partner require sensitive, competent nursing care. The young woman may choose to terminate the pregnancy or carry it to term. She may place the infant up for adoption or elect to keep the baby. The nurse can play a vital role in helping the client make informed decisions and in supporting her, both physically and emotionally, in carrying out her chosen option.

Adolescent Sexual Development

Many factors contribute to teenage sexual activity: peer pressure, sex-oriented media, minimum or no parental supervision, mobility, and a transient society that discourages neighbors from knowing one another (Corbett and Meyer, 1987; McAnarney and Hendee, 1989a). This young, inexperienced population is thus enticed to sexual activity without adequate preparation (Holder, 1987). For many there is no turning back.

Risk-taking behavior and the need to explore new roles and new experiences occur at a time when cognitive development has not yet reached the point where teenagers can make judgments that will keep them out of trouble (Goleman, 1987). Belief in their own invulnerability persuades teenagers that they can take risks safely. In one study (Goleman, 1987), adolescents were found to anticipate that the risk of pregnancy from unprotected intercourse *decreases* with each subsequent occurrence. Further, perception of risks may fade in face of peer pressure (e.g., use of condoms is rejected regardless of risk of pregnancy if peers' view of their use is negative). Worries about long-term consequences are nonexistent; only the immediate experience matters (Sachs, 1986; Goleman, 1987). Adolescent sexuality, masturbation, homosexuality, sexual activity, and myths shared with adults are discussed in Chapter 4.

ADOLESCENT CHOICES

A major task of the adolescent is to develop cognitive ability, the ability to think through alternatives and to make abstractions (Yoos, 1987). The underlying cognitive level may account for the "apparent irrationality" of adolescent decision making in sexual behavior (Yoos, 1987). The adolescent may fail to translate knowledge into behavior because of the manner in which the information is given, a manner ill suited to the adolescent's stage of cognitive development (Yoos, 1987).

Adolescents are faced with making decisions about sexuality in the early teens. Regardless of their decision-making abilities, adolescents will need factual information relative to sexuality, intercourse, and parenthood on which to base decisions. The **sexual decision-making** tree in Fig. 27-1 represents a process of sexual decision making. Unfortunately young teenagers use **denial** as a coping mechanism. They can *deny* the significance of what they hear.

Peer group pressure to initiate sexual activity is strong in present-day teen culture. It can supersede the influence of parents or older friends. Often teenagers feel that once virginity has been lost, they have nothing more to lose. Abstinence needs positive reinforcement, but if abstinence is not to be, the next decision for the teenager is whether to use contraception.

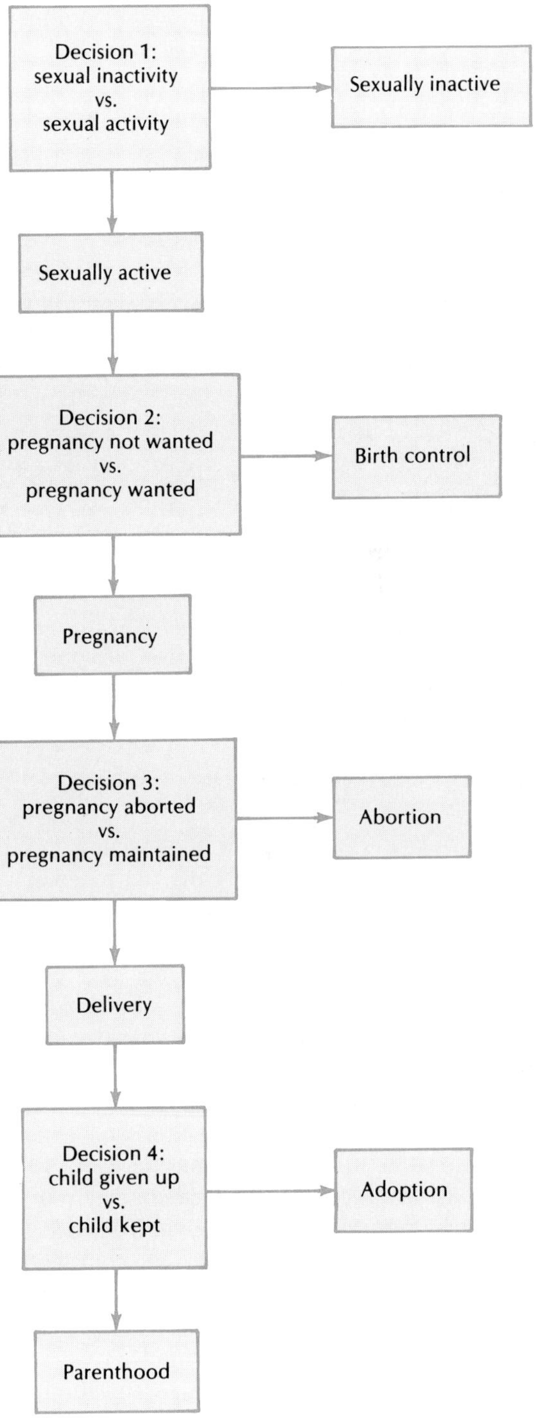

Fig. 27-1 Decision tree for adolescent sexual decision making. (From Kreipe RE. In McAnarney E, editor: Premature adolescent pregnancy and parenthood, New York, 1983, Grune & Stratton, Inc. Reprinted by permission.)

Contraception

There are significant numbers of adolescents, especially those over the age of 16 years, who would benefit from information on contraception (Emans and Grimes, 1987; McAnarney and Hendee, 1989,b). In a study conducted at a Planned Parenthood clinic it was found that the average 14-year-old engaged in sexual activity for 4.8 months before taking contraceptive precautions, while the 17-year-old risked 10.4 months of unprotected intercourse (Kornfield, 1985). Fear of parental discovery of contraception is a major reason why adolescents will delay seeking contraceptive services for a year or more after initiating sexual intercourse (Zelnik, 1983).

Fear of pregnancy and a decision to continue to be sexually active is the primary reason why adolescents seek contraceptive services. Oral contraceptives are usually the contraceptive of choice because "the pill" is not as directly associated with sexual intercourse as barrier methods (Chapter 6). Barrier methods are described by adolescents as messy and disturbing pleasure. However, current public education regarding "safe sex" and the significant protection against sexually transmitted diseases afforded by condoms and foam may change the adolescent's use of them.

The female adolescent is the decision-maker concerning sexual relationships, pregnancy risks, and contraception. The sexual behavior of the average adolescent female is seldom promiscuous. Few adolescents have more than two or three partners before marriage. Most have a single partner in a monogamous relationship (Corbett and Meyer, 1987).

Factors that influence adolescent contraceptive use are as follows:

1. Patterns of sexual activity. Frequency of intercourse, number of partners, and cooperation between the adolescent partners.
2. Contraceptive services. Access, staff attitudes, flexibility of appointment schedules, and costs.

Examples of factors contributing to nonuse of contraceptives include:

1. Erroneous beliefs regarding conception and a feeling of immunity to pregnancy risk.
2. Fear of exposure and peer disapproval or punishment by parents.
3. Belief that contraceptives are dangerous and harmful—exaggerated fears of side effects.
4. Partners who are unsupportive, uncommitted, or who have a negative attitude toward contraception. Some believe that the use of contraception decreases sexual spontaneity or runs counter to their religious beliefs.

Abortion

Once pregnancy occurs, the adolescent is faced with the choice of abortion or carrying the pregnancy. Denial of the pregnancy or a lack of decision-making skills results in delay in informing parents until the pregnancy is well advanced. The teenager who vacillates regarding abortion often makes a decision to have her baby in a roundabout way. Options need to be presented in a nonjudgmental manner to ensure the young person's freedom of choice.

The adolescent may not choose to involve her family in her decision to elect abortion (Holder, 1987). In some states a judge is appointed to determine if the teenager is mature enough to make the decision for herself. In other states, adolescents are considered "mature minors" and may consent to abortion as they may to any other procedures. Where there is doubt of the young adolescent's capacity to understand and give consent to an abortion, parental notification may be considered. However, in cases where the physician or social worker suspects that the pregnant adolescent is the victim of incest or sexual abuse within the household or extended family, parental notification may place her at additional risk. It is generally believed that a great many pregnant 12 to 14-year-olds are such victims and are not participants in sexual relationships with age-appropriate boyfriends (Holder, 1987; Zdanuk, Harris, and Wisian, 1987). In such cases, child abuse agencies may need to become involved.

Adoption

If the adolescent mother chooses to have her child, she can either keep the baby or release the infant for adoption. If adoption is contemplated, discussion of the adoption process should begin in the prenatal period (see general nursing care plan, p. 807). The adolescent is encouraged to talk freely of her feelings, both for and against the process. If possible, the girl's family and the father of the baby are part of the group that help her with her decision. The adolescent needs to be assured that what she is doing is positive and that feelings of sadness and of frustration are bound to occur.

After the baby is born, the young mother may or may not wish to see the baby or to know its sex. It is generally agreed that releasing a child is facilitated if one grieves for an *actual loss* rather than a *fantasy* one; however, the mother has the right to make her own choice. She can be given the information about the infant's health (e.g., "your baby is healthy and strong"), since it may affect her response to her own feelings of self-worth.

It is essential to help the young woman cultivate a positive attitude toward potential future pregnancies. "Subconsciously she may compensate for the loss of this infant by producing another as soon as possible, by drifting into new relationships while seeking support during her grief, by making unreasonable demands on subsequent children, or by becoming overly protective of subsequent offspring" (Polit and Kahn, 1986).

Today the teenager and her parent need to be informed of the possibility that the infant given for adoption may, as an adult, seek to identify her or his biologic parents. It is now a recognized practice to provide adoptive parents with all pertinent biologic knowledge that may affect the infant. It is also helpful for the child to know of psychosocial "successes" in her or his biologic family—musical ability, sports prowess, scientific success—all of which can be part of the adopted baby's history and a source of pride.

The grief of the young mother at her loss has to be balanced with the need of her infant for continued care and nurturing. The experience of relinquishing her child "for the child's good" may be the young woman's first major autonomous decision in her life and as such is an important step toward maturity (Arms, 1983).

Parenthood

Carrying the pregnancy and keeping the baby is also an option in adolescent sexual decision making (see

Fig. 27-1). When this choice is made, the health care giver, community resources, and the family must be mobilized to assist the adolescent parent. Research findings suggest that children born to adolescent mothers are at greater risk for behavioral, social, intellectual, and perhaps even physical retardation than are children born to older mothers (Stockard, 1986; White-Traut and Pabst, 1987). In 1979, McAnarney et al reported that the younger the adolescent mother, the less likely she was to display maternal behaviors such as touching, synchrony with the baby, vocalization, or closeness. In later research, McAnarney et al (1986) reported that adolescent mothers are less likely to be accepting, cooperative, accessible, and sensitive to their children's needs.

❑ ADOLESCENT PREGNANCY AND PARENTHOOD

Many adults have difficulty understanding the high incidence of adolescent pregnancy when contraception and elective abortion are available. Ignorance about conception and contraception or fear of discovery if contraception is sought and used may be factors. Or perhaps, for their own reasons, some deliberately select pregnancy and motherhood.

Each day more than 3000 teenagers in the United States become pregnant (Stockard, 1986). Each year 1 of 11 adolescent females becomes pregnant; about one third of these are by adolescent males. Every year slightly more than 1 million pregnancies occur to females between the ages of 15 and 19 years. Teenage pregnancy and fertility rates (1987) vary widely among the states, but the average is 11.2 per 1000 aged 15 to 19. Of these pregnancies, 38.7% ended in abortion and 13.4% were estimated to have ended by miscarriage. The remainder (47.9%) were carried to the birth of a preterm or term infant; 4% of these mothers relinquished their babies for adoption (Nakashima, 1986). Overall, the teenage pregnancy rate for the 15 to 19-year-old age group has slightly decreased, while the birth rate for the 10 to 14-year-old age group has comparably increased (Johnson, 1986). Among the developed nations, the United States has the highest fertility and abortion rates for adolescent females and a very poor standing in adolescent neonatal mortality (Blum, 1987; Lee and Corpuz, 1988).

Consequences

The **physiologic consequences** of early adolescent pregnancy seem to be less than previously proposed (McAnarney and Hendee, 1989a). However, for the early adolescent, anemia, preeclampsia, cephalopelvic disproportion (CPD), and placental abruption persist as pregnancy sequelae (Blum, 1987). The maternal mortality from pregnancy complications among females under age 15 years who give birth is much higher (approximately 2.5 times higher) than that for mothers aged 20 to 24 (Stockard, 1986). There is a question of whether age or the adolescent's psychosocial development is the major determinant of the most frequent sequelae for the infant: low birth weight, birth trauma, and preterm birth (Elster, 1984). The incidence of low-birth-weight babies born to adolescents is reported to be as high as 20% (American Academy of Pediatrics, 1989a). Factors other than maternal age are also implicated in poor outcome. They include inadequate prenatal care and life-style (e.g., use of drugs, smoking, drinking, exposure to sexually transmitted disease), which are known contributors to poor perinatal outcome (Elster, 1984; Mansfield, 1987; Lee and Corpuz, 1988).

Adolescents, even those in early adolescence, who receive excellent prenatal care, including nutritional guidance, have been found not to be at greater risk than older adolescents or adult women who are of similar socioeconomic status, marital status, and race. While high-quality comprehensive prenatal care can limit the physiologic complications experienced by adolescent mothers and their children, such health services are often unavailable. Even if these services are accessible, they often are not used by the adolescent until relatively late in pregnancy (Stockard, 1986; Blum, 1987).

Personal costs of adolescent childbearing are well known. Although most adolescents have the strengths needed to cope successfully with the developmental crises of adolescence, usually they have not yet developed the strengths and skills required of a woman during pregnancy. Social and environmental resources may be limited as well. The adolescent is often without social acceptance of her pregnancy and parenthood, a supportive husband, a stable home, and some financial security. After delivery, adolescent parents face many obstacles to economic and social success (Blum, 1987; Spivak and Weitzman, 1987). Married or not, the adolescent mother may be ill prepared for the responsibilities she is about to assume.

Data from the National Longitudinal Survey of Work Experience of Youth indicate that among young women who become pregnant, drop out of school, and subsequently are delivered of an infant, only 53% have completed their high school requirements by the age of 26 years (Blum, 1987). This compares with a high school completion rate of 95% for women 20 to 26 years of age who bore no children (Mott and Marsiglio, 1985). *Adolescent pregnancy seems to be the primary reason for females to terminate their education prematurely.* A lifetime of lost advantages may result if she lacks the educational criteria to enter the labor force. The adolescent who moves away from home and family may suffer increased loneliness, isolation, and poor self-image. The adolescent mother who marries because she is pregnant is predisposed to divorce (i.e., one out of two such marriages ends in divorce) (Corbett and Meyer, 1987).

The **public cost** of teenage pregnancy is staggering (Stockard, 1986; Blum, 1987). Stickle (1981) reported a 26.4% incidence of low-birth-weight (LBW) infants among mothers under 18 who lacked proper prenatal care. Mothers under 15 are twice as likely to have preterm or LBW infants. Infants at risk as a result of LBW, preterm birth, or intrauterine growth retardation (IUGR) impose a tremendous cost on society. Initial care in intensive care units is expensive. Sequelae to LBW and IUGR, such as mental retardation, cerebral palsy, and epilepsy, add to society's cost.

During 1986 the United States spent $17.93 billion on all families that had been started when the mother was an adolescent, which calculates to an average exceeding $18,000 per year per child born to an adolescent for each of the first 18 years of life (Blum, 1987; Haffner, 1987). This amount represents outlays for Aid to Families with Dependent Children (AFDC), Medicaid, Women and Infant Care (WIC), and food stamps.

Motivation

The personal reasons adolescents give for becoming pregnant vary widely. They include the effect of family relationships, use of coping mechanisms, love and commitment to one another, and the enhancement of self-concept. Some adolescents may have faulty relationships within the family. It may be that in mother-daughter conflicts the daughter uses pregnancy to act out her rebellion or as a statement of her growing sexuality as opposed to her mother's declining sexuality. For others there may be a search for nurturance from a mother or father who failed to provide it during an earlier stage of development.

Some adolescents living in certain ethnic and multigenerational families know that their offspring will be warmly welcomed into the family. In a few instances the pattern for early adolescent pregnancy out of wedlock is a familiar and accepted one. There appears to be a warm, supportive relationship that, once the initial shock to the family system is resolved, results in supportive and nurturing care for the adolescent and her infant.

Pregnancy may function as a coping mechanism. For young girls living in poverty, having babies is one form of economic survival. The allotments of money, food stamps, medical and dental care, and special schooling provided by the government may help them establish their economic, as well as personal, independence. In reality, however, the adolescent's concept of wealth is usually distorted, and a cycle of poverty can be established or perpetuated.

Some adolescents view the child to be born as an ally for themselves, someone who will love them in spite of adversity and who will act as a supportive person. The infant's need to be dependent, to be nurtured, and to be viewed as a person apart is not recognized. The young mother's disappointment and bewilderment over her infant's normal behavior can lead to bitterness and eventual neglect.

Researchers have found a significant love relationship in some teenage couples (Elster and Panzarine, 1983). They report that a crisis during the pregnancy often arose in the relationship between the father of the baby and the girl's parents. Of those adolescents who keep their children, a substantial number eventually marry; the premarital sexual relationship was part of a longer commitment to one another.

Pregnancy can serve as a rite of passage into adulthood and irrefutable evidence of sexual identity and attractiveness. Some adolescents become pregnant as a result of experimentation with genital sex or sexual intercourse. Many teenagers assume this is a normal part of peer activity. Still other teenagers seem to have little or no respect for themselves or their bodies. One nursing student who worked with school-age mothers remarked:

> I was appalled by their passivity. They seemed to feel that another person had every right to do things to their bodies. I feel what is needed most is for them to value themselves, to see the beauty of their own bodies, and not to allow themselves to be destroyed.

Whereas self-esteem is important as a psychosocial variable, it also has strong implications for health care beliefs and practices (Brack, 1988).

Cultural Beliefs

A country such as the United States represents a mosaic of social, ethnic, and racial groups. No culture in the United States promotes premarital pregnancy and childbirth, especially among adolescents. Each group rears its young to accept and act on beliefs considered important to the particular group. As a result, individuals' beliefs vary considerably, as do the resulting actions. Health care providers need to view the client's situation from the client's perspective. Sensitivity to differences must be reflected in nursing care plans, educational materials, and outreach programs to increase the likelihood that the needs of all clients are met (Hendricks, 1988).

Horn (1983) investigated the differences in the beliefs of three groups of young women in the United

States (native-born Indian women, black women, and white women) concerning (1) prevention of pregnancy and contraception, (2) the significance of being a mother at an early age, and (3) the kinds of support systems available within their social networks. These beliefs were found to be influential in their becoming pregnant, as well as during their pregnancies. Horn found that although all the women were knowledgeable about contraception, beliefs dictated its use: "not until after the first baby is born," "use of birth control pills and IUD not acceptable because menstrual cycle is altered," or "religious belief prevented or encouraged use." The significance of becoming a mother at an early age also differed: "there is a value in early pregnancy—it validates one's feminine role"; "it (pregnancy) is not highly desired but accepted"; and "early motherhood is not valued; it is seen as a failure." With reference to expectations that support would be available, the first two groups believed that it would be, but the third group did not expect assistance (and did not receive it).

Speraw (1987) reported on a cross-cultural perspective of adolescents' perceptions of pregnancy. The results of her study suggest that there are distinct, measurable differences in the ways adolescents from differing backgrounds perceive their pregnancies and the effects of pregnancy on their lives. Adolescents who participated identified themselves as white, black, Hispanic, or Pacific Asian. Response themes within groups had many similarities, but in only a few areas was total or near total agreement found. In no group were answers so alike that they could be classified as characteristic of any one group. Perception of pregnancy was individual and dependent on many variables, only one of which was culture.

Findings showed that within the black community, high value was placed on children and motherhood, and strong family support was usually given. Most negative reactions centered on changes experienced within their bodies. High regard was also felt by Hispanic subjects. However, perceived family support was nonexistent or mixed. Responses of white subjects indicated reluctance to accept their pregnancies and reflected feelings of guilt and regret. Pacific Asian subjects offered no clear initial response to pregnancy, made statements related to the idea of fate, and were least likely to list "family" as the source of support. Many subjects from this group were sent away from home in disgrace; there was an expressed need to maintain the family's good name in the community that overrode the need of the adolescent to feel loved or accepted.

In Speraw's study (1987) adolescents described life changes that were pregnancy related. Necessary clothing changes, social isolation from peers (all groups) and from family (Pacific Asian adolescents, especially), modified recreational activities (no motor bike rides), and altered relationships were concerns. The best part of pregnancy and motherhood was given as "just to have something." The anticipated "worst" part of motherhood was "mothering," concern about child abuse, worry, long hours, loss of freedom, and "being disappointed by your child like you disappointed your parents."

❑ DEVELOPMENTAL TASKS

Psychosocial Developmental Tasks of Adolescence

The psychosocial **developmental tasks** of adolescence are interrupted by pregnancy. As with other developmental sequences, there are critical periods when interference can have traumatic effects. The younger the adolescent when she becomes pregnant, the greater will be the trauma. For the 12- to 14-year-old female, pregnancy can be a fearful experience. Because of the extreme youth of these younger adolescents, society tends to respond in a more protective way, and there seems to be a generalized effort to minimize the trauma. The 15- to 17-year-old female, with her mixture of childlike and adult behavior and her more overt conflicts with parents, seems to arouse more societal anger and resentment, perhaps because both family and society must respond in a responsible way to behavior they are at a loss to control. The 18- to 20-year-old female is viewed somewhat as an adult who, with a modicum of support, can fend more adequately and who can assume that major responsibility for her offspring.

The following developmental tasks may be interrupted by pregnancy in adolescence:

1. ***Achievement of new and more mature relations with age mates of both sexes***

The pregnant adolescent may find herself isolated from her peer group. Within some social groups, parents will try to prevent contact between their teenagers and one who has become pregnant—an attempt to proclaim societal condemnation of adolescent behavior. In some areas regular school attendance must be discontinued, which effectively limits meetings with peers. The pregnant adolescent has contact largely with other pregnant teenagers, her boyfriend if he remains available to her, and relatives. Thus the practice time and arena for developing social relationships are limited.

2. ***Achievement of a feminine social role***

In one sense pregnancy confers overt adult sexuality on the teenager, and the feminine role is achieved. In another sense, adolescent pregnancy tends to limit the feminine role to one of procreation. Opportunities for social development of feminine potential are either abandoned or are set aside until early or middle adulthood.

This delay in role maturation is a primary concern for nurses and should be considered when implementing any plan of action. The frustration the adolescent already feels is compounded further by current trends that allow a multitude of life-style choices for women (e.g., single/married, career/homemaker [Hayes, 1987]).

3. ***Acceptance of her physique and effective use of the body***

Adolescents are experiencing a period of rapid change in physical growth and become acutely conscious of their bodies and body sensations. The symptoms of pregnancy can cause the teenager much dismay. The frequent urination of early and late pregnancy may be "treated" by restricting fluid intake. This restriction increases the likelihood of severe constipation or bladder infections.

The increase in melanin causes deepening of color in the areolar tissue of the breasts, the formation of the mask of pregnancy, and the appearance of the linea nigra. These changes may be viewed by the adolescent as stigmas. The increased mucoid vaginal secretions may be thought to be caused by infection and may increase her anxiety and fear. Increased sensitivity of the breasts can be a source of discomfort and anxiety. The fatigue of early pregnancy, compounding the fatigue experienced by many adolescents, can cause the adolescent to assume that she is ill.

Until late adolescence, body image is still formative. By midpregnancy the enlarging abdomen and the increasing size of breasts and buttocks may prompt the teenager to try to control her appearance by dieting, with adverse consequences to fetal health and her own growth needs. The shift in the center of gravity as body posture changes to accommodate the protuberant abdomen causes back strain and lack of balance. These are aggravated by the disparity between the rate of growth of the skeleton and the muscles supporting it; the muscles are not strong enough (even in the nonpregnant state) to maintain correct posture. The effects may be severe if the teenager feels compelled to compete in strenuous activities (including dancing) or to wear nonsupportive shoes because of her need to belong to her peer group. Symptoms of abnormalities, vaginal bleeding, and dizziness are sometimes concealed until serious conditions develop.

It is one thing for a woman who is knowledgeable and secure to accept and cope with the symptoms of pregnancy. For the adolescent whose pregnancy does not have full social approval and whose baby may not be welcomed, the discomforts of pregnancy can assume major proportions. Unfortunately to some they are seen as punishment for their illicit or "sinful" behavior.

4. ***Achievement of independence from parents and other adults***

A teenager's move toward independence comes to an end when she becomes pregnant, and she is compelled to turn to her family for nurturance just as she did as a young child. Even with the support provided by social agencies, the school-age mother-to-be finds it almost impossible to separate herself from her family. With that support comes a reestablishment of family dominance and dependency.

For example, a 15-year-old-girl cannot make a decision relative to the continuing care of her infant without family concurrence. She is not able to provide such care for her child unless some adult is willing to provide shelter and assistance for them both. If this support is not forthcoming, the younger teenager must examine other options (e.g., foster care or giving the child up for adoption). The pregnancy may, however, serve as a catalyst to force the family to examine its relationships. In many instances the pregnancy has been a means of resolving parent-child conflicts in a more growth-responsive way.

Although certain areas of independence are curtailed, others may be substituted. The teenager who assumes responsibility may emerge from this life experience as one who can function in an interdependent manner with adults. These responsibilities include attendance at prenatal care classes, following an adequate dietary regimen, and participating in parenting skills groups.

For some adolescents the forced contact with a caring health professional during pregnancy may have a dramatic effect and provide a role model. As one 16-year-old girl expressed it:

> ■ The only thing that was okay with it all was that I met F ______ (nursing counselor). She likes me—well, I know she does. Even when I got rough, she'd be there. I never knew grown people were like that, that they cared about me. I would like to be like her, not a nurse, but like someone who loves people.

5. ***Establishment of a life-style that is personally and socially satisfying***

A prerequisite of a satisfying life-style is the opportunity to make thoughtful and informed choices in the areas of career, sexual relationships, marriage, family interdependence, and parenthood. Because of interruptions in schooling, many teenagers who might realistically have had other career goals are relegated to occupations that are not commensurate with their capabilities and temperament. Some never overcome this disadvantage; others must postpone any formal preparations until much later in life.

Precipitate marriage by pregnant adolescents has a reported failure rate of 50% (Corbett and Meyer, 1987). This results because the adolescent is unprepared for the give-and-take of such a close relationship, beset by economic problems, and living in inadequate housing (often with parents or inlaws). Often the adolescent has no time for the "fun" of growing up. Thus participants in early marriage tend to experience desertion or divorce, intensifying their sense of alienation and defeat. For the early adolescent, pregnancy and parenthood are seen as unrelated to sexual behavior. Thus, pregnancy comes as a surprise. Parenthood is something that happens to parents, from whom the younger teenager is seeking to establish independence.

The older adolescent, being less egocentric and more capable of problem solving, often is able to face the reality of pregnancy and parenthood in an adult manner. She can seek assistance from social agencies in her own right. She may find, however, that the care of a child without the emotional and economic support of another caring adult means altering career plans.

6. ***Acquisition of a set of values (an ethical system) that will serve as a guide to socially responsible behavior***

Many adolescents do not accept responsibility for becoming pregnant, nor do they develop into concerned, responsible parents. They have failed to act in a socially responsible manner. However, by assuming adult responsibilities associated with pregnancy and parenthood, some adolescents emerge as stronger, other-centered individuals. For those who are unable to be helped or who are not helped to use this experience as a time of maturation, pregnancy may become a coping mechanism, albeit an inadequate one, to solve the problems of the moment. For this group recidivism (repeat of unmarried pregnancy) is more prevalent, and the adolescent who sought to become independent through sexual activity remains a dependent person.

Psychosocial Developmental Tasks of Pregnancy

In common with older pregnant women, the adolescent faces certain developmental tasks directly related to becoming a parent. Her response to the implications and challenges of these tasks reflects her cognitive level (Chapter 4). Adolescents are in the period of transition between the inductive reasoning of late childhood (concrete operations) and the deductive reasoning of the older individual (formal operations). For an adolescent whose thoughts are circumscribed by the "here and now" and "seeing is believing," movement toward the "there and then" and predictions of the future may be limited. The old saying that "you cannot put an old head on young shoulders" holds true.

1. ***Accepting the biologic reality of pregnancy***

The usual response of the adolescent is **denial.** Anxiety about the response of her family or boyfriend will often delay her seeking of outside support. Adolescents have reported that sharing their suspicions of pregnancy with their parents was the most difficult part of their pregnancy and assumed crisis proportions. Many parents also have reported how emotionally distraught their daughter became. Evidently the idea of being pregnant comes with a sense of surprise and disbelief: "I can't believe it is happening to me," "I didn't think I could get pregnant; I'm too young," "I keep thinking it is some awful dream and I will wake up." The sense of denial is so profound that the girl experiences genuine shock at the consequences of her sexual behavior. Denial is also one means to create time to reevaluate her situation. Recognition that she can no longer control the size and appearance of her body heightens her sense of vulnerability and increases the feelings of alienation imposed by the pregnancy.

The end result of the denial of the reality of pregnancy is the postponement of medical care, to the detriment of both the adolescent and her fetus. Abortion as an option may have to be ruled out because of the advanced stage of pregnancy. Infection, drug ingestion, and inadequate nutrition may have already traumatized the fetus. Once the pregnancy is confirmed and care has been initiated, the adolescent, whatever her age, needs help in assuming the responsibility for continuing the care.

2. ***Accepting the reality of the unborn child***

The second task relating to acceptance of the reality of the unborn child develops in the same manner with the adolescent as with the older woman. The idea of a healthy, happy, cuddly baby who will love and obey the parent seems a common fantasy. The young adolescent can be enthusiastic about how she will dress her baby, take her baby out for walks, and bathe and play with the baby. In fantasy the infant acquires a doll-like form, but the care of the baby cannot be set aside as can the care of a doll. The realities of infant care are not faced. The all-consuming nature of child care—the problems with alleviating crying, feeding the infant, and washing clothes—can prove frustrating and may result in nonnurturing behavior toward the child. The concept of the infant's growth and development into first a toddler, then a preschooler, next a school-age child, and an adolescent does not occur to them. They tend to be centered in the present.

3. ***Accepting the reality of parenthood***

Being a parent implies being loving, concerned, and capable of providing the nurturing care an infant needs. It is the most difficult task for adolescents, as it is for many adult pregnant women. The desire for knowledge about childcare activities, nutritional needs of infants, and infant growth and development is evidenced in this group as in any other. One is impressed by the *desire* of the adolescent to be a good mother. The young adolescent is limited in her ability to fulfill the commitment to her child. This results from her meager life experiences, her own need to grow and develop, and her inability to cope with abstractions and to solve problems on the basis of inference and projection (Yoos, 1987).

The older adolescent is more likely to project herself into the future. She can see herself and her infant more readily as separate entities with differing needs. She is more able to fantasize about her child as a preschooler or even a teenager. However, in spite of her greater ability to propose solutions to problems and follow through on suggestions, the family she will create will remain one of the most vulnerable in our society.

Developmental Tasks of Parenthood. The developmental tasks of parenthood include reconciling the imagined with the actual child, becoming adept in caregiving activities, being aware of the infant's needs, and establishing oneself and one's infant as a family. These tasks will be as important to the new adolescent parent's schema as to the adult's (see also Chapters 20 and 21).

NUTRITION

Within the United States the age group with the poorest and most unsatisfactory nutrition status is the adolescent between the ages of 10 and 16 (Corbett and Meyer, 1987). Nutrition requirements are at their highest during this period of rapid weight gain and linear growth. The diet of many adolescents is high in fats, sugar, and salt. These diets ("fast foods") are particularly low in vitamins C and A, folic acid, and fiber. Other deficiencies include riboflavin, thiamin, calcium, iron, and zinc. Although these nutritional imbalances are related to other diseases in later life, this discussion focuses on immediate reproductive consequences. These diets are responsible for such common nutritional concerns as overnutrition and undernutrition and iron deficiency anemia. *Iron deficiency anemia* is seen in 5% to 15% of adolescents, with increased incidence in the black population.

The adolescent's appetite is responsive to many competing influences. Desire for slimness, prevention of acne, wearing of braces, fast foods, food fads, and use of drugs affect nutrition. Nicotine and alcohol consumption alter the appetite by displacing food in the diet. These drugs can lead to nutritional deficiency by changing the transport, metabolism, and storage of nutrients.

Thiamin, riboflavin, and niacin are necessary for energy metabolism. Folacin is important for DNA metabolism. Vitamin B_{12}, vital to the rapid growth of cells during adolescence, is important for fat, protein, and carbohydrate metabolism.

Many adolescents begin to use oral contraceptives (OCs) during the growth spurt. OCs alter the metabolism of proteins, carbohydrates, lipids, and some vitamins and minerals (Chapter 11) regardless of the adequacy of the dietary intake. No clinical manifestations result and routine supplementation is not indicated. However, should vitamin B_6 deficiency be associated with mental depression, supplementation (1.5 mg B_6 per day) or discontinuation of OCs may be considered. Fluid retention increases body weight, a side effect to which many adolescents object.

The use of OCs should be discouraged in the young adolescent who smokes or has a family history of atherosclerotic disease. The health care provider may need to consider monitoring lipid levels for those with such risk factors.

Nutrition During Pregnancy

Nutrition requirements include those of a normal adolescent as well as the growth and development of maternal and fetal tissues. Nutrition inadequacies are to be expected. Early detection and timely intervention of undernourishment may prevent or minimize negative effects of inadequate nutrition on the fetus. Poor nutrition and poverty have been implicated in complications of preeclampsia, anemia, CPD, and low-birth-weight infants.

Adolescent diets restricted out of concern for appearance or by denial of pregnancy can be hazardous to both adolescent and fetal growth and development. For optimum fetal growth the adolescent needs to reach a critical body weight. This point is reached when the woman achieves a weight in *excess of 10% above ideal body weight* by term gestation. This approximates the requirement for adult women: 25 to 30 pounds if the woman is at ideal body weight for height and age at the time of conception. Deficiency in weight must be corrected (see also Chapter 11). Then the 25 to 30 pounds should follow. However, most adolescents, regardless of weight at time of conception, gain less than 25 pounds.

There is a direct correlation between *inadequate weight gain* and LBW infants. Inadequate preconception weight, gestation length, and gynecologic age (≤ 2 years) also influence birth weight. *Gynecologic age* equals the age of the female at conception minus her age at menarche; that is, if the adolescent's present age is 14 and her menarche occurred at age 12, her gynecologic age is 2.

The outcome for the fetus may not be reflected in lowered birth weight alone. Research indicates that ***brain growth*** takes place in an orderly sequence, as does growth of other organs. The first-phase hyperplasia (growth by increase in the number of cells) takes place prenatally. The second-phase hypertrophy (growth by increase in cell size), in combination with hyperplasia, is the growth pattern noted in the first 6 months of life. Maternal malnutrition may therefore contribute to a reduced complement of brain cells in the fetus, and the mother's lack of knowledge of the nutrition requirements of her newborn compounds the problem. The adolescent's concern about her changing body image may cloud her better judgment with regard to food selection and overall nutritional status during pregnancy.

During the adolescent's growth spurt the recommended daily allowances (RDAs) for pregnancy may be insufficient to meet maternal and fetal needs. Factors such as the adolescent's stage of growth, activity level, and physical and mental health may add to or subtract from her nutritional needs (Tables 27-1 and 27-2). Pregnancy increases the need for certain nutri-

Table 27-1 Recommended Daily Dietary Allowance in Calories (Kilocalories)* for Females

Age (Years)	Weight Kg	Weight (lb)	Height Cm	Height (In)	Calories per Kg	Calories per Day
11-14	46	101	157	62	47	2200
15-18	55	120	163	64	40	2200
19-24	58	128	164	65	38	2200
25-50	63	138	163	64	36	2200
51+	65	143	160	63	30	1900
Pregnant						
First trimester						+0†
Second trimester						+300‡
Third trimester						+300‡
Lactating						
First 6 months						+500§
Second 6 months						+500§

Subcommittee on the Tenth Edition of the RDAs, Food and Nutrition Board, Commission on Life Sciences, National Research Council—10th rev. ed: Recommended dietary allowances, Washington, DC, 1989, National Academy Press.
*Based on light to moderate activity.
†If weight is at or above standard for height and age.
‡Based on pregnancy gain of 12.5 kg and infant birth weight of 3.3 kg.
§Plus 650 calories if weight is below standard for age and height.

Table 27-2 Sample Menus for Pregnant Adolescents

	Day 1	Day 2
Breakfast	1 cup unsweetened ready-to-eat cereal with 1 cup 2% milk ¾ cup orange juice	2 pancakes, 1 medium waffle or 1 slice French toast 2 Tbsp syrup 1 cup 2% milk
Snack	1 blueberry muffin 1 cup 2% milk	2 graham crackers 1 6 oz can apple juice
Lunch	1 cheeseburger (fast food) 1 banana Carrot sticks 1 cup 2% milk	3 slices pizza 1 apple Small salad 1 Tbsp dressing 1 cup 2% milk
Snack	1 apple 3 Tbsp peanut butter Caffeine-free soda*	½ cup cottage cheese dip Raw vegetables Caffeine-free soda*
Dinner	1 cup spaghetti with meat sauce Salad 2 Tbsp dressing 1 roll ½ cup chocolate pudding 1 glass water†	3 oz baked chicken 1 cup rice 1 cup green beans 1 roll 1 ice cream sandwich 1 glass water†
Snack	1 slice angel-food cake ½ cup fresh or frozen fruit, no sugar added	3 cups popcorn 1 glass diet ginger ale
	Kilocalories = 2515‡	Kilocalories = 2568‡

*Sample diets should include foods that clients normally consume and therefore provide teaching opportunities about better choices (Example: cola vs. caffeine-free drink).
†Encourage adequate water consumption daily—6 to 8 glasses.
‡Kilocalorie calculations are based on the maximum allowance for growth; however, the best indication that a pregnant adolescent is eating sufficient kilocalories is to monitor weight gain throughout pregnancy. If inadequate or excess weight gain occurs, consultation with a registered dietitian is recommended.

ents that are already deficient in nonpregnant adolescents: kilocalories, protein, iron, folic acid, vitamin C, and other vitamins and minerals. Controversy regarding the need to increase and supplement dietary calcium continues. Most sources support this increase to facilitate mineralization of the fetal skeleton, meet the adolescent's growth needs, and support lactation. A dietary intake of 1200 mg per day is needed.

Newborn Feeding. Initially many adolescents respond negatively to the idea of *breastfeeding*. Fear of permanent alteration in the breasts, a view of breastfeeding as "dirty," other misconceptions, or a lack of role models may inhibit any woman. Peer reactions or negative responses from the spouse or boyfriend are other factors.

Formula-feeding is often the method chosen. The child's nutrition and freedom from infection will depend on the mother's good hygiene in preparation and storage of the formula and in feeding practices.

NURSING CARE

Many interacting biologic and social factors affect the quality of human reproduction, and these in turn are influenced by the preconceptional, maternity, and neonatal care that is made available. The adolescent and her offspring are particularly vulnerable to the risks inherent in pregnancy and parenthood. This is a result of circumstances characteristic of her age group, such as psychologic immaturity, economic dependency, or delayed medical care, and political ineffectiveness. Parental education, age, and parity have been associated with injuries of children. The adolescent's neuromuscular immaturity, impulsivity, use of chemical substances, and lack of safety precautions (i.e., risk-taking behaviors) affect her parenting behaviors (Blum, 1987).

The infants of young teenagers demonstrate a 30% lower birth-weight (accompanied by brain and vital organ immaturity) and a 100% increase in infant mortality (Miller and Miller, 1983). With a quality health care system, early prenatal diagnosis, continued health care and follow-up, adequate nutrition, and education, some of the poor sequelae attributed to the mother's youth have been decreased. For these reasons the care of the adolescent parent requires the concerted effort of physicians, nurses, nutritionists, and social workers. The team approach has proved to be effective in the care of young teenage mothers.

Assessment

An accurate assessment occurs within an atmosphere of trust, understanding, and confidentiality (Fullar, 1986). The nurse must maintain objectivity. A nonjudgmental approach and skillful communication techniques are needed to put the adolescent at ease in expressing her feelings and concerns.

Several areas must be assessed. These include the adolescent mother's health status, developmental level, knowledge base and perceived needs, support systems, and parenting characteristics and abilities. Careful assessment is needed to identify learning and care needs.

Health Status

A thorough health history with a review of systems is needed (Chapter 10). Physical examination and laboratory tests add to the data base. During puberty the vaginal epithelium is thin. Therefore it is more vulnerable to irritation and infection. The adolescent who begins sexual activity at an early age and has an increased number of sexual partners is at greater risk for sexually transmitted diseases (STDs) and associated conditions. Contact vaginitis can result from perfumed soap, powders, and sprays; colored, perfumed toilet paper; and tight jeans or other garments.

Nutrition assessment is essential (Chapter 11). Nutrition problems stemming from the current "in" diet for teenagers can compromise both the mother and fetus. The life-style of many pregnant teenagers includes abuse of alcohol, smoking, and substance abuse and dependence. STDs (Chapter 23) are common risks in this group. These behaviors compromise general health and affect nutrition (Chapters 11 and 28). Adolescent females are at greater risk for scoliosis, which is related to adolescent growth patterns, nutrition, and psychosocial factors.

Immunization status is assessed. Immunizations such as those against diphtheria, tetanus, polio, measles, mumps, and rubella need to be renewed every 10 years. Vision and dental screening must also be considered.

The cardiorespiratory systems must be assessed. If the adolescent smokes, she is asked about a productive chronic cough and shortness of breath, which are indicative of small airway disease. In the presence of severe pleuritic pain with right-upper-quadrant tenderness under the rib cage the young sexually active female is assessed for Fitz-Hugh and Curtis syndrome. This syndrome accompanies perihepatitis that is secondary to gonococcal or nongonococcal pelvic inflammatory disease (PID). Cervical cytology is required to rule out severe dysplasia or even carcinoma in situ (Corbett and Meyer, 1987).

Careful determination of baseline blood pressure is necessary since teenagers have lower systolic and diastolic pressures than older women. A teenager could be in serious jeopardy for eclampsia with a blood pressure reading of 140/90. Chronic hypertension is found in 1% to 2% of adolescents.

During labor and delivery the young teenager (11 to 14 years) suffers from dystocia more commonly than the older teenager or woman. Therefore the incidence of cesarean delivery is higher. Prematurity, small-for-gestational age (SGA), and fetal perinatal mortality are also increased. The risk of maternal mortality is 60% higher for pregnant teenagers under age 15 than for women in their early twenties (Carey, McCann-Sanford, and Davidson, 1983).

Psychosocial Status

Psychosocial screening includes assessment for reactions to pregnancy, depression, or suicide. For many adolescents the pregnancy results in a private grief that is not publicly displayed. The primary language spoken, the school grade completed, and the literacy of the adolescent are also important factors to assess. If possible, it should be determined if the expectant mother is the victim of sexual abuse or incest, which has been found to be the most common cause of pregnancy in those under 15 years of age (Corbett and Meyer, 1987; Holder, 1987; Zdanuk, Harris, and Wisian, 1987).

Effective interaction with the adolescent requires an understanding of the level of psychosocial development and tasks of this age group (Chapter 4). The psychosocial development of the teenager reflects the three stages (early, middle, and late) of adolescence. These stages roughly approximate chronologic age but more precisely are characterized by predominant drives, moods, and abilities (Sahler, 1983; Fullar, 1986). Hatcher (1976) described five aspects of personality development that have proved to be good indicators of the adolescent's overall developmental level. The five aspects are as follows:

1. The identity of parent most related to conflicts
2. The quality and style of her relationships with others
3. Her view of herself
4. Her major defense mechanisms
5. Her goals and interests

Sahler (1983) applied these findings to **readiness for the task of childbearing.**

Significant factors to consider include the adolescent's cognitive status and time orientation, egocentricity, body image, dependency, and peer and spouse relationships. The adolescent is assessed for her knowledge of reproduction, sexual functioning, and her own sexuality. Basic knowledge of these factors is important to help the pregnant adolescent understand more readily the additional changes during pregnancy.

Support Systems

There appears to be a direct relationship between the amount of social support and prenatal course and evidence of appropriate maternal behavior (Mercer, 1985; Fullar, 1986). Emotional support is seen by the young mothers as being the most important type of support, especially if provided by the mother's family of origin (Colletta and Gregg, 1981).

The pregnant adolescent and mother is particularly sensitive to the attitudes and actions of persons in her support system (Mercer, 1985). These people include parents, boyfriends or husbands, and health personnel. Pregnant adolescents become introverted. Often they become distanced from their sexual partners, who may not understand this as a normal stage in accepting the pregnancy. Mercer (1985) notes that assessment of the following can provide a basis for supportive care:

1. How the mother perceives her role
2. Who is helpful to her
3. How she views her infant

Many pregnant teenagers come from socially and economically deprived families. Appropriate use of health care facilities and compliance with preventive health care measures may not be part of their perception of what health care is or of how to maintain good health.

Parenting Abilities

Studies to date have not produced conclusive evidence to show there are major attitudinal differences between adolescent and adult mothers. However, some differences in parenting behaviors are beginning to be documented. For example, adolescents, although providing warm and attentive physical care, appear to use less verbal interaction than do older parents (McAnarney et al, 1986).

Jones et al (1980) and Mercer (1983) found that adult mothers were significantly more responsive to their newborn infants than were younger mothers, regardless of race or of socioeconomic or marital status. Other researchers have confirmed clinical observations that some adolescents use aggressive, inappropriate behaviors, for example, poking and pinching their infants. These behaviors are rarely seen in adult mothers (Lawrence et al, 1981). The negative attitudes may reflect the adolescent's self-centeredness and level of cognitive development. Excessive child abuse by adolescent mothers has not been substantiated by research. It may be that neglect, secondary to lack of knowledge, is a more pronounced feature of parenting disorders in the adolescent (Taylor et al, 1983).

Parenting ability is based on a parent's sensitivity to the infant's needs. Many factors can affect sensitivity, including stress, level of cognitive development, knowledge, infant responses, and support systems. The adolescent mother's age and grade in school influence her behavior toward her infant (Ruff, 1987).

The adolescent's ability to function in a mothering role is affected by the level of stress she is experiencing. Adolescents are exposed to many stresses as they undertake the tasks and responsibilities of parenthood, a role that in our culture is traditionally reserved for adults who are financially and educationally secure. Stress can affect the quality of a person's functioning, making her insensitive to other needs. Adolescents' reactions to perceived stress depend on the quality of their support systems, their self-esteem, and their ability to solve problems directly.

The responses of teenage mothers to their infant's responses parallel those of the adult mother (Chapter 20). Adolescents certainly respond to positive feedback from their infants. They are pleased when their infants recognize them and prefer them over others. However, studies do indicate that adolescents perceive their infants as more temperamentally difficult than do adult mothers (Field et al, 1980).

The adolescent's knowledge of child development is usually limited. This lack may directly affect parental sensitivity by influencing the mother's perception, interpretation, and responsiveness to infant cues (Elster et al, 1983).

Teenage parents have been found to expect too much of their children too soon. A study of adolescent couples revealed that they consistently underestimated the age at which their child could accomplish certain behaviors, for example, sitting alone at 12 weeks (mothers) or at 6 weeks (fathers) (DeLissovoy, 1973). Jarrett (1982) found a similar lack of knowledge. In addition, teenage parents were found to possess inaccurate knowledge of their offspring's cognitive, social, and language development.

Nursing Diagnoses

The information gathered during physical examinations, interviews, and laboratory analysis of specimens is analyzed, and nursing diagnoses are formulated. Nursing diagnoses relevant to the pregnant adolescent might include the following:

Potential for fetal injury related to
- Inadequate placental perfusion secondary to preeclampsia

Knowledge deficit related to
- Nutritional needs of the mother and baby during pregnancy
- Infant growth and development

Potential altered health maintenance related to
- Substance abuse
- Socioeconomic deficits

Situational low self-esteem related to
- Inability to relate to own mother
- Nonsupportive support systems

Planning

The plan of care reflects the adolescent mother's need for increased surveillance, complying with health care measures, and feelings of positive self-worth. The care begins as early as possible in the prenatal period and extends through the formative period of the new family.

The ***goals*** for care of pregnant adolescents parallel those for care of all pregnant women: to assist them in experiencing a physically safe and emotionally satisfying pregnancy and to promote optimum health in their offspring. Care of teenage mothers also includes the following goals:

1. The mother receives early and continued prenatal care
2. The mother receives comprehensive obstetric, psychosocial, parenting, and outreach services in one setting
3. The mother receives creative forms of health care delivery to maximize services to all pregnant adolescents and their families

Implementation

It is important that persons who work with pregnant adolescents have come to terms with their own sexuality to be able to maintain a nonjudgmental approach. They must be genuinely interested in the adolescent, as well as being enthusiastic, warm, caring individuals able to view adolescents as young persons involved in an exciting growth period. They need to accept the adolescent as someone willing to respond to a concerned adult and who basically wants to be accepted and successful. Nurses need to be able to listen and to respond with honest answers, to be available when needed, and to be capable of accepting repeated "testing" by the adolescent. They need to be able to create a safe and stable environment that engenders trust. Such an environment will enable the professional to determine the adolescent's real problems and to set realistic goals. Accepting some behavior as typically adolescent and not as acting-out or hostile reactions to pregnancy will enable the caregiver to maintain concern for the population served and to remain committed on an individual basis.

Nurses who work with pregnant adolescents need to be knowledgeable concerning (1) the physical attributes of the adolescent and her developmental needs, (2) the adolescent's maturational level relative to personality and cognitive development, (3) maternal responses to pregnancy and the adolescent's interpretation of them, and (4) the cues that indicate stress in the adolescent and difficulties in parenting.

Nurses need to be adept in using a variety of teaching strategies (Fullar, 1986). Group discussions are effective because adolescents have a strong need for peer contact and acceptance. However, because of the immaturity of the participants the nurse will often need to act as leader. Question boxes and anonymous pretests are devices that reveal gaps in knowledge or belief in myths. Demonstrations by the nurse, with group members exhibiting the same skill, are an effective means of assessing the teenager's abilities. Creative approaches, including peer education and computer games, actively involve teenagers in self-care with good results. As counselors and advocates, nurses are concerned with the adolescent's ability to make decisions, to explore the risks and consequences of her actions, and to assume responsibility for her behavior. Some of the techniques used to encourage growth in these areas include having the adolescent set up a discussion group, decorate a child care space, select a menu, plan a day for herself and her infant, and talk over solutions to problems. Independent function is encouraged; the nurse acts as a catalyst in solving problems, but the problem solving belongs to the adolescent.

Another area in which the adolescent requires assistance is in helping her separate herself from her baby so that she can see the child's unique needs. Information relative to child development and to infant caregiving is basic to this goal.

Nurses can act as role models for adolescent parents in the care of themselves and their infants. Areas particularly important to emphasize to the mother are healthy life-styles, cleanliness, and good eating habits. The nurse can help the young mother become skillful in taking care of the daily needs of her infant. The nurse's physical assessment skills can be taught to the parent so that she becomes more knowledgeable about her child's needs.

Community Support

Before 1960 the care of pregnant adolescents was centered in maternity residences for unmarried mothers, operated in many cases by either the Salvation Army or the Florence Crittendon organizations. In the 1960s and 1970s the age of the mother, rather than the "legitimacy" aspects of the parenthood, became the focus of attention. As a result, community programs with a triad of services—medical, social, and educational—were established.

Because of the circumstances of adolescent pregnancy, programs specifically addressing the problems of the adolescent are being developed across the country (Appendix I). Clinics for adolescents are better equipped to provide health care services responsive to the teenager's unique needs (Nathanson and Becker, 1985). They also provide for supportive associations with the father of the child and with the girl's parents or other authority figures. They utilize a multidisciplinary team of nurse-midwives, physicians, nurses, nutritionists, and social workers. The outcomes of lower recidivism and increased birth weights are two indicators of their effectiveness.

Pregnancy

The adolescent is considered to be at risk during her pregnancy. There is an increase in scheduled prenatal visits. Effort is expended to encourage prompt attendance at the clinic; lapses in attendance are followed up by telephone calls or personal contacts.

Prenatal Classes. The content of prenatal classes is chosen with the adolescent's needs in mind. Content relating to maternal adaptations during pregnancy should be presented in terms of how the adolescent can adjust to changes (Fig. 27-2). For example, exercises to promote posture, the care of skin, hair, and nails, and hygiene for increased perspiration and vaginal secretions are discussed. Concrete examples of "what to do" and "what not to do" are needed. Orientation in the present makes it difficult for the adolescent to anticipate the baby's needs.

Teaching requires flexibility, good humor, ingenuity, and at times, ego strength. Standard approaches are not likely to appeal to adolescents. Probably they will not have anyone with whom to attend the classes. Films that depict a loving couple experiencing classes and birth may cause the unpartnered adolescent to "tune out." The teacher needs to be friendly and welcoming and may need to sit near the adolescent. Teaching must consider the early adolescent's short attention span; the teaching pace is brisk and interesting. Role-playing allows the expectant mother to become a part-

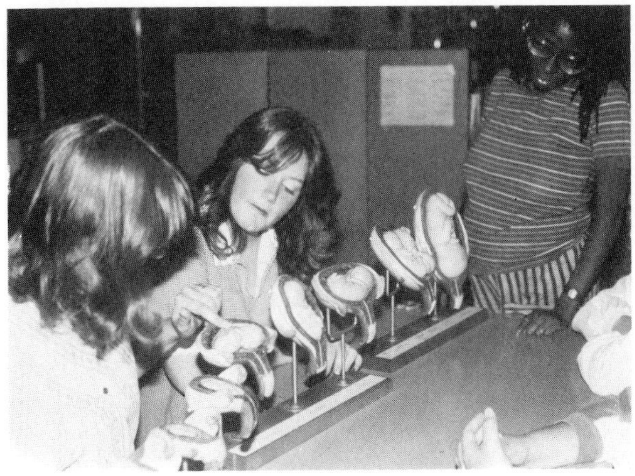

Fig. 27-2 Teenage expectant mothers learn about maternal adaptations to pregnancy. (Courtesy Marjorie Pyle, RNC, Lifecircle, Costa Mesa, Calif.)

ner in her own care. Audiovisual methods allow her to "be there" without actually being there, giving her an option to pace the input.

Information about what happens during labor and delivery and how pain is controlled requires considerable emphasis. Opportunities to discuss feelings and fears with other adolescents who have experienced birth are welcome. Basic information about sex and reproduction is needed to ensure accuracy of the adolescent's knowledge in this area. Birth control information should be included in prenatal classes and presented realistically and nonjudgmentally. Adolescents welcome information about infant care but need help to see the usefulness of information given about child growth and development.

Support and Information Groups. Besides clinics, another type of adolescent health care program designed especially for the pregnant and parenting teen is attracting the attention of various health care providers. These support and information groups are most often community based and coordinated by professional staff and volunteers, but they have self-help and peer assistance as the primary helping method. Generally group meetings are held on a weekly to monthly basis. Prenatal participants may be invited to join as early as the pregnancy is confirmed or up to the time of delivery. For the groups that also have parenting as a component, teen parents and their babies may join at any time.

Other individuals in need of support and information are parents of pregnant and parenting teens. Informally, they have always shared their common problems and tried to learn of workable solutions to their new life situations. Recently, "grandma" groups, composed of mothers of participants of teen groups, have been meeting formally to learn how to better cope, adapt, and grow through their experiences (Lutheran, 1989).

Each adolescent health care program will vary in structure and content depending on the organization or agency sponsoring the program. Some programs, such as MELD's Young Moms (MYM), the teen mom support and information group sponsored by Minnesota Early Learning Design (MELD), are prepackaged with curricular materials, staff training, and technical assistance provided to the purchaser of the program (Ellwood, 1987). Other programs such as Teen Club, a part of Rochester Adolescent Maternity Program (RAMP), admits teens starting at 28 weeks of pregnancy and even helps them learn some basic health care skills, such as measuring and recording blood pressures, weights, fundal height, fetal heart rate, and fetal position (Fullar et al, 1988).

Young Parents Young People (YPYP) was established in St. Louis to help meet a rising need in that

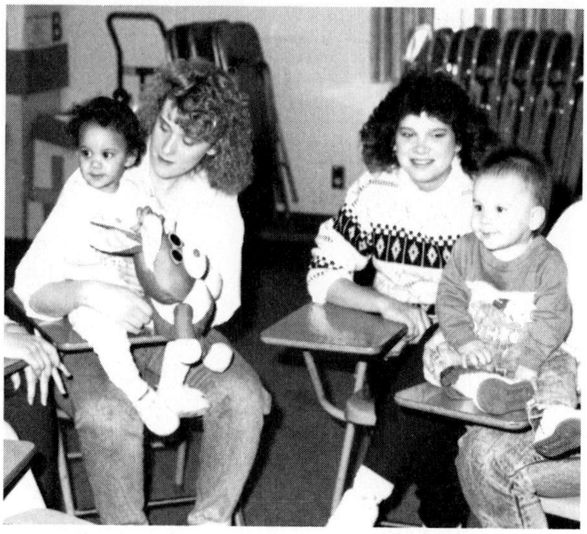

Fig. 27-3 A meeting of pregnant and parenting adolescents belonging to the support and information group, Young Parents Young People (St. Louis).

community. Again, the primary feature is self-help and peer assistance for pregnant and parenting teens under the direction of a nurse educator/researcher who is assisted by community volunteers (Lutheran, 1989). As with the other programs, the desired outcome is fulfillment of social and emotional support needs and assimilation of health care information for successful personal development and parenting (Fig. 27-3). There are a number of self-help and peer assistance programs throughout the country and some of these are listed in Appendix I. Each has been designed to meet the specific needs of adolescent parents by providing services and cooperating with other resource agencies in the community.

Labor and Delivery

The adolescent in labor should have the support of a knowledgeable coach, whether husband, boyfriend, parent, or nurse. Many teenagers come to labor lacking preparation; they are fearful and often alone. If they are admitted early in the first stage, teaching about relaxation with contractions, ambulation, side-lying positions, and comfort measures can be accomplished (Unit III). The teenager's rights to grant informed consent and to refuse treatments must be continually acknowledged (Morrissey, Hofmann, and Thrope, 1986; Holder, 1987). This is also true of her right to be informed of her progress and of both her own and her infant's health status. Recognizing the rights of youthful parents fosters their self-esteem and personal development.

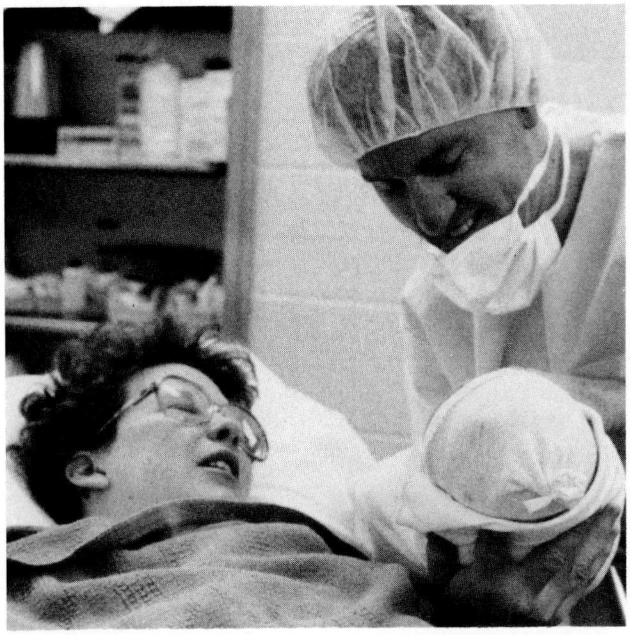

Fig. 27-4 Nurse acquaints young mother with newborn son after cesarean delivery.

Today many adolescents keep their infants and are responsive to the staff's sharing in their delight and joy (Fig. 27-4). For these young parents, efforts to promote parent-child attachment are particularly important.

The Postpartum Period

Physically the adolescent mother will require the same care as any woman who has delivered an infant. Increased emphasis on teaching self-care and breast examination is warranted. Explicit directions as to follow-up care for herself and her infant are required. The need for continued assessment of her parenting abilities during the postdelivery period is essential if needed support is to be forthcoming. Although the nurse may be responsive to cues of parenting ability evidenced in the prenatal period, these findings are not as predictive as the cues noted during the reality phase of parenthood.

If possible the young mother and her child are placed in a rooming-in accommodation so that the process of mothering the child can be started as early as possible. This support needs to be sustained after the mother and child return home. The process of continued care should include home visit and group sessions for discussion of infant care or parenting problems. Research indicates that outreach programs concerned with parent-child interactions, child injuries, and instances of failure to thrive and that provide prompt and effective community intervention do prevent more serious subsequent problems (Ellwood, 1987).

Parenting education needs must be met for the increased number of adolescents who are bearing and raising children. Inexperience and a lack of knowledge about caring for children (i.e., limited knowledge of growth and development, use of physical punishment for controlling child behavior, and suboptimum social stimulation), are probable causes of problems demonstrated by infants of adolescent mothers.

To enhance learning, motivation to learn must be strengthened, and the content taught must be relevant. The learner must recognize a need for information or learning will not occur. Howard and Sater (1985) reported on self-perceived health education needs of 66 adolescent mothers. White, Hispanic, and black females were almost equally represented in this group of 14- to 18-year-old participants. Their educational level varied from 7 to 12 years. The care of the infant was rated the area of primary concern. Ways to make the baby feel loved (90.9%), to protect the baby from accidents (89.4%), and to take care of a sick baby (86.4%) topped the list of perceived learning needs.

The adolescent who has an infant who was born prematurely or who is SGA may find it extremely difficult to reconcile this tiny, scrawny infant with her fantasized baby. Her feelings of helplessness when she contemplates the care of a healthy term infant are compounded when she is introduced to her child in the intensive care unit. It may be impossible for her to perceive herself as mothering such an infant. The additional care needed by the infant can overwhelm the coping mechanisms she had built up so trustingly in the prenatal period. The consequent alienation of mother and infant may never be overcome. Intensive teaching and continuous support programs are essential if both the young mother and her vulnerable infant are not to be overwhelmed.

As noted earlier the young adolescent may not be able to establish a family unit for herself or her child. The interdependence possible in such a unit is denied her. If the young mother and her child are incorporated into the older family unit, the process in which she was moving from dependent to interdependent behavior must be adjusted to accommodate an essentially dependent individual. Persons who provide counseling that involves the parents of the young mother seek to set realistic goals for developing the independence of the adolescent. Topics for open discussions among all persons concerned should include infant care responsibilities, the teenager's need to continue her education, and her need to work toward maturity. The adolescent's parents will need support as well, since they face a new set of responsibilities and tasks. They, too, in a sense, must adjust a fantasy to an actual child.

When assistance is given to a young mother, efforts are made to determine her feelings toward her infant, the quality of the interaction between mother and infant, her knowledge of or attitude toward infant care activities, and her understanding of her infant's growth and developmental needs. Many young mothers pattern their practice on what they themselves experienced. It is vital, therefore, to determine the kind of support that those close to these young mothers are able or prepared to give and the kinds of community aid that can supplement this support. The use of a questionnaire reassures the adolescent that there are concerns common to herself and others.

A general nursing care plan for teenage pregnancy is shown on pp. 807-810.

Evaluation

The maternity nurse needs to evaluate the care she provides to the adolescent client to see how effective her nursing actions have been. As with all pregnant women, the plan of care may have to be revised to meet the unique needs of the individual adolescent client. The maternity nurse has the responsibility of becoming involved in the increasing health needs of the teenage mother.

❑ ADOLESCENT FATHER

The Children's Defense Fund (1988) reported that in 1985, approximately 20% of the infants born to adolescent mothers had fathers under 20 years of age. Thirty-six percent of the infants were born to fathers between 20 and 24 years of age. Studies consistently report that the unwed father is approximately 3 years older than the adolescent unwed mother (Felice et al, 1987). As a matter of routine health history, a determination of health status needs to be made for each adolescent male parent (American Academy of Pediatrics, 1989b).

The effect of pregnancy and parenthood on adolescent fathers has recently become an area of nursing concern. Three major factors have prompted interest in the problems of these young parents.

1. The critical role of the father in the development of a child has been shown (Parke et al, 1980; Lamb, 1981).

2. Health programs have been developed that consider the needs of both the adolescent mother and the adolescent father (Berland, 1987).

3. The role of the father in the birth process has changed. Fathers are now encouraged to be participants in birth. Responsibilities and rights of fathers are more accepted. For example, the federal government expects the unwed mother to attempt to gain child support from the father of the child before it will grant financial assistance (Moore, 1981). A father has the legal right to petition for custody of his child if the mother wishes to place the baby for adoption. Regardless of the length or even the existence of marriage between teen parents, significant numbers of young men remain involved with their children (Stengel, 1985).

Berland (1987) attempted to establish a young fathers' support group. He assumed that he could entice the fathers to attend by persuading the mothers. He found that the mothers often are powerless in their relationships with the father of the baby. For various reasons, other mothers did not wish to have the fathers involved. When the fathers were reached, Berland found that among his subjects, their children's welfare was not as important as their own personal development. Relating to female friends was as far as they could manage. They appeared unready for parenthood.

Nursing Care

Basic to good nursing care is the awareness and appreciation of cultural differences and their implications related to fathering and fatherhood. Results of research reveal that cultural diversity must be addressed in outreach programs for teenage fathers if they are to be effective (Hendricks, 1988).

The adolescent father, as well as the adolescent mother, is faced with the immediate developmental crises of completing the developmental tasks of adolescence and making a transition to parenthood. If the young couple marry, a third stress is added—transition to marriage. In a study of adolescent fathers from three different ethnic groups; white, black, and Mexican American, there was no difference noted by group for the stability of a relationship with their child's mother. Within 6 months of the birth of the infant, up to 24% of the relationships surveyed suffered abandonment, abuse, separation, or divorce (Felice, 1987). The long-range effects of premature parenthood are related to delayed educational and vocational attainment and to lack of stability in a permanent relationship with the infant's mother.

Some unwed fathers voluntarily accompany their pregnant partners to prenatal appointments. Some clinic staffs make it clear that they expect the pregnant adolescent to bring her partner to the clinic and that he will take an active role in the birth process. Assuming that the father is available and that the mother wants him to take an active role, data that are needed for inclusion of the young father in all aspects of the care are based on the assessment of four areas. These areas include (1) the future of the couple together, (2) the adequacy of coping, (3) educational and vocational goals,

General Nursing Care Plan

ADOLESCENT PREGNANCY

ASSESSMENT	NURSING DIAGNOSIS (ND), PLAN/GOAL (P/G)	RATIONALE/ IMPLEMENTATION	EVALUATION
Previous obstetric history. Knowledge regarding: pregnancy, childbirth, parenthood. Cultural beliefs. Financial status. View of pregnancy. Does client want to continue with the pregnancy? Does client want to be a parent or release child for adoption?	ND: Knowledge deficit related to choices regarding pregnancy, childbirth experience, and parenthood. P/G: Client will learn about pregnancy, childbirth, and parenthood. P/G: Client will make her choice to maintain or abort the pregnancy, keep the child, or place the child for adoption.	*Information presented in a sensitive, accepting environment enhances learning:* Examine own views regarding sexuality to be able to maintain nonjudgmental approach. Listen and give honest answers. Accept and expect repeated testing from the adolescent. Create a safe and stable environment that engenders trust. Evaluate which of the three stages of development the adolescent is experiencing. Teach the adolescent about pregnancy choices, childbirth, and parenthood. Utilize group teaching as a means for learning and establishing teen support. Encourage questions and verbalization of fears or concerns. Compliment teen on well-thought-out questions and reference to learned issues. Encourage support person to attend and participate in prenatal care. Refer to childbirth and parenthood class, community support and information groups.	Client learns about her pregnancy choices, childbirth experience; and parenthood. Client makes a choice with which she is comfortable. Client is able to effectively utilize community resources or support from family or friends.
Teen's support systems: boyfriend, peers, family.	ND: Altered family process related to situational crises of adolescent pregnancy. P/G: Client will be able to verbalize expectations of support persons and accept available support.	*Understanding her needs and how support systems may or may not help assists the adolescent in making decisions:* Encourage family members to verbalize questions and concerns. Provide time and opportunity for client to verbalize what she needs/wants from support persons.	Client is able to recognize and effectively utilize support from family and friends. Client and support person attend preparation classes. Client and support person utilize information relating to her physical symptoms.

Continued.

General Nursing Care Plan—cont'd

ASSESSMENT	NURSING DIAGNOSIS (ND), PLAN/GOAL (P/G)	RATIONALE/ IMPLEMENTATION	EVALUATION
		Encourage support person to attend and participate in prenatal care. Reinforce specific healthy behaviors. Refer to childbirth and parenting classes. Provide teaching and assistance to support persons as needed.	
Client's knowledge of community out-reach services.	ND: Knowledge deficit regarding availability of community resources and how to access them. P/G: Client and/or support persons will understand purpose, availability, and how to use community resources. P/G: Client and/or support persons will seek assistance from available community resources.	*Learning about available community resources and how to utilize them increases potential for support:* Provide accurate and current information. Accompany client as appropriate. Make initial contact for client if requested. Offer all appropriate options. Evaluate transportation needs and assist as needed. Encourage use of resources throughout pregnancy, postpartum, and childrearing.	Client and family recognize and use appropriate community services. Client verbalizes positive feelings about using resources.
Teen's current obligations (school, work, home). Accessibility to health care. Coping mechanisms/ strategies client uses.	ND: Ineffective individual coping, related to situational crises of teen pregnancy. P/G: Client will learn the importance of early and continuous prenatal care. P/G: Client will keep her appointments and participate in her care. P/G: Client will use appropriate coping mechanisms	*Prenatal care is associated with healthier outcomes for the client and family:* Provide consistency of caregivers. Explain the need to closely monitor her pregnancy. Create safe, stable environment. Evaluate transportation needs to health care center. Schedule appointments around school or work activities. Use creative forms of health care delivery to maximize services. Note maternal responses to pregnancy and the adolescent's interpretation of them. Provide obstetric, psychosocial, and outreach services in one setting, if possible.	Client attends prenatal care. Client participates in her plan of care. Client demonstrates healthy, appropriate coping strategies. Client keeps regularly scheduled appointments.

General Nursing Care Plan—cont'd

ASSESSMENT	NURSING DIAGNOSIS (ND), PLAN/GOAL (P/G)	RATIONALE/ IMPLEMENTATION	EVALUATION
		Offer teen as many choices as possible and encourage her to take an active role in her plan of care.	
Determine answers to the following: How do you feel about yourself? How do you feel about pregnancy? How do you feel about becoming a mother? What are your goals for the future? Support system.	ND: Body image disturbance, situational low self-esteem, altered role performance, related to pregnancy. ND: Potential for altered growth and development related to concurrent adolescence and pregnancy. ND: Potential for social isolation from family or peers related to pregnancy. P/G: Client will discuss concerns and feelings about pregnancy. P/G: Client will identify her support system. P/G: Client will continue to develop in her stage of adolescence during her pregnancy. P/G: Client will adjust appropriately to new/altered roles.	*A positive self-concept supports healthy growth and development:* Show interest in client, her thoughts and feelings. Provide private place to talk and discuss matters in an unhurried manner. Encourage verbalization. Identify support system with teen. Evaluate teen's adolescent stage to counsel and support her in achieving her developmental tasks. Compliment teen on her appearance, verbalization of feelings, and learning. Refer to outside resources, guidance counselor, tutor. Clarify family's ideas about role delineation.	Client verbalizes her concerns and feelings about pregnancy. Client identifies her support system. Client develops in her own stage of maturity. Client plans for and progresses toward chosen goals for the future.
Assess for teen's use of: alcoholic beverages, smoking, street drugs. Ask if teen's close friends use alcohol, drugs, or tobacco products (see substance abuse, Chapter 24). Assess for teen's use of laxatives, diuretics, and over-the-counter drugs.	ND: Altered health maintenance related to substance abuse. ND: Potential for injury (maternal and fetal) related to substance abuse. ND: Potential for infection related to intravenous drug abuse. P/G: Client will learn how substance abuse will effect herself and her baby during pregnancy. P/G: Client will avoid nonprescribed drugs, smoking, and alcoholic beverages during pregnancy. P/G: Client will not use drugs to alter normal pregnancy weight gain and body changes.	*Substance abuse compromises maternal-fetal well-being:* Explain the dangers of substance abuse to the pregnant woman and fetus. Utilize group teaching to promote peer support against substance abuse. Examine with teen her current peer group and their influence with the use of drugs, smoking, and alcohol. Involve support person in plan to reduce, then eliminate substance abuse. Refer teen to social services and a "quit smoking" or addiction program.	Client learns about the effects of substance abuse on pregnancy. Client avoids nonprescribed drugs, smoking, and alcoholic beverages during pregnancy. Client enters a drug rehabilitation program as necessary.

Continued.

General Nursing Care Plan—cont'd

ASSESSMENT	NURSING DIAGNOSIS (ND), PLAN/GOAL (P/G)	RATIONALE/ IMPLEMENTATION	EVALUATION
How many meals are eaten daily? Who prepares the meals? Cultural and religious influences on food. Knowledge of the four basic food groups. Client's food likes/dislikes. Does she take vitamins? Financial status. (See assessment, Chapter 10). (Does she qualify for WIC?)	ND: Knowledge deficit related to nutritional needs of the mother and fetus during pregnancy. ND: Altered nutrition: less than body requirements, related to increased nutrient requirements during pregnancy and adolescence. P/G: Client will learn about the nutritional needs of pregnancy. P/G: Client will design sample meals that are balanced with the basic food groups. P/G: Client will gain weight appropriate to stage of pregnancy.	*The client's knowledge about nutrition during pregnancy increases her ability to meet nutritional needs that support maternal-fetal well-being:* Review the four basic food groups. Instruct on the importance of adequate nutrition during pregnancy. Examine cultural and financial considerations. Refer to financial support agencies for low income cases (welfare, WIC). Mutually select foods to meet nutrition needs, personal preferences, budget requirements, and seasonal availability. Assist client in designing sample menus. Teach client how to prepare foods to ensure optimum nutritive value.	Client verbalizes understanding of instruction. Client prepares sample menus that meet the daily nutrition requirements during pregnancy. Client keeps a food diary. Client gains weight appropriately during pregnancy.
Has adolescent cared for a child before? Who will be assisting in child care? Support system. Knowledge of infant needs.	ND: Knowledge deficit related to infant care activities, growth patterns, and developmental needs. P/G: Client will learn infant care activities, growth pattern, and developmental needs. P/G: Client will identify her support system for child care. P/G: Infant will remain healthy and grow and develop normally	*Knowledge of infant care activities, growth patterns, and developmental needs assists in the development of parenting skills:* Identify baseline knowledge. Begin infant care activities instruction during prenatal period. Involve support person in teaching sessions. Focus teaching toward adolescent's maturity and cognitive level. Refer client to parenthood classes. Refer to and make initial contact with social services for a future resource person if problems arise in child care.	Client learns infant care activities, growth patterns, and developmental needs. Client identifies her support system. Client's self-esteem increases with increase in skill. Client verbalizes acceptance of assistance from support system. Infant remains healthy, free of symptoms of neglect or abuse, and meets growth and development expectations.

and (4) the adequacy of health education knowledge (Elster, 1982; Elster and Lamb, 1982).

Adolescent fathers (as all fathers) need support to discuss their emotional responses to the pregnancy. These may include pleasure, ambivalence, or anger. The fathers' feelings of guilt, powerlessness, or bravado deserve recognition, since these may have negative consequences for both parents and children (Berland, 1987). Caparulo and London (1981) characterize them as "adolescents first, fathers second." Counseling needs to be reality oriented. Topics such as child care and expense, parenting skills, and the father's role in the birth experience need to be explored. In addition, teenage fathers often need to have myths and fallacies replaced with sound knowledge of both male and female reproductive anatomy and physiology and birth control options (Scott et al, 1988; Westney et al., 1988).

The adolescent mother's partner, as well as her family, have an impact on how she will deal with her pregnancy, labor and delivery, and subsequent parenthood. The adolescent partner may continue to be involved in an ongoing relationship with the young mother. In many instances he plays an important role in the decisions she faces in pregnancy. He may influence her decision to continue the pregnancy or have an abortion and to keep the child or place the child for adoption. Depending on his relationship with his own parents and with the parents of the mother, he may be encouraged to take an active role as a prospective father, or he may be rejected and forced to withdraw from the situation altogether.

The nurse supports the young father by helping him develop realistic perceptions of his role as "father to a child." The nurse encourages his use of coping mechanisms that are not detrimental to his, his partner's, or his child's well-being. The nurse encourages him to enlist support from parents, professionals, and agencies/organizations as he deems appropriate. Promoting mutual responsibility for birth control is a constant necessity.

SUMMARY

Much has still to be done before the problems of adolescent pregnancy and its sequelae for infant, mother, family, and society in general are solved. Cooperative effort on personal, local, and national levels is mandatory. Further investigation of biopsychosocial etiologic factors is imperative if long-term and short-term effects of physical/mental morbidities related to adolescent pregnancy are to be reduced. In spite of the development of many successful programs, adolescent pregnancy remains the most pressing problem in maternity and gynecologic nursing care today.

KEY CONCEPTS

- Adolescents vary considerably depending on age and life experiences.
- Adolescents see their world in far different terms than do adults: their major task is the development of cognitive ability.
- Cognitive development influences sexual decision making.
- Increasingly, poverty, life-style, and risk-taking behaviors are implicated in adolescent morbidity, with associated sequelae of pregnancy and other major health problems.
- Physiologic consequences and personal and public costs of adolescent pregnancy and parenthood are staggering.
- The adolescent's perception of pregnancy and parenthood is individual and dependent on many variables.
- The developmental tasks of adolescents are interrupted by pregnancy.
- Poor nutrition and poverty have been implicated in physiologic consequences to the adolescent mother and her fetus and newborn.
- Adolescents' reactions to perceived stress depend on the quality of their support systems, their self-esteem, and their skill in problem identification and problem solving.
- Adolescents can develop trusting relationships with helping professionals whom they respect.
- The adolescent's knowledge of child development is usually limited.
- Standard approaches to prenatal and postpartum teaching are not appropriate or appealing for most adolescents.

LEARNING ACTIVITIES

1. Ask to be assigned to a newly delivered adolescent mother. Sit down with her and jointly plan a day for herself and her infant after discharge home.
2. Explain how each of the following adolescent developmental tasks may be interrupted by pregnancy:
   A. Acceptance of one's physique and effective use of the body.
   B. Achievement of independence from parents and other adults.
   C. Acquisition of a set of values that will serve as a guide to socially responsible behavior.
3. Make a list of your personal feelings about adolescent pregnancy.
   A. Identify your biases and values.
   B. Make a list of your responses as a professional to the issues of adolescent pregnancy.
   C. Analyze the relationship between your personal and professional values as it affects your care of the adolescent couple experiencing pregnancy.

References

American Academy of Pediatrics, Committee on Adolescence: Adolescent pregnancy, Pediatrics 83:132, 1989a.

American Academy of Pediatrics, Committee on Adolescence: Care of adolescent parents and their children, Pediatrics 83:138, 1989b.

Arms S: To love and let go, New York, 1983, Alfred A Knopf, Inc.

Berland A: Young fathers' support group, Pediatr Nurs 13(4):255, 1987.

Blum R: Contemporary threat to adolescent health in the United States, JAMA 257(24):3390, 1987.

Brack CJ, Orr DP, and Ingersoll G: Pubertal maturation and adolescent self-esteem, J Adolesc Health Care, 9:280, 1988.

Caparulo F and London K: Adolescent fathers: adolescents first, fathers second, Issues in Health Care of Women 3:23, 1981.

Carey W, McCann-Sanford T, and Davidson E, Jr: Adolescent age and obstetric risk. In McAnarney E, editor: Premature adolescent pregnancy and parenthood, New York, 1983, Grune & Stratton, Inc.

Children's Defense Fund Reports 9(10):1, 1988.

Colletta ND and Gregg CH: Adolescent mothers' vulnerability to stress, J Nerv Ment Dis 169:50, 1981.

Corbett M and Meyer JH: The adolescent and pregnancy, Boston, 1987, Blackwell Scientific Publications, Inc.

DeLissovoy V: Child care by adolescent parents, Child Today 2:23, 1973.

Ellwood A: Prove to me that MELD works. In Weiss H and Jacobs F, editors: Evaluating family programs, Boston, Harvard Family Research Project, 1987.

Elster AB: Effects of pregnancy and parenthood on adolescent fathers and implications for clinical intervention, J Calif Perinatal Assoc 2(2):44, 1982.

Elster AB: The effect of maternal age, parity, and prenatal care on perinatal outcome in adolescent mothers, Am J Obstet Gynecol 149(8):845, 1984.

Elster AB and Lamb ME: Adolescent fathers: a group potentially at risk for parenting failure, Infant Ment Health J 3:148, 1982.

Elster AB and Panzarine S: Teenage fathers: a trajectory of stress over time. Presented at the Society for Adolescent Medicine, New Orleans, Oct 29, 1983.

Elster AB et al: Parental behavior of adolescent mothers, Pediatrics 71:494, 1983.

Emans SJ and Grimes DA: Contraceptive choice for teenagers, JAMA 257(24):3419, 1987.

Felice ME et al: Clinical observations of Mexican-American, caucasian, and black pregnant teenagers, J Adolesc Health Care 7:305, 1987.

Field TM et al: Teenage, lower-class black mothers and their preterm infants: an intervention of developmental follow-up, Child Dev 51:426, 1980.

Fullar SA: Care of postpartum adolescents, MCN 11(6):398, 1986.

Fullar SA et al: A small group can go a long way, MCN 13:414, 1988.

Goleman D: Why teenagers are reckless, San Francisco Chronicle Dec 2, 1987.

Hatcher SL: Understanding adolescent pregnancy and abortion, Primary Care 3:407, 1976.

Hayes CD: Risking the future: adolescent sexuality, pregnancy, and childbearing, Washington, DC, 1987, National Academy Press.

Hendricks LE: Outreach with teenage fathers: a preliminary report on three ethnic groups, Adolescence 23(91):711, 1988.

Holder AR: Minors' rights to consent to medical care, JAMA 257(24):3400, 1987.

Horn B: Cultural beliefs and teenage pregnancy, Nurs Pract 8:35, Sept, 1983.

Howard JS and Sater J: Adolescent mothers: self-perceived health education needs, JOGN Nurs 14(5):399, 1985.

Jarrett GE: Childrearing patterns of young mothers: expectations, knowledge, and practices, MCN 7(2):119, 1982.

Johnson KA: Building health programs for teenagers, Washington, DC, May, 1986, Children's Defense Fund.

Jones FA et al: Maternal responsiveness of primiparous mothers during the postpartum period: age differences, Pediatrics 65:579, 1980.

Kornfield R: Who's to blame: adolescent sexual activity, J Adolesc 8(1):17, 1985.

Lamb ME: Fathers and child development: an integrative overview. In Lamb ME, editor: The role of the father in child development, New York, 1981, Wiley-Interscience.

Lawrence RA et al: Aggressive behaviors in young mothers: markers of future morbidity? Pediatr Res 15:443, 1981.

Lee K and Corpuz M: Teenage pregnancy: trend and impact on rates of low birth weight and fetal, maternal, and neonatal mortality in the United States, Clin Perinatol 15(4):929, 1988.

Lutheran charities grant expands parents programs Saint Louis Lutheran 43(2):4, 1989.

Mansfield PK: Teenage and midlife childbearing update: implications for health educators, Health Educ 18(4):18, 1987.

McAnarney ER and Hendee WM: Adolescent pregnancy and its consequences, JAMA 262(1):74, 1989a.

McAnarney ER and Hendee WM: The prevention of adolescent pregnancy, JAMA 262(1):78, 1989b.

McAnarney ER et al: Premature parenthood: a preliminary report of adolescent mother-infant interaction, Pediatr Res 13:328, 1979.

McAnarney E et al: Interaction of adolescent mothers and their 1-year-old children, Pediatrics 78:585, 1986.

Mercer RT: Assessing and counseling teenage mothers during the perinatal period, Nurs Clin North Am 18(2):293, 1983.
Mercer R: Relationship of birth experience to later mothering behaviors, J Nurse Midwife 30:204, July/Aug, 1985.
Miller EK and Miller KA: Adolescent pregnancy, a model for intervention, Personnel and Guidance 62:15, 1983.
Moore KA: Government policies related to teenage family formation and functioning: an inventory. In Ooms T, editor: Teenage pregnancy in a family context: implications for policy, Philadelphia, 1981, Temple University Press.
Morrissey JM, Hofmann SD, and Thrope JC: Consent and confidentiality in the health care of children and adolescents: a legal guide, New York, 1986, Free Press.
Mott F and Marsiglio W: Early childbearing and the completion of high school, Fam Plann Perspect 17:234, 1985.
Nakashima I: Adolescent pregnancy in practice of pediatrics, Philadelphia, 1986, Harper & Row, Publishers, Inc.
Nathanson CA and Becker MH: The influence of client-provider relationships on teenage women's subsequent use of contraception, Am J Pediatr Health 75:33, 1985.
Parke RD et al: The adolescent father's impact on the mother and child, J Soc Issues 36:88, 1980.
Polit D and Kahn J: Early subsequent pregnancy among economically disadvantaged teenage mothers, Am J Public Health 76(2):167, 1986.
Ruff CC: How well do adolescents mother? MCN 12(4):249, 1987.
Sachs B: Reproductive decisions in adolescence, IMAGE: J Nurs Scholarship 18(2):69, 1986.
Sahler OJ: Adolescent mothers: how nurturant is their parenting? In McAnarney ER, editor: Premature adolescent pregnancy and parenthood, New York, 1983, Grune & Stratton, Inc.
Scott CS et al: Hispanic and black American adolescents' beliefs relating to sexuality and contraception, Adolescence 23(91):667, 1988.
Speraw S: Adolescents' perceptions of pregnancy: a cross-cultural perspective, West J Nurs Res 9(2):180, 1987.
Spivak H and Weitzman M: Social barriers faced by adolescent parents and their children, JAMA 258(11):1500, 1987.
Stengel R: The missing father myth, Time, p 88, Dec 9, 1985.
Stickle G: Overview of incidence, risks and consequences of adolescent pregnancy and childbearing, Birth Defects 17(3):5, 1981.
Stockard R: Facing the facts on adolescent pregnancy, NAACOG Newsletter 13(9):1, 1986.
Taylor B et al: Teenage mothering, admission to hospital, and accidents during the first five years, Arch Dis Child 58:6, 1983.
Westney OE et al: The effects of prenatal education intervention on unwed prospective adolescent fathers, J Adolesc Health Care 9:214, 1988.
White-Traut RC and Pabst MK: Parenting of hospitalized infants by adolescent mothers, Pediatr Nurs 13(20:97, 1987.
Yoos L: Adolescent cognitive and contraceptive behaviors, Pediatr Nurs 13(4):247, 1987.
Zdanuk JM, Harris CC, and Wisian NL: Adolescent pregnancy and incest: the nurse's role as counselor, JOGN Nurs 16(2):99, 1987.
Zelnick M: Sexual activity among adolescents: perspectives of a decade. In McAnarney ER, editor: Premature adolescent pregnancy and parenthood, New York, 1983, Grune & Stratton, Inc.

Bibliography

Baisch MJ, Fox RA, and Goldberg BD: Breast-feeding attitudes and practices among adolescents, J Adolesc Health Care 10:41, 1989.
Bearinger L and Gephart J: Priorities for adolescent health: recommendations of a national conference, MCN 12(3):161, 1987.
Burke PJ: Adolescent's motivation for sexual activity and pregnancy prevention, Issues Compr Pediatr Nurs 10:161, 1987.
Davidson J and Grant C: Growing up is hard to do . . . in the AIDS era, MCN 13(5):352, 1988.
DuRant RH and Sanders JM: Sexual behavior and contraceptive risk taking among sexually active adolescent females, J Adolesc Health Care 10:1, 1989.
Giblin PT: Pregnant adolescents' health information needs J Adolesc Health Care 7:168, 1986.
McAnarney E: Children having babies, Am J Dis Child 141:1053, 1987.
Mercer RT: First-time motherhood: experiences from teens to forties, New York, 1986, Springer Publishing Co, Inc.
Panel on adolescent pregnancy and childbearing, National Research Council: Risking the future: adolescent sexuality, pregnancy and childbearing, Washington, DC, 1987, National Academy Press.
Panzarine S: Teen mothering: behavior and interventions, J Adolesc Health Care 9:443, 1988.
Szydlo VL: Approaching an adolescent about a pelvic exam, Am J Nurs 88(11):1502, 1988.

CHAPTER

28 The Newborn at Risk

Irene M. Bobak

Learning Objectives

Correctly define the key terms listed.

Discuss the nursing process relative to a newborn at risk.

Develop a nursing care plan for a newborn with respiratory distress.

Explain the importance of temperature support and regulation.

Discuss nursing care related to nutrition, feeding, and elimination.

Explore the emotional aspects of care of the high-risk newborn and the family.

Discuss the nursing process relative to newborns according to gestational age and weight.

Discuss complications associated with preterm birth or dystocia.

Describe the nursing process relative to newborns for birth trauma and for sequelae to a diabetic pregnancy.

Describe the nursing process relative to a newborn with infection and drug dependence.

Compare and contrast Rh and ABO incompatibility.

Develop a general plan of care for the prevention, identification, and management of hyperbilirubinemia in any newborn.

Review prenatal diagnosis and present assessment strategies during the postnatal period to aid in diagnosis of congenital disorders.

Develop nursing care plans for newborns with selected complications presented in this chapter.

Key Terms

ABO incompatibility
α-fetoprotein
appropriate-for-gestational age (AGA)
birth trauma (injuries)
bronchopulmonary dysplasia (BPD)
cardiomyopathy
cold stress
congenital anomalies
congenital rubella syndrome
Coombs' test
fetal alcohol syndrome (FAS)
fetal hyperinsulinism
fetal tobacco syndrome
hemolytic disease of newborn
high-risk parenting
hydrocephalus
hydramnios
inborn errors of metabolism
infants of diabetic mothers (IDMs)
infants of gestational diabetic mothers (IGDMs)
"kangaroo method"
kernicterus
large-for-gestational age (LGA)
low birth weight (LBW)
macrosomia
meconium aspiration syndrome (MAS)
necrotizing enterocolitis (NEC)
newborns at risk
newborn maturity rating and classification
newborn stimulation
nonnutritive suckling
nosocomial infections
oligohydramnios
perinatal asphyxia
prolonged pregnancy
PROM
postmature
postterm
premature
preterm
readiness for interaction
respiratory distress syndrome (RDS)
retinopathy of prematurity (ROP)
sepsis
septicemia
septic shock
small-for-gestational age (SGA)
term
TORCH
withdrawal syndrome

The compromised newborn or newborn at risk is one whose intact survival is in jeopardy. "Normal" values and parameters vary with the newborn's level of maturity and developmental problems. Assessment and therefore supportive care are complicated further by the newborn's inability to speak and by nonspecific, generalized responses to dysfunctional problems. Assessment rests heavily on historical data provided by the mother and obstetric team and on current levels of knowledge related to gestational age and disorders of the newborn. Planning and implementation of the nursing process with the newborn at risk focus on the physiologic maintenance of warmth, respiration, and nutrition.

Assessment for factors that place the newborn at risk is presented in Chapter 22. The box below summarizes these factors. For greater ease in studying the content that follows some terms will be defined. Classification of newborns according to *gestational age* is as follows (Fig. 28-1):

Preterm or premature Born before completion of 37 weeks' gestation, regardless of birth weight.

Term Born between the beginning of the thirty-eighth week and the end of the forty-second week of gestation.

Postterm Born after completion of the forty-second week of gestation.

Postmature Born after completion of the forty-second week of gestation and have experienced the effects of progressive placental insufficiency.

The *weight* of the newborn has a normal range for each gestational week (Figs. 28-1 and 28-2). Variations in weight may occur in the preterm, term, postterm, or postmature newborn. Classification of newborns by weight is as follows:

Large-for-gestational age (LGA) Weight is above the 90th percentile (or two or more standard deviations above the norm) at any week.

Appropriate-for-gestational age (AGA) Weight falls between the 10th and 90th percentile for infant's age.

Small-for-gestational age (SGA) Weight is below the 10th percentile (or two or more standard deviations below the norm).

Low birth weight (LBW) Weight of 2500 g or less at birth. These newborns are considered to have had either less than the expected rate of intrauterine growth or a shortened gestation period. Preterm birth and LBW commonly occur together (e.g., <32 weeks and <1200 g birth weight). **Intrauterine growth retardation (IUGR)** is the term used to describe the fetus whose rate of growth does not meet expected norms.

Common causes of LGA newborns include glucose intolerance of pregnancy, true maternal diabetes mellitus, maternal overnutrition, and heredity. SGA newborns may be the result of maternal smoking, hypertensive states, undernutrition, anemia, or nephritis. In addition, the birth of an SGA newborn may be associated with multifetal gestation, a discordant twin pregnancy, or congenital anomalies. High altitude, rubella, or intrauterine infection may predispose a woman to the birth of an SGA newborn. Fetal malnutrition, IUGR, and chronic fetal distress are other processes that may result in the birth of newborns who are SGA.

The care of the newborn at risk has become highly

FACTORS THAT PLACE THE NEWBORN AT RISK

FACTORS THAT PLACE NEWBORN IN HIGH-RISK CATEGORY

- Newborns continuing or developing signs of respiratory distress syndrome (RDS) or other respiratory distress
- Asphyxiated newborns (Apgar score of less than 6 at 5 minutes); resuscitation required at birth
- Preterm newborns; dysmature newborns
- Newborns with cyanosis or suspected cardiovascular disease; persistent cyanosis
- Newborns with major congenital malformations requiring surgery; chromosomal anomalies
- Newborns with convulsions, sepsis, hemorrhagic diathesis, or shock
- Meconium aspiration syndrome
- Central nervous system (CNS) depression for longer than 24 hours
- Hypoglycemia
- Hypocalcemia
- Hyperbilirubinemia

FACTORS THAT PLACE NEWBORN IN MODERATE-RISK CATEGORY

- Dysmaturity
- Low birth weight
- Apgar score of less than 5 at 1 minute
- Feeding problems
- Multifetal gestation (e.g., twins)
- Transient tachypnea
- Hypomagnesemia or hypermagnesemia
- Hypoparathyroidism
- Failure to gain weight
- Jitteriness or hyperactivity
- Cardiac anomalies not requiring immediate catheterization
- Heart murmur
- Anemia
- CNS depression for less than 24 hours

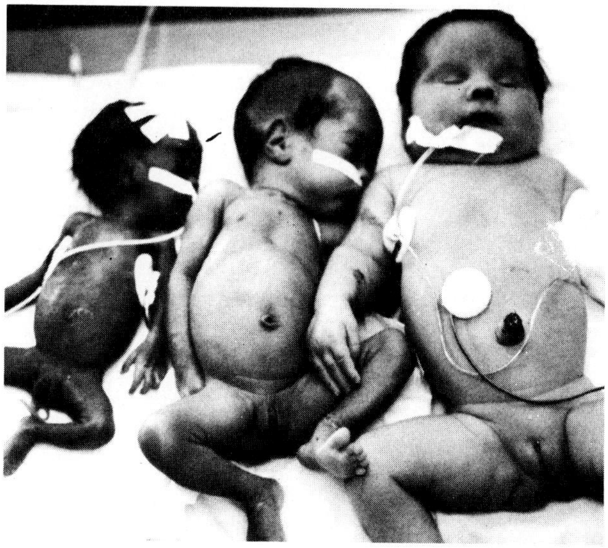

A

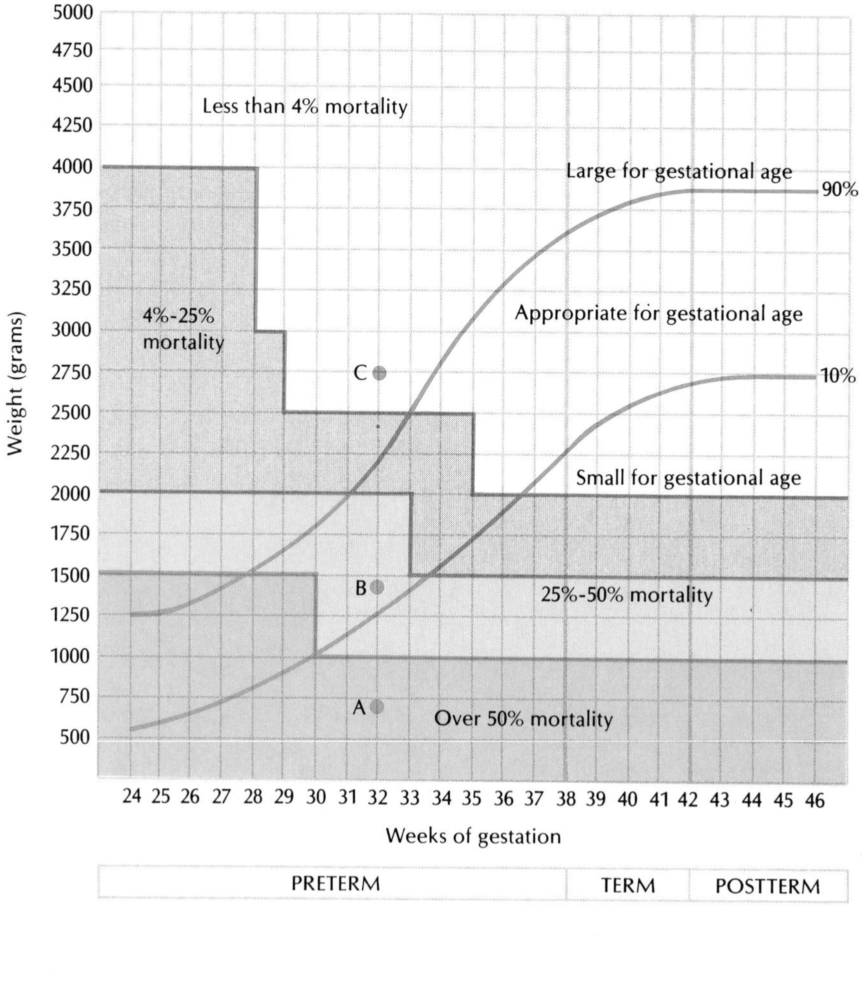

B

Fig. 28-1 **A,** Three babies of same gestational age, with weights of 600, 1400, and 2750 g, respectively, from left to right. Their weights are plotted in **B,** at points *A, B,* and *C.* **B,** Intrauterine growth status for gestational age and according to appropriateness of growth. Weights of infants shown in **A,** are plotted at points *A, B,* and C. (**A,** From Korones SB: High-risk newborn infants; the basis for intensive nursing care, ed 4, St Louis, 1986, The CV Mosby Co. **B,** Courtesy Mead Johnson & Co, Evansville, Indiana. Modified from Battaglia FC and Lubchenco LO: J Pediatr 71:59, 1967.)

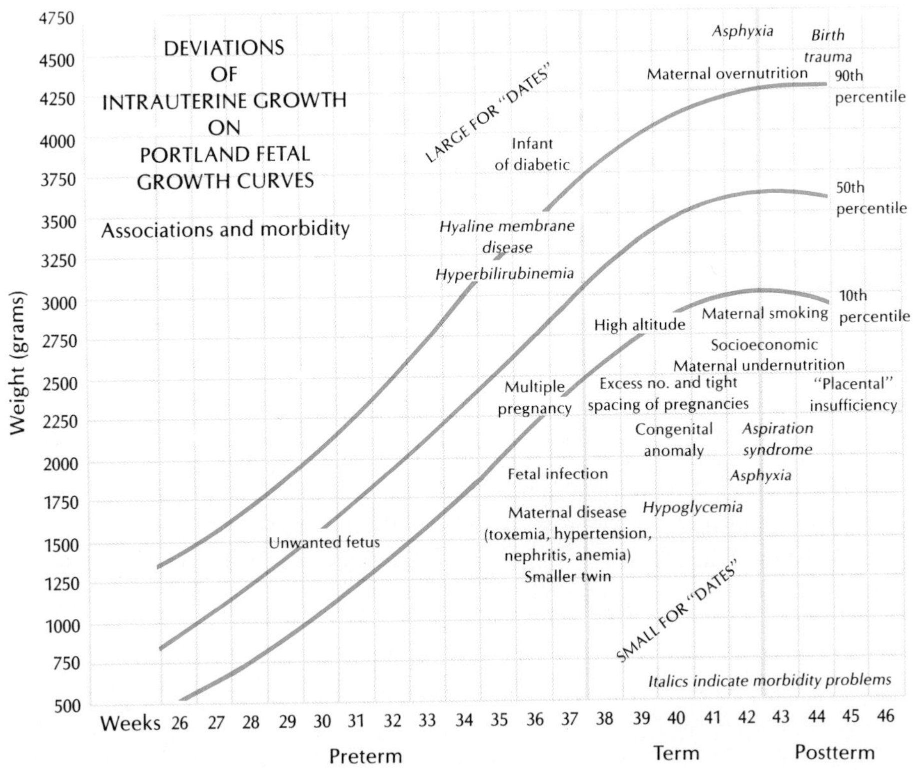

Fig. 28-2 Important associations and morbidity factors of accelerated or reduced fetal growth above 90th percentile and below 10th percentile for gestational age using Portland curves. Fetal growth data obtained from 40,000 single, white, middle-class infants born at *sea level.* (Modified from Babson SG et al: Diagnosis and management of the fetus and neonate at risk, ed 4, St Louis, 1980, The CV Mosby Co.)

specialized and is beyond the scope of this text.* The following discussion presents general content relevant to the care of the newborn at risk. Care of newborns with selected risk factors is discussed. *The nurse's actions can influence the health care team to keep the family's childbearing experience in focus rather than concentrating solely on the risk factors and their management.*

Transport to a Regional Center

Hospitals that are not staffed or equipped to care for the mother and fetus or newborn at high risk arrange for their immediate transfer to a specialized perinatal or tertiary care center (Fanaroff and Martin, 1987). Transfer of the gravida carrying a fetus at risk has two distinct advantages: (1) the mother and newborn are not separated so that attachment is facilitated, and (2) neonatal morbidity and mortality are decreased. It is not always possible to transport the mother before delivery for a variety of reasons (e.g., imminent delivery, lack of prior diagnosis). Therefore it is necessary for physicians and nurses to have the necessary skills and equipment for accurate diagnosis and emergency intervention to stabilize the client's physical condition and to maintain it until transport can be effected.

Parents of newborns who have been transported to regional centers need support, since attachment is interrupted. Parents who are physically separated from their newborns feel a loss of control after the transport team gives them a quick glimpse of the baby and they see wires, equipment, and tubes attached to the newborn (Merenstein and Gardner, 1989). Before they are transported to regional centers, newborns at risk must be stabilized. Attention is given to six basic physiologic areas: temperature regulation and support; oxygen needs and ventilation; acid-base balance; fluid needs; glucose needs; and vital signs (Sandman, 1989).

❑ GENERAL CARE OF THE COMPROMISED NEWBORN

Maintenance of Respirations. Any newborn with respiratory difficulty is in jeopardy.* The newborn's response to prompt, appropriate treatment bears a direct relationship to the cause, degree of maturity, and other medical problems.

Breathing is a new experience. In priority of care, it ranks second only to the control of massive hemor-

*See References and Bibliography. Most facilities have developed modular study guides and manuals for procedures and for laboratory values and their management.

*See discussion on techniques for suctioning the newborn, oxygen therapy, and resuscitation in Chapter 17.

rhage. Because of its high priority and its challenging nursing aspects, considerable space in the delivery room is devoted to the initiation and maintenance of respirations. The alert nurse often is the pivotal point between functional and dysfunctional survival for the newborn in respiratory distress.

Assessment

Prebirth Events

A review of pregnancy and labor records may reveal that the fetus had been at risk for intrauterine hypoxia and **meconium aspiration syndrome (MAS)**. Two fetal responses to intrauterine hypoxia are the passage of meconium through a relaxed anal sphincter and reflex gasping. Hypoxia-induced gasping draws amniotic fluid and any particulate matter contained in the fluid deep into the tracheobronchial tree. At birth, more aspiration may occur, and symptoms of respiratory distress often appear.

An interruption in the oxygen supply to the fetus may result from maternal conditions such as hypertension, anemia, chronic disease, or postterm gestation (Glassanos and Giles, 1986; Turnage, 1989). Several intrapartum events are associated with meconium aspiration. These include prolonged labor, fetal heart rate (FHR) decelerations, fetal bradycardia, and passage of thick meconium early in labor. Preterm or LBW newborns are more at risk for MAS. Atelectasis occurs after partial or complete obstruction of the airway. In addition, atelectasis in MAS may result from the displacement of surfactant by the free fatty acids found in meconium (Clark et al, 1987).

Postbirth Events

The newborn in distress at birth is immediately identifiable. In addition, some newborns who at birth appear pink and vigorous, with good muscle tone and respiratory rates and rhythms within normal range, become distressed soon afterward. Respiratory difficulty, with cyanosis and retractions such as occur after aspiration or tension pneumothorax, may appear suddenly. More commonly, respiratory difficulty follows a progressive sequential pattern: the ***respiratory rate*** initially may increase without a change in rhythm. Flaring of the nares and expiratory grunt are also early signs of respiratory distress. The ***apical pulse*** increases in rate. ***Retractions,*** depending on the cause, may begin as subcostal and xiphoid and then progress upward to intercostal, suprasternal, and supraclavicular retractions (Fig. 28-3). The ***color*** changes from pink to circumoral pallor, to circumoral cyanosis, and then to generalized cyanosis; acrocyanosis deepens. ***Respiratory effort*** and

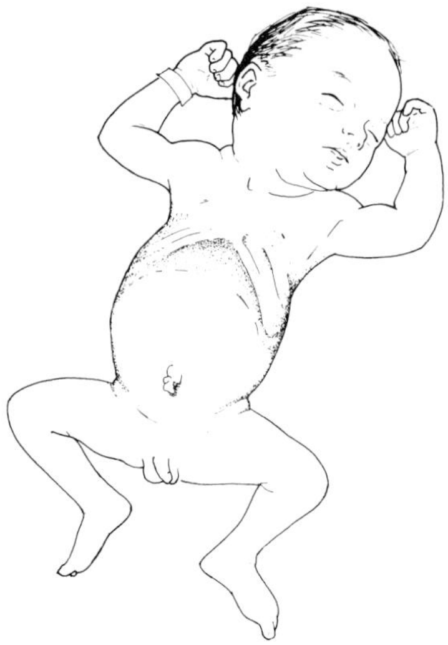

Fig. 28-3 Retraction: substernal, subcostal, and intercostal retractions are evident. (Courtesy Ross Laboratories, Columbus, Ohio.)

deepening distress are indicated by the following (Fig. 28-4):

1. Chin tug (chin is pulled down [and mouth opens wider] as auxiliary muscles of respiration are activated).
2. Abdominal seesaw breathing patterns (Figs. 16-2 and 28-3).
3. Increased number of apneic episodes.

If the newborn is hypoxic, the ***temperature*** may begin to drop. (Avoid rapid warming of the newborn; it may evoke apneic episodes.) An accurate and timely ***blood pressure*** reading can assist in the early diagnosis of cardiorespiratory disease and in the monitoring of fluid therapy. Blood pressure readings are obtained by the Doppler method or electronic monitor. A blood pressure cuff of appropriate size must be used. A too wide cuff results in a false low reading; an overly narrow cuff will give a false elevated reading. For the newborn a cuff of about 2.5 to 3 cm (1 in) wide and 7.5 cm (3 in) long is usually adequate.

The stethoscope should have a pediatric-sized diaphragm for maximum skin contact and localization of sounds. The stethoscope is applied with firm pressure but not so much pressure that transmission of sound and vibrations is compromised.

The Doppler instrument and electronic monitoring device (on a biometric console) are more accurate methods for determining blood pressure. However, this type of equipment is not available in all hospitals or community health settings.

The monitor displays the systolic and diastolic value, the mean systolic/diastolic pressure (the reading

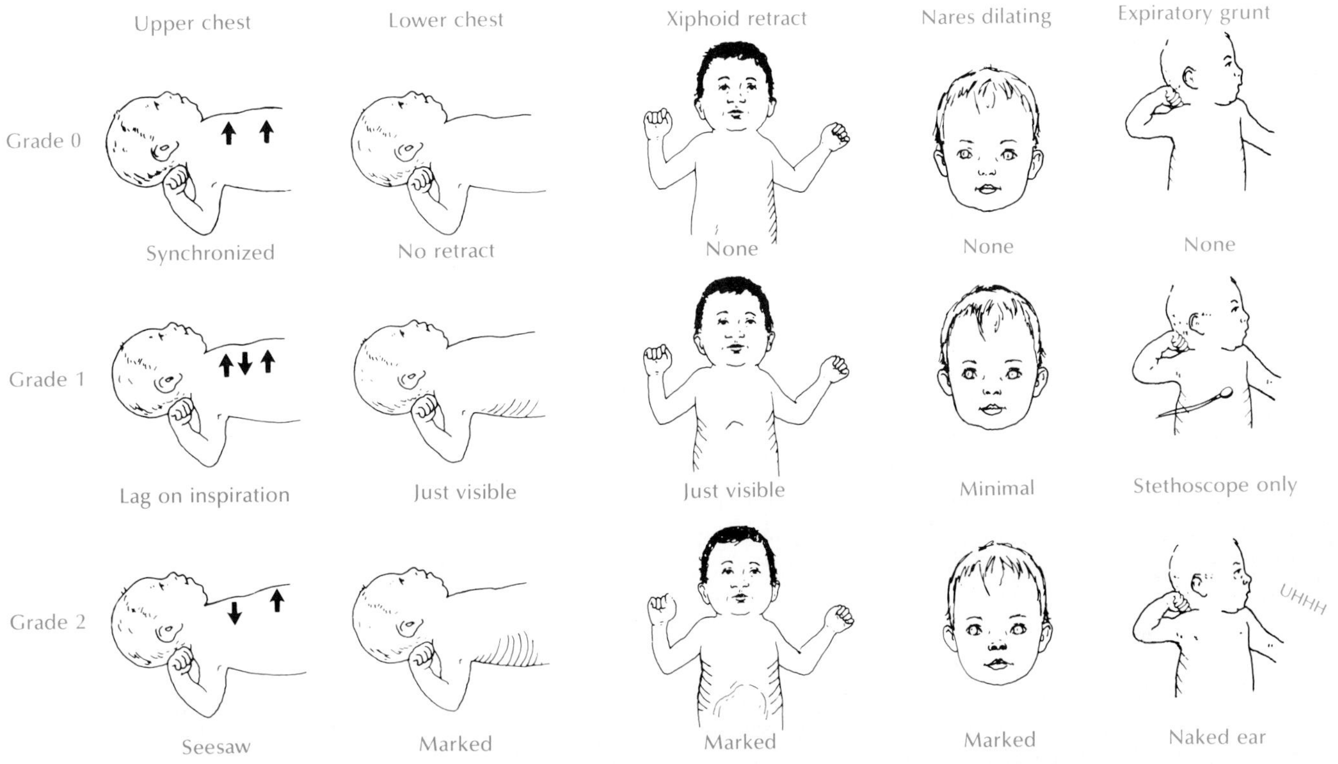

Fig. 28-4 Observation of retractions. Silverman-Anderson index of respiratory distress is determined by grading each of five arbitrary criteria: *grade 0* indicates no difficulty; *grade 1,* moderate difficulty; and *grade 2,* maximum respiratory difficulty. Retraction score is sum of these values; total score of 0 indicates no dyspnea, whereas total score of 10 denotes maximum respiratory distress. (Modified from Silverman W and Anderson D: Pediatrics 17:1, 1956.)

is midway between the diastolic and systolic pressures), and the newborn's heart rate. The existing standard normal range for the mean pressure for newborns weighing 2500 g (5½ lb) or more is 30 to 60 mm Hg.

Nursing Diagnoses

Examples of nursing diagnoses for the newborn with respiratory distress include the following:

Ineffective breathing pattern related to
- Immaturity
- Cold stress

Ineffective airway clearance related to
- Newborn anatomy, immobility, and increased secretions
- Meconium aspiration
- Immaturity or congenital disorder

Impaired gas exchange related to
- Immaturity (e.g., insufficient surfactant)
- Respiratory depression secondary to narcosis or acidosis

Planning

During the important planning step, goals are set to meet the unique needs of the high-risk newborn. The goals are prioritized. Nursing actions are selected to meet the goals. Before nursing care is implemented, the nurse plans carefully to assure that the care provided is goal directed.

Goals include the following:

1. Newborn's respirations are maintained
2. Newborn does not develop bronchopulmonary dysplasia or retinopathy of prematurity (retrolental fibroplasia)
3. Newborn's metabolism meets needs of repair, maintenance, and growth
4. Newborn's respiratory needs of all tissues are met (e.g., blood gases and acid-base balance are maintained within normal limits)
5. Newborn's congenital dysfunctions or anomalies are recognized early, and appropriate treatment is initiated

6. Parents cope constructively with the situation and relating to the newborn as a person

Implementation

Supportive Measures

The newborn's respiratory efforts may be supported by careful *positioning.* When the newborn is supine, the arms will be at the sides, flexed, and slightly abducted. Diapers, if used, are pinned loosely. The prone position recently has been shown to improve respiratory effort, increase PaO_2, and diminish the work of respiration.

Suctioning assists the newborn in maintaining a patent airway. An unobstructed airway usually decreases the newborn's labored breathing by improving ventilation. (See discussion of suctioning procedures in Chapter 17.)

A *thermoneutral environment* is essential for metabolic homeostasis. **Cold stress** is detrimental to the well-being of any infant, especially the infant at risk. For a discussion of thermogenesis and the prevention of cold stress, see Chapters 16 and 17.

Nutrition and feeding of the newborn in respiratory distress are as much a challenge for the nurse as for the newborn. The extra work of breathing taxes the infant's energy reserves and demands greater caloric input. Breastfeeding and formula-feeding are not appropriate for the newborn in distress. The newborn in severe distress may require gavage feeding exclusively. Total parenteral nutrition (TPN) may be required for the newborn who cannot tolerate gavage feedings (see p. 827).

For the newborn in no respiratory distress who can formula feed, a softer nipple with an adequate opening is used (e.g., when the bottle is inverted, fluid should drip at 1 drop per second). Some newborns can breastfeed when both mother and child receive supportive guidance (Chapter 18). The airway must be cleared before and during feeding as necessary. Moreover, the infant is "bubbled" (burped) before feedings.

If the newborn is feeding at the breast, the nurse remains at the bedside with a bulb syringe at hand. This provides reassurance for the mother and avoids a buildup of tension, which might be transferred from mother to infant. Should the infant gag or choke, the nurse can show the mother how to manage such a situation.

Oxygen Therapy

Oxygen therapy may be lifesaving, but its administration must be carefully monitored, as with any medication. The administration of oxygen to newborns requires clinical judgment supported by laboratory determinations (Fanaroff and Martin, 1987). Use of oxygen may be hazardous, resulting in retinopathy of prematurity (retrolental fibroplasia) and bronchopulmonary dysplasia. See the discussion on oxygen therapy (Chapter 17), retinopathy of prematurity (retrolental fibroplasia), and bronchopulmonary dysplasia (p. 847).

When a newborn requires supplemental oxygen, despite its potential hazards, the delivery of oxygen is carefully controlled and monitored. Small increases in ambient oxygen can be delivered directly into the incubator. A head box within the incubator is used when oxygen concentrations exceed 30%. The head box more accurately provides the correct concentration while simultaneously limiting significant fluctuations in oxygen, especially when the incubator portholes are opened. Some incubators have an automatic cut-off mechanism when ambient oxygen reaches a preset level. These controls cannot be relied on independently. The ambient oxygen concentration is checked at regular intervals by a paramagnetic oxygen analyzer or continuously monitored by means of an oxygen electrode. To prevent cold stress and drying of respiratory mucosa, oxygen delivered to a newborn is warmed and humidified. Periodic measurement of PaO_2, hemoglobin, and pH, in addition to close clinical observation, is the most reasonable and accurate approach to minimizing the risk of both hyperoxic and hypoxic insults to a newborn (Fanaroff and Martin, 1987).

Continuous Positive Airway Pressure. Continuous positive airway pressure (CPAP) is most commonly administered through nasal prongs or an endotracheal tube (oral or nasal). The purpose of this technique is to reduce the work of breathing. CPAP increases alveolar volume. It employs the same principle as the expiratory grunt (a physiologic adaptation to trap air within the lungs, keeping alveoli open to prevent atelectasis on expiration). CPAP also increases functional residual capacity, improves oxygenation, and decreases pulmonary shunting.

Transcutaneous Oxygen Tension Monitoring. Accurate noninvasive transcutaneous (tc) oxygen tension ($tcPo_2$) monitoring is feasible on a continuous basis. Electrodes are applied to a hairless and greaseless site, and an airtight contact with the skin is secured. The electrode application site is changed every 4 hours to avoid burns. The distinct advantage of this method is that the data are available on a moment-to-moment basis (Fanaroff and Martin, 1987; Merenstein and Gardner, 1989).

Extracorporeal Membrane Oxygenation. Extracorporeal membrane oxygenation (ECMO) is an innovative technique that offers promise as a means of supporting life during intractable respiratory failure in selected infants (Fanaroff and Martin, 1987). Perfusion and gas exchange are accomplished by means of a cardiopulmonary bypass through a membrane lung. This allows the heart and lungs to recover at low ventilator settings and inspired oxygen concentrations. This experimental approach may decrease acute and chronic lung disease. Despite the technical challenge and staff time expenditure involved in its delivery, ECMO is considered a useful option for respiratory failure in several major neonatal centers (Fanaroff and Martin, 1987).

Evaluation

Small improvements such as the slight downward adjustment in the administration of oxygen can represent major milestones in the status of the newborn. Successful weaning from ventilatory support systems and development of parental attachment to the infant are signs that goals are being achieved. The nurse can be reasonably assured that goals have been achieved when assessment years later shows no evidence of adverse sequelae (e.g., respiratory, visual, or neurobehavior impairment in the child) and no dysfunctional family processes directly attributable to the child's early illness.

❑ TEMPERATURE SUPPORT AND REGULATION

Assessment

In the non-cold-stressed newborn measuring *axillary temperature* is the safest, most practical means of monitoring deep body temperature. However, in the cold-stressed newborn, metabolism of brown fat in the axillary area may result in misleadingly high readings.

A *thermistor probe* or transducer taped to the skin is designed to provide accurate temperature readings for the newborn under an overhead radiant heat source or in a Servo-Control incubator. When only a single skin temperature is to be sensed, the thermistor probe is attached to the skin between the umbilicus and the pubis. Least favored attachment sites are over bony prominences (one of the least vasoreactive body regions) or extremities (one of the most vasoreactive regions). False temperature measures will occur if the probe is attached near heat-producing transcutaneous gas-monitoring transducers or over areas of bruised or burned skin (Fanaroff and Martin, 1987).

Skin temperature usually decreases first in the cold-stressed newborn. Therefore the infant's body and extremities are touched to assess for coolness or warmth. The newborn is also assessed for physiologic ***signs of cold stress.*** The stronger, more mature newborn responds by increased physical activity and crying. In other newborns, respiratory rate often increases. Color changes may be noted in any newborn. These include deepening acrocyanosis, appearance of generalized cyanosis, and mottling of the skin (cutis marmorata). In a male with descended testes, the cremasteric reflex is activated; that is, on exposure to cold, the testes are pulled up into the inguinal canal.

The sigmoid colon bends at a right angle to itself at a depth of 3 cm. Inserting a ***rectal thermometer*** to a depth of less than 5 cm (2 in) may not accurately reflect core temperature (Fanaroff and Martin, 1987). Insertion of the thermometer to 5 cm to obtain an accurate reading risks perforation of the rectum. Rectal perforation carries a mortality of approximately 70% in reported cases (Merenstein and Gardner, 1989). Therefore routine use of a glass rectal thermometer or an electronic probe is contraindicated for the newborn, even after rectal patency has been demonstrated.

Nursing Diagnoses

Examples of nursing diagnoses related to temperature support and regulation include the following:

Ineffective thermoregulation, related to
- Immaturity
- Congenital disorder

Potential altered body temperature related to
- Environmental factors leading to hypothermia or hyperthermia
- Disease processes such as infection
- Fluid deficit secondary to hypovolemia
- Physiologic immaturity of newborn

Planning

During the important planning step, goals are set in client-centered terms. Whenever possible, parents are included in the planning. The goals are prioritized. Nursing actions are selected to meet the goals.

Goals may include the following:
1. The newborn's skin temperature is maintained between 36.1° and 36.7° C (97° to 98° F).*
2. The newborn experiences no apneic spells.
3. The newborn gains adequate weight.
4. The newborn does not develop sequelae of cold stress (i.e., sclerema, oxygen deprivation to tis-

*See discussions on techniques for regulating warmth and humidity in infant's environment and for maintaining thermoneutral environment in Chapter 17.

sues, metabolic acidosis, hypoglycemia, abnormal blood gases, and dysfunction of CNS).

Implementation

Nursing care is planned and implemented to prevent or minimize cold stress. Nursing actions to support thermoregulation include quickly drying the newborn immediately after birth in a warm, absorbent blanket, taking particular care to dry and cover the head (one fourth of body length). The nurse prevents cold air from blowing over the newborn's face because receptors in facial skin are extremely sensitive to cold. The wrapped newborn is placed in warm incubator, Kreisselmann, or other heated carrier. The newborn may be placed unwrapped under a radiant heat source or under plastic wrap to reduce insensible water loss (Fig 28-5). All procedures and observations when infant is unwrapped are done in incubator, under radiant heat, on warm surface, etc. All surfaces and materials touching a newborn are kept warm. The nurse's hands should be warm when handling a newborn. Oxygen or air is warmed before it is administered to a newborn.

The equipment needs to be maintained in excellent operative condition. The nurse needs to know procedures and rationale for procedures. Equipment is plugged in and operative. The thermostat is set on the control panel. The probe is placed in contact with the skin, and the portholes and lid are closed. The incubator is placed away from windows, fans, and air-conditioning units. Bassinets are placed away from drafts or sources of heat or cold. The newborn's temperature is measured periodically to check the accuracy of the equipment.

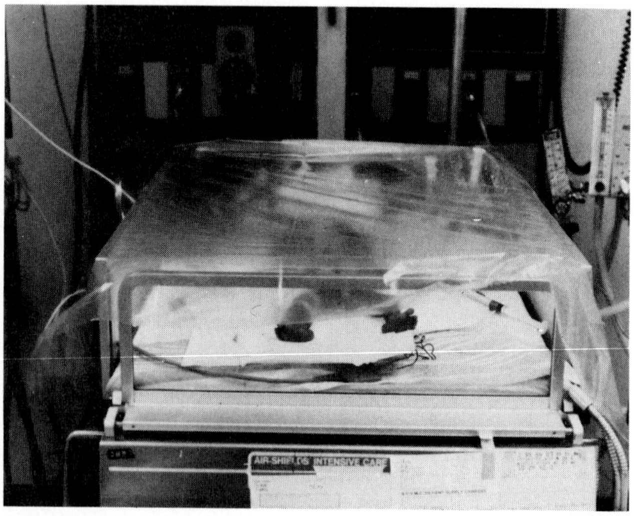

Fig. 28-5 Infant under plastic wrap to ensure a draft-free environment. (Photography by Anne Kunke, San Jose, Calif. From Whaley LF and Wong DL: Essentials of pediatric nursing, ed 3, St Louis, 1989, The CV Mosby Co.)

Abdominal skin temperatures are maintained at 36.1° to 36.7° C (97° to 98° F), and axillary temperature is maintained at 36.5° C (97.7° F). Any rise in temperature over 37.3° C (99° F) or drop of 0.6° to 1° C (1° to 2° F) is reported. If the newborn's temperature is too low or too high, the environment is altered to return the newborn to the desired body temperature. The nurse checks and readjusts the thermostat setting as necessary and checks to see that the equipment is plugged into an electrical outlet.

The thermistor probe is reapplied if it is wet or detached. Incubator portholes are closed. On incubator portholes with plastic sleeve covers, the sleeve is kept on its track. The newborn's clothing and blankets are adjusted as necessary. The placement of the incubator or bassinet is changed as needed to prevent temperature changes from elements such as drafts and sunlight.

Warming the Hypothermic Newborn. Rapid warming or cooling may produce apneic spells and acidosis in a newborn. Therefore the warming process is increased slowly over a period of 2 to 4 hours.*

The nurse places the newborn in an incubator and sets the temperature on the control panel at 1.2° C (2° F) above skin temperature, even if the skin temperature is lower than normal. When the skin temperature reaches the predetermined temperature, the incubator temperature is reset. The process is repeated until an abdominal skin temperature of 36.5° C (97.7° F) is achieved.

Evaluation

The nurse can be assured that care was effective if the newborn's temperature stabilizes within normal limits, apneic episodes do not occur, and sequelae of cold stress do not develop. The plan of care evolves to meet the changing needs of the newborn.

❑ MAINTENANCE OF NUTRITION AND FLUID AND ELECTROLYTE BALANCE

The feeding and nutrition of the newborn at risk warrant careful consideration. The extent to which nutrition needs are met is directly related to the newborn's immediate and long-range well-being. For example, if the low-birth-weight newborn with low glycogen stores is not fed promptly, the resultant symp-

*Rapid warming is elected by some authors: Kaplan and Eidelman (1984).

tomatic or asymptomatic hypoglycemia may seriously damage carbohydrate-dependent brain cells.

Caloric, nutrient, and fluid requirements of the newborn at risk may be greater for many reasons. Preterm or dysmature (malnourished) newborns usually have limited stores. Depletion of stores occurs in the newborn who is stressed by one or a combination of factors, including such conditions as increased respirations or respiratory effort, insensible fluid loss by evaporation when the newborn is under radiant heat or during phototherapy, and a hypothermic environment. The immaturity of the body system affects nutrient requirements. Other newborns at nutritional risk include those of any gestational age who have perinatal asphyxia, a gastrointestinal (GI) anomaly, severe neurologic abnormalities, or other conditions that prevent feeding via the oral route. Newborns with cleft lip and/or palate are at nutritional risk, even though they may otherwise be healthy. GI tract losses occur through vomiting, diarrhea, and dysfunctional absorption. Renal system losses are caused by inability to concentrate urine and maintain an adequate rate of urea excretion, as well as by an inadequate response to antidiuretic hormone (ADH). Growth demands also affect nutrient requirements.

Assessment

Nutritional, fluid, and electrolyte assessment of the newborn includes assessment of general appearance, blood glucose level, weight changes, state of hydration, elimination patterns, GI function, and tolerance of feedings. The feedings may be oral, gavage (feeding by tube), or parenteral. The newborn is observed for lethargy, jitteriness, color (pallor, cyanosis, or other undesirable findings), increasing occurrence of apnea and bradycardia after initiation of feedings, and abdominal distension (Fig. 28-6).

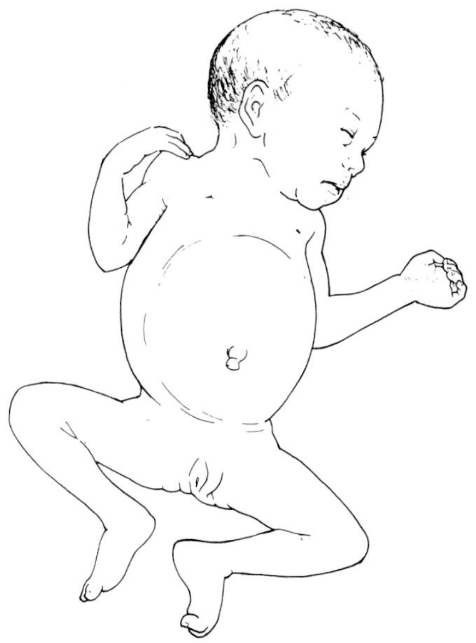

Fig. 28-6 Abdominal distension. (Courtesy Ross Laboratories, Columbus, Ohio.)

Blood Glucose and Calcium

Hypoglycemia during the early newborn period has been defined as *whole blood glucose* concentrations of less than 35 mg/dl in the term newborn and less than 25 mg/dl in the preterm newborn; or alternatively, as a *plasma concentration* of less than 40 mg/dl (term) and 30 mg/dl (preterm). At birth, the newborn abruptly loses its glucose supply. Glucose levels fall normally over the first hours after birth. Since hypoglycemia may be asymptomatic, a blood-glucose test (Dextrostix, Clinistix) (see Fig. 17-11) should be done on admission and at 4 hours of age. More frequent monitoring is required if the newborn is in an at-risk group (LGA [insulin-dependent mother], SGA, or LBW). Hypoglycemia in SGA infants calls for prompt action, since these newborns lack stores of fat or glycogen to mobilize glucose. Stressed newborns are also at risk for the development of hypoglycemia. Stress may include prenatal exposure to β-agonist agents for tocolysis for preterm labor, perinatal asphyxia, cold stress, maternal disease such as maternal diabetes, or any acute illness in the newborn (e.g., sepsis, respiratory distress) (Merenstein and Gardner, 1989).

The newborn is also observed for signs of hypoglycemia. These signs include feeding difficulty, hunger; lethargy; apnea, irregular respiratory effort; cyanosis; weak, high-pitched cry; jitteriness, twitching, eye-rolling, seizures (Table 28-1)

Hypocalcemia (less than 7 mg/dl) is strongly associated with newborns of diabetic mothers, perinatal asphyxia, trauma, LBW, and preterm birth. Symptoms

Table 28-1 **Comparison of Newborn Jitteriness and Seizures**

Normal Newborn Jitteriness	Newborn Seizure
Dominant movement tremor	Clonic jerking that cannot be stopped by flexing the affected limbs
No ocular movement	Ocular movement
Highly sensitive to stimulation	Not sensitive to stimulation
Persists for about 4 days after birth	Persists beyond 4 days after birth

include edema, apnea, intermittent cyanosis, and abdominal distension. Hypocalcemia must be considered if therapy for hypoglycemia is ineffective. ***Jitteriness*** is one symptom of hypoglycemia and of hypocalcemia (see Table 28-1). In many newborns, jitteriness remains despite therapy and cannot be explained by hypoglycemia or hypocalcemia (Fanaroff and Martin, 1987).

Weight and Hydration

Weight is obtained at least daily, at the same time of day and on the same scale, with the newborn nude. In the early postnatal period, weight loss is to be expected. The limits of acceptable weight loss over the first 3 to 4 days of extrauterine life are: (1) preterm newborn, 12% or less of birth weight (e.g., 184 g or less in the newborn with a birth weight of 1530 g); (2) term newborn of appropriate weight for gestational age, 10% or less of birth weight; (3) newborn weighing 4500 g (9 lb 14 oz) or more, 15% or less of birth weight; and (4) SGA gestational age newborn, 5% or less of birth weight.

Most of the early weight loss can be accounted for by loss of fluid. As much as 80% to 85% of the preterm (at 28 to 34 weeks of gestation) newborn's body weight consists of water, and even the term newborn is 70% water. Most of this water lies within the extracellular compartment, which shrinks in size during the early postnatal period, as some of the fluid is excreted. In addition to this normal fluid loss and weight loss caused by passage of meconium, other causes of weight loss can include:

1. Insensible water loss (IWL), which represents evaporative losses that occur largely through the skin and respiratory tract. Total IWL ranges from 1.75 to 3.6 ml/kg/hour. Respiratory losses are reduced by humidification of the oxygen-enriched gases that are used for respiratory support. Skin losses are greatest in preterm newborns at the youngest gestational and postnatal ages (i.e., the newborn at 24 weeks of gestation will have greater losses than the one born at 30 weeks, and the newborn will generally have greater losses at 4 days of age than at 8 days). *The preterm newborn has a greater body surface area (BSA) in proportion to body size than does the term newborn,* and the term newborn has a proportionally greater BSA than the child or adult. The large BSA, coupled with thin skin, increases IWL. Use of radiant warmers and phototherapy increase IWL, while incubators help conserve body fluids.
2. Inadequate fluid intake. While inadequate fluid intake may occur as a result of the inability to tolerate oral or gavage feedings, it is often a consequence of deliberate fluid restriction. Many physicians prefer to restrict fluids for the first few days of life to reduce the possibility of fluid overload, which increases the likelihood of continued shunting of blood though the ductus arteriosus and heart failure.
3. Polyuria associated with glycosuria, especially in newborns receiving TPN (p. 827).
4. Vomiting, diarrhea, ostomy output, etc.

Elimination Patterns

Assessment of urinary elimination includes noting the frequency of urination, the specific gravity of the urine, and the presence or absence of glucosuria and proteinuria. In newborns receiving intravenous (IV) therapy, the volume of urine should be determined by collecting all urine in a bag. An alternative method is the weighing of all diapers when dry and again when wet and subtracting the difference. Evaporative losses cause this method to yield falsely low values, especially in newborns under radiant warmers. The newborn should be observed for *signs of fluid volume excess* (edema, bulging fontanelle, crackles [rales] in lungs) and *fluid volume deficit* (depressed fontanelle, poor skin turgor, dry mucous membranes with no fluid bubbles under the tongue). Stools are assessed for frequency and consistency, color, and presence of blood.

Gastrointestinal Function and Tolerance of Feedings

The nurse assists the physician in determining the newborn's readiness for and tolerance of feedings given by any route. Presence or absence of bowel sounds, character of any bowel sounds, appearance of the abdomen (distended abdomen; tight, shiny skin or discolored skin over the abdomen; visible loops of bowel), abdominal tenderness, and abdominal girth are assessed. Absent or hypoactive bowel sounds indicate ileus, while hyperactive and high-pitched bowel sounds often accompany GI obstruction. Abdominal girth is measured over the umbilicus, or another location on the abdomen is marked with a pen to enable repeated measurements to be made consistently.

Any vomiting or regurgitation should be recorded, along with the estimated volume, appearance, forcefulness, and time in relation to feeding. Bilious (gold or green) vomitus is presumed to be associated with intestinal obstruction until proven otherwise. Feedings should be discontinued and the physician notified immediately if bilious vomiting occurs.

The type of feeding (formula, breast milk, TPN, IV fluid) is recorded along with the route of delivery and the volume given. Tolerance of oral feedings is assessed by observing the newborn's attempts at sucking and the length of time required for feeding, especially for preterm newborns and those with cleft lip or palate. Also, any signs of distress, such as elevated respiratory rate, cyanosis, or choking during feeding should be noted. In monitoring gavage feedings, the residual volume in the stomach before the feeding and signs of distress during the feeding are noted. In monitoring TPN, it is especially important to evaluate the newborn's serum glucose and electrolytes and state of hydration, as well as to stay alert for *signs of sepsis* (i.e., increasing apnea, difficulty maintaining body temperature, lethargy).

Newborns at risk often undergo prolonged periods of nothing by mouth (NPO), when their hunger cries and pains are not relieved. Although pacifiers are soothing, these babies may learn that sucking and satiety are not related. Neonatal intensive care unit (NICU) babies also undergo many aversive stimuli around and within the mouth (i.e., oral intubation; oral and endotracheal tube suction; intermittent gavage) that result in touch aversion of the mouth and a hypersensitive gag reflex. The newborn may display an acquired or developmental sucking defect or feeding difficulty as a result (Merenstein and Gardner, 1989).

Necrotizing Enterocolitis

Necrotizing enterocolitis (NEC) is usually a disease of preterm and LBW newborns but may be seen in term newborns (Merenstein and Gardner, 1989). Although its precise cause is unknown, it appears to follow hypoxic-ischemic injury to the mucosa of the intestinal tract (Amspacher, 1989; Hodson and Truog, 1989). NEC appears in about 5% of newborns in intensive care nurseries.

Mucosal injury may be a result of **perinatal asphyxia.** Perinatal events that contribute to fetal asphyxia include preeclampsia-eclampsia, multifetal gestation, placenta previa, placenta abruptio, prolapsed cord, bradycardia, and FHR deceleration. Postnatal apnea, polycythemia, hyperosmolar feedings, GI infection (bacterial or viral), RDS, exchange transfusion, or severe cardiopulmonary disease place the newborn at risk for NEC. There is often a history of umbilical artery catheterization. Vasospasm can occur from placement of an umbilical arterial catheter. NEC is rare in newborns fed only fresh breast milk and in newborns who have not yet been milk-fed (Hodson and Truog, 1989). Maternal medical conditions that stress the fetus include infection, urinary tract infection, diabetes mellitus, and rupture of membranes 24 hours or more before birth (Amspacher, 1989).

Signs of developing NEC are nonspecific, which is characteristic of many newborn disease processes. Abdominal distension is probably the most common and regularly encountered sign. Temperature instability and jaundice may appear. The newborn's color is poor. Apneic periods increase in number. Commonly, there are gastric residuals of 2 ml or more before feedings. The stool may show occult blood (positive guaiac test). Commonly there is an associated thrombocytopenia. Diagnosis is confirmed by x-ray examination of the GI tract.

The best treatment is prevention of the risk factors listed above. Proper obstetric monitoring and intervention will minimize perinatal asphyxia. When perinatal asphyxia is unavoidable, delaying milk feedings for several days may be beneficial. Treatment of *polycythemia* (a central hemotocrit of 65% or more) with exchange transfusion may help prevent NEC.

The incidence of NEC is lower in newborns fed *fresh breast milk* than in newborns fed formula. The mechanism for protection with breastfeeding is not thoroughly understood. Fresh breast milk has immunologic benefits (Amspacher, 1989). If breast milk must be stored, plastic bags or bottles should be used: white blood cells in milk adhere to glass. Freezing or refrigeration diminishes the number of macrophages and the viability of leukocytes, reducing or eliminating the antibacterial properties of fresh breast milk.

Treatment is supportive. A neutral thermal environment is maintained. Oral or tube feedings are discontinued to rest the GI tract. Parenteral therapy (often by TPN) is begun. If present, shock is treated, and acidosis and abnormal coagulation are corrected. Antibiotic therapy may be instituted, and surgery is performed when necessary. Therapy may be prolonged, and recovery may be delayed by adhesions, complications of bowel resection (malabsorption), and intolerance of oral feedings.

Nursing Diagnoses

Examples of nursing diagnoses related to nutrition and elimination include the following:

Altered nutrition, less than body requirements, related to

- Problems of immaturity or newborn disorder

Fluid volume deficit or overload related to

- Immaturity or newborn disorder

Ineffective breathing pattern related to

- Sudden abdominal distension

Planning

During the important planning step, goals are set in client-centered terms. Parents are encouraged to be involved to the extent they feel ready. The goals are prioritized. Nursing actions are selected to meet the goals.

Goals include the following:

1. The newborn experiences:
   a. Minimum respiratory distress; no aspiration or aspiration pneumonia.
   b. Minimum expenditure of energy.
   c. No hypoglycemic or hypocalcemic reactions.
   d. Acceptable fluid-electrolyte balance.
   e. No abdominal distension.
   f. No trauma to tissues of the gastrointestinal tract.
   g. No diarrhea or vomiting.
2. The newborn's sucking satisfaction is maximized.
3. The newborn receives adequate nutrition to:
   a. Meet resting metabolic requirements.
   b. Provide sufficient energy to perform physical activity.
   c. Counter losses through gastrointestinal and urinary tracts.
   d. Achieve a steady pattern of appropriate weight gain
4. Parent-child relationship is fostered in the following ways:
   a. Parent begins to participate in the feeding process in light of the newborn's physical capabilities and the parent's desired degree of involvement.
   b. Newborn begins to associate feeding and eating with pleasure as she or he develops a sense of trust.
   c. At discharge parents are comfortable with the feeding method needed, whether feeding is by breast, bottle, gavage, or the parenteral route.

Implementation

Nourishment Types and Schedules

The feeding solution and feeding schedule of the newborn at risk are based on several criteria. The newborn's birth weight, pattern of weight gain or loss, estimated gestational age, and physical condition are factors. Pharyngeal coordination (sucking and swallowing reflexes present and coordinated), fatigability, malformations, and amount of urine excreted per hour must be taken into account. Laboratory values such as nitrogen balance, electrolyte imbalance, glucose level, serum bilirubin level, and others also influence the type and schedule of feeding. Variants that influence the feeding of the newborn at risk include fluid volume given, caloric requirements, mode of feeding, and feeding solution (breast milk, predigested formula [elemental or regular], or parenteral solutions).

Enteral Formulas. Various formulas are available. These vary in calory, protein, and mineral content (Chapter 18). Regular formulas provide 20 calories/ounce, approximately the same caloric density as human milk. Many formulas contain 24 calories/ounce to meet rapid growth needs. Caloric density can be further increased for newborns with cardiac or renal failure or other conditions necessitating fluid restriction. 'Premature' formulas generally contain higher levels of protein, sodium, calcium, phosphorus, and other minerals than regular formulas. Much interest has been generated by the finding that milk from mothers delivering before term is richer in protein, sodium, and certain other nutrients than milk from mothers delivering at term. These differences would seem to indicate that preterm milk is uniquely tailored to meet the needs of preterm newborns. However, nutrient levels in milk from preterm mothers decline rapidly over the first 3 to 4 weeks after delivery and soon resemble those in term milk. Rapidly growing preterm newborns have developed zinc deficiency and rickets as a result of lack of calcium and phosphorus when fed only their mother's milk. Commercial fortifiers are available to increase the nutritional content of human milk. Breast milk or formula may be fed by continuous flow with a pump and feeding tube inserted into the stomach or jejunum or by intermittent gavage or nipple.

Feeding Methods

Oral Feedings. Oral feedings are used whenever possible. However, newborns generally lack a coordinated suck and swallow mechanism until 32 to 34 weeks of gestational age. Thus nipple feedings are unsafe until the newborn reaches a combined gestational and postnatal age of at least 32 to 34 weeks. Nipple feedings are usually avoided in the newborn with a respiratory rate greater than 60/minute because of the increased danger of pulmonary aspiration. Furthermore, some stressed newborns may fail to gain weight when given nipple feedings because the effort required causes rapid exhaustion, which leads to cessation of feeding. Use of smaller nipple sizes sometimes alleviates this problem. These newborns may benefit from gavage feedings given either continuously or intermittently.

Early feeding is avoided if the newborn had low Apgar scores at birth. Early feeding of asphyxiated newborns may be an important cause of NEC (p. 825). In the absence of asphyxia, however, feedings within 6 hours of birth may be advantageous. Newborns given such feedings tend to have less weight loss and lower serum bilirubin levels. Oral feedings often begin with sterile water. Feedings are advanced by increasing the amount of fluid *or* the number of calories/30 ml (1 oz) at any one feeding. During the feeding the newborn's tolerance is observed. Too rapid advancement may lead to vomiting, diarrhea, abdominal distension, and apneic episodes. Regurgitation at any age can occur and predispose the newborn to aspiration pneumonia.

Gavage (Tube) Feedings. Gavage feedings are given by orogastric, nasogastric, or nasojejunal tubes. Where gavage feedings are expected to be required for prolonged periods, a gastrostomy tube may be placed into the stomach through an external incision through the abdomen (see pediatric text for more details). Newborns given a pacifier during gavage feedings have been found to gain weight more rapidly (Bernbaum et al, 1983).* **Nonnutritive suckling** during gavage and between feedings is associated with better oxygenation; quieter, more restful behavior; and increased readiness for nipple feedings. Sucking on a pacifier satisfies the newborn's sucking needs and may facilitate early learning that satiety and sucking are associated. However, nutritive and nonnutritive suckling are *not* alike. Because the newborn vigorously sucks on a pacifier does not mean the baby will be able to suckle nutritively, since the expressive and swallow phases have not been present in nonnutritive suckling. This is often confusing to most parents and many professionals (Merenstein and Gardner, 1989).

Procedure 28-1 and Fig. 28-7 describe gavage feedings using orogastric and nasogastric insertion. The neonatal intensive care nurse involves the parents in the actual feeding or teaches them how to give gavage feedings if the child will require such feedings after going home.

Total Parenteral Nutrition. Total parenteral nutrition (TPN) refers to the administration of a nutritionally adequate solution consisting of glucose, amino acids, minerals, and vitamins through an indwelling catheter in the superior vena cava (Fig. 28-8), umbilical artery, or peripheral vein. This feeding method is used to provide nutrition for newborns who cannot tolerate adequate feedings via the enteral route for extended periods. Insertion of the catheter may be done in the operating room. The prescribed mixture is ordered from the pharmacy; nothing else should be added. The catheter is used only for the prescribed mixture; it is not to be used for blood or medications. The bottle, tubing, and millipore filter are changed every 24 hours. The dressing around the catheter insertion site is changed aseptically as directed by hospital protocol. The newborn's weight is monitored daily, at the same time, on the same scale, and before feeding. For stimulation, the newborn is provided with a pacifier (see nonnutritive suckling, above), a mobile, and newborn stimulation

*One-piece commercially made pacifiers are recommended. Makeshift pacifiers have been implicated as aspiration hazards (Miluncheck and McArtor, 1986).

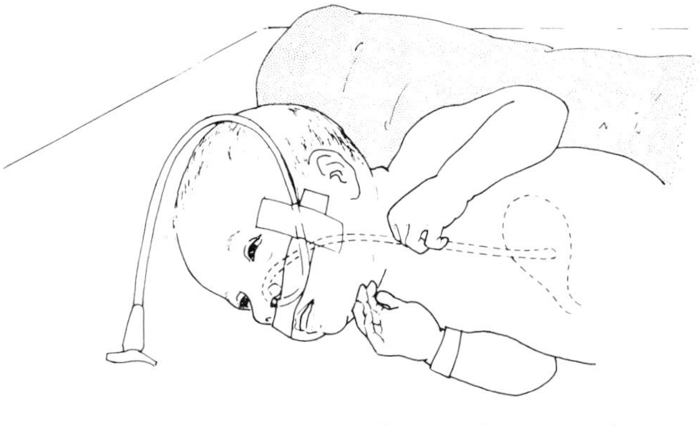

Fig. 28-7 Indwelling gavage tube: nasal route. Infant is propped on right side to facilitate emptying of stomach into small intestine. Note rolled towel for support. (See also Fig. 17-2.)

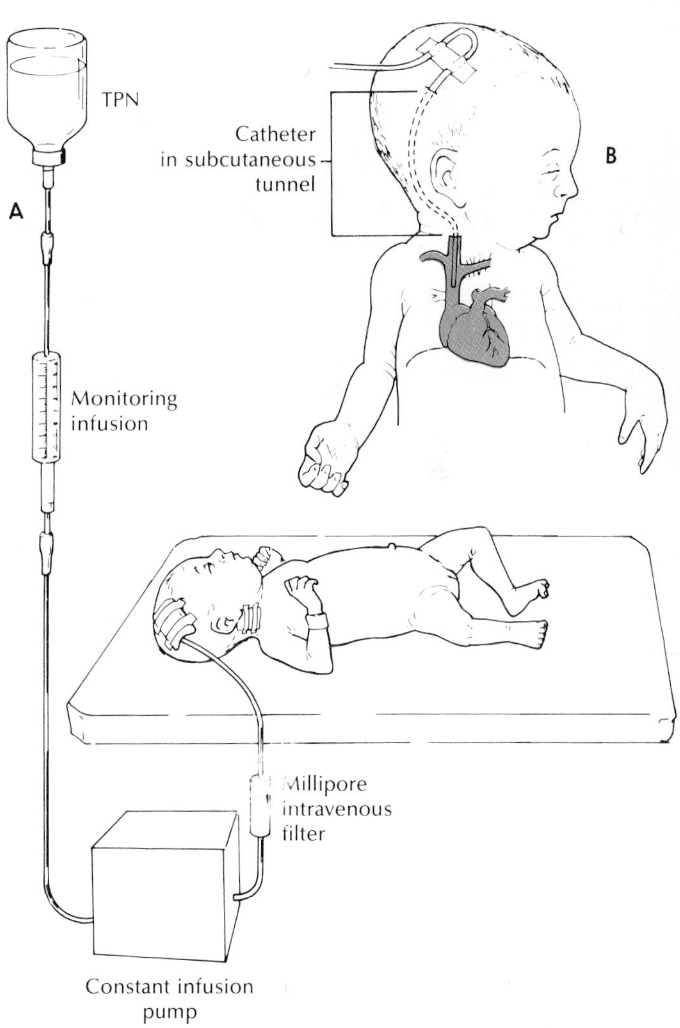

Fig. 28-8 **A,** Total parenteral nutrition (TPN). **B,** Close-up to show infusion site and internal placement of catheter into the descending vena cava. Parenteral nutrition is often used in conjunction with other forms of feeding, particularly when weaning to oral feedings.

PROCEDURE 28-1
GAVAGE FEEDING

DEFINITION
A procedure in which a tube is passed through the nose or mouth into the stomach to feed a newborn with weak sucking, uncoordinated sucking and swallowing, or respiratory distress.

PURPOSE
To meet the nutrition and fluid needs of the newborn who cannot suck.

EQUIPMENT
Sterile feeding tube: Silastic, polyurethane, or plastic, rounded tips; sizes 3½ to 8, newborn lengths; clearly calibrated syringe for feeding; stethoscope and sterile medication syringe without needle; sterile water for lubrication; feeding formula; medications; feeding pump and pump tubing if feeding is continuous.

NURSING ACTIONS	RATIONALE
Identify newborn and check physician's orders.	Provides the right therapy for the right client.
Wash hands before and after touching newborn or equipment; glove prn.	Prevents nosocomial infection and implements universal precautions.
Oral insertion: intermittent or indwelling catheter:	***Orogastric insertion:***
Position newborn: head of mattress up one notch, folded towel under shoulders to slightly extend neck.	Opens oropharynx. Extends and straightens esophagus.
Select size 8 F feeding tube.	Adequate size for feeding less apt to fold over or curl up.
Measure distance between bridge of nose, to earlobe, and then to lower end of xiphoid process. Mark distance with 5 cm (2 in) thin strip of paper tape. Fold tape over tube, leaving two long ends with which to secure tube when it is in place.	Determines length necessary to reach into stomach without folding back on itself. Facilitates anchoring tubing if it is to be indwelling. Paper tape is usually less irritating to skin.
Lubricate tube in sterile water.	Prevents trauma and infection.
Pass tube along base of tongue, advancing it into esophagus as newborn swallows.	Offers less risk of vagal stimulation or of accidental entry into trachea. Stimulates esophageal peristalsis and opens cardiac sphincter.
Test placement of tube (see below).	Avoids introduction of formula, vitamins, and medicines into trachea or esophagus.
Aspirate and measure any residual feeding in stomach. Decrease volume of feeding by amount of residual obtained, or follow physician's order.	Avoids overfeeding. Excessive fluid in stomach suggests intestinal obstruction, hypomotility, or delayed gastric emptying.
Slowly pour warmed formula into syringe barrel and allow it to flow by gravity into stomach. Hold reservoir 15 to 20 cm (6 to 8 in) above newborn's head. If gravity flow is too rapid, lower syringe, or insert plunger into syringe, and inject *slowly.* Feeding time should approximate that of nipple feedings (20 minutes or about 1 ml/min).	Rapid entry of formula into stomach causes rapid rebound response with regurgitation, thus increasing danger of aspiration or abdominal distension, which compromises respiratory effort.
Do not allow level of formula to go below neck of syringe.	Prevents entry of air into stomach to minimize risks of regurgitation and distension.
Observe newborn's response.	Prevents respiratory distress. Assists gastrointestinal functioning.
Follow formula with specific amount of sterile water.	Clears tubing of formula, ensuring that entire dose is administered.
Pinch tubing (or clamp it off) and withdraw it rapidly.	Prevents entry of air into stomach. Creates vacuum to hold fluid in tubing to prevent dripping it into trachea on withdrawal.
Nasal route: intermittent or indwelling catheter:	***Nasogastric insertion:***
Position as for oral route.	Opens oropharynx. Extends and straightens esophagus.
Select size 3½ to 5 F feeding tube.	Adequate size for feeding and small enough to allow breathing space around it, since newborns are obligate nose breathers.

PROCEDURE 28-1—cont'd

NURSING ACTIONS	RATIONALE
If indwelling plastic tube, change every 2 or 3 days (48 to 72 hours) or more frequently if otitis is present, alternating sides of nares.	Prevents infection, irritation; excess mucus, ulceration, bleeding. Polyurethane and Silastic tubes are less irritating and can be left in place longer.
Observe infant for respiratory distress.	If tube causes distress, remove it. Use oral route.
May be preferred route for indwelling tube for continuous drip feeding.	Very small preterm infant often tolerates feeding better by continuous drip, stomach is not overloaded.
Measure distance from bridge of nose to earlobe, and then to xiphoid process (just beyond tip of sternum). Mark spot with 5 cm (2 in) thin strip of paper tape, and overlap tube, leaving ends free.	Provides adequate length to reach stomach without curling. Facilitates anchoring of tubing. Decreases risk of skin irritation from tape.
Lubricate with sterile water.	Prevents tissue trauma.
Insert tube, holding it horizontally until it reaches back of nares; then lift tubing slightly and continue to advance. Allow infant to swallow tube while it is being advanced.	Accommodates to bend in back of nares and minimizes direct tissue damage. Stimulates peristalsis and opens cardiac sphincter.
Continue as for oral route.	Same as for oral route.
Use one or more of the following tests to determine proper placement:	
Use sterile syringe to inject 0.5 ml of air through catheter into stomach. Simultaneously, listen for sound of air bubbling or "growling" in stomach with stethoscope over epigastric region.	Sound of air bubbling confirms tube placement in stomach.
Listen with stethoscope first over the epigastrium and then on each side of the anterior chest.	The sound of rushing air heard over the anterior chest should be considerably diminished in intensity compared with that heard over the epigastrium.
Aspirate small amount of stomach contents.	Aspiration of stomach contents confirms proper placement of tube.
Check pH to verify that fluid was obtained from stomach.	Highly acidic pH usually indicates gastric origin.
Nursing care after feedings:	
Burp or bubble newborn. With left hand, support infant's head and shoulders. Raise infant to sitting position and lean infant onto right hand. Right hand supports newborn's chest with palm and jaw with thumb and forefinger. Gently rub back with left hand.	Increases comfort and prevents regurgitation.
Position on right side with small rolled drape or towel (Fig. 28-7), or prone position.	Facilitates stomach emptying; protects against pulmonary aspiration of stomach contents if vomiting or regurgitation occurs.
Postpone postural drainage and percussion for a minimum of 1 hour after feeding.	Promotes retention of feeding.
Avoid feeding within an hour before a laboratory test for blood glucose.	Promotes accurate reading in laboratory tests.
Record the following: Amount of residual gastric aspirate. Type and amount of feeding, medicine. Time of feeding. Newborn response: fatigue, peaceful sleep, abdominal distension, respiratory distress, type and amount of vomiting or regurgitation; heart and respiratory rate.	Provides basis for evaluation and readjustment of feeding regimen. Facilitates communication among personnel.

pictures. The newborn should be held if physiologic condition permits. Holding during feeding simulates the interaction enjoyed by an orally-fed newborn and the caregiver.

The newborn is observed for complications associated with TPN: local skin infection around the insertion site, septicemia, blood vessel thrombosis, obstruction or dislodgment of the catheter, and cardiac symptoms such as arrhythmia. *Candida* septicemia is common. Complications of the infusion solution include glucosuria, dehydration, acidosis, hyperglycemia, fluid excess, and electrolyte imbalance.

As the newborn's condition improves, fluids may be offered by nipple. As the oral feeding is increased and tolerated, the amount given by infusion is decreased.

Feeding the Newborn with Cleft Lip and Palate. The baby born with a cleft lip and palate may be normal in every other way. Surgical repair on the lip is usually done soon after birth if possible to assist parents in the attachment process with their newborn. The palate is usually repaired some months later. The nurse may be called to feed the newborn during the early neonatal period or to teach the parent to do so. Procedure 28-2 and Fig. 28-9 are presented to assist the nurse in feeding the newborn and to serve as a guide for teaching the parent(s).

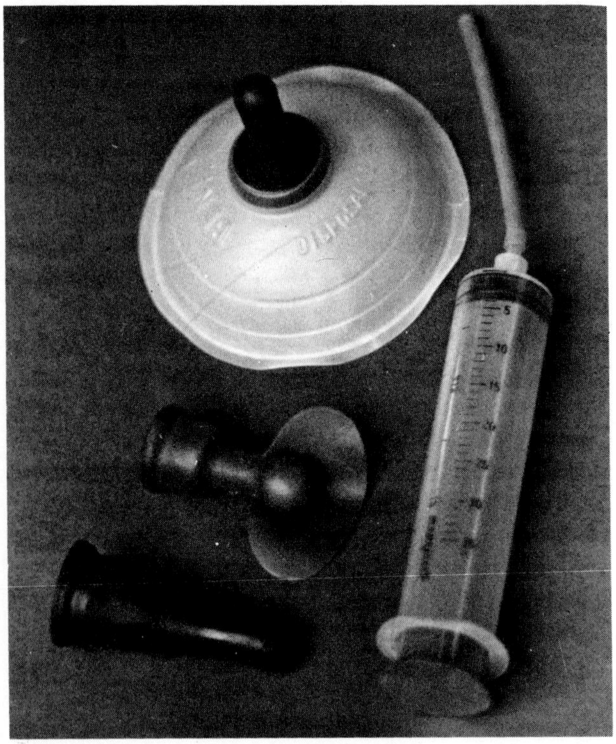

Fig. 28-9 Some devices used to feed infant with cleft palate. *Clockwise,* lamb's nipple, flanged nipple, special nurser, and syringe with rubber tubing (Brecht feeder). (From Whaley, LF, and Wong, DL: Essentials of pediatric nursing, ed. 3. St Louis, 1989, The CV Mosby Co.)

Fluid and Electrolyte Balance

Fluid and electrolyte requirements may need to be met by the intravenous route. Fluid requirements are calculated in ml/kg of body weight per day. For the first day of life, 60 to 100 ml/kg may be ordered; for day 2, 100 to 120 ml/kg; and for day 3, 120 to 150 ml/kg may be ordered. Fluid amounts may be increased if the newborn is receiving phototherapy or is under a radiant heater. Less fluid may be needed by the newborn if a heat shield is used, humidified oxygen is being given, or the environment is humid. The amount of fluid is calculated by the physician and is based on the nurse's observations of the newborn's general condition and weight gain or loss.

Monitoring fluid volume replacement is a major nursing responsibility. The newborn's hydration is evaluated every hour. The weight of the naked newborn is assessed every 8, 12, or 24 hours on the same scale and before feeding. Early signs of ***dehydration*** include a urine volume of less than 1 ml/kg/hr and specific gravity of 1.012 or more. Dehydration is evident by a weight loss greater than 2% of body weight in 24 hours, poor skin turgor, fever, sunken fontanels, soft sunken eyeballs, dry mucous membranes, and increases in hematocrit (10% or more) and serum protein (6 g/dl or more). Shock is a late finding.

Early signs of ***overhydration*** include a urine volume that exceeds 3 ml/kg/hr with a specific gravity of 1.008 or less. Overhydration is evident by a weight gain greater than 2% of body weight within 24 hours, subcutaneous edema, and decreases in hematocrit (10% or less) and serum protein (4 g/dl or less). The specific gravity assists in assessing the fluid the newborn is receiving, as well as kidney function. Presence of glucose in the urine indicates an excessive glucose load in the intravenous infusate. Pulmonary crackles (rales) and edema and cardiac decompensation are late signs.

The flow rate must be precise to avoid underhydration or overhydration. A number of continuous infusion pumps are available for use exclusively for pediatric intravenous fluid administration. For administering a very small amount over a specific time (e.g., 1 ml/hr or less), precision-controlled syringe pumps may be preferred. Careful periodic assessment by the nurse is important. Over-reliance on the accuracy of the machine can result in the infusion of too much or too little fluid or infiltration of tissues if the needle is out of the blood vessel. ***A deficiency or excess of fluid is not made up by changing the rate of flow without consulting with the physician.*** Possible complications of fluid overload or deficit, or fluctuations in electrolytes or glucose can result.

PROCEDURE 28-2

FEEDING NEWBORN WITH CLEFT LIP AND PALATE

DEFINITION

Congenital defects characterized by a fissure(s) in the palate and upper lip, resulting from the failure to fuse during embryonic development (p. 895).

PURPOSE

To facilitate feeding when newborn has difficulty creating a vacuum and sucking.
To prevent aspiration of feeding.
To prevent discomfort from increased amount of swallowed air.

EQUIPMENT (FIG. 28-9)

Lamb's nipple; Duckey nipple with flange; Brecht feeder; or rubber-tipped Asepto syringe.

NURSING ACTIONS	RATIONALE
Identify client and check physician's orders.	Provides the right therapy for the right newborn.
Wash hands before and after touching client or equipment. Glove, prn.	Prevents nosocomial infection and implements universal precautions.
Prepare thickened formula as ordered, usually with dried rice cereal.	Increases gravity flow of fluid into stomach and prevents aspiration.
Choose appropriate nipple:	Assists newborn in creating a vacuum during sucking and to encourage development of normal sucking pattern.
Lamb's nipple.	Carries formula past the defect.
Duckey nipple with flange.	Covers the defect.
Brecht feeder, rubber-tipped Asepto syringe, other special feeders.	Allows caregiver to regulate the rate of flow, thus preventing the newborn from becoming exhausted before consuming adequate formula.
Enlarge hole in nipple as needed.	Permits passage of thickened formula.
Check newborn for clear airway.	Minimizes possibility of aspiration.
During feeding check newborn for the following signs: aspiration—choking and cyanosis; swallowed air—abdominal distension.	Prevents abdominal distension and aspiration that can compromise respirations.
Hold newborn in upright position.	Minimizes possibility of aspiration and return of fluid through nose and aids swallowing.
Interact with newborn: talk and make eye contact with her or him.	Stimulates psychosocial development. If mother sees nurse doing this, it may facilitate her acceptance of the newborn.
Burp or bubble newborn frequently, at least every ounce.	Removes air that is swallowed when there is unnatural passage between nose and mouth. Technique increases newborn's comfort and minimizes regurgitation and aspiration.
When feeding with a rubber-tipped Asepto syringe, place rubber tip on top of and to side of newborn's tongue.	Prevents tip of syringe from entering cleft in palate. Facilitates feeding.
Offer feeding slowly.	Allows newborn time to swallow.

NOTE: The newborn with a cleft lip only may be able to feed well with a regular or "preemie" nipple. The newborn with a cleft lip usually can breastfeed successfully. The newborn with a cleft palate has more difficulty breastfeeding, because the defect interferes with formation of a seal around the breast. Breastfeeding may sometimes be possible, however, particularly if a mother who has breastfed a similar newborn is available to serve as a resource.

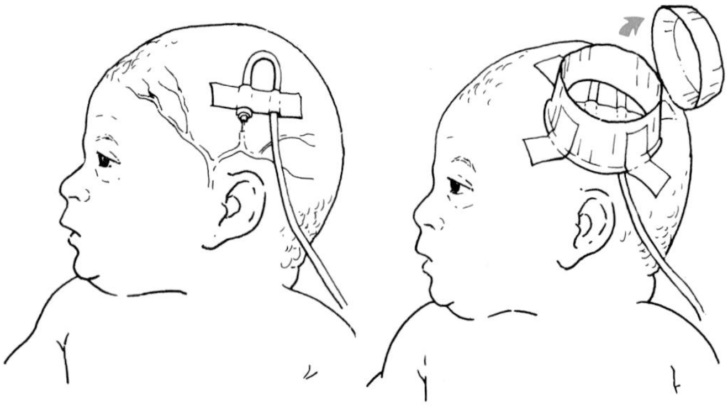

Fig. 28-10 **A,** Venipuncture of scalp vein. **B,** Paper cup protecting venipuncture site.

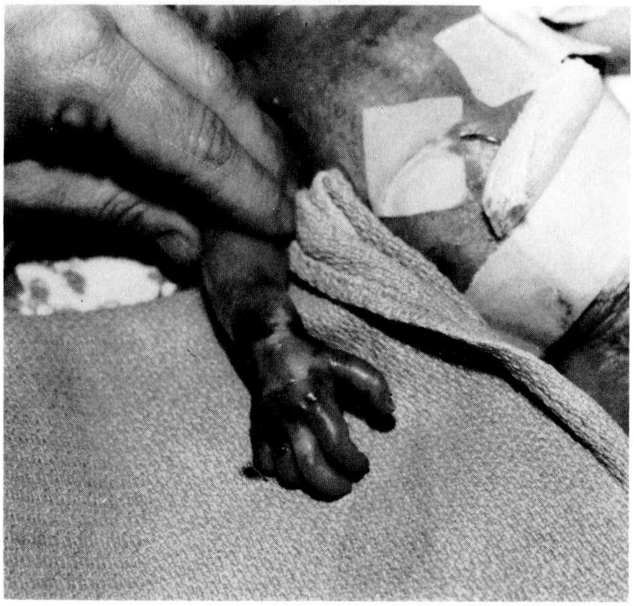

Fig. 28-11 Intravenous infiltration in small infant can cause severe ischemia. (Courtesy Mount Zion Hospital and Medical Center, San Francisco.)

The insertion site is monitored carefully to maintain tissue integrity. A scalp-vein (butterfly) needle, size 21 or 23 gauge, is used with flex-winged tabs that are easily secured to the skin. For long-term therapy, a 22- or 24-gauge over-the-needle catheter is preferred. A medicine cup (paper) or other appliance can be used to protect the insertion site (Fig. 28-10). Sandbags, rolled towels or small blankets assure proper body alignment and restrain the newborn's movements, thus protecting the insertion site.

Clear, porous tape, compared with the more adhesive tapes, permits inspection of the site and minimizes tissue trauma. The surrounding tissue is assessed for trauma, color, and temperature. If the needle is in a scalp vein, the face and head are assessed for symmetry of contour and movement. If the needle is in an extremity, that extremity is compared with the corresponding extremity. Possible complications include infection, thrombophlebitis, and cellulitis (Fig. 28-11).

The nurse records the type of fluid being infused, the amount absorbed every hour and amount scheduled to have been absorbed, the amount of fluid remaining in the fluid chamber, the flow rate, and the newborn's condition. Intravenous tubing is changed every 24 hours and the time is noted. After the intravenous fluid is discontinued, the newborn is observed for hypoglycemia and adequacy of nutrition and hydration.

❑ EMOTIONAL ASPECTS OF CARE

Newborns at risk who are not in acute distress or who are convalescing have at least the same emotional and developmental needs that the normal term newborn has. It may be difficult to meet the needs of the infant at risk. The newborn who needs intravenous therapy, nasogastric feedings, heel-stick samples, oxygen by plastic hood, or CPAP cannot be cuddled, fondled, or played with as can the term infant. Instead she or he must experience many painful stimuli, including numerous intrusive procedures, such as having electronic leads taped to and removed from the chest wall. The view through the plastic walls of the incubator is blurred, a cacophony of sounds (e.g., motors, hiss of oxygen) penetrates the infant's closed-in world, and overhead bright lights deny diurnal and nocturnal rhythms.

Without adequate attention to emotional and developmental needs, the newborn may begin to show signs of great anxiety and tension, including the following:

- Failure to thrive (slow or absent recovery, growth, weight gain)
- Looking away from or to the side of the people who are caring for her or him
- Absent, weak, or infrequent crying (as if to say, "What's the use?")

These are a result of being exposed to life-support measures while being separated from the constant presence of one mothering and comforting person.

Communication Patterns

Newborns communicate with the world around them in various ways. Developing skill in reading these cues is essential for the nurse to individualize a plan of care that maximizes the neonate's potential for healing and growth. Newborns thrive on stimulation. However, the compromised neonate may be overwhelmed by too much stimulation. ***Cues of readiness for interaction*** include an overall appearance of relaxation. The neonate looks at the caregiver's face and appears to listen.

Cues of a newborn who is overstimulated and needs timeout from interaction include color changes (e.g., pale or flushed). The infant may hiccough, gag, or spit up. The breathing pattern changes. Muscle tone changes. Frequent startles and tremors may be seen. The newborn uses several methods to cope with overstimulation. Nurses and parents alike benefit from being on the alert for these cues. The coping strategies include ways to decrease the intensity of incoming cues (avoiding eye contact), to take time away from interaction (yawning, becoming drowsy, and sneezing), and to provide self-gratification (thumb sucking). These strategies allow the child to avoid overload and loss of energy.

Several methods are available to the nurse to *reduce* the neonate's *incoming stimuli.* Swaddling the infant (when possible), propping the newborn with rolled diapers, covering the crib with a blanket, and organizing care to allow for long stretches of rest in between treatments are a few. DO NOT DISTURB signs on the crib remind people to give the infant time to rest.

Newborn Stimulation

Newborn stimulation needs to be adjusted to the developmental level and tolerance of each neonate (Merenstein and Gardner, 1989). Newborns in the early stages of development (less than 33 weeks) respond to stimulation with jerky limb extension, hyperflexion, and irregular vital signs. Stimulation for this group is kept to a minimum. They need to be handled with slow, sure motions. Their heads are supported and limbs held close to their body when changing their position. This type of support reduces motor disorganization and stress. At age 34 to 36 weeks the newborn will respond to visual and auditory stimuli in an alert state. At age 36 to 40 weeks newborns are ready to respond to the caregiver's efforts to stimulate them.

The newborn's sense of trust develops when she or he learns the feel, sound, and smell of the same mothering person who provides comfort and who removes uncomfortable stimuli (e.g., hunger, wet or soiled clothing). The newborn even learns to anticipate these happenings and soon learns that cries bring this mothering person. These conditions cannot be duplicated in the nursery, but some modifications often can be made in the nursing care plan. In the technologic environment of the intensive care nursery (Fig. 28-12), nursing's focus must be on people, not on equipment. The possibilities are limited only by the parameters of human creativity.

When the newborn is ready for stimulation, the nurse has many options. Time from treatments can be scheduled to stroke the newborn's skin. The parents may be encouraged to touch their newborn through portholes. Mobiles and decals that can be changed frequently may be placed inside the incubator. The nurse can respond to the newborn's efforts to cry by reassuring her or him and offering a pacifier while stroking the skin and talking.

A

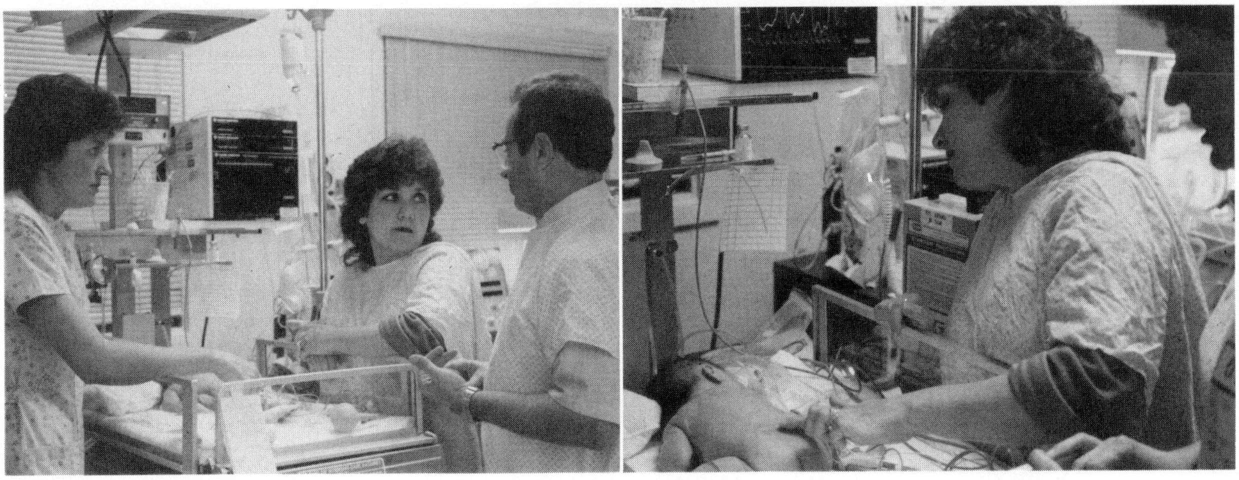

B

Fig. 28-12 Mother in special care nursery. **A,** Mother listens intently as physician keeps her informed of her baby's condition and progress. Nurse stands by for support. **B,** Note mother's tentative, tender fingertip touch as she begins to explore her baby. (Courtesy Nanci Newell, Fountain Valley Community Hospital, Fountain Valley, Calif.)

When the newborn can tolerate being out of the incubator, even for short periods, the nurse can remove, cuddle and rock, and sing to the newborn. This activity is beneficial, especially during feedings—even when feeding by gavage or gastrostomy. If possible, the newborn may be taken out of the incubator and held to raise bubbles of air from the stomach. If the mother or father is able to visit frequently, both parent and newborn will benefit immeasurably from this activity.

If the newborn must have feedings by gavage or gastrostomy, the nurse can offer a pacifier during the feeding process (in the absence of respiratory distress). This will provide sucking satisfaction, and the newborn will begin to associate this pleasant, self-gratifying, and self-initiated activity with the comforting feeling of a filling stomach.

The nurse can talk, sing, and hum to the newborn whenever possible. However loud talking and excessive discordant noise should be avoided (Fanaroff and Martin, 1987). Some nurseries permit the placement of wind-up musical toys in the incubator or crib.

The newborn can be held so that she or he can see the caregiver's face. Eye contact can be established as the nurse talks or sings to the newborn. Even if the newborn is undergoing phototherapy, there can be some periods when therapy is interrupted. The protective eye patches can be removed so that the newborn can see the nurse's or the parent's face during periodic, short comforting sessions.

The Human Incubator: "Kangaroo Method"
Vivian Wahlberg

In Western cultures, preterm newborns are usually cared for in a technically advanced environment—an incubator—to conserve warmth and energy for repair, maintenance, and growth. Thus these newborns are separated from their mothers. They are faced with many technologic treatments and procedures, such as gavage feedings and biometric monitoring. However, in Colombia, South America, it has been possible for recently born healthy preterm newborns to be cared for by their mothers. The newborns are tucked inside their mother's blouses in a head-up position and are breastfed as soon as their condition is stable (Ress, 1984; Anderson, Marks, and Wahlberg, 1986). Here, in the "human incubator," the newborns have all they need in a natural way: skin-to-skin contact, humidity, nourishment, warmth, and love. Because of its marsupial nature, this initial care of the preterm newborn by the mother has become known around the world as the **"kangaroo method"** (Fig. 28-13). It originated in 1979 in Bogota, Colombia. Reports in 1983 by the founders of the program showed dramatic decreases in mortality, morbidity, and parental abandonment. This method is in sharp contrast to the care of preterm newborns in North America and Europe.

The Programma Ambulatorio de Prematuros arose out of severe economic restraints and problems with

A

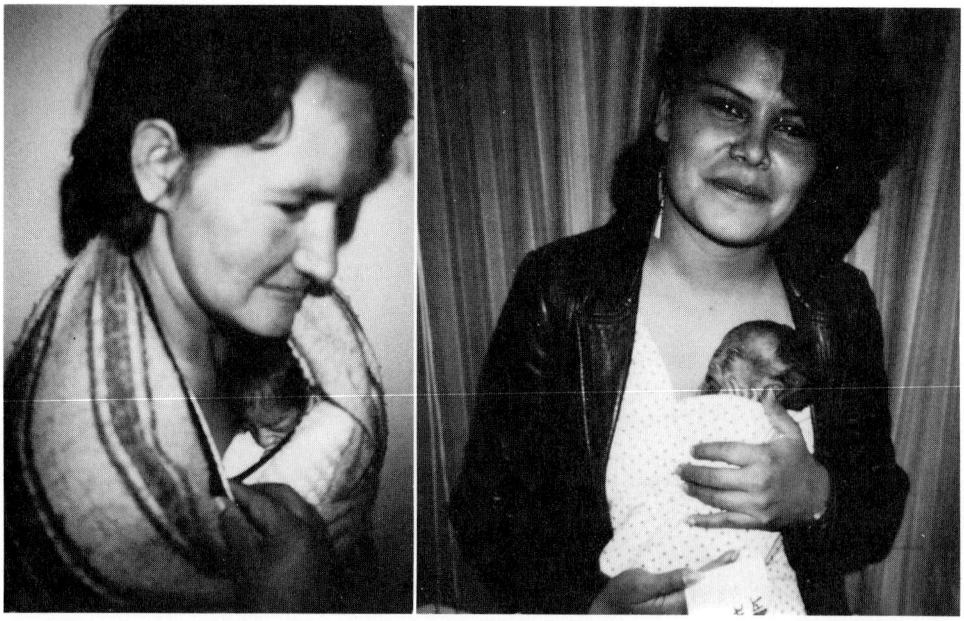

B

Fig. 28-13 The kangaroo method. **A,** Infant snuggled inside wrap. **B,** Infant inside mother's blouse in skin-to-skin contact. (Bogota, Columbia, S.A.). (Courtesy Vivian Wahlberg, R.N., C.M., Dr. Med. Sc., Karolinska, Stockholm.)

nosocomial and cross-infections, but is based on a deep respect for natural processes. Premature newborns in satisfactory clinical condition, no matter how small, are not kept in intensive care units. Instead they go directly to their mothers as early as 2 to 3 hours after birth and most are discharged within 12 to 24 hours after birth. Mother and newborn remain together 24 hours a day.

It has been observed in Colombia, Sweden, and England that the continuity of closeness and mutual stimulation between the mother and preterm newborn has reciprocal effects. Mothers reported feelings of emotional harmony and a psychologic sense of oneness with their newborns. Because the newborn's head is in an upright position, the risk of a "pathologic flat" head (seen in many preterm newborns) is not observed. In this upright position the risk of regurgitation and aspiration is minimized.

Parental Support

The nurse as support person and teacher shapes the environment and makes the caregiving more responsive to the needs of parents and newborn. Nurses' actions as support persons and teachers are a part of the first phase of the parents' adjustment to the birth of the compromised newborn. Nurses are instrumental in helping parents learn who their newborn is and to recognize behavioral cues in her or his development.

As soon as possible the parents should see and touch the newborn so they can begin to acknowledge the reality of the event and reaffirm the newborn's true appearance and condition. They will need encouragement to begin working through the psychologic tasks imposed by the preterm delivery.

A nurse or physician should be present when the parents visit the newborn. They can help parents "see" the newborn rather than focus on the equipment. The significance and function of the apparatus that surround the newborn should be explained to them. The nurse or physician should explain the characteristics normal for a newborn of their baby's gestational age. In this way parents do not compare their child with a full-term healthy newborn. The nurse or physician can encourage the parents to express their feelings about the pregnancy, labor, and delivery, and can assess the parents' perceptions of the newborn to determine the appropriate time for them (especially the mother) to become actively involved in care. Parents who have negative feelings about the pregnancy or the newborn at risk need support. The parents' feelings can be acknowledged as valid, including the burden they are experiencing financially and emotionally and their understandable feelings toward the newborn. (See Parenting Disorders discussion, p. 843.)

Soon after delivery, the parents are given the opportunity to meet the newborn in the *en face* position (Fig. 20-6), to touch the newborn, and to see her or his favorable characteristics. As soon as possible, depending primarily on her physical condition, the mother is encouraged to visit the nursery at will and help with the newborn's care. When she cannot be physically present, the staff devises appropriate methods to keep the family in almost constant touch with the newborn.

Some hospitals have instituted a parents' club for parents of infants in intensive care nurseries. These clubs encourage parents experiencing the same anxiety and grief to share their feelings. An "older" member often takes over a new member and provides additional support. Incorporating these actions into the newborn's care plan acknowledges and supports nature's design by engaging and maintaining a bond between the mother and newborn. This assures the newborn the continued care she or he needs for physical and emotional survival at the optimum level.

Discharge Planning

Early discharge of some preterm newborns is possible. The nurse's assessment, counseling, and teaching skills are invaluable for the success of home follow-up of newborns after early hospital discharge . Brooten (1986) studied a group of newborns who were discharged before they weighed 2200 g (4 lb 3½ oz), as long as they met specific criteria. The early-discharge (experimental) group received home follow-up care provided by a perinatal nurse-specialist. The nurse-specialist met with the parents soon after the baby's birth; once a week during the baby's hospitalization; and during the first week after discharge and at 1, 9, 12, and 18 months. The nurse was in contact with the parents by telephone at least 3 times a week for the first 2 weeks and weekly thereafter for 8 weeks.

The findings from this study demonstrated that programs of early-hospital discharge for low-birth-weight newborns can potentially decrease iatrogenic illness and **nosocomial** (hospital-acquired) **infections**, enhance parent-newborn interaction, and decrease hospital costs for care.

From a nursing perspective the most important findings were reported as follows: there were no newborns with failure to thrive because of parental neglect; there was no reported physical abuse of newborns; and there were no foster placements among the babies in the early-discharge group observed by the nurse-specialist.

Adequate discharge planning for the newborn at risk and follow-up arrangements should include general pediatric care, visiting nurse service, parenting classes and training in cardiopulmonary resuscitation (Chapter 17). This is especially true for young or psychosocially high-risk parents (Merenstein and Gardner, 1989). Referrals to county social service departments should be made for single mothers who are eligible for Aid to Families of Dependent Children and Medicaid. For newborns with special problems (spina bifida, cerebral palsy, or Down's syndrome), referrals should be made for special programs. These programs provide services for the newborns and support groups for parents. Parents whose newborns have special medical needs (gavage feedings, tracheostomy or colostomy care, or oxygen) should be evaluated by the medical and nursing personnel. This evaluation will help determine community resources (equipment, supplies, or emergency care) and make appropriate referrals. Home nursing care and homemaker services are sometimes covered by medical insurance. Home visits may be necessary to provide actual nursing activities and to relieve parents from the emotional burden inherent in caring for a newborn with medical problems. For newborns who are developmentally disabled, stimulation programs and follow-up programs provided by many hospitals that have newborn intensive care units are extremely valuable. Locating babysitters who will care for a child with special problems can be an overwhelming task for parents. Cultivating a resource list for parents and suggesting that parents exchange services with each other can be helpful. Graduate parents (parents of children discharged from the NICU) and nurses can provide a useful service to parents in this situation. Lastly, parents should be referred to appropriate funding agencies (Handicapped or Crippled Children's Program, Medicaid, or Social Security Disability) that provide financial assistance.

Cardiopulmonary Resuscitation. Parents must be able to administer cardiopulmonary resuscitation (CPR) to their newborn before his or her discharge (Chapter 17). Preterm newborns are 8 to 10 times more likely than term newborns to develop sudden infant death syndrome (SIDS). Further, newborns discharged from a neonatal intensive care unit are about twice as likely to die unexpectedly during the first year of life as are newborns in the general population (Rehm, 1983). The phone number to be dialed in case of emergency should be posted near the parents' phone.

Evaluation

Nursing care is evaluated to determine if the nursing goals have been met. Success can be measured by small steady increments in weight gain, fluid and electrolyte balance, and absence of GI distress. Initiation and maintenance of oral feedings are reassuring to parents and nurses. Parental success and satisfaction with the feeding process and the infant's response to it are indicators that goals are being met.

❑ GESTATIONAL AGE AND BIRTHWEIGHT

Newborns at risk for *gestational age* and *weight problems* exhibit physiologic and pathologic states related to the degree of maturity. Modern technology has contributed to the improved survival rate and overall health of *preterm* newborns, but problems remain. These relate to the appearance of "new" diseases such as necrotizing enterocolitis (NEC) (p. 825) and the survival of newborns born so small that their expectancy of a "quality life" is questionable. The plan of care for the preterm newborn must include an understanding of newborn behavior. Nursing care emphasizes the need for parental support to give the newborn her or his best chance for a healthy, happy life.

Preterm Newborn

Preterm birth is responsible for almost two thirds of newborn deaths. The newborn born before term does not possess the growth and development necessary for uncomplicated adjustment to extrauterine life, and prospects for survival or good health may be severely compromised. Newborns weighing more than 2500 g (5½ lb) and delivered after 37 weeks of pregnancy have the best prospects of survival.

The preterm newborn is at risk because of immaturity of organ systems and lack of reserves. The morbidity and mortality occurring with preterm newborns are higher 'o· three to four times than those of older newborns of comparable weight (see Fig. 28-2). The potential problems and care needs of the preterm newborn of 2000 g differ from those of the term, postterm, or postmature newborn of equal weight (Philip, 1987).

Preterm newborns are at a distinct disadvantage when they face the transition from intrauterine to extrauterine life. *The degree of disadvantage depends primarily on their level of maturity.* Physiologic disorders and anomalous malformations affect their response to treatment as well. In general, the closer they are to the normal term newborn in gestational age and weight, the easier will be their adjustment to the external environment.

Assessment

Gestational Age. Physical examination procedures to determine gestational age are based on the procedure devised by Dubowitz et al (1970). Ideally the tests are performed between 2 and 8 hours of age. For the first hour the newborn is recovering from the stress of birth, and this is reflected in muscle movements; for example, the arm recoil is slower in a fatigued newborn. After 48 hours some responses change significantly.

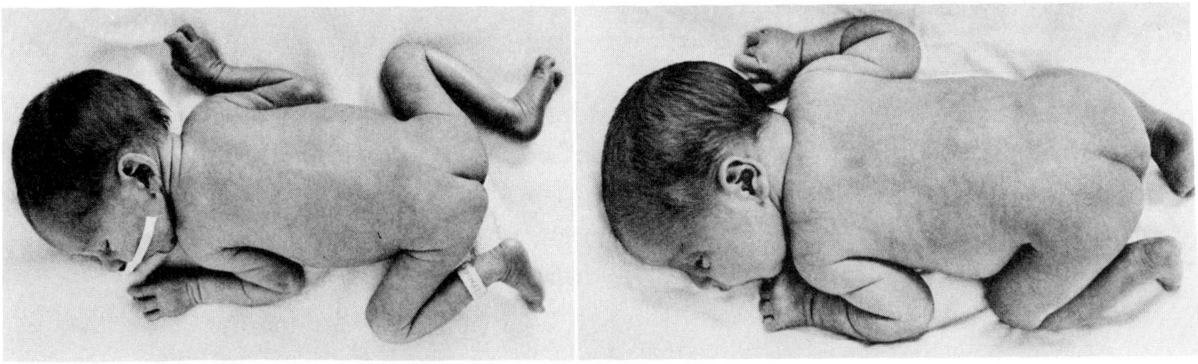

Fig. 28-14 **A,** In prone position, preterm infant lies with pelvis flat and legs splayed like a frog's. **B,** Normal full-term infant lies with his limbs flexed, pelvis raised, and knees usually drawn under abdomen. (Courtesy Mead Johnson & Co, Evansville, Indiana.)

The plantar creases on the soles of the feet appear to increase in number and become visible as the skin loses fluid and dries. See Figs. 28-14 to 28-18 and Tables 28-2 and 28-3 for the clinical estimation of gestational age (maturity). Fig. 28-19, p. 844, is an example of **newborn maturity rating and classification** (estimation of gestational age by maturity rating).

Potential Problems of Preterm Newborn. An accurate assessment of gestational age is a good indicator of the problems a preterm newborn is likely to experience (Philip, 1987). The clinical problems occurring in the preterm newborn and their physiologic bases are summarized in Table 28-4.

Text continued on p. 842.

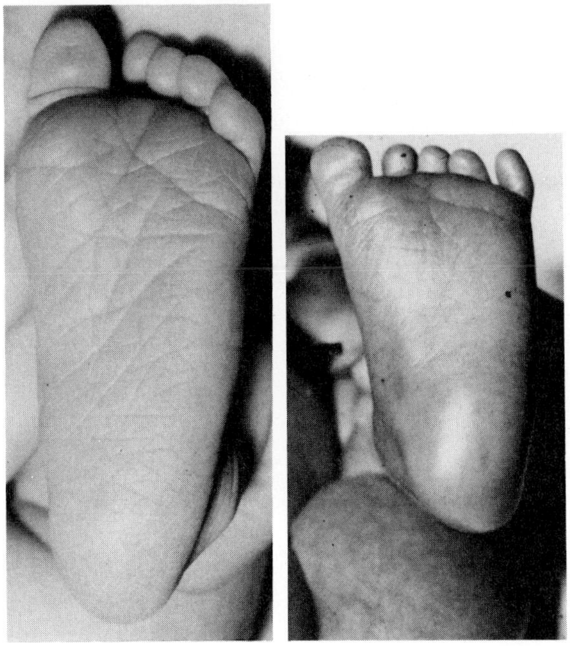

Fig. 28-15 **A,** Normal sole creases of full-term newborn. **B,** Sole of foot of preterm infant. As infant loses interstitial fluid after birth, creases become apparent even in preterm infants. Therefore assessment needs to be done in first 2 hours after birth.

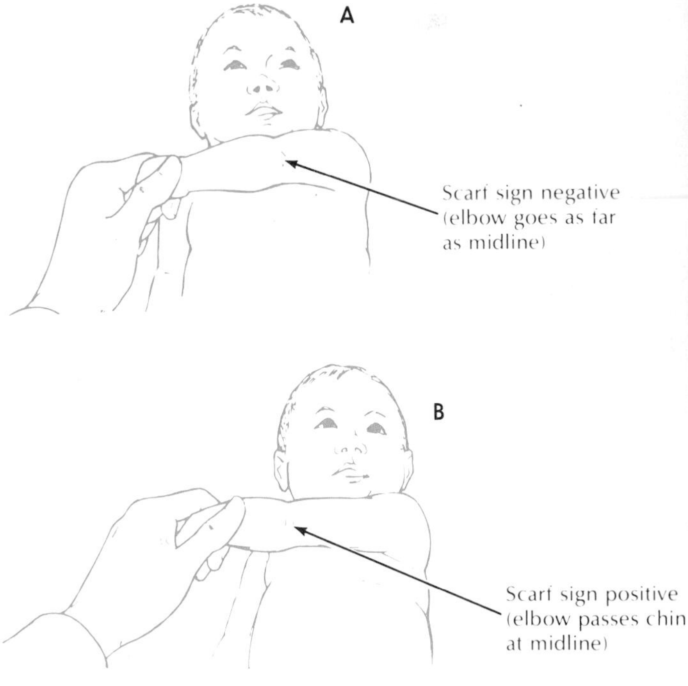

Fig. 28-16 Assessment of gestational age in term newborn, **A,** and preterm newborn, **B.**

Table 28-2 Elaboration of Physical Maturity Scales

Criterion	Findings and Assigned Scores: 0	1	2	3	4	Infant Score*
SKIN						_____
Edema	Edema evident over hands and feet; pitting seen over tibia	Pitting edema over tibia	No edema obvious	—	—	
Texture and opacity	Gelatinous, transparent; veins seen especially over abdomen	Visible veins; thin, smooth	Few larger veins seen, especially over abdomen; medium-thick smooth skin	Veins rarely seen; some thickening and superficial cracking	No vessels; parchmentlike, thick, cracking; if leathery, very cracked, and wrinkled, give score of 5	
Color	Dark red (infant is quiet for evaluation)	Pink	Pale pink	Pale; pink mainly over palms, soles, lips, and ears		
LANUGO	None	Abundant over body; long; thick	Thinning, especially over lumbosacral area	Bald areas; thinning over other areas	Mostly bald of lanugo; at least half of back bald	_____
PLANTAR CREASES	No creases seen	Faint red marks on upper half of sole	Red marks obvious over more than upper half; deeper lines over less than one third	Indentations noticeable over more than one third; lines seen over two thirds	Creases cover entire sole (see Fig. 28-15)	_____
BREAST	Nipple barely perceptible; no palpable breast tissue	Flat, smooth areola present around well-defined nipple; some breast tissue	Stippled areola but edge flat; 1-2 mm breast bud	Stippled areola with edges raised; 3-4 mm breast bud	Full areola; 5-10 mm breast bud; may have breast milk	_____
EAR FORM						_____
Cartilage	Pinna flat, soft, easily folded	Slight incurving of pinna; soft, easily folded; slow recoil	Well-incurved pinna; soft; ready recoil	Upper pinna well curved; formed and firm to edge; instant recoil	Thick cartilage; ear stiff	
GENITALS						_____
Male	No testes in scrotum and no rugae over scrotum	—	Testes descending; few rugations	Testes within scrotum; good rugae	Scrotum pendulous with rugae covering scrotum	
Female	Prominent clitoris and labia minora; labia majora do not cover labia minora	—	Labia majora and labia minora equally prominent	Labia majora appear large; labia minora, small	Labia majora completely cover clitoris and labia minora	
					TOTAL	_____

*Highest score possible = 25

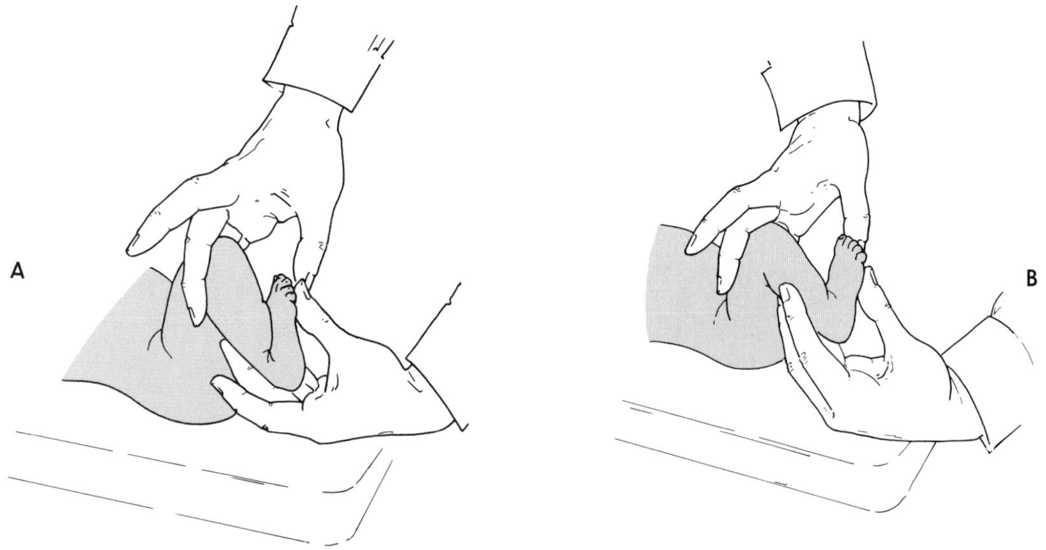

Fig. 28-17 Ankle dorsiflexion. **A,** Angle of 0 degrees in term newborn. **B,** Angle of 20 degrees in the preterm newborn.

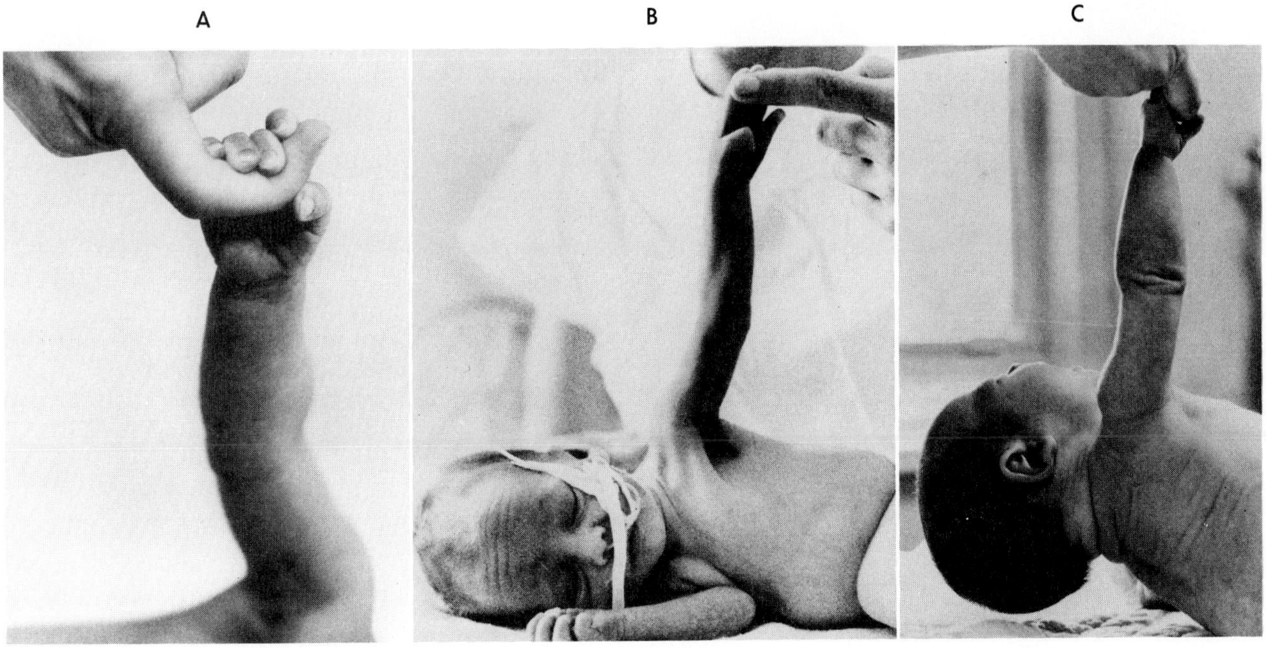

Fig. 28-18 **A,** Primitive grasp reflex present in all normal newborns usually weakens and disappears after 3 months. When palm is stimulated by finger, infant will grasp it. Full-term infant reinforces grip as finger is drawn upward. Dorsum of hand should not be touched, since this excites opposite reflex, and hand opens. **B,** Grasp reflex present in preterm infant is distinct from that noted in term infant. Grip can be obtained and arm drawn upward, but when traction is applied, grip opens and there is much less muscle tension. **C,** Once grasp is obtained in term infant, grip is reinforced when the arm is drawn upward. There is progressive tensing of muscles until baby hangs momentarily. (**B** and **C,** Courtesy Mead Johnson & Co, Evansville, Indiana.)

Table 28-3 Elaboration of Neuromuscular Maturity Scales*

Criterion	Method of Assessment	0
Posture (see Fig. 28-14)	Position: supine Activity: quiet Assessment: extension and flexion of arms, hips, legs	Complete extension 
Square swindow (wrist)†	Position: supine Method: with thumb supporting back of arm below wrist, apply gentle pressure with index and third fingers on dorsum of hand; do not rotate infant's wrist Assessment: angle formed between hypothenar eminence and forearm	Very premature (<30 weeks) 90° 
Arm recoil	Position; supine Method; flex forearms on upper arms for 5 sec; pull on hands to full extension and release Assessment: degree of flexion	No recoil; arms remain extended 180° 
Popliteal angle	Position: supine; pelvis on flat, firm surface Method: flex leg on thigh; then flex thigh on abdomen; holding knee with thumb and index finger, extend leg with index finger of other hand behind ankle Assessment: degree of angle behind knee	Complete extension; very premature 180° 
Scarf sign (see Fig. 28-16)	Position: supine Method: support head in midline with one hand; pull hand to opposite shoulder Assessment: position of elbow in relation to midline	Elbow to opposite arm like scarf around neck 

*Compare combined scores for physical and neuromuscular maturity to the "maturity rating" scores and read estimated weeks of gestational age. Estimate of gestational age obtained is accurate only to plus or minus 2 weeks. After gestational age is estimated, infant's length, weight, and head circumference are entered on appropriate graphs. All three measurements should fall within same approximate range, for example, all within SGA, LGA, or AGA. If one measurement is excessively large (falling into LGA range) and other two fall into SGA range, growth deviation should be assessed. **X**, First examination; **O**, second examination.
†Counterpart: ankle dorsiflexion (see Fig. 28-17).

Table 28-3 Elaboration of Neuromuscular Maturity Scales—cont'd

Finding and Assigned Scores					Infant Score	
1	2	3	4	5	X	0
Extension of arms; slight flexion of hips, legs 	Extension of arms 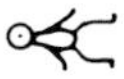	Slight flexion of arms; full flexion of legs 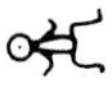	Complete flexion 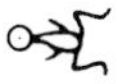	—	______	______
Premature (30-35 weeks) 60° 	Premature (30-35 weeks) 45° 	Maturing (35-38 weeks) 30° 	Term: hand lies flat on ventral surface of forearm 0°	—	______	______
—	Some recoil; sluggish response 100°-180° 	Maturing (35-38 weeks) 90°-100° 	Brisk recoil to complete flexion >90° 	—	______	______
Premature (30-35 weeks) 160° 	Premature (30-35 weeks) 130° 	Maturing (35-38 weeks) 110° 	Maturing (35-38 weeks) 90° 	Extension is resisted >90° 	______	______
Elbow beyond midline of thorax 	Elbow just beyond midline 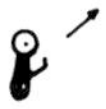	Elbow at midline 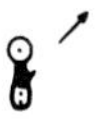	Elbow does not reach midline 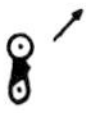	—	______	______

Continued.

Table 28-3 Elaboration of Neuromuscular Maturity Scales

Criterion	Method of Assessment	0
Heel to ear	Position: supine, pelvis is kept flat on surface Method: pull foot up toward ear on same side; do not hold knee Assessment: distance of foot from ear and degree of extension of knee	Toes touch ear; leg completely extended (180°) 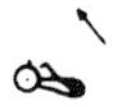

Parental Adaptation to Preterm Newborn

Parents who experience a preterm birth have a totally different experience from parents giving birth to a full-term newborn (Sammons and Lewis, 1985). Preterm delivery does not permit the parents to complete the psychologic and emotional growth of a 40-week-gestation pregnancy. The parents are often overwhelmed by feelings of failure, loss, fear, and sadness. The newborn is small, immature, often physically unattractive, and sick. The newborn has none of the cute, appealing behaviors of a full-term newborn. He or she is not alert, does not suck, and may be too compromised to be held at all. Because of these differences, parental attachment and adaptation to the parental role will be different also.

Parental Tasks. Parents face a number of psychologic tasks before effective relationships and parenting patterns can evolve. These tasks include the following:

1. *Anticipatory grief over the potential loss of their newborn.* The parent grieves (Chapter 29) in preparation for the newborn's possible death, although the parent clings tenuously to the hope that the newborn will survive. This begins during labor and lasts until the newborn dies or shows evidence of surviving.
2. *Acceptance by the mother of her failure to deliver a healthy, full-term newborn.* Grief and depression typify this phase, which persists until the newborn is out of danger and is expected to survive.
3. *Resumption of the process of relating to the newborn.* As the baby begins to improve—gains weight, feeds by nipple, and is weaned from the incubator—the parent can begin the process of developing attachment that was interrupted by the newborn's precarious condition at birth (Als and Brazelton, 1981).
4. *Learning how this newborn differs in special needs and growth patterns.* Another parental task is to learn, understand, and accept this newborn's caregiving needs and growth and development expectations (Sammons and Lewis, 1985).
5. *Adjusting the home environment to the needs of the newborn.* Grandparents and brothers and sisters also react to the birth of the preterm newborn. Parents must reconcile the grief of grandparents and the bewilderment and anger of brothers and sisters at the disproportionate amount of parental time absorbed by the newborn.

Parental Responses. Two different approaches noted by Newman (1980) are *coping through commitment* and *coping through distance.* With the first approach parents take each day as it comes, recognizing and accepting the lessened responses of their newborn and noting the gradual progress in their newborn's condition. With the second approach the parents pull away from emotional attachment to the newborn; they postpone becoming attached until the newborn is in better health.

Table 28-3 Elaboration of Neuromuscular Maturity Scales—cont'd

Finding and Assigned Scores					Infant Score	
1	2	3	4	5	X	0
Toes almost reach face (130°) 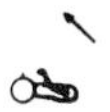	Knees flexed (110°) 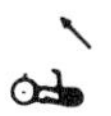	Knees flexed (90°) 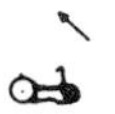	Knees flexed popliteal angle is less than 90° 	—	______	______
			NEUROMUSCULAR MATURITY TOTALS		______	______
			PHYSICAL MATURITY TOTALS		______	______
			(see Table 28-2)		______	______
			COMBINED SCORE		______	______

See Fig. 28-19 for Maturity Rating.

Parents have been observed to progress through stages as they spend more time with their newborns. In the first stage they maintain an *en face* position, stroking and touching their newborn (Figs. 28-20 and 28-21, p. 846). In the second stage they assume some newborn care activities—feeding, bathing, changing. In the third stage the newborn becomes a person and is seen as a whole child (Schraeder, 1980). Sosa and Grua (1982) reported a personal communication with Brazelton in which he correlated parental behaviors with the previously noted three stages. In the first stage parents ask about *chemical data,* such as "What is his bilirubin today?" In the second stage they note their baby yawning, sneezing, hiccoughing, *reflexes* that mark their newborn as human. At this time the newborn is still not "claimed." In later stages they note their *newborn's responses* to them and begin to feel that "this child is mine" and part of our family. Parents take on the role of advocate for their child (Sammons and Lewis, 1985).

Newborn Responsiveness. The preterm newborn's states of consciousness are more labile than the term newborn's. The quiet alert state is less evident and unpredictable. Field (1979) noted that if a mother concentrated her interactions on imitation of the newborn's behavior, the newborn was increasingly attentive and interested. Too-active an involvement in child care tended to result in the newborn becoming disinterested and glancing away (gaze aversion). One young mother noted that "gentle stroking of his head caused him to look at her." (She also reported that even at age 7 years, gentle head stroking calmed her child.)

Parenting Disorders. The incidence of physical and emotional abuse is greater toward the newborn who, by virtue of prematurity or illness, was separated from the mother for a period after birth (Fomufod, 1976). Physical abuse includes varying degrees of poor nutrition and poor hygiene. Emotional abuse ranges from subtle to outright dislike of the child. There may be preferential treatment for brothers and sisters, nagging, extremely high expectations of the child, and various other types of overt or covert negative responses by one or both parents.

Factors surrounding the birth may predispose parents to subconsciously or overtly reject the child. These factors might include parental pain and anxiety, a heavy financial burden for the newborn's care, unresolved anticipatory grief, threat to self-esteem, or unwanted pregnancy. The goal of the helping professionals is to reduce the incidence of child abuse and neglect.

Nursing Diagnoses

To formulate nursing diagnoses, the nurse must analyze data obtained from continuous monitoring of the newborn and from observation of and discussions with the parents. The diagnoses may be physical, cognitive, or psychologic. Examples of diagnoses are as follows:

Ineffective breathing pattern (newborn) related to
- Inadequate chest expansion, secondary to newborn's position or immaturity

Parental knowledge deficit related to
- Feeding the newborn

Situational low self-esteem (parent) related to
- Mother's feelings of inadequacy in caring for the newborn

Planning

The physiologic problems of immature body systems govern the plan of care of these newborns. The newborn is faced with many emergency treatments and procedures. Nursing care during this time of crisis is a critical factor in the newborn's chances for survival

NEWBORN MATURITY RATING and CLASSIFICATION

ESTIMATION OF GESTATIONAL AGE BY MATURITY RATING

Symbols: X - 1st Exam O - 2nd Exam

NEUROMUSCULAR MATURITY

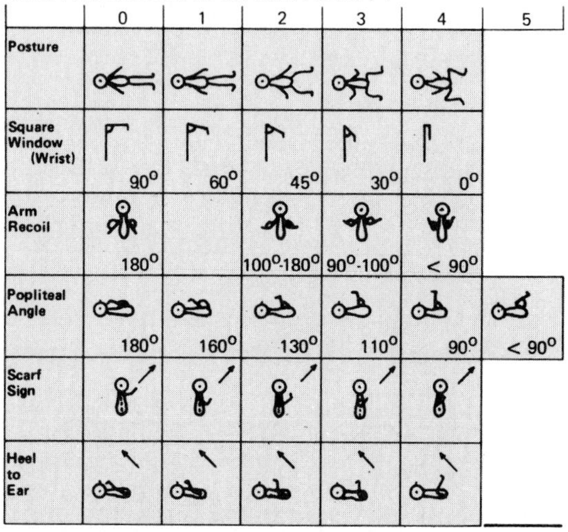

	0	1	2	3	4	5
Posture						
Square Window (Wrist)	90°	60°	45°	30°	0°	
Arm Recoil	180°		100°-180°	90°-100°	< 90°	
Popliteal Angle	180°	160°	130°	110°	90°	< 90°
Scarf Sign						
Heel to Ear						

PHYSICAL MATURITY

	0	1	2	3	4	5
SKIN	gelatinous red, transparent	smooth pink, visible veins	superficial peeling &/or rash, few veins	cracking pale area, rare veins	parchment, deep cracking, no vessels	leathery, cracked, wrinkled
LANUGO	none	abundant	thinning	bald areas	mostly bald	
PLANTAR CREASES	no crease	faint red marks	anterior transverse crease only	creases ant. 2/3	creases cover entire sole	
BREAST	barely percept.	flat areola, no bud	stippled areola, 1–2 mm bud	raised areola, 3–4 mm bud	full areola, 5–10 mm bud	
EAR	pinna flat, stays folded	sl. curved pinna, soft with slow recoil	well-curv. pinna, soft but ready recoil	formed & firm with instant recoil	thick cartilage, ear stiff	
GENITALS Male	scrotum empty, no rugae		testes descending, few rugae	testes down, good rugae	testes pendulous, deep rugae	
GENITALS Female	prominent clitoris & labia minora		majora & minora equally prominent	majora large, minora small	clitoris & minora completely covered	

Score is obtained by adding totals from Tables 37-1 and 37-2.

Gestation by Dates ______________ wks

Birth Date ____________ Hour ____________ am/pm

APGAR ____________ 1 min ____________ 5 min

MATURITY RATING

Score	Wks
5	26
10	28
15	30
20	32
25	34
30	36
35	38
40	40
45	42
50	44

SCORING SECTION

	1st Exam=X	2nd Exam=O
Estimating Gest Age by Maturity Rating	______ Weeks	______ Weeks
Time of Exam	Date ______ Hour ______ am/pm	Date ______ Hour ______ am/pm
Age at Exam	______ Hours	______ Hours
Signature of Examiner	______ M.D.	______ M.D.

Fig. 28-19 Newborn maturity rating and classification. (Mead Johnson & Co, Evansville, Indiana. Scoring section adapted from Ballard JL et al: Pediatr Res 11:374, 1977. Figures modified from Sweet AY: Classification of the low-birth-weight infant. In Klaus MH and Fanaroff AA: Care of the high-risk infant, Philadelphia, 1977, WB Saunders Co.)

Table 28-4 Preterm Newborn's Potential Problems and Their Physiologic Bases

Potential Problem	Physiologic Bases
Initiating and maintaining respirations	Paucity of functional alveoli; incomplete aeration of lungs caused by deficient surfactant Smaller lumen and greater collapsibility or obstruction of respiratory passages Weakness of respiratory musculature Insufficient calcification of bony thorax Absent or weak gag reflex Immature and friable capillaries in brain and lungs Few functional alveoli in newborns less than 24 weeks' gestational age
Maintaining body temperature	Large surface area in relation to body weight (mass) Absent or poor reflex control of skin capillaries (no shiver response) Small, inadequate muscle mass activity; absent or minimum flexion of extremities Meager insulating subcutaneous fat Friable capillaries and immature temperature regulating center in brain
Maintaining adequate nutrition	Mechanical feeding problems ▪ Absent or weak sucking and swallowing reflexes; unsynchronized ▪ Absent or weak gag and cough reflexes ▪ Small stomach capacity ▪ Immature cardiac sphincter (stomach) ▪ Lax abdominal musculature Absorption and assimilation problems ▪ Paucity of stored nutrients: vitamins A and C; calcium, phosphorus, iron; loss of fat and fat-soluble vitamins in stool ▪ Immature absorption, decreased amount of hydrochloric acid ▪ Impaired metabolism (enzyme systems) or enzyme pathology
Maintaining CNS function	Birth trauma: damage to immature structures Fragile capillaries and impaired coagulation process; prolonged prothrombin time Recurrent anoxic episodes Tendency toward hypoglycemia
Maintaining renal function	Impaired renal clearance of metabolites and drugs Inability to maintain acid-base, fluid, and electrolyte homeostasis Impaired ability to concentrate urine Paucity of stored nutrients from mother
Resisting infection	Paucity of stored immunoglobulins from mother Impaired ability to synthesize antibodies Thin skin and fragile capillaries near surface Impaired ability to muster white blood cells
Resisting hematologic problems	Increased capillary friability and permeability Low plasma prothrombin levels (increased tendency to bleed) Relatively slowed erythropoietic activity in bone marrow Relatively increased rate of hemolysis Loss of blood for laboratory specimens
Maintaining musculoskeletal integrity	Weak, underdeveloped muscles Immature skeletal system (bones, joints) Meager subcutaneous fat with its cushioning effect
Maintaining retinal integrity	Immature vascular structures in retina Need for oxygen therapy

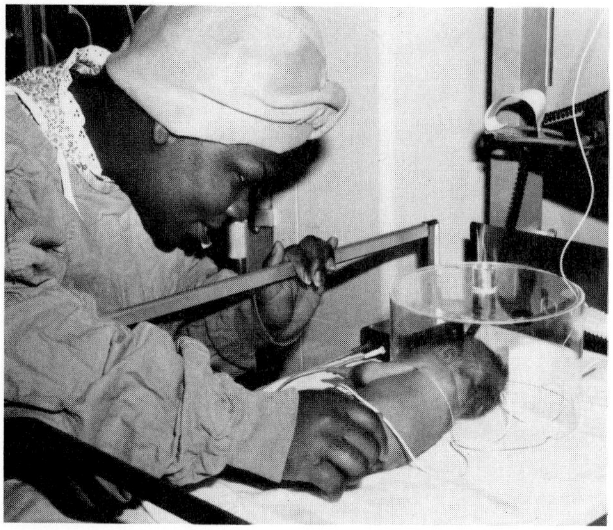

Fig. 28-20 Mother interacting with her baby using touch. Oxygen hood and overhead warmer are being used in place of incubator.

and in the parents' eventual relationship with their child.

Goals should include the following:

1. The newborn's physiologic functioning and adequate nutrition are maintained.
2. Hematologic problems are minimized.
3. Infection, retinal problems, and trauma to immature musculoskeletal system are prevented.
4. Newborn attachment to parents begins.
5. Parents perceive the child as potentially normal (if this is medically substantiated).
6. Parents provide care comfortably and experience pride and satisfaction in the care of the newborn.
7. Parents organize their time and energies to meet the love, attention, and care needs of the other members of the family and themselves as well.

Implementation

The extrauterine environment of the preterm newborn must approximate a healthy intrauterine environment for the normal sequence of growth and development to continue. The provision of such an environment is the basis for care of the preterm newborn. Medical and nursing personnel and respiratory therapists work as a team to provide the intensive care needed. Nursing actions are based on knowledge of the *physiologic problems* (Table 28-4) *imposed on the preterm newborn and on the newborn's need to conserve energy for repair, maintenance, and growth* (see General Care of the Compromised Newborn, p. 817).

Respiratory Distress Syndrome

Respiratory distress syndrome (**RDS**) is a leading cause of morbidity and mortality among preterm newborns. It affects about 20,000 newborns each year in North America. Generally the smaller the preterm newborn, the higher the mortality. RDS is seen almost exclusively in preterm newborns, but occasionally a full-term newborn is affected.

The central problem in RDS is progressive ***atelectasis*** (alveolar collapse), which results from the development of a hyaline membrane within the newborn's terminal bronchial tree, that is, within the alveolar ducts and the alveoli. It occurs within a few hours after birth. The *hyaline membrane* is composed in part of fibrin derived from the pulmonary circulation and is not the

A

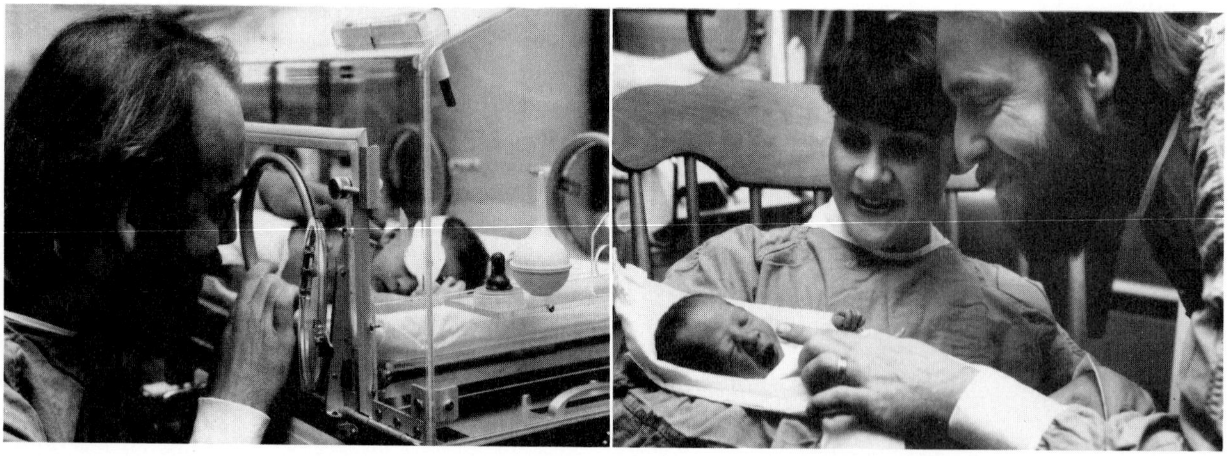

B

Fig. 28-21 Father interacts with his baby. **A,** Stroking baby's back. **B,** Touching baby with fingertip.

result of aspirated fluid or an irritant. Accompanying problems such as hypoxia, metabolic and respiratory acidosis, and pulmonary hypoperfusion with right-to-left shunting (i.e., persistent fetal circulation) are secondary to atelectasis.

The cause of RDS is still unknown. The role of surfactant in preventing alveolar collapse at the end of expiration has been established. A deficiency in surfactant production may be the basis for RDS.

A deficiency in surfactant forces the newborn to work to reexpand the lungs with each inspiration. The result is fatigue, depletion of energy reserves, hypoxia and hypercapnia, progressive atelectasis, and diminishing lung compliance (or increasing "stiffness"). *Factors that impair the production of surfactant* are hypoxia, acidosis, and reduced pulmonary blood circulation. Thus a vicious cycle is established. The normal newborn expends more calories and consumes more oxygen to breathe than does the adult. For the newborn in respiratory distress this expenditure may be as much as six times that of the normal term newborn.

RDS may be apparent at birth. The newborn often has a low Apgar score and commonly requires resuscitation and ventilatory assistance. Other symptoms generally appear within the first 6 hours. Initially expiratory grunting and nasal flaring are evident. As the disease progresses, tachypnea (60 breaths/min or more), retractions, and even cyanosis in room air may be noted. Hypotension and shock may be evident. Apneic pauses replace the expiratory grunting. An arterial PO_2 of 40 mm Hg or less in room air is a constant finding.

The diagnosis is confirmed by x-ray films, blood tests for pH, serum nonprotein nitrogen (NPN), potassium, and phosphorus. Tests for arterial blood gases are also used as diagnostic indicators for RDS.

Formerly, if the newborn with RDS survived the first 48 to 72 hours, the clinical condition improved slowly until recovery at about 10 to 12 days. Newer methods and equipment have sustained the severely affected newborn beyond 72 hours. Because of the more serious effects of the disease, death still may occur several weeks after birth. Therefore a guarded prognosis is given for several weeks.

Treatment. A thermoneutral environment is provided so the newborn's body temperature is maintained at 36.5° C (97.6° F). Gentle handling is necessary; this newborn is disturbed as little as possible. The newborn's caloric intake must be sufficient to prevent catabolism (40 kcal/kg/24 hr or more). Blood is replaced if an excessive amount is lost, usually as a result of samples taken for laboratory analysis. Serum bilirubin levels are controlled by phototherapy, exchange transfusion, or both. Low serum albumin levels, hypoxia, and acidosis interfere with the albumin's binding to bilirubin and therefore subject these newborns to kernicterus at low serum bilirubin levels (10 mg/dl or less) (see discussion of hyperbilirubinemia, p. 879).

Specific respiratory therapies are employed. Oxygen (60% or less) is administered by means of a hood (Fig. 28-20). Continuous positive airway pressure (CPAP) may be administered by means of an intratracheal tube, face mask, nasal prongs, or hood. Continuous negative airway pressure (CNAP) may be needed. CNAP is a respirator that works in the same manner as CPAP but exerts negative pressure on the newborn's body while the head is exposed. The newborn may breathe room air or an air-oxygen mix by means of a mask or prongs. Intermittent positive end expiratory pressure (PEEP) may be used.

New medical methods include the use of artificial surfactant or extracorporeal membrane oxygenation (ECMO) with a modified heart-lung machine (Bartlett et al, 1985). Artificial surfactant or surfactant obtained from exogenous sources may be administered. In recent years a number of controlled clinical trials of artificial surfactant in preterm newborns have clearly shown its effectiveness, both as a preventative and as a therapy for RDS (Merritt et al, 1986; Gitlin et al, 1987). These studies used either human surfactant from amniotic fluid or a bovine-based preparation. Adverse side effects have been minimal to absent in the acute management of affected newborns. Active research into a synthetic, protein-free material, which has been proved effective in animals, is under way. A bovine extract is expected to be commercially available soon. Surfactant replacement can then become routine care for the preterm newborn in the delivery room (Lawson, 1987; Hodgman, 1987).

Complications of Oxygen Therapy

Bronchopulmonary dysplasia (BPD) and **retinopathy of prematurity (ROP)** (previously called retrolental fibroplasia) are diseases of prematurity secondary to oxygen therapy (Bancalari and Gerhardt, 1986). Both conditions are relatively "new" disorders, recognized since the advent of methods of administering high concentrations of oxygen beginning in the 1940s. Although oxygen therapy may be lifesaving and occasionally must be given in high concentrations for extended periods, it is also potentially hazardous and must be administered judiciously. Other conditions besides BPD and ROP have become apparent. The mechanical creation of positive pressure in the lungs has increased the incidence of "air leaks." Use of oxygen apparatuses has also resulted in nasal, tracheal or pharyngeal perforation or inflammation.

Bronchopulmonary Dysplasia. BPD is a common concomitant of lung disorders in newborns, primarily preterm newborns, in which focal areas of emphysema develop in the lungs. The cause is unknown, but the condition may develop as a sequela to alveolar damage caused by lung disease, use of high oxygen concentrations, and the prolonged use of CPAP or PEEP (Bancalari and Gerhardt, 1986). Symptoms of respiratory distress, tachypnea, and increased effort appear. It is difficult to wean the newborn from the positive pressure ventilator. This finding may be the first indication of the disease process.

The first sign that the newborn is recovering from BPD is a decreasing dependence on oxygen therapy. Recovery may take several months. Mortality is between 30% and 50%; death may occur after the infant has been discharged from the hospital.

Retinopathy of Prematurity. The retinal changes in ROP were first described in 1942. The condition has been related to the use of high levels of oxygen and prolonged oxygen therapy. Judicious use of oxygen therapy and monitoring of PaO_2 levels have reduced the incidence of ROP, but the disease has not been eradicated.

PaO_2 between 50 and 70 mm Hg may be within safe limits. (The recently developed transcutaneous oxygen tension monitor [$tcPO_2$] is a noninvasive device that provides continuous oxygen tension values.) The most crucial period for toxic levels to occur is during the recovery phase from RDS and other respiratory distress. The exact level at which arterial oxygen tension becomes toxic and causes ROP is unknown.

Oxygen tensions that are too high for the level of retinal maturity initially result in vasoconstriction. After oxygen therapy is discontinued, neovascularization occurs in the retina and vitreous, with capillary hemorrhages, fibrotic resolution, and possible retinal detachment. Cicatricial (scar) tissue formation and consequent visual impairment may be mild or severe. The entire disease process in severe cases may take as long as 5 months to evolve. Examination by an ophthalmologist before discharge and a schedule for repeat examinations thereafter are recommended.

Evaluation

Evaluation of the care given preterm infants and their families has to be multidimensional (Montgomery and Williams-Judge, 1986). In some families the infant dies despite all medical and nursing knowledge and skill. In other families the sequelae of preterm birth result in newborns who will face lifetime disability. For these families evaluation criteria relate to the concepts of loss, grief, and self-concept (see Chapter 29). For many other newborns and families the immediate threat to well-being is overcome by intensive neonatal care.

Small-for-Gestational-Age, Low-Birth-Weight Newborns

Newborns whose birth weight falls below the tenth percentile expected at term, for reasons other than heredity, are considered at high risk (mortality greater than 10%) (Korones 1986). Fetal growth retardation is attributable to causes such as deficient supply of nutrients (intrauterine malnutrition), intrauterine infections, and congenital malformations.

Intrauterine growth retardation (IUGR) related to malnutrition will be discussed here. Two types of growth retardation are identified by the examination of cellular characteristics: IUGR may result from hypoplasia, a *deficient number of cells,* each containing the normal amount of cytoplasm. IUGR may also result from an adequate number of cells, each of which is diminished in size because of the *reduced amount of cytoplasm.*

Several physical findings are characteristic of the *growth-retarded newborn:*

- Generally has normal skull, but reduced dimensions of rest of body make skull look inordinately large
- Reduced subcutaneous fat
- Loose and dry skin
- Diminished muscle mass especially over buttocks and cheeks
- Sunken abdomen (scaphoid) as opposed to being normally well rounded
- Thin, yellowish, dry, and dull umbilical cord (normal cord is gray, glistening, round, and moist)
- Sparse scalp hair
- Wide skull sutures (inadequate bone growth)

The infant who is SGA as a result of intrauterine nutritional deficiency faces a number of physiologic problems, such as meconium aspiration syndrome, hypoglycemia, and heat loss.

Hypoglycemia is commonly encountered in SGA newborns, whether term or preterm. The incidence may be as high as 40%. Hypoglycemia in LBW newborns is considered to be a glucose level of 20 mg/dl of blood or less. This disorder may occur anytime from birth until day 4 of life. If it is untreated, neurologic sequelae can be anticipated. Blood glucose levels are monitored by laboratory biochemical study and reagent tests.

Diminution of subcutaneous fat and a large body surface compared with body weight subject the SGA newborn to problems in thermoregulation. Cold stress jeopardizes recovery from asphyxia. The meagerness of fat and glycogen reserves increases such a newborn's vulnerability to cold and other stress.

Nursing care of the SGA newborn is based on the clinical problems present. The nursing care related to those problems is the same as for the preterm newborn (see Implementation, p. 846).

Postterm Newborn

Postterm, or *postdate,* refers to gestation prolonged beyond 42 *completed* weeks from the first day of the last menstrual cycle (**prolonged pregnancy**). *Postmaturity,* however, implies progressive placental insufficiency resulting in a dysmature newborn. *Not all postterm newborns are postmature* (see p. 815).

Weights of postmature newborns usually fall within the normal range for gestational age. However, because of severe deteriorating metabolic exchange in the aging placenta, the newborn may be SGA. Fetal malnutrition and hypoxia result in the wasted appearance of this dysmature newborn.

These newborns have a higher-than-normal incidence of fetal distress and perinatal death. The normal-appearing newborns do well if fetopelvic disproportion (FPD) does not develop because of their increased size. A breakdown of newborn deaths associated with prolonged pregnancy reveals that about one third occurred during pregnancy; approximately one half occurred during labor and delivery; and about one sixth during the puerperium.

After confirmation of prolonged pregnancy the physician determines the protocol for delivery. A *trial of labor* by induction may be ordered (Chapter 26). The postmature fetus (AGA or SGA) may tolerate the stress of labor poorly as a result of increasing placental insufficiency. Indices of fetal jeopardy are late FHR deceleration patterns with a slow return to the baseline rate, meconium-stained amniotic fluid, oligohydramnios, and a fetal scalp blood pH of 7.2 or less. Cephalopelvic or fetopelvic disproportion complicates some postterm labors. The oversized fetus may be exposed to excessive trauma during vaginal delivery, such as fractures and intracranial hemorrhage, and to asphyxia during labor. If induction is unsuccessful, if labor is unsatisfactory, or if fetal distress develops, cesarean delivery follows.

During the antepartum period the nurse contributes to the assessment for identification of a prolonged pregnancy and often conducts nonstress tests to monitor fetal well-being. Identification and management of maternal reactions are important components of the nursing care plan. Emotional response of the woman can reflect feelings of fatigue, frustration, and anger as the pregnancy "never seems to end." She may experience negative feelings about her ability to cope and her "normalcy as a woman." Fears for the safety of her baby and the baby's future development can arise.

Intrapartum nursing care of the fetus is the same as for all other labors (Unit III). It may be similar to that needed for fetopelvic disproportion and dystotic labor (Chapter 26). Parental fears are recognized, and support is offered. After birth, the neonate is assessed in the same manner as all newborns (Chapter 16).

Assessment

Most postterm and postmature newborns are oversized but otherwise normal, with advanced development and bone age.

A postterm newborn will have some but not necessarily all of the following physical characteristics:

- Generally has normal skull, but reduced dimensions of rest of body make skull look inordinately large
- Dry, cracked skin (desquamating), parchmentlike at birth
- Nails of hard consistency extending beyond fingertips
- Profuse scalp hair
- Subcutaneous fat layers depleted, leaving skin loose and giving an "old person" appearance
- Long and thin body contour
- Absent vernix
- Often meconium staining (golden yellow to green) of skin, nails, and cord
- May have an alert, wide-eyed appearance symptomatic of chronic intrauterine hypoxia

Nursing Diagnoses

The postterm newborn's size and condition will determine whether the nursing diagnoses suitable for the "normal" newborn or those formulated for the preterm newborn are appropriate. Examples include the following:

Ineffective airway clearance related to
- Meconium aspiration syndrome

Potential hypothermia related to
- Depleted stores of subcutaneous fat

Potential for injury (permanent disability) related to
- Birth trauma

Potential for injury secondary to hypoglycemia related to
- Depleted glycogen stores

Planning

Physiologic problems of postmaturity are reflected in the plan of care. ***Immediate goals*** are the initiation and maintenance of respiration, maintenance of body temperature and nutrition, prevention of CNS trauma and infection, and identification and treatment of birth trauma. The ***long-term goal*** is to prevent or minimize adverse sequelae to postmaturity.

Implementation

Immediate care is similar to that given to preterm newborns (Affonso and Harris, 1980). Procedures to support physiologic function (e.g., respiration, body temperature, nutrition) are discussed in Chapters 17 and 18, and on p. 846.

Evaluation

The nurse can be assured that care was effective when the goals for care have been met. Evaluation of the degree to which the long-term goal is achieved is delayed beyond the period of infancy.

❑ NEWBORN BIRTH TRAUMA

Birth trauma is any physical injury sustained by a neonate during labor and delivery. Such injuries still represent an important source of neonatal morbidity. Therefore the clinician should consider the broad spectrum of birth injuries in the differential diagnosis of neonatal clinical disorders (Fanaroff and Martin, 1987).

Most birth trauma may be preventable at least in theory. Careful attention to risk factors and the appropriate planning of delivery should reduce the incidence of such injuries to a minimum. Ultrasonography allows for antepartum diagnosis of macrosomia, hydrocephalus, and unusual presentations. Particular pregnancies may then be delivered by controlled elective cesarean delivery to avoid significant birth trauma (Merenstein and Gardner, 1989).

Often a small percentage of significant birth traumas may be unavoidable and occur despite skilled and competent obstetric care. Some injuries cannot be anticipated until the specific circumstances are encountered during delivery. Emergency cesarean delivery may provide a last-minute salvage, but in these circumstances the injury may truly be unavoidable. The same injury might be caused in several ways. Thus a cephalhematoma could be the result of an obstetric technique such as forceps delivery or vacuum extraction, or the same injury may occur as a result of the pressure of the fetal skull against the maternal pelvis.

Many injuries are minor and readily resolve in the neonatal period without treatment. Other traumas require some degree of intervention. A few are serious enough to be fatal.

The nurse's contributions to the welfare of the newborn begin with early observation and accurate recording. The prompt reporting of signs indicative of deviations from normal permits early initiation of appropriate therapy.

Assessment

Several factors predispose an infant to birth trauma (Fanaroff and Martin, 1987; Merenstein and Gardner, 1989). *Maternal* factors include uterine dysfunction that leads to prolonged or precipitous labor, preterm or postterm labor, and cephalopelvic disproportion. Injury may result from dystocia caused by *fetal* macrosomia, multifetal gestation, abnormal or difficult presentation (not caused by maternal uterine or pelvic conditions), and congenital anomalies. *Intrapartum events* that can result in scalp injury include the use of intrapartum monitoring of FHR and collection of fetal scalp blood for acid-base assessment. *Obstetric delivery techniques* can cause injury. Forceps delivery, vacuum extraction, version and extraction, and cesarean delivery are all potential contributory factors.

The Apgar score may alert the caregiver to birth trauma. Flaccid muscle tone, regardless of cause, increases the risk of joint dislocations and separation during the birth process. Flaccid tone in extremities may be traced to nerve plexus injuries or long-bone fractures. A weak or hoarse cry is characteristic of laryngeal nerve palsy as a result of excessive traction on the neck during delivery. Marked bruising of the skin may preclude accurate assessment for color.

A complete physical assessment of the newborn is performed soon after birth (Chapter 16). LGA newborns may be preterm, term, postmature, or postterm; or children of diabetic (or prediabetic) mothers (see Figs. 28-1 and 28-2). Each of these categories has special concerns. Regardless of coexisting potential problems, the oversized newborn or the newborn too large for the maternal pelvis is at risk by virtue of size alone. Birth trauma, especially associated with breech or shoulder presentation, is a serious hazard for the oversized newborn. Asphyxia or CNS injury or both may also occur.

An oversized infant traditionally has been one who weighs 4000 g (8 lb 13 oz) or more at birth. About 10% of newborns are of this weight, and about 2% weigh 4500 g (9 lb 15 oz) or more. Moreover, most of these newborns have other proportionately larger measurements. Many are delivered well after the estimated date of delivery (EDD). Since evidence of birth trauma may not be apparent at the initial examination, assessment continues during each contact with the neonate.

Nursing Diagnoses

The nursing diagnoses will depend on the particular injury incurred. The following are therefore presented as examples only.

Parents

Knowledge deficit related to
- The injury
- Cause of injury
- Management and therapy
- Prognosis

Anticipatory grieving related to
- Possible sequelae to the birth injury

Spiritual distress related to
- Occurrence of birth injury

Newborn

Potential for impaired physical mobility related to
- Brachial plexus injury

Potential impaired gas exchange related to
- Diaphragmatic paralysis (partial or complete)

Planning

Meeting the unique needs of the birth-injured newborn requires constant vigilance. Goals are established and prioritized. Nursing actions are selected in light of the particular disorder and individual needs of the infant and family.

The overall ***goals*** for care of newborns with birth trauma are as follows:

1. The newborn's premonitory or early sequelae of trauma are diagnosed and effects are minimized
2. The newborn's injury or its sequelae are treated promptly and appropriately when possible
3. The parents initiate a positive parent-child relationship
4. The parents' (family's) educational needs regarding the injury and its management are met

Implementation

Soft Tissue Injuries

Caput succedaneum is a localized edematous swelling of the scalp that persists for a few days after birth and then disappears. It has no pathologic significance (see Fig. 16-4, *A*).

Cephalhematoma is a collection of blood from ruptured blood vessels between the periosteum and surface of the parietal bone (see Fig. 16-4, *B*, and discussion in Chapter 16). The swelling may appear unilaterally or bilaterally and disappears gradually in 2 to 3 weeks. Occasionally hyperbilirubinemia may result from breakdown of the accumulated blood.

Subconjunctival and retinal hemorrhages result from rupture of capillaries from increased intracranial pressure during birth. They clear within 5 days after birth and usually present no problems. However, parents need reassurance about their presence.

Erythema, ecchymoses, petechiae, abrasions, lacerations, and *edema* of buttocks and extremities may be present. Localized discoloration may appear over presenting or dependent parts. Ecchymoses and edema appear as bruises anywhere on the body. They can appear on the presenting part or from the application of forceps. They can result from manipulation of the infant's body during delivery.

Bruises and ecchymoses over the face may be the result of face presentation (Fig. 28-22). The skin over the entire head may be ecchymotic and covered with petechiae as a result of a tight nuchal cord. Petechiae, or pinpoint hemorrhagic areas, acquired during birth may extend over the upper trunk and face. These lesions are benign if they disappear within 2 days of birth and no new lesions appear. Ecchymoses and petechiae may be signs of a more serious disorder, such as *thrombocytopenic purpura.* If they do not disappear spontaneously in 2 days, the physician is notified. To differentiate hemorrhagic areas from skin rashes and discolorations, the nurse blanches the skin with two fingers. Because extravasated blood remains within the tissues, petechiae and ecchymoses do not blanch.

Trauma secondary to dystocia occurs over the presenting part; forceps injury occurs at the site of application of the instrument. Forceps injury commonly has

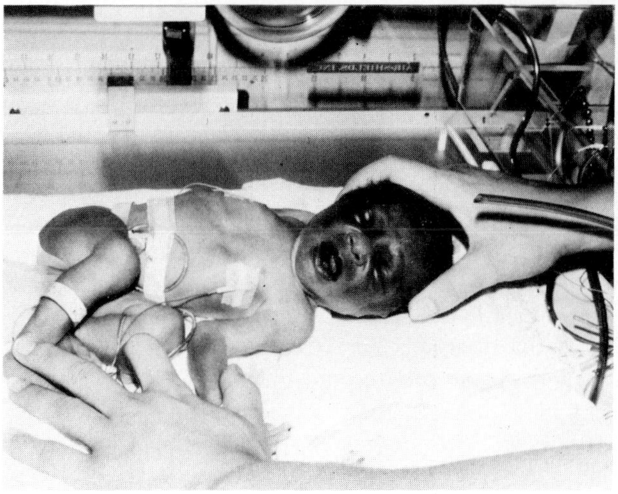

Fig. 28-22 Marked bruising of the entire face of 1490 g female born vaginally after face presentation. Less severe ecchymoses were present on the extremities. Despite use of phototherapy from the first day, icterus resulting from breakdown of the accumulated blood was noted on the third day, and exchange transfusions were required on the fifth and sixth days. (From Fanaroff AA and Martin RJ, editors: Behrman's neonatal-perinatal medicine, ed 4, St Louis, 1987, The CV Mosby Co.)

a linear configuration across both sides of the face outlining the placement of the forceps. The affected areas are kept clean to minimize the risk of secondary infection. These injuries usually resolve spontaneously within several days with no specific therapy. The increased use of padded forceps blades may reduce the incidence of these lesions significantly (Fanaroff and Martin, 1987).

Accidental lacerations may be inflicted with a scalpel during cesarean delivery. These cuts may occur on any part of the body but are most often found on the scalp, buttocks, and thighs. Usually they are superficial, needing only to be kept clean. Butterfly adhesive strips will hold the edges of more serious lacerations together. Rarely, sutures are needed.

Skeletal Injuries

The newborn's immature, flexible *skull* can withstand a great degree of deformation (molding) before fracture results. Considerable force is required to fracture the newborn's skull. Location of the fracture determines whether it is insignificant or fatal. If an artery lying in a groove on the undersurface of the skull is torn as a result of the fracture, increased intracranial pressure will ensue (p. 854). Unless a blood vessel is involved, linear fractures (which account for 70% of all fractures for this age group) heal without special treatment. The soft skull may become indented without laceration of either the skin or the dural membrane. These depressions, or "ping-pong ball" indentations, may occur during difficult deliveries from pressure of the head on the bony pelvis (Fig. 28-23). They can also occur as a result of injudicious application of forceps.

The *clavicle* is the bone most often fractured during delivery. Generally the break is in the middle third of the bone. Dystocia, particularly shoulder impaction, may be the predisposing problem. *Limitation of motion of the arm, crepitus of the bone, and no Moro's reflex on the affected side are diagnostic.* Except for use of gentle rather than vigorous handling, there is no accepted treatment for fractured clavicle. The figure-eight bandage appropriate for the older child should not be used for the newborn. The prognosis is good.

The *humerus and femur* are other bones that may be fractured during a difficult delivery. Fractures in newborns generally heal rapidly. Immobilization is accomplished with slings, splints, swaddling, and other devices.

The parents need support in handling these infants because they are often fearful of hurting them. Parents are encouraged to practice handling, changing, and feeding the affected newborn in the nursery under the guidance of personnel. This will increase their confidence and knowledge and facilitate attachment. A plan for follow-up therapy is developed with the parents so that the times and arrangements for therapy are workable and acceptable to them.

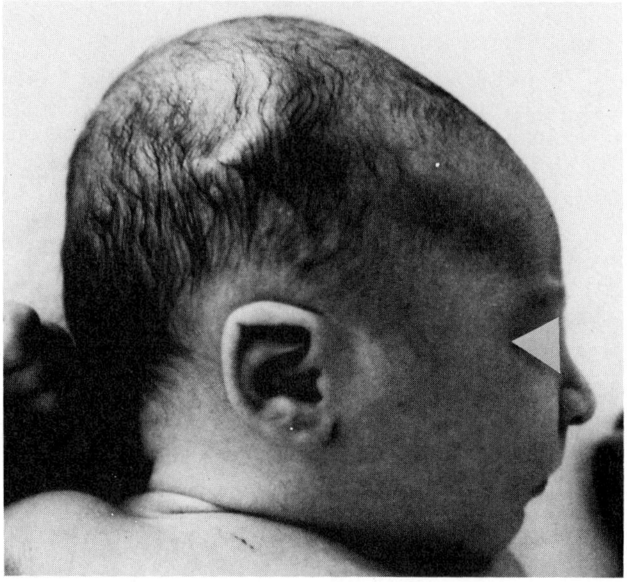

Fig. 28-23 Depressed skull fracture in a full-term male delivered after rapid (1 hour) labor. The infant was delivered by occipitoanterior presentation after rotation from occipitoposterior position. (From Fanaroff AA and Martin RJ, editors: Behrman's neonatal-perinatal medicine, ed 4, St Louis, 1987, The CV Mosby Co.)

Peripheral Nervous System Injuries

Erb-Duchenne paralysis (upper arm brachial paralysis) is the most common type of paralysis associated with a difficult delivery (Fig. 28-24). Typical symptoms are a flaccid arm with the elbow extended and the hand rotated inward, negative Moro's reflex on the affected side, sensory loss over the lateral aspect of the arm, and an intact grasp reflex.

Treatment consists of intermittent immobilization, proper positioning, and exercise to maintain the range of motion of joints. Gentle manipulation and range-of-motion exercises are delayed until about the tenth day to prevent additional injury to the brachial plexus.

Immobilization may be accomplished with a brace or splint or by pinning the infant's sleeve to the mattress. The infant should be positioned for 2 or 3 hours at a time in the following manner: abduct the arm 90 degrees; externally rotate the shoulder; flex the elbow 90 degrees; and supinate the wrist with the palm directed slightly toward the face (Fig. 28-25). The arm should be freed periodically for good skin care. About the tenth day, gentle massage and range-of-motion exercises are begun to prevent contractures.

A 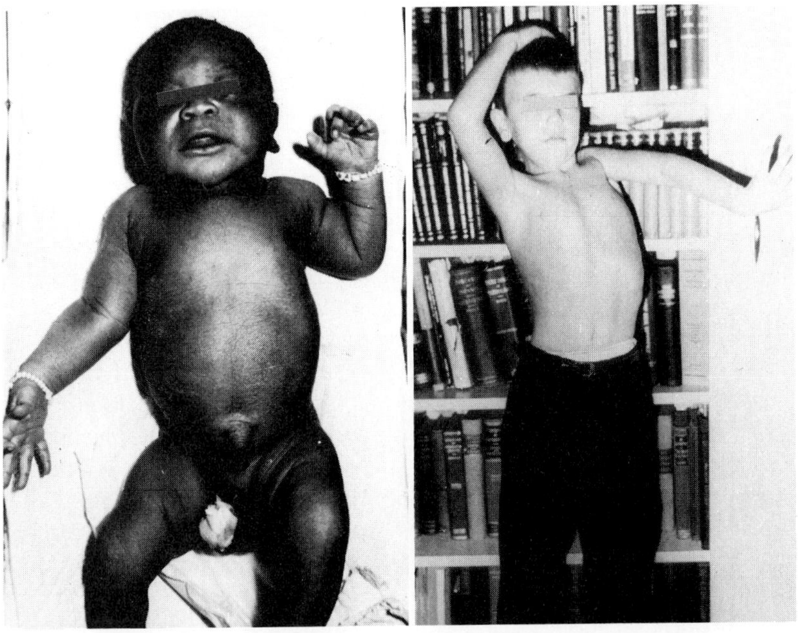 B

Fig. 28-24 **A,** Erb-Duchenne paralysis in newborn infant. Right upper extremity failed to participate in Moro's reflex. Recovery was complete. **B,** Residual of Erb-Duchenne paralysis. Left arm was short; it could not be raised above level shown. (From Shirkey HC, editor: Pediatric therapy, ed 6, St Louis, 1975, The CV Mosby Co.)

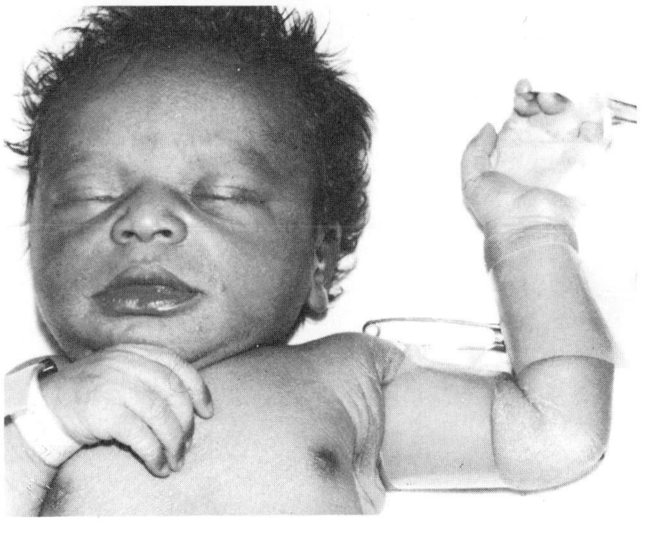

Fig. 28-25 Recommended corrective positioning for treatment of Erb-Duchenne paralysis. Note abduction and external rotation at shoulder, flexion at elbow, supination of forearm, and slight dorsiflexion at wrist. (From Behrmann RE, editor: Neonatology: diseases of the fetus and infant, St Louis, 1973, The CV Mosby Co.)

Damage to the lower plexus, *Klumpke's palsy,* is less common. With lower arm paralysis, the wrist and hand are flaccid, the grasp reflex is absent, deep tendon reflexes are present, and dependent edema and cyanosis may be apparent (in the affected hand). Treatment consists of placing the hand in a neutral position, padding the fist, and gently exercising the wrist and fingers.

Parents are taught to position and immobilize the arm or wrist or both. They can gently massage and manipulate the muscles to prevent contractures while the arm is healing. If edema or hemorrhage is responsible for the paralysis, the prognosis is good and recovery may be expected in a few weeks. If laceration of the nerves has occurred and healing does not result in return of function within a few months (3 to 6 months or 2 years at the most), surgery may be indicated; however, little or no function will develop.

Facial paralysis (Fig. 28-26) is generally caused by misapplication of forceps with pressure by one blade against the facial nerve during delivery. The face on the affected side is flattened and unresponsive to the grimace of crying or stimulation, and the eye will remain open. Moreover, the forehead will not wrinkle. Often the condition is transitory, resolving within hours or days of birth. Permanent paralysis is rare.

Treatment involves careful, patient feeding; prevention of damage to the cornea of the open eye; and supportive care of the parents. Commonly the infant looks

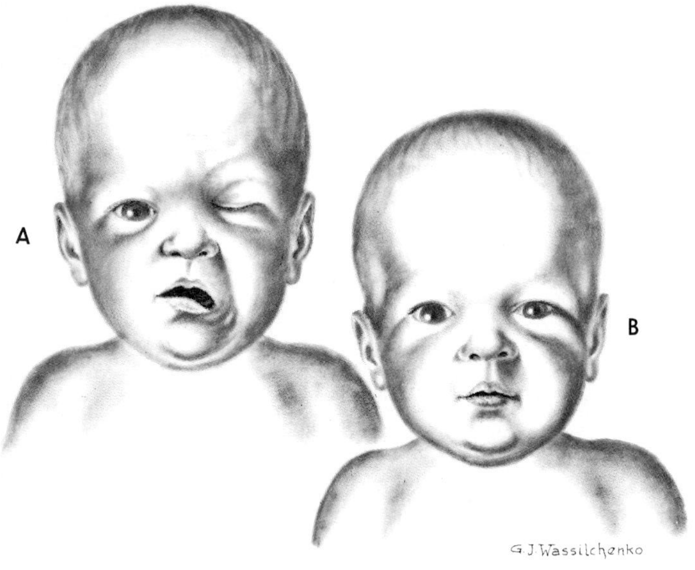

Fig. 28-26 **A,** Paralysis of right side of face 15 minutes after forceps delivery. Absence of movement on affected side is especially noticeable when infant cries. **B,** Same infant 24 hours later. (From Whaley LF and Wong DL: Essentials of pediatric nursing, ed 3, St Louis, 1989, The CV Mosby Co.)

grotesque, especially when crying. Feeding may be prolonged, with the milk flowing out of the newborn's mouth around the nipple on the affected side. The mother will need understanding and sympathetic encouragement while learning how to feed and care for the infant, as well as how to hold and cuddle the baby.

Phrenic nerve injury almost always occurs as a component of brachial plexus injury. Injury to the phrenic nerve results in diaphragmatic paralysis. Cyanosis and irregular thoracic respirations with no abdominal movement on inspiration are characteristic of paralysis of the diaphragm. Babies with diaphragmatic paralysis usually require mechanical ventilatory support, at least for the first few days after birth. Occasionally this support is essential for several weeks until corrective surgery can be performed.

Central Nervous System Injuries

Intracranial hemorrhage as a result of birth trauma is more likely to occur in the full-term, LGA infant. The hemorrhage occurs into the brain substance or as a subdural hematoma. The latter is the principal manifestation of intracranial hemorrhage. The signs and symptoms of intracranial hemorrhage are:

1. ***Separation of the sutures***
2. ***Bulging of the anterior fontanel***

Subdural hematoma is seen with relative infrequency today because of the remarkable improvements in obstetric care in recent years.

Hypoxia and hypovolemia are the most common causes of intracranial hemorrhage. Hemorrhage from hypoxia occurs in the subarachnoid space or in the ventricles of the brain. *These intracranial hemorrhages, seen most commonly in preterm infants, are not related to trauma.* The symptomatology varies. Abnormal respiration with cyanosis; hypotonia; reduced responsiveness (lethargy); irritability; a high-pitched, shrill cry; tense fontanel; twitching (see Table 28-1); or convulsions may be noted.

General treatment consists of elevation of the head several inches higher than the hips, warmth, oxygen to relieve cyanosis, and administration of intravenous fluids or other suitable means of meeting the newborn's food and fluid needs. Minimum handling to promote rest should guide nursing care.

The treatment of subdural hemorrhage is aspiration or surgical removal of the blood collection. Repeated subdural taps for the evacuation of subdural blood is indicated whether or not the separation of sutures widens, the head size is increasing, and the fontanel is bulging.

Spinal cord injuries may occur during manipulation of the newborn's body during breech extraction. Injury occurs when considerable traction force is required to deliver the shoulders or head or both. This injury is rarely seen today.

Evaluation

The nurse can be assured that care has been effective if the goals for care have been met. Risk factors such as large fetal size and unusual presentations are identified before delivery. Mode of delivery is selected to prevent birth trauma. If injury is sustained, prompt identification permits early initiation of appropriate therapy. On a long-term basis, care has been effective if there are no residual adverse sequelae to birth injury as the child grows and develops.

❑ INFANTS OF DIABETIC MOTHERS

Metabolic abnormalities of diabetes in pregnancy adversely affect embryonic and fetal development. Good diabetic control (Chapter 24) during critical embryonic development is possible for the woman whose glucose intolerance is known *and* well controlled before pregnancy. However, gestational diabetes is diagnosed after the crucial period of organogenesis is over. Consequently, the risk of hydramnios and congenital anomalies is greater for the woman with gestational diabetes. Correction of the metabolic abnormalities and individualizing the timing of delivery can minimize the incidence of stillbirths and neonatal deaths (Fanaroff and Martin, 1987). The mechanism of the process leading to problems from conception through birth is as follows.

In early pregnancy, fluctuations in blood glucose and episodes of ketoacidosis are thought to cause congenital anomalies. Later in pregnancy, when the mother's pancreas cannot release sufficient insulin to meet increased demands, maternal hyperglycemia results. The high levels of glucose cross the placenta and stimulate the fetal pancreas to release insulin. The combination of the increased supply of maternal glucose and other nutrients and increased fetal insulin (**fetal hyperinsulinism**) results in excessive fetal growth called **macrosomia.** Hyperinsulinemia accounts for most of the problems seen. In addition, poor diabetic control or superimposed maternal infection adversely affects the fetus. *Normally, maternal blood has a more alkaline pH than does fetal blood* (with its excess of CO_2). This phenomenon encourages exchange of O_2 and CO_2 across the placental membrane. When the maternal blood is more acidotic than the fetal blood, no CO_2 or O_2 exchange occurs at the level of the placenta. The mortality for the unborn baby resulting from an episode of maternal ketoacidosis may be as high as 50% or greater (Fanaroff and Martin, 1987).

Prepregnancy and Prenatal Period. There is some indication that some neonatal conditions—macrosomia, hypoglycemia, hypocalcemia, hyperbilirubinemia, and perhaps fetal lung immaturity—may be eliminated or the incidence decreased by maintaining control over maternal glucose levels within narrow limits (Fuhrmann et al, 1983).

Infants with major congenital anomalies are born to diabetic women two to three times more often than they are to women in the general obstetric population. These anomalies most commonly arise during the first 7 weeks of embryonic life, before most women come under prenatal care and before metabolic control is normalized. Poor diabetic control in early pregnancy as evidenced by elevated maternal hemoglobin A_{1c} (≥ 8.5) is associated with an increased risk of major structural malformations. There is a growing body of evidence that the establishment of euglycemia before *conception* and *through the first trimester* will reduce the incidence of congenital anomalies to approximately that of the general obstetric population.

Maternal lack of food intake and dehydration act in concert to promote the production of ketone bodies and to decrease their rate of eventual excretion. Disturbances in oral intake coupled with nausea and vomiting set the stage for a ketoacidotic episode. Maternal acidosis is often reflected in uterine hyperactivity, together with a loss of FHR variability or the appearance of late decelerations. Hospitalization is required to prevent preterm birth or stillbirth. Metabolic stability is achieved with insulin, calories, fluids, and electrolytes.

Labor and Delivery. Perinatal management focuses on maternal hydration-calorie-insulin balance, adequate fetal perfusion and oxygenation, and prevention of maternal stress. Fetal hypoxia and acidosis can initiate or aggravate RDS. Careful assessment of labor identifies a dystotic labor early so that appropriate interventions may be implemented for a safe vaginal or abdominal birth. Infusions given to the mother that contain dextrose require insulin to minimize the risk of fetal postnatal hypoglycemia and hyperbilirubinemia.

Postpartum Period. No single physiologic or biochemical event can explain the diverse clinical manifestations seen in the **infants of diabetic mothers (IDMs)** or **infants of gestational diabetic mothers (IGDMs).** For the conditions described previously, and those listed and discussed below the same principles of management pertain, whether they occur in the IDM or any other newborn. These conditions include macrosomia and birth trauma, congenital anomalies, hypoglycemia, hypocalcemia, lung immaturity—RDS, hyperbilirubinemia, hyperviscosity of blood, and cardiomyopathy.

Assessment

The mother's health and obstetric record is reviewed (Chapter 24). Observation and physical examination of the newborn reveals the conditions associated with pregnancies complicated by diabetes mellitus. Appropriate laboratory tests are performed.

Macrosomia

At birth the typical infant who is LGA has a round, cherubic ("tomato" or cushingoid) face, chubby body, and plethoric appearance (Fig. 28-27). This infant is ***macrosomic.*** The infant has enlarged viscera (hepatosplenomegaly, splanchnomegaly, cardiomegaly) and increased body fat (Fig. 28-28). The placenta and umbilical cord are larger than average. The brain is the only organ that is not enlarged. IDMs may be LGA but physiologically immature.

Insulin has been implicated as the primary growth hormone for intrauterine development. Maternal diabetes results in elevated maternal levels of amino acids and free fatty acids along with hyperglycemia. As the nutrients cross the placenta, the fetal pancreas responds by producing insulin to match the fuel supply. The resulting accelerated protein synthesis, together with a deposition of excessive glycogen and fat stores, is responsible for the typical macrosomic infant. This is the infant most at risk for the neonatal complications of hypoglycemia, hypocalcemia, hyperviscosity, and

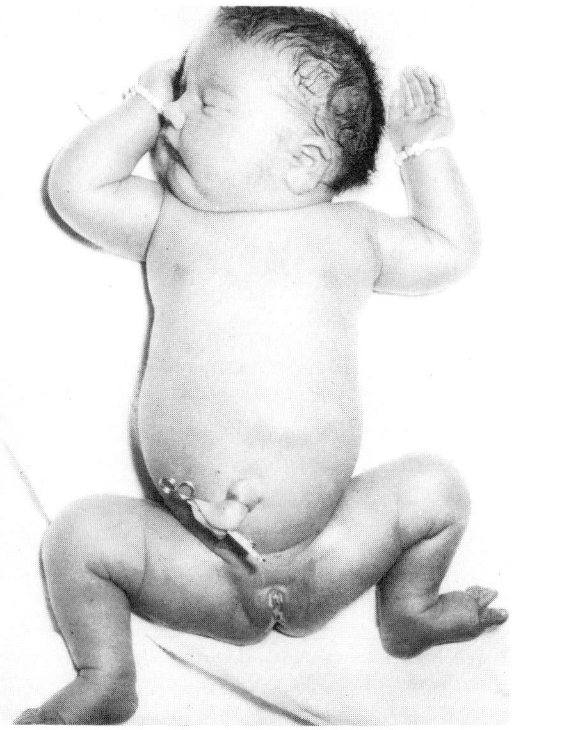

Fig. 28-27 "During their first 24 or more extrauterine hours they lie on their backs, bloated and flushed, their legs flexed and abducted, their tightly closed hands on each side of their head, the abdomen prominent and their respiration sighing. They convey a distinct impression of having had so much food and fluid pressed upon them by an insistent hostess that they desire only peace so that they may recover from their excesses." (From Shirkey HC, editor: Pediatric therapy, ed 6, St Louis, 1980, The CV Mosby Co; Quotation from Whaley LF and Wong DF: Essentials of pediatric nursing, ed 3, St Louis, 1989, The CV Mosby Co.)

hyperbilirubinemia. *The excessive amounts of metabolic fuels presented to the fetus from the mother and the consequent fetal hyperinsulinism are now understood to represent the basic pathologic mechanism in the diabetic pregnancy* (Fanaroff and Martin, 1987).

Macrosomia (LGA infants) occurs in about 20% to 40% of class A, B and C diabetic pregnancies. Clinical efforts can only be focused on the control of maternal plasma glucose concentrations. With good prenatal care and control of diabetes mellitus, the incidence of macrosomia can be decreased.

The excessive size of these infants can and often does lead to dystocia because of fetopelvic disproportion. These infants, who may be born vaginally or by cesarean delivery after a trial of labor, may incur birth trauma.

Birth Trauma and Perinatal Asphyxia

Birth trauma (secondary to macrosomia or to method of delivery) and perinatal asphyxia occur in 20% of IGDMs and 35% of IDMs. Examples of birth trauma include cephalhematoma; paralysis of the facial nerve (seventh cranial nerve) (Fig. 28-26); fracture of the clavicle or humerus (Fig. 28-28); brachial plexus paralysis, usually Erb-Duchenne (upper right arm) paralysis; and phrenic nerve paralysis, invariably associated with diaphragmatic paralysis. (See general nursing care plan, p. 859.)

Congenital Anomalies

Congenital anomalies occur in about 6% of IDMs. Their incidence is two to four times that for normal controls. The incidence is greatest among the SGA newborns. IUGR leading to SGA infants is seen in IDMs with severe vascular disease. The most commonly occurring anomalies include CNS—anencephaly, encephalocele, meningomyelocele, hydrocephalus; caudal regression syndrome (CRS)—sacral agenesis with weakness or deformities of the lower extremities, malformation and fixation of the hip joints, and shortening or deformity of the femurs (Fig. 28-29); tracheoesophageal fistula; and congenital heart malformations or cardiomyopathy. Hypertrichosis on the pinnae has recently been added to the list of characteristic clinical features (Fanaroff and Martin, 1987).

Neonatal small left colon syndrome occurs in some IDMs and IGDMs. Neonatal small left colon syndrome is suspected when failure to pass meconium, abdominal distension, and bile-stained vomitus are noted. Contrast enemas show a markedly diminished caliber of the left colon from the splenic flexure. The syndrome is transient (Fanaroff and Martin, 1987).

Cardiomyopathy

The incidence of congenital heart lesions in these infants is five times higher than in the general population. Other lesions include transposition of the aorta and pulmonary artery, ventricular septal defects, and coarctation of the aorta. Maternal diabetic control is correlated with the incidence of lesions. Poor control is defined as maternal blood glucose greater than 300 mg/dl with glycosuria, ketonuria, or occasional ketoacidosis. Good control is defined as the maintenance of maternal blood glucose between 100 mg and 120 mg/dl. Careful diabetic management, especially in the second and third trimesters, decreases the severity of these lesions.

All IDMs need careful observation for **cardiomyopathy;** 50% of IDMs have cardiomegaly or congestive

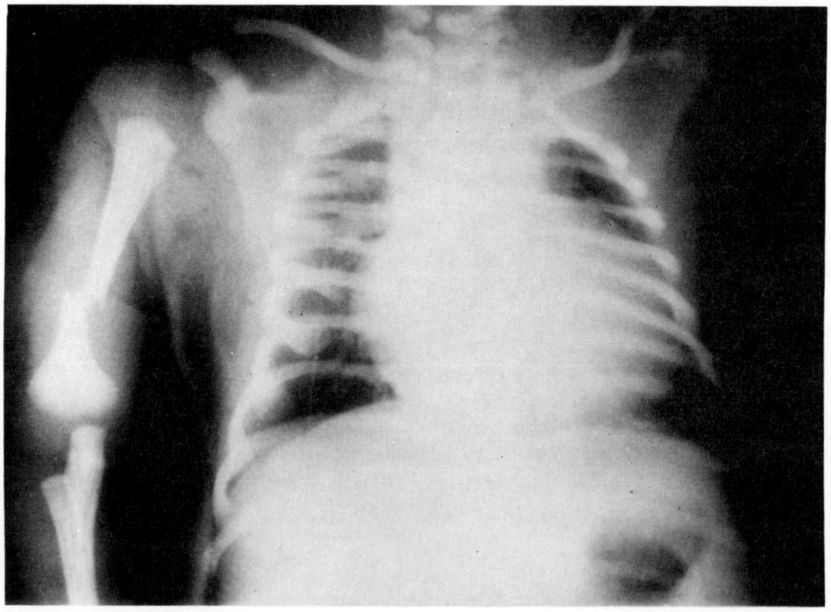

Fig. 28-28 Chest roentgenogram of a vaginally delivered full-term infant (4.7 kg) of a diabetic mother. Note cardiomegaly, hepatomegaly, congested lung fields, and fractures of the right humerus and left clavicle. (From Fanaroff AA and Martin RJ, editors: Behrman's neonatal-perinatal medicine, ed 4, St Louis, 1987, The CV Mosby Co.)

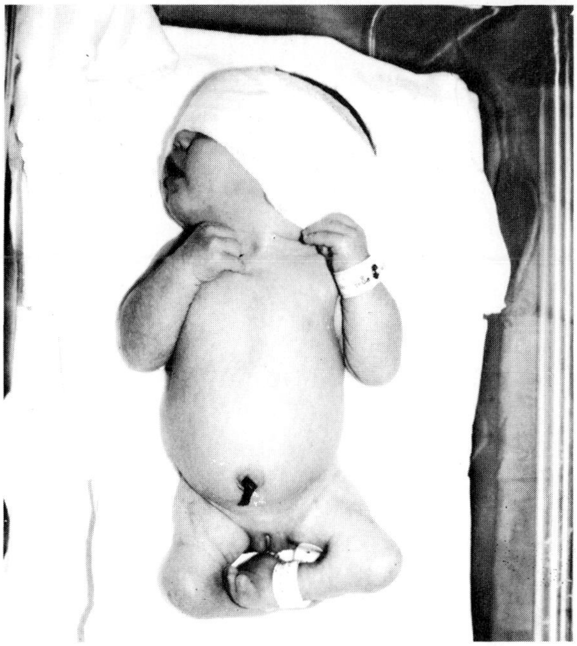

Fig. 28-29 Infant of diabetic mother with caudal regression syndrome (sacral agenesis). (From Fanaroff AA and Martin RJ, editors: Behrman's neonatal-diseases of the fetus and infant, ed 4, St Louis, 1987, The CV Mosby Co.)

heart failure within 7 days of birth. Two types of cardiomyopathy are contrasted here. Clinicians must be alert to correctly identify the type of lesion so that appropriate therapy is instituted. Both types are associated with respiratory symptoms and congestive heart failure (Fanaroff and Martin, 1987). Hypertrophic cardiomyopathy (HCM) is treated with a β-adrenergic blocker (e.g., propranolol to decrease contractility and heart rate). Nonhypertrophic cardiomyopathy (NHCM) is treated with a cardiotonic (e.g., digoxin to increase contractility and decrease heart rate). Hypoglycemia/hypocalcemia and polycythemia are treated (Gutgesell et al, 1980; Fanaroff and Martin, 1987). The abnormality usually resolves in 3 to 12 months.

Hypoglycemia and Hypocalcemia

In hypoglycemia and hypocalcemia (p. 823) separation of the placenta suddenly interrupts the constant infusion of glucose. The high level of circulating glucose at the time the umbilical cord is severed falls rapidly in the presence of fetal hyperinsulinism. *Asymptomatic* or symptomatic hypoglycemia occurs within the first 1 to 3 hours after birth. Hypocalcemia occurs in 30% of IDMs.

Respiratory Difficulty

IDMs or IGDMs manifest a greater incidence of RDS than is found in normal infants of comparable gestational age. Synthesis of surfactant may be delayed because of the high fetal serum level of insulin (Philip, 1987). Fetal lung maturity as evidenced by a ***L/S ratio of 2 to 1 is not reassuring if the mother has diabetes mellitus or gestation-induced diabetes mellitus.*** For the infants of such mothers, an L/S ratio of 3 to 1 or more or the presence of ***phosphatidylglycerol*** in the amniotic fluid is more indicative of adequate lung maturity.

Respiratory distress without RDS also occurs. Transient tachypnea or "wet lung" syndrome is a cause of respiratory distress (Pernoll, Benda, and Babson, 1986; Fanaroff and Martin, 1987).

Hyperbilirubinemia

Hyperbilirubinemia develops in 50% of newborns of 32 to 34 weeks' gestation, and 15% of newborns born at 37 weeks' gestation manifest this condition (p. 879). Many newborns are plethoric because of polycythemia. *Polycythemia* increases blood viscosity, thereby impairing circulation. In addition, this increased number of red blood cells to be hemolyzed increases the potential bilirubin load that the newborn must clear. The excessive red blood cells are produced in extramedullary foci (liver and spleen) in addition to the usual sites in bone marrow. Therefore both liver function and bilirubin clearance may be adversely affected.

Nursing Diagnoses

Following are examples of nursing diagnoses:

Newborn

Potential for injury related to
- Metabolic effects of maternal condition
- Hypoglycemia, hypocalcemia, hyperbilirubinemia, hyperviscosity of blood
- Birth trauma

Potential for ineffective gas exchange related to
- Lung immaturity
- Cardiomyopathy

Ineffective thermoregulation related to
- Physiologic immaturity

Parents/Family

Anxiety, fear, or powerlessness related to
- Uncertainty regarding newborn's prognosis

Self-esteem disturbance
- Experience of an "abnormal" pregnancy and compromised newborn

Knowledge deficit related to
- Newborn's condition, management, and prognosis

Planning

Ideally, planning for the newborn of a diabetic mother begins during the antenatal period. Pediatric staff are present at the birth. For each child an individualized plan of care is developed.

Goals for the infant and family may include:

1. For the newborn: a birth without trauma or injury and a neonatal period without sequelae to trauma or pregnancy complicated by maternal diabetes mellitus.
2. For the family: an understanding of diabetes mellitus or the birth injury and willing compliance with management. If the newborn exhibits a disorder or dies, the grieving process is initiated.

Implementation

Implementation of care depends on the newborn's particular problems. General care of the compromised newborn is addressed earlier in this chapter. A general nursing plan for newborns of diabetic mothers follows.

Evaluation

The nurse can be assured that care has been effective if the goals of care are achieved. Prepregnancy counseling and excellent client collaboration in prenatal care and control of diabetes mellitus result in reduced congenital anomalies and macrosomia; the newborn is AGA, born at term, and suffers no sequelae seen in infants exposed to poorly controlled diabetes mellitus during pregnancy.

❑ NEONATAL INFECTIONS

Sepsis continues to be one of the most significant causes of fetal wastage and neonatal morbidity and mortality. The newborn is uniquely susceptible to infection. Maternal immunoglobulin IgM does not cross the placenta. IgA and IgM require time to reach optimum levels after birth. Phagocytosis is less efficient. Serum complement levels are inadequate. Serum complement (C1 through C6) is involved in immunologic reactions (Chapter 5), some of which kill or lyse bacteria and enhance phagocytosis. Dysmaturity seen with IUGR, LBW, and preterm and postterm birth further compromises the newborn's immune system. Special precautions for preventing infection, as well as prompt

General Nursing Care Plan

COMPLICATIONS OF INFANTS OF DIABETIC MOTHERS

ASSESSMENT	NURSING DIAGNOSIS (ND), PLAN/GOAL (P/G)	RATIONALE/ IMPLEMENTATION	EVALUATION
Review prenatal records, especially noting: maternal glucose control, ultrasound results for growth, nonstress test results, amniocentesis (L/S ratio, phosphatidylglycerol). Assess newborn for: Respiratory distress, and congenital anomalies or disorders. Birth trauma (cephalhematoma, paralysis of the facial nerve, fracture of the clavical).	ND: Ineffective breathing pattern related to lung immaturity as manifested by respiratory distress. ND: Ineffective breathing pattern related to secretions or meconium in airway after birth. P/G: Infant will maintain an open airway and show no signs of respiratory distress.	*An open airway must be maintained:* Have oxygen and resuscitative equipment available. Note and report signs of respiratory distress. Monitor breath sounds every 15 minutes for 6 hours. Position newborn on side, with head slightly lower and neck slightly extended.	Newborn maintains an open airway and respiratory distress is prevented or treated quickly.
Meconium aspiration (amniotic fluid is stained, or if skin, nails, or cord is stained).		Suction newborn's mouth and nose as necessary and report meconium-stained secretions.	Newborn suffers no birth trauma; or, trauma is promptly identified and treated with no adverse sequelae.
Gestational age, weight (LGA, AGA, SGA), and degree of maturity		Report and evaluate any birth trauma or congenital anomaly that might interfere with adequate ventilation. Treat newborn as premature, regardless of weight, until gestational age and respiratory maturity are established.	Newborn's gestational age is correctly determined and appropriate care is initiated.
Assess for hypoglycemia (p. 823).	ND: Potential for injury related to hypoglycemia. ND: Altered nutrition: less than body requirements, related to hypoglycemia. P/G: Newborn will maintain acceptable blood glucose levels and remain free from signs of hypoglycemia.	*Brain damage can result from hypoglycemia:* Observe and report signs of hypoglycemia. If suck and swallow reflex is intact, feed according to hospital protocol. Feedings should be in small frequent amounts beginning at 1 hour of age. Administer intravenous fluids as ordered if unable to feed. Report blood glucose <30 mg/dl; physician may administer 10% glucose in water intravenously.	Newborn suffers no hypoglycemic episodes. Newborn suffers no brain damage from hypoglycemia.
Assess for hypocalcemia (p. 823). After 48 hours classic symptoms of tetany may be noted.	ND: Potential for injury related to hypocalcemia. P/G: Newborn will maintain acceptable blood calcium levels.	*Tetany can result if hypocalcemia is not treated:* Observe and report signs of hypocalcemia.	Newborn suffers no episodes of hypocalcemia. Newborn has no episodes of tetany.

Continued.

General Nursing Care Plan—cont'd

ASSESSMENT	NURSING DIAGNOSIS (ND), PLAN/GOAL (P/G)	RATIONALE/ IMPLEMENTATION	EVALUATION
		Obtain intravenous access for calcium gluconate 10% solution as ordered (no scalp vein sites).	
Assess for polycythemia between 6 and 24 hours of life (if present). If polycythemia is present, closely monitor for hyperbilirubinemia.	ND: Potential for injury related to polycythemia. P/G: Newborn does not suffer complications of polycythemia.	*Polycythemia can impair circulation and hyperbilirubinemia may result:* Obtain blood for complete blood cell count (CBC) and report results. See hyperbilirubinemia care plan, p. 885.	Newborn will not suffer effects of polycythemia.
If newborn is suffering sequelae to a pregnancy complicated by diabetes mellitus: Assess parent-newborn interactions. Assess educational needs for child care. See perinatal loss care plan, p. 914.	ND: Knowledge deficit related to care of an IDM. ND: Anxiety, fear, grieving, powerlessness, situational low self-esteem, spiritual distress, ineffective individual or family coping, altered family processes—related to having and caring for a child with a birth defect. P/G: Parents will verbalize understanding of the explained congenital anomalies or birth trauma and their effects or complications to the child's well-being. P/G: Parents will verbalize feelings and concerns regarding their newborn.	*Parents need assistance in adjusting to and caring for a child with an anomaly or transient birth injury:* Explain all procedures to parents. Explain congenital anomalies or birth trauma and their effects on newborn. Answer questions and correct misconceptions. Encourage open communication. Demonstrate newborn care activities. Schedule appointments for lab studies and follow-up physical examination. Refer to outside resources (child care, homemaker, clergy, home health).	Parents verbalize understanding of instructions. Parents express feelings and concerns about their newborn. If newborn has an anomaly or dies, parents experience appropriate grief response. Parents learn how to care for their newborn.

recognition when it occurs, are necessary for optimum management of the newborn.

Newborn infections may be acquired in utero, during delivery, during resuscitation, and from within the nursery. Prenatal acquisition occurs by organisms placentally transferred directly into the fetal circulatory system and from infected amniotic fluid (e.g., herpes simplex virus [HSV], cytomegalovirus [CMV], rubella). Microorganisms ascend from the vagina and pass through the cervix. The membranes become infected and possibly rupture. Infection of the fetal skin and respiratory or GI tract may result.

During delivery contact with an infected birth canal can result in generalized or local infection. The upper airway and GI tract are again the principal pathways for generalized infections. The conjunctiva and oral cavity are the usual sites of local infection.

Postnatal infection may be acquired during resuscitation, usually from contamination of indwelling catheters or endotracheal tubes. Nursery-acquired (nosocomial) infections may be transferred to the newborn by hands of personnel or spread from contaminated equipment. The umbilicus is a receptive site for cutaneous infection leading to sepsis (Pernoll, Benda, and Babson, 1986; Fanaroff and Martin, 1987).

Certain pathogens may cause abortion, stillbirth, intrauterine infection, congenital malformations and acute disease. These pathogens may also cause chronic infection, with subtle manifestations that may be recognized only after a prolonged period. It is important to recognize the manifestations of infections in the neonatal period not only to treat the acute infection but also to anticipate the potential implication for the subsequent growth and development of the infant.

Septicemia refers to a generalized infection in the blood stream. Septicemia, a common type of sepsis, affects between 1 in 500 to 1 in 1600 newborns. Pneumonia is the most common form of neonatal infection and one of the most important causes of perinatal death (Fanaroff and Martin, 1987). Bacterial meningitis affects one in 2500 live-born infants. Gastroenteritis is sporadic, depending on epidemic outbreaks. Local infections such as conjunctivitis and omphalitis occur commonly but incidence rates are unavailable. Incidence rates of specific infections are given in the text when available. Infection continues to be a significant factor in fetal and neonatal morbidity and mortality.

Assessment

The *prenatal record* is reviewed for risk factors associated with and signs and symptoms suggestive of infection. Maternal vaginal or perineal infection may be transmitted directly to the infant during passage through the birth canal. Psychosocial history and history of sexually transmitted diseases (STDs) may strongly suggest possible acquired immunodeficiency syndrome (AIDS), hepatitis B, or CMV infection. There may be an association between poverty and lack of prenatal care and amniotic fluid infection (Cerase, 1989).

The *perinatal events* are also reviewed. Premature rupture of membranes (**PROM**) may be secondary to maternal or intrauterine infection. Ascending infection may occur after prolonged rupture of membranes, prolonged labor, or intrauterine fetal monitoring. Resuscitation requiring intubation and deep suctioning may result in infection. The newborn's gestational age, maturity, birth weight, and gender all affect the incidence of infection. Sepsis occurs about twice as often in boys as in girls and results in a higher mortality in boys. The newborn is assessed for skin abscesses, rashes, cellulitis, and other indications of infection.

During the *postnatal period* the time of onset of suspicious signs is noted. Onset within the first 48 hours of life is more commonly associated with prenatal or perinatal predisposing factors. Onset after 2 or 3 days more commonly reflects disease acquired at or subsequent to delivery (Fanaroff and Martin, 1987).

The earliest clinical ***signs of neonatal sepsis*** are characterized by a lack of specificity. The nonspecific signs include lethargy, poor feeding, poor weight gain, or irritability. Or, the nurse or parent may also simply note that the newborn is just not doing as well as before. Differential diagnosis may be confounded because of the similarity of signs of sepsis to noninfectious neonatal problems such as anemia or hypoglycemia. Additional clinical and laboratory information and appropriate cultures supplement the findings described.

Primary or secondary involvement of any organ system adds to the clinical signs. Hypothermia is as common as hyperthermia (fever) in response to infection. Tachypnea or apnea, cyanosis, tachycardia or bradycardia, and hypotension may be noted. Focal neurologic signs, tremors, seizures, or a full (bulging) fontanel are seen in septic newborns even without meningitis. Other signs may be vomiting, abdominal distension, diarrhea, jaundice, pallor, or petechiae. Necrotizing enterocolitis may develop (p. 825). Jaundice occurs within the first 24 hours in the absence of hemolytic disease. Hemorrhage may be an associated sign in sepsis, which may be preceded or accompanied by focal infections such as omphalitis or conjunctivitis, or skin abscesses.

Laboratory studies are performed. Specimens for cultures include samples of blood, umbilical stump, naso-oropharynx, ear canals, skin, cerebrospinal fluid (CSF), stool, and urine. Increased direct (conjugated) bilirubin levels may be found, especially if the infecting microorganism is gram negative. Blood studies are performed to determine the presence of anemia, increased white blood cell count (WBC), or decreased red blood cell count (RBC) (an ominous sign). C-reactive protein may or may not be elevated (Chapter 5).

Vigilant assessment (e.g., parenteral fluid infusion) continues during and after treatment (p. 831). The newborn continues to be assessed for sequelae to septicemia.

Before the advent of antibiotics, 90% of newborns with sepsis died. Antibiotic therapy decreased mortality to between 13% and 45% depending on the causative organism.

Sequelae to septicemia include meningitis, pyarthrosis, and septic shock. ***Meningitis,*** a common sequela, may be evidenced by a bulging anterior fontanel (see discussion of signs of increased intracranial pressure, p. 854). Systemic antibiotics may not diffuse into CSF. Intrathecal infusion of a drug such as polymyxin may be initiated.

Pyarthrosis, which may affect any joint, usually localizes in the hips. Limitation in joint movement is one of the few signs of this condition.

Septic shock results from the toxins released into the bloodstream. The most common sign is a drop in blood pressure—a vital sign commonly overlooked in the care of the newborn. Other signs are rapid, irregular respirations and pulse (similar to septicemia in general).

Nursing Diagnoses

Any number of nursing diagnoses are possible depending on the newborn's gestational age and birth weight, the organ systems involved, and the nature of the infection. Following are examples of nursing diagnoses:

Newborn

Potential for infection related to
- Need for resuscitation or inhalation therapy
- Need for indwelling umbilical catheters, TPN, parenteral fluids
- Intrauterine electronic fetal monitoring
- Dysmaturity, IUGR, gestational age

Ineffective thermoregulation related to
- Infection

Impaired tissue integrity related to
- Need for multiple supportive measures (e.g., biometric monitoring, TPN, inhalation therapy)

Pain related to
- Need for multiple supportive measures

Parents/Family

Anxiety, fear, or anticipatory grieving related to
- Uncertainty about newborn's prognosis

Potential altered parenting related to
- Feelings of inadequacy in caring for the infant

Powerlessness or spiritual distress related to
- Perinatal events or newborn's condition

Knowledge deficit related to
- Newborn's condition, its course, and management

Planning

Planning begins with the development of standards for preventive measures in nurseries and protocols for diagnosis and treatment of infections. Individual assessment findings are utilized to plan care for each newborn. Parents and family are encouraged to participate in planning.

Goals include:

1. The newborn remains free of sepsis
2. If therapy is necessary, the newborn suffers no harmful sequelae
3. Parents form attachment to newborn
4. Parents' maintain self-esteem
5. Staff establishes caring relationship with parents to foster their trust and to encourage continuing, active, positive interactions of family with members of health care system

Implementation

Preventive Measures

Virtually all controlled clinical trials have demonstrated that effective ***handwashing*** is responsible for the prevention of nosocomial infection in nursery units (Fanaroff and Martin, 1987). Nursing is directly or indirectly responsible for minimizing or eliminating environmental sources of infectious agents in the nursery. Measures to be taken include careful and thorough cleaning, frequent replacement of used equipment (e.g., changing intravenous tubing per hospital protocol, cleaning resuscitation and ventilation equipment), and disposal of excrement and linens in an appropriate manner. Overcrowding must be avoided in nurseries.

The *skin,* its secretions, and normal flora are natural defense mechanisms that protect against invading pathogens. The American Academy of Pediatrics (1988) supports a ***dry skin cleansing technique.*** The benefits of this approach are reduction of heat loss by exposure, decrease in skin trauma, limitation of exposure to agents with unknown toxicity, and reduction in nursing time. Initial cleansing is delayed until the newborn's temperature has stabilized. Sterile cotton sponges and sterile water or a mild nonmedicated soap are used to remove blood from the infant's face and head and meconium from the perineal area. The rest of the body is not cleansed unless a part is grossly soiled. The vernix caseosa is left in place. No single method of *cord* care has been shown to prevent colonization and subsequent disease. Alcohol, triple dye, or an antimicrobial agent is applied locally (Fanaroff and Martin, 1987; Merenstein and Gardner, 1989).

Curative Measures

Breastfeeding or feeding the newborn fresh breast milk from the mother is encouraged. Protective mechanisms exist in breast milk. Colostrum contains agglutinins that are active against gram-negative bacteria. Human milk contains iron-binding protein that exerts a bacteriostatic effect on *Escherichia coli,* it also contains macrophages and lymphocytes. The vulnerability of newborns to common mucosal pathogens such as respiratory syncytial virus (RSV) may be reduced by passive transfer of maternal immunity in colostrum and breast milk (also see discussion of NEC, p. 825). See Chapter 18 for assisting mothers with breastfeeding, maintenance of lactation until the newborn can breastfeed, and expression and storage of breast milk.

The mother's knowledge of the importance of her breast milk for the compromised newborn and her active involvement in this aspect of care benefits her in several ways as well. Bonding with the newborn is facilitated. Self-concept and self-esteem are enhanced. Coping skills may be strengthened; if the infant succumbs, the mother's healthy grieving may be facilitated. If the mother cannot breastfeed or provide breast milk, the nurse provides support during the mother's formula-feeding or other activity with the infant. The parents' activity with the infant is supported and appropriately guided and praised to achieve the benefits desired.

Emphasis is placed on following reliable surveillance to identify infection in newborns so that prompt isolation and appropriate therapy is instituted.

Eye and umbilical cord prophylaxis is discussed in Chapter 17. Monitoring *intravenous infusion* rate (p. 831) and administering *antibiotics* are the nurse's responsibility. It is important to administer the prescribed dose of antibiotic within 1 hour after it is prepared to avoid loss of drug stability. If the intravenous fluid the newborn is receiving contains electrolytes, vitamins, or other medications, *do not* add antibiotics. The antibiotic (or other medication) may be deactivated or may form a precipitate. Instead, piggyback another bottle of the prescribed fluid to be infused and attach its tubing with a three-way stopcock to the needle at the infusion site. Remember to include the number of milliliters of fluid used from the piggyback bottle when calculating the newborn's intake.

Care must be taken when *suctioning secretions* from the newborn's oropharynx or trachea. These secretions may be infected. Clinicians who use mouth-suction-activated devices are potentially at risk for getting some of these secretions in their own mouths. Though no cases of virus transmission via this route have been documented, enough concern exists to make it seem prudent to use wall or bulb suction devices.

Isolation procedures are implemented according to hospital policy as indicated. See Chapter 23 for universal precautions. The reader is reminded that changes in isolation protocols are occurring rapidly. Continuing education and inservices are suggested for the nurse to remain updated.

Rehabilitative Measures

Rehabilitative measures will vary with the individual need of the newborn. Some newborns will need to be weaned from ventilatory support systems. Those who suffer sequelae such as mental retardation will require a knowledgeable family and supportive community resources. Other children will require corrective care for problems with dentition, vision, and hearing.

Evaluation

The nurse can be reasonably assured that care was effective if the goals for care are achieved. Sepsis is prevented. Or, if infection occurs, early signs are recognized and appropriate therapy is begun. No harmful sequelae develop to either the infection or its management. Parents are able to initiate a healthy attachment to their newborn and their self-esteem is maintained.

TORCH Infections

The occurrence of certain maternal infections during early pregnancy is well known to be associated with various congenital malformations and disorders (Chapter 23). The most common and best understood infections are represented by the acronym **TORCH,** for toxoplasmosis, other, rubella, cytomegalic virus, and herpes simplex (see box below). Herpes simplex may result in a severe systemic illness in newborns that is often fatal. Survivors of herpetic infection may have residual neurologic defects and chorioretinitis. The other congenital infections may also result in an encephalopathy with various anomalies, including microcephaly, chorioretinitis, intracranial calcifications, microphthalmia, and cataracts. To a certain extent the varied clinical manifestations of these infections overlap, but a specific diagnosis can be made by the constellation of clinical findings, as well as specific antibody studies (Fanaroff and Martin, 1987).

Toxoplasmosis. Toxoplasmosis is a multisystem disease caused by the protozoan *Toxoplasma gondii.* Cats who hunt infected birds and mice harbor the parasite and excrete the infective oocysts in their feces. Human infection follows hand-to-mouth contact, such as after disposal of cat litter or after handling or ingesting raw meat from cattle or sheep that grazed in contaminated fields.

About 30% of women who contract toxoplasmosis during gestation transmit the disease to their offspring. The diagnosis of toxoplasmosis in the newborn is supported by elevated cord blood serum IgM.

About 60% to 75% of affected newborns are asymptomatic. The clinical features of toxoplasmosis resemble CMID in mother and infant. Both diseases are responsible for serious perinatal mortality and morbidity: 10% to 15% die; 85% have severe psychomotor problems or mental retardation by 2 to 4 years; and 50% have visual problems by 1 year.

Severe toxoplasmosis is associated with preterm birth, growth retardation, microcephalus or hydrocephalus, microphthalmia, chorioretinitis, CNS calcifi-

TORCH INFECTIONS AFFECTING NEWBORNS

T Toxoplasmosis
O Other: syphilis, varicella, group B β-hemolytic streptococcus, chlamydial infections, hepatitis B, HIV
R Rubella
C CMV infections or cytomegalic inclusion disease (CMID)
H Herpes simplex

cation, thrombocytopenia, jaundice, and fever. Some clinical manifestations do not develop until later in life.

Treatment of toxoplasmosis during pregnancy is problematic. Pyrimethamine is the first-choice drug against *T. gondii.* However, it may be teratogenic, especially during the first trimester (Fanaroff and Martin, 1987). Sulfonamide therapy is effective, but the drug must be discontinued before delivery and even-exchange transfusion of the newborn may be necessary to avoid kernicterus. This may occur because sulfa drugs have a greater albumin-binding affinity than bilirubin, which may rise after delivery to critical levels. The newborn may be treated with pyrimethamine, but folinic acid supplement will be required to reduce the toxicity of the drug. Regrettably, encysted (intramuscular) forms of *T. gondii* cannot be eradicated by any therapy and they may cause recurrence of the disease.

Hepatitis B Virus Infection. Hepatitis B virus (HBV), the most common etiologic agent of viral hepatitis, is implicated in 24% to 40% of cases. HBV infection during pregnancy is *not* associated with an increase in malformations, stillbirths, or IUGR; however, there is about a 32% increase in risk for preterm birth (Fanaroff and Martin, 1987). The transmission rate of HBV to the newborn is high (Hodson and Truog, 1989). Transmission occurs transplacentally, serum to serum, and by contact with contaminated urine, feces, saliva, semen, or vaginal secretions during delivery. Infants are most commonly infected during birth or in the first few days of life. The rate of transmission is highest when the mother contracts the virus immediately before delivery. Transmission may possibly occur through breast milk, but formula-fed infants also become antigen positive at the same or higher rate. Diagnosis is made by viral culture of amniotic fluid, presence of hepatitis B surface antigen, and by the presence of IgM in cord or baby's serum.

Neonatal and fetal effects are serious. Preterm birth exposes the neonate to the problems of prematurity. Infants may be asymptomatic at birth or show evidence of acute hepatitis with changes in liver function. Infants are at high risk of developing chronic hepatitis, cirrhosis of the liver, or liver cancer even years later (NAACOG, 1986).

The newborn is initially treated with H-BIG 0.5 ml intramuscular (IM) injection within the first 12 hours of life, or with immune serum globulin. H-BIG vaccine, given in a course of three doses induces antibodies in 90% of recipients. The second dose is given at 1 month; and the third dose is given at 6 months (Merenstein and Gardner, 1989). The vaccine should protect the child for up to 9 years. After the newborn has been cleansed thoroughly and has received the vaccine, breastfeeding may be allowed.

The Public Health Service defines women at high risk for hepatitis B as women who are Indochinese refugees, of Asian descent, or born in Haiti or South Africa; women with a history of liver disease; women who have occupational exposure to the HBV, such as laboratory technologists, nurses, and physicians; and women who work with mentally retarded individuals. Intravenous drug abusers, prostitutes, and household contacts of hepatitis B carriers are also at high risk (Rubella/hepatitis, 1986).

There is now overwhelming evidence that screening pregnant women for hepatitis B surface antigen (HBsAg) will identify carriers of HBV (Marwick, 1987). Perinatal transmission of the virus can be reduced to 5% to 10% by using a series of immunizations (Blocking, 1987). Screening all pregnant women for HBsAg would result in as many as 140 cases of acute neonatal hepatitis and as many as 1400 cases of chronic liver disease being prevented yearly per 100,000 pregnant women screened in the high risk groups, at a net annual savings of as much as $765 million (Arevalo and Washington, 1988).

Syphilis. Congenital and neonatal syphilis has reemerged in recent years as a significant health problem. Nationwide in 1987, 35,398 cases were reported. This represents an increase of 30% from the year before (Syphilis, 1988). The nationwide rate stands at 14.7 cases per 100,000; this is the highest figure since 1950. One significant cause for the increase may be the increase in prostitution by younger women who accept "crack"—a form of cocaine that can be smoked—as payment for sex, particularly in large urban regions (Morningstar and Chitwood, 1987) (Chapter 25).

Fetal infestation with the spirochete *Treponema pallidum* is blocked by Langhans' layer in the chorion until this layer begins to atrophy between 16 and 18 weeks' gestation. If spirochetemia is untreated, it will result in fetal death by midtrimester abortion or stillbirth in one out of four cases. All newborns in whom the infection occurs before 7 months' gestation are affected. Only 60% are affected if the infection occurs late in pregnancy. If maternal infection is adequately treated before the eighteenth week, newborns seldom demonstrate signs of the disease. Although treatment after the eighteenth week may cure fetal sphirochetemia, pathologic changes may not be prevented completely.

Because the fetus becomes infected after the period of organogenesis (first trimester), maldevelopment of organs does not result. Congenital syphilis may stimulate preterm labor, but there is no evidence that it causes IUGR. Stigmas of congenital syphilis (Fig. 28-30) may include inflammatory and destructive changes in the placenta; in organs such as the liver, spleen, kidneys, and adrenal glands; and in bone covering and marrow. Disorders of the CNS, teeth, and cornea may

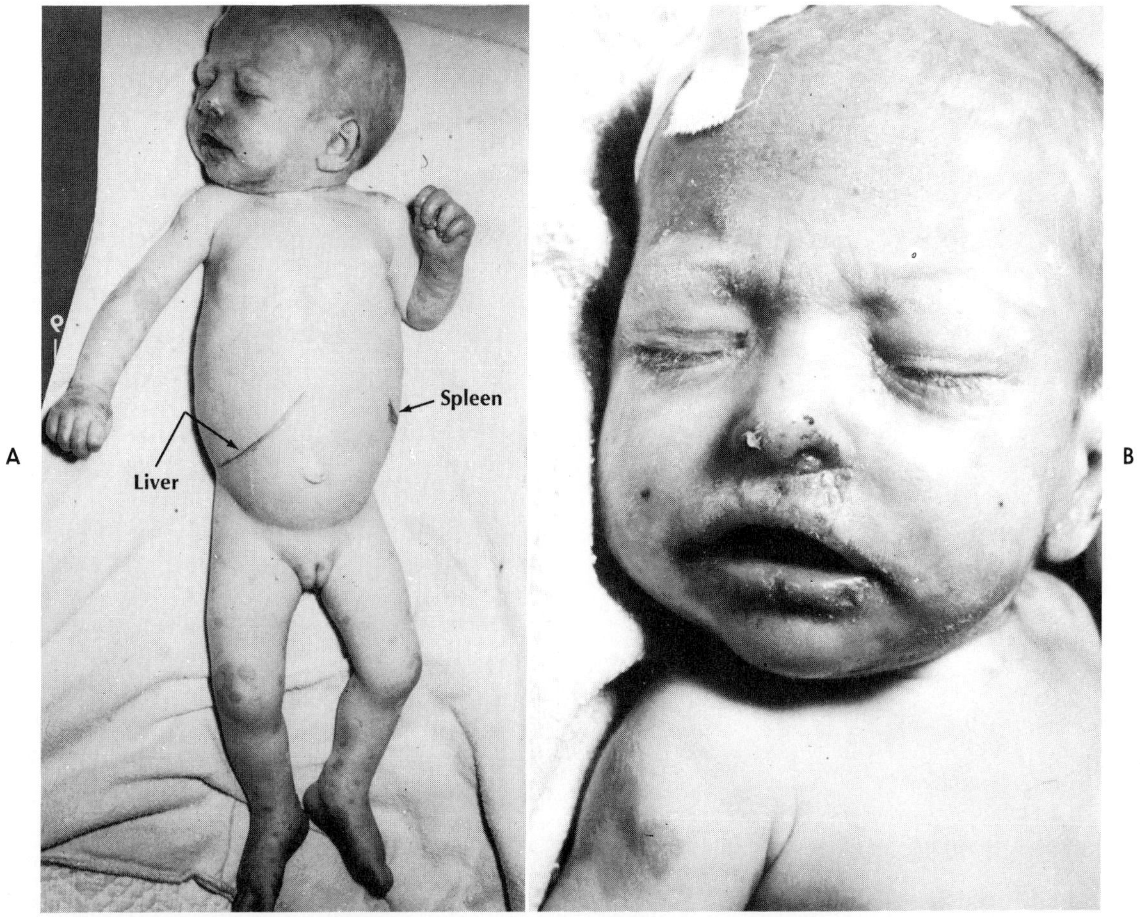

Fig. 28-30 Early congenital syphilis apparent at birth, which corresponds to secondary syphilis in the adult. (Late congenital syphilis corresponding to tertiary syphilis, becomes apparent after 2 years of age.) **A,** Cutaneous lesions of congenital syphilis. Lines drawn on body indicate hepatosplenomegaly. No destruction of bridge of nose (common finding in congenital syphilis) is noted on this infant. **B,** Rhinitis (snuffles) resulting in rhagades and excoriation of upper lip. Red-colored rash is around mouth and on chin. (From Shirkey HC, editor: Pediatric therapy, ed 6, St Louis, 1980, The CV Mosby Co.)

not become evident until several months after birth.

Assessment. The most severely affected newborns may be ***hydropic*** (edematous) and ***anemic,*** with enlarged liver and spleen. Hepatosplenomegaly is probably secondary to extramedullary hematopoietic activity stimulated by the severe anemia.

In some cases signs of congenital syphilis do not appear until late in the neonatal period. In these newborns early signs, such as poor feeding, slight hyperthermia, and snuffles, may be nonspecific. ***Snuffles*** refers to the copious clear serosanguineous mucous discharge from the obstructed nose. A mucopurulent discharge indicates secondary infection, usually by streptococci or staphylococci.

By the end of the first week of life, in untreated cases, a copper-colored maculopapular ***dermal rash*** appears. The rash is characteristically first noticeable on the palms of the hands, soles of the feet, and diaper area, and around the mouth and anus. The maculopapular lesions may become vesicular and confluent and extend over the trunk and extremities. ***Condylomas*** (elevated wartlike lesions) may be seen around the anus. Rough, cracked mucocutaneous lesions of the lips heal to form circumoral radiating scars known as ***rhagades.***

Other involvement results in exfoliation (separation, flaking) of nails and loss of hair. Iritis and choroiditis are characteristic of infection of the eyes. Nephrotic syndrome secondary to renal infection, hepatitis with ***jaundice,*** lymphadenopathy, inflammation of the pancreas, testes, and colon, and a pseudoparalysis of the extremities may be noted. Laboratory tests may show a pleocytosis (usually lymphocytosis) and elevated CSF protein levels.

By 3 months of age, in 90% of infants (treated or

untreated), periostitis and metaphyseal osteochondritis may be demonstrated by roentgenography. These bone lesions generally disappear by 10 months of age regardless of whether the infant receives antibiotic treatment.

After the physician determines that congenital syphilis is possible, the CSF (obtained by lumbar puncture) is examined with the FTA-ABS test (Chapters 5 and 23). If results are inconclusive, the physician will probably opt to treat the child as if the disease existed.

Medical Management. If the mother had been adequately treated before delivery and serologic testing of the newborn does not show syphilis, generally the newborn is not treated with antibiotics. In this case the newborn is checked for antibody titer (received from the mother via the placenta) every 2 weeks for 3 months, at which time the test result should be negative. Some physicians recommend antibiotic therapy for asymptomatic or inconclusive cases.

For antibiotic treatment to be effective, an "adequate" blood level must be maintained for an "adequate" period. Suggested medication protocol in the presence of symptomatic systemic disease differs from author to author and physician to physician. After 12 hours of antibiotic therapy, the child is not considered contagious. It is generally accepted that erythromycin is the substitute antibiotic of choice for newborns sensitive to penicillin.

Prognosis and Sequelae. In general, treatment of syphilis is more effective if it is begun early rather than late in the course of the disease. However, a recurrence rate of 5% can be expected. Even adequate treatment of congenital syphilis after birth does not always prevent late (5 to 15 years after initial infection) complications. Potential complications include neurosyphilis, deafness, Hutchinson's teeth (notched incisors), saber shins, joint involvement, saddle nose (depressed bridge), gummas (soft, gummy tumors) over the skin and other organs, and interstitial keratitis (inflammation of the cornea). The failure of therapy with the persistence of spirochetes in the eyes is not unusual. Antibiotics penetrate ocular tissue poorly. Mortality from congenital syphilis during early childhood is uncommon.

Rubella Infection. Congenital rubella infection is a major concern. The last epidemic in the United States occurred in 1964 and 1965. Of the 30,000 affected pregnancies, 20,000 resulted in infants with **congenital rubella syndrome,** and 10,000 fetal deaths or therapeutic abortions were recorded (Fanaroff and Martin, 1987). Since vaccination was begun in 1969, congenital rubella cases have been drastically reduced. Rubella immunity should be confirmed in all women before pregnancy (Chapter 5). Confirmation is determined either by verification of rubella immunization or by serologic determination of rubella-specific IgM in cord or baby's serum since history of rubella infection is unreliable. Diagnosis is possible with viral cultures of amniotic fluid, placenta or newborn's throat, urine, or spinal fluid.

Congenital rubella is not a static disease. More than two thirds of infected infants show no apparent involvement at birth, but they develop consequences years later. Central and peripheral *hearing defects,* the most common result, appear to be progressive after birth. The major teratogenic effects of rubella involve the *cardiovascular* system (pulmonary artery hypoplasia, patent ductus arteriosus, and coarctation of the aortic isthmus) and *cataract* formation. Multiple other abnormalities commonly occur. These disorders include intrauterine and postnatal growth retardation, thrombocytopenic purpura (Fig. 28-31), dermal erythropoiesis, interstitial pneumonia, bony radiolucencies, retinopathy, and hepatosplenomegaly. Severe infections may result in fetal death. Delayed effects are manifested as thyroid dysfunction, diabetes mellitus, growth hormone deficiency, and progressive rubella panencephalopathy (Fanaroff and Martin, 1987).

The risk of a congenitally infected infant varies with the gestational age of the fetus when maternal infection

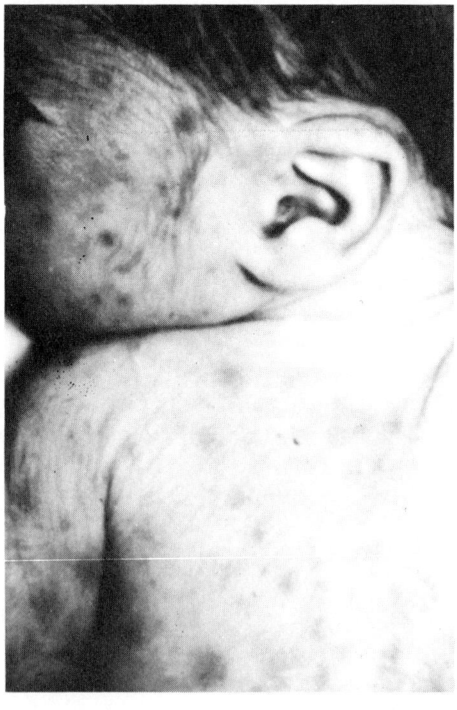

Fig. 28-31 Newborn with congenital rubella syndrome, showing multiple purpuric lesions over face, trunk, and upper arm. (From Fanaroff AA and Martin RJ, editors: Behrman's neonatal-perinatal medicine: diseases of the fetus and infant, ed 4, St Louis, 1987, The CV Mosby Co.)

occurs. Anomalies are most severe if the mother contracts the virus during the first trimester.

The rubella virus has been cultured in babies for 1 to 1½ years after delivery. These infants are a serious source of infection to susceptible individuals, particularly potentially or actually pregnant women. Extended pediatric isolation is mandatory until the noncontagious stage of rubella has been reached. (Isolate newborn until pharyngeal mucus and urine are free of virus.)

For maternal vaccination in the puerperium, see Chapter 21. The use of Rh immune globulin does not interfere with effective rubella immunization.

Cytomegalovirus Infection. Cytomegalic inclusion disease (CMID) is a disorder caused by one or more of at least six strains of cytomegalovirus (CMV). CMV is deoxyribonucleic acid (DNA) virus of the herpes family. Maternal viremia during pregnancy may result in abortion, stillbirth, or congenital or neonatal CMID in a live-born infant. It is the most common cause of congenital viral infections in humans, occurring in 1% of all newborns (Fanaroff and Martin, 1987). It is always a severely crippling disease in the infant.

Maternal infection with CMV may begin as a mononucleosis-like syndrome. However, in the majority of adults, the onset of the disease is uncertain. It may remain subclinical for years. Respiratory transmission is the major vector, but the virus has been recovered from semen, vaginal secretions, urine, or feces, and from bank blood. Maternal CMID may be diagnosed serologically. Many women have antibody evidence of CMID. Women at risk for CMV infection include those who work in, or have children in, day care centers, institutions for the mentally retarded, or certain health fields (nursery, dialysis, laboratories, oncology).

The newborn with classic, full-blown CMID displays IUGR and has microcephaly. The newborn has a petechial rash, jaundice, and hepatosplenomegaly. Anemia, thrombocytopenia, and hyperbilirubinemia are to be expected. Intracranial, periventricular calcification often will be noted on x-ray films. Inclusion bodies ("owl's eye" figures) in cells sedimented from freshly voided urine or in liver biopsy specimens are typical. Elevated cord blood IgM is suggestive evidence of disease. The virus may be isolated from urine or saliva of the newborn. Differential diagnosis includes other causes of jaundice, syphilis (positive VDRL), toxoplasmosis (positive Sabin-Feldman dye test), hemolytic disease of the newborn (positive Coombs' test), or coxsackie virus infection (culture).

Despite the extensive, endemic nature of the disease in women and men and its potential for havoc in perinatal life, critically affected newborns are only occasionally delivered. Milder forms of the disease may often result when the fetus is affected late in pregnancy. CMV can be transmitted through breast milk while the mother is experiencing acute CMV syndrome. Severe mental and physical handicaps mark virtually all infants who survive CMID.

Infants who are asymptomatic at birth are at risk for late sequelae. Hearing loss may not be apparent until after the first year of life. Chorioretinitis, microcephaly, mental retardation, and neuromuscular deficits may occur by 2 years of age. Some children are at risk for a defect in tooth enamel, resulting in severe caries.

No reasonable prevention or specific therapy exists for mother or infant (Fanaroff and Martin, 1987). Repeated pregnancies may be complicated by CMV infection.

Herpes Simplex Virus Infection. Herpes simplex virus (HSV) infections among newborns are being diagnosed more frequently. HSV infection is estimated to occur in as many as 1 in every 4000 to 5000 deliveries (Fanaroff and Martin, 1987).

The herpes viruses belong to a group of DNA viruses that cause latent infection, last for the lifetime of the individual, and result in periodic recurrences. Pregnancy increases both the frequency of infection and the persistence of the virus.

The newborn may acquire the virus by any of four modes of transmission:

1. Transplacental infection
2. Ascending infection by way of the birth canal
3. Direct contamination during passage through an infected birth canal
4. Direct transmission, from infected personnel or family

Transplacental transmission of HSV infection may occur during maternal viremia. However, an ascending transcervical infection first involves the intact fetal membranes causing chorioamnionitis. This infection then is likely to be the *cause of rupture of membranes*, rather than the sequel to rupture of membranes. Ascending transcervical infection of intact membranes may account for the triple rate of spontaneous abortions in the first 20 weeks of gestation with genital HSV infections, the development of neonatal infections despite cesarean birth with intact membranes, and the high rate of preterm birth (Brown et al, 1987). Transcervical infection can be accelerated by fetal monitoring electrodes. The electrodes break the fetal skin barrier and increase the risk of infection. Still the majority of infants show no evidence of infection in utero.

Congenital infection is rare. Congenital infection is marked by in utero destruction of normally formed organs. Affected newborns are growth retarded. They have severe psychomotor retardation with intracranial calcifications, microcephaly, hypertonicity, and seizures. They suffer eye involvement, including microphthalmia, cataracts, chorioretinitis, blindness, and retinal dysplasia. Some infants have patent ductus arteriosus, limb anomalies, and recurrent skin vesicles, with a short life expectancy.

Most newborns are infected directly during passage through the birth canal. The risk of infection during vaginal delivery in the presence of genital herpes has not been clearly delineated. It may be as high as 40% to 60% with active infection at term. Primary maternal infections after 32 weeks' gestation carry a higher risk (50%) for the fetus and newborn than recurrent infections (4%) (Fanaroff and Martin, 1987; Petit, 1987). The transmission rate of chronic vaginal herpes from the pregnant woman to her newborn is low, 8% or less (Bennett, 1987; Prober, 1987). Passive intrauterine immunity to herpes may be responsible. If the mother is asymptomatic at delivery, detectable infection may not be found in the newborn.

Probably 10% of infants are infected postnatally. These infections occur most commonly via either airborne infection or direct contact with virus from labial lesions (cold sores) on the mother, father, or nursery personnel.

Clinically, neonatal infections have been classified as disseminated, with or without CNS involvement, or localized. Localized infections may involve the CNS, the eyes, the skin, or the oral cavity and occur in nearly one third of the infants.

Disseminated infections may involve virtually every organ system but predominantly the liver, adrenal glands, and lungs. The infants exhibit initial symptoms usually in the first week of life, but sometimes in the second week, with signs of bacterial sepsis or shock.

Clinical manifestations include skin vesicles in about 50% of infants (Fig. 28-32). Death results from progression of CNS involvement, respiratory distress and pneumonitis, shock, disseminated intravascular coagulation (DIC), and bleeding. Overall, the mortality without antiviral therapy is 82%.

Localized infections usually become apparent during the second to the fourth week of life. Lethargy, poor feeding, irritability, and focal or generalized seizures may be the initial manifestations. Half of the infants have skin vesicles, but some infants will never have mucocutaneous lesions. About 40% of infants die by 6 months of age from progressive neurologic deterioration. About the same percent survive with severe neurologic sequelae, including blindness.

Ocular involvement may occur alone and may be secondary to either HSV-1 or HSV-2. Ocular disease may not be discovered for months. Microphthalmia, cataracts, optic atrophy, and corneal scarring may result from chorioretinitis, keratitis, and retinal hemorrhage.

Management. Care of all newborns begins with parental prevention of genital infections. Spermicidal foams kill the virus, and condoms offer some protection against direct contact with lesions in the sexual partner. Maternal oral or intravenous acyclovir does shorten the viral shedding time but its effect on fetal safety is unknown. Therefore this agent is not recommended during pregnancy (Fanaroff and Martin, 1987).

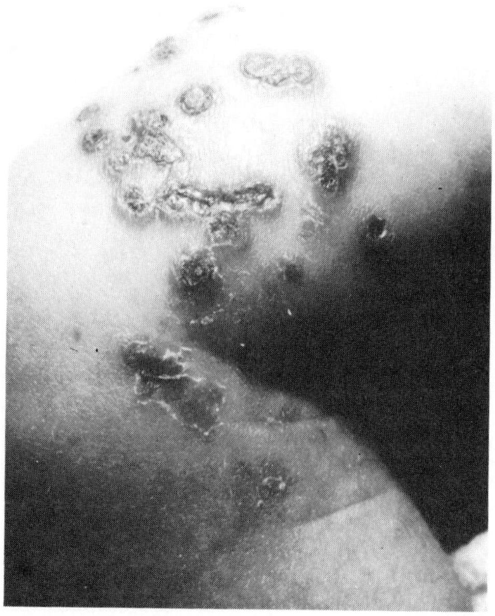

Fig. 28-32 Neonatal herpesvirus infection. (From Fanaroff AA and Martin RJ, editors: Behrman's neonatal-perinatal medicine: diseases of the fetus and infant, ed 4, St Louis, 1987, The CV Mosby Co.)

Antepartum maternal cultures and antibody screening do not predict the infant's risk of exposure to HSV at delivery. The best time and route of delivery are still controversial. There is consensus that infants should be delivered by cesarean surgery when an active herpes infection is present at the onset of labor and the amniotic membranes have been ruptured less than 4 to 6 hours, regardless of whether the infection is primary or recurrent. Because of the possibility of transplacental and ascending transcervical infection, the mother must be informed that even cesarean delivery gives no guarantee that the baby will be free from infection (Fanaroff and Martin, 1987). Fetal scalp monitors are avoided.

During the postpartum period the nurse's main function is to teach the mother about the disease, recognition of lesions, and prevention of its transmission during care of the infant. Initially all newborns should be isolated. Both gown and gloves should be worn by persons in contact with newborns, until the results of the maternal cultures are determined negative. Nursery personnel with cold sores should practice strict handwashing and wear a mask. However there is no evidence to require their actual removal from the nursery (Fanaroff and Martin, 1987).

The newborn's eyes, oral cavity, and skin are inspected carefully for the presence of any lesions. Cultures are obtained from the mouth, the eyes, and any possible lesions. Circumcision is delayed until the infant is discharged. The infant may be discharged with the mother if the infant's cultures are negative. The mother is advised about the need for weekly pediatric appointments throughout the first month. As long as there are no suspicious lesions on the mother's breasts, breastfeeding is allowable (Merenstein and Gardner, 1989). For the infant at risk, prophylactic topical eye ointment (vidarabine) is ordered to be administered for 5 days for prevention of keratoconjunctivitis.

Other than general supportive measures, the only therapy shown to have a significant effect on outcome is vidarabine, although a trial of acyclovir currently is being evaluated. There is no hyperimmune globulin available for use and there is little evidence to support the use of globulin (Fanaroff and Martin, 1987). Any newborn who has lesions, is shedding virus, or has suspicious symptoms with a history of exposure to the virus should be treated immediately. Vidarabine is ordered in mg/kg/day. Therapy usually extends over 10 days. Vidarabine therapy has been credited with reduction in the mortality for disseminated herpes infection.

Chlamydial Infection. *Chlamydia trachomatis* is an ***intracellular bacterium*** that causes ***neonatal conjunctivitis*** and ***pneumonia.*** The conjunctivitis (congestion and edema) with minimum discharge develops 1 to 2 weeks after birth. If chlamydial disease is not treated, chronic follicular conjunctivitis with conjunctival scarring and corneal neovascularization may result. Newborns with pneumonitis exhibit prolonged staccato cough, tachypnea, mild hypoxemia, and eosinophilia (Merenstein and Gardner, 1989).

If prenatal screening reveals infection with *C. trachomatis,* treatment of the mother is deferred until the early postpartum period to avoid exposing the fetus to the therapy. After delivery the mother is treated with tetracycline, 500 mg orally 4 times each day for 7 to 14 days. The newborn is also treated with tetracycline, 6 mg/kg/24 hr for 7 days, and ointment or solution of tetracycline is instilled into the conjunctival sac every 2 to 4 hours for 2 to 4 days. Sulfacetamide (10%) drops or ointment may be used instead.

Prognosis is generally good. Ideally, the condition is diagnosed early, and both mother and newborn are treated in the immediate postpartum period.

Human Immunodeficiency Virus—Acquired Immunodeficiency Syndrome. Maternal infection with the retrovirus, human immunodeficiency virus (HIV), is presented in Chapter 23. The focus of this discussion is the newborn at risk for infection with HIV. The Public Health Service estimates that by 1991 about 3000 children will have the disease, and without new efficacious drug therapy, virtually all will die (Human, 1987). Pediatric acquired immunodeficiency syndrome (AIDS) cases account for 1.4% of reported AIDS cases in the United States, but the numbers are expected to grow (Harris, 1986). The populations at risk for acquiring HIV have been identified (Chapter 23). Some women are unaware that they are in a high-risk group; these women are unaware that their sexual partners engage in high-risk behaviors (Landesman et al, 1987; HIV, 1987).

Transmission of HIV from the mother to the infant occurs transplacentally at various gestational ages, perinatally via maternal blood and secretions, and postnatally through breast milk or through other close contact (Fanaroff and Martin, 1987; Pyun et al, 1987).

Routine screening and counseling of all pregnant women is sparking considerable controversy (Landesman et al, 1987). Comparisons are being made between the frequency of perinatally transmitted AIDS with that of other perinatal diseases for which screening standards already exist. For example, the incidence of perinatally contracted herpes is between 1 in every 4000 to 5000 births to 1 in every 7500 to 10,000 births (Monif and Hardt, 1985), congenital rubella occurs once in every 300,000 births (Public 1987), and neural tube defects occur once in every 1000 births (Main and Mennuti, 1986). In one hospital in New York City, however, an HIV transmission rate of 33%, or 1 in every 150 births, was reported (Landesman et al, 1987).

The Centers for Disease Control (CDC) has issued guidelines for counseling and antibody testing (Public 1987). Several issues are being debated regarding routine screening. Many issues touch the core of the social fabric of the United States. These issues include the populations who have been identified to be at risk, including *victims of child abuse;* the adequacy and availability of social services, education and health care systems; the volatile issue of therapeutic abortion; the option of avoiding future pregnancies (Facing, 1987); and the reliability of current tests for HIV.

Diagnosis. *Diagnosis* of HIV infection in the newborn is the subject of intense research. Pyun et al (1987) studied specific antibody responses by the neonate. Gravidas infected with HIV produce IgG antibodies. The IgG crosses the placenta to the fetus. Therefore cord blood is positive for antibody when tested by enzyme-linked immunosorbent assay (ELISA) or Western blot techniques. Because of their physiologically depressed immune response, newborns generally produce a less vigorous and more limited antibody response to HIV infection (Pahwa et al, 1986; Harnish et al, 1987; Johnson, Nair, and Alexander, 1987). The presence of

HIV in the newborn currently must be verified either by culture or by demonstration of the presence of antigen (Harnish et al, 1987). Pyun et al (1987) were able to demonstrate the early appearance of anti-HIV antibody of the IgM and later of the IgG3 class, suggesting perinatal infection.

Diagnosis is assisted by physical examination for stigmas of the *AIDS dysmorphia syndrome* (Klug, 1986; Marian et al, 1986). The dysmorphia resembles that seen in fetal alcohol syndrome. The history of each woman must be scrutinized for other possible teratogenes (e.g., alcohol abuse.) The neonate may be preterm or SGA. The cranial and facial abnormalities that have been noted include microcephaly, a prominent box-like forehead, an increase in outer and inner canthal distance, mild slant to the eyes, a broad, flattened nasal bridge, a prominent triangular philtrum, and patulous lips.

The occurrence of an *opportunistic infection* in the newborn may alert the caregiver to the presence of HIV infection or assist in the confirmation of the diagnosis of HIV infection. In pediatrics, the presence of lymphoid interstitial pneumonitis is now considered a criterion for diagnosis (Fanaroff and Martin, 1987). The presence of oral candidiasis (thrush) that is refractory to administration of topical antifungal agents carries a high index of suspicion for HIV infection (Prenatal, 1987).

Infected infants are usually symptomatic before 1 year of age with signs that are seen in adults. These signs include lymphadenopathy, hepatosplenomegaly, chronic diarrhea, interstitial pneumonitis, and persistent thrush. In addition, infants have failure to thrive, recurrent severe bacterial infections, and occasionally recurrent enlargement of the parotid glands. *Pneumocystis carinii* has occurred in 70% and Kaposi's sarcoma in 5% of affected children. Viral infection caused by CMV and Epstein-Barr virus is commonly observed in children with AIDS. Bacterial sepsis also may be an initial manifestation (Fanaroff and Martin, 1987).

Infants who exhibit signs of HIV infection at birth tend to expire within a month. The disease progression has been slower and the mortality lower in infants with a later onset.

Management. *Management* begins by implementing universal precautions and precautions for invasive procedures (Chapter 23) to prevent further transmission of HIV (Jackson et al, 1987; Public, 1987). Circumcision in males is avoided. Umbilical cord stumps are cleaned meticulously every day until healing is complete. Therapy includes prophylactic γ-globulin, antimicrobial medications specific for the infections encountered, and corticosteroids in the presence of lymphoid interstitial pneumonitis. Azidothymidine (AZT) and ribavirin cross the brain barrier and may result in increase in weight and in the number of T-helper cells. For general care of the compromised newborn, see p. 817.

Counseling regarding the care of the women themselves, the family's care of the infant, and future pregnancies challenges the caregiver. Self-care involves avoiding at-risk behaviors during sexual encounters, avoiding substance abuse (Chapter 25), and avoiding future pregnancies. Regardless of proven risks and mass media education, "safe sex" practices have not been implemented by many people for a variety of reasons, including denial (Leishman, 1987).

The public health community has become aware that women who know that they carry HIV antibody still become pregnant for many reasons. These include denial of risk, desire to have a family despite the risk, and many more complex sociocultural considerations (Prenatal, 1987).

Some parents are opting to place the infected infants in foster homes despite the low risk for transmission among members of the same household. Social services are required in these cases. If the parent chooses to keep the infant, home health care is arranged. For more information and updated information parents are offered the following resource: The National AIDS Hotline, 1-800-342-AIDS.

The family must be counseled about vaccinations. The child will not receive live vaccines against childhood diseases such as measles,* mumps, and rubella. The child will receive sabin polio vaccination, vaccination against pertussis and diphtheria, and tetanus toxoid.

Oral Thrush. Oral thrush, or mycotic stomatitis, is caused by *Candida albicans*. This infection results from direct contact with a contaminated birth canal, hands (mother's or others'), feeding equipment, breast, or bedding. The appearance of white plaques on the oral mucosa, gums, and tongue is characteristic. The white patches are easily differentiated from milk curds; the patches cannot be removed and tend to bleed when touched. In most cases the infant does not seem to be discomforted by the infection. A few newborns seem to have some difficulty swallowing.

Infants who are sick, debilitated, or receiving antibiotic therapy are more susceptible. Those with conditions such as cleft lip or palate, neoplasms, and hyperparathyroidism seem to be more vulnerable to mycotic infection.

The objectives of management are to eradicate the causative organism, control exposure to *C. albicans*,

*In the wake of six severe measles cases among children infected with the AIDS virus, federal health officials have reversed their earlier stand and recommend measles vaccinations for children with AIDS (Measles, 1988).

and improve the infant's resistance. Interventions include maintenance of scrupulous cleanliness to prevent reinfection (nursing personnel, parents, others.) Good hand-washing technique is always essential. Clean surfaces should be provided for newborns (newborn is never placed directly on sheets on which the mother has been sitting). Proper cleanliness of the equipment and environment is ensured. The compromised newborn's physiologic function must be supported.

Medications are administered as ordered. Aqueous solution of gentian violet (1% to 2%) is applied with swab to oral mucosa, gums, and tongue. (Guard against permanent stain on skin, clothes, equipment. Warn parents about purple staining of baby's mouth.)

Nystatin (Mycostatin) is instilled into the newborn's mouth with a medicine dropper. Give infant sterile water to wash out milk before giving nystatin. Nystatin may also be swabbed over mucosa, gums, or tongue.

To give *oral medication by medicine dropper,* position the infant's head to the side or support the infant in a semi-Fowler's position. Insert the dropper into the oral cavity so that the tip rests against the cheek, alongside the tongue. Wait until the infant begins to suck on the dropper, then squeeze the rubber end slowly until the dropper is empty.

Gonorrhea. The incidence of gonococcal infection in gravidas has ranged from 2.5% to 7.3% in recent studies (Fanaroff and Martin, 1987). With this high incidence, it is not surprising that neonatal infection with *Neisseria gonorrhoeae* occurs frequently. After rupture of membranes, ascending infection can result in orogastric contamination of the fetus. The organism may also invade mucosal surfaces, such as the conjunctiva (ophthalmia neonatorum, Chapter 17), rectal mucosa, and pharynx. Contamination may occur as the infant passes through the birth canal or it may occur postnatally from an infected adult. Neonatal gonococcal arthritis, septicemia, meningitis, vaginitis, and scalp abscesses also occur.

Endocervical cultures for *N. gonorrhoeae* should be obtained routinely during pregnancy and appropriate treatment instituted when necessary to prevent fetal-neonatal infection. The newborn with a mild infection often recovers completely with appropriate treatment (Chapter 23). Occasionally infants die in the early neonatal period from overwhelming infection.

❑ SUBSTANCE ABUSE

Perinatal risk is also created by certain maternal behaviors. Maternal habits hazardous to the fetus and newborn are drug addiction, smoking, and alcohol abuse. Occasional withdrawal reactions have been reported in newborns of mothers who use to excess such drugs as barbiturates, alcohol, or amphetamines. Serious reactions are seen in newborns whose mothers abuse psychoactive drugs (Chapter 25) or are treated with methadone. Almost 50% of pregnancies of women addicted to opioids result in LBW infants who are not necessarily preterm. Alcohol is a teratogen. Maternal ethanol abuse during gestation creates a readily identifiable fetal alcohol syndrome (FAS).

The adverse effects of exposure of the fetus to drugs are variable. They include transient behavioral changes such as fetal breathing movements or irreversible effects such as fetal death, IUGR, structural malformations, or mental retardation. Maternal use of drugs may be for the pharmacologic control of disease process (e.g., insulin) or for symptomatic relief of benign problems (e.g., aspirin). It has been shown that 92% to 100% of all obstetric clients take at least one physician-prescribed drug, and 65% to 80% also take self-prescribed drugs. In addition to the therapeutic use of drugs the nontherapeutic use of drugs, such as alcohol, nicotine, or narcotics, poses threats to fetal well-being. Critical determinants of the effect of the drug on the fetus include the specific drug, the dosage, the route of administration, the genotype of the mother or fetus, and the timing of the drug exposure (Chapter 25). Figs. 28-33 and 7-13 show critical periods in human embryogenesis and the teratogenic effects of drugs.

Assessment

Assessment of the newborn requires a review of the mother's prenatal record. A medical and social history of drug abuse and detoxication is noted. Some obstetric complications are seen in pregnancies complicated by substance abuse. The obstetric events include PROM, amnionitis, preterm labor, precipitous labor, abruptio placentae, placenta previa, and spontaneous abortion. Perinatal and neonatal mortality and morbidity are also seen. There is an increase in stillbirths and in the births of newborns diagnosed with IUGR, LBW, or preterm.

The woman who is addicted to narcotics may have infections that compound the risk to the infant. These infections include hepatitis, septicemia, and STDs, including AIDS (Niebyl, 1988).

The nurse is commonly the first to observe the signs of drug dependence in the newborn. The nurse's observations help the physician differentiate between drug dependence and other conditions: tracheoesophageal fistula, CNS disorder, sepsis, hypoglycemia, and electrolyte imbalance.

The newborn is assessed using the guidelines discussed in Chapter 16. The newborn's gestational age and maturity are noted (p. 836). In utero exposure to some drugs results in observable malformations or dys-

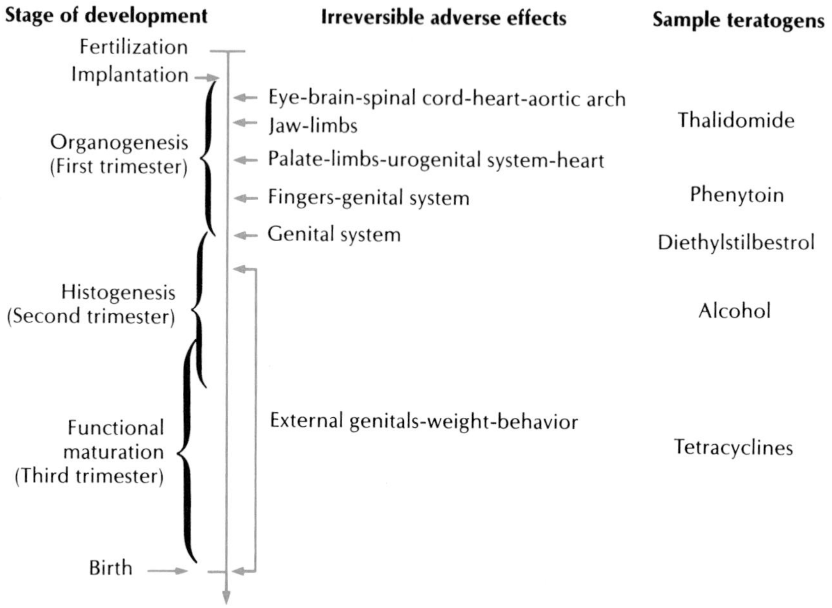

Fig. 28-33 Critical periods in human embryogenesis. (From Fanaroff A and Martin R, editors: Behrman's neonatal-perinatal medicine: diseases of the fetus and infant, ed 4, St Louis, 1987, The CV Mosby Co.)

morphia. Neonatal behavior may be suspect. Lethargy, decreased visual alertness and auditory response to the Brazelton Neonatal Behavioral Assessment Scale (BNBAS), or withdrawal symptoms are noted. Urine screening may be used to identify substances abused by the mother. Since many women are polydrug users, the newborn infant may initially exhibit a confusing complex of signs.

Nursing Diagnoses

Nursing diagnoses will depend on the assessment findings and are tailored to the individual needs of the newborn and the family. Following are examples of nursing diagnoses:

Newborn

Potential for infection related to
- Maternal risk behaviors
- PROM

Altered growth and development related to
- Effects of maternal substance abuse

Sleep pattern disturbance related to
- Drug withdrawal

Parent(s)

Actual or potential altered parenting related to
- Continuation of substance abuse or detoxification program
- Guilt for infant's condition
- Inability to cope with care needs of a special infant

Knowledge deficit related to
- Care needs of an affected infant

Planning

Planning for care of the newborn presents a challenge to the health care team. Parents are included in the planning for the care of the newborn and are also encouraged to plan for their own care. A multidisciplinary approach is needed that includes home health or community resource people.

Goals are stated in client-centered terms and include the following:

1. Newborn suffers no adverse sequelae to drug withdrawal
2. Malformations and dysfunction are identified and appropriate curative and rehabilitative measures are instituted
3. Parent(s) comes to terms with the newborn's condition and its management.

Implementation

Education and social support to prevent the abuse of drugs is the ideal approach. However, given the scope of the drug abuse problem, total prevention is unrealistic.

Nursing care of the drug-dependent newborn involves supportive therapy for fluid and electrolyte balance, nutrition, infection control, and respiratory care. Medications are given as ordered. The newborn's narcotic withdrawal signs may require a schedule of weaning from the drug. Phenobarbital, 6 mg/kg/24 hr IM, may be ordered to be given or 2 mg orally 4 times a day for 3 or 4 days; the dose is reduced by one third every 2 days for about 2 weeks, at which time treatment is discontinued. Paregoric may be ordered to be given 2 to 4 drops/kg orally every 4 to 6 hours initially to as much as 20 to 30 drops/kg orally every 4 to 6 hours, depending on the symptomatology.

Swaddling, holding, reducing stimuli, and feeding as necessary may be helpful in easing withdrawal. See general nursing care plan, pp. 874-875.

Drug dependence in the newborn is physiologic, not psychologic, so there is thought to be no predisposition to dependence later in life. However, the psychosocial environment in which the infant is raised may predispose to addiction.

The mother requires considerable support. Her need for and her abuse of drugs results in a decreased capacity to cope. The newborn's withdrawal signs and decreased consolability stress her coping abilities even further. Home health care, treatment for addiction, and education are important considerations. Sensitive exploration of the woman's options for the care of her infant and herself and for future fertility management may help her see that she has choices. Through this approach, respect is communicated to her as a person who can make responsible decisions.

Evaluation

Final evaluation may not be possible. Goals may be met to some extent on a short-term basis. However, both the infant and the parent have long-term needs. The extent to which goals are met may not be known for years.

Alcohol

Reference to the association between fetal malformation and maternal alcoholism can be found in Greek and Roman mythology. Laws in Carthage and Sparta forbade consumption of alcohol by couples on their wedding night to prevent the conception of children with defects. Documentation of the **fetal alcohol syndrome (FAS)** can be found in the literature since the early part of the eighteenth century. The incidence of FAS in the United States is about 2.2 per 1000 live births and worldwide it is 1.9/1000 births (Abel and Sokol, 1988; Niebyl, 1988).

Table 28-5 Risks Associated with Maternal Alcohol Ingestion

Amount of Alcohol	Risks
Two or more drinks daily	IUGR
Includes:	
2 mixed drinks, 1 oz. liquor each	Immature motor activity Increased rate of anomalies
2 glasses of wine, 5 oz. each	Decreased muscle tone
2 beers, 12 oz. each	Poor sucking pressure Increased rate of stillbirths Decreased placental weight
Five or more drinks on occasion	Increased risk of structural brain abnormalities
Six or more drinks daily	FAS

From McCarthy P: Am J Primary Health Care 8:34, 1983. Copyright the Nurse Practitioner: The American Journal of Primary Health Care.

Predictable patterns of fetal and neonatal dysmorphogenesis are attributed to severe, chronic alcoholism in women who continue to drink heavily during pregnancy (Davis and Keith, 1983). The pattern of growth deficiency begun in prenatal life persists after delivery, especially in the linear growth rate, rate of weight gain, and growth of head circumferences (Zuspan, 1984). Table 28-5 summarizes the risks associated with maternal alcohol ingestion.

Ocular structural anomalies are common findings (Fig. 28-34). Limb anomalies and a variety of cardiocirculatory anomalies, especially ventricular septal defects, pose problems for the child. Mental retardation

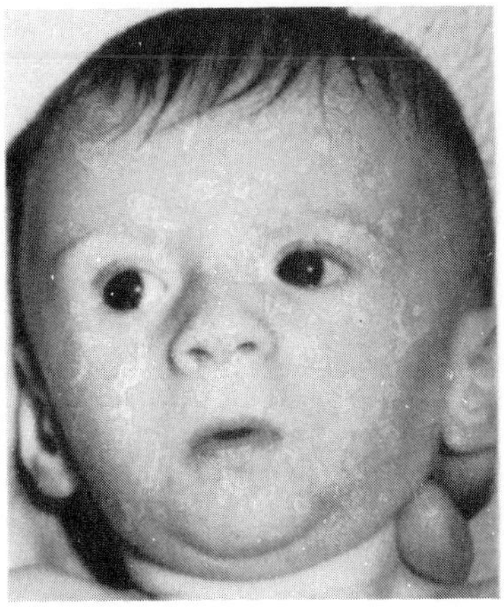

Fig. 28-34 Fetal alcohol syndrome. (Courtesy Dr. Charles Linder, Medical College of Georgia. From Goodman RM and Gorlin RJ: Atlas of the face in genetic disorders, ed 2, St Louis, 1977, The CV Mosby Co.)

General Nursing Care Plan

NEWBORN DRUG WITHDRAWAL

ASSESSMENT	NURSING DIAGNOSIS (ND), PLAN/GOAL (P/G)	RATIONALE/ IMPLEMENTATION	EVALUATION
Note maternal drug history: length of drug habit; drug use during pregnancy; time and type of last drug taken. Assess patency of respiratory system: Note cough, swallow, and gag reflex. Note sneezing and nasal stuffiness. Note amount and color of mucus. Assess for congenital defects (esophageal atresia).	ND: Ineffective airway clearance related to mucous or anatomic obstruction. P/G: Infant will maintain an open airway and possess no anatomic or mucous obstruction.	*An open airway is essential:* Have resuscitative equipment available. Aspirate mouth and nose as indicated. Assess breath sounds frequently. Report tachypnea or signs of respiratory distress. Feed slowly in small amounts. Keep head elevated during feeding.	Infant maintains open airway and breathes easily.
Assess for respiratory distress. Note onset and duration of tachypnea respiratory rate > 60/minutes. Note heart rate frequently during tachypnea episodes. Note presence of respiratory distress (retractions, flaring of nostrils, apnea). Note color—pallor or cyanosis. Note mottling. Note symptoms indicating pathology (heart disease).	ND: Impaired gas exchange related to drug withdrawal effects. P/G: Newborn will be able to maintain adequate ventilation by own respiratory effort.	*Ventilation is essential for life:* Place newborn on cardiopulmonary monitor. Position for respiratory distress (head of bed elevated, prone, or side-lying). Report any increasing distress that alters heart rate or blood pressure. Provide oxygen therapy. Monitor blood gas values or transcutaneous oxygen and carbon dioxide values. Resuscitate and intubate as needed.	Infant able to maintain oxygen intake and respirations by own effort. Symptomatology indicates adequate perfusion of tissues.
Note hyperactive Moro's reflex: Symmetric or asymmetric. Moderately or markedly exaggerated. Has medication affected reflex? Does newborn have high-pitched cry? Does crying stop or increase with soothing?	ND: Sensory/perceptual alterations related to withdrawal as manifested by increased sensitivity to stimuli. ND: Pain related to withdrawal effects. P/G: Infant will relax when stimuli reduced or infant is medicated.	*CNS excitability must be reduced:* Group care to allow for uninterrupted rest. Decrease environmental stimuli. Medicate or sedate as ordered. Swaddle infant with blankets, cuddle, and hold close.	Infant relaxes and sleeps. Crying diminishes.
Note tremors: Note occurrence with stimuli. Note location of tremors. Note degree of tremors. Observe for seizures: onset, origin, body involvement, clonic, tonic, (or both), eye deviations, skin color.	ND: Sensory/perceptual alterations related to withdrawal as manifested by seizures. ND: Potential for injury related to seizures. P/G: Newborn will recover from seizures with minimal or no sequelae.	*Newborn must be protected from injury during seizures:* Record and report frequency and duration of seizures. Medicate or sedate as ordered. Have resuscitative equipment available.	Newborn recovers from seizures with minimal or no sequelae.

General Nursing Care Plan—cont'd

ASSESSMENT	NURSING DIAGNOSIS (ND), PLAN/GOAL (P/G)	RATIONALE/ IMPLEMENTATION	EVALUATION
Note CNS signs: bulging fontanel at rest, increased head circumference, widely spaced sutures, fixation of gaze without blinking.			
Note inability to sleep for long intervals. Assess sleep pattern. Assess effects of medication. Note yawning—onset and frequency.	ND: Sleep pattern disturbance related to withdrawal effect. P/G: Infant will be able to remain asleep for 3 to 4 hours.	*Rest is essential to well-being and growth:* Organize care to provide long rest periods. Reduce environmental stimuli. Swaddle infant with blankets, cuddle, or hold close.	Newborn remains asleep for 3 to 4 hour periods.
Note suck, swallow, and gag reflex. Note "frantic" suck response. Assess sucking with different types of nipples. Assess for sucking blisters on lip or arms. Assess for causes of poor feeding (esophageal atresia, immaturity, hypoglycemia, sepsis). Note occurrence and frequency of regurgitation. Note intake and output (I&O).	ND: Altered nutrition: less than body requirements, related to inability to ingest or retain food. P/G: Newborn will ingest and retain sufficient nutrients to promote growth.	*Nutrition is essential to well-being and growth:* Feed small, frequent amounts. Position nipple in mouth so sucking is effective. Keep head elevated during and after feeding. Avoid handling between feeding. Medicate between feedings if possible. Monitor I&O. Correlate intake with condition, growth, and therapy. Protect arms with shirt to prevent sucking blisters. Offer safety pacifier.	Newborn ingests and retains sufficient nutrients for growth.
Note signs of dehydration weight loss, sunken eyes and fontanel, poor skin turgor. Note characteristics of emesis or diarrhea (estimate fluid loss, color).	ND: Fluid volume deficit related to inability to retain fluids. P/G: Newborn will maintain adequate hydration and not demonstrate signs of dehydration.	*Fluid and electrolyte balance is essential to well-being:* Monitor I&O. Weigh every 8 hours or more often if vomiting and diarrhea continue. Give supplementary fluids if indicated for dehydration. Obtain blood for electrolyte levels as ordered.	Newborn ingests and retains sufficient fluid, or parenteral infusions provide sufficient fluids.
Note reddened areas over bony prominences. Note areas of skin breakdown. Note skin scratches.	ND: Impaired skin integrity related to withdrawal symptoms as manifested by excessive movement causing abrasions of the skin. ND: Potential for injury related to infection. P/G: Newborn will maintain intact skin free from infection.	*Skin integrity is essential to protect against infection:* Change position frequently. Provide skin care to reddened areas. Pad pressure areas with clothing. Keep fingernails trimmed. If skin is excoriated, treat for possible infection.	Newborn's skin will remain intact and free from infection.

(IQ of 79 or below at 7 years of age), and fine motor dysfunction (poor hand-to-mouth coordination, weak grasp) add to the handicapping problems that maternal alcoholism can impose. Genital abnormalities are seen in daughters of alcoholic mothers. Two thirds of newborns with FAS are girls; the cause of this altered sex birth ratio is unknown. Severe and chronic alcoholism (ethanol toxicity), not maternal malnutrition, is responsible for the severity and consistency of postdelivery performance problems (Fanaroff and Martin, 1987). High alcohol levels are lethal to the developing embryo. Lower levels cause brain and other malformations (McCarthy, 1983). Long-term prognosis (no studies are available as yet) is discouraging even in an optimum psychosocial environment, when one considers the combination of growth failure and mental retardation.

Alcohol effects, however, depend not only on the amount of alcohol consumed but on the interaction of quantity, frequency, type of alcohol, and other drug abuse. Other drugs such as cigarettes, caffeine, and marijuana may potentiate the fetal effects of alcohol consumption during gestation (Fanaroff and Martin, 1987).

The newborn of a mother who abuses alcohol is faced with a number of clinical problems. Identification of the problems leads to the medical diagnosis of FAS. The newborn may suffer respiratory distress related to prematurity, neurologic damage, and a "floppy" epiglottis and small trachea. Tracheal-epiglottal anomalies may cause cardiopulmonary arrest. Feeding difficulties are related to prematurity, poor sucking ability, and possible cleft palate. The newborn may exhibit brain dysfunction, microcephaly, and grand mal seizures.

Nursing care involves many of the same strategies used for the care of preterm infants (p. 817). Special efforts are made to involve the parents in their child's care and encourage opportunities for parent-child attachment. The application of the nursing process to the care of a newborn with FAS is presented in the specific nursing care plan on p. 877.

Heroin

Heroin crosses the placenta. Of infants born to heroin-addicted mothers, 50% are LBW, and 50% of these newborns are SGA. Heroin may have a direct growth-inhibiting effect on the fetus. There is an increased rate of stillbirths but not of congenital anomalies.

Detoxification is not advised before 14 weeks' gestation because of a potential risk of spontaneous abortion, and it is also not advised after the thirty-second week because of possible withdrawal-induced fetal distress (Niebyl, 1988).

Heroin withdrawal occurs in 50% to 75% of infants born to addicted mothers, usually within the first 24 to 48 hours of life. The signs depend on the length of maternal addiction, the amount of drug taken, and the time of injection before birth. The infant whose mother is on methadone may not demonstrate signs of withdrawal until a week or so after birth. The symptoms of newborns whose mothers used heroin or methadone are similar in nature. Initially the infant may be depressed. The **withdrawal syndrome** may consist of a combination of any of the following signs. The newborn may be jittery and hyperactive. Commonly the newborn's cry is shrill and persistent. The infant may yawn or sneeze frequently. The tendon reflexes are increased, but the Moro's reflex is decreased (Bartlett and Davis, 1980; Merker, Higgins, and Kinnard, 1985). The neonate may exhibit poor feeding and sucking, tachypnea, vomiting, diarrhea, hypothermia or hyperthermia, and sweating. In addition, an abnormal sleep cycle with absence of quiet sleep and disturbance of active sleep has been described in these infants (Fanaroff and Martin, 1987).

If withdrawal is not treated, the infant may develop fever, vomiting, diarrhea, dehydration, apnea, and convulsions. Death may follow. Therapy is individualized. Dehydration and electrolyte imbalance are prevented or treated. Usually one of the following drugs is ordered: phenobarbital; paregoric (compound tincture of opium); or diazepam, singly or in combination.

The long-term effect on these newborns is now being studied. Researchers have found that "many serious" mental and physical problems are evident in the child's first few months of life, as well as "numerous indications . . . [of] serious abnormalities in the brain structure that will not be revealed until later years" (Howard, 1986).

Methadone

Methadone, a synthetic opiate, has been the therapy of choice for heroin addiction since 1965. By blocking the euphoric effects, it reduces the craving for heroin. It does cross the placenta. An increasing number of infants have been born to methadone-maintained mothers, who seem to have better prenatal care and a somewhat better life-style than those taking heroin (Fanaroff and Martin, 1987). Multiple drug abuse, however, is a problem for many. The drugs include alcohol, barbiturates, tranquilizers, and other psychoactive drugs. Many are heavy smokers as well. Methadone withdrawal occurs in about 70% to 90% of newborns born to these women. Methadone withdrawal resembles heroin withdrawal syndrome, but tends to be more severe and prolonged. The incidence of seizures is higher, however. Seizures usually occur

Specific Nursing Care Plan

FETAL ALCOHOL SYNDROME (FAS)

Baby Albert was born 3 hours ago. His birth weight was 2464 g (5½ lb). His mother, age 24, drank heavily during pregnancy. Albert exhibits clinical problems of FAS (microcephaly, hypotonia, irritability, poor suck, and increased respiratory effort). Both his mother and father are anxious to care for their baby.

ASSESSMENT	NURSING DIAGNOSIS (ND), PLAN/GOAL (P/G)	RATIONALE/ IMPLEMENTATION	EVALUATION
Increased respiratory effort. Note respiratory distress. Note apnea of prematurity with associated bradycardia. Monitor for seizure activity. Monitor cardiopulmonary response to distress: mottling, cool extremities, bradycardia, hypotension. Assess breath sounds frequently.	ND: Ineffective breathing pattern related to FAS. P/G: Albert will maintain a patent airway. P/G: Albert will be able to maintain adequate ventilation by his own respiratory effort.	*A patent airway and adequate ventilation are essential to life:* Place on cardiopulmonary monitor (set close alarm limits). Place Albert in position where he exhibits least distress (prone or side). Suction mouth and nose as necessary. Have resuscitative equipment available. Implement seizure precautions.	Albert maintains a patent airway. Albert maintains adequate ventilation through his own respiratory effort.
Irritability. Poor suck. Assess suck, gag, and swallow reflex. Observe for potential aspiration (gagging, choking, cyanosis). Assess I&O.	ND: Altered nutrition: less than body requirements, related to irritability and poor suck. P/G: Albert will ingest and retain nutrients sufficient for growth.	*Nutrition is essential to well-being and growth:* Elevate Albert's head during and after feeding. Feed in small frequent amounts. Evaluate different nipples for feeding. Burp well after feeds. Oral gavage feed as necessary. Obtain daily weight, maintain strict I&O. Keep suction ready to use; aspirate nares as circumstances require.	Albert takes and retains enough nutrients for growth.
Microcephaly, hypotonia, irritability, poor suck. Observe for other signs of brain dysfunction (tremulousness, hyperacusis).	ND: Altered family processes related to need to care for and love a child with a handicap. ND: Knowledge deficit related to infant's birth anomalies and their potential sequelae. P/G: Albert will be successfully cared for by his parents. P/G: Parents will learn about infant's special needs.	*Parent-child attachment is essential for well-being of parent and child:* Encourage frequent parental visits to the special care nursery and promote physical contact with Albert. Teach parents about Albert's anomalies and their possible sequelae. Help parents verbalize their concerns. Be realistic when discussing Albert's potential for future development. Involve the parents in Albert's care (diapering, holding, bathing). Refer to outside resources (e.g., infant developmental/ stimulation programs).	Parents learn about Albert's anomalies and their possible effects on the child's future. Parents recognize and eventually accept Albert's handicaps. Parents verbalize their concerns. Parents learn child-care activities. Parents utilize community resources prn.

between days 7 and 10. The infants exhibit a disturbed sleep pattern similar to that seen in heroin withdrawal. The newborns have higher birth weight and most are AGA. No increased incidence of congenital anomalies is seen.

Late-onset withdrawal occurs at 2 to 4 weeks and may continue for weeks or months. A higher incidence of SIDS has also been reported in these infants.

Therapy for methadone withdrawal is similar to that for heroin withdrawal. The few follow-up studies of these infants that are available reveal a higher incidence of hyperactivity, learning and behavior disorders, and poor social adjustment (Fanaroff and Martin, 1987). See the nursing care plan for newborn drug withdrawal, p. 874.

Marijuana

Marijuana is thought to be the most abused drug in the United States with an estimated 20 million users. It crosses the placenta. Its use during pregnancy may result in a shortened gestation and a higher incidence of precipitate labor (<3 hours) (Niebyl, 1988). Some investigators have found a higher incidence of meconium staining (Greenland et al, 1984; Fanaroff and Martin, 1987; Niebyl, 1988). No increased incidence of congenital complications or effects on the infant's growth and physical parameters specific to marijuana use alone have been identified. However, when used with alcohol, decreased birth weight and a five-fold increase in risk for FAS is expected. Long-term follow-up studies on exposed infants are needed.

Cocaine

Cocaine is another commonly used drug in all social classes. It is the most powerfully addictive drug available (Chapter 25). Commonly it is used along with other drugs such as marijuana and alcohol. Its use is credited with a higher incidence of spontaneous abortion and abruptio placentae secondary to frequent episodes of vasospastic hypertension. It crosses the placenta and is found in breast milk. No congenital anomalies or effects on the infant's growth and physical parameters have been identified specific to cocaine.

Cocaine-dependent newborns often experience a significant and agonizing withdrawal syndrome that can last 2 to 3 weeks (Landry and Smith, 1987). The withdrawal signs have some of the same characteristics as heroin withdrawal. Irritability, marked jitteriness, rapid changes in mood, and hypersensitivity to noise and external stimuli characterize the infants. They exhibit poor feeding, irregular sleep patterns, tachypnea, tachycardia, and often diarrhea. Chasnoff et al (1985) identified significant depression in interactive behavior and a poor organization response to environmental stimuli.

The infants exposed to cocaine are typically lethargic, almost catatonic. They have visual attention problems in that they are unable to focus on their parent's face. These children often have been subjected to numerous small strokes because of abrupt changes in their mothers' blood pressure during pregnancy (Howard, 1986). Renal problems, lack of coordination, developmental retardation, and perhaps visual problems may be related. There may be an increased risk for SIDS. See the nursing care plan for newborn drug withdrawal, p. 874.

Phencyclidine (Angel Dust)

Phencyclidine (PCP) is one of the most dangerous of the available abused drugs. It may have extremely unpredictable, bizarre, and violent effects, especially when combined with crack (cocaine free base) (a combination known as "space base") (Chapter 25). PCP increases the risk of injury to the user and therefore also to her passively dependent fetus. The user may be unaware that she is using PCP since it is commonly misrepresented as another drug of abuse or mixed with other drugs.

PCP crosses the placenta and is found in breast milk. Literature about newborns is limited. The infants exposed to PCP appear to be alert, active babies. "Their mothers often think they are smarter. They hold their heads up faster. . . . But, in fact, it is abnormal behavior. Although we aren't sure why, the tone of the muscles in the head is of the kind that we see in [children with] cerebral palsy," a disorder of the CNS characterized by spastic paralysis or other forms of defective motor ability (Bean, 1986).

Miscellaneous Substances

Methamphetamine ("ice") is one of the most potent stimulants available (for discussion of maternal use, see p. 743). It is used commonly by adolescents and young adults. The fetal and neonatal effects of maternal use of methamphetamines in pregnancy are not well known. The effects appear to be dose related. LBW, preterm birth, and perinatal mortality may be consequences of higher doses used throughout pregnancy. Newborns may be drowsy, jittery, and experience respiratory distress soon after birth. Lethargy may continue for several months, along with frequent infections, and poor weight gain. Emotional disturbances and delays in gross and fine motor coordination may be seen during early childhood.

Phenobarbital is another commonly abused drug in all social classes. It crosses the placenta readily and is subsequently found in high levels in the fetal liver and brain. Because of its slow metabolic rate, when withdrawal does occur, onset is generally at 2 to 14 days after birth and duration is about 2 to 4 months. Irritability, crying, hiccoughs, and sleepiness mark the initial response. During the second stage the infant is extremely hungry, regurgitates and gags frequently, and demonstrates episodic irritability, sweating, and a disturbed sleep pattern.

Treatment consists of swaddling, frequent feedings, and protection from noxious external stimuli. If there is no improvement with these methods, the newborn should be given phenobarbital and then slowly withdrawn from this drug after control of symptoms (Fanaroff and Martin, 1987).

Caffeine has not been implicated as a teratogen in humans. After controlling for smoking and other habits (including alcohol consumption), demographic characteristics, and medical history, Linn et al (1982) found no relationship between coffee consumption and any adverse outcomes of pregnancy (Niebyl, 1988). The FDA (1980) suggests that "prudence dictates that pregnant women and those who may become pregnant avoid caffeine-containing products or use them sparingly."

Tobacco

Cigarette smoking in pregnancy has been found to be associated with birth weight deficits of up to 250 g for a full-term neonate (Stein and Sussler, 1984; Fanaroff and Martin, 1987). Maternal cigarette smoking is implicated in 21% to 39% of LBW infants. The rate of preterm birth is increased. Nicotine and continine, the two pharmacologically active substances in tobacco, are found in higher concentrations in infants whose mothers smoke (Luck et al, 1982). These substances can be secreted in breast milk for up to 2 hours after the mother has smoked. Cigarette smoke contains over 2000 compounds including carbon monoxide, dioxin, cyanide, and cadmium. Long-term studies show residual effects beyond the neonatal period (Niebyl, 1988). Deficits in growth, intellectual and emotional development, and behavior have been documented (DHHS 1983; Naeye and Peters, 1984).

The **fetal tobacco syndrome** is a diagnostic term applicable to infants who fit the following criteria (Nieberg et al, 1985):

1. The mother smoked five or more cigarettes a day throughout pregnancy.
2. The mother had no evidence of hypertension during pregnancy, specifically: (a) no preeclampsia and (b) documentation of normal blood pressure at least once after the first trimester.
3. The newborn has symmetric growth retardation at term (up to or greater than 37 weeks), defined as (a) a birth weight less than 2500 g and (b) a ponderal index ([weight in g]/[length in m]) greater than 2.32.
4. There is no other obvious cause of IUGR (e.g., congenital infection or anomaly).

Pregnant women need to be aware of the deleterious effects of smoking on their unborn baby's health. Mothers (and all others) need to refrain from smoking while near their newborn infant. Several studies have reported a positive association between maternal smoking and SIDS (Niebyl, 1988). It is not clear whether this association reflects in utero exposure or passive exposure postnatally, or both.

❑ HYPERBILIRUBINEMIA

The yellow discoloration of the skin and other organs caused by accumulation of bilirubin is termed *jaundice* or *icterus*. Jaundice in the newborn, a common sign of potential trouble, is primarily caused by unconjugated bilirubin, a breakdown product of hemoglobin (Hgb), after its release from hemolysed red blood cells (RBCs). The challenge of neonatal jaundice is to distinguish physiologic jaundice from a serious clinical pathologic condition.

Hyperbilirubinemia has a variety of etiologic factors. The main focus of this section is isoimmune hemolytic disease of the newborn secondary to Rh or ABO incompatibility (see Immunology, Chapter 5). A serious sequela of Rh incompatibility is erythroblastosis fetalis. Antibodies from the mother cross the placenta into fetal blood. Maternal antibodies attach to fetal RBCs and initiate a process that ends in hemolysis. Hemolysis of fetal RBCs leads to anemia and hyperbilirubinemia. Anemia decreases O_2 and CO_2 transport. It also favors movement of fluid out of the vascular bed to the extravascular compartment causing hypovolemia and edema. Elevated levels of serum unconjugated bilirubin result in the deposit of this pigment in body cells. Unconjugated bilirubin is cytotoxic to certain body cells; in the skin it is recognized as jaundice.

Rh Incompatibility

During antibody studies in the 1940s, it was observed that the injection of RBCs of rhesus monkeys into rabbits caused the production of an antiserum that agglutinated the RBCs of these monkeys and of most humans as well. Consequently RBCs that could be agglutinated by this specific antiserum possessed the rhesus (Rh) antigen and were called ***Rh positive.*** Those RBCs that did not possess the Rh factor (antigen) could not be agglutinated and were called ***Rh negative.***

Subsequently it was discovered that the Rh factor is not a single antigen but a complex blood system with a number of variants.

Soon after the Rh factor was reported, it was found that erythroblastosis fetalis, hydrops fetalis, and icterus gravis—variations of **hemolytic disease of the newborn**—were caused by the hemolysis of fetal Rh-positive RBCs by specific antibodies from an Rh-negative mother.

Between 10% and 15% of marriages of white persons will involve Rh-incompatible partners. About 5% of black couples will be Rh incompatible. It is rare that an Oriental couple will be similarly affected.

Not all Rh-positive men are homozygous for the Rh factor, nor will all children of Rh-positive men married to Rh-negative women be Rh positive. About 50% of the progeny of Rh-positive men who are heterozygous will be Rh positive; the remainder will be Rh negative. Rh negative offspring are in no danger because they are compatible with their mothers.

Effects of sensitization are seen in subsequent pregnancies. The placenta of the seriously affected fetus is larger than normal. Increased villous size, persistence of Langerhans' cells, and foci of erythropoiesis are apparent. Commonly the amniotic fluid is yellowish, that is, pigment stained from the decomposition of bilirubin.

Severe Rh incompatibility results in marked fetal hemolytic anemia. The placenta clears the released blood pigments fairly well, however, so that only in extreme cases (such as icterus gravis) is the fetus icteric (yellow, or jaundiced). The ***marked anemia*** leads to cardiac decompensation, cardiomegaly, hepatomegaly, and splenomegaly. Edema, ascites, and hydrothorax develop. Severe anemia may lead to hypoxia. Intrauterine or early neonatal death may occur.

Once delivery has occurred, the erythroblastotic newborn becomes icteric (in severe cases, within 30 minutes after birth) because it cannot excrete the considerable residue of RBC hemolysis. Yellowish pigmentation of cerebral basal nuclei, hippocampal cortex, and subthalamic nuclei often develops (kernicterus).

ABO Incompatibility

ABO incompatibility is more common than Rh incompatibility, but the effects are generally less severe in the affected infant. ABO incompatibility occurs when type A, B, or AB fetal RBCs cause a type O mother to develop specific antibodies. These anti-A and anti-B antibodies are transferred across the placenta to the mother's fetus. In this situation even the firstborn infant may be affected. The newborn may show a weakly positive direct Coombs' test (p. 881, and Chapter 5). Cord bilirubin is usually less than 4 mg/100 ml and any hyperbilirubinemia can usually be treated with phototherapy as outlined in Chapter 17 and Fig. 17-14. Exchange transfusions are required in occasional cases only. Ongoing hemolysis may cause anemia, jaundice, and kernicterus and justifies serial hematocrit studies until stable.

Kernicterus

Kernicterus refers to bilirubin encephalopathy that results from the deposit of bilirubin, especially within the brain stem and basal ganglia. The yellow staining (jaundice of the brain tissue) and necrosis of neurons result from unconjugated bilirubin. Unconjugated bilirubin is readily capable of crossing the ***blood-brain barrier*** because of its high lipid solubility. Kernicterus may occur in certain newborns with no apparent clinical jaundice. Only one sequela in survivors is specific: ***choreoathetoid cerebral palsy.*** Other sequelae, such as mental retardation and serious sensory disabilities, may reflect hypoxic, vascular, or infectious injury that is often associated with kernicterus. About 70% of newborns who develop kernicterus die in the neonatal period.

The perinatal events that enhance the development of hyperbilirubinemia also increase the likelihood that kernicterus will develop, perhaps even in the presence of mild to moderate unconjugated hyperbilirubinemia. The perinatal events include hypoxia, asphyxia, acidosis, hypothermia, hypoglycemia, bacterial infection, certain medications, and hypoalbuminemia. These conditions interfere with conjugation or compete for albumin-binding sites.

Clinical manifestations of kernicterus commonly first appear between 2 and 6 days after birth. *Kernicterus is never present at birth.* Symptomatology changes as the disease process progresses. Four phases are recognized:

1. ***Phase one:*** the newborn is hypotonic and lethargic and exhibits a poor sucking reflex and depressed or absent Moro's reflex (some infants die during this phase).
2. ***Phase two:*** the newborn develops spasticity and hyperreflexia, often becomes opisthotonic, has a high-pitched cry, and may be hyperthermic. The newborn may convulse.
3. ***Phase three:*** at about 7 days of age, the newborn's spasticity lessens and may disappear.
4. ***Phase four:*** after the first month of life, the infant develops sequelae (e.g., spasticity, athetosis, partial or complete deafness, or mental retardation).

Rh_0(D) Human Immune Globulin

The more severe forms of isoimmune hemolytic disease result from Rh_0D^u group incompatibility. This form of hemolytic disease of the newborn occurred in

0.5% to 1% of all pregnancies in North America before prophylactic $Rh_0(D)$ human immune globulin (RhoGAM) became available in the mid-1960s. Many children died or were seriously affected. Since immunization of Rh-negative women against this antigen began, the incidence of severe erythroblastosis has been drastically reduced.

Prophylaxis for Rh isoimmunization involves the use of Rh immune globulin as a preventive measure against Rh isoimmunization. It is not a treatment for Rh-negative women who are already sensitized, because ***it has no effect against antibodies already present in the maternal bloodstream.*** An injection of ***$Rh_0(D)$ immune globulin provides passive immunity,*** which is transient and therefore will not affect a subsequent pregnancy. $Rh_0(D)$ immune globulin (RhIG) prepares RBCs containing the Rh antigen for lysis by phagocytes, before the recipient's immune system is activated to produce antibodies. ***Production of one's own antibodies provides active immunity*** (Chapter 5).

Antibodies formed by an active immune response remain within the individual's bloodstream, presumably for life. RhIG given to an $Rh_0(D)$-negative woman who is already sensitized would accomplish no purpose. Therefore it is recommended only for non-sensitized Rh-negative women at risk of developing Rh isoimmunization. Given to any Rh-positive person, an injection of RhIG would result in hemolysis of RBCs.

Assessment

Prenatal

Risk factors from the prenatal record are identified. The severity of physiologic jaundice differs greatly between *Oriental* and other ethnic populations. The mean serum levels of unconjugated bilirubin in Chinese, Japanese, Korean, and American Indian full-term newborns are between 10 and 14 mg/dl, or approximately double those for other non-Oriental populations. The incidence of bilirubin toxicity is also increased (Fanaroff and Martin, 1987).

Maternal infections often precede neonatal hyperbilirubinemia. Bacterial (e.g., syphilis), viral (e.g., rubella) and protozoal (e.g., toxoplasmosis) infections have a direct association. Maternal ingestion of sulfonamides or salicylates close to delivery affect the newborn's ability to remove bilirubin. Medical conditions such as *maternal diabetes mellitus* predispose the newborn to hyperbilirubinemia (Pernoll, Benda, and Babson, 1986).

Maternal blood type and Rh place the woman at risk for *isoimmunization* (Chapter 5), which subsequently jeopardizes future pregnancies. *Women who are Rh negative are* at risk for developing antibodies to the Rh factor, a process called isoimmunization, or sensitization. To develop antibodies, the mother will need to have been innoculated with Rh-positive RBCs. Therefore the woman's history is investigated for events that can lead to innoculation. These events include (1) transfusion with Rh-positive blood, (2) spontaneous or elective abortions ≥ 8 gestational weeks, (3) previous pregnancy(s) with an Rh-positive fetus, (4) amniocentesis for any reason, and (5) premature separation of the placenta (the latter is often difficult to identify).

Sensitization of the mother occurs promptly after an incompatible blood transfusion (improperly typed [Rh-positive] blood). Hematopoiesis (formation and development of blood cells) begins in the embryo during the sixth week after conception (i.e., during the eighth week after the last menstrual period [LMP]). Therefore a woman who has experienced one or more abortions 2 months or more since her LMP or has given birth has received innoculations of fetal blood generally at the time of placental separation.

During amniocentesis, the needle may cause localized damage to the single layer of cells that separates maternal and fetal circulation in the placenta, thus allowing some fetal RBCs into maternal circulation. If any of these events have occurred, the woman's record is checked for documentation of prophylaxis for isoimmunization (see p. 883). The postnatal course(s) of a previous baby(s) is also assessed for evidence of maternal isoimmunization. Rh-negative women who receive prenatal care have blood drawn to screen for the presence of antibodies to antigens such as the Rh factor (i.e., the Hemantigen screen and Coombs' test). The *Hemantigen test* also screens for other less common RBC-antigens such as Kell, Duffy, and Kidd. Fortunately, serious fetal damage from these factors is unlikely.

Results of the indirect **Coombs' test** are reviewed. In this test the ***maternal blood*** serum is mixed with Rh-positive RBCs. The test is positive (maternal antibodies are present) if Rh-positive RBCs agglutinate (clump). The dilution of the specimen of blood at which clumping occurs (if it does occur) determines the titer (level of maternal antibodies). The titer determines the degree of maternal sensitization (isoimmunization). If the titer reaches 1:16, an amniocentesis for delta optical density (ΔOD) analysis is performed (Perry, Parer, and Inturrisi, 1986).

The first amniocentesis is usually performed between 18 weeks' (in the case of a high antibody titer and any previously affected fetuses) and 24 weeks' gestation (in the case of a low fixed antibody titer and any previously unaffected fetuses) (Perry, Parer, and Inturrisi, 1986). ΔOD is a spectrophotometric (color) analysis test (Chapter 22). This test determines the amount of bilirubin in the amniotic fluid.

Maternal blood type O may also place the newborn at risk (p. 880).

Perinatal

The perinatal record is reviewed for conditions that are associated with increased RBC destruction in the newborn and that may increase susceptibility (particularly from the immature infant) to the neurotoxic effect of bilirubin by (1) enhancing its passage across the blood-brain barrier and (2) reducing cellular integrity (Fanaroff and Martin, 1987). These factors include (1) perinatal asphyxia with a pH under 7.20, (2) an unstable physiologic condition of the newborn indicated by an Apgar score of 3 or less at 5 minutes, (3) hypothermia (temperature less than 35° C [95° F]), (4) deterioration of the newborn's condition as indicated by clinical signs, and (5) hypoglycemia (also leads to acidosis).

All of these conditions adversely affect metabolism. Compromised metabolism in the newborn delays or interferes with bilirubin conjugation into a water-soluble form for excretion in urine and stool. Although the precise effects of these insults are undetermined, the increased risk to the newborn may be sufficient to justify treatment at lower levels of bilirubin.

Postnatal

The newborn who has severe ***erythroblastosis fetalis*** may initially exhibit yellow-stained vernix or umbilical cord. The infant may have *hydrops fetalis*. Signs of this manifestation of severe hemolytic anemia include edema, pleural and pericardial effusions, and ascites; all of which indicate cardiac failure (many of these infants are stillborn). Placental enlargement is seen with severe disease.

Preterm birth, LBW, and immaturity affect the newborn's ability to process bilirubin. *Immaturity* of, or defects in, the *glucuronyl transferase enzyme system* delays or interferes with the conjugation of bilirubin. Hepatic cell damage caused by infection or drugs also interferes with that enzyme system.

Sequestered blood accounts for elevated bilirubin levels. Blood is sequestered (trapped or confined) in cephalhematomas, ecchymoses, and hemangiomas. As the blood is hemolyzed, levels of serum bilirubin rise.

Newborn Jaundice

Approximately 50% of all full-term newborns are visibly jaundiced (yellowish in color) during the first 3 days of life. Serum bilirubin levels less than 5 mg/dl usually are not reflected in visible skin jaundice.

Physiologic hyperbilirubinemia (jaundice) (p. 507) characterized by a progressive increase in serum levels of unconjugated bilirubin from 2 mg/dl in cord blood to a mean peak of 6 mg/dl by 72 hours of age, followed by a decline to 5 mg/dl by day 5, and not exceeding 12 mg/dl. These serum values are within the normal physiologic limitations of the healthy term newborn who was not exposed to perinatal complications (such as hypoxia). No bilirubin toxicity develops.

Pathologic hyperbilirubinemia cannot be defined solely in terms of serum concentrations of unconjugated bilirubin. Pathologic hyperbilirubinemia refers to that level of serum bilirubin at which a particular newborn will sustain lesions in the brain tissue (kernicterus), renal tubular cells, intestinal mucosa, and pancreatic cells.

Every newborn is assessed for jaundice and hyperbilirubinemia. Findings are assessed from physical and behavioral examination and laboratory tests. The *blanch test* assists in the differentiation of cutaneous jaundice from skin color. To do the test, apply pressure with the thumb over a bony area (e.g., forehead) for several seconds to empty all the capillaries in that spot. If jaundice is present the blanched area will look yellow before the capillaries refill. The conjunctival sacs and buccal mucosa are assessed, especially in darker-skinned infants. It is preferable to assess for jaundice in daylight, because there is possible distortion of color from artificial lighting, reflection from nursery walls, and the like.

The nurse notes the newborn's behavior. Changes in feeding and sleeping patterns, pallor, and dark color of stools and urine accompany hyperbilirubinemia. Neurologic signs of kernicterus are presented on p. 880.

Laboratory results add to the data base. Blood type, Rh factor, hemoglobin, hematocrit, and Coombs' test results identify maternal-fetal RBC incompatibility and erythroblastosis fetalis.

Laboratory reports that support the diagnosis of hyperbilirubinemia follow*:

1. Serum bilirubin levels increasing more than 5 mg/dl/24 hr
2. Full-term newborn: serum bilirubin level greater than 12 mg/dl, which represents the upper limit of peak concentration of physiologic jaundice (Chapter 16)
3. LBW newborn: serum bilirubin levels of 10 to 12

*For the normal full-term newborn, serum bilirubin of 12 to 15 mg/dl is the cut-off point for phototherapy and 20 mg/dl for exchange transfusion. For sick or preterm newborns, it is best to prevent *any* rise in serum bilirubin altogether; no level can be regarded as "safe" in view of the possibility of opening the blood-brain barrier and the vulnerability of brain cells resulting from disease processes and inadequate energy reserves. For the sick or preterm newborn, phototherapy is advisable for visible jaundice, and exchange transfusion for serum bilirubin of 15 mg/dl (Wu et al, 1985).

mg/dl, even though the peak concentration of "physiologic jaundice" is 15 mg/dl
4. Preterm newborn: all visible jaundice, even with serum bilirubin levels as low as 5 mg/dl

Blood from the umbilical cord is sent to the laboratory to establish the blood type and Rh status. Occasionally an Rh-positive infant is wrongly typed as Rh-negative because of so-called blocking antibodies covering the affected newborn's RBCs.

A direct **Coombs' test** is performed with neonatal cord blood. The newborn's RBCs are "washed" and mixed with Coombs' serum. The test is positive (maternal antibodies are present) if the infant's RBCs agglutinate. The dilution of the specimen of blood at which agglutination occurs (if it does occur) determines the titer of maternal antibodies in fetal serum. The titer determines the degree of maternal sensitization. If the titer is 1:64, an exchange transfusion is indicated.

Increased erythropoiesis with many nucleated RBCs are seen in hemolytic anemia of a progressive type. Hypoglycemia may be present and treated to avoid additional CNS insult (p. 823).

Transcutaneous bilirubinometry is a screening test for newborn jaundice based on the relationship between the yellow color of the skin and total serum bilirubin level. This rapid, noninvasive transcutaneous procedure uses a spectrophotometric hand-held fiberoptic instrument that illuminates the skin and measures the intensity of its yellow color. The intensity of color is then displayed as a number that correlates with serum bilirubin concentration; it is *not* an absolute estimate of total bilirubin. This test screens for those jaundiced newborns with rising bilirubin levels whose condition may need further diagnostic investigation.

The small probe of the bilirubinometer is applied firmly against the newborn's skin over a bony surface of the forehead or the sternum. The photoprobe is held against the skin with enough pressure to blanch the skin. Then a pulse of light is transmitted through the skin to the subcutaneous tissues and the reflected color is recorded within a few seconds.

Skin pigmentation *does affect* the readings. Correlations between transcutaneous bilirubin index and serum bilirubin levels have been established for Japanese infants, American white infants, and American black infants at term. The different values for the preterm or LBW newborn of each racial group are not yet available. The instrument is not suitable for monitoring the newborn during or immediately after phototherapy or exchange transfusion.

Nursing Diagnoses

Following are examples of nursing diagnoses for newborns at risk from hyperbilirubinemia:

Potential for injury to neurons and cells in the kidney, pancreas, and intestine related to
- Hyperbilirubinemia

Impaired gas exchange related to
- Hemolytic anemia

Potential fluid volume deficit related to
- Phototherapy

Potential for parental anxiety related to
- Hyperbilirubinemia, its management, and potential sequelae

Planning

Hospital protocols for care of hyperbilirubinemia are developed as a collaborative effort of the health care team. The health care team utilizes hospital protocols or standards when individualizing care for the infant and parents.

Goals for care are stated in client-centered terms and include the following:
1. Prenatal and perinatal risk factors are identified and intervention implemented where appropriate
2. The newborn remains free of hyperbilirubinemia and its sequela—kernicterus
3. The newborn suffers minimum or no sequelae from hyperbilirubinemia and any necessary treatment
4. Parents understand newborn's condition, therapies, and possible sequelae

Implementation

Preventive Measures

Prevention is the primary focus of care. The nurse is not responsible for typing and cross-matching blood and blood products. However, the nurse is responsible for checking the product to be administered against the physician's order and the woman's blood type and Rh status.

Prenatal control of diabetes mellitus, prevention of infection, avoidance of sulfonamides and aspirin (when possible), and prevention of preterm birth reduce perinatal risks. Prevention of or prompt appropriate therapy for perinatal asphyxia, acidosis, cold stress, and hypoglycemia will decrease the newborn's risk of severe hemolytic disease and of susceptibility to neurotoxicity of bilirubin. Early feeding is initiated to stimulate the gastrocolic reflex to remove bilirubin through stooling (Chapter 17).

Prophylaxis for Rh isoimmunization is now available.

Antenatal Administration of $Rh_0(D)$ Immune Globulin (Human). Rh sensitization is possible during pregnancy if the cellular layer separating fetal and maternal circulations is disrupted and fetal blood enters the maternal bloodstream. The cellular layer may be disrupted during amniocentesis or by placental abruption. For the woman who is $Rh_0(D)$ negative D^u (allemorph variant) negative, and Coombs' negative, RhIG administered during the antenatal period after amniocentesis, at about 28 weeks' gestation and again within 72 hours after delivery can further reduce the incidence of maternal isoimmunization.

Postnatal Administration of $Rh_0(D)$ Immune Globulin (Human). The United States Public Health Service recommendations are as follows:

1. RhIG is given only to a woman after delivery or abortion who is $Rh_0(D)$ negative and D^u negative and whose fetus is $Rh_0(D)$ positive or D^u positive. ***It is never given to an infant or father.***
2. RhIG is not useful in a woman who has Rh antibodies.
3. RhIG should be given intramuscularly, not into fatty tissue or intravenously.

Prevention of isoimmunization of an Rh-negative woman to the Rh factor in her fetus is now possible in over 95% of cases. Prophylaxis is achieved by administering RhIG within 72 hours of evacuation of the uterus (by spontaneous or elective abortion or more advanced pregnancy).

Jaundice may not be apparent before the baby is discharged. Some baby's have sequestered blood (e.g., cephalhematoma). Therefore, especially if the mother is discharged with the infant soon after delivery, parents need to learn how to identify jaundice and know when to notify the physician (Locklin, 1987). See guidelines for client teaching: hyperbilirubinemia in Chapter 17.

Curative Measures

Hyperbilirubinemia occurs in approximately 50% of normal newborns. *Phototherapy* is conducted in the normal newborn nursery, usually for physiologic hyperbilirubinemia (see guidelines for client teaching, p. 510 and Fig. 17-14). A nursing care plan for an infant with hyperbilirubinemia is on p. 885.

Some fetuses are candidates for *intrauterine transfusion*. The ***blood type used for transfusion is $Rh_0(D)$ negative and (usually) group 0.*** Only blood that is negative for CMV, hepatitis, and HIV is used (Perry, Parer, and Inturrisi, 1986). The RBC transfusion counteracts the anemia and cardiac decompensation is thus forestalled. The second transfusion is administered 10 days later, followed by transfusions every 3 weeks until delivery.

Exchange transfusion may be required in the immediate neonatal period. The nurse is alert to the fact that a significant risk for morbidity and a mortality risk of 0.1% to 1.0% exist with exchange transfusions. It is time consuming and expensive as well.

An exchange transfusion is accomplished by alternately removing a small amount of the newborn's blood and replacing it with a like amount of donor blood. Depending on the infant's size, maturity, and condition, amounts of 5 to 20 ml at a time are slowly exchanged. The total amount of blood exchanged approximates 170 ml/kg of body weight (80 ml/lb) or 75% to 85% of the infant's total blood volume. During the procedure, the staff observes infection control precautions for invasive procedures (Chapter 23).

Rehabilitative Measures. Planning for rehabilitative measures is necessary if kernicterus occurs. The family will need the services from many community resources to care for the affected child. An interdisciplinary approach that includes social services must be taken.

Evaluation

On a short-term basis care can be considered to be effective if unconjugated serum bilirubin levels do not reach or exceed toxic levels. These levels are arbitrarily set at $\geq$ 5 mg/dl/24 hr, $\geq$ 12 mg/dl in term newborns, and $\geq$ 15 mg/dl in preterm newborns. Parents understand and are able to cope with hyperbilirubinemia and its management. Long-term evaluation of effective care rests in the absence of sequelae to hyperbilirubinemia (e.g., minimal brain dysfunction).

❑ CONGENITAL ANOMALIES

The desired and expected outcome of every wanted pregnancy is a normal, functioning infant with a good intellectual potential. Fulfillment of this hope depends on numerous factors, both hereditary and environmental. Probably all human characteristics have a genetic component, including those that produce unpleasant symptoms or unwelcome physical abnormalities that impair the fitness of the individual. Some diseases are produced through the action of a single gene or the combined action of many genes inherited from the parents; others are the result of the action of the environment on the genetic composition of the individual. A disease or disorder that can be transmitted from generation to generation is termed *genetic* or *hereditary* (Chapter 7). A *congenital* disorder is one that is present at birth and can be caused by genetic or environmental factors or both.

Each year 250,000 infants are born with significant structural and functional disorders. Major congenital

Specific Nursing Care Plan

HYPERBILIRUBINEMIA

Bret Jackson is a 34-week-gestation preterm infant born to a 26-year-old mother who came to the hospital 9 cm dilated in active labor. Bret was born via spontaneous vaginal delivery with Apgar scores of 6 and 8. He has been cared for in the Special Care Nursery in a 40% oxyhood with mild retractions, occasional tachypnea and nasal flaring. Phototherapy was initiated 24 hours ago for a bilirubin level of 9.7 mg/dl, however, this morning's lab results are significantly higher at 14.0 mg/dl.

ASSESSMENT	NURSING DIAGNOSIS (ND), PLAN/GOAL (P/G)	RATIONALE/ IMPLEMENTATION	EVALUATION
14.0 mg/dl serum bilirubin level. Assess color and consistency of stools; dark, concentrated urine. Assess for increasing pallor. Assess skin color in daylight and not artificial light, if possible. Assess signs of kernicterus: diminished Moro's reflex, poor suck, vomiting, hypotonia, high-pitched cry, lethargy, seizures. Obtain blood for testing as ordered (bilirubin, hemoglobin and hematocrit, liver function tests, blood incompatibility studies, etc.).	ND: Potential for injury related to hyperbilirubinemia. P/G: Bret's hyperbilirubinemia is treated promptly and he will demonstrate no signs of kernicterus.	*Hyperbilirubinemia may cause irreversable brain damage:* Obtain IV access and monitor IV infusion (adequate hydration is essential for bilirubin excretion). Maintain phototherapy as ordered (keep eyes patched and expose as much skin surface to light as possible, see p. 510). Test strength of bili lights while Bret is under phototherapy according to hospital and manufacturer policy. Note neurologic signs of kernicterus and report immediately. Set-up, assist, and monitor Bret during an exchange transfusion as indicated and ordered.	Bret's bilirubin levels decline with treatment and he demonstrates no signs of kernicterus or any iatrogenic complications of IV therapy, phototherapy, exchange transfusion, etc.
Assess parent's knowledge of hyperbilirubinemia, its treatment, and possible sequelae.	ND: Knowledge deficit related to hyperbilirubinemia, its treatment, and complications. P/G: Parents learn about their newborn's condition, therapies, and possible sequelae. P/G: Parents participate in maintaining the treatment regimen.	*Knowledge increases one's sense of control and enhances coping:* Explain the different causes of hyperbilirubinemia and their potential sequelae. Explain the treatment modalities. Encourage parents to take an active role in the treatment plan (e.g., keeping eye patches in place and full skin exposed to light while under phototherapy, etc.). Encourage questions, feelings, or concerns.	Parents verbalize understanding of instruction. Parents participate in maintaining the treatment regimen.

defects are now the leading cause of death in term births where perinatal care is of good quality. With the decrease in other causes of neonatal mortality, they now account for over 25% of all deaths.

The seriousness of this community health problem is reflected in the more than 6 million hospital days and $200 billion a year allocated to the care and treatment of these newborns. Prevention and detection procedures are being improved continuously. Methods of promoting the availability of these services to populations at risk challenge the community health care systems. An interdisciplinary team approach is imperative to provide holistic care: surgery, rehabilitation, and education of the child and social, psychologic, and financial assistance to the parents. Parental disappointment and disillusion and the nurse's own negative feelings toward (or stigmatization of) the infant's disorder add to the complexity of nursing care.

Assessment

Prenatal Diagnosis

Recently refined testing procedures are available to monitor the development of the fetus. Prenatal diagnostic techniques such as amniocentesis, ultrasound, **α-fetoprotein** measurements (AFP), chorionic villi sampling (CVS), percutaneous umbilical cord blood sampling (PUBS), and gene probes contribute to the data base (Chapter 22). Although they comprise a valuable adjunct to prenatal care, these tests do not achieve 100% accuracy in detecting congenital defects (Main and Mennuti, 1986; Cohen, 1987; Kogan, Doherty, and Gitschier, 1987; Lewis and Mocarski, 1987; Routine, 1987). Some women choose to continue the pregnancy after positive identification of a congenital problem. The prenatal record is reviewed for documentation of parental wishes for the level of aggressiveness of management they would consider for the care of the newborn.

Despite the status and availability of current technology, not all congenital disorders are or can be anticipated. The historical and medical information in the prenatal record is reviewed for factors that are associated with congenital disorders. These factors include various medical, surgical, and social conditions and their treatments, maternal infection, maternal endocrine and metabolic disorders, and maternal substance abuse.

Perinatal Diagnosis

Many congenital anomalies require intervention soon after birth. Careful observations will identify most of these conditions.

Assessment of the volume of amniotic fluid can provide important data. An excessive amount of amniotic fluid, **hydramnios,** is commonly associated with congenital anomalies in the newborn. The newborn should be examined closely at the earliest possible time. In the presence of hydramnios, any of the following may be suspected: cephalocaudal malformations, such as hydrocephalus, microcephaly, anencephaly, and spina bifida; orogastrointestinal malformations, such as cleft palate, esophageal atresia with or without a tracheal fistula, pyloric stenosis, volvulus, and imperforate anus; miscellaneous conditions, such as Down's syndrome, congenital heart disease, deformed extremities, and infants of diabetic or prediabetic mothers; and preterm birth.

Oligohydramnios (an insufficient amount of amniotic fluid) is primarily associated with those anomalies of the urinary tract that preclude normal micturition in utero. As a rule, renal agenesis or renal dysplasia is involved. Urethral stenosis has also been reported to be associated with oligohydramnios. Anomalies of the earlobes, rather than agenesis of the ear, are sometimes associated with renal abnormalities and are not direct results of oligohydramnios. Potter's syndrome (renal agenesis) is the classic example of an association between oligohydramnios and renal anomalies. It includes a typical facies that involves abnormal earlobes.

Postnatal Diagnosis

An Apgar score and minimal assessment are completed as they are for each newborn after birth (see Fig. 17-1, p. 484). Any deviations from normal are reported to the physician immediately.

Respiratory System. Screening for congenital anomalies of the respiratory tract is necessary even for the infant who is apparently normal at birth. Respiratory distress at birth or shortly thereafter may be the result of lung immaturity or anomalous development. Congenital laryngeal web and bilateral choanal atresia (Fig. 28-35) are readily apparent at birth. Both require emergency surgery. Respiratory distress caused by diaphragmatic hernia and tracheoesophageal fistula appear immediately or may be delayed depending on the severity of the defect.

Neurologic System. Neurologic signs may reflect hidden congenital anomalies as well as numerous other conditions. Many neonatal responses are nonspecific. Each sign, such as high-pitched cry, hypotonia, jitteriness, low-set ears, and microcephaly or hydrocephaly, must be evaluated carefully before appropriate therapy can be instituted.

Some neural tube defects are obvious at first glance. The three main defects are anencephaly, spina bifida (which includes occult and visible meningocele and my-

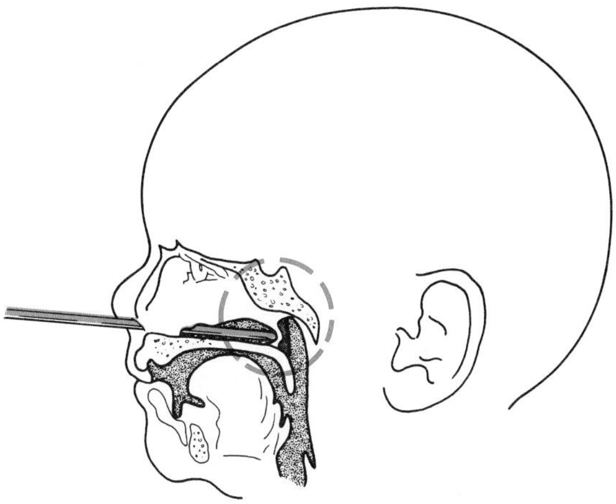

Fig. 28-35 Choanal atresia. Posterior nares are obstructed by membrane or bone either bilaterally or unilaterally. Infant becomes cyanotic at rest. With crying, newborn's color improves. Nasal discharge is present. Snorting respirations are often observed with increased respiratory effort. Newborn may be unable to breathe and eat at same time. Diagnosis is made by noting inability to pass small feeding tube through one or both nares. (Courtesy Ross Laboratories, Columbus, Ohio.)

elomeningocele), and encephalocele (p. 893). These are defects in midline closures. If a neural tube defect is identified, the infant may have one or more of the other malformations in this group: cleft lip and palate, tracheoesophageal atresia and/or fistula, and diaphragmatic hernia.

Cardiovascular System. Severe congenital cardiovascular disorders often are evident immediately after birth, for example, severe cyanotic heart disease. These newborns usually are transferred directly to special nurseries or pediatric units. Some problems, such as a small patent ductus arteriosus or a minimal coarctation of the descending aorta, become apparent only as the infant is exposed to stresses such as growth demands of later infancy and early childhood, or infection. In about 75% of cases cardiovascular anomalies are unexpected.

Cardiovascular defects occur in 3 of every 1000 births. Congenital heart disease is implicated in approximately 50% of deaths from malformations during the first year of life. The etiologic factors are still unclear, although a familial tendency is evident in many cases. Coexisting congenital defects are common in newborns with cardiovascular anomalies. Maternal disease during pregnancy has been implicated. Symptoms characteristically are first evident after the umbilical cord is severed. The newborn's *cry* is weak and muffled or loud and breathless. The newborn may be *cyanotic*. Cyanosis is usually generalized, it increases in the supine position, and is often unrelieved by oxygen. Cyanosis usually deepens with crying. The gray dusky color may be mild, moderate, or severe. Other infants may be *acyanotic,* pale, with or without mottling with exertion (such as crying).

The newborn's *activity level* varies from restless to lethargic. The newborn may be unresponsive except to pain. The arms may be flaccid when eating. *Posturing* is significant. Hypotonia and flaccidity may be evident, even when sleeping. There may be hyperextension of the neck or opisthotonos. The newborn may be dyspneic when supine. Persistent *bradycardia* (below 120 bpm or less than 30 bpm from the normal baseline for a duration of 10 minutes or more [Tucker, 1988]) or persistent *tachycardia* (above 160 bpm) may be noted.

Respirations are counted when the newborn is asleep. Findings may include tachypnea (60 respirations per minute or more), retractions with nasal flaring or tachypnea, and dyspnea with diaphoresis or grunting. Diaphoresis is an uncommon response in the normal newborn. Respirations may be gasping followed in 2 or 3 minutes by respiratory arrest if not treated promptly. Grunting may occur with exertion, such as crying or feeding by nipple.

These findings must be reported immediately. Children showing these types of signs are not cared for in the normal newborn nursery. They require prompt definite diagnosis and immediate appropriate therapy in a tertiary care pediatric unit.

Gastrointestinal System. Screening for gastrointestinal tract malformations is performed on a routine basis for all infants. Abdominal wall defects are apparent at birth. Omphalocele and gastroschisis are discussed on pp. 892 and 927. Intestinal obstruction; which occurs in about 1 in 3000 newborns, may occur in the presence of diaphragmatic hernia (p. 890). A scaphoid (sunken) abdomen usually indicates a diaphragmatic hernia. A distended abdomen is particularly noteworthy in H-type tracheoesophageal fistula. These conditions require immediate surgery and are discussed later in this chapter.

Other malformations are apparent when further assessment is made. Malformations such as esophageal atresia and imperforate anus are discussed on pp. 891 and 892.

Urogenital System. Careful notation of perinatal events and observations such as oligohydramnios and absence of voiding aids in the identification and confirmation of existing congenital anomalies. In cases of ambiguous genitals (p. 897), there is an urgent association between the parent-child relationship and the identification of the infant's sex. The identity of the newborn must be established as quickly as possible to facilitate initiation of a positive parent-child relationship. Exstrophy of the bladder or the cloaca is rare (p. 897).

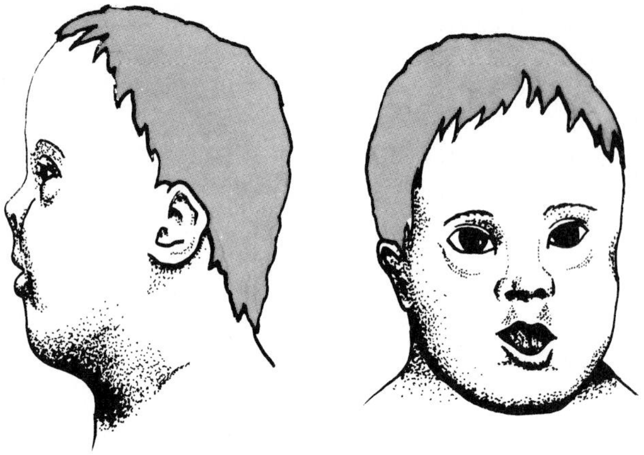

Fig. 28-36 Clinical features of Down's syndrome.

Multiple-system Anomalies. Some newborns have multiple congenital anomalies. A syndrome refers to a recognized pattern of malformations. The most familiar is Down's syndrome (Fig. 28-36). Diagnosis is confirmed early in the neonatal period.

Down's syndrome is most often the result of trisomy of a Group G (number 21) chromosome. The average incidence is 1:500. Major clinical manifestations include the following: brachycephaly with flat occiput; inner epicanthal folds; small ears, nose, and mouth with protruding tongue; muscular hypotonia; broad, short hands with stubby fingers and simian palmar crease (Fig. 28-37); broad stubby feet with wide space between big and second toes; mental retardation; and variable life expectancy.

Five congenital anomalies require emergency surgery. These conditions and other malformations are presented under Implementation in this section. Although the surgery is the physician's responsibility, considerable nursing care is involved.

Genetic Diagnosis

Most diagnostic procedures for detection of genetic disorders are implemented after birth at any time from the postdelivery period through adulthood. The number and variety of these tests are too extensive to include here; therefore only those employed most frequently in the newborn period will be discussed.

Biochemical Tests. The most widespread use of postdelivery testing for genetic disease is the routine screening of newborns for inborn errors of metabolism such as phenylketonuria (PKU) (Appendix G), which is mandatory in most states in the United States. **Inborn errors of metabolism** is a term applied to a large group of disorders caused by a metabolic defect that results from the absence of or change in a protein, usually an enzyme, because of gene action. These defects can involve any substrate produced from protein, carbohydrate, or fat metabolism. Inborn errors of metabolism are recessive disorders and, as such, require that the individual receive a defective gene from each parent. The parents are usually unaffected, because their normal, dominant gene directs the synthesis of sufficient protein to meet their metabolic needs under normal circumstances. With new biochemical techniques it is now possible to detect the presence of the abnormal gene in an increasing number of these disorders.

PKU results from a deficiency of the enzyme phenylalanine dehydrogenase. The test for PKU is not valid until the newborn has ingested an ample amount of the amino acid phenylalanine, a constituent of both human and cow's milk (Chapter 18). The child with this disorder will have blond hair, blue eyes, and fair skin. A diet low in phenylalanine is ordered to prevent the severe mental retardation and bizarre behavior seen in untreated cases.

Galactosemia, caused by a deficiency of the enzyme galactose-1-phosphate uridyl transferase, results in the inability to convert galactose to glucose. Galactosemia can be detected by measuring blood levels of galactose in the urine of affected newborns who have ingested milk containing galactose. Failure to thrive, mental retardation, cataracts, jaundice, hepatomegaly, and cirrhosis of the liver are manifestations in untreated cases. Therapy consists of the elimination of galactose from the diet.

In recent years many states in the United States have required routine screening for *hypothyroidism.* Thyroxine (T_4) is measured from a drop of blood obtained from a heel stick at 2 to 5 days of age. At this time the normally expected increase in T_4 is lacking in newborns with hypothyroidism. Untreated affected individuals develop cretinism. The same blood sample can be used to test for all three of these metabolic disorders—PKU, galactosemia, and hypothyroidism (see Fig. 17-11).

Cytologic Studies. In most instances disorders resulting from chromosomal abnormalities can be diagnosed by clinical manifestations alone. Occasionally an infant is born whose clinical appearance is only suggestive. In these cases cytologic studies are more often carried out to confirm or rule out a tentative diagnosis. Sometimes all that is required are sex chromatin or fluorescent staining techniques. These stains can be prepared from any cells in the body. The most easily obtained and therefore the most commonly used are mucosal cells scraped from the inside of the cheek, placed on a glass slide, prepared, and stained (buccal smear).

Preparation of a karyotype (see Fig. 7-1) requires cells in the process of cell division. The most commonly used cells are those obtained from bone marrow, skin, or peripheral blood. The cells are grown in culture media. Division is arrested at the stage when cells are best visualized, then stained, photographed, and arranged in a karyotype for assessment. A karyotype is also requested in cases in which the sex of the infant is in doubt, since the assignment of a gender constitutes a social emergency (p. 897).

Two examples of chromosome abnormalities are Turner's and Klinefelter's syndromes. The child with *Turner's syndrome* is a female with the genetic designation of 45,X. She will have short stature, webbed neck, low posterior hairline, shield-shaped chest with widely spaced nipples, and lymph edema of hands and feet. This female is sterile. The child with *Klinefelter's syndrome* is a male whose genetic designation may be 47,XXY or 48,XXYY. This male is tall with long legs, has hypogenitalism, and is sterile. He may have deficient male secondary sexual characteristics and may demonstrate aberrant behavior.

Dermatoglyphics. The pattern formed by dermal ridges early in development is largely genetically determined by many genes on many chromosomes. Therefore addition or deletion of genetic material will produce alterations in the loops, swirls, and arches of the finger and toe prints, in the palm lines, and in the flexion creases on palms of the hands and soles of the feet. Characteristic dermatoglyphic patterns have been noted in almost all the chromosomal abnormalities such as Down's syndrome (see simian line, Fig. 28-37).

Characteristic palm creases have also been noted in a significant number of children with rubella syndrome and leukemia. The Sydney line (Fig. 28-37) has been observed more frequently in children with rubella syndrome than in children in a control group. Also this line is seen in approximately 15% of children with leukemia. Certain fingerprint patterns may be found in persons who suffer cardiac valvular problems later in life.

Many other diagnostic studies may be performed in the neonatal period to detect or rule out genetic defects, for example, x-ray studies for a variety of structural defects of bone and for gastrointestinal, renal, and neurologic disorders. Meconium ileus in the newborn is often the first manifestation of cystic fibrosis.

Parental Responses. Parental responses are carefully assessed. Signs and symptoms of initial grief responses are expected (Chapter 29). The family's understanding of the information presented to them is assessed on an ongoing basis. The family's comprehension of the proposed management and risks, and of alternative courses of action are evaluated. The family's feelings about proposed management and their role in posttherapy care are explored. The family's emotional, social, and financial resources must be considered.

Nursing Diagnoses

Following are examples of nursing diagnoses to direct the care of newborns with congenital abnormalities.

Newborn

Potential for injury or death related to
- Presence of a congenital disorder

Potential for infection related to
- Anomaly or its treatment

Potential for impaired gas exchange, nutrition, or mobility related to
- Congenital anomaly

Potential for altered growth and development related to
- Inborn error of metabolism

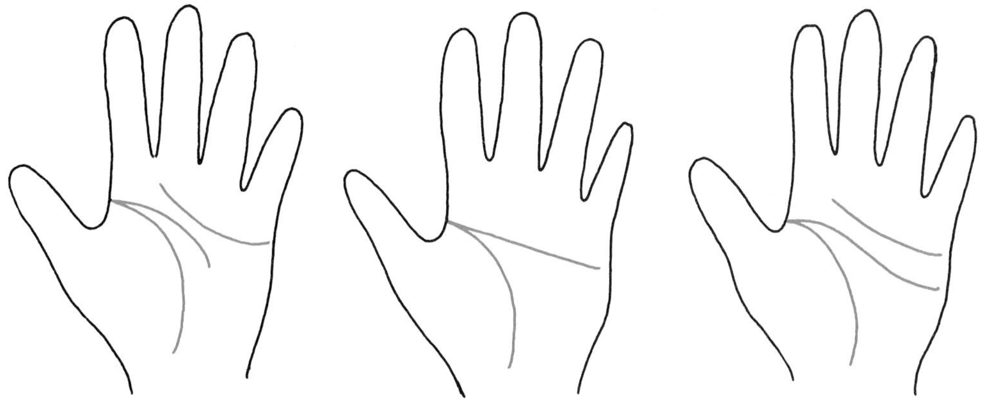

Fig. 28-37 Dermatoglyphic examples of flexion creases on palm. *Left,* normal; *center,* simian line; *right,* Sydney line. (From Whaley LF: Understanding inherited disorders, St Louis, 1974, The CV Mosby Co.)

Parents/Family

Dysfunctional grieving or spiritual distress related to
- Birth of a child with a defect

Potential for ineffective individual/family coping related to
- Birth of a child with a defect

Anxiety related to
- Uncertainty of prognosis or own ability to care for child

Knowledge deficit related to
- Cause
- Management
- Alternative courses of action
- Community resources
- Prognosis
- Care needed by child after discharge

Planning

Planning for the care of a newborn with a congenital defect begins before the birth of the infant. Hospital protocols and standards of care are established so that definitive and prompt therapy is facilitated. Parents are involved in the plan for care to the extent possible. For some disorders, a collaborative health team approach that includes specialists (e.g., orthodontists, physical therapists, geneticists) and community services representatives is needed.

Goals are stated in client-centered terms for the newborn and parents.

1. The newborn's disorder is recognized and appropriate therapy is initiated promptly
2. The newborn suffers no adverse sequelae to the disorder or its management
3. The parents understand the newborn's condition, its management and possible sequelae, as well as the anticipated prognosis
4. The parents choose a course of action commensurate with their family's values and goals

Implementation

General Preoperative and Postoperative Care

The newborn withstands the stress of surgery surprisingly well, provided it is done as soon after birth as feasible and the facilities available for care are adequately equipped and staffed. The medical-nursing team must be specially trained to anticipate and meet the newborn's physiologic needs. The surgical team consists of the radiologist, surgeon, anesthesiologist, and nurse. Diagnostic studies are kept to a minimum, and consideration of the newborn's immaturity is kept in mind.

The infant is transported to the operating room in an incubator with a self-contained power pack for the continuous provision of warmth. The infant is accompanied by an intensive care nursery nurse. Preanesthesia preparation includes hydration, administration of preoperative medications (usually minute amounts of atropine), insertion of an endotracheal tube, and gastric emptying.

During the operation, blood loss is constantly monitored. Blood is replaced milliliter for milliliter because the newborn's remarkable ability to maintain blood circulation through vasoconstriction means that vital signs remain unaltered until sudden and complete collapse occurs as the compensatory system is overtaxed. Temperature is maintained by positioning the infant on a thermal mattress and draping suitably.

Once the operation is completed, the infant is returned to the intensive care nursery. The first hour after the procedure is a crucial one; constant surveillance of recovery from the anesthesia is imperative. Body temperature is maintained between 36.1° and 36.7° C (97° and 98° F); optimum temperature is 36.5° C (97.6° F). An open airway is maintained by means of positioning of the head, suctioning, and use of high humidity. If the respiratory rate increases, suctioning is indicated. Oxygen dosage is prescribed on the basis of arterial blood gas values (such as Po_2). Fluid-electrolyte balance is monitored. Intravenous replacement is given as ordered. Postural drainage and percussion are ordered as necessary. The infant is turned from side to side to equalize pressure areas. An indwelling gastric catheter attached to intermittent suction removes gastric secretions. Removal of gastric contents prevents their possible aspiration because the infant's cough reflex is inadequate.

Common Surgical Emergencies

The following five congenital anomalies account for more than 90% of surgical emergencies of the newborn:

1. Diaphragmatic hernia
2. Tracheoesophageal anomalies
3. Omphalocele
4. Intestinal obstruction
5. Imperforate anus

Diaphragmatic Hernia. Diaphragmatic hernia is the most urgent of the neonatal emergencies. Incomplete embryonic development of the diaphragm allows herniation of abdominal viscera into the thoracic cavity (Fig. 28-38). The defect and herniation may be minimal and easily reparable or the defect may be so extensive that the viscera present in the thoracic cavity during embryonic life precluded the normal development of pulmonary tissue. Most cases involve a posterolateral defect, usually on the left. The extent of the defect

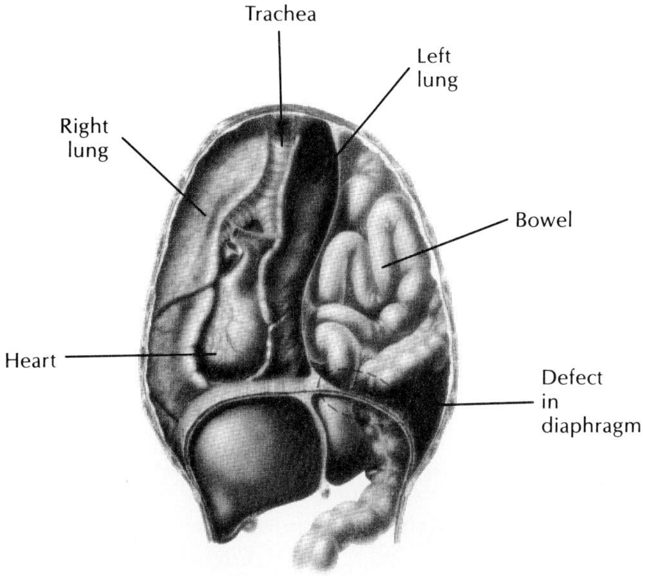

Fig. 28-38 Diaphragmatic hernia. (Courtesy Ross Laboratories, Columbus, Ohio.)

and the severity and timing of the symptomatology determine the seriousness of the problem.

Signs that are suspicious of extensive diaphragmatic herniation can be assessed by the nurse. Signs include the following: constant respiratory distress from birth that becomes increasingly severe as bowels fill with air, large or asymmetric chest contour, dullness to percussion on affected side, bowel sounds heard in thoracic cavity, and diminished breath sounds.

Prompt surgical repair is imperative after correction of acidosis, insertion of a nasogastric tube and aspiration, and oxygen therapy. The prognosis depends largely on the degree of pulmonary development and the success of diaphragmatic closure. Prognosis in severe cases is guarded.

Tracheoesophageal Anomalies. Esophageal atresia is an urgent congenital anomaly. Various types are recognized, depending on the presence or absence of an associated tracheoesophageal fistula, the site of the fistula, and the point and degree of esophageal obstruction (Fig. 28-39). The most common variety is associated with moderate hydramnios.

The following signs are suspicious for atresia with or without tracheoesophageal fistula: excessive oral secretions with drooling; progressive respiratory distress as unswallowed secretions spill over into trachea; and feeding intolerance. In feeding intolerance, choking, coughing, and cyanosis follow even a small amount of fluid taken by mouth. Soon after the first feeding is initiated, there is regurgitation of unaltered formula (unmixed with stomach secretions or bile).

Nursing actions are supportive. In the presence of excessive oral secretions and respiratory distress, ***do not feed the infant orally*** before consulting physician. In the presence of abdominal distension, place the newborn in semi-Fowler's position and raise the head 30 degrees or more (infant seat may be used). This position facilitates respiratory efforts and discourages reflux (spillage) of stomach secretions into the respiratory tree, with resultant chemical bronchitis and pneumonitis. On physician's order or per standing orders,

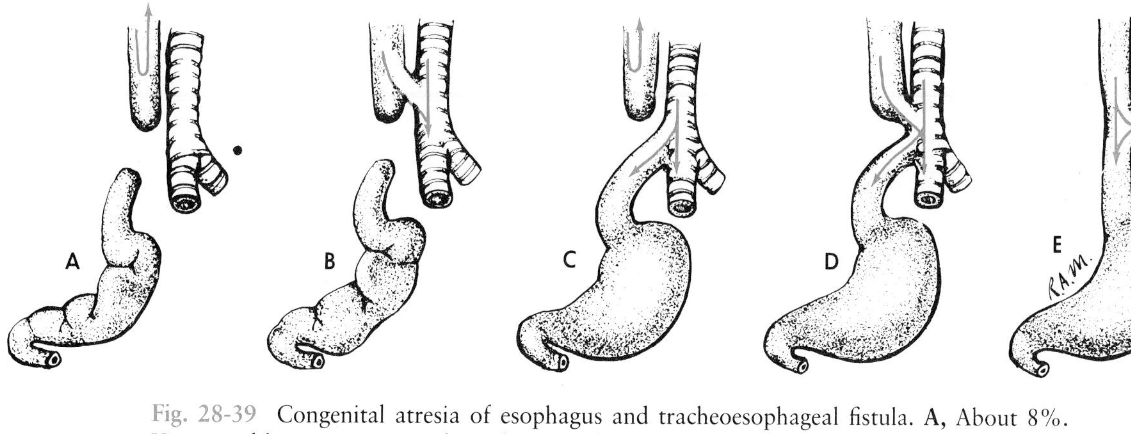

Fig. 28-39 Congenital atresia of esophagus and tracheoesophageal fistula. **A,** About 8%. Upper and lower segments of esophagus end in blind sac. **B,** Less than 1%. Upper segment of esophagus ends in atresia and connects to trachea by fistulous tract. Infant may drown with first feeding. **C,** About 87%. Upper segment of esophagus ends in blind pouch; lower segment connects with trachea by small fistulous tract. **D,** Less than 1%. Both segments of esophagus connect by fistulous tracts to trachea. Infant may drown with first feeding. **E,** About 4%. Esophagus is continuous but connects by fistulous tract to trachea; known as *H-type.* (From Whaley LF and Wong DL: Essentials of pediatric nursing, ed 3, St Louis, 1989, The CV Mosby Co.)

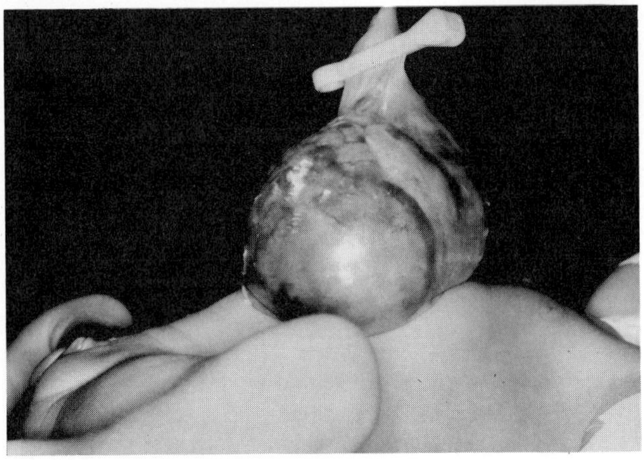

Fig. 28-40 Omphalocele containing liver. (Courtesy John R Campbell, MD, University of Oregon Health Sciences Center, Portland, Oregon.)

insert a suction tube into the blind pouch. Connect the tube to low, intermittent suction.

Surgical correction of the anomaly is mandatory. The prognosis depends on the degree of maturity of the newborn and the presence of a fistula or pneumonia. Cardiac and other gastrointestinal anomalies commonly are associated with esophageal atresia.

Omphalocele. Omphalocele is a herniation noted at birth in which part of the intestine protrudes through a defect in the abdominal wall at the umbilicus (Fig. 28-40). Failure of migration of the midgut in embryonic development probably is responsible for omphalocele. The protruding bowel is covered only by a thin, transparent membrane composed of amnion.

Prompt closure of defects of less than 5 cm in diameter usually is successful. Larger defects may require closure in stages. The general prognosis is related to associated anomalies.

There is usually only a short span of time between the infant's birth and surgical intervention. Planning for the provision of support to the parents in an essential aspect of nursing care. In addition to the usual preoperative orders, preparation of the infant for surgery includes protecting the defect from infection, rupture, and drying. The physician prescribes that the omphalocele be protected by one of the following:

1. Sterile towels or sponges kept moist with sterile saline solution that has been warmed to body temperature.
2. Protective sterile petrolatum dressings and a firm plastic or metal dome covering.

Intestinal Obstruction. Congenital jejunal or ileal obstruction is suspected when distension and bile-stained or fecal vomiting occur in a newborn in the first 24 to 48 hours of life. Normal meconium stool is not passed. Although this condition is uncommon, premature infants and those with other anomalies may be affected.

Nursing care is supportive: stop oral feedings and monitor intravenous therapy (see p. 831); prevent aspiration and suction gastric contents on physician's order (indwelling catheter to low, intermittent suction may be ordered); place infant in semi-Fowler's position to facilitate respiration. Prompt surgery usually provides good results.

Imperforate Anus. Imperforate anus is a congenital disorder that is more common in infant boys than infant girls (Fig. 28-41). About 85% of affected girls will have developed a small fistula (Fig. 28-42), but this is rare in boys. The obstruction may be of the low type

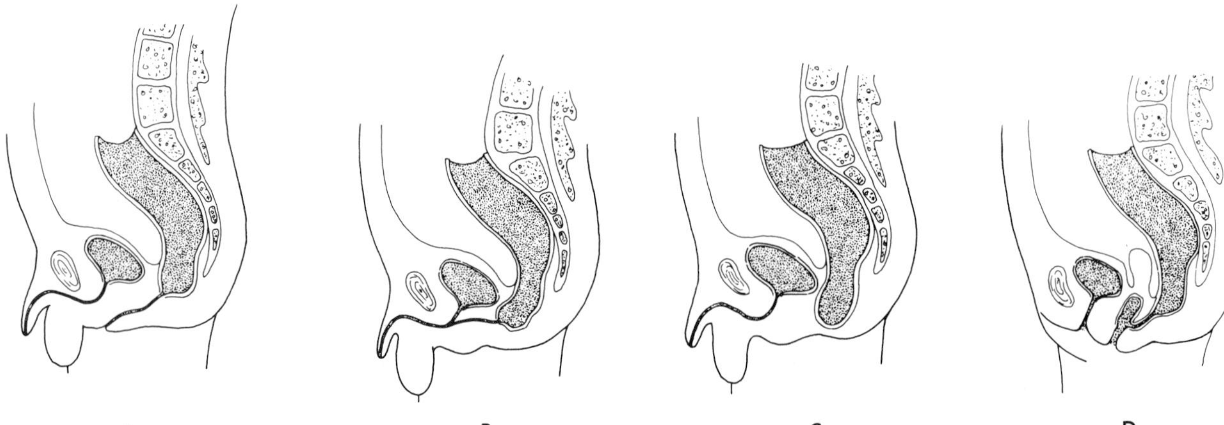

Fig. 28-41 Types of imperforate anus. Anal sphincter muscle may be present and intact. **A,** High lesion opening onto perineum through narrow fistulous tract. **B,** High lesion ending in fistulous tract to urinary tract. **C,** Low lesion in bowel passes through puborectal muscle. **D,** High lesion ending in fistulous tract to vagina.

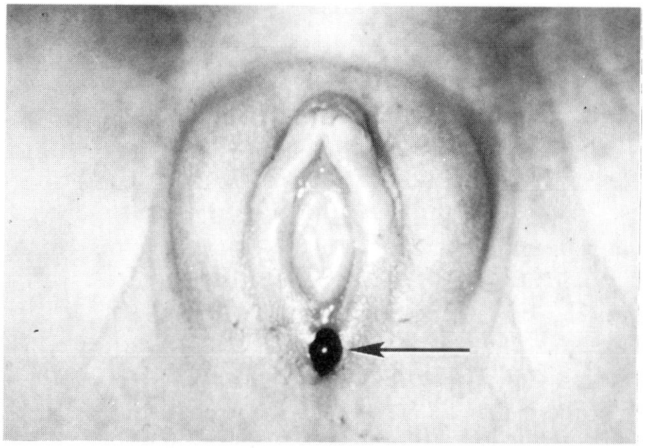

Fig. 28-42 Imperforate anus; fourchette fistula. Note meconium draining through fistula. *Arrow* indicates meconium exiting via fistulous tract. (Courtesy John R Campbell, MD, University of Oregon Health Sciences Center, Portland, Oregon.)

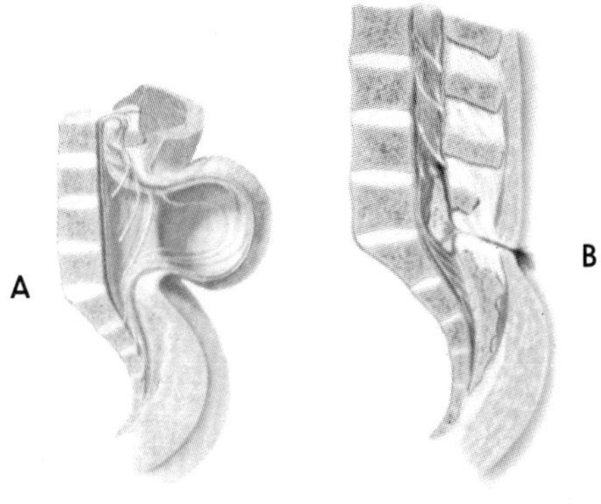

Fig. 28-43 **A,** Myelomeningocele. **B,** Dermal sinus tract with dermoid cyst, often associated with spina bifida occulta. Note also tuft of hair. (Courtesy Ross Laboratories, Columbus, Ohio.)

(anal membrane) or the high type (anal or rectal atresia).

Since continence for a lifetime may be dependent on the proper corrective surgery, a pediatric surgeon is consulted at once. Surgery may be as simple as an incision of an anal membrane. With anorectal agenesis, a prompt colostomy will be necessary. Continence, on the other hand, is dependent on several factors, including sacral anomalies and proper surgery.

Common Malformations

Meningomyelocele. ***Meningomyelocele,*** a neural tube defect, is a herniation of part of the meninges (containing CSF and CNS tissue) through a defect in the vertebral column or skull. The defect often occurs in the lower back (Fig. 28-43). In the accompanying spinal malformation, ***spina bifida,*** the meningomyelocele extrudes through the opening of the spinal column. The opening is the result of a congenital absence of one or more vertebral arches. Occasionally a familial history (5% recurrence rate) of this anomaly is identified. Most cases are of unknown (infectious?) origin. A ***meningocele*** is also a herniation of the meninges. A meningocele contains CSF but does not contain CNS tissue (cord or nerve roots). Prenatal diagnosis of neural tube defects (meningomyelocele, meningocele, anencephaly) is now possible (Chapter 22).

If the neonate is born with a large defect, the nurse aids in preventing its rupture and infection before surgery. Protection of the defect includes the following actions:

1. Position with care.
   a. Position prone or side-lying with rolled towels to prevent pressure or injury to defect, thereby preventing portal of entry for infectious agents.
   b. Change position every hour to prevent pressure areas.
   c. If physician permits infant to be held, exercise caution to avoid injury to defect.
2. Provide skin care: skin around defect is cleansed and dried carefully to prevent breakdown, which would establish a portal of entry for infectious agents. Apply physician-ordered dressings, ointments, and so on.

The nurse assists in the diagnosis of a hidden defect (e.g., **spina bifida occulta**) (Fig. 28-43, *B*). The nurse assesses neurologic function and notes the following: paralysis of lower extremities, flaccidity and spasticity of muscles below defect, and sphincter control (character and number of voidings and stools; leakage of urine and stool).

Surgical repair often can be done in the neonatal period. If other anomalies, such as **hydrocephalus,** are present, delayed correction may be elected. Permanent impairment of neuromuscular function below the level of the defect depends on the amount of CNS tissue involved. In severe cases, voluntary and involuntary functions are absent. The prognosis is guarded. Only about 60% of cases are operable. Many of these children die or achieve only partial function. Hydrocephalus ultimately develops in virtually all of these infants.

The parents will need considerable support and instruction regarding the infant's care. In some instances parents may require assistance in placing the child in a special care facility.

Congenital Hydrocephalus. Congenital hydrocephalus is macrocephaly caused by abnormal enlargement of the cerebral ventricles and skull. Head enlargement is the result of increased intraventricular CSF pressure. This condition is accompanied by enlargement of the head, prominence of the forehead, "setting sun" sign of the eyes, atrophy of the brain, weakness, and convulsions as the condition worsens. Congenital hydrocephalus is encountered in approximately 1 in 2000 fetuses (about 12% of all malformations). Several types are known. Spina bifida occurs in approximately one third of infants born with hydrocephalus.

Surgery is usually performed soon after birth. If surgical shunting is not accomplished, increasing intracranial pressure, evidenced by palpably widening fontanels and sutures, lethargy, irritability, vomiting, or high-pitched shrill cry, results in irreversible neurologic damage.

Nursing actions appropriate to the needs of a newborn with hydrocephalus include careful documentation of ongoing observations. Meticulous skin care is necessary to prevent pressure areas and infection of the skin of the head. Lamb's wool, sheepskin, or a flotation mattress is used under the infant. Frequent position changing and keeping the newborn clean and dry helps maintain skin integrity and health.

The newborn's heavy head is supported carefully when being held or turned. The method, amount, and frequency of feeding are chosen to accomodate the infant's tolerance and energy level. Care is taken to prevent vomiting and subsequent aspiration. Nonnutritive sucking, touching, and cuddling needs are met.

Damaged or destroyed brain tissue cannot be restored. Spontaneous arrest of hydrocephalus may occur, but often surgical shunting may be required to eliminate excess CSF. Despite arrest of the process, serious mental retardation and neurologic sequelae are common.

Anencephaly and Microcephaly. Anencephaly and microcephaly are congenital fetal deformities in which the head is considerably smaller than normal. In anencephaly there is complete or partial absence of the brain and of the overlying skull. Because the pituitary gland is absent or vestigial, the adrenal cortex is diminutive (for lack of adrenocorticotropic hormone [ACTH] stimulation). About 70% of anencephalic infants are girls. This condition is commonly accompanied by hydramnios. The cause of anencephaly is unknown, but multiple environmental factors have been postulated. A 3% recurrence rate in familial histories has been noted. Anencephaly is incompatible with life; warmth and fluid are provided until the neonate's death, which is usually before the end of the first 24 hours after birth.

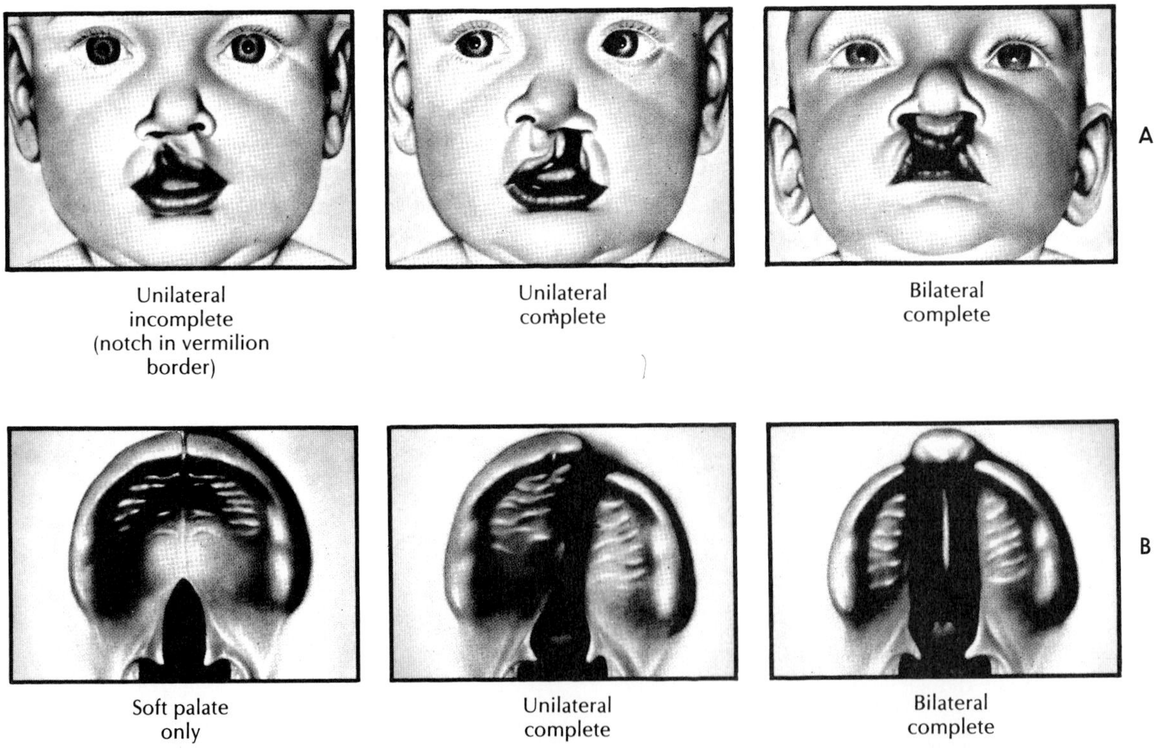

Fig. 28-44 **A,** Cleft lip. **B,** Cleft palate. (Courtesy Ross Laboratories, Columbus, Ohio.)

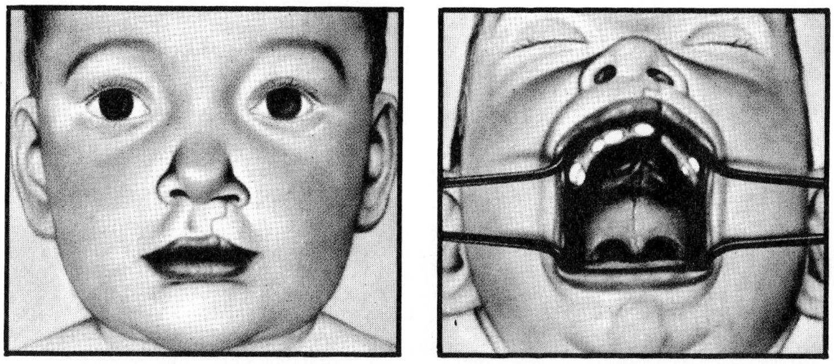

Fig. 28-45 Surgical repair of **A,** unilateral complete cleft lip and **B,** unilateral complete cleft palate. (Courtesy Ross Laboratories, Columbus, Ohio.)

In microcephaly the head generally is well formed but small. X-ray exposure of the woman may result in fetal microcephaly. Rubella, CMV, and perhaps other infectious processes are the causes in some cases. Microcephalic infants require specific nursing care and medical observation to appraise the extent of psychomotor retardation that almost always accompanies this abnormality. The nurse's supportive role with parents is considerable.

Cleft-lip or Palate. Cleft lip or palate is a common congenital midline fissure, or opening, in the lip or palate; one or both deformities may occur (Fig. 28-44). The incidence is approximately 1 in 700 white newborns and 1 in 2000 black newborns. Polygenetic factors are causative in some cases, but fetal viral infection, maternal corticosteroid therapy, radiation, dietary influence, and hypoxia have been associated factors. The combination of cleft lip and palate affects more male than female infants.

Treatment requires special feeding techniques, for example, the use of uniquely designed nipples (Procedure 28-2). Cleft lip repair may be done soon after delivery if the newborn is free of infection, in good condition, and weighs 2500 g (5 lb, 9 oz). Cleft lip repair (Fig. 28-45, *A*) is best done when the infant weighs 4500 g (10 lb) or more since there is more tissue to work with. Advantages of earlier labial (lip) repair include facilitating a positive parent-child relationship and permitting the infant to learn to use and strengthen musculature around the mouth. Infants with palatolabial fissures often look grotesque and repulsive to the parents. After repair and with collaborative health team support, the mother commonly is able to assume responsibility for the newborn's care until palatal repair is feasible (Fig. 28-45, *B*). Repair is done usually between 16 and 24 months of age (9 kg [20 lb] body weight or more). The plastic surgeon, pediatrician, orthodontist, hospital and community nurses, speech therapist, and social worker make up the collaborative health team that has made possible the effective treatment available today. Until repair of the palate is performed, a prosthesis is fitted to aid the infant's feeding and speech development and to reduce respiratory tract infections.

Musculoskeletal Disorders. The two most common musculoskeletal deviations seen in the neonatal period are congenital dysplasia of the hip and congenital clubfoot. Both conditions are easily recognized. Early detection and definitive treatment are mandatory for successful correction. Delay makes repair more difficult and prognosis less favorable.

Congenital Hip Dysplasia. Also known as *congenital dislocation of the hip,* this often hereditary disorder occurs more commonly in girls (Fig. 28-46) because of the structure of the pelvis. In this condition the acetabulum is abnormally shallow. The head of the femur becomes dislocated upward and backward to lie on the dorsal aspect of the ilium. The pressure of the displaced femoral head may form a false acetabulum on the ilium. A stretched joint capsule results, and ossification of the femoral head is delayed.

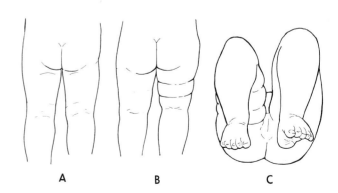

Fig. 28-46 Congenital dysplasia of hip. **A,** Normal gluteal and popliteal skin creases. **B,** Abnormal skin creases and asymmetry of skin folds. **C,** Apparent shortening of femur. Femur head is displaced. (Courtesy Ross Laboratories, Columbus, Ohio.)

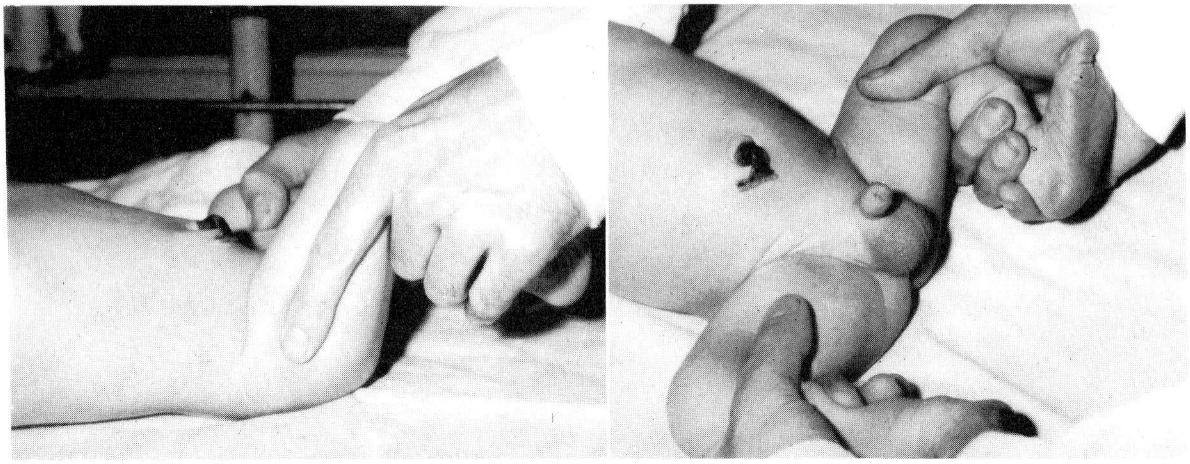
A B

Fig. 28-47 Method of assessing for hip dysplasia using Ortolani's maneuver. **A,** Examiner's middle fingers are placed over greater trochanter and thumbs over inner thigh opposite lesser trochanter. **B,** Gentle pressure is exerted to further flex thigh on hip, and thighs are rotated outward. If hip dysplasia is present head of femur can be felt to slip forward in acetabulum and slip back when pressure is released and legs returned to their original position. A click is sometimes heard (Ortolani's sign).

Before dislocation occurs, reduced movement, splinting of the affected hip, limited abduction, and asymmetry of the hip may be noted. After dislocation, all these signs will be present, together with the external rotation and shortening of the leg. A clicking sound may be noted on gentle forced abduction of the leg (Ortolani's sign, Fig. 28-47), and a bulge of the femoral head is felt or seen (Fig. 28-46, *B*). X-ray films will reveal a deformity in congenital dysplasia of the hip.

Treatment involves pressing the femoral head into the acetabulum to form an adequate socket before ossification is complete. The following methods are possible:

1. Thick diapers to abduct and externally rotate leg and flex hip (pin anterior flaps of diapers under posterior flaps).
2. Frejka pillow (apply diapers and plastic pants, and then apply pillow). Later this appliance will be followed by a spica cast in most instances to maintain abduction, extension, and internal rotation, usually with the infant in a "frog-leg" position.

Talipes Equinovarus. Talipes equinovarus, or clubfoot, is a congenital fixed deformity in which the foot is twisted out of shape or position. The heel is turned inward from the midline of the leg, the sole of the foot is flexed at the ankle joint, and the Achilles tendon is shortened.

Before the infant is 2 months old, often during the first days of life, successive plaster casts are applied first to correct the heel inversion and adduction of the forefoot and later, the equinus deformity. The prognosis depends on the extent of the deformity and the response to progressive orthopedic treatment.

Phocomelia. Phocomelia, or "seal-like limbs," is a developmental anomaly typified by absence of the arms or legs, or both, or stunting of the extremities. In the early 1960s the drug ***thalidomide*** was implicated as the causative agent for the limb deformities of many thousands of infants, especially in Germany. As a result the U.S. FDA tightened its regulations governing drug approval. Painfully apparent was evidence that drugs ingested during pregnancy may have tragic implications for fetal development. Thalidomide (and perhaps imipramine [Tofranil]) is a cause of this condition. Sporadic cases of congenital amputation or stunting are of unknown cause. The child born with these deformities requires special care.

Supportive care of the parents must begin at the birth of the child and continue for years. After the initial grief reaction, the parents need information regarding the rehabilitative and psychosocial components of their child's care.

Polydactyly. Extra digits on the hands or feet occur occasionally (Fig. 28-48). In some instances polydactyly is hereditary. If there is little or no bone involvement, the extra digit is tied with silk suture soon after birth. The finger falls off within a few days, leaving a small scar. When there is bone involvement, surgical repair is indicated.

Genitourinary Tract Anomalies. Abnormally low-set or misshapen ears may indicate other, often

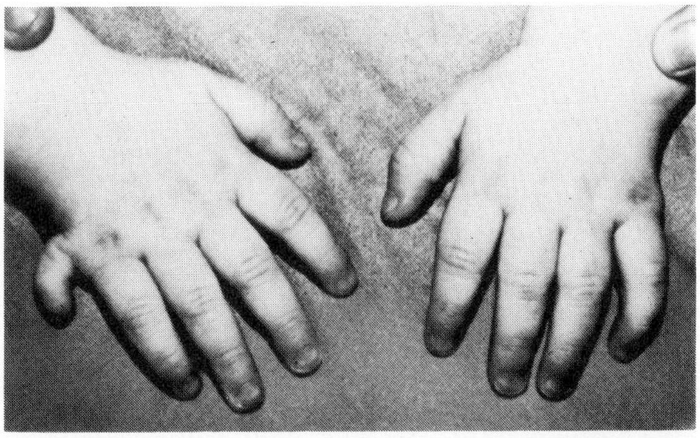

Fig. 28-48 Polydactyly: supernumerary digit of right hand. Most common congenital anomaly of upper extremity and is occasionally seen in conjunction with other congenital malformation. (Courtesy Mead Johnson & Co, Evansville, Indiana.)

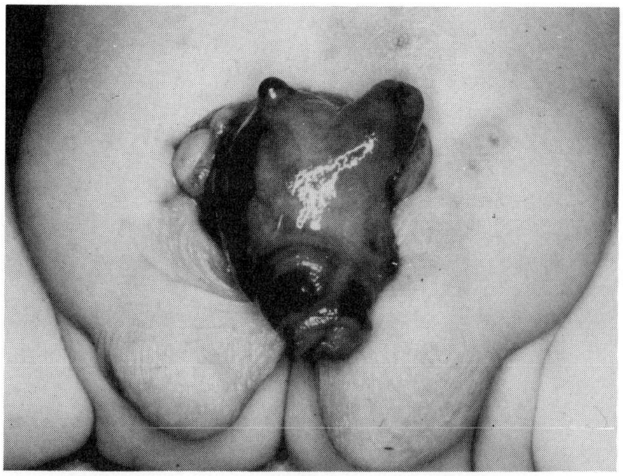

Fig. 28-49 Exstrophy of bladder. (Courtesy Edward S Tank, MD, Division of Urology, University of Oregon Health Sciences Center, Portland, Oregon.)

genitourinary, anomalies (such as renal agenesis) (see Fig. 16-13).

Exstrophy of the Bladder. Exstrophy of the bladder (Fig. 28-49) is a congenital anomaly of unknown cause. With this anomaly a separation of the symphysis pubis and anterior abdominal wall structures results in exteriorization of the bladder trigone and surrounding mucosa. The exposed mucosa is deep red, has numerous folds, and is sensitive to touch. A direct passage of urine to the outside occurs. Associated anomalies, such as undescended testes, inguinal hernia, absence of the vagina, or bowel defects, should be sought. Surgical correction, often elimination of the bladder and construction of an ileal conduit, is rarely justified in the neonatal period. A prosthesis for collection of the urine and protection of the bladder may be employed.

Nursing management in the presence of exstrophy of the bladder focuses on the prevention of urinary tract infection and ulceration of adjacent skin from the constant seepage of urine. The child's touching and cuddling needs are met. Parents require considerable support and teaching to care for the defect if surgery is scheduled when the infant is several weeks or months of age.

Hypospadias and Epispadias. Hypospadias is a developmental anomaly in which the urethral meatus is placed lower than normal. In an infant boy the meatus opens in the midline of the undersurface of the penis or on the perineum. In an infant girl the meatus opens into the vagina. This condition tends to be hereditary.

Epispadias, also occurring in both sexes but predominating in boys, is a congenital absence of the upper urethral wall. In girls it is often associated with exstrophy of the bladder. In boys the meatal opening is located anywhere along the dorsum (upper side) of the penis.

Most instances of hypospadias are minor and require no corrective surgery. Pronounced defects require extensive urethroplasty. If needed, surgery is completed before the boy enters school so that he can urinate from a standing position like other boys. The more serious defects often coexist with other, multiple anomalies.

Nursing management of the physical care of the infant with hypospadias is the same as that for the normal infant. Should urethroplasty be required, no circumcision is done, since the foreskin is used in the surgical procedure. The parents are taught how to care for the urethral meatus and foreskin to prevent infection and promote cleanliness.

Sexual Ambiguity. Sexual ambiguity in the newborn (Fig. 28-50) often is discovered by the nurse, who is usually the first one to perform a physical assessment. The obstetrician is still concentrating on the mother during the third stage of labor.

Erroneous or abnormal sexual differentiation may be a genetic aberration (for example, congenital adrenal hypoplasia), or it may be caused by maternal problems (such as steroid sex hormone therapy for threatened abortion). It is imperative to establish the genetic sex and the sex of child rearing as soon as possible. Early identification is imperative to save embarrassment of reporting the birth of a (genetic) male who in fact is a female or the opposite. Early determination of genetic sex is important to permit the surgical correction of anomalies before an individual or social pattern

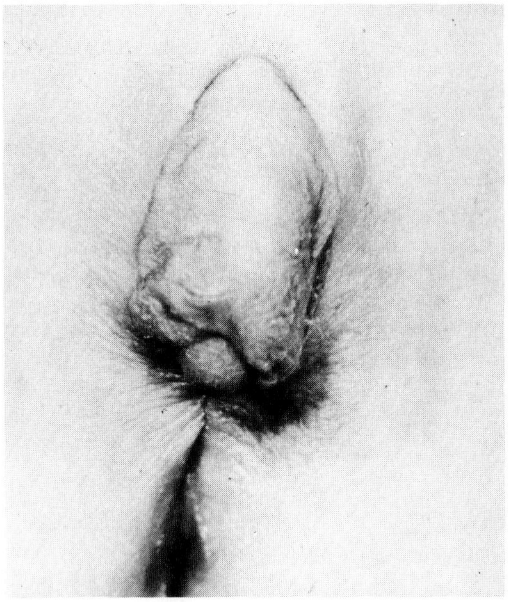

Fig. 28-50 Ambiguous external genitals (e.g., structure can be an enlarged clitoral hood and clitoris or a malformed penis). (Courtesy Edward S Tank, MD, Division of Urology, University of Oregon Health Sciences Center, Portland, Oregon.)

is set. Prompt consultation with a surgeon who is experienced in the area of intersexuality should be arranged without delay. Meanwhile parents need supportive care as they await the decision.

Teratoma. Teratoma, a solid or semisolid neoplasm, is composed of the three embryonal tissue types (ectoderm, mesoderm, entoderm). A teratoma in the newborn may occur in the skull, mediastinum, or abdomen. A solid or semisolid tumor in the sacral area also may prove to be a teratoma. It is protected by sterile dressings before surgical removal. Many teratomas diagnosed in the newborn are malignant. If the lesion cannot be removed entirely by surgery, x-ray therapy and chemotherapy are used. Long-term survival rate for infants with sacrococcygeal teratoma is 85% after surgical removal in the neonatal period. The survival rate is only 50% if surgery is delayed until the infant is more than 1 month old. Rectal and anal function can always be preserved.

Genetic Disease

At the present time there is no cure for genetic disease, although remedies can be implemented to prevent or reduce the harmful effects of a few disorders. Structural defects can sometimes be modified to produce normal or near-normal function. Research is continually being carried out in the hope that methods can be devised to influence or change the genes directly, thereby preventing the disease process. However, at this time the major thrust in therapy is modification of the internal or external environment to minimize the effects of the disease. Rapid advances in the field of plastic and reconstructive surgery have reduced the impact of many functional and cosmetically displeasing physical defects. In some hereditary disorders, supplying the missing product that cannot be synthesized prevents the undesirable effects, for example, thyroid extract for hereditary cretinism, corticosteroids for adrenogenital syndrome, insulin for diabetes mellitus, and administration of missing blood factors for the hemophilias.

Diet modification may be required for infants with some inborn errors of metabolism. For example, a low phenylalanine diet reduces the harmful effects of that protein in phenylketonuria (PKU). Some female children successfully treated for PKU are now of reproductive age and present unique management challenges to caregivers (p. 706). Other examples are substitution of lactose-free products for milk fed to infants and children with galactosemia, and use of a diet low in branched chain amino acids for infants and children with maple syrup urine disease.

Parental Support. Clarifying information and misunderstanding of information are important nursing functions. A newly diagnosed disorder often implies the implementation of a therapeutic regimen. For example, the disorder in question may be an inborn error of metabolism such as PKU or galactosemia that requires consistent and rigid adherence to a diet. The family may need help to secure the necessary formula and counseling from dietetic services. The importance of maintaining the diet, especially keeping an adequate supply of special preparations and avoiding unauthorized substitutions, must be impressed on the family.

Referral to appropriate agencies is another essential part of the follow-up management. Many organizations and foundations help provide services and equipment for affected children, for example, the Cystic Fibrosis Foundation and the Muscular Dystrophy Association. Early Infant Stimulation Foundation programs are available for a child born with Down's syndrome. There are also numerous parent groups with whom the family can share experiences and derive mutual support from other families with a similar problem. Nurses need to become familiar with services available in their community that provide assistance and education to families with these special problems (Appendix I).

Probably the most important of all nursing functions is providing *emotional support* to the family during all aspects of the care of the child born with a defect or disorder. Feelings that are generated under the real or imagined threat posed by a genetic disorder are as varied as the persons being counseled. Responses may include all stress reactions, such as apathy, denial, anger, hostility, fear, embarrassment, grief, and loss of self-esteem (Chapter 29).

Parents benefit from seeing before and after pictures of other babies born with this defect. Coupled with other verbal and nonverbal supportive care, this visual reassurance is effective. Parents can be referred to other parents (or organizations of parents such as the Cleft Palate Club) for continuing mutual support.

Guilt and self-blame are universal reactions. Many look on the disorder as a stigma—especially if the disorder is visible to others. Persons involved with the family are often able to dispel fears and even absolve the family from guilt simply by explaining the random nature of cell division and segregation. Parents may derive comfort from knowing that everyone carries defective genes, which, when combined with the same genes in a partner, can produce undesirable consequences. Old wives' tales, superstitions, and long-held misconceptions are all factors that may influence a client's reaction to a disorder. Obstacles such as religious beliefs, intellectual level, and prior attitudes toward the disease affect the way in which families respond.

The attitude of other family members and relatives can have a significant impact on some persons—especially in situations where the blame can be pinpointed (such as a dominant or an X-linked disorder). Recessive disorders are less likely to cause blaming, since both partners carry the defective gene. Unfortunately most families tend to view a congenital disorder as a cause for shame. Its presence in a family may be cause to alter plans for marriage or childbearing even when the probability of recurrence is no more than a random risk. The way a family views the probability of recurrence varies tremendously. For example, one family will consider a 10% risk as reassuring, whereas another may consider it too great a risk to contemplate marriage or childbearing.

The nature of a newborn's condition also influences the way families respond to a disorder. Factors such as the severity or chronicity of a disease, the age of onset, the threat of early death, a lengthy period of deterioration, presence or absence of pain, mental retardation, or cosmetic disfiguration all determine the impact that a condition will produce in a family. One family may risk having a child with a disorder that produces a minor defect or even an early death but will not risk having a child with a lifelong physical or mental disability.

Sometimes counselors and other health personnel create barriers through their own attitudes toward a specific disease. It is often difficult to be nonjudgmental and objective in all instances. Nurses may intentionally or unintentionally influence families in making decisions. This is especially true when the client's intellectual level makes it difficult or impossible for that person to comprehend the ramifications of a situation. Even persons who can repeat information accurately often fail to grasp its significance in their case. Families may pressure the nurse to make decisions for them with questions such as, "What would you do if you were me?"

Families and individuals need ongoing education, guidance, and support (Sammons and Lewis, 1985; Johnson, 1986). They should be given the facts and possible consequences and all the assistance they need in problem solving, but the final decision regarding a course of action must be their own.

Evaluation

Care is evaluated by assessing the degree to which goals have been met. On the short-term basis, care has been effective if the neonate's disorder has been treated appropriately and the condition has stabilized within normal limits; when the parents have begun to cope with the situation, initiate attachment to the newborn, and mobilize family support; and when appropriate community services have become involved therapeutically. Long-term evaluation is more difficult and is more relevant to pediatric and adult health care.

SUMMARY

The woman, her family, and the newborn at risk are highly vulnerable. Protection of the newborn by maintenance of a warm environment, adequate oxygen, and safety is an important part of the nurse's care. The newborn's nutrition, fluid and electrolyte, and elimination needs must be monitored and met carefully. The family of the woman experiencing a high-risk pregnancy, labor, and delivery and the birth of a newborn at risk requires skilled nursing care.

KEY CONCEPTS

- The nurse's primary contribution to the welfare of the newborn begins with early observation, accurate recording, and prompt reporting of signs indicative of deviations from normal.
- Nurses' skills in interpreting data, making decisions, and initiating therapy of the newborn at risk before transfer to an NICU are crucial to the infant's survival.
- The newborn at risk has special problems caused by immaturity, alterations in functioning of systems, and metabolic balances.
- Birth injuries range from those that are minor and resolve without treatment to those few that are serious enough to result in death.
- Prepregnancy planning and good diabetic control coupled with tight diabetic control during pregnancy may prevent the embryonic/fetal/neonatal conditions associated with pregnancies complicated by diabetes mellitus.
- Infection in the newborn may be acquired in utero, during delivery, during resuscitation, and from within the nursery.
- Injection of Rho(D) immune globulin to Rh-negative and Coombs'-negative women bestows passive immunity and minimizes the possibility of isoimmunization.
- Rehabilitative measures must be included in the plan for care for the newborn and the parent to offer the infant an opportunity for optimum growth and development after discharge.
- Involvement of the family (including spouse or sexual partner, parents, children, or other close relatives living with or near the woman) and community resources must be considered in the implementation of care for the newborn suffering the effects of conditions such as maternal infection or drug dependence, sequelae to gestational age or birth weight, and congenital anomalies.

LEARNING ACTIVITIES

1. For students with no previous experience with intensive care units: in groups of two, walk into an intensive care nursery (ICN) as if you were new parents of a newborn who was just admitted. Bring a notebook with you. Limit your visit to 30 minutes, but stay the *full* 30 minutes. Individually, jot down your observations, keeping the following in mind: describe your "gut reactions"; what do you notice first?; using all of your senses, make one observation for each item you observed; stand beside one newborn and focus in on everything you see within 15 cm (6 in) of the neonate; spend 15 minutes comparing notes with your partner.
2. Develop a general nursing care plan for the parents starting with the birth of a newborn at risk until the mother (who is reasonably healthy) is discharged from the hospital.
3. Have students "buddy up" with an ICN nurse for 1 clinical day. The clinical observation day should follow an orientation to the ICN so that the student can focus in on the experience to be described. Choose any of the following:
   a. Observe a complete physical assessment. Compare with the routine physical assessments in the well-baby nursery.
   b. Describe the newborn's willingness to interact with caregivers and to engage in eye-to-eye contact. Note your reactions to the neonate. Discuss implications for nursing care of the newborn and family, based on your findings.
   c. Calculate the percentage of weight gain and loss for three newborns at risk. Identify probable causes and describe nursing actions.
   d. Observe nursing care related to maintenance of respirations, temperature, and nutrition and elimination.
4. Choose a newborn at risk. Identify ethical issues involved. Discuss the identified issues (using content regarding ethical issue decision making in Chapter 3) from the following perspectives:
   a. As the professional nurse working with the newborn and family.
   b. As the parent.
   c. As the taxpayer/legislator who must decide how best to allocate funds among a variety of community needs.
5. In the clinical setting or in the laboratory, demonstrate techniques such as oxygen administration and application of thermistor probes, and monitoring of parenteral fluid administration.

References

General Care/Temperature Support/Maintenance of Nutrition/Emotional Aspects of Care

Amspacher KA: Necrotizing enterocolitis: the never-ending challenge, J Perinat Neonat Nurs 3(2):58, 1989.
Anderson GC, Marks EA, and Wahlberg V: Kangaroo care for premature infants, Am J Nurs 86(7):807, 1986.
Bernbaum JC et al: Non-nutritive sucking during gavage feeding enhances growth and maturation in premature infants, Pediatrics 71:41, 1983.

Brooten D et al: A randomized clinical trial of early hospital discharge and home follow-up of very-low-birth-weight infants, N Engl J Med 315:934, 1986.
Clark DA et al: Surfactant displacement by meconium free fatty acids: an alternative explanation for atelectasis in meconium aspiration syndrome, J Pediatr 110:765, 1987.
Fanaroff AA and Martin RJ, editors: Neonatal-perinatal medicine: diseases of the fetus and infant, ed 4, St Louis, 1987, The CV Mosby Co.
Galassanos MR and Giles RM: Perinatal and neonatal asphyxia and nursing management. In Angelini D, editor: Perinatal/neonatal nursing: a clinical handbook, Boston, 1986, Blackwell Scientific Publications, Inc.
Hodson WA and Truog WE: Critical care of the newborn, ed 2, Philadelphia, 1989, WB Saunders Co.
Kaplan M and Eidelman AT: Improved prognosis in severely hypothermic newborn infants treated by rapid rewarming, J Pediatr 105:468, 1984.
Merenstein GB and Gardner SL: Handbook of neonatal intensive care, ed 2, St Louis, 1989, The CV Mosby Co.
Milluncheck E and McArtor R: Fatal aspiration of a makeshift pacifier, Pediatrics 77:369, March, 1986.
Rehm R: Teaching cardiopulmonary resuscitation to parents, MCN 8:411, Nov/Dec, 1983.
Ress PE: Saving underweight babies in Bogota, Secretariat News 39(13):7, 1984 (United Nations Headquarters, New York).
Sandman K: Emergency stabilization in transport of the critically ill neonate, Crit Care Nurse 8(6):14, 1989.

Gestational Age and Birthweight

Affonso D and Harris T: Postterm pregnancy: implications for mother and infant, challenge for the nurse, JOGN Nurs 9:139, 1980.
Als H and Brazelton TB: A new model of assessing the behavioral organization in preterm and full term infants, J Am Acad Child Psychiatry 20:239, 1981.
Bancalari E and Gerhardt T: Bronchopulmonary dysplasia, Pediatr Clin North Am 33:1, 1986.
Bartlett RH et al: Extracorporeal circulation in neonatal respiratory failure: a prospective randomized study, Pediatrics 76:479, 1985.
Dubowitz LMS et al: Gestational age of the newborn, J Pediatr 77:1, 1970.
Field TM: Interaction patterns of preterm and term infants. In Field TM, editor: Infants born at risk, Jamaica, NY, 1979, Spectrum Publications.
Fomufod AK: Low birthweight and early neonatal separation as factors in child abuse, J Nat Med Assoc 68:106, 1976.
Gitlin JD et al: Randomized controlled trial of exogenous surfactant for the treatment of hyaline membrane disease, Pediatrics 79:31, 1987.
Hodgman JE: Neonatology, JAMA 258(16):2254, 1987.
Korones S: High-risk newborn infants: the basis for intensive nursing care, ed 4, St Louis, 1986, The CV Mosby Co.
Lawson EE: Exogenous surfactant therapy to prevent respiratory distress syndrome, J Pediatr 110:492, 1987.
Merritt TA et al: Prophylactic treatment of very premature infants with human surfactant, N Engl J Med 315:785, 1986.
Montgomery LA and Williams-Judge S: An anticipatory support program for high-risk parents, Neonatal Network 5:33, Aug, 1986.
Newman L: Parent perceptions of their low birth weight infant, Pediatrician 9:182, 1980.
Philip A: Neonatology: a practical guide, ed 3, Philadelphia, 1987, WB Saunders Co.
Sammons W and Lewis J: Premature babies: a different beginning, St Louis, 1985, The CV Mosby Co.
Schraeder BD: Attachment and parenting despite lengthy intensive care, MCN 5:37, 1980.
Sosa R and Grua P: Perinatal responses to normal and premature birth experiences, J Calif Perinat Assoc 2:36, 1982.
Turnage CS: Meconium aspiration syndrome, J Perinat Neonat Nurs 3(2):69, 1989.

Birth Trauma

Fanaroff AA and Martin RJ, editors: Neonatal-perinatal medicine: diseases of the fetus and infant, ed 4, St Louis, 1987, The CV Mosby Co.
Merenstein GB and Gardner SL: Handbook of neonatal intensive care, ed 2, St Louis, 1989, The CV Mosby Co.

Infants of Diabetic Mothers

Fanaroff AA and Martin RJ, editors: Neonatal-perinatal medicine: diseases of the fetus and infant, ed 4, St Louis, 1987, The CV Mosby Co.
Fuhrmann D et al: Prevention of congenital malformations in infants of insulin-dependent mothers, Diabetes Care 6:219, 1983.
Gutgesell HP et al: Characterization of the cardiomyopathy in infants of diabetic mothers, Circulation 61:441, 1980.
Pernoll ML, Benda GI, and Babson SG: Diagnosis and management of the fetus and neonate at risk: a guide for team care, ed 5, St Louis, 1986, The CV Mosby Co.
Philip A: Neonatology: a practical guide, ed 3, Philadelphia, 1987, WB Saunders Co.

Neonatal Infections

American Academy of Pediatrics, American College of Obstetricians and Gynecologists: Guidelines of perinatal care ed 2, Oak Grove Village, Ill, 1988, American Academy of Pediatrics.
Arevalo JA and Washington AE: Cost-effectiveness of prenatal screening and immunization for hepatitis B virus, JAMA, 259(3):365, 1988.
Bennett EC: Sexually transmitted diseases: current approaches, NAACOG Newletter 14(8):1, 1987.
Blocking hepatis B birth transmission, Med World News 28:17, 1987.
Brown AA et al: Effects on infants of a first episode of genital herpes during pregnancy, N Engl J Med 317(2):1249, 1987.
Cerase PA: Neonatal sepsis, J Perinat Neonat Nurs 3(2):48, 1989.
Facing the complex issues of pediatric AIDS: a public health perspective JAMA 258(19):2736, 1987 (editorial).
Fanaroff AA and Martin RJ, editors: Neonatal-perinatal medicine: diseases of the fetus and infant, ed 4, St Louis, 1987, The CV Mosby Co.
Harnish DG et al: Early detection of HIV infection in a newborn, N Engl J Med 316:272, 1987.
Harris M: S.F. Panel's Report: abortion urged in AIDS pregnancies, The San Francisco Chronicle, Jan 4, 1986.
HIV infection and childhood sexual abuse, JAMA 259(15):2235, 1988 (letter).
Hodson WA and Truog WE: Critical care of the newborn, ed 2, Philadelphia, 1989, WB Saunders Co.
Human immunodeficiency virus infection in women, JAMA 257(15):2074, 1987 (editorial).

Jackson MM et al: Clinical savvy: why not treat all body substances as infectious? Am J Nurs 87(9):1137, 1987.

Johnson JP, Nair P, and Alexander S: Early diagnosis of HIV infection in the neonate, N Engl J Med 316:273, 1987.

Klug RM: AIDS beyond the hospital: part two of a CE feature—children with AIDS, Am J Nurs 86(10):1126, 1986.

Landesman S et al: Serosurvey of human immunodeficiency virus infection in parturients, JAMA 258(19):2701, 1987.

Leishman K: Heterosexuals and AIDS: the second stage of the epidemic, The Atlantic Monthly, p 39, Feb, 1987.

Main D and Mennuti M: Neural tube defects: issues in prenatal diagnosis and counseling, Obstet Gynecol 67:1, 1986.

Marion RW et al: Human T cell lymphotrophic virus type III (HTLV-III) embryopathy: a new dysmorphia syndrome, Am J Dis Child 140:638, 1986.

Marwick C: Routine screening considered to end perinatal hepatitis transmission, JAMA 257(15):1999, 1987.

Measles shots advised for kids with AIDS, San Francisco Chronicle, April 4, 1988.

Merenstein GB and Gardner SL: Handbook of neonatal intensive care, ed 2, St Louis, 1989, The CV Mosby Co.

Monif G and Hardt W: Management of herpetic vulvovaginitis in pregnancy, Semin Perinatol 7:16, 1985.

Morningstar PJ and Chitwood DD: How women and men get cocaine: sex role stereotypes and acquisition patterns, J Psychoactive Drugs 19(2):135, 1987.

Pahwa S et al: Spectrum of human T-cell lymphotropic virus type III infection in children: recognition of symptomatic, asymptomatic, and seronegative patients, JAMA 255:2299, 1986.

Pernoll ML, Benda GI, and Babson SG: Diagnosis and management of the fetus and neonate at risk: a guide for team care, ed 5, St Louis, 1986, The CV Mosby Co.

Petit C: Stanford researchers find flaw in herpes test, San Francisco Chronicle, p 24, Jan 29, 1987.

Prenatal care and HIV screening, JAMA 258(19):2693, 1987 (letter to editor).

Prober CG: Low risk of herpes simplex virus infections in neonates exposed to the virus at the time of vaginal delivery to mothers with recurrent genital herpes simplex virus infections, N Engl J Med 316:240, 1987.

Public Health Service guidelines for counseling and antibody testing to prevent HIV infection and AIDS, MMWR 36:509, 1987.

Pyun KH et al: Perinatal infection with human immunodeficiency virus: specific antibody responses by the neonate, N Engl J Med 317(10):611, 1987.

Rubella/hepatitis B precautions advised, NAACOG Newsletter 13(4):April, 1986.

Syphilis cases up 35 percent in state, San Francisco Chronicle, p 4A, Jan 29, 1988.

Substance Abuse

Abel EL and Sokol RJ: Incidence of fetal alcohol syndrome and economic impact of FAS-related anomalies, Drug Alcohol Depend, 1988.

Bartlett D and Davis A: Recognizing fetal alcohol syndrome in the nursery, JOGN Nurs 9:23, 1980.

Bean Y: Report of ongoing research on the infants of mothers using cocaine and PCP, Los Angeles Times, January, 1986.

Chasnoff IJ et al: Cocaine use in pregnancy, N Engl J Med 313:666, 1985.

Davis RP and Keith L: Fetal alcohol syndrome: incurable but preventable, Contemp OB/GYN 21(3):57, 1983.

DHHS: The health consequences of smoking for women: a report of the Surgeon General, Pub No 410-889/1284, Washington, DC, 1983, Department of Health and Human Services

Fanaroff AA and Martin RJ: Neonatal-perinatal medicine: diseases of the fetus and infant, ed 4, St Louis, 1987, The CV Mosby Co.

Food and Drug Administration: Caffeine and pregnancy, FDA Drug Bulletin, 10:19, 1980.

Greenland S et al: The effects of marijuana use during pregnancy. I. A preliminary epidemiology study, Am J Obstet Gynecol 150:23, 1984.

Howard J: Report of ongoing research on the infants of mothers using cocaine and PCP, Los Angeles Times, January, 1986.

Landry M and Smith DE: CRACK: anatomy of an addiction, part 2, Calif Nurs Rev 9(3):28, 1987.

Linn S et al: No association between coffee consumption and adverse outcomes of pregnancy, N Engl J Med 306:141, 1982.

Luck W et al: Nicotine and cotinine: two pharmacologically active substances as parameters for the strain on fetuses and babies of mothers who smoke, J Perinatal Med 10:107, 1982.

McCarthy P: Fetal alcohol syndrome, Nurse Practitioner: Am J Primary Health Care 8:34, 1983.

Merker L, Higgins P, and Kinnard E: Assessing narcotic addiction in neonates, Pediatr Nurs 11:177, 1985.

Naeye RL and Peters EC: Mental development of children whose mothers smoked during pregnancy, Obstet Gynecol 64:60, 1984.

Nieberg L et al: The fetal tobacco syndrome JAMA 253:2998, 1985 (commentary).

Niebyl JR: Drug use in pregnancy, ed 2, Philadelphia, 1988, Lea & Febiger.

Stein ZA and Sussler M: Intrauterine growth retardation: epidemiological issues and public health significance, Semin Perinatal 8:5, 1984.

Zuspan FP: When drugs and alcohol complicate pregnancy, Contemp OB/GYN 24(1):35, 1984.

Hyperbilirubinemia and Congenital Anomalies

Cohen FL: Neural tube defects: epidemiology, detection, and prevention, JOGN Nurs 16(2):105, 1987.

Fanaroff AA and Martin RJ, editors: Neonatal-perinatal medicine: diseases of the fetus and infant, ed 4, St Louis, 1987, The CV Mosby Co.

Johnson SH: Nursing assessment and strategies for the family at risk: high-risk parenting, ed 2, Philadelphia, 1986, JB Lippincott Co.

Kogan SC, Doherty M, and Gitschier J: An improved method for prenatal diagnosis of genetic diseases by analysis of amplified DNA sequences, N Engl J Med 317:985, 1987.

Lewis C and Mocarski V: Obstetric ultrasound: application in a clinic setting, JOGN Nurs 16(1):56, 1987.

Locklin M: Assessing jaundice in full-term newborns, Pediatr Nurs 13(1):15, 1987.

Main DM and Mennuti MT: Neural tube defects: issues in prenatal diagnosis and counselling, Obstet Gynecol 67:1, 1986.

Pernoll ML, Benda GI, and Babson SG: Diagnosis and management of the fetus and neonate at risk: a guide for team care, ed 5, St Louis, 1986, The CV Mosby Co.

Perry SE, Parer JT, and Inturrisi M: Intrauterine transfusion for severe isoimmunization, MCN 11(3):182, 1986.

Routine prenatal genetic screening, N Engl J Med 317(22):1407, 1987 (editorial).
Sammons WA and Lewis JM: Premature babies: a different beginning, St Louis, 1985, The CV Mosby Co.
Tucker S: Pocket nurse guide to fetal monitoring, St Louis, 1988, The CV Mosby Co.
Wu PY et al: Transcutaneous bilirubinometry: factors affecting the correlation of TcB index and serum bilirubin, J Perinatol 5:41, Summer, 1985.

Bibliography

General

Blackburn S and Lowen L: Impact of an infant's premature birth on the grandparents and parents, JOGN Nurs 15(2):173, 1986.
Brooten D: RN follow-up plan helps high-risk infants, Am Nurse, Feb, 1988.
Censullo M: Home care of the high-risk newborn, JOGN Nurs 15:146, March/April, 1986.
Consolvo CA: Relieving parental anxiety in the care-by-parent unit, JOGN Nurs 15:154, March/April, 1986.
Franck LS: A national survey of the assessment and treatment of pain and agitation in the neonatal intensive care unit, JOGN Nurs 16(6):384, 1987.
Gennaro S: Anxiety and problem-solving ability in mothers of premature infants, JOGN Nurs 15:160, March/April, 1986.
Grabauskas P et al: Helping the parents after a baby's death, RN, p 31, Aug, 1987.
Harrison LL and Twardosz S: Teaching mothers about their preterm infants, JOGN Nurs 15:165, March/April, 1986.
Human milk and the premature baby, Nutr Rev 46:287, 1988.
Keating SB and Kelman GB: Home health care nursing: concepts and practice, Philadelphia, 1988, JB Lippincott Co.
Kemp V and Page C: Maternal prenatal attachment in normal and high-risk pregnancies, JOGN Nurs 16(3):179, 1987.
Korones SB: High-risk newborn infants: the basis for intensive nursing care, ed 4, St Louis, 1986, The CV Mosby Co.
Moen JE et al: Axillary versus rectal temperatures in preterm infants under radiant warmers, JOGN Nurs 16(5):348, 1987.
Moore MC: Total parenteral nutrition for infants, Neonatal Network 6(2):33, 1987.
NAACOG: Ethical decision making in OGN nursing practice, OGN Nurs Pract Res, R26, Oct 1987, The Association. (The Nurses Association of the American College of Obstetricians and Gynecologists, 409 Twelfth Street, SW, Washington, DC, 20024-2191, 202/638-0026)
Sadler ME: When your patient's baby dies before birth, RN, p 28, Aug, 1987.
Stevenson DK, Frankel LR, and Benitz WE: Immediate management of the asphyxiated infant: facilitating the cardiorespiratory transition from fetus to newborn, J Perinatol 7(3):221, 1987.
Weibley TT, Adamson M, and Clinkscales N: Gavage tube insertion in the premature infant, MCN 12(1):24, 1987.
Whaley LF and Wong DL: Essentials of pediatric nursing, ed 3, St Louis, 1989, The CV Mosby Co.
Young LY, Creighton DE, and Suave RS: The needs of families of infants discharged home with continuous oxygen therapy, JOGN Nurs 17(3):187, 1988.

Preterm Infant

Clinical News: Breast is best—for preemies too, Am J Nurs 87(11):1403, 1987.
Fanaroff AA and Martin RJ: Neonatal-perinatal medicine: diseases of the fetus and infant, ed 4, St Louis, 1987, The CV Mosby Co.

Infants with Problems Related to Gestational Age and Weight

Fay MJ: The positive effects of positioning, Neonatal Network 6(5):23, 1988.
Gangitano E: Protocol: hypoglycemia, J Perinatology 7(1):72, 1987.
Kleinman JC and Kessell SS: Racial differences in low birth weight: trends and risk factors, N Engl J Med 317:749, Sept, 1987.
Meier P and Wilks S: The bacteria in expressed mothers' milk, MCN 12(6):420, 1987.
Sims ME, Jasani N, and Hodgman JE: Care of very low birth weight infants with neonatal nurse clinicians, J Perinatology 7(1):55, 1987.

Birth Injuries and Infants of Diabetic Mothers

Grabauskas P et al: Helping the parents after a baby's death, RN, p 31, Aug, 1987.
Kemp VH and Page CK: The psychosocial impact of a high-risk pregnancy on the family, JOGN Nurs 15(3):232, 1986.
Korones SB: High-risk newborn infants: the basis for intensive nursing care, ed 4, St Louis, 1986, The CV Mosby Co.
Troy P et al: Sibling visiting in the NICU, Am J Nurs 88(1):68, 1988.
Whaley LF and Wong DL: Nursing care of infants Essentials of pediatric nursing, ed 3, St Louis, 1989, The CV Mosby Co.

Neonatal Infections

Becker L and Lagomarsino W: Isolation guidelines for perinatal patients: creating a new protocol, MCN 12(6):400, 1987.
Bromberg MH and Hsia LS: Rubella in the perinatal period, J Perinat Neonat Nurs 1(4):24, 1988.
California Nurses Association (CNA): Infection control precautions, (Correspondence) Sept, 1987, The Association.
Cohen SP: Bacterial sepsis in the very low birth weight infant, J Perinat Neonat Nurs 1(4):66, 1988.
Gershon A: Chickenpox: how dangerous is it? Contemp OB/GYN 31(3):41, 1988.
Gordin PC: Candida infection in the very low birth weight infant, J Perinat Neonat Nurs 1(4):47, 1988.
Ippolito C and Gives RM: AIDS and the newborn, J Perinat Neonat Nurs 1(4):78, 1988.
Kaunitz AM et al: Prenatal care and HIV screening, JAMA 258(19):2693, 1987.
Klein ME: Hepatitis B virus: perinatal management, J Perinat Neonat Nurs 1(4):12, 1988.
Marecki MA: *Chlamydia trachomatis:* a developing perinatal problem, J Perinat Neonat Nurs 1(4):1, 1988.
Marvin C and Slevin A: Chlamydia—cause, prevention, and cure, MCN 12(5):318, 1987.
Minkoff HL et al: Pregnancies resulting in infants with acquired immunodeficiency syndrome: description of the antepartum, intrapartum, and postpartum course, Obstet Gynecol 69:285, 1987.

Minkoff HL et al: Follow-up of mothers of children with AIDS, Obstet Gynecol 87:288, 1987.
MMWR Supplement: Recommendations for prevention of HIV transmission in health-care settings, MMWR 36:2S, Aug, 1987.
Samson LF: Perinatal viral infection and neonates, J Perinat Neonat Nurs 1(4):56, 1988.
Stear LA and Elinger SS: Understanding acquired immunodeficiency syndrome: implications for pregnancy, J Perinat Neonat Nurs 1(4):April, 1988.
Treatment of sexually transmitted diseases, Med Lett 32(810):5, 1990.
Troy P et al: Sibling visiting in the NICU, Am J Nurs 88(1):68, 1988.

Substance Abuse

Bingue N et al: Cocaine teratogenicity in humans, J Pediatr 110:93, 1987.
Dixon SD, Coen RW, and Crutchfield S: Visual dysfunction in cocaine-exposed infants, Pediatr Res 21:359, 1987 (abstract).
MacGregor S et al: Cocaine use during pregnancy: adverse perinatal outcome, Am J Obstet Gynecol 157(3), 686, 1987.
Oro AS and Dixon SD: Perinatal cocaine and methamphetamine exposure: maternal and neonatal correlates, J Pediatr 111(4):571, 1987.
Silver H et al: Addiction in pregnancy: high risk intrapartum management and outcome, J Perinatol 7(3):178, 1987.
Woods J, Plessinger M, and Clark K: Effect of cocaine on uterine blood flow and fetal oxygenation, JAMA 257:957, 1987.

Hyperbilirubinemia and Congenital Anomalies

Censullo M: Home care of the high-risk newborn, JOGN Nurs 15:146, March/April, 1986.
Consolvo CA: Relieving parental anxiety in the care-by-parent unit, JOGN Nurs 15:154, March/April, 1986.
Erlen JA and Holzman IR: Anencephalic infants: should they be organ donors? Pediatr Nurs 14(1):60, 1988.
Gross SJ et al: Sacrococcygeal teratoma: prenatal diagnosis and management, Am J Obstet Gynecol 156(2):393, 1987.
Harris SR: Early detection of cerebral palsy: sensitivity and specificity of two motor assessment tools, J Perinat 7(1):11, Winter, 1987.
Kemp V and Page C: Maternal prenatal attachment in normal and high-risk pregnancies, JOGN Nurs 16(3):179, 1987.
Segal S et al: The death of a child—parents' views of professional support, Can Med Assoc 134:38, Jan 1, 1986.
Whaley LF and Wong DL: Essentials of pediatric nursing, ed 3, St Louis, 1989, The CV Mosby Co.

Resources for Down's Syndrome

The National Association for Down's Syndrome, Dept. N83, Box 63, Oak Park, Ill, 60303, and the Down's syndrome Congress, Dept N83, 1640 W Roosevelt Rd, Chicago, Ill, 60608. For additional help, contact national and local associations for the mentally retarded.

CHAPTER

29 Loss and Grief

Irene M. Bobak

Learning Objectives

Correctly define the key terms listed.

Describe common behavioral and somatic manifestations of the grief response.

Formulate at least five examples of appropriate nursing diagnoses related to grief.

Describe how the nurse helps meet the special needs of the woman and her family experiencing loss and grief.

Develop criteria to evaluate nursing care for grieving clients.

Evaluate possible reactions of the nurse when caring for clients experiencing loss and grief.

Key Terms

acceptance
acute mourning
anticipatory grief
bargaining
bereavement
developing awareness
dysfunctional grieving
grieving process
replacement child
resolution
role-playing
shock and disbelief
validating loss

Perinatal bereavement is a significant situational crisis for the parents, their family, and the family's social network (Krone, 1988). A death when birth is expected is a powerful loss, devastating to parents' hopes and expectations. The experience of perinatal death (or birth of a child with a defect) is a *personal and physical loss* for parents—a part of themselves, their spirit, and their future is gone forever (Krone, 1988). It is also a *social loss*—loss of self-esteem in not meeting societal expectations of producing a healthy child. Experienced maternity nurses recognize the need to be prepared to meet the grief and grieving needs of women and their families.

Pregnancy and birth constitute an identity crisis situation in which everything is expected to proceed normally. During this natural transition in the woman's life cycle, she examines and actively relates to her femininity, sexuality, and capacity for motherhood. An unnatural or unexpected interruption in the process poses a real or potential threat to a woman's self-esteem and femininity. Possible threats to maternal health include abortion (spontaneous, elective, or therapeutic), nonmarital pregnancy, preterm or postterm delivery, birth trauma, placing the baby for adoption, stillbirth, neonatal death, or the birth of a child with a defect.

When expectations of birth and joy are replaced by loss, the nurse's role is critical. Nurses must be able to cope constructively with their responses to loss and grief to meet the woman's needs. As in any crisis situation, the nurse's problems may be reactivated by those presented by the woman and her family. The nurse also becomes vulnerable as these internal conflicts emerge while helping the woman cope with her problems.

❑ GRIEF REACTION

When an individual experiences a loss, the person's reactions follow a somewhat predictable pattern. Grieving, **bereavement,** or mourning are terms used to describe the expected reactions that follow a loss or a perceived threat of a loss. The **grieving process** has been described by Lindemann (1944) and Kübler-Ross (1969). Their interpretations of the grieving process may be compared as follows:

Lindemann (Three Phases)	Kübler-Ross (Five Stages)
1. Shock and disbelief	1. Denial and isolation: "No, not me!"
	2. Anger: "Why me?"
	3. **Bargaining:** "If I . . ."
2. Developing awareness and acute mourning	4. Depression and acute grief: "How can I . . ."
3. Resolution or acceptance	5. Acceptance: "I can, I must."

Lindemann's three phases of grieving are explained further.

Shock and Disbelief. During the period immediately after the loss, the person struggles with the reality of the event and may even deny its existence. This is the **shock and disbelief** phase. This natural shielding is a sign of psychologic health. Mental symptoms may include restlessness, confusion, and apathy. The following somatic manifestations are common: dizziness, lightheadedness or syncope, pallor, perspiration, tachycardia, palpitations, and nausea and other gastrointestinal tract symptoms. Sensations of somatic distress seem to occur in waves and last from 20 to 60 minutes. The somatic manifestations include a tendency to sighing respirations, complaints of lack of strength and exhaustion, and an alteration in appetite and in the taste of food.

Developing Awareness and Acute Mourning. During the **developing awareness** and **acute mourning** phase, reality of the loss begins to penetrate awareness; interest in daily affairs, established relationships, and activity diminishes. Feelings of sadness, yearning, self-depreciation, depression, guilt, helplessness, and hopelessness surface. Yearning for that which was lost may take the form of intense information-seeking. Intense feelings of loneliness or emptiness, a strong urge to cry, and preoccupation with the loss are common. Blame may be internalized or projected onto others. *Anger and frustration* are common characteristics. Exhaustion and shortness of breath may occur occasionally.

Resolution or Acceptance. Recovering from grief may take a year or longer, although the acute period lasts approximately 6 weeks. With **resolution,** or **acceptance,** of the grieving process, the person gradually resumes daily activities, reestablishes pre-crisis relationships in light of the crisis event, forms new relationships, and becomes less preoccupied with the loss.

❑ NURSING CARE

The critical period for intervention is in the immediate crisis period. The goal of crisis intervention is to help the woman and her family begin *now* to grieve appropriately. The nurse must be aware of individual differences and cultural proscriptions for mourning and the expression of grief when assessing the appropriateness of the grief response.

Assessment

Nurses can anticipate a wide range of unique responses from the bereaved (Carter, 1989). Many factors influence the client's individual reaction. The person's level of growth and development, experience with past losses, and perception of loss affect one's concept of loss. The meanings that people attribute to birth and death are highly individualized (Swanson-Kauffman, 1988). Cultural and spiritual beliefs may promote or hinder the expression and resolution of grief. Societal expectations about sex role behavior influence the expression of grief, with women generally more open in expression than men. The nature of the relationship one has with a significant other affects how one grieves if the other dies or has a loss. Socioeconomic factors are important because they affect the availability of resources for coping with loss.

Data are gleaned from available prenatal, intranatal, and postnatal records. The woman's age is important since a child's or adolescent's needs are different from those of a middle-aged woman. The woman is assessed for variables that affect her responses (e.g., analgesia, fatigue, discomfort, lack of sleep, concurrent medical or surgical condition). The woman's obstetric history is reviewed: gravidity, parity, any difficulty in conceiving, abortion (elective or spontaneous).

Bereaved clients (i.e., parents, grandparents, siblings) are observed for *signs and symptoms* of grieving. The findings are compared with those characteristic of shock and disbelief and developing awareness and acute mourning. The client may be quiet, composed, upset, or crying. Denial may be evident in comments such as "I just don't believe it." Anger toward the staff or others is possible: "Why do I have to feel any pain? Give me something *now*!"; "If only the doctor had. . . ."; "If I had only. . . ."

Clients are assessed for their level of *understanding of the grieving process.* Previous experiences with loss and coping mechanisms that were effective are identified.

External support systems are explored. The nurse assesses the availability of relatives, whether their behavior and presence are supportive, and whether they are interested and able to be there to provide emotional support and physical comfort. Some clients have access to support from community sources such as work, school, and church. The nurse assesses the level of the client's expressed anxiety. What is her or her family's understanding of what is happening?

The family's desire and need to see or hold the lost fetus/newborn is determined. The family's need to have clergy, nurse, physician, or others present during the viewing is noted. Desire for baptism or other ceremony is assessed. The nurse assesses the parents' reactions as they face the need to tell their older child, children, other family members, and friends.

A checklist (Fig. 29-1) can be developed to assist with assessment. Assessment findings are used to develop and implement a plan of care since the assess-

Checklist for Assisting Parents Experiencing Perinatal Loss

Date/Time	Check ( ) to Indicate Completion	Signature
	( ) Inform all shift personnel of loss	
	( ) Prior to viewing, discuss baby's appearance with family (skin color, anomalies)	
	Provide Memories	
	( ) Saw baby after delivery ______Mother ______Father	
	( ) Touched/held baby ______Mother ______Father	
	( ) Repeat request to see baby again ______Mother ______Father	
	( ) Photos of baby ______unclothed ______with blanket ______with family	
	( ) Given option to bathe and dress baby ______Yes ______No	
	( ) Crib card ( ) ID bracelets ( ) Footprints	
	( ) Lock of hair ( ) Memory book	
	Post Delivery Options	
	( ) Requested baptism _________Yes _________No Performed by: ______________________________	
	( ) Discussed burial options (hospital, funeral*) ______Mother ______Father	
	( ) Discussed transfer off Perinatal Unit	
	( ) Discussed autopsy ____Yes ____No	
	( ) Offered genetic studies ____Yes ____No	
	( ) Discussed informing siblings and friends*	
	( ) Discuss availability of parent-to-parent support group*	
	( ) Discuss common emotional/physical reactions to loss	
	Resource Material	
	( ) Rainbow phamplet	
	( ) Sibling coloring book	
	( ) Funeral fact sheet	
	( ) Community resource list	
	( ) Bibliography of books on grieving/loss	
	( ) Grieving booklet	
	*Written resource available	

Fig. 29-1 Resolve Through Sharing: Checklist for assisting parent(s) experiencing stillbirth or newborn death.

ment process validates for the clients that grief reactions are normal and help is available.

Nursing Diagnoses

Nursing diagnoses may include physiologic and psychosocial problems related to grieving or problems occurring in the grieving process itself. Examples of nursing diagnoses include the following:

Anxiety or situational low self-esteem related to
- Lack of understanding of the grieving process

Ineffective individual (or family) coping related to
- Perinatal death of fetus or newborn or mother

Knowledge deficit related to
- Loss and the grieving process

Altered family processes/parenting related to
- Loss of a family member, maternal morbidity, or birth of a child with a disorder

Powerlessness related to
- Loss and grief

Sleep pattern disturbance related to
- Grieving process

Spiritual distress (distress of the human spirit) related to
- Loss and grieving process

Altered sexual patterns related to
- Physiologic healing and grieving
- Inability to produce a healthy baby
- Desire to quickly replace baby who has died

Planning

During this important step, goals are set in client-centered terms. The goals are prioritized. Nursing actions are selected to meet the goals.

Goals may include the following:

1. The woman retains a positive sense of self-esteem and self-worth as a woman, mother, and sexual being
2. The woman and family appraise the situation realistically (e.g., ambivalent or negative feelings toward the pregnancy did not cause the loss)
3. The woman and family receive anticipatory guidance regarding components of the grieving process and possible reactions of family and friends
4. The woman and her family can verbalize their feelings and an understanding of the grieving process
5. The woman and her family rehearse (role play) approaches to communicate loss to family and friends
6. The woman and her family are able to utilize community and family resources for support
7. The woman and her family verbalize satisfaction with the support received from caregivers
8. Religious beliefs of the woman and her family are respected.

Implementation

Mothers and families look to the hospital staff to meet their needs. Having had an unfortunate maternity experience, these mothers may suffer a severe blow to their sense of worth associated with the ability to give life. Their role concept, self-esteem, and femininity may be diminished. Nursing interventions that assist the grieving family in coping with this ego-threatening experience may foster a healthy mourning process and can be incorporated easily within the busiest nursing assignment.

Regardless of the specific loss experienced, some nursing actions are appropriate to all. Therapeutic communication techniques help the mother and family understand the meaning of the loss, share feelings, and move less stressfully through the grieving process. Interventions to maintain the client's self-esteem involve active listening, responding positively to requests, maintaining confidentiality, providing physical comfort and support, and meeting spiritual needs. Involvement in decision-making increases the parent's sense of power and control. A checklist (see Fig. 29-1) reminds the nurse of topics to cover, encourages client participation in decision-making, and validates for the bereaved that their reactions reflect a normal response to grief.

Physical Comfort

Coping with grief and recovering from childbirth exact a heavy toll on the mother's resources. She may be recovering from an abdominal incision or an episiotomy or laceration repair. Hemorrhoids are a common source of discomfort. Afterpains and engorgement serve as reminders of having given birth (see Chapter 18 for initiation and maintenance of lactation if the mother is providing milk for a compromised newborn.) Nonpharmacologic comfort measures are implemented first (Chapter 21). Hands-on interventions provide tangible evidence of caring. Analgesics are employed judiciously; sleeping pills do not guarantee restful sleep and may even delay the grieving process. Although the grieving process often makes sleep difficult and appetite nonexistent, adequate rest and diet must be assured to replenish the mother's vitality.

Emotional Comfort

A nurturing, supportive network is one of the most critical factors in healthful grieving (Ilse and Furrh,

1988). Many interventions provide emotional support directly or indirectly. *Knowledge of the grieving process,* open communication, and involvement in decision-making are emotionally supportive. Individuals experiencing a loss need to understand grief reactions to help dispel fear of the unknown and know that their feelings are 'normal.' In addition, the nurse needs to educate the family's support system about the dynamics of grief, what to expect, and how they can help (Ilse and Furrh, 1988). Parents need to feel that those around them know that it is natural for them to feel sad, weepy, and easily distracted. Nurses should convey to parents that grieving takes time and that they may never really "get over it," although the pain does ease with time; good memories then tend to persist.

When nursing and medical staff act as role-models by being able to communicate comfortably and openly about death and grief reactions and feelings, the family may be better able to face and cope with their situation. Through role-modeling, the nurse can foster *open communication* between parents and family and staff. Therefore they do not have to divert energy to keeping up a front. Open communication in a supportive environment gives permission to grieve, validates appropriateness of grieving here and now in a manner acceptable to them, and gives permission to speak of death. People experiencing loss may need to ask the same questions repeatedly from the same or other people. Answers may need to be brief, given frequently, and offered with patience and understanding. Information is given clearly and in understandable terms. Sentences are kept short and simple.

Verbal repetition of the experience helps one cope with a situation and integrate it into one's perception of self in a nonthreatening manner. The nurse must indicate genuine interest and a willingness to sit and listen actively and objectively to the woman and family. The nurse encourages and assists verbalization of any of the following: feelings of loss or being cheated; fear that woman may not be able to ever carry a pregnancy and give birth to a healthy term newborn or that there is something 'wrong' with her; any feelings, actions, or lack of action that the woman or family may believe caused the incident; and reflections on previous pregnancies, labors, or any grief experience. Nurses need to be prepared for the anger and self-blame parents may feel. Parents may not be able to work through their anger before discharge; some parents return or write many months later to apologize for their behavior and to thank those who were able to see beyond their anger and help them with their needs.

Participation in decision-making helps dispel the feelings of powerlessness and being 'out of control.' The mother needs to be consulted as to whether she prefers to spend her postpartum recovery on the maternity unit. Some mothers believe that being on the maternity unit will assist them in working through their grief. Others believe that it would be unbearable to hear babies crying and see other mothers holding their newborns. Another issue concerns the nursery and layette that had been prepared for the expected child. Sometimes family members believe that it is important to take down the nursery before the mother returns home. Many mothers relate how helpful it was for them to personally pack and store the clothes and equipment themselves.

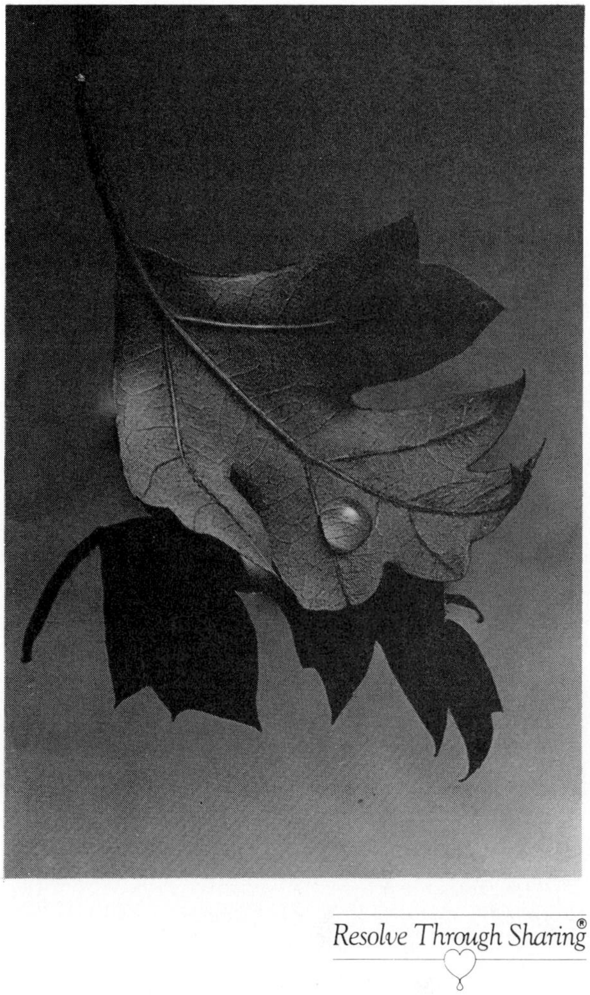

Fig. 29-2 Door card for room of mother who has experienced perinatal loss. (© Resolve Through Sharing.)

If a woman has suffered a perinatal loss, this fact needs to be communicated to hospital staff and volunteers. Some hospitals place a symbol such as a photograph of a leaf and tear drop (Fig. 29-2) or a heart with a tear drop on the door of the woman's room. In this way, staff and volunteers can be prevented from inadvertently making inappropriate comments such as, "Did you have a boy or a girl?" or "Did you wish to order photographs of your baby?"

Validating Loss

Validating loss is promoted by having the parents and family view the fetus/newborn. The *family is prepared* for seeing and holding their baby. They are asked if they want others to be with them (e.g., clergy, nurse). They are prepared for the appearance and feel of their baby. *Care of the body* after death requires respectful handling. The baby is usually removed to a work area. All instruments are removed and the baby is bathed as necessary. The baby is weighed, measured, identified (e.g., identification bands, footprints), and photographed. Any obvious defects of the fetus/newborn can be covered creatively (e.g., a cap to cover anencephaly); parents can undo the blankets should they wish to see all of the baby. Parents commonly find at least one positive characteristic to remember (e.g., "she had such a beautiful mouth"). After viewing her spontaneously aborted 12 week fetus, one mother exclaimed, "Oh *he's* perfect, just perfect. I thought *it* would be a monster!"

The parents are profoundly affected by the *manner and attitudes of those around them,* especially the medical and nursing personnel. Parents are sensitive to and respond quickly to nonverbal cues from others that may connote nonacceptance, revulsion, or blame. Voice inflections, facial expressions, or the posture of the nurse who witnesses parental grief reactions or views the body are quickly noted and internalized. Therefore the nurse should cradle the baby in her arms and carry the body to the parents' arms.

If the mother or family does not want to see the fetus or newborn at this time, the photograph and other mementoes are stored with the chart. Often the family requests to see the photographs at a later date. Occasionally, parents request to have their baby brought from the morgue several days after delivery. The baby looks best immediately after birth. The parents and family should be encouraged to view the baby soon after delivery.

A *private space* is provided, but the physician, nurse, clergy, or other chosen friends or relatives stay close by for support per the parents' wishes. Facial tissues and fresh water and glasses are supplied. The nurse gives permission for family to cry by actions such as supplying tissues, and by saying things such as "It's worth crying over." Some facilities have a Perinatal Loss Committee, which can be called on to attend the family at this time.

Keepsakes are assembled (Furrh and Copley, 1989). Parents find comfort in having keepsakes such as the photographs, a lock of hair, certificate with footprints, identification bands, or the blanket that has been used to wrap the newborn. The blanket will retain the odor of the soap and powder used after the bath.

The rite of baptism is particularly significant to Roman Catholic, some Episcopalian, and Greek Orthodox religious groups. Conditional baptism is used when tissue is to be baptized following an abortion—only the initial words are changed to, "If you can be baptized . . .". A stillborn or live born baby that dies is baptized in the conventional manner. The parents are included in the baptism if they desire. They may actually perform the baptism. They may wish to contact their own clergy to perform the rite. Water is poured down the head or other skin surface and the following words are spoken, "I baptize you, Jane Doe, in the name of the Father, of the Son, and of the Holy Spirit." Notation of the baptism and who performed it is made on the record. Parents are encouraged to name the fetus/newborn. *Naming* provides further validation of the existence and subsequent loss of the baby.

Teaching

Knowledge about any situation helps dispel fear of the unknown, misconceptions, and fantasy. Knowledge supports ego strength. The physician may have explained the obstetric problem, medical condition, or genetic factors implicated. However, grief influences one's ability to hear, understand, and retain. Therefore the nurse fills in gaps in information and clarifies misconceptions of what the bereaved heard. The nurse helps the family formulate questions for the physician regarding cause of the loss and prospects for future childbearing. In some instances, there is no identifiable cause.

Many women experience ambivalent feelings about being pregnant. Coincident loss of the pregnancy may precipitate a guilt reaction for real or imagined negative thoughts. Many women do not follow directions for their care to the letter (e.g., some do not take their iron supplement regularly, and some have an alcoholic beverage at least once during pregnancy.) Other women have gone against a cultural proscription their mother or family had warned them about.

If perinatal loss is the result of cocaine or other substance abuse, the mother and family require professional counseling. These mothers are often acutely aware of the adverse effects of substance use. Some may already be on the long list of those awaiting space in a rehabilitation unit.

Discharge Planning

Parents and family can be invited to participate in a discharge planning conference. The opportunity to participate helps educate, as well as alleviate feelings of powerlessness. Topics to cover include anticipatory guidance for expectations of self, siblings, and grandparents; consideration of a memorial service; coping strategies for interactions with family and friends; community resources; and follow-up care.

Expectations of Self. Physical symptoms that parents may continue to experience include sleep problems with fatigue, anorexia, muscle aches and "knots," gastrointestinal symptoms, and palpitations.

Psychologic or emotional symptoms that parents may experience include an inability to concentrate for long on any one activity (i.e., their minds may wander or they may feel everything is whirling around in their heads) and pressure in the head. People commonly express the fear of "going crazy" when they experience reactions that they do not expect or understand. Parents may fear being alone, wish to go away somewhere, or become over-concerned about or disinterested in their older children. Irritability with or disinterest in the other children may compound guilt feelings.

The mother may hold her abdomen and state she feels "empty" and that her arms "ache to hold a baby." The parents are cautioned against a rapid subsequent conception and birth of a child to replace this one that was lost. The **replacement child** (like the surviving co-twin, p. 913) would be born into a time of confusion and fear (Swanson-Kauffman, 1988). If grief over the loss of one child is not addressed, the replacement child may ironically become the focus of the parents' rage, depression, or fears (Swanson-Kauffman, 1988).

Siblings. Siblings may feel that the parent or parents lied to them about the coming of a new baby. The older child may feel that it is her or his fault that the baby died because she or he may not have wanted a new sibling now, or because she or he wanted a boy but got a girl, so the girl died. Older siblings may act out their feelings in other ways. Older children may need verbal explanations as well as assistance in voicing feelings and thoughts. Discussion about the fetal or newborn death, as well as death in general, should be an open subject in the family. The cause of the death should be openly presented so that the child may cope with any existing feelings of guilt. It is difficult for children to see their mother or family unhappy. Though it may take a great deal of maternal effort, it may help siblings if their mother acknowledges that they are not the cause of the tears—"Mom is sad and crying because your baby sister/brother has died; you haven't done anything to cause her/him to die. Even though mom is very sad, she loves you very much."

A small child who cannot understand verbal explanations needs demonstrations of love and affection to provide reassurance and security. He may be unable to express frightening thoughts that he is experiencing. Occasionally the small child may resort to misbehavior to draw attention or may cling excessively to his parents. Euphemisms such as, "The baby went away (or to sleep)" or "God took him" are usually meant to help the child, but more often they can be threatening. The family is encouraged to discuss the event openly with adolescent children. Regardless of the way parents handle the reaction to death or the birth of an infant with a disorder, some older siblings may manifest their inner disturbance in nightmares, bed-wetting, school problems, or other ways.

Grandparents. A nursing care plan is incomplete without an assessment and plan for action regarding grandparental responses. Grandparents are also touched by the loss of a pregnancy or newborn or the birth of a newborn at risk. Grandparents can be supportive to the young family, having the natural response to protect their offspring. For others, death of a grandchild or birth of a grandchild who is less than perfect seems to lower their self-esteem. They may resort to blaming the young parents or their child's spouse for acts of omission or commission in precipitating the problem with remarks such as, "We've never had this happen in *our* family before—ever." Other comments commonly heard include, "The women in *our* family have never had problems having babies" and "I told him (her) that nothing good would come of this marriage (relationship)." Comments such as these from members of the parents' families may mask hidden feelings. Such feelings might include inadequacy about themselves, feelings of helplessness in the situation, or concern that there may be no grandchild and therefore no "immortality" for them. Many other emotional reactions are possible.

The nurse must avoid the pitfall of taking sides. The nurse provides patience, tact, and warm sympathy. This is coupled with efforts to help family members identify and explore feelings, clarify misconceptions, and provide simple, cogent explanations that may contribute to the comfort, strength, and unity of the entire family.

Family and Friends. Another hurdle is facing others—the older children, family, and friends. Even during the hospital stay, parents experience society's discomfort. Subtle or blatant expressions of social isolation are evident. The cards, flowers, and other gifts of congratulation are sparse if the newborn is born with a defect or is in danger of dying. Commonly the cheery forms of congratulations come from those unaware of the "situation." Telephone conversations are guarded. Even medical personnel, unhappily, may shun these parents. Families may be insinuating blame on each other.

The entire health team and community resources such as clergy must accept the task of helping parents reenter the outside world. One simple technique is *role-playing*. The anticipated meetings with the other children, family, and friends are acted out. Another approach is to discuss how parents will handle the curiosity of friends, acquaintances, and strangers. These techniques help in several ways. First, by anticipating the words and reactions of others, they verbalize their own. Second, the practice augments their store of coping strategies. Both techniques may uncover feelings that can be dealt with here and now, although resolution of these feelings may not come until much later. Each encounter may serve to strengthen coping mechnisms and bring the resolution of feelings a step closer.

Funeral or Memorial Services. Many support groups and parents who have experienced a perinatal loss encourage parents to have a funeral or memorial service. These rituals facilitate formal "leave-taking." Family and friends can acknowledge the reality of the loss and publicly express their sorrow. Even if the mother requires extended hospitalization after the delivery of the baby, it is helpful to encourage the family to include her in arrangements for the funeral or memorial service. Families often appreciate having the primary nurse attend the service (Ilse and Furrh, 1988).

Resource Referrals. As with other losses, most parents who have experienced a perinatal loss derive a special support from others who have experienced a similar loss. National organizations such as Pregnancy and Infant Loss Center, SHARE, Resolve, Compassionate Friends, AMEND, and Resolve Through Sharing offer support for parents experiencing a perinatal loss (Appendix I). The parents or family may consider other referrals: spiritual leader, family planning, psychiatric social worker, or genetic counselor. In the case of maternal loss (p. 916) additional services may be needed: child care, homemaker service, home health care.

Well-intentioned "Reassurance". The nurse may be unaware of personal struggles with reactions to grief. The nurse may resort to reassuring and comforting the bereaved individual or individuals in a manner that does not foster a healthy grieving response. ***Some commonly heard responses given by physicians, nurses, and well-meaning friends should be avoided:***

- "There was a reason why God wanted this baby."
- "It's God's will. We have to have faith that it was for the best."
- "It's probably better this way. This often happens when the baby has something wrong with it."
- "You are so young. There's time for more."
- "Be thankful you have those other lovely children at home. They'll be a solace and comfort to you."
- "Be grateful you found out now (in early pregnancy) that there's a problem before it's a real baby."

These comments minimize the event for the family. *This* baby is important *now*. The mother (and family) needs to talk about *this* baby. She does not want or need to focus on her other children or any suggestions for substitutes for her loss.

Certain behaviors give the message that to face grief is "bad" for a person and to avoid facing it is better for all concerned. An example might be avoiding talking about the lost child, quelling tears, and forbidding the parents to see and hold the fetus/newborn.

Somehow it is thought that to avoid an issue is the healthiest and easiest way. It does prevent "scenes." Out of sight is out of mind. But out of sight is not out of the bereaved parent's mind. The mother has felt life. She has developed a relationship with the child through shared internal physical sensation and fantasy. The father (and other family members) has also begun attachment to the expected child and anticipated parenthood. If the child lives for a few hours or days after birth, the parent's relationship with the child has progressed even further. Even after delivery the hormones that sustain an attachment between mother and child are still present. The physical signs and discomforts that occur during the normal postpartum period also exist. At home are the baby clothes and furniture, family, and friends, awaiting the hoped-for new arrival. Resolution of grief is important *now* and can be a healthy growth-inducing process.

Evaluation

Evaluation of the effectiveness of nursing actions is somewhat more difficult when working with loss and grief. The grieving response takes a considerable period. The nurse's contact with the family may be limited. The nurse must rely on the knowledge that supportive and understanding care is significant to the family's successful resolution of their loss.

For many parents, resolution of the loss of a child is not possible. For them, the goal is integration of the loss into their life experience.

❑ LOSS OF THE FETUS OR NEWBORN

Conception affirms the woman's ability to initiate her biologic role. Any event that interferes with her ability to carry a normal fetus to term causes her to question her biologic intactness. The event may be perceived as an assault to the woman's self-concept and feelings of self-worth. She may feel cheated. Many women experience ambivalent feelings toward the idea of pregnancy; many harbor thoughts of self-abortion. Coincident loss of the pregnancy may precipitate a guilt reaction for real or imagined negative thoughts or actions.

Negative Outcome from Perinatal Diagnosis

Chorionic villi sampling (CVS), percutaneous umbilical blood sample (PUBS), and amniocentesis may identify a fetus with a defect (Chapter 22). The identification of a fetus with a defect precipitates a significant crisis for prospective parents (VanPutte, 1988). The parents face family and friends who may have sufficient negative feelings about the diagnosis and therefore may not be as supportive of the parents. The subject of abortion is controversial for many. Some parents keep their situation a secret, thus limiting availability of support systems. Regardless of whether the diagnosis and subsequent selective abortion are kept secret, the experience may be one of the loneliest losses experienced in a lifetime (VanPutte, 1988). The parents who decide to continue the pregnancy will require a multidisciplinary plan of care (Chapter 28).

Spontaneous Abortion and Ectopic Pregnancy

For the woman who has a history of difficulty in conceiving and carrying a pregnancy to viability (about 24 weeks), negative feelings about herself as a complete woman may be expected. Nursing care of such a woman and her family should focus on helping them verbalize their feelings openly and honestly. Sympathetic, active listening by the nurse may help the woman in retaining or regaining her self-esteem and feelings of self-worth (Wall-Haas, 1985).

One woman who suffered spontaneous abortion submitted these "thoughts on being a habitual aborter" (Zlomke, 1986):

> The term 'habitual aborter' is an insidious one, and one which I believe no woman should ever hear. It is a phrase which implies that she could have control over her life if she would only exert herself, as though she were a smoker or a nail biter. The truth is that she has lost all control over her life. With the death of each baby a little more of her future dies until she finally can bear it no longer and gives up. The pain is so great that even after having had a healthy baby since my last miscarriage, I notice that I wrote this whole paragraph in the third person.

Fetal Death

Fetal movements may cease before the onset of labor, that is, between 20 weeks and term. The mother may deny a lack of fetal activity: "Maybe he's just asleep . . . he's quiet sometimes." She may call the physician for reassurance that everything is all right. Subsequently she may be admitted to the hospital for tests of fetal status. Even in light of evidence from the tests and clinical symptoms, some women cling tenaciously to the hope that the infant will be born alive and well.

Other women acknowledge fetal death by a change in their behavior. One woman arrived on a maternity unit in active labor. A review of her chart showed that she had kept all her clinic appointments until 4 weeks before labor. She stated she was feeling well and described her labor so far. She said nothing as the nurse checked for the fetal heart rate (FHR). When none were heard, the nurse inquired about fetal activity. Quietly and unemotionally, the mother replied, "They stopped a month ago."

Occasionally it is the nurse who responds with denial. The nurse may rationalize the absence of FHR and funic and uterine souffles as "positional," "too much noise in the room," "defective fetoscope," and the like. The nurse may choose to avoid the woman or to avoid open communication on the subject. The nurse has several therapeutic alternatives available (see specific nursing care plan, p. 914).

Intranatal Fetal or Newborn Death. FHR may be lost late in the first stage of labor or during the second stage. The atmosphere in the labor unit becomes tense and subdued. There is a sudden change from joyful anticipation to dread. Silence accompanies the birth. Resuscitative measures are attempted. All persons present focus on the newborn. Shock and disbelief are experienced by parents and staff alike.

The supportive role of the nurse in the care of parents who experience the death of their infant during labor and delivery is presented in the specific nursing care plan for the family following the death of a fetus on p. 914.

Nurse and Parent Reactions and Interactions. The nurse may undergo a period of self-recrimination relevant to her own behavior surrounding the incident, for example: Could the physician have been called earlier? Were the fetal heart tones really there and was the rate normal when they were last checked? Was it judicious to give that last medication at the time it was given? Were there any clues earlier? Did the nursing care (ability to assess labor and the maternal-fetal condition during labor, ability to resuscitate) cause the fetal or neonatal death? The nurse's self-examination can undermine self-confidence as a nurse. In their search for answers and to vent angry feelings, the mother and family may also probe. Nurses may perceive the questioning as challenges to their capabilities as nurses. At times like this even the most competent and self-assured nurse may need peer or other support to identify feelings and verbalize them and to regain perspective.

Perinatal Death of a Twin

The death of a twin before, during, or after birth imposes on parents a very confusing and ambivalent induction into parenthood (Swanson-Kauffman, 1988).

Specific Nursing Care Plan

PARENTS EXPERIENCING FETAL DEATH

Ann, age 27, gestational week 20, was admitted to the labor floor after complaining of severe abdominal cramping and leaking small amounts of pink vaginal discharge. Ann and her husband are placed in a private examining room. As the nurse enters the room she hears Ann state, "I don't want to lose this baby—I feel so close to it now that I have felt it move—I'm scared." After several unsuccessful trials of drug therapy to cease labor, and cessation of the FHR, Ann is being prepared for her imminent delivery. The physician is currently reviewing the assessment with Ann and her husband and explaining choices of anesthesia for delivery.

ASSESSMENT	NURSING DIAGNOSIS (ND), PLAN/GOAL (P/G)	RATIONALE/ IMPLEMENTATION	EVALUATION
Ann's response is one of being scared and upset. Spouse is at bedside listening to Ann's feelings. Ask if Ann wishes anyone else at the hospital as a support person and make effort to contact individual.	ND: Powerlessness related to loss and grief. ND: Potential ineffective individual (or family) coping related to death of a fetus. P/G: Ann will verbalize her needs and discuss her concerns and feelings.	*Therapeutic communication and assistance with physical needs can enhance coping skills:* Introduce yourself and immediately indicate your awareness of the situation. ("This is a very difficult and sad time for you.") Encourage and assist verbalization of feelings. Be cognizant of own nonverbal messages. Provide physical care and meet dependency needs in thoughtful and unhurried manner.	Ann verbalizes her immediate needs to the nurse or through her husband. Spouse is able to remain at bedside as a support to Ann. Mother (family) openly communicate their concerns and reactions.
Persistent preterm labor despite drug therapy. Pink serous vaginal discharge. 20 week gestation fetus (nonviable). No FHR noted. Parents informed by physician of imminent delivery of a stillborn fetus. Assess parents' understanding of cause of fetal loss and choices regarding anesthesia and the birth process.	ND: Knowledge deficit related to fetal loss. ND: Knowledge deficit related to the birth process. P/G: Ann will ask questions about the cause of fetal death. P/G: Ann will make an informed decision regarding choice of anesthesia for delivery	*Knowledge is ego-strengthening:* Act as advocate to physician in regard to woman's questions concerning cause of death and events she will experience during delivery. Fill in gaps in information and clarify misconceptions. Respect Ann's choice of anesthesia. Prepare the parent(s) for the following: (a) Silence and tension at delivery. (b) Sight of still, pale, or reddish infant; infant's peeling skin and markedly molded head.	Ann asks questions about the cause of fetal loss. Ann chooses a method of anesthesia for delivery. Ann and husband express satisfaction with care received.

Specific Nursing Care Plan—cont'd

ASSESSMENT	NURSING DIAGNOSIS (ND), PLAN/GOAL (P/G)	RATIONALE/ IMPLEMENTATION	EVALUATION
Assess the couple's desire to hold or see the fetus. Assess for desire to have the fetus baptized.	ND: Potential anxiety related to initiating the grieving process. ND: Potential ineffective individual or family coping related to initiating the grieving process. ND: Potential spiritual distress (distress of the human spirit) related to loss and grief. P/G: The couple will identify and validate the loss that will permit the grieving process to begin.	*Many parents experiencing a loss need to see or hold the fetus to identify and validate the loss:* If mother, spouse, or relatives wish to see or hold infant: (a) Prepare family for sight of fetus, and identify individuals for viewing. (b) Bathe and wrap the infant. (c) Provide privacy for viewing and stay close by for support. (d) Give permission to cry, (giving tissues) by saying, "It's a sad time, and it's OK to cry." Arrange for baptism if desired and record event in progress notes.	Ann and her husband initiate the grieving process. Ann and her husband identify their support system. Family expresses satisfaction in viewing and holding infant. Baptism or other religious rite is performed.
Assess any previous loss the couple might have had and identify effective coping mechanisms and support systems utilized.	ND: Knowledge deficit related to grief and grieving. P/G: The couple will receive anticipatory guidance regarding components of the grief process.	*Knowledge of the normal grieving process validates the couples responses as normal:* Explain characteristic patterns of the grief response. Identify and examine any previous effective coping mechanisms. Identify couple's support system.	The couple verbalizes understanding of grief reactions.

They must attend to birth and death certificates, a baptism and a funeral, and both congratulations and condolences. "Well-meaning" people make unsupportive statements such as "at least you are blessed with one baby." Parents must grieve the loss of the baby to whom they began to attach early in pregnancy and the loss of the fantasies surrounding being parents of twins. The parents have a need to grieve the dead twin even as they are trying to attach to the surviving twin. If grieving is repressed or set-aside, it lingers just beneath the surface only to resurface, perhaps as a maladaptive parenting behavior with the survivor (e.g., overprotection, abuse, emotional abandonment).

In some respects, nursing care of parents after the death of the twin is similar to that after the loss of a singleton: provide an accepting atmosphere, create memories, handle the baby with respect and compassion. There are several differences, however. The life and subsequent death of the twin must be acknowledged. The parents can be encouraged to give the dead twin a name and consider a funeral or other meaningful ceremony (Swanson-Kauffman, 1988). The parents can be referred to support groups (Appendix I) or parent books on perinatal loss. Parents will need these resources later as they consider dilemnas such as how to tell the surviving twin about the co-twin's existence. Parents will need assistance in relating to the surviving twin so that he or she will get the message that "you are special" and not "you are not enough" (Swanson-Kauffman, 1988). To the parents, the surviving twin remains a constant reminder of what could have been.

Birth of a Compromised Newborn

The birth of a preterm newborn or newborn with a disorder is a shattering experience for parents and a disturbing experience for those who attended the birth (Chapter 28). Parents feel devastated and inadequate; anticipated joy ends in despair and confusion. A flurry of activity often follows such a birth. The child may then be examined by specialists, often at a facility far from the mother's hospital. Physicians and others (e.g., clergy) may talk with the parents. The natural order of postdelivery psychologic tasks is disrupted, and the new parents are in crisis. The nurse is in a unique and critical position. Of all the members of the health care team, the nurse alone can be available 24 hours a day. A nurse can help plan for discharge and postdischarge care. Although clinical intervention will vary with each situation, in every case, nurses must establish themselves as caring, knowledgeable, resourceful persons.

Parents may express feelings of shame and embarrassment lest they be carrying a "bad" gene or are responsible for exposure to a devastating environmental agent (e.g., stripping paint off an old crib with methylene chloride and repainting it in a poorly ventilated space). Others are anxious to fix the blame somewhere. Many women remember transient (or persistent) negative feelings about the pregnancy or baby and interpret the birth of a child with a disorder as punishment for their real or imagined transgressions.

The nurse's role must be supportive. This includes preparing parents for what to expect and allowing for **anticipatory grief,** listening actively, and assisting with the formulation of questions and the ventilation of feelings. Skillfully executed, the nurse's supportive function aids parents in decision-making and in self-acceptance regarding their decisions (e.g., surgical corrective surgery or institutionalization of the impaired child).

❑ LOSS OF THE MOTHER

Maternal death is rarely encountered. The death of a mother during the perinatal period is an unexpected tragedy. Even if the mother had been designated as "high risk," maternal death sends ripples of shock throughout the maternity unit. "Death of the mother completely disrupts the family structure and often leaves the father with the care of a baby at a time when his emotional reserves are lowest" (Johnson, 1986). For the family the sense of loss and grief is enormous.

Childbirth is viewed as a normal physiologic event. When the mother dies, the survivors may respond in a wide variety of ways. The newborn infant may be targeted as the cause of the mother's death. Family members who feel that the newborn is somehow responsible may find it difficult to develop a positive, caring relationship with the child. The loss leaves the father emotionally drained at this time when the newborn and older children need him most. In the back of his mind, he may experience guilt for his role in family planning. He may wonder how the family can manage financially regardless of whether the wife had contributed to the family income.

Families have a need to know why the event occurred. Consent for autopsy is usually given. The physician may gain more information with which to discuss the maternal death with the family.

Grandparents feel the loss intensely as well. Parents expect that their children will survive them in the "natural order" of things. The death of their daughter is a break in the continuity. Furthermore the maternal grandparents may be faced with the possibility that the husband will remarry and thus create a distance between them and their grandchild.

Denial is the prominent defense mechanism used intermittently by children of all ages. Denial is used even though intellectually death is comprehended. The pain of coming to grips with the loss extends over a long period. For varying lengths of time there is hope and expectation that the loved one will return.

The time to offer counseling is at the time when a death occurs, before conflicts and anxieties have resulted in behavior difficulties or symptom formation. Important areas involve helping the bereaved around burial services. This includes clarifying with the parent the importance of discussing the nature of the illness so that the child can achieve his own differentiation and supporting the bereaved in their grief so that they in turn can allow the expression of grief in their children (Sahler, 1978).

Working with the family who suffers this type of loss is challenging but also potentially rewarding.

Children Under 5 Years of Age

There is a special necessity for preventive work with children under 5 when a parent dies. Children under 5 form the most vulnerable age group (Sahler, 1978). Such children depend solely on parental support for their ego development and mastery of the instinctual drives. Their reality testing is limited. They are easily overwhelmed with anxiety. Their capacity to verbalize is not fully developed. They need adult help in identifying feelings. Symptoms of anxiety and inner stress are prone to take the form of physical activity (e.g., regressive behaviors, over or under activity, or psychosomatic symptoms).

Adolescent Reactions

Because of greater ego maturity, the normal adolescent is better able to cope with the finality of death. The predominant task of adolescence is to move toward independence, to free oneself from close dependence on parents. Adolescents need repeated attempts to break away, to try various activities outside the family. Although critical of and hostile to parents at times, adolescents have an option to return and be cared for. When one parent is no longer available to meet this need for comfort and care, the struggle toward independence may be disrupted. Guilt is common. The child wonders if the parent might have lived if he had done something different (e.g., been nicer, not rebelled so much).

The relationship between the adolescent and the surviving parent needs consideration. The living parent may be preoccupied with his own grief. Thus the adolescent is doubly deprived. Attempts to console the father may be met with anger and irritation. The adolescent may turn away with a sense of being a failure. The potential for suicide often arises in the adolescent group. Many develop a renewed interest in immortality. Deutsch (1967) has made the point that as the adolescent struggles with intense anxieties, she or he is confronted with one of life's sharpest paradoxes—namely, that on the threshold of a new life, she or he feels the threat of death.

Adolescents are struggling with their sexual identity as well. The death of their mother during childbirth can have a negative effect on both the female and male adolescent. Open communication is essential in helping the adolescent identify these feelings and differentiate herself or himself from the deceased (Sahler, 1978).

Adults often mourn at a faster pace than children. When the two generations are out of phase in their grieving, a sensitive nurse is aware that children may be confused, especially if the father remarries. The nurse can play a supportive role by alerting the family to expect this reaction. The adolescent needs much emotional support and opportunities to verbalize her or his concerns so that misconceptions about death can be clarified.

Dysfunctional Grieving

Dysfunctional grieving is defined as the failure to grieve. The nursing diagnosis of dysfunctional grieving is supported by the identification of defining characteristics. Failure to grieve may be marked by mild chronic depression, withdrawal from friends and/or normal activities, regressive behaviors, and constricted affect. The person may display "acting out" behavior such as continued hostility toward the staff, the spouse, or the maternal or paternal family. Marked or persistent guilt feelings regarding the event may be evident. Somatic complaints may be described. The person may avoid any discussion of the event or of any affectively charged topic.

The format for the nursing care plan is similar to that for "normal grieving." The nurse *assesses* the person's current affective state, past coping style, degree of relatedness with others, and degree of insight into the present situation. Disturbing topics of conversation or experience are identified. The degree of stress being experienced is estimated.

The nurse *plans* interventions with specific client-centered *goals* in mind. The goals include that the client will begin to experience grieving in a supportive environment; demonstrate normal grieving behaviors (e.g., variability in affect, ambivalence toward and preoccupation with the lost object); and describe a return to normal physiologic functioning (e.g., hunger, activity, sleep).

Implementation of the nursing care plan proceeds in an unhurried manner within an atmosphere of acceptance. The nurse listens attentively, encourages verbalization, refrains from criticizing, and provides appropriate reassurance (e.g., "emotional pain will decrease with time"). The nurse describes usual expressions of grief to validate their normalcy. The nurse can discuss various tension reduction or coping behaviors that may assist in grief recovery (e.g., active relaxation, activity with others).

To *evaluate* the client's response to intervention, the nurse assesses the degree to which goals are being met. The client will begin to display "normal" grief behaviors, experience the return of normal physiologic functions (e.g., hunger and appetite, activity, sleep, elimination), and display the reestablishment of mutually acceptable relatedness with others.

SUMMARY

Nurses are expected to provide physical care, comfort, understanding, and emotional support to the individual and family who experience loss. The nurse needs to have a grasp of the developmental aspects of the concept of death, the stages and processes associated with grief, and community resources available. The individual's values, beliefs, and experiences influence the cognitive aspects of dying. It is important to assess one's viewpoints and attitudes toward death, since these often transfer over into the caregiving situation. Nurses must recognize that there are limitations and immense emotional strains that pervade nursing the bereaved. Nurses caring for the bereaved benefit from a professional support system of their own. Touching and sharing another's experience of loss can be threatening but also rewarding.

KEY CONCEPTS

- Parent-infant affectional bonds develop early in a pregnancy.
- The duration of a pregnancy preceding a perinatal loss does not necessarily influence the severity of the grieving response.
- An unnatural or unexpected interruption of a pregnancy poses a potential threat to a woman's self-esteem.
- All family members of a baby who dies, including the siblings, are affected by a perinatal loss.
- When expectations of birth and joy are replaced by loss and sadness, the nurse's role is critical.
- An understanding of loss and common manifestations of the grieving process are fundamental to the implementation of the nursing process.
- Therapeutic communication techniques can help parents understand the meaning of their loss and share their feelings.
- Though guidelines can be given to facilitate a couple's grieving response, one needs to remember that each individual grieves in a unique way.
- Nurses are also vulnerable when caring for clients experiencing loss and grief.

LEARNING ACTIVITIES

1. Discover what community resources and support groups exist to assist parents who have experienced:
   A. A preterm birth.
   B. Birth of an imperfect child.
   C. A fetal death.
2. After viewing a film on death and grieving, discuss the kinds of behavior the group observed of the grieving person.

   Inexperienced students may be quite uncomfortable in situations of grief and loss. Exercises should focus on developing self-awareness of feelings regarding loss and how these feelings can transfer to parents. Activities that are beneficial are:
   A. Develop a role-playing situation wherein a student acts as a nurse assisting parents of an imperfect child. Anticipate meetings with older children, families, and friends.
   B. Invite a speaker from a local support group to describe her or his work with parents and families.

References

Carter SL: Themes of grief, Nurs Res 38(6):354, 1989.

Deutsch H: Selected problems of adolescence, Monogr Ser Psychoanal Study Child no 3, 1967, International Universities Press, Inc.

Furrh CB and Copley R: One precious moment: what you can offer when a newborn infant who dies, Nurs'89 19(9):52, 1989.

Ilse S and Furrh CB: Development of a comprehensive follow-up care plan after perinatal and neonatal loss, J Perinat Neonat Nurs 2(2):23, 1988.

Johnson SH: Nursing assessment and strategies for the family at risk: high-risk parenting, ed 2, Philadelphia, 1986, JB Lippincott Co.

Krone C and Harris CC: The importance of infant gender and family resemblance within parents' perinatal bereavement process: establishing personhood, J Perinat Neonat Nurs 2(2):1, 1988.

Kübler-Ross E: On death and dying, New York, 1969, Macmillan Publishing Co.

Lindemann E: Symptomatology and management of acute grief, Am J Psychol 101:141, 1944.

Sahler OJ, editor: The child and death, St Louis, 1978, The CV Mosby Co.

Swanson-Kauffman K: There should have been two: nursing care of parents experiencing the perinatal death of a twin, J Perinat Neonat Nurs 2(2):78, 1988.

VanPutte AW: Perinatal bereavement crisis: coping with negative outcomes from prenatal diagnosis, J Perinat Neonat Nurs 2(2):12, 1988.

Wall-Haas CL: Women's perceptions of first trimester spontaneous abortion, JOGN Nurs 14(1):50, 1985.

Zlomke E: Personal correspondence, Spring, 1986.

Bibliography

Archer DN and Smith AC: Sorrow has many faces, Nurs'88 18(5):43, 1988.

Arms S: To love and let go, New York, 1983, Alfred A Knopf, Inc.

Blackburn S and Lowen L: Impact of an infant's premature birth on the grandparents and parents, JOGN Nurs 15:173, March/April, 1986.

Bright PD: Adolescent pregnancy and loss, Matern Child Nurs J 16(1):1, 1987.

Cole D: It might have been: mourning the unborn, Psychology Today (7):64, 1987.

Dickason EJ, Schultz MO, and Silverman BL: Maternal-infant nursing care, St Louis, 1990, The CV Mosby Co.

Freitag-Koonitz MJ: Parents' grief reaction to the diagnosis of their infant's severe neurologic impairment and static encephalopathy, J Perinat Neonat Nurs 2(2):45, 1988.

Gifford BJ and Cleary BB: Supporting the bereaved, 90(2):49, 1990.

Grabauskas P et al: Helping the parents after a baby's death, RN, p 31, Aug, 1987.

Green D: Prenatal diagnosis: when reality shatters parents' dreams, Nurs '88 18(2):61, 1988.

Grubb-Phillips CA: Intrauterine fetal death: the maternal bereavement experience, J Perinat Neonat Nurs 2(2):34, 1988.

Howard JC and Nyari DM: Traumatic fetal death: dimensions of critical care nursing 8(4):217, 1989.

Iams JD and Zuspan FP: Zuspan and Quilligan's manual of obstetrics and gynecology, St Louis, 1990, The CV Mosby Co.

Kavanaugh K: Infants weighing less than 500 grams at birth: providing parental support, J Perinat Neonat Nurs 2(2):58, 1988.

Leff PT: Here I am, Ma: the emotional impact of pregnancy loss on parents and health-care professionals, Family Systems Medicine 5(1):105, 1987.

Maguire DP and Skoolicas SJ: Developing a bereavement follow-up program, J Perinat Neonat Nurs 2(2):67, 1988.

Malcolm N and Wooten B: It's hard to say Goodbye, Can Nurse 83(4):27, 1987.

Merenstein GB and Gardner SL: Handbook of neonatal intensive care, ed 2, St Louis, 1989, The CV Mosby Co.

Mina CF: A program for helping grieving parents, MCN 10:118, March/April, 1985.

Neithercut C, Pacek C, and Sparks M: Helping the parents after a baby's death, RN, p 31, Aug, 1987.

Novak S: In moments of crisis, MCN 13(5):349, 1988.

Poe AH: Legal and ethical issues. Premature labor: a perinatal dilemma, J Prof Nurs 5(5):242, 1989.

Raff BS: Nursing care of high-risk infants and their families: introduction, JOGN Nurs 15:141, March/April, 1986.

Raff BS: The use of homemaker-home health aids' perinatal care of high-risk infants, JOGN Nurs 15:142, March/April, 1986.

Ransohoff-Adler M: When newborns die: do we practice what we preach? J Perinat 4(3):311, 1989.

Sadler ME: When your patient's baby dies before birth, RN, p 28, Aug, 1987.

Schaffer P: When your baby has died . . . practical suggestions and emotional support for grieving parents. Montana Perinatal Program, Montana Dept. of Health and Environmental Sciences, July, 1987.

Snyder DJ: Peer group support for high-risk mothers, MCN 13(2):114, 1988.

Steele K: Caring for parents of critically ill neonates during hospitalization: strategies for health care professionals, MCN 16(1):13, 1986.

Whitaker CM: Death before birth, Am J Nurs 86:156, Feb, 1986.

Woolsey SF: Support after sudden infant death, Am J Nurs 88(10):1348, 1988.

Glossary

abdominal Belonging or relating to the abdomen and its functions and disorders.

a. delivery Birth of a child through a surgical incision made into the abdominal wall and uterus; cesarean delivery.

a. gestation Implantation of a fertilized ovum outside the uterus but inside the peritoneal cavity.

abortion Termination of pregnancy before the fetus is viable and capable of extrauterine existence, usually less than 21 to 22 weeks' gestation (or when the fetus weighs less than 600 g).

complete a. Abortion in which fetus and all related tissue have been expelled from the uterus.

criminal a. Termination of pregnancy performed by unqualified people usually under septic conditions. Women may resort to this if therapeutic abortions are unavailable.

elective a. Termination of pregnancy chosen by the woman that is not required for her physical safety.

habitual (recurrent) a. Loss of three or more successive pregnancies for no known cause.

incomplete a. Loss of pregnancy in which some but not all the products of conception have been expelled from the uterus.

induced a. Intentionally produced loss of pregnancy by woman or others.

inevitable a. Threatened loss of pregnancy that cannot be prevented or stopped and is imminent.

missed a. Loss of pregnancy in which the products of conception remain in the uterus after the fetus dies.

septic a. Loss of pregnancy in which there is an infection of the products of conception and the uterine endometrial lining, usually resulting from attempted termination of early pregnancy.

spontaneous a. Loss of pregnancy that occurs naturally without interference or known cause.

therapeutic a. Pregnancy that has been intentionally terminated for medical reasons.

threatened a. Possible loss of a pregnancy; early symptoms are present (e.g., the cervix begins to dilate).

voluntary a. See *abortion, elective.*

abortus Fetus usually less than 21 weeks' gestational age and under 600 g.

abruptio placentae Partial or complete premature separation of a normally implanted placenta.

abstinence Refraining from sexual intercourse periodically or permanently.

accreta, placenta See *placenta accreta.*

acidosis Increase in hydrogen ion concentration resulting in a lowering of blood pH below 7.35.

acini cells Milk-producing cells in the breast.

acme Highest point (e.g., of a contraction).

acrocyanosis Peripheral cyanosis; blue color of hands and feet in most infants at birth that may persist for 7 to 10 days.

acromion Projection of the spine of the scapula (forming the point of the shoulder); used to explain the presentation of the fetus.

adnexa Adjacent or accessory parts of a structure.

uterine a. Ovaries and fallopian tubes.

adult respiratory distress syndrome (ARDS) Set of symptoms including decreased compliance of lung tissue, pulmonary edema, and acute hypoxemia. The condition is similar to respiratory distress syndrome of the newborn.

afibrinogenemia Absence or decrease of fibrinogen in the blood such that the blood will not coagulate. In obstetrics, this condition occurs from complications of abruptio placentae or retention of a dead fetus.

afterbirth Lay term for the placenta and membranes expelled after the birth or delivery of the child.

afterpains Painful uterine cramps that occur intermittently for approximately 2 or 3 days after delivery and that result from contractile efforts of the uterus to return to its normal involuted condition.

AGA Appropriate (weight) for gestational age.

agenesis Failure of an organ to develop.

alae nasi Nostrils.

albuminuria Presence of readily detectable amounts of albumin in the urine.

alkalosis Abnormal condition of body fluids characterized by a tendency toward an increased pH, as from an excess of alkaline bicarbonate or a deficiency of acid.

amniocentesis Procedure in which a needle is inserted through the abdominal and uterine walls into the amniotic fluid; used for assessment of fetal health and maturity and for therapeutic abortion.

amnion Inner membrane of two fetal membranes that form the sac and contain the fetus and the fluid that surrounds it in utero.

amnionitis Inflammation of the amnion, occurring most frequently after early rupture of membranes.

amniotic Pertaining or relating to the amnion.

a. fluid Fluid surrounding fetus derived primarily from maternal serum and fetal urine.

a. sac Membrane "bag" that contains the fetus before delivery.

amniotomy Artificial rupture of the fetal membranes (AROM).

analgesia Lack of pain without loss of consciousness.

analgesic Any drug or agent that will relieve pain.

android pelvis Male type of pelvis.

anencephaly Congenital deformity characterized by the absence of cerebrum, cerebellum, and flat bones of skull.

anesthesia Partial or complete absence of sensation with or without loss of consciousness.
anomaly Organ or structure that is malformed or in some way abnormal with reference to form, structure, or position.
anovulatory Failure of the ovaries to produce, mature, or release eggs.
anoxia Absence of oxygen.
antenatal Occurring before or formed before birth.
antepartal Before labor.
anterior Pertaining to the front.
  a. fontanel See *fontanel, anterior.*
anthropoid pelvis Pelvis in which the anteroposterior diameter is equal to or greater than the transverse diameter.
antibody Specific protein substance developed by the body that exerts restrictive or destructive action on specific antigens, such as bacteria, toxins, or Rh factor.
anticipatory grief Grief that predates the loss of a beloved object.
antigen Protein foreign to the body that causes the body to develop antibodies. Examples: bacteria, dust, Rh factor.
Apgar score Numeric expression of the condition of a newborn obtained by rapid assessment at 1, 5, and 15 minutes of age; developed by Dr. Virginia Apgar.
apnea Cessation of respirations for more than 10 seconds associated with generalized cyanosis.
Apt test Differentiation of maternal and fetal blood when there is vaginal bleeding. It is performed as follows: Add 0.5 ml blood to 4.5 ml distilled water. Shake. Add 1 ml 0.25N sodium hydroxide. Fetal and cord blood remains pink for 1 or 2 minutes. Maternal blood becomes brown in 30 seconds.
areola Pigmented ring of tissue surrounding the nipple.
  secondary a. During the fifth month of pregnancy, a second faint ring of pigmentation seen around the original areola.
artificial insemination Introduction of semen by instrument injection into the vagina or uterus for impregnation.
asphyxia Decreased oxygen and/or excess of carbon dioxide in the body.
  fetal a. Condition occurring in utero, with the following biochemical changes: hypoxemia (lowering of Po_2), hypercapnia (increase in Pco_2), and respiratory and metabolic acidosis (reduction of blood pH).
  a. livida Condition in which the infant's skin is characteristically pale, pulse is weak and slow, and reflexes are depressed or absent; also known as *blue asphyxia.*
  a. pallida Condition in which the infant appears pale and limp and suffers from bradycardia (80 beats/min or less) and apnea.
aspiration pneumonia Inflammatory condition of the lungs and bronchi caused by the inhalation of vomitus containing acid gastric contents.
aspiration syndrome See *meconium aspiration syndrome.*
ataractic Drug capable of promoting tranquility; a tranquilizer.
atelectasis Pulmonary pathosis involving alveolar collapse.
atony Absence of muscle tone.
atresia Absence of a normally present passageway.
  biliary a. Absence of the bile duct.
  choanal a. Complete obstruction of the posterior nares, which open into the nasopharynx, with membranous or bony tissue.
  esophageal a. Congenital anomaly in which the esophagus ends in a blind pouch or narrows into a thin cord, thus failing to form a continuous passageway to the stomach.
attachment Relationship between two persons (e.g., a parent and a child).
attitude Body posture or position.
  fetal a. Relation of fetal parts to each other in the uterus (e.g., all parts flexed, all parts flexed except neck is extended, etc.).
autoimmunization Development of antibodies against constituents of one's own tissues (e.g., a man may develop antibodies against his own sperm).
autosomes Any of the paired chromosomes other than the sex (X and Y) chromosomes.
axis Line, real or imaginary, about which a part revolves or that runs through the center of a body.
  pelvic a. Imaginary curved line that passes through the centers of all the anteroposterior diameters of the pelvis.
azoospermia Absence of sperm in the semen.

bacteremic shock Shock that occurs in septicemia when endotoxins are released from certain bacteria in the bloodstream.
bag of waters Lay term for the sac containing amniotic fluid and fetus.
ballottement (1) Movability of a floating object (e.g., fetus). (2) Diagnostic technique using palpation: a floating object, when tapped or pushed, moves away and then returns to touch the examiner's hand.
Bandl's ring Abnormally thickened ridge of uterine musculature between the upper and lower segments that follows a mechanically obstructed labor, with the lower segment thinning abnormally.
Barr body (sex chromatin) Chromatin mass located against the inner surface of the nucleus in females, possibly representing the inactive X chromosome.
Bartholin's glands Two small glands situated on either side of the vaginal orifice that secrete small amounts of mucus during coitus and that are homologous to the bulbourethral glands in the male.
basalis, decidua See *decidua basalis.*
Bell's palsy See *palsy, Bell's.*
bicornuate uterus Anomalous uterus that may be either a double or single organ with two horns.
biliary atresia See *atresia, biliary.*
bilirubin Yellow or orange pigment that is a breakdown product of hemoglobin. It is carried by the blood to the liver, where it is chemically changed and excreted in the bile or is conjugated and excreted by the kidneys.
Billings method See *ovulation method.*
bimanual Performed with both hands.
  b. palpation Examination of a woman's pelvic organs done by placing one hand on the abdomen and one or two fingers of the other hand in the vagina.
biopsy Removal of a small piece of tissue for microscopic examination and diagnosis.
blastoderm Germinal membrane of the ovum.

b. vesicle Stage in the development of a mammalian embryo that consists of an outer layer, or trophoblast, and a hollow sphere of cells enclosing a cavity.

blood-brain barrier Obstruction that prevents passage of certain substances from blood into brain tissue.

bloody show Vaginal discharge that originates in the cervix and consists of blood and mucus; increases as cervix dilates during labor.

body image Person's subjective concept of his or her physical appearance.

bonding See *attachment.*

born out of asepsis (**BOA**) Pertaining to birth without the use of sterile technique.

Bradley method Preparation for parenthood with active participation of father and mother.

Braxton Hicks sign Mild, intermittent, painless uterine contractions that occur during pregnancy. These contractions occur more frequently as pregnancy advances but do not represent true labor.

Braxton Hicks version One of several types of maneuvers designed to turn the fetus from an undesirable position to a more acceptable one to facilitate delivery.

Brazelton assessment Criteria for assessing the interactional behavior of a newborn.

breakthrough bleeding Escape of blood occurring between menstrual periods; may be noted by women using chemical contraception (birth control pill).

breast milk jaundice See *jaundice, breast milk.*

breech presentation Presentation in which buttocks and/or feet are nearest the cervical opening and are born first; occurs in approximately 3% of all deliveries.

complete b.p. Simultaneous presentation of buttocks, legs, and feet.

footling (incomplete) b.p. Presentation of one or both feet.

frank b.p. Presentation of buttocks, with hips flexed so that thighs are against abdomen.

bregma Point of junction of the coronal and sagittal sutures of the skull; the area of the anterior fontanel of the fetus.

brim Edge of the superior strait of the true pelvis; the inlet.

bronchopulmonary dysplasia Emphysematous changes caused by oxygen toxicity.

brown fat Source of heat unique to neonates that is capable of greater thermogenic activity than ordinary fat. Deposits are found around the adrenals, kidneys, and neck, between the scapulas, and behind the sternum for several weeks after birth.

bruit, uterine Sound of passage of blood through uterine blood vessels, synchronous with fetal heart rate.

caked breast See *engorgement.*

Candida vaginitis Vaginal, fungal infection; moniliasis.

capsularis, decidua See *decidua capsularis.*

caput Occiput of fetal head appearing at the vaginal introitus preceding delivery of the head.

c. succedaneum Swelling of the tissue over the presenting part of the fetal head caused by pressure during labor.

carrier Individual who carries a gene that does not exhibit itself in physical or chemical characteristics but that can be transmitted to children (e.g., a female carrying the trait for hemophilia, which is expressed in male offspring).

caudal anesthesia Type of regional anesthesia used in childbirth in which the anesthetic agent is injected into the caudal area of the spinal canal through the sacral hiatus, affecting the caudal nerve roots and thereby anesthetizing the cervix, vagina, and perineum. Medication does not mix with cerebrospinal fluid (CSF).

caul Hood of fetal membranes covering fetal head during delivery.

centesis Suffix pertaining to a surgical puncture or perforation.

cephalhematoma Extravasation of blood from ruptured vessels between a skull bone and its external covering, the periosteum. Swelling is limited by the margins of the cranial bone affected (usually parietals).

cephalic Pertaining to the head.

c. presentation Presentation of any part of the fetal head.

cephalopelvic disproportion (**CPD**) Condition in which the infant's head is of such a shape, size, or position that it cannot pass through the mother's pelvis.

cervical cap (**custom**) Individually fitted contraceptive covering for the cervix.

cervical mucus method See *ovulation method.*

cervical os "Mouth" or opening to the cervix.

cervicitis Cervical infection.

cervix Lowest and narrow end of the uterus; the "neck." The cervix is situated between the external os and the body or corpus of the uterus, and its lower end extends into the vagina.

cesarean delivery Birth of a fetus by an incision through the abdominal wall and uterus.

cesarean hysterectomy Removal of the uterus immediately after the cesarean delivery of an infant.

Chadwick's sign Violet color of mucous membrane that is visible from about the fourth week of pregnancy; caused by increased vascularity of the vagina.

chloasma Increased pigmentation over bridge of nose and cheeks of pregnant women and some women taking oral contraceptives; also known as *mask of pregnancy.*

choanal atresia See *atresia, choanal.*

cholelithiasis Presence of gallstones in the gallbladder.

chorioamnionitis Stimulated by organisms in the amniotic fluid, which then become infiltrated with polymorphonuclear leukocytes.

chorion Fetal membrane closest to the intrauterine wall that gives rise to the placenta and continues as the outer membrane surrounding the amnion.

chorionic villi See *villi, chorionic.*

chromosome Element within the cell nucleus carrying genes and composed of DNA and proteins.

circumcision Excision of the male's prepuce (foreskin).

cleft lip Incomplete closure of the lip; harelip.

cleft palate Incomplete closure of the palate or roof of mouth; a congenital fissure.

clitoris Female organ analogous to male penis; a small, ovoid body of erectile tissue situated at the anterior junction of the vulva.

prepuce of the c. See *prepuce of the clitoris.*

coitus Penile-vaginal intercourse.

c. interruptus Intercourse during which penis is withdrawn from vagina before ejaculation.

colostrum Yellow secretion from the breast containing mainly serum and white blood corpuscles preceding the onset of true lactation 2 or 3 days after delivery.

complement Naturally occurring blood component that is a factor in the destruction of bacteria.

complete abortion See *abortion, complete.*

complete breech presentation See *breech presentation, complete.*

conception Union of the sperm and ovum resulting in fertilization; formation of the one-celled zygote.

conceptional age In fetal development, the number of completed weeks since the moment of conception. Because the moment of conception is almost impossible to determine, conceptional age is estimated at 2 weeks less than gestational age.

conceptus Embryo or fetus, fetal membranes, amniotic fluid, and the fetal portion of the placenta.

condom Mechanical barrier worn on the penis for contraception; "rubber."

confinement Period of childbirth and early puerperium.

congenital Present or existing before birth as a result of either hereditary or prenatal environmental factors.

conjoined twins See *twins, conjoined.*

conjugate

- **diagonal c.** Radiographic measurement of distance from *inferior border* of SP to sacral promontory; may be obtained by vaginal examination; 12.5 to 13 cm.
- **true c.** (**c. vera**) Radiographic measurement of distance from *upper margin* of symphysis pubis (SP) to sacral promontory; 1.5 to 2 cm less than diagonal conjugate.

conjunctivitis Inflammation of the mucous membrane that lines the eyelids and that is reflected onto the eyeball.

contraception Prevention of impregnation or conception.

contraction ring See *Bandl's ring.*

Coombs' test Indirect: determination of Rh-positive antibodies in maternal blood; direct: determination of maternal Rh-positive antibodies in fetal cord blood. A positive test result indicates the presence of antibodies or titer.

coping mechanism Any effort directed at stress management. It can be task oriented and involve direct problem-solving efforts to cope with the threat itself or be intrapsychic or ego defense oriented with the goal of regulating one's emotional distress.

copulation Coitus; sexual intercourse.

corpus Discrete mass of material; body.

- **c. cavernosum** Term referring to one of two cylinders of spongy tissue within the penis or tissue within the clitoris that engorges with blood during sexual excitement resulting in erection.
- **c. luteum** Yellow body. After rupture of the graafian follicle at ovulation, the follicle develops into a yellow structure that secretes progesterone in the second half of the menstrual cycle, atrophying about 3 days before sloughing of the endometrium in menstrual flow. If impregnation occurs, this structure continues to produce progesterone until the placenta can take over this function.
- **c. spongiosum** One of the spongy cylinders of tissue within the penis; has a protective function.

cotyledon One of the 15 to 28 visible segments of the placenta on the maternal surface, each made up of fetal vessels, chorionic villi, and an intervillous space.

couvade Custom whereby the husband goes through mock labor while his wife is giving birth.

Couvelaire uterus See *uterus, Couvelaire.*

CPAP Continuous positive airway pressure.

cradle cap Common seborrheic dermatitis of infants consisting of thick, yellow, greasy scales on the scalp.

craniotabes Localized softening of cranial bones.

creatinine Substance found in blood and muscle; measurement of levels in maternal urine correlates with amount of fetal muscle mass and therefore fetal size.

crib death Unexpected and sudden death of an apparently normal and healthy infant that occurs during sleep and with no physical or autopsic evidence of disease. Also referred to as sudden infant death syndrome (SIDS).

cri-du-chat syndrome Rare congenital disorder recognized at birth by a kittenlike cry, which may prevail for weeks, then disappear. Other characteristics include low birth weight, microcephaly, "moon face," wide-set eyes, strabismus, and low-set misshaped ears. Infants are hypotonic; heart defects and mental and physical retardation are common. Also called cat-cry syndrome.

crowning Stage of delivery when the top of the fetal head can be seen at the vaginal orifice.

cryptochidism Failure of one or both of the testicles to descend into the scrotum. Also called undescended testis.

cul-de-sac of Douglas Pouch formed by a fold of the peritoneum dipping down between the anterior wall of the rectum and the posterior wall of the uterus; also called *Douglas' cul-de-sac, pouch of Douglas,* and *rectouterine pouch.*

Cullen's sign Faint, irregularly formed, hemorrhagic patches on the skin around the umbilicus. The discolored skin is blue-black and becomes greenish brown or yellow. Cullen's sign may appear 1 to 2 days after the onset of anorexia and the severe, poorly localized abdominal pains characteristic of acute pancreatitis. Cullen's sign is also present in massive upper gastrointestinal hemorrhage, ruptured ectopic pregnancy.

curettage Scraping of the endometrium lining of the uterus with a curet to remove the contents of the uterus (as is done after an inevitable or incomplete abortion) or to obtain specimens for diagnostic purposes.

cutis marmorata Transient vasomotor phenomenon occurring primarily over extremities when the infant is exposed to chilling. It appears as a pink or faint purple capillary outline on the skin. Occasionally it is seen if the infant is in respiratory distress.

cyesis Pregnancy.

cystocele Bladder hernia; injury to the vesicovaginal fascia during labor and delivery may allow herniation of the bladder into the vagina.

cytology The study of cells, including their formation, origin, structure, function, biochemical activities, and pathology.

death Cessation of life.

- **fetal d.** Intrauterine death. Death of a fetus weighing 500 g or more of 20 weeks' gestation or more.
- **infant d.** Death during the first year of life.
- **maternal d.** Death of a woman during the childbearing cycle.
- **neonatal d.** Death of a newborn within the first 28 days after birth.

perinatal d. Death of a fetus of 20 weeks' gestation or older or death of a neonate 28 days old or younger.
decidua Mucous membrane, lining of uterus, or endometrium of pregnancy that is shed after giving birth.
d. basalis Maternal aspect of the placenta made up of uterine blood vessels, endometrial stroma, and glands. It is shed in lochial discharge after delivery.
d. capsularis That part of the decidual membranes surrounding the chorionic sac.
d. vera Nonplacental decidual lining of the uterus.
decrement Decrease or stage of decline, as of a contraction.
delivery Expulsion of the child with placenta and membranes by the mother or their extraction by the obstetric practitioner.
abdominal d. See *abdominal delivery.*
ΔOD_{450} (read delta OD_{450}) Delta optical density (or absorbance) at 450 nm, obtained by spectral analysis of amniotic fluid. This prenatal test is used to measure the degree of hemolytic activity in the fetus and to evaluate fetal status in women sensitized to Rh(D).
deoxyribonucleic acid (DNA) Intracellular complex protein that carries genetic information, consisting of two purines (adenine and guanine) and two pyrimidines (thymine and cytosine).
dermatoglyphics Study of skin ridge patterns on fingers, toes, palms of hands, and soles of feet.
DES Diethylstilbestrol, used in treating menopausal symptoms. Exposure of female fetus predisposes her to reproductive tract malformations and (later) dysplasia.
desquamation Shedding of epithelial cells of the skin and mucous membranes.
developmental crisis Severe, usually transient, stress that occurs when a person is unable to complete the tasks of a psychosocial stage of development and is therefore unable to move on to the next stage.
developmental task Physical or cognitive skill that a child must accomplish during a particular age period in order to continue developing, as walking, which precedes the development of sense of autonomy in the toddler period.
diaphragmatic hernia Congenital malformation of diaphragm that allows displacement of the abdominal organs into the thoracic cavity.
diastasis recti abdominis Separation of the two rectus muscles along the median line of the abdominal wall. This is often seen in women with repeated childbirths or with a multiple gestation (triplets, etc.). In the newborn it is usually due to incomplete development.
DIC Disseminated intravascular coagulation.
Dick-Read method An approach to childbirth based on the premise that fear of pain produces muscular tension, producing pain and greater fear. The method includes teaching physiological processes of labor, exercise to improve muscle tone, and techniques to assist in relaxation and prevent the fear-tension-pain mechanism.
dilatation of cervix Stretching of the external os from an opening a few millimeters in size to an opening large enough to allow the passage of the infant.
dilatation and curettage (D and C) Vaginal operation in which the cervical canal is stretched enough to admit passage of an instrument called a *curet.* The endometrium of the uterus is scraped with the curet to empty the uterine contents or to obtain tissue for examination.
discordance Discrepancy in size (or other indicator) between twins.
disparate twins See *twins, disparate.*
dizygotic Related to or proceeding from two zygotes (fertilized ova).
dizygous twins See *twins, dizygous.*
Döderlein's bacillus Gram-positive bacterium occurring in normal vaginal secretions.
dominant trait Gene that is expressed whenever it is present in the heterozygous gene state (e.g., brown eyes are dominant over blue).
Douglas' cul-de-sac See *cul-de-sac of Douglas.*
Down's syndrome Abnormality involving the occurrence of a third chromosome, rather than the normal pair (trisomy 21), that characteristically results in a typical picture of mental retardation and altered physical appearance. This condition was formerly called *mongolism* or *mongoloid idiocy.*
dry labor Lay term referring to labor in which amniotic fluid has already escaped. A "dry birth" does not exist.
Dubowitz assessment Estimation of gestational age of a newborn, based on criteria developed for that purpose.
ductus arteriosus In fetal circulation, an anatomic shunt between the pulmonary artery and arch of the aorta. It is obliterated after birth by a rising Po_2 and change in intravascular pressures in the presence of normal pulmonary function. It normally becomes a ligament after birth but in some instances remains patent.
ductus venosus In fetal circulation, a blood vessel carrying oxygenated blood between the umbilical vein and the inferior vena cava, bypassing the liver. It is obliterated and becomes a ligament after birth.
Duncan's mechanism Delivery of placenta with the maternal surface presenting, rather than the shiny fetal surface.
dura (dura mater) Outermost, toughest of the three meninges covering the brain and spinal cord.
dys- Prefix meaning abnormal, difficult, painful, faulty.
dysmaturity See *intrauterine growth retardation (IUGR).*
dysmenorrhea Difficult or painful menstruation.
dysmorphogenesis Development of ill-shaped or malformed structures.
dyspareunia Painful sexual intercourse.
dystocia Prolonged, painful, or otherwise difficult delivery or birth because of mechanical factors produced by either the passenger (the fetus) or the passage (the pelvis of the mother) or because of inadequate powers (uterine and other muscular activity).
placental d. Difficulty in the delivery of the placenta.

ecchymosis Bruise; bleeding into tissue caused by direct trauma, serious infection, or bleeding diathesis.
eclampsia Severe complication of pregnancy of unknown cause and occurring more often in the primigravida; characterized by tonic and clonic convulsions, coma, high blood pressure, albuminuria, and oliguria occurring during pregnancy or shortly after delivery.
ectoderm Outer layer of embryonic tissue giving rise to skin, nails, and hair.

ectopic Out of normal place.
  e. pregnancy Implantation of the fertilized ovum outside of its normal place in the uterine cavity. Locations include the abdomen, fallopian tubes, and ovaries.

EDC Expected date of confinement; "due date."

effacement Thinning and shortening or obliteration of the cervix that occurs during late pregnancy or labor or both.

effleurage Gentle stroking used in massage.

ejaculation Sudden expulsion of semen from the male urethra.

elective abortion See *abortion, elective.*

embolus Any undissolved matter (solid, liquid, or gaseous) that is carried by the blood to another part of the body and obstructs a blood vessel.

embryo Conceptus from the second or third week of development until about the eighth week after conception, when mineralization (ossification) of the skeleton begins. This period is characterized by cellular differentiation and predominantly hyperplastic growth.

endocervical Pertaining to the interior of the canal of the cervix of the uterus.

endocrine glands Ductless glands that secrete hormones into the blood or lymph.

endometriosis Tissue closely resembling endometrial tissue but aberrantly located outside the uterus in the pelvic cavity. Symptomatology may include pelvic pain or pressure, dysmenorrhea, dyspareunia, abnormal bleeding from the uterus or rectum, and sterility.

endometrium Inner lining of the uterus that undergoes changes caused by hormones during the menstrual cycle and pregnancy; decidua.

engagement In obstetrics, the entrance of the fetal presenting part into the superior pelvic strait and the beginning of the descent through the pelvic canal.

engorgement Distension or vascular congestion. In obstetrics, the process of swelling of the breast tissue brought about by an increase in blood and lymph supply to the breast, which precedes true lactation. It lasts about 48 hours and usually reaches a peak between the third and fifth postdelivery days.

engrossment Sustained involvement of a parent with an infant.

entoderm Inner layer of embryonic tissue giving rise to internal organs such as the intestine.

entrainment Phenomenon observed in the microanalysis of sound films in which the speaker moves several parts of the body and the listener responds to the sounds by moving in ways that are coordinated with the rhythm of the sounds. Infants have been observed to move in time to the rhythms of adult speech but not to random noises or disconnected words or vowels. Entrainment is thought to be an essential factor in the process of maternal-infant bonding.

epicanthus Fold of skin covering the inner canthus and caruncle that extends from the root of the nose to the median end of the eyebrow; characteristically found in certain races but may occur as a congenital anomaly.

episiotomy Surgical incision of the perineum at the end of the second stage of labor to facilitate delivery and to avoid laceration of the perineum.

epispadias Defect in which the urethral canal terminates on dorsum of penis or above the clitoris (rare).

Epstein's pearls Small, white blebs found along the gum margins and at the junction of the soft and hard palates. They are a normal manifestation and are commonly seen in the newborn. Similar to Bohn's nodules.

epulis Tumorlike benign lesion of the gingiva seen in pregnant women.

equilibrium A state of balance or rest owing to the equal action of opposing forces, as calcium and phosphorus in the body. In psychiatry, a state of mental or emotional balance.

Erb-Duchenne paralysis Paralysis caused by traumatic injury to the upper brachial plexus, occurring most commonly in childbirth from forcible traction during delivery. The signs of Erb's paralysis include loss of sensation in the arm and paralysis and atrophy of the deltoid, the biceps, and the branchialis muscles. Also called Erb's palsy.

ergot Drug obtained from *Claviceps purpurea,* a fungus, which stimulates the smooth muscles of blood vessels and the uterus, causing vasoconstriction and uterine contractions.

erythema toxicum Innocuous pink papular neonatal rash of unknown cause, with superimposed vesicles appearing within 24 to 48 hours after birth and resolving spontaneously within a few days.

erythroblastosis fetalis Hemolytic disease of the newborn usually caused by isoimmunization resulting from Rh incompatibility or ABO incompatibility.

escutcheon Pattern of distribution of pubic hair.

esophageal atresia See *atresia, esophageal.*

estradiol An estrogen.

estriol Major metabolite of estrogen that increases during the second half of pregnancy with an intact fetoplacental unit (normal placenta, normal fetal liver and adrenals) and normal maternal renal function.

estrogen Female sex hormone produced by the ovaries and placenta.

eutocia Normal or natural labor or birth.

exchange transfusion Replacement of 75% to 85% of circulating blood by withdrawing the recipient's blood and injecting a donor's blood in equal amounts, the purposes of which are to prevent an accumulation of bilirubin in the blood above a dangerous level, to prevent the accumulation of other by-products of hemolysis in hemolytic disease, and to correct anemia.

expulsive Having the tendency to drive out or expel.
  e. contractions Labor contractions that are characteristic of the second stage of labor.

extension Straightening of a body part; opposite of flexion.

extrauterine Occurring outside the uterus.
  e. pregnancy Ectopic pregnancy in which the fertilized ovum implants itself outside the uterus.

facies Pertaining to the appearance or expression of the face; certain congenital syndromes typically present with a specific facial appearance.

FAD Fetal activity determination.

failure to thrive Condition in which neonate's or infant's growth and development patterns are below the norms for age.

fallopian tubes Two canals or oviducts extending laterally from each side of the uterus through which the ovum travels, after ovulation, to the uterus.

false labor Uterine contractions that do not result in cervical dilatation, are irregular, are felt more in front, often do not last more than 20 seconds, and do not become longer or stronger.

false pelvis The part of the pelvis superior to a plane passing through the linea terminalis.

Ferguson's reflex Reflex contractions of the uterus after stimulation of the cervix.

ferning (arborization) test The appearance of a fernlike pattern in dried smears of uterine cervical mucus, indicating the presence of estrogen.

- **ovulation f. t.** Test in which cervical mucus, placed on a slide, dries in a branching pattern in the presence of high estrogen levels at the time of ovulation.
- **pregnancy f. t.** Test in which cervical mucus, placed on a slide, does not dry in a branching pattern because of high levels of progesterone along with estrogen.

fertility Quality of being able to reproduce.

fertility rate Number of births per 1000 women aged 15 through 44 years.

fertilization Union of an ovum and a sperm.

fetal Pertaining or relating to the fetus

- **f. alcohol syndrome** Congenital abnormality or anomaly resulting from maternal alcohol intake above 3 oz. of absolute alcohol per day. It is characterized by typical craniofacial and limb defects, cardiovascular defects, intrauterine growth retardation, and developmental delay.
- **f. attitude** See *attitude, fetal.*
- **f. asphyxia** See *asphyxia, fetal.*
- **f. death** See *death, fetal.*
- **f. distress** Evidence such as a change in the fetal heartbeat pattern or activity indicating that the fetus is in jeopardy.
- **f. lie** Relation of the fetal spine to the maternal spine; i.e., in vertical lie, maternal and fetal spines are parallel and the fetal head or breech presents; in transverse lie, fetal spine is perpendicular to the maternal spine and the fetal shoulder presents.
- **f. presentation** The part of the fetus that presents at the cervical os.

fetofetal transfusion See *parabiotic syndrome.*

α-fetoprotein (AFP) Fetal antigen; elevated levels in amniotic fluid associated with neural tube defects.

fetotoxic Poisonous or destructive to the fetus.

fetus Child in utero from about the eighth week after conception, until birth.

fibroid Fibrous, encapsulated connective tissue tumor, especially of the uterus.

fimbria Structure resembling a fringe, particularly the fringelike end of the fallopian tube.

fissure Groove or open crack in tissue.

fistula Abnormal tubelike passage that forms between two normal cavities, possibly congenital or caused by trauma, abscesses, or inflammatory processes.

flaccid Having relaxed, flabby, or absent muscle tone.

flaring of nostrils Widening of nostrils (alae nasi) during inspiration in the presence of air hunger; sign of respiratory distress.

flexion In obstetrics, resistance to the descent of the baby down the birth canal causes the head to flex, or bend, so that the chin approaches the chest. Thus the smallest diameter (suboccipitobregmatic) of the vertex presents.

fluid, amniotic See *amniotic fluid.*

follicle Small secretory cavity or sac.

- **graafian f.** Mature, fully developed ovarian cyst containing the ripe ovum. The follicle secretes estrogens, and after ovulation, the corpus luteum develops within the ruptured graafian follicle and secretes estrogen and progesterone.

follicle-stimulating hormone (FSH) Hormone produced by the anterior pituitary during the first half of the menstrual cycle. Stimulates development of the graafian follicle.

fomites Nonliving material on which disease-producing organisms may be conveyed (e.g., bed linen).

fontanel Broad area, or soft spot, consisting of a strong band of connective tissue contiguous with cranial bones and located at the junctions of the bones.

- **anterior f.** Diamond-shaped area between the frontal and two parietal bones just above the baby's forehead at the junction of the coronal and sagittal sutures.
- **mastoid f.** Posterolateral fontanel usually not palpable.
- **posterior f.** Small, triangular area between the occipital and parietal bones at the junction of the lambdoidal and sagittal sutures.
- **sagittal f.** Soft area located in the sagittal suture, halfway between the anterior and posterior fontanels; may be found in normal newborns and in some neonates with Down's syndrome.
- **sphenoid f.** Anterolateral fontanel usually not palpable.

footling (incomplete) breech presentation See *breech presentation, footling.*

foramen ovale Septal opening between the atria of the fetal heart. The opening normally closes shortly after birth, but if it remains patent, surgical repair usually is necessary.

foreskin Prepuce, or loose fold of skin covering the glans penis.

fornix Any structure with an arched or vaultlike shape.

- **f. of the vagina** Anterior and posterior spaces, formed by the protrusion of the cervix into the vagina, into which the upper vagina is divided.

Fowler's position Posture assumed by client when head of bed is raised 18 or 20 inches and individual's knees are elevated.

frank breech presentation See *breech presentation, frank.*

fraternal twins Nonidentical twins that come from two separate fertilized ova.

frenulum Thin ridge of tissue in midline of undersurface of tongue extending from its base to varying distances from the tip of the tongue.

Friedman's curve Labor curve; pattern of descent of presenting part and of dilatation of cervix; partogram.

frigidity Archaic term designating a woman's inability to achieve orgasm; orgasmic dysfunction.

FSH See *follicle-stimulating hormone.*

fulguration Destruction of tissue by means of electricity.

fundus Dome-shaped upper portion of the uterus between the points of insertion of the fallopian tubes.

funic souffle See *souffle, funic.*

funis Cordlike structure, especially the umbilical cord.

galactosemia Inherited, autosomal recessive disorder of galactose metabolism, characterized by a deficiency of the enzyme galactose-1-phosphate uridyl transferase.

gamete Mature male or female germ cell; the mature sperm or ovum.

gastroschisis Abdominal wall defect at base of umbilical stalk.

gastrostomy Surgical creation of an artificial opening into the stomach through the abdominal wall, performed to feed a client when oral feeding is not possible.

gate control theory Proposed in 1965 by Melzack and Wall, this theory explains the neurophysical mechanism underlying the perception of pain.

gavage Feeding by means of a tube passed to the stomach.

gender identity The sense or awareness of knowing to which sex one belongs. The process begins in infancy, continues throughout childhood, and is reinforced during adolescence.

gene Factor on a chromosome responsible for hereditary characteristics of offspring.

genetic Dependent on the genes. A genetic disorder may or may not be apparent at birth.

genetic counseling Process of determining the occurrence or risk of occurrence of a genetic disorder within a family and of providing appropriate information and advice about the courses of action that are available, whether care of a child already affected, prenatal diagnosis, termination of a pregnancy, sterilization, or artificial insemination is involved.

genitalia Organs of reproduction.

genotype Hereditary combinations in an individual determining physical and chemical characteristics. Some genotypes are not expressed until later in life (e.g., Huntington's chorea); some hide recessive genes, which can be expressed in offspring; and others are expressed only under the proper environmental conditions (e.g., diabetes mellitus appearing under the stress of obesity or pregnancy).

gestation Period of intrauterine fetal development from conception through birth; the period of pregnancy.
  abdominal g. See *abdominal gestation.*

gestational age In fetal development, the number of completed weeks counting from the first day of the last normal menstrual cycle.

glabella Bony prominence above the nose and between the eyebrows.

glans penis Smooth, round head of the penis, analogous to the female glans clitoris.

glomerulonephritis Noninfectious disease of the glomerulus of the kidney, characterized by proteinuria, hematuria, decreased urine production, and edema.

glycosuria Presence of glucose (a sugar) in the urine.

gonad Gamete-producing, or sex, gland; the ovary or testis.

gonadotropic hormone Hormone that stimulates the gonads.

Goodell's sign Softening of the cervix, a probable sign of pregnancy, occurring during the second month.

gossypol Oral contraceptive produced from cotton plants; currently in experimental stage of use by males in the United States.

graafian follicle (vesicle) See *follicle, graafian.*

gravid Pregnant.

grieving process A complex of somatic and psychological symptoms associated with some extreme sorrow or loss, specifically the death of a loved one.

grunt, expiratory Sign of respiratory distress (hyaline membrane disease [respiratory distress syndrome, or RDS] or advanced pneumonia) indicative of the body's attempt to hold air in the alveoli for better gaseous exchange.

gynecoid pelvis Pelvis in which the inlet is round instead of oval or blunt; heart shaped. Typical female pelvis.

gynecology Study of the diseases of the female, especially of the genital, urinary, and rectal organs.

habitual (recurrent) abortion See *abortion, habitual.*

habituation An acquired tolerance from repeated exposure to a particular stimulus. Also called negative adaptation; a decline and eventual elimination of a conditioned response by repetition of the conditioned stimulus.

habitus Indications in appearance of tendency or disposition to disease or abnormal conditions.

harlequin sign Rare color change of no pathologic significance occurring between the longitudinal halves of the neonate's body. When infant is placed on one side, the dependent half is noticeably pinker than the superior half.

Hawthorne effect A general beneficial effect on a person or group of people as a result of a therapeutic encounter with a health care provider or as a result of a change in the environment (lighting, temperature, type of room [family-centered versus four-bed unit]).

Hegar's sign Softening of the lower uterine segment that is classified as a probable sign of pregnancy and that may be present during the second and third months of pregnancy and is palpated during bimanual examination.

hematocrit Volume of red blood cells per deciliter (dl) of circulating blood; packed cell volume (PCV).

hematoma Collection of blood in a tissue; a bruise or blood tumor.

hemoconcentration Increase in the number of red blood cells resulting from either a decrease in plasma volume or increased erythropoiesis.

hemoglobin Component of red blood cells consisting of globin, a protein, and hematin, an organic iron compound.
  h. electrophoresis Test to diagnose sickle cell disease in newborns. Cord blood is used.

hemorrhagic disease of newborn Bleeding disorder during first few days of life based on a deficiency of vitamin K.

hereditary Pertaining to a trait or characteristic transmitted from parent to offspring by way of the genes; used synonymously with *genetic.*

hermaphrodite Person having genital and sexual characteristics of both sexes.

heterologous insemination Insemination in which the semen specimen is provided by an anonymous donor. The procedure is used primarily in cases where the husband is sterile.

heterozygous Having two dissimilar genes at the same site, or locus, on paired chromosomes (e.g., at the sites for eye color, one chromosome carrying the gene for brown, the other for blue).

high risk An increased possibility of suffering harm, damage, loss, or death.

Homans' sign Early sign of phlebothrombosis of the deep veins of the calf in which there are complaints of pain when the leg is in extension and the foot is dorsiflexed.

homoiothermic Referring to the ability of warm-blooded animals to maintain internal temperature at a specified level regardless of the environmental temperature. This ability is not fully developed in the human neonate.

homologous Similar in structure or origin but not necessarily in function.

homologous insemination Insemination in which the semen specimen is provided by the husband. The procedure is used primarily in cases of impotence or when the husband is incapable of sexual intercourse because of some physical disability.

homozygous Having two similar genes at the same locus, or site, on paired chromosomes.

hormone Chemical substance produced in an organ or gland that is conveyed through the blood to another organ or part of the body, stimulating it to increased functional activity or secretion. See specific hormones.

hour-glass uterus Uterus in which a segment of circular muscle fibers contracts during labor. The resultant "constriction ring" dystocia is characterized by lack of progress in spite of adequate contractions; by pain experienced prior to palpation of a uterine contraction and persisting after the observer feels the contraction end; and by recession of the presenting part during a contraction, instead of descent of the presenting part.

hyaline membrane disease (HMD) Disease characterized by interference with ventilation at the alveolar level, theoretically caused by the presence of fibrinoid deposits lining alveolar ducts. Membrane formation is related to prematurity (especially with fetal asphyxia) and insufficient surfactant production (L/S ratio less than 2:1). Otherwise known as *respiratory distress syndrome (RDS)*.

hydramnios (polyhydramnios) Amniotic fluid in excess of 1.5L; often indicative of fetal anomaly and frequently seen in poorly controlled, insulin-dependent, diabetic pregnant women even if there is no coexisting fetal anomaly.

hydrocele Collection of fluid in a saclike cavity, especially in the sac that surrounds the testis, causing the scrotum to swell.

hydropic Dropsical or pertaining to edema; abnormal accumulation of serous fluid in the body tissues and cavities.

hydrops fetalis Most severe expression of fetal hemolytic disorder, a possible sequela to maternal Rh isoimmunization; infants exhibit gross edema (anasarca), cardiac decompensation, and profound pallor from anemia and seldom survive.

hymen Membranous fold that normally partially covers the entrance to the vagina in the virgin.

hymenal caruncles Small, irregular bits of tissue that are remnants of the hymen.

hymenal tag Normally occurring redundant hymenal tissue protruding from the floor of the vagina that disappears spontaneously in a few weeks after birth.

hymenotomy Surgical incision of the hymen.

hyperbilirubinemia Elevation of unconjugated serum bilirubin concentrations.

hyperemesis gravidarum Abnormal condition of pregnancy characterized by protracted vomiting, weight loss, and fluid and electrolyte imbalance.

hyperesthesia Unusual sensibility to sensory stimuli, such as pain or touch.

hyperplasia Increase in number of cells; formation of new tissue.

hyperreflexia Increased action of the reflexes.

hypertrophy Enlargement, or increase in size, of existing cells.

hyperventilation Rapid, shallow (or prolonged, deep) respirations resulting in respiratory alkalosis: a decrease in H^+ concentration and P_{CO_2} and an increase in the blood pH and the ratio of $NaHCO_3$ to H_2CO_3. Symptoms may include faintness, palpitations, and carpopedal (hands and feet) muscular spasms. Relief may result from rebreathing in a paper bag or into one's cupped hands to replace the CO_2 "blown off" during hyperventilation.

hypochlorhydria Diminished secretion of hydrochloric acid.

hypofibrinogenemia Deficient level of a blood clotting factor, fibrinogen, in the blood; in obstetrics, it occurs following complications of abruptio placentae or retention of a dead fetus.

hypogastric arteries Branches of the right and left iliac arteries carrying deoxygenated blood from the fetus through the umbilical cord, where they are known as *umbilical arteries*, to the placenta.

hypoglycemia Less-than-normal amount of glucose in the blood, usually caused by administration of too much insulin, excessive secretion of insulin by the islet cells of the pancreas, or by dietary deficiency.

hypospadias Anomalous positioning of urinary meatus on undersurface of penis or close to or just inside the vagina.

hypotensive drugs Drugs that lower the blood pressure.

hypothalamus Portion of the diencephalon of the brain forming the floor and part of the lateral wall of the third ventricle. It activates, controls, and integrates the peripheral autonomic nervous system, endocrine processes, and many somatic functions, as body temperature, sleep, and appetite.

hypothenar Fleshy elevation on the ulnar (little finger) side of the palm of the hand. Also called *hypothenar eminence*.

hypotonia Reduced tension; relaxation of arteries. Also, loss of tonicity of the muscles or intraocular pressure.

hypoxemia Reduction in arterial P_{O_2} resulting in metabolic acidosis by forcing anaerobic glycolysis, pulmonary vasoconstriction, and direct cellular damage.

hypoxia Insufficient availability of oxygen to meet the metabolic needs of body tissue.

hysterectomy Surgical removal of the uterus.

- **panhysterectomy** Removal of entire uterus, but ovaries and tubes remain.
- **subtotal h.** Removal of fundus and body of the uterus, but the cervical stump remains.
- **total h.** Removal of entire uterus, including the cervix, but the ovaries and tubes remain.

hysterosalpingography Recording by x-ray of the uterus and uterine tubes after injecting them with radiopaque material.

hysterotomy Surgical incision into the uterus.

iatrogenic Caused by a physician's words, actions, or treatment.

icterus neonatorum Jaundice in the newborn.

idiopathic respiratory distress syndrome (hyaline membrane disease) Severe respiratory condition found almost exclusively in preterm infants and in some infants of diabetic mothers regardless of gestational age. See also *hyaline membrane disease (HMD)*.

IDM Infant of a diabetic mother.
IgA Primary immunoglobulin in colostrum.
IgG Transplacentally acquired immunoglobulin that confers passive immunity against the infections to which the mother is immune.
IgM Immunoglobulin neonate can manufacture soon after birth. Fetus produces it in the presence of amnionitis.
iliopectineal line Bony ridge on the inner surface of the ilium and pubic bones that divides the true and false pelvises; the brim of the true pelvic cavity; the inlet.
implantation Embedding of the fertilized ovum in the uterine mucosa; nidation.
impotence Archaic term designating a man's inability, partial or complete, to perform sexual intercourse or to achieve orgasm; erectile dysfunction.
inborn error of metabolism Hereditary deficiency of a specific enzyme needed for normal metabolism of specific chemicals (e.g., deficiency of phenylalanine hydroxylase results in phenylketonuria [PKU]; a deficiency of hexosaminidase results in Tay-Sachs disease).
incompetent cervix Cervix that is unable to remain closed until a pregnancy reaches term, because of a mechanical defect in the cervix resulting in dilatation and effacement usually during the second or early third trimester of pregnancy.
incomplete abortion See *abortion, incomplete.*
increment An increase, or buildup, as of a contraction.
induced abortion See *abortion, induced.*
induction Artificial stimulation or augmentation of labor.
inertia Sluggishness or inactivity; in obstetrics, refers to the absence or weakness of uterine contractions during labor.
inevitable abortion See *abortion, inevitable.*
infant A child who is under 1 year of age.
infertility Decreased capacity to conceive.
infiltration Process by which a substance such as a local anesthetic drug is deposited within the tissue.
inhalation analgesia Reduction of pain by administration of anesthetic gas. Occasionally given during the second stage of labor. Consciousness is retained to allow the woman to follow instructions and to avoid the adverse effects of general anesthesia.
inlet Passage leading into a cavity.
  pelvic i. Upper brim of the pelvic cavity.
internal os Inside mouth or opening.
interstitial cell-stimulating hormone (ICSH) Hormone that stimulates production of testosterone; analogous to LH in the female.
intertuberous diameter Distance between ischial tuberosities. Measured to determine dimension of pelvic outlet.
intervillous space Irregular space in the maternal portion of the placenta, filled with maternal blood and serving as the site of maternal-fetal gas, nutrient, and waste exchange.
intrapartum During labor and delivery.
intrathecal Within the subarachnoid space.
intrauterine device (IUD) Small plastic or metal form placed in the uterus to prevent implantation of a fertilized ovum.
intrauterine growth retardation (IUGR) Fetal undergrowth of any etiology, such as deficient nutrient supply or intrauterine infection, or associated with congenital malformation.
introitus Entrance into a canal or cavity such as the vagina.
intromission Insertion of one part or object into another (e.g., introduction of penis into vagina).
intussusception Prolapse of one segment of bowel into the lumen of the adjacent segment.
in utero Within or inside the uterus.
in vitro fertilization Fertilization in a culture dish or test tube.
inversion Turning end for end, upside down, or inside out.
  i. of the uterus Condition in which the uterus is turned inside out so that the fundus intrudes into the cervix or vagina, caused by a too vigorous removal of the placenta before it is detached by the natural process of labor.
involution (1) Rolling or turning inward. (2) Reduction in size of the uterus after delivery and its return to its normal size and condition. See *retraction.*
isoimmune hemolytic disease Breakdown (hemolysis) of fetal/neonatal Rh-positive RBCs because of Rh antibodies formed by an Rh-negative mother who had been previously exposed to Rh-positive RBCs.
isoimmunization Development of antibodies in a species of animal with antigens from the same species (e.g., development of anti-Rh antibodies in an Rh-negative person).
ITP Abbreviation for idiopathic thrombocytopenic purpura.

jaundice Yellow discoloration of the body tissues caused by the deposit of bile pigments (unconjugated bilirubin); icterus.
  breast milk j. Yellowing of infant's skin from pregnanediol (in mother's milk) inhibition of enzyme (glucuronyl transferase) necessary for conjugation of bilirubin.
  pathologic j. Jaundice usually first noticeable within 24 hours after birth; caused by some abnormal condition such as an Rh or ABO incompatibility and resulting in bilirubin toxicity (e.g., kernicterus)
  physiologic j. Jaundice usually occurring 48 hours or later after birth, reaching a peak at 5 to 7 days, gradually disappearing by the seventh to tenth day, and caused by the normal reduction in the number of red blood cells. The infant is otherwise well.

Kahn test Precipitation or flocculation test for the diagnosis of syphilis.
karyotype Schematic arrangement of the chromosomes within a cell to demonstrate their numbers and morphology.
Kegel exercises Exercises to strengthen the pubococcygeal muscles.
kernicterus Bilirubin encephalopathy involving the deposit of unconjugated bilirubin in brain cells, resulting in death or impaired intellectual, perceptive, or motor function, and adaptive behavior.
kin group People related by blood or marriage.
Klumpke's palsy Atrophic paralysis of forearm.

labia Lips or liplike structures.
  l. majora Two folds of skin containing fat and covered with hair that lie on either side of the vaginal opening and from each side of the vulva.
  l. minora Two thin folds of delicate, hairless skin inside the labia majora.
labor Series of processes by which the fetus is expelled from the uterus; parturition; childbirth.

laceration Irregular tear of wound tissue; in obstetrics, it usually refers to a tear in the perineum, vagina, or cervix caused by childbirth.
lactase Enzyme necessary for the digestion of lactose.
lactation Function of secreting milk or period during which milk is secreted.
lactogen Drug or other substance that enhances the production and secretion of milk.
lactogenic Stimulating the production of milk.
l. hormone Gonadotropin produced by anterior pituitary and responsible for promoting growth of breast tissue and lactation; prolactin; luteotropin.
lactose intolerance Inherited absence of the enzyme lactose.
lactosuria Presence of lactose in the urine during late pregnancy and during lactation. Must be differentiated from glycosuria.
Lamaze method Method of psychophysical preparation for childbirth developed in the 1950s by a French obstetrician, Fernand Lamaze. It requires classes, practice at home, and coaching during labor and delivery.
lambdoid Having the shape of the Greek letter lambda.
l. suture Suture line extending across the posterior third of the skull, separating the occipital bone from the two parietal bones, and forming the base of the triangular posterior fontanel.
laminaria tent Cone of dried seaweed that swells as it absorbs moisture. Used to dilate the cervix nontraumatically in preparation for an induced abortion or in preparation for induction of labor.
lanugo Downy, fine hair characteristic of the fetus between 20 weeks' gestation and birth that is most noticeable over the shoulder, forehead, and cheeks but is found on nearly all parts of the body except the palms of the hands, soles of the feet, and the scalp.
laparoscopy Examination of the interior of the abdomen by inserting a small telescope through the anterior abdominal wall.
large for dates (large for gestational age [LGA]) Exhibiting excessive growth for gestational age.
lecithin A phospholipid that decreases surface tension; surfactant.
lecithin/sphingomyelin ratio Ratio of lecithin to sphingomyelin in the amniotic fluid. This is used to assess maturity of the fetal lung.
Leopold's maneuver Four maneuvers for diagnosing the fetal position by external palpation of the mother's abdomen.
let-down reflex Oxytocin-induced flow of milk from the alveoli of the breasts into the milk ducts.
leukorrhea White or yellowish mucous discharge from the cervical canal or the vagina that may be normal physiologically or caused by pathologic states of the vagina and endocervix (e.g., *Trichomonas vaginalis* infections).
LH See *luteinizing hormone (LH)*.
libido Sexual drive.
lie Relationship existing between the long axis of the fetus and the long axis of the mother. In a longitudinal lie, the fetus is lying lengthwise or vertically, whereas in a transverse lie the fetus is lying crosswise or horizontally in the mother's uterus.
ligation Act of suturing, sewing, or otherwise tying shut.
tubal l. Abdominal operation in which the fallopian tubes are tied off and a section is removed to interrupt tubal continuity and thus sterilize the woman.
lightening Sensation of decreased abdominal distention produced by uterine descent into the pelvic cavity as the fetal presenting part settles into the pelvis. It usually occurs 2 weeks before the onset of labor in nulliparas.
linea nigra Line of darker pigmentation seen in some women during the latter part of pregnancy that appears on the middle of the abdomen and extends from the symphysis pubis toward the umbilicus.
linea terminalis Line dividing the upper (false) pelvis from the lower (true) pelvis.
lithotomy position Position in which the woman lies on her back with her knees flexed and abducted thighs drawn up toward her chest.
live birth Birth in which the neonate, regardless of gestational age, manifests any heartbeat, breathes, or displays voluntary movement.
lochia Vaginal discharge during the puerperium consisting of blood, tissue, and mucus.
l. alba Thin, yellowish to white, vaginal discharge that follows lochia serosa on about the tenth postdelivery day and that may last from the end of the third to the sixth postdelivery week.
l. rubra Red, distinctly blood-tinged vaginal flow that follows delivery and lasts 2 to 4 days after delivery.
l. serosa Serous, pinkish brown, watery vaginal discharge that follows lochia rubra until about the tenth postdelivery day.
L/S ratio (lecithin/sphingomyelin ratio) Test for fetal lung maturity.
lunar month Four weeks (28 days).
lutein Yellow pigment derived from the corpus luteum, egg yolk, and fat cells.
l. cells Ovarian cells involved in the formation of the corpus luteum and that contain a yellow pigment.
luteinizing hormone (LH) Hormone produced by the anterior pituitary that stimulates ovulation and the development of the corpus luteum.
luteotropin (LTH) Lactogenic hormone; prolactin; an adenohypophyseal hormone.
lysozyme Enzyme with antiseptic qualities that destroys foreign organisms and that is found in blood cells of the granulocytic and monocytic series and is also normally present in saliva, sweat, tears, and breast milk.

maceration (1) Process of softening a solid by soaking it in a fluid. (2) Softening and breaking down of fetal skin from prolonged exposure to amniotic fluid as seen in a postterm infant. Also seen in a dead fetus.
macroglossia Hypertrophy of tongue or tongue large for oral cavity; seen in some preterm neonates and in neonates with Down's syndrome.
macrophage Any phagocytic cell of the reticuloendothelial system including Kupffer cell in the liver, splenocyte in the spleen, and histocyte in the loose connective tissue.
macrosomia Large body size as seen in neonates of diabetic or prediabetic mothers; macrosomatia.
malpractice Professional negligence that is the proximate

cause of injury or harm to a client, resulting from a lack of professional knowledge, experience, or skill that can be expected in others in the profession or from a failure to exercise reasonable care or judgment in the application of professional knowledge, experience, or skill.

mammary gland Compound gland of the female breast that is made up of lobes and lobules that secrete milk for nourishment of the young. Rudimentary mammary glands exist in the male.

manic depressive psychosis Major affective disorder characterized by episodes of mania and depression. One or the other phase may be predominant at any given time; one phase may appear alternately with the other; or elements of both phases may be present simultaneously. Also called bipolar disorder.

mask of pregnancy See *chloasma.*

mastalgia Breast soreness or tenderness.

mastectomy Excision, or removal, of the mammary gland.

mastitis Inflammation of mammary tissue of the breasts.

maternal mortality Death of a woman related to childbearing.

maturation (1) Process of attaining maximum development. (2) In biology, a process of cell division during which the number of chromosomes in the germ cells (sperm or ova) is reduced to one half the number (haploid) characteristic of the species.

maturational crisis Crisis that arises during normal growth and development, e.g., puberty.

meatus Opening from an internal structure to the outside (e.g., urethral meatus).

mechanism Instrument or process by which something is done, results, or comes into being; in obstetrics, labor and delivery.

meconium First stools of infant: viscid, sticky; dark greenish brown, almost black; sterile; odorless.

m. aspiration syndrome Function of fetal hypoxia: with hypoxia, the anal sphincter relaxes and meconium is released; reflex gasping movements draw meconium and other particulate matter in the amniotic fluid into the infant's bronchial tree, obstructing the air flow after birth.

m. ileus Lower intestinal obstruction by thick, puttylike, inspissated meconium that may be the result of deficiency of trypsin production in the newborn with cystic fibrosis.

m.-stained fluid In response to hypoxia, fetal intestinal activity increases and anal sphincter relaxes, resulting in the passage of meconium, which imparts a greenish coloration.

meiosis Process by which germ cells divide and decrease their chromosomal number by one half.

-melia Pertaining to a limb or part of a limb or extremity, as in amelia (absence of a limb) or phocomelia (absence of part of arms or legs).

membrane Thin, pliable layer of tissue that lines a cavity or tube, separates structures, or covers an organ or structure; in obstetrics, the amnion and chorion surrounding the fetus.

membrane rupture Tearing of the fetal membranes (amnion and chorion) with the release of amniotic fluid.

menarche Onset, or beginning, of menstrual function.

meningomyelocele Saclike protrusion of the spinal cord through a congenital defect in the vertebral column.

menopause From the Greek word *men* (month) and *pausis* (to stop), the actual permanent cessation of menstrual cycles.

menorrhagia Abnormally profuse or excessive menstrual flow.

menses (menstruation) Periodic vaginal discharge of bloody fluid from the nonpregnant uterus that occurs from the age of puberty to menopause.

mentum Chin, a fetal reference point in designating position (e.g., "Left mentum anterior" [LMA], meaning that the fetal chin is presenting in the left anterior quadrant of the maternal pelvis).

mesoderm Embryonic middle layer of germ cells giving rise to all types of muscles, connective tissue, bone marrow, blood, lymphoid tissue, and all epithelial tissue.

metritis Inflammation of the endometrium and myometrium.

metrorrhagia Abnormal bleeding from the uterus, particularly when it occurs at any time other than the menstrual period.

microcephaly Congenital anomaly characterized by abnormal smallness of the head in relation to the rest of the body and by underdevelopment of the brain, resulting in some degree of mental retardation.

micrognathia Abnormal smallness of mandible or chin.

midwife One who practices the art of helping and aiding a woman to give birth.

milia Unopened sebaceous glands appearing as tiny, white, pinpoint papules on forehead, nose, cheeks, and chin of a neonate that disappear spontaneously in a few days or weeks.

milk-leg See *phlegmasia alba dolens.*

miscarriage Spontaneous abortion; lay term usually referring specifically to the loss of the fetus between the fourth month and viability.

missed abortion See *abortion, missed.*

mitleiden Suffering along with.

mitosis Process of somatic cell division in which a single cell divides, but both of the new cells have the same number of chromosomes as the first.

mittelschmerz Abdominal pain in the region of an ovary during ovulation, which usually occurs midway through the menstrual cycle. Present in many women, mittelschmerz is useful for identifying ovulation, thus pinpointing the fertile period of the cycle.

molding Overlapping of cranial bones or shaping of the fetal head to accommodate and conform to the bony and soft parts of the mother's birth canal during labor.

mongolian spot Bluish gray or dark nonelevated pigmented area usually found over the lower back and buttocks present at birth in some infants, primarily nonwhite. The spot fades by school age in black or Oriental infants and within the first year or two of life in other infants.

mongolism See *Down's syndrome.*

moniliasis Infection of the skin or mucous membrane by a yeast-like fungus, *Candida albicans;* see *thrush.*

monitrice One trained in psychoprophylactic methods an who supports women during labor.

monosomy Chromosomal aberration characterized by the al sence of one chromosome from the normal diploid compl ment.

monozygotic Originating or coming from a single fertiliz ovum, such as identical twins.

monozygous twins See *twins, monozygous.*

mons veneris Pad of fatty tissue and coarse skin that overlies the symphysis pubis in the woman and that, after puberty, is covered with short curly hair.

Montgomery's glands tubercles Small, nodular prominences (sebaceous glands) on the areolas around the nipples of the breasts that enlarge during pregnancy and lactation.

morbidity (1) Condition of being diseased. (2) Number of cases of disease or sick persons in relationship to a specific population; incidence.

morning sickness Nausea and vomiting that affect some women during the first few months of their pregnancy; may occur at any time of day.

Moro's reflex Normal, generalized reflex in a young infant elicited by a sudden loud noise or by striking the table next to the child, resulting in flexion of the legs, an embracing posture of the arms, and usually a brief cry. Also called startle reflex.

mortality (1) Quality or state of being subject to death. (2) Number of deaths in relation to a specific population; incidence.

- **fetal m.** Number of fetal deaths per 1000 births (or per live births). See also *death, fetal.*
- **infant m.** Number of deaths per 1000 children 1 year of age or younger.
- **maternal m.** Number of maternal deaths per 100,000 births.
- **neonatal m.** Number of neonatal deaths per 1000 births (or per live births). See also *death, neonatal.*
- **perinatal m.** Combined fetal and neonatal mortality. See also *death, perinatal.*

morula Developmental stage of the fertilized ovum in which there is a solid mass of cells resembling a mulberry.

mosaicism Condition in which some somatic cells are normal, whereas others show chromosomal aberrations.

mucous membrane Specialized thin layer of tissue lining certain cavities and passages that is kept moist by the secretion of mucus.

multigravida Woman who has been pregnant two or more times.

multipara Woman who has carried two or more pregnancies to viability, whether they ended in live infants or stillbirths.

multifetal pregnancy Pregnancy in which there is more than one fetus in the uterus at the same time; multiple pregnancy.

mutation Change in a gene or chromosome in gametes that may be transmitted to offspring.

Naegele's rule Method for calculating the estimated date of confinement (EDC), or "due date."

natal Relating or pertaining to birth.

navel Depression in the center of the abdomen, where the umbilical cord was attached to the fetus; umbilicus.

necrotizing enterocolitis (NEC) Acute inflammatory bowel disorder that occurs primarily in preterm or low-birth-weight neonates. It is characterized by ischemic necrosis (death) of the gastrointestinal mucosa that may lead to perforation and peritonitis.

negligence Commission of an act that a prudent person would not have done or the omission of a duty that prudent person would have fulfilled, resulting in injury or harm to another person. In particular, in a malpractice suit a professional person is negligent if harm to a client results from such an act or such a failure to act, but it must be proved that other prudent persons of the same profession would ordinarily have acted differently under the same circumstances.

neonatal hypovolemic shock Cardiovascular collapse due to a diminished volume of circulating fluid in the cardiovascular system.

neonatal mortality Statistical rate of infant death during the first 28 days after live birth, expressed as the number of such deaths per 1,000 live births in a specific geographic area or institution in a given period of time.

neonatology Study of the neonate.

neutral temperature range That grouping of environmental conditions in which the neonate's oxygen consumption is at a minimum and temperature is within normal limits.

nevus Natural blemish or mark; a congenital circumscribed deposit of pigmentation in the skin; mole.

- **n. flammeus** Port-wine stain; reddish, usually flat, discoloration of the face or neck. Because of its large size and color, it is considered a serious deformity.
- **n. vasculosus (strawberry hemangioma)** Elevated lesion of immature capillaries and endothelial cells that regresses over a period of years.

nidation Implantation of the fertilized ovum in the endometrium, or lining, of the uterus.

nondisjunction Failure of homologous pairs of chromosomes to separate during the first meiotic division or of the two chromatids of a chromosome to split during anaphase of mitosis or the second meiotic division. The result is an abnormal number of chromosomes in the daughter cells.

nonshivering thermogenesis Infant's method of producing heat by increasing metabolic rate.

nonstress test (NST) Evaluation of fetal response (fetal heart rate) to natural contractile uterine activity or to an increase in fetal activity.

nosocomial Pertaining to a hospital.

nulligravida Woman who has never been pregnant.

nullipara Woman who has not yet carried a pregnancy to viability.

nursing practitioner Registered nurse who has additional education to practice nursing in an expanded role.

obstetrix Midwife; from *obstare,* to stand before.

occipitobregmatic Pertaining to the occiput (the back part of the skull) and the bregma (junction of the coronal and sagittal sutures) or anterior fontanel; the smallest diameter of the fetal head.

occiput Back part of the head or skull.

oligohydramnios Abnormally small amount or absence of amniotic fluid; often indicative of fetal urinary tract defect.

oliguria Diminished secretion of urine by the kidneys.

omphalic Concerning or pertaining to the umbilicus.

omphalitis Inflammation of the umbilical stump characterized by redness, edema, and purulent exudate in severe infections.

omphalocele Congenital defect resulting from failure of closure of the abdominal wall or muscles and leading to hernia of abdominal contents through the navel.

oocyte Primordial or incompletely developed ovum.
operculum Plug of mucus that fills the cervical canal during pregnancy.
ophthalmia neonatorum Infection in the neonate's eyes usually resulting from gonorrheal or other infection contracted when the fetus passes through the birth canal (vagina).
opisthotonos Tetanic spasm resulting in an arched, hyperextended position of the body.
oral GTT Test for blood sugar following oral ingestion of a concentrated sugar solution.
orchitis Inflammation of one or both of the testes, characterized by swelling and pain, often caused by mumps, syphilis, or tuberculosis.
orgasmic platform Congestion of the lower vagina during sexual intercourse.
orifice Normal mouth, entrance, or opening, to any aperture.
os Mouth, or opening.
 external o. (o. externum) External opening of the cervical canal.
 internal o. (o. internum) Internal opening of the cervical canal.
 o. uteri Mouth, or opening, of the uterus.
ossification Mineralization of fetal bones.
-otomy Combining form meaning cutting, incision, section.
outlet Opening by which something can exit.
 pelvic o. Inferior aperture, or opening, of the true pelvis.
ovary One of two glands in the female situated on either side of the pelvic cavity that produces the female reproductive cell, the ovum, and two known hormones, estrogen and progesterone.
ovulation Periodic ripening and discharge of the unimpregnated ovum from the ovary, usually 14 days prior to the onset of menstrual flow.
 o. method Evaluation of cervical mucus throughout the menstrual cycle; ovulation occurs just after the appearance of the peak mucus sign; Billings method.
ovum Female germ, or reproductive cell, produced by the ovary; egg.
oxygen toxicity Oxygen overdosage that results in pathologic tissue changes (e.g., retinopathy of prematurity, bronchopulmonary dysplasia).
oxytocics Drugs that stimulate uterine contractions, thus accelerating childbirth and preventing postdelivery hemorrhage. They may be used to increase the let-down reflex during lactation.
oxytocin Hormone produced by the posterior pituitary that stimulates uterine contractions and the release of milk in the mammary gland (let-down reflex).
 o. challenge test (OCT) Evaluation of fetal response (fetal heart rate) to contractile activity of the uterus stimulated by exogenous oxytocin (Pitocin).

$Paco_2$ Partial pressure of carbon dioxide in arterial blood.
palsy Permanent or temporary loss of sensation or ability to move and control movement; paralysis.
 Bell's p. Peripheral facial paralysis of the facial nerve (cranial nerve VII), causing the muscles of the unaffected side of the face to pull the face into a distorted position.
 Erb's p. See *Erb-Duchenne paralysis.*
Pao_2 Partial pressure of oxygen in arterial blood.
Papanicolaou (Pap) smear Microscopic examination using scrapings from the cervix, endocervix, or other mucous membranes that will reveal, with a high degree of accuracy, the presence of premalignant or malignant cells.
para Term used to refer to past pregnancies that reached viability regardless of whether the infant(s) was dead or alive at birth.
parabiotic syndrome Fetofetal blood transfer caused by placental vascular anastomoses occurring in a small plethoric twin (polycythemia) and one pale twin (anemia).
parity Number of pregnancies that reached viability.
parturient Woman giving birth.
parturition Process or act of giving birth.
patent Open.
pathogen Substance or organism capable of producing disease.
pathologic hyperbilirubinemia High (toxic) levels of serum bilirubin due to a disease process causing hemolysis (e.g., Rh incompatibility); jaundice apparent within first 24 hours.
pathologic jaundice See *jaundice, pathologic.*
patulous Open or spread apart.
peak mucus sign Lubricative, cloudy-to-clear-egg white cervical mucus occurring under high estrogen levels close to time of ovulation; ferns; good spinnbarkheit.
pedigree Shorthand method of depicting family lines of individuals who manifest a physical or chemical disorder.
pelvic Pertaining or relating to the pelvis.
 p. axis See *axis, pelvic.*
 p. inlet See *inlet, pelvic.*
 p. outlet See *outlet, pelvic.*
pelvimetry Measurement of dimensions and proportions of the pelvis to determine its capacity and ability to allow the passage of the fetus through the birth canal.
pelvis Bony structure formed by the sacrum, coccyx, innominate bones, and symphysis pubis, and the ligaments that unite them.
 android p. See *android pelvis.*
 anthropoid p. See *anthropoid pelvis.*
 false p. Pelvis above the linea terminalis and symphysis pubis.
 gynecoid p. See *gynecoid pelvis.*
 platypelloid p. See *platypelloid pelvis.*
 true p. Pelvis below the linea terminalis.
penis Male organ used for urination and copulation.
peridural anesthesia Injection of anesthetic outside the dura mater (anesthetic does not mix with spinal fluid); epidural anesthesia.
perinatal Of or pertaining to the time and process of giving birth or being born.
perinatal period Period extending from the twentieth or twenty-eighth week of gestation through the end of the twenty-eighth day after birth.
perinatologist Physician who specializes in fetal and neonatal care.
perineum Area between the vagina and rectum in the female and between the scrotum and rectum in the male.
periodic breathing Sporadic episodes of cessation of respirations for periods of 10 seconds or less not associated with cyanosis commonly noted in preterm infants.
periods of reactivity (newborn infant) *First period* (within 30

minutes after birth): brief cyanosis, flushing with crying; rales, nasal flaring, grunting, retractions; heart sounds loud, forceful, irregular; alert; mucus; no bowel sounds; followed by period of sleep. *Second period* (4 to 8 hours after birth): swift color changes; irregular respiratory and heart rates; mucus with gagging; meconium passage; temperature stabilizing.

petechiae Pinpoint hemorrhagic areas caused by numerous disease states involving infection and thrombocytopenia and occasionally found over the face and trunk of the newborn because of increased intravascular pressure in the capillaries during delivery.

pH Hydrogen ion concentration.

phenotype Expression of certain physical or chemical characteristics in an individual resulting from interaction between genotype and environmental factors.

phenylketonuria (**PKU**) Recessive hereditary disease that results in a defect in the metabolism of the amino acid phenylalanine caused by the lack of an enzyme, phenylalanine hydroxylase, that is necessary for the conversion of the amino acid phenylalanine into tyrosine. If PKU is not treated, brain damage may occur, causing severe mental retardation.

phimosis Tightness of the prepuce, or foreskin, of the penis.

phlebitis Inflammation of a vein with symptoms of pain and tenderness along the course of the vein, inflammatory swelling and acute edema below the obstruction, and discoloration of the skin because of injury or bruise to the vein, possibly occurring in acute or chronic infections or after operations or childbirth.

phlebothrombosis Formation of a clot or thrombus in the vein; inflammation of the vein with secondary clotting.

phlegmasia alba dolens Phlebitis of the femoral vein with thrombosis leading to a venous obstruction, causing acute edema of the leg, and occurring occasionally after delivery; also called *milk-leg.*

phocomelia Developmental anomaly characterized by the absence of the upper portion of one or more limbs so that the feet or hands or both are attached to the trunk of the body by short, irregularly shaped stumps, resembling the fins of a seal.

phototherapy Utilization of lights to reduce serum bilirubin levels by oxidation of bilirubin into water-soluble compounds that are then processed in the liver and excreted in bile and urine.

physiologic hyperbilirubinemia Hemolysis of excessive fetal RBCs in the early neonatal period; jaundice not apparent during first 24 hours. Levels are nontoxic to the individual.

physiologic jaundice See *jaundice, physiologic.*

pica Unusual craving during pregnancy (e.g., of laundry starch, dirt, red clay).

pinna Ear cartilage.

placenta Latin, flat cake; afterbirth; specialized vascular disc-shaped organ for maternal-fetal gas and nutrient exchange. Normally it implants in the thick muscular wall of the upper uterine segment.

- **abruptio p.** See *abruptio placentae.*
- **battledore p.** Umbilical cord insertion into the margin of the placenta.
- **circumvallate p.** Placenta having a raised white ring at its edge.
- **p. accreta** Invasion of the uterine muscle by the placenta, thus making separation from the muscle difficult if not impossible.
- **p. previa** Placenta that is abnormally implanted in the thin, lower uterine segment and that is typed according to proximity to cervical os: total—completely occludes os; partial—does not occlude os completely; and marginal—placenta encroaches on margin of internal cervi-
- **p. succenturiata** Accessory placenta.

placental Pertaining or relating to the placenta.

- **p. dysfunction** Failure of placenta to meet fetal needs and requirements; placental insufficiency.
- **p. dystocia** See *dystocia, placental.*
- **p. infarct** Localized, ischemic, hard area on the fetal or maternal side of the placenta.
- **p. souffle** See *souffle, placental.*

platypelloid pelvis Broad pelvis with a shortened anteroposterior diameter and a flattened, oval, transverse shape.

plethora Deep beefy red coloration ("boiled lobster" hue) of a newborn caused by an increased number of blood cells (polycythemia) per volume of blood.

podalic Concerning or pertaining to the feet.

- **p. version** Shifting of the position of the fetus so as to bring the feet to the outlet during labor.

polycythemia Increased number of erythrocytes per volume of blood, which may be caused by large placental transfusion, fetofetal transfusion, or maternal-fetal transfusion, or it may be due to hypovolemia resulting from movement of fluid out of vascular into interstitial compartment.

polydactyly Excessive number of digits (fingers or toes).

polygenic Pertaining to the combined action of several different genes.

polyhydramnios See *hydramnios.*

polyuria Excessive secretion and discharge of urine by the kidneys.

position Relationship of an arbitrarily chosen fetal reference point, such as the occiput, sacrum, chin, or scapula on the presenting part of the fetus to its location in the front, back, or sides of the maternal pelvis.

positive sign of pregnancy Definite indication of pregnancy (e.g., hearing the fetal heartbeat, visualization and palpation of fetal movement by the examiner, sonographic examination).

posterior Pertaining to the back.

- **p. fontanel** See *fontanel, posterior.*

postmature infant Infant born at or after the beginning of week 43 of gestation or later and exhibiting signs of dysmaturity.

postnatal Happening or occurring after birth (newborn).

postpartum Happening or occurring after birth (mother).

precipitate delivery Rapid or sudden labor of less than 3 hours' duration beginning from onset of cervical changes to completed birth of neonate.

preeclampsia Disease encountered during pregnancy or early in the puerperium characterized by increasing hypertension, albuminuria, and generalized edema; pregnancy-induced hypertension (PIH): toxemia.

pregnancy Period between conception through complete delivery of the products of conception. The usual duration of pregnancy in the human is 280 days, 9 calendar months, or 10 lunar months.

abdominal p. See *abdominal gestation.*
ectopic p. See *ectopic pregnancy.*
extrauterine p. See *extrauterine pregnancy.*

premature infant Infant born before completing week 37 of gestation, irrespective of birth weight; preterm infant.

premenstrual syndrome Syndrome of nervous tension, irritability, weight gain, edema, headache, mastalgia, dysphoria, and lack of coordination occurring during the last few days of the menstrual cycle preceding the onset of menstruation.

premonitory Serving as an early symptom or warning.

prenatal Occurring or happening before birth.

prepartum Before delivery; prior to giving birth.

prepuce Fold of skin, or foreskin, covering the glans penis of the male.
p. of the clitoris Fold of the labia minora that the glans clitoris.

presentation That part of the fetus which first enters the pelvis and lies over the inlet: may be head, face, breech, or shoulder.
breech p. See *breech presentation.*
cephalic p. See *cephalic presentation.*

presenting part That part of the fetus which lies closest to the internal os of the cervix.

pressure edema Edema of the lower extremities caused by pressure of the heavy pregnant uterus against the large veins; edema of fetal scalp after cephalic presentation (caput succedaneum).

presumptive signs Manifestations that suggest pregnancy but that are not absolutely positive. These include the cessation of menses, Chadwick's sign, morning sickness, and quickening.

preterm infant See *premature infant.*

previa, placenta See *placenta previa.*

primigravida Woman who is pregnant for the first time.

primipara Woman who has carried a pregnancy to viability without regard to the child's being dead or alive at the time of birth.

primordial Existing first or existing in the simplest or most primitive form.

probable signs Manifestations or evidence which indicates that there is a definite likelihood of pregnancy. Among the probable signs are enlargement of abdomen, Goodell's sign, Hegar's sign, Braxton Hicks' sign, and positive hormonal tests for pregnancy.

prodromal Serving as an early symptom or warning of the approach of a disease or condition (e.g., prodromal labor).

progesterone Hormone produced by the corpus luteum and placenta whose function is to prepare the endometrium of the uterus for implantation of the fertilized ovum, develop the mammary glands, and maintain the pregnancy.

prolactin See *lactogenic hormone.*

prolapsed cord Protrusion of the umbilical cord in advance of the presenting part.

proliferative phase of menstrual cycle Preovulatory, follicular, or estrogen phase of the menstrual cycle.

promontory of the sacrum Superior projecting portion of the sacrum at the junction of the sacrum and the L-5.

prophylactic Pertaining to prevention or warding off of disease or certain conditions; condom, or "rubber."

prostaglandin (PG) Substance present in many body tissues; has a role in many reproductive tract functions.

proteinuria Excretion of protein into urine.

prudent person One who acts wisely, judiciously. See *negligence.*

pruritus Itching.

pruritus gravidarum Itching of the skin caused by pregnancy.

pseudocyesis Condition in which the woman has all the usual signs of pregnancy, such as enlargement of the abdomen, cessation of menses, weight gain, and morning sickness, but is not pregnant; phantom or false pregnancy.

pseudopregnancy See *pseudocyesis.*

psychoprophylaxis Mental and physical education of the parents in preparation for childbirth, with the goal of minimizing the fear and pain and promoting positive family relationships.

ptyalism Excessive salivation.

puberty Period in life in which the reproductive organs mature and one becomes functionally capable of reproduction.

pubic Pertaining to the pubis.

pubis Pubic bone forming the front of the pelvis.

pudendal block Injection of a local anesthetizing drug at the pudendal nerve root in order to produce numbness of the genital and perianal region.

pudendum External genitalia of either sex; Latin, "that of which one should be ashamed."

puerperal sepsis Infection of the pelvic organs during the postdelivery period; childbed fever.

puerperium Period of time following the third stage of labor and lasting until involution of the uterus takes place, usually about 3 to 6 weeks.

quickening Maternal perception of fetal movement; usually occurs between weeks 16 and 20 of gestation.

RDS See *respiratory distress syndrome (RDS).*

recessive trait Genetically determined characteristic that is expressed only when present in the homozygotic state.

reflex Automatic response built into the nervous system that does not need the intervention of conscious thought (e.g., in the newborn, rooting, gagging, grasp).

regional block anesthesia Anesthesia of an area of the body by injecting a local anesthetic to block a group of sensory nerve fibers.

regurgitate Vomiting or spitting up of solids or fluids.

residual urine Urine that remains in the bladder after urination.

respiratory distress syndrome (RDS) Condition resulting from decreased pulmonary gas exchange, leading to retention of carbon dioxide (increase in arterial P_{CO_2}). Most common neonatal causes are prematurity, perinatal asphyxia, and maternal diabetes mellitus; hyaline membrane disease (HMD).

restitution In obstetrics, the turning of the fetal head to the left or right after it has completely emerged from the introitus as it assumes a normal alignment with the infant's shoulders.

resuscitation Restoration of consciousness or life in one who is apparently dead or whose respirations or cardiac function or both have ceased.

retained placenta Retention of all or part of the placenta in the uterus after delivery.

retraction (1) Drawing in or sucking in of soft tissues of chest, indicative of an obstruction at any level of the respiratory tract from the oropharynx to the alveoli. (2) Retraction of uterine muscle fiber. After contracting, the muscle fiber does not return to its original length but remains slightly shortened, a unique attribute of uterine muscle that aids in preventing postdelivery hemorrhage and results in involution.

retroflexion Bending backward

r. of the uterus Condition in which the body of the womb is bent backward at an angle with the cervix, whose position usually remains unchanged.

retrolental fibroplasia (RLF) *Retinopathy of prematurity* associated with hyperoxemia, resulting in eye injury and blindness.

retroversion Turning or a state of being turned back.

r. of the uterus Displacement of the uterus; the body of the uterus is tipped backward with the cervix pointing forward toward the symphysis pubis.

retrovirus A single piece of RNA surrounded by a protein coat, or envelope. A unique enzyme, reverse transcriptase, allows this RNA retrovirus to go backward, *against the 'flow of life.'* The RNA becomes a piece of DNA, which infects the cell's DNA nucleus and remains in the cell until its death. (The normal flow of genetic information in life is from DNA to RNA to protein.)

Rh factor Inherited antigen present on erythrocytes. The individual with the factor is known as *positive* for the factor.

rhythm method Contraceptive method in which a woman abstains from sexual intercourse during the ovulatory phase of her menstrual cycle and at least 3 days before and 1 day after the ovulation date.

ribonucleic acid (RNA) Element responsible for transferring genetic information within a cell; a template, or pattern.

risk factors Factors that cause a person or a group of people to be particularly vulnerable to an unwanted, unpleasant, or unhealthful event.

Ritgen maneuver Procedure used to control the delivery of the head.

role playing Psychotherapeutic technique in which a person acts out a real or simulated situation as a means of understanding intrapsychic conflicts.

rooming-in unit Maternity unit designed so that the newborn's crib is at the mother's bedside or in a nursery adjacent to the mother's room.

rooting reflex Normal response in newborns when the cheek is touched or stroked along the side of the mouth to turn the head toward the stimulated side, to open the mouth, and to begin to suck. The reflex disappears by 3 to 4 months of age but in some infants may persist until 12 months.

rotation In obstetrics, the turning of the fetal head as it follows the curves of the birth canal downward.

Rubin's test Transuterine insufflation of the fallopian tubes with carbon dioxide to test their patency.

rugae Folds of vaginal mucosa.

sac, amniotic See *amniotic sac.*

sacroiliac Of or pertaining to the sacrum and ilium.

sacrum Triangular bone composed of five united vertebras and situated between L-5 and the coccyx; forms the posterior boundary of the true pelvis.

saddle block anesthesia Type of regional anesthesia produced by injection of a local anesthetic solution into the cerebrospinal fluid intrathecal (subarachnoid) space in the spinal canal.

sagittal suture Band of connective tissue separating the parietal bones, extending from the anterior to the posterior fontanel.

salpingo-oophorectomy Removal of a fallopian tube and an ovary.

scaphoid abdomen Abdomen with a sunken interior wall.

Schultze's mechanism Delivery of the placenta with the fetal surfaces (shiny in appearance) presenting (archaic).

sclerema Hardening of skin and subcutaneous tissue that develops in association with such life-threatening disorders as severe cold stress, septicemia, and shock.

scrotum Pouch of skin containing the testes and parts of the spermatic cords.

sebaceous glands Oil-secreting glands found in the skin.

secondary areola See *areola, secondary.*

secretory phase of menstrual cycle Postovulatory, luteal, progestational, premenstrual phase of menstrual cycle; 14 days in length.

secundines Fetal membranes and placenta expelled after childbirth; afterbirth.

semen Thick, white, viscid secretion discharged from the urethra of the male at orgasm; the transporting medium of the sperm.

sensitization Development of antibodies to a specific antigen.

septic abortion See *abortion, septic.*

shake test "Foam" test for lung maturity of fetus; more rapid than determination of L/S ratio.

Sims' position Position in which the client lies on the left side with the right knee and thigh drawn upward toward the chest.

singleton Pregnancy with a single fetus.

situational crisis Crisis that arises suddenly in response to an external event or a conflict concerning a specific circumstance. The symptoms are transient, and the episode is usually brief.

small for dates (small for gestational age [SGA]) Refers to inadequate growth for gestational age.

smegma Whitish secretion around labia minora.

souffle Soft, blowing sound or murmur heard by auscultation.

funic s. Soft, muffled, blowing sound produced by blood rushing through the umbilical vessels and synchronous with the fetal heart sounds.

placental s. Soft, blowing murmur caused by the blood current in the placenta and synchronous with the maternal pulse.

uterine s. Soft, blowing sound made by the blood in the arteries of the pregnant uterus and synchronous with the maternal pulse.

sperm Male sex cell. Also called spermatozoon.

spermatogenesis Process by which mature spermatozoa are formed, during which the diploid chromosome number (46) is reduced by half (haploid, 23).

spermicide Chemical substance that kills sperm by reducing their surface tension, causing the cell wall to break down by a bactericidal effect or by creating a highly acidic environment. Also called spermatocide.

spina bifida occulta Congenital malformation of the spine in which the posterior portion of laminas of the vertebras fails to close but there is no herniation or protrusion of the spinal cord or meninges through the defect. The newborn may have a dimple in the skin or growth of hair over the malformed vertebras.

spinnbarkheit Formation of a stretchable thread of cervical mucus under estrogen influence at time of ovulation.

splanchnic engorgement Excessive filling or pooling of blood within the visceral vasculature that occurs following the removal of pressure from the abdomen, e.g., birth of a child, removal of an excess of urine from bladder (1000 ml), removal of large tumor.

spontaneous abortion See *abortion, spontaneous.*

square window Angle of wrist between hypothenar prominence and forearm; one criterion for estimating gestational age of neonate.

station Relationship of the presenting fetal part to an imaginary line drawn between the ischial spines of the pelvis.

sterility (1) State of being free from living microorganisms. (2) Complete inability to reproduce offspring.

sterilization Process or act that renders a person unable to produce children.

stillborn Born dead.

striae gravidarum (**"stretch marks"**) Shining reddish lines caused by stretching of the skin, often found on the abdomen, thighs, and breasts during pregnancy. These streaks turn to a fine pinkish white or silver tone in time in fair-skinned women and brownish in darker-skinned women.

subinvolution Failure of a part (e.g., the uterus) to reduce to its normal size and condition after enlargement from functional activity (e.g., pregnancy).

subtotal hysterectomy See *hysterectomy, subtotal.*

succedaneum See *caput succedaneum.*

supine hypotension Shock; fall in blood pressure caused by impaired venous return when gravid uterus presses on ascending vena cava, when woman is lying flat on her back; vena caval syndrome.

surfactant Phosphoprotein necessary for normal respiratory function that prevents the alveolar collapse (atelectasis). See also *lecithin* and *L/S ratio.*

suture (1) Junction of the adjoining bones of the skull. (2) Operation uniting parts by sewing them together.

symphysis pubis Fibrocartilaginous union of the bodies of the pubic bones in the midline.

syndactyly Malformation of digits, commonly seen as a fusion of two or more toes to form one structure.

synostosis Articulation by osseous tissue of adjacent bones; union of separate bones by osseous tissue.

taboo Proscribed (forbidden) by society as improper and unacceptable.

tachypnea Excessively rapid respiratory rate (e.g., in neonates, respiratory rate of 60 breaths/min or more).

talipes equinovarus Deformity in which the foot is extended and the person walks on the toes.

telangiectasia Permanent dilatation of groups of superficial capillaries and venules.

telangiectatic nevi (**"stork bites"**) Clusters of small, red, localized areas of capillary dilatation commonly seen in neonates at the nape of the neck or lower occiput, upper eyelids, and nasal bridge that can be blanched with pressure of a finger.

teratogenic agent Any drug, virus, or irradiation, the exposure to which can cause malformation of the fetus.

teratogens Nongenetic factors that cause malformations and disease syndromes in utero.

teratoma Tumor composed of different kinds of tissue, none of which normally occur together or at the site of the tumor.

term infant Live infant born between weeks 38 and 42 of completed gestation.

testis One of the glands contained in the male scrotum that produces the male reproductive cell, or sperm, and the male hormone testosterone; testicle.

tetany, uterine Extremely prolonged uterine contractions.

therapeutic abortion See *abortion, therapeutic.*

thermogenesis Creation or production of heat, especially in the body.

thermoneutral environment Environment that enables the neonate to maintain a body temperature of 36.5° C (97.7° F) with minimum use of oxygen and energy.

threatened abortion See *abortion, threatened.*

thrombocytopenia Abnormal hematologic condition in which the number of platelets is reduced, usually by destruction of erythroid tissue in bone marrow owing to certain neoplastic diseases or to an immune response to a drug.

thrombocytopenic purpura Hematologic disorder characterized by prolonged bleeding time, decreased number of platelets, increased cell fragility, and purpura, which result in hemorrhages into the skin, mucous membranes, organs, and other tissue.

thromboembolism Obstruction of a blood vessel by a clot that has become detached from its site of formation.

thrombophlebitis Inflammation of a vein with secondary clot formation.

thrombus Blood clot obstructing a blood vessel that remains at the place it was formed.

thrush Fungal infection of the mouth or throat characterized by the formation of white patches on a red, moist, inflamed mucous membrane and is caused by *Candida albicans.*

toco- (toko-) Combining form that means childbirth or labor.

tocolytic drug Drug used to suppress preterm labor.

tocotransducer Electronic device for measuring uterine contractions.

tongue-tie Congenital shortening of the frenulum, which, if severe, may interfere with sucking and articulation; a rare condition.

TORCH organisms Organisms that damage the embryo or fetus; acronym for *t*oxoplasmosis, *o*ther (e.g., syphilis), *r*ubella, *c*ytomegalovirus, and *h*erpes simplex.

torticollis Congenital or acquired stiff neck caused by shortening or spasmodic contraction of the neck (sternocleidomastoid) muscles that draws the head to one side with the chin pointing in the other direction; wryneck.

total hysterectomy See *hysterectomy, total.*

toxemia Term previously used for hypertensive states of pregnancy.

tracheoesophageal fistula Congenital malformation in which there is an abnormal tubelike passage between the trachea and esophagus.

transition Last phase of first stage of labor; 8 to 10 cm dilatation.

translocation Condition in which a chromosome breaks and all or part of that chromosome is transferred to a different part of the same chromosome or to another chromosome.

Trichomonas vaginitis Inflammation of the vagina caused by *Trichomonas vaginalis,* a parasitic protozoon and characterized by persistent burning and itching of the vulvar tissue and a profuse, frothy, white discharge.

trimester Time period of 3 months.

trisomy Condition whereby any given chromosome exists in triplicate instead of the normal duplicate pattern.

trophoblast Outer layer of cells of the developing blastodermic vesicle that develops the trophoderm or feeding layer which will establish the nutrient relationships with the uterine endometrium.

tubal ligation See *ligation, tubal.*

tubercles of Montgomery Small papillae on surface of nipples and areolae that secrete a fatty substance that lubricates the nipples.

twins Two neonates from the same impregnation developed within the same uterus at the same time.

- **conjoined t.** Twins who are physically united; Siamese twins.
- **disparate t.** Twins who are different (e.g., in weight) and distinct from one another.
- **dizygous t.** Twins developed from two separate ova fertilized by two separate sperm at the same time; fraternal twins.
- **monozygous twins** Twins developed from a single fertilized ovum; identical twins.

ultrasonography High frequency sound waves to discern fetal heart rate or placental location or body parts.

umbilical cord (funis) Structure connecting the placenta and fetus and containing two arteries and one vein encased in a tissue called *Wharton's jelly.* The cord is ligated at birth and severed; the stump falls off in 4 to 10 days.

umbilicus Navel, or depressed point in the middle of the abdomen that marks the attachment of the umbilical cord during fetal life.

urachus Epithelial tube connecting the apex of the urinary bladder with the allantois. Its connective tissue forms the median umbilical ligament.

urethra Small tubular structure that drains urine from the bladder.

urinary frequency Need to void often or at close intervals.

urinary meatus Opening, or mouth, of the urethra.

uterine Referring or pertaining to the uterus.

- **u. adnexa** See *adnexa, uterine.*
- **u. bruit** Abnormal sound or murmur heard while auscultating the uterus.
- **u. ischemia** Decreased blood supply to the uterus.
- **u. prolapse** Falling, sinking, or sliding of the uterus from its normal location in the body.
- **u. souffle** See *souffle, uterine.*

uterus Hollow muscular organ in the female designed for the implantation, containment, and nourishment of the fetus during its development until birth.

- **Couvelaire u.** Interstitial myometrial hemorrhage following premature separation (abruptio) of placenta. A purplish-bluish discoloration of the uterus and boardlike rigidity of the uterus are noted.
- **inversion of the u.** See *inversion of the uterus.*
- **retroflexion of the u.** See *retroflexion of the uterus.*
- **retroversion of the u.** See *retroversion of the uterus.*

vagina Normally collapsed musculomembranous tube that forms the passageway between the uterus and the entrance to the vagina.

vaginismus Intense, painful spasm of the muscles surrounding the vagina.

varices (varicose veins) Swollen, distended, and twisted veins that may develop in almost any part of the body but are most commonly seen in the legs, caused by pregnancy, obesity, congenital defective venous valves, and occupations requiring much standing.

vasectomy Ligation or removal of a segment of the vas deferens, usually done bilaterally to produce sterility in the male.

VDRL test Abbreviation for Venereal Disease Research Laboratory test, a serological flocculation test for syphilis.

vernix caseosa Protective gray-white fatty substance of cheesy consistency covering the fetal skin.

version Act of turning the fetus in the uterus to change the presenting part and facilitate delivery.

- **podalic v.** See *podalic version.*

vertex Crown or top of the head.

- **v. presentation** Presentation in which the fetal skull is nearest the cervical opening and born first.

viable Capable of living, such as a fetus that has reached a stage of development, usually 24 weeks, which will permit it to live outside the uterus.

villi Short, vascular processes or protrusions growing on certain membranous surfaces.

- **chorionic v.** Tiny vascular protrusions on the chorionic surface that project into the maternal blood sinuses of the uterus and that help to form the placenta and secrete hCG.

voluntary abortion See *abortion, elective.*

vulva External genitalia of the female that consist of the labia majora, labia minora, clitoris, urinary meatus, and vaginal introitus.

Wharton's jelly White, gelatinous material surrounding the umbilical vessels within the cord.

witch's milk Secretion of a whitish fluid for about a week after birth from enlarged mammary tissue in the neonate, presumably resulting from maternal hormonal influences.

womb See *uterus.*

X chromosome Sex chromosome in humans existing in duplicate in the normal female and singly in the normal male.

X linkage Genes located on the X-chromosome.

Y chromosome Sex chromosome in the human male necessary for the development of the male gonads.

zona pellucida Inner, thick, membranous envelope of the ovum.

zygote Cell formed by the union of two reproductive cells or gametes; the fertilized ovum resulting from the union of a sperm and an ovum.

Appendices

A The Pregnant Patient: Bill of Rights

The Pregnant Patient has the right to participate in decisions involving her well-being and that of her unborn child, unless there is a clear-cut medical emergency that prevents her participation. In addition to the rights set forth in the American Hospital Association's "Patient's Bill of Rights" (which has also been adopted by the New York City Department of Health), the Pregnant Patient, because she represents *two* patients rather than one, should be recognized as having the additional rights listed below.

1. *The Pregnant Patient has the right,* prior to the administration of any drug or procedure, to be informed by the health professional caring for her of any potential direct or indirect effects, risks, or hazards to herself or her unborn or newborn infant which may result from the use of a drug or procedure prescribed for or administered to her during pregnancy, labor, birth or lactation.

2. *The Pregnant Patient has the right,* prior to the proposed therapy, to be informed, not only of the benefits, risks and hazards of the proposed therapy, but also of known alternative therapy, such as available childbirth education classes which could help to prepare the Pregnant Patient physically and mentally to cope with the discomfort or stress of pregnancy and the experience of childbirth, thereby reducing or eliminating her need for drugs and obstetric intervention. She should be offered such information early in her pregnancy in order that she may make a reasoned decision.

3. *The Pregnant Patient has the right,* prior to the administration of any drug, to be informed by the health professional who is prescribing or administering the drug to her that any drug she receives during pregnancy, labor and birth, no matter how or when the drug is taken or administered, may adversely affect her unborn baby, directly or indirectly, and that there is no drug or chemical which has been proven safe for the unborn child.

4. *The Pregnant Patient has the right,* if cesarean section is anticipated, to be informed prior to administration of any drug, and preferably prior to her hospitalization, that minimizing her and, in turn, her baby's intake of nonessential preoperative medicine, will benefit her baby.

5. *The Pregnant Patient has the right,* prior to the administration of a drug or procedure, to be informed if there is *no* properly controlled follow-up research which has established the safety of the drug or procedure with regard to its direct and/or indirect effects on the physiological, mental and neurological development of the child exposed, via the mother, to the drug or procedure during pregnancy, labor, birth or lactation (this would apply to virtually all drugs and the vast majority of obstetric procedures).

6. *The Pregnant Patient has the right,* prior to the administration of any drug, to be informed of the brand name and generic name of the drug in order that she may advise the health professional of any past adverse reaction to the drug.

7. *The Pregnant Patient has the right* to determine for herself, without pressure from her attendant, whether she will accept the risks inherent in the proposed therapy or refuse a drug or procedure.

8. *The Pregnant Patient has the right* to know the name and qualifications of the individual administering a medication or procedure to her during labor or birth.

9. *The Pregnant Patient has the right* to be informed, prior to the administration of any procedure, whether that procedure is being administered to her for her or her baby's benefit (medically indicated) or as an elective procedure (for convenience or teaching purposes).

10. *The Pregnant Patient has the right* to be accompanied during the stress of labor and birth by someone she cares for, and to whom she looks for emotional comfort and encouragement.

11. *The Pregnant Patient has the right* after appropriate medical consultation to choose a position for labor and for birth which is least stressful to her baby and to herself.

12. *The Obstetric Patient has the right* to have her baby cared for at her bedside if her baby is normal, and to feed her baby according to her baby's needs rather than according to the hospital regimen.

From Haire DB: The Pregnant Patient's Bill of Rights, J Nurs Midwife 20:29, Winter, 1975. This article is not reproduced here in its entirety.

13. *The Obstetric Patient has the right* to be informed in writing of the name of the person who actually delivered her baby and the professional qualifications of that person. This information should also be on the birth certificate.

14. *The Obstetric Patient has the right* to be informed if there is any known or indicated aspect of her or her baby's care or condition which may cause her or her baby later difficulty or problems.

15. *The Obstetric Patient has the right* to have her and her baby's hospital medical records complete, accurate and legible and to have their records, including Nurses' Notes, retained by the hospital until the child reaches at least the age of majority, or, alternatively, to have the records offered to her before they are destroyed.

16. *The Obstetric Patient,* both during and after her hospital stay, has the right to have access to her complete hospital medical records, including Nurses' Notes, and to receive a copy upon payment of a reasonable fee and without incurring the expense of retaining an attorney.

It is the obstetric patient and her baby, not the health professional, who must sustain any trauma or injury resulting from the use of a drug or obstetric procedure. The observation of the rights listed above will not only permit the obstetric patient to participate in the decisions involving her and her baby's health care, but will help to protect the health professional and the hospital against litigation arising from resentment or misunderstanding on the part of the mother.

❑ RESPONSIBILITIES

In addition to understanding her rights the Pregnant Patient should also understand that she too has certain responsibilities. The Pregnant Patient's responsibilities include the following:

1. *The Pregnant Patient is responsible* for learning about the physical and psychologic process of labor, birth, and postpartum recovery. The better informed expectant parents are the better they will be able to participate in decisions concerning the planning of their care.

2. *The Pregnant Patient is responsible* for learning what comprises good prenatal and intranatal care and for making an effort to obtain the best care possible.

3. *Expectant parents are responsible* for knowing about those hospital policies and regulations that will affect their birth and postpartum experience.

4. *The Pregnant Patient is responsible* for arranging for a companion or support person (husband, mother, sister, friend, etc.) who will share in her plans for birth and who will accompany her during her labor and birth experience.

5. *The Pregnant Patient is responsible* for making her preferences known clearly to the health professional involved in her care in a courteous and cooperative manner and for making mutually agreed-upon arrangements regarding maternity care alternatives with her physician and hospital in advance of labor.

6. *Expectant parents are responsible* for listening to their chosen physician or midwife with an open mind, just as they expect him or her to listen openly to them.

7. Once they have agreed to a course of health care, *expectant parents are responsible,* to the best of their ability, for seeing that the program is carried out in consultation with others with whom they have made the agreement.

8. *The Pregnant Patient is responsible* for obtaining information in advance regarding the approximate cost of her obstetric and hospital care.

9. *The Pregnant Patient* who intends to change her physician or hospital is responsible for notifying all concerned, well in advance of the birth if possible, and for informing both of her reasons for changing.

10. In all their interactions with medical and nursing personnel, *the expectant parents should* behave toward those caring for them with the same respect and consideration they themselves would like.

11. During the mother's hospital stay *the mother is responsible for* learning about her and her baby's continuing care after discharge from the hospital.

12. After birth, *the parents should* put into writing constructive comments and feelings of satisfaction and or dissatisfaction with the care (nursing, medical and personal) they received. Good service to families in the future will be facilitated by those parents who take the time and responsibility to write letters expressing their feelings about the maternity care they received.

APPENDIX

B NAACOG's Standards for Obstetric, Gynecologic, and Neonatal Nursing

❑ I: NURSING PRACTICE

STANDARD: Comprehensive obstetric, gynecologic, and neonatal (OGN) nursing care is provided to the individual, family, and community within the framework of the nursing process.

INTERPRETATION: The nurse is responsible for decisions and actions within the domain of nursing practice. Comprehensive nursing care includes helping the person meet physical, psychosocial, spiritual, and developmental needs. Systematic use of the nursing process, which encompasses assessment, nursing diagnosis, planning, implementation, and evaluation will meet the patient's needs. Individualized nursing care is best achieved by collaboration with patient, family, and other members of the health-care team. Complete and accurate documentation of all nursing care and patient response is essential for continuity of care and for meeting legal requirements. The nurse must promote a safe and therapeutic environment for the individual, family, and community.

❑ II: HEALTH EDUCATION

STANDARD: Health education for the individual, family, and community is an integral part of obstetric, gynecologic, and neonatal nursing practice.

INTERPRETATION: The nurse is responsible for providing pertinent information to the individual, family, and community so they may participate in and share responsibility for their own health promotion, maintenance, and restorative care. The nurse plans, implements, and evaluates health education based on principles of teaching and learning. To enhance health care and promote continuity of health education, the nurse uses the educational resources within the community and collaborates with other health-care providers.

Health education should be documented and evaluated. Evaluation is based on individualized goals and set criteria.

❑ III: POLICIES AND PROCEDURES

STANDARD: The delivery of obstetric, gynecologic, and neonatal nursing care is based on written policies and procedures.

INTERPRETATION: Policies and procedures define the boundaries of nursing practice within the health-care setting and indicate the qualifications of personnel authorized to perform OGN nursing procedures. The qualifications may include educational preparation and/or certification. The policies and procedures should be in accordance with the philosophy of the agency, state nurse practice act, governmental regulations, and other applicable standards or regulations.

A multidisciplinary framework should be used in writing policies and procedures. Policies and procedures should be evaluated on an ongoing basis and revised as necessary. The policies and procedures should be readily accessible to the health-care providers within the health-care setting.

❑ IV: PROFESSIONAL RESPONSIBILITY AND ACCOUNTABILITY

STANDARD: The obstetric, gynecologic, and neonatal nurse is responsible and accountable for maintaining knowledge and competency in individual nursing practice and for being aware of professional issues.

INTERPRETATION: Maintaining both the knowledge and skills required to achieve excellence in OGN nursing is incumbent upon the nurse. The nurse should be cognizant of changing concepts, trends, and scientific advances in OGN care. Updating knowledge and skills is achievable through formal education, professional continuing education, and the use of or participation in nursing research. Knowledge of specialty nursing can be recognized through certification.

The nurse should be aware of governmental policies and legislation affecting health care and nursing practice. Participating in legislative and regulatory processes is appropriate for the nurse.

Responsibilities defined in written position descriptions and performance demonstrated by the OGN nurse should be regularly evaluated and documented. In addition, criteria for the evaluation of OGN nursing practice should be drawn from applicable statutes, the ethics of the profession, and current standards of practice.

❑ V: PERSONNEL

STANDARD: Obstetric, gynecologic, and neonatal nursing staff are provided to meet patient care needs.

INTERPRETATION: The obstetric, gynecologic, and neonatal nursing management determines the staff required for the provision of individualized nursing care commensurate with demonstrated patient needs, appropriate nursing interventions, qualifications of available nursing personnel, and other factors that must be considered. These factors may include nursing care needs; number of deliveries; number and types of surgical procedures; average inpatient census; volume of ambulatory patients; percentage of high-risk patients; educational, emotional, and economic needs of the patients; provision for staff continuing education; medical staff coverage, ancillary services available; size and design of facilities; responsibilities of nursing staff; and ongoing research.

Personnel in each OGN unit should be directed by a registered nurse with educational preparation and clinical experience in the specific OGN area of practice. This nurse is responsible for management of nursing care and supervision of nursing personnel.

When nursing, medical, or other specialty students are assigned to the unit for clinical experience, their roles and responsibilities should be clearly defined in writing. Nursing students should not be included in the unit's staffing plan.

Written position descriptions that identify standards of performance for OGN nurses should be developed and used in periodic personnel evaluations. Documentation should reflect each nurse's participation in orientation and verify knowledge and expertise in those skills required for OGN nursing practice. Orientation and evaluation of personnel for whom the registered nurse is held accountable should be documented as well.

Written policies for the reassignment of OGN nursing personnel should exist to accommodate both increases and decreases of inpatient days and ambulatory visits. The policies should include a contingency plan for staffing during peak activity periods.

C NANDA-Approved Nursing Diagnoses (Through the 9th Conference, 1990)

Activity intolerance
Activity intolerance, potential
Adjustment, impaired
Airway clearance, ineffective
Anxiety
Aspiration, potential for
Body image disturbance
Body temperature, altered, potential
Breastfeeding, ineffective
Breathing pattern, ineffective
Cardiac output, decreased
Communication, impaired verbal
Constipation
Constipation, colonic
Constipation, perceived
Coping, defensive
Coping, family: potential for growth
Coping, ineffective family: compromised
Coping, ineffective family: disabling
Coping, ineffective individual
Decisional conflict (specify)
Denial, ineffective
Diarrhea
Disuse syndrome, potential for
Diversional activity deficit
Dysreflexia
Family processes, altered
Fatigue
Fear
Fluid volume deficit (1)
Fluid volume deficit (2)
Fluid volume deficit, potential
Fluid volume excess
Gas exchange, impaired
Grieving, anticipatory
Grieving, dysfunctional
Growth and development, altered
Health maintenance, altered
Health seeking behaviors (specify)
Home maintenance management, impaired
Hopelessness
Hyperthermia
Hypothermia
Incontinence, bowel
Incontinence, functional
Incontinence, reflex
Incontinence, stress
Incontinence, total
Incontinence, urge
Infection, potential for
Injury, potential for
Knowledge deficit (specify)
Mobility, impaired physical
Noncompliance (specify)
Nutrition, altered: less than body requirements
Nutrition, altered: more than body requirements
Nutrition, altered: potential for more than body requirements
Oral mucous membrane, altered
Pain
Pain, chronic
Parental role conflict
Parenting, altered
Parenting, altered, potential
Personal identity disturbance
Poisoning, potential for
Post-trauma response
Powerlessness
Rape-trauma syndrome
Rape-trauma syndrome: compound reaction
Rape-trauma syndrome: silent reaction
Role performance, altered
Self care deficit, bathing/hygiene
Self care deficit, dressing/grooming
Self care deficit, feeding
Self care deficit, toileting
Self-esteem disturbance
Self-esteem, chronic low
Self-esteem, situational low
Sensory/perceptual alterations (specify) (visual, auditory, kinesthetic, gustatory, tactile, olfactory)
Sexual dysfunction

Sexuality patterns, altered
Skin integrity, impaired
Skin integrity, impaired, potential
Sleep pattern disturbance
Social interaction, impaired
Social isolation
Spiritual distress (distress of the human spirit)
Suffocation, potential for
Swallowing, impaired
Thermoregulation, ineffective
Thought processes, altered
Tissue integrity, impaired
Tissue perfusion, altered (specify type) (renal, cerebral, cardiopulmonary, gastrointestinal, peripheral)
Trauma, potential for
Unilateral neglect
Urinary elimination, altered patterns
Urinary retention
Violence, potential for: self-directed or directed at others

APPENDIX

D Nursing Responsibilities in Implementing Intrapartum Fetal Heart Rate Monitoring

With the publication of the new position on fetal heart rate monitoring from The American College of Obstetricians and Gynecologists, as reflected in the 1988 *Guidelines for Perinatal Care.*[1] NAACOG finds it necessary to clarify the nursing responsibilities in implementing intrapartum fetal heart rate monitoring.

The primary goal of perinatal care is to ensure optimal maternal and neonatal outcomes. The intrapartum period represents a time of risk for the parturient and the fetus. An assessment of fetal heart rate (FHR) has long been recognized as a vital aspect of evaluating fetal well-being during the stresses of labor and birth. Two techniques of fetal heart rate assessment are auscultation and electronic fetal heart monitoring. Each method has its advantages and limitations necessitating individualized decision-making for appropriate use. The method of fetal heart rate monitoring selected and the frequency of FHR evaluation should be based on consideration of maternal–fetal risk factors and the availability of nursing personnel skilled in the monitoring techniques. The patient's preference should be carefully considered.

Nurses who perform fetal heart rate monitoring are responsible for their actions and will be held to the established standards of care as defined by their professional organizations, the standards of practice in their institutions, and the laws governing practice in their states.

❑ METHODOLOGY

Auscultation. Auscultation of the fetal heart rate is an auditory assessment procedure which, when properly performed, allows the evaluation of the FHR both during and immediately following the stress of a uterine contraction. Further, auscultation between contractions establishes the baseline FHR. Auscultation as a primary technique of fetal heart rate surveillance requires a thorough knowledge of the basic principles of fetal heart and uterine physiology and pathophysiology. Clinical experience in the recognition of and the response to significant FHR changes is required. The validation of competency in the use of this technique must be in accordance with established institutional policy.

Recently ACOG indicated that auscultation of the fetal heart at 15-minute intervals during the active phase of the first stage of labor and at 5-minute intervals during the second stage is equivalent to electronic fetal monitoring (EFM) when risk factors are present during labor or when intensified monitoring is elected. For low-risk patients, the suggested auscultation frequency remains unchanged at 30 minutes in active first stage labor and 15 minutes in second stage labor. Therefore, for the high-risk patient, and for the low-risk patient in the second stage of labor, if auscultation is prescribed as the primary technique of fetal heart rate surveillance, a minimum of a 1:1 nurse-fetus ratio is required.

Electronic Fetal Monitoring. EFM is an auditory and visual assessment procedure which provides continuous data for evaluation of uterine activity and fetal heart responses, including baseline heart rate, variability, and fetal heart rate change over time. Further, EFM produces a continuous printed record. The use of EFM requires knowledge of its equipment and thorough knowledge of the basic principles of fetal heart and uterine physiology and pathophysiology. Nurses who use EFM must be able to recognize fetal heart rate patterns, beat-to-beat variability, and uterine activity. Fetal monitoring patterns have been given descriptive names (e.g., accelerations and early, late, or variable decelerations). Nurses should use these terms in written chart documentation and verbal communication. When a change in fetal heart rate patterns is noted, the nurse should also document a subsequent return to normal patterns.

The patient medical record should include observations and assessments of fetal heart rate and characteristics of uterine activity as well as specific actions taken when changes in fetal heart rate patterns are observed. The monitor tracing is a legal part of the medical record and should include identifying information about the patient as well as times and events related to the patient's ongoing care.

After the identification of a nonreassuring pattern, the nurse is responsible for initiating appropriate nursing interventions, as indicated by the pattern identified, and for notifying a physician. Once the physician is notified of a nonreassuring pattern, the nurse can expect the physician to respond. An institutional policy should be established for the nurse to follow in the event the physician is unable to respond in a timely fashion.

Core competencies in fetal heart rate monitoring have been published by NAACOG.[2] Competency validation of this expertise must be in accordance with established institutional policy.[3] Standards for staffing when EFM is the primary method of monitoring are found in the NAACOG OGN Nursing Practice Resource *Considerations for Nurse Professional Staffing in Perinatal Units* and in AAP/ACOG *Guidelines for Perinatal Care.*[1,4]

❑ EVALUATION AND DOCUMENTATION

The institution should establish policies and procedures which define evaluation and documentation of fetal heart rate monitoring. In developing policies and procedures, the institution should address the following:

- Method(s) for assessment (EFM, auscultation, or a combination of both)
- Maternal–fetal risk factors
- Stage of labor
- Frequency of assessment
- Qualifications of health-care providers performing assessments
- Nurse–fetus ratios
- Methods of documentation

Documentation of the evaluation of FHR monitoring information during labor is applicable regardless of the method of monitoring selected, and may be accomplished in narrative nurses' notes and/or by the use of comprehensive flow sheets at the time of assessment. Documentation may also be achieved by the use of abbreviated nurses' notes with follow-up summary nurses' notes at intervals specified by institutional policy. The format for abbreviated notes may include initialing the EFM tracing, annotating the EFM tracing, or annotating basic flow sheets.

Suggested frequencies for interval evaluation of FHR information have been addressed in the recent ACOG position. For the high-risk patients being monitored with auscultation during the active phase of the first stage and during the second stage of labor, intervals for both the evaluation and recording of FHR information are suggested at 15 and 5 minutes, respectively. For the same group of patients being monitored electronically, evaluation of the tracing is suggested at the same intervals.

For low-risk patients being monitored with auscultation, the suggested intervals for evaluation and recording remain unchanged at 30 and 15 minutes in the first and second stages of labor, respectively. An interval frequency for evaluation of the tracing for this same group of patients being monitored electronically was not suggested.

Evaluation of FHR information may take place at the intervals suggested above or more frequently as necessitated by the individual patient care situation. Written documentation of these FHR evaluations, however, may occur at longer intervals in narrative, abbreviated, and/or summary formats in accordance with institutional policy and procedure.

❑ CONFLICT RESOLUTION

The potential for conflict exists in terms of professional judgment and decision-making regarding which method of monitoring is best for a particular patient in a given situation. Institutional policies and procedures must provide a mechanism that will allow nurses the flexibility to decline to implement the prescribed method of fetal heart rate monitoring if any question exists regarding the ability to meet the required staffing ratios or if the methodology is beyond the individual nurse's expertise. Ultimately, the responsibility for implementing the prescribed method of fetal heart rate monitoring remains with the prescriber. In the event of differences of opinion among professionals regarding the ability to implement the prescribed method, the established institutional policy for the resolution of the conflict should be followed.

References

1. American Academy of Pediatrics and The American College of Obstetricians and Gynecologists: Guidelines for perinatal care, ed 2, Washington, DC, 1988.
2. NAACOG: Electronic fetal monitoring: nursing practice competencies and educational guidelines, Washington, DC, 1986.

3. NAACOG: Competency validation. Resource book from Essentials of electronic fetal monitoring, NASCOG. 1988. Videotape.
4. NAACOG. Considerations for professional nurse staffing in perinatal units, OGN Nursing Practice Resource, Washington, DC, 1988.

This statement replaces the Joint ACOG/NAACOG Statement on Electronic Fetal Monitoring published in January 1986 by NAACOG.

APPENDIX

E Standard Laboratory Values: Pregnant and Nonpregnant Women

	Nonpregnant	Pregnant
HEMATOLOGIC VALUES		
Complete Blood Count (CBC)		
Hemoglobin, g/dl	12-16*	10-14*
Hematocrit, PCV, %	37-47	32-42
Red cell volume, ml	1600	1900
Plasma volume, ml	2400	3700
Red blood cell count, million/mm^3	4-5.5	4-5.5
White blood cells, total per mm^3	4500-10,000	5000-15,000
Polymorphonuclear cells, %	54-62	60-85
Lymphocytes, %	38-46	15-40
Erythrocyte sedimentation rate, mm/h	≤	30-90
MCHC, g/dl packed RBCs (mean corpuscular hemoglobin concentration)	30-36	No change
MCH/(mean corpuscular hemoglobin per picogram [less than a nanogram])	29-32	No change
MCV/μm^3 (mean corpuscular volume per cubic micrometer)	82-96	No change
Blood Coagulation and Fibrinolytic Activity†		
Factors VII, VIII, IX, X		Increase in pregnancy, return to normal in early puerperium; factor VIII increases during and immediately after delivery
Factors XI, XIII		Decrease in pregnancy
Prothrombin time (protime)	60-70 sec	Slight decrease in pregnancy
Partial thromboplastin time (PTT)	12-14 sec	Slight decrease in pregnancy and again decrease during second and third stage of labor (indicates clotting at placental site)
Bleeding time	1-3 min (Duke) 2-4 min (Ivy)	No appreciable change
Coagulation time	6-10 min (Lee/White)	No appreciable change
Platelets	150,000 to 350,000/mm^3	No significant change until 3-5 days after delivery, then marked increase (may predispose woman to thrombosis) and gradual return to normal
Fibrinolytic activity		Decreases in pregnancy, then abrupt return to normal (protection against thromboembolism)
Fibrinogen	250 mg/dl	400 mg/dl

*At sea level. Permanent residents of higher levels (e.g., Denver) require higher levels of hemoglobin.
†Pregnancy represents a hypercoagulable state.

Continued.

	Nonpregnant	Pregnant
Mineral/Vitamin Concentrations		
Vitamin B_{12}, folic acid, ascorbic acid	Normal	Moderate decrease
Serum proteins		
Total, g/dl	6.7-8.3	5.5-7.5
Albumin, g/dl	3.5-5.5	3.0-5.0
Globulin, total, g/dl	2.3-3.5	3.0-4.0
Blood sugar		
Fasting, mg/dl	70-80	65
2-hour postprandial, mg/dl	60-110	Under 140 after a 100 g carbohydrate meal is considered normal
CARDIOVASCULAR DETERMINATIONS		
Blood pressure, mm Hg	120/80*	114/65
Pulse, rate/min	70	80
Stroke volume, ml	65	75
Cardiac output, L/min	4.5	6
Circulation time (arm-tongue), sec	15-16	12-14
Blood volume, ml		
Whole blood	4000	5600
Plasma	2400	3700
Red blood cells	1600	1900
Chest x-ray studies		
Transverse diameter of heart	—	1-2 cm increase
Left border of heart	—	Straightened
Cardiac volume	—	70 ml increase
HEPATIC VALUES		
Bilirubin total	Not more than 1 mg/dl	Unchanged
Serum cholesterol	110-300 mg/dl	↑ 60% from 16-32 weeks of pregnancy; remains at this level until after delivery
Serum alkaline phosphatase	2-4.5 units (Bodansky)	↑ from week 12 of pregnancy to 6 weeks after delivery
Serum globulin albumin	1.5-3.0 g/dl 4.5-5.3 g/dl	↑ slight ↓ 3.0 g by late pregnancy
RENAL VALUES		
Bladder capacity	1300 ml	1500 ml
Renal plasma flow (RPF), ml/min	490-700	Increase by 25%, to 612-875
Glomerular filtration rate (GFR), ml/min	105-132	Increase by 50%, to 160-198
Nonprotein nitrogen (NPN), mg/dl	25-40	Decreases
Blood urea nitrogen (BUN), mg/dl	20-25	Decreases
Serum creatinine, mg/kg/24 hr	20-22	Decreases
Serum uric acid, mg/kg/24 hr	257-750	Decreases
Urine glucose	Negative	Present in 20% of gravidas
Intravenous pyelogram (IVP)	Normal	Slight to moderate hydroureter and hydronephrosis; right kidney larger than left kidney

*For the woman about 20 years of age
10 years of age: 103/70.
30 years of age: 123/82.
40 years of age: 126/84.

APPENDIX

F Human Fetotoxic Chemical Agents

Maternal Medication	Reported Effects on Fetus or Neonate
ANALGESICS	
Indomethacin (Indocin)	Prolongs gestation (monkey); in neonates, used to close patent ductus arteriosus
Narcotics	70% of maternal level; death, apnea, depression, bradycardia, hypothermia
Salicylates	Death in utero; hemorrhage, methemoglobinemia, ↓ albumin-binding capacity, salicylate intoxication, difficult delivery,? prolonged gestation
ANESTHESIA	
Conduction	Indirect effect of maternal hypotension; direct effect—convulsions, death, acidosis, bradycardia, myocardial depression, fetal hypotension, methemoglobinemia
Paracervical	Methemoglobinemia, fetal acidosis, bradycardia, neurologic depression, myocardial depression
ANTICOAGULANTS	
Coumarins	Fetal death, hemorrhage, calcifications
ANTICONVULSANT AGENTS	
Barbiturates	Irritability and tremulousness 4-5 months after delivery; hemorrhage, enzyme inducer
Phenytoin and barbiturate	Congenital malformations, cleft lip and palate, congenital heart disease (CHD), CNS and skeletal anomalies, failure to thrive, enzyme inducer, hemorrhage
ANTIMICROBIALS	All antimicrobials cross placenta
Ampicillin	↓ Maternal urinary and plasma estriol levels
Chloramphenicol	Crosses placenta with no reported effect; interferes with biotransformation of tolbutamide, phenytoin, biohydroxycoumarin (i.e., hypoglycemia may occur if used in combination)
Chloroquine	Death, deafness, retinal hemorrhage
Erythromycin	Possible hepatic injury
Nitrofurantoin	Megaloblastic anemia, G6PD deficiency
Novobiocin	Hyperbilirubinemia
Streptomycin	Therapeutic levels reached, nerve deafness
Sulfonamides	Icterus, hemolytic anemia, kernicterus, ? growth retardation, thrombocytopenia
Tetracycline	Placental transfer after 4 months' gestation; enamel hypoplasia, delay in bone growth, ? congenital cataract
ANTITUBERCULOSIS	
Isoniazid	Toxic blood level in fetus; no reported effect; mother should be on pyridoxine supplement
Pyridoxine	*See* vitamins

Modified from Babson SG et al: Diagnosis and management of the fetus and neonate at risk: a guide for team care, ed 4, St Louis, 1980, The CV Mosby Co; and Perinatal pharmacology, Mead Johnson Symposium and Perinatal and Developmental Medicine (no 5), Vail, Colo, 1974.

Maternal Medication	Reported Effects on Fetus or Neonate
CANCER CHEMOTHERAPEUTIC AGENTS	
Aminopterin 6-Mercaptopurine Methotrexate	Abortion, congenital anomalies (first trimester); combination of drugs detrimental to fetus; skeletal and cranial malformations, hydrocephalus; questionable long-term effects = slow somatic growth; ovarian agenesis; ↓ immune mechanisms
CARDIOVASCULAR AGENTS	
Digitoxin	Placental transfer, no reported effect
Propranolol	Indirect effect of delay in cervical dilatation
CHOLINESTERASE INHIBITORS	Myasthenia-like symptoms for 1 week; muscle weakness in 10% to 20% of infants
Cigarette smoking	Effect equal to number of cigarettes smoked; ↑ incidence of stillbirth; lowbirth weight; ? effect on later somatic growth and mental development; reduction in O_2 transport to fetus
DIURETICS	
Ammonium chloride Thiazide	Maternal and fetal acidosis; thrombocytopenia, hemorrhage, hypoelectrolytemia, convulsions, respiratory distress, death, hemolysis
DRUGS OF ABUSE (usually multiple drugs consumed)	
Alcohol	Blood level equal to mother's; convulsions, withdrawal syndrome, hyperactivity, crying, irritability, poor sucking reflex, low birth weight; cleft palate, ophthalmic malformation, malformation of extremities and heart; poor mental performance, microencephaly, small-for-dates, growth deficiency
Barbiturates	Withdrawal symptoms, convulsions, onset immediately after birth or at 2 weeks of age
Cocaine	Placenta abruptio, preterm labor
"Ice"-methamphetamine	Preterm labor, IUGR, abnormal sleep patterns, poor feeding, tremors, hypertonia.
LSD (lysergic acid)	Chromosome breakage, limb and skeletal anomalies
Narcotics Heroin Methadone	Small-for-dates, 4% to 10% mortality, habituation, withdrawal symptoms, convulsions, sudden death, indirect effect of maternal complications (i.e., infection, hepatitis venereal disease), ? permanent effect on somatic growth
HORMONES	
Androgens Estrogens Progestins	Labioscrotal fusion before week 12; after 12 weeks, phallic enlargement: ? other anomalies; ? ↑ bilirubin, vaginal cancer; cleft lip and palate, CHD; tracheoesophageal fistula and atresia; cancer and prostate, testes, and bladder
Corticosteroids	Adrenal insufficiency, cleft palate, small-for-dates infant
Ovulatory agents	? Anencephaly, ? chromosomal abnormalities in abortus, multiple pregnancy
PSYCHOTROPIC DRUGS	
Diazepam (Valium)	High fetal levels; hypotonia, poor sucking reflex, hypothermia; ↑ low Apgar score; ↑ resuscitation, ↑ assisted deliveries; dose related
Lithium carbonate	Neonatal serum levels reach adult toxic range; lethargy, cyanosis for 10 days; teratogenic—dose related
RADIATION	Microencephaly, mental retardation, many unknown effects; nondisjunction of chromosomes
SEDATIVES	
Barbiturate	Apnea, depression, depressed EEG, poor sucking reflex, slow weight gain; concentration of drug in brain; enzyme inducer = lower bilirubin level
Bromides	Growth failure, lethargy, dilated pupils, dermatitis, hypotonia, ? effect on mental development
Magnesium sulfate	Neonatal blood level does not correlate with clinical condition; respiratory depression, hypotonia, convulsions, death; exchange transfusion may be required
Paraldehyde	Apnea, depression
Thalidomide	Administered between days 34-50 of gestation causes phocomelia, malformation of cord, angiomas of face, CHD, intestinal stenosis, eye defects, absence of appendix

Maternal Medication	Reported Effects on Fetus or Neonate
TOXINS	
Carbon monoxide	Stillbirth, brain damage equal to anoxia
Heavy metals	
Arsenic	Concentrated in brain
Lead	Abortion, growth retardation, congenital anomalies, sterility
Mercury	Cerebral palsy, mental retardation, convulsions, involuntary movements, defective vision; mother asymptomatic
Naphthalene	Hemolysis
VITAMINS	
A and D	Congenital anomalies
K (water-soluble analogs)	Icterus, anemia, kernicterus
Pyridoxine	Withdrawal seizures

G Standard Laboratory Values in the Neonatal Period

1. HEMATOLOGIC VALUES		Neonatal	
Clotting factors			
Activated clotting time (ACT)		2 min	
Bleeding time (Ivy)		1-8 min	
Clot retraction		Complete 1-4 hr	
Fibrinogen		150-300 mg/dl*	
	Term		Preterm
Hemoglobin (g/dl)	17-19		15-17
Hematocrit (%)	57-58		45-55
Reticulocytes (%)	3-7		Up to 10
Fetal hemoglobin (% of total)	40-70		80-90
Nucleated RBC/mm^3 (per 100 RBC)	200(0.05)		(0.2)
Platelet count/mm^3	100,000-300,000		120,000-180,000
WBC/mm^3	15,000		10,000-20,000
Neutrophils (%)	45		47
Eosinophils and basophils (%)	3		
Lymphocytes (%)	30		33
Monocytes (%)	5		4
Immature WBC (%)	10		16

2. BIOCHEMICAL VALUES		Neonatal
Bilirubin, direct		0-1 mg/dl
Bilirubin, total	Cord:	<2 mg/dl
	Peripheral blood: 0-1 day	6 mg/dl
	1-2 day	8 mg/dl
	3-5 day	12 mg/dl
Blood gases	Arterial:	pH 7.31-7.45
		P_{CO_2} 33-48 mm Hg
		P_{O_2} 50-70 mm Hg
	Venous:	pH 7.28-7.42
		P_{CO_2} 38-52 mm Hg
		P_{O_2} 20-49 mm Hg
α_1-fetoprotein		0
Fibrinogen		150-300 mg/dl

3. URINALYSIS

Volume: 20-40 ml excreted daily in the first few days; by 1 week, 24 hr urine volume close to 200 ml
Protein: may be present in first 2-4 days
Casts and WBCs: may be present in first 2-4 days
Osmolarity (mOsm/L): 100-600
pH: 5-7
Specific gravity: 1.001-1.020

1 to 5 from Pierog SH and Ferrara A: Medical care of the sick newborn, ed 2, St Louis, 1976, The CV Mosby Co.
*dl refers to deciliter (1 dl = 100 ml); this conforms to the SI system: international measurements that have been standardized.

4. CARDIORESPIRATORY DETERMINATIONS

Blood pressure at birth
- Term: systolic, 78 mm Hg; diastolic, 42 mm Hg
- Preterm: systolic, 50-60 mm Hg; diastolic 30 mm Hg

Respiratory rate: 30-60 min

Heart rate, fetus
- Baseline: 120-160/min
  - Tachycardia: >160 bpm (with maternal complications)
  - Bradycardia: <120 bpm (with maternal hypotension and hypoxia)
  - Acceleration: tachycardia >160 bpm with uterine contraction—normal (usually)
- Beat-to-beat variability: disappears with fetal distress
- With uterine contraction
  - Early deceleration: bradycardia with onset of contraction—benign
  - Variable deceleration: bradycardia due to cord compression—usually benign
  - Late deceleration: bradycardia after lag period due to fetal hypoxia—ominous sign

Heart rate, term infant: 140 ± 20 bpm

5. URINE SCREENING TESTS FOR INBORN ERRORS OF METABOLISM

Benedict's test: for reducing substances in the urine—glucose, galactose, fructose, lactose; phenylketonuria, alkaptonuria, tyrosyluria, and tryosinosis may give positive Benedict's test.

Ferric chloride test: an immediate, green color for phenylketonuria, histidinemia, and tyrosinuria, a gray to green color for presence of phenothiazines, isoniazid, red to purple color for presence of salicylates or ketone bodies.

Dinitrophenylhydrazine test: for phenylketonuria, maple syrup urine disease, Lowe's syndrome.

Cetyltrimethyl ammonium bromide test: for mucopolysaccharides: immediate positive reaction in gargoylism (Hurler's syndrome); delayed, moderately positive reaction for Marfan's, Morquio-Ullrich, and Murdoch syndromes.

Metachromatic stain (or *urine sediment):* Granules: (free or as inclusion bodies in cells) are seen in metachromatic leukodystrophy; may also be seen rarely in Tay-Sachs and other lipid diseases of the central nervous system.

Amino acid chromatography: Aminoaciduria may be normal in newborns; chromatography may be helpful to detect hypophosphatasia and argininosuccinicaciduria.

Diaper test, Phenistix test, and *Dinitrophenyl-hydrazine (DNPH) test:* simple, inexpensive tests for PKU (phenylketonuria): used for screening; most useful when infant is at least 6 weeks of age.

6. BLOOD SERUM PHENYLALANINE TESTS

Guthrie inhibition assay methods: drops of blood placed on filter paper; laboratory uses bacterial growth inhibition test; phenylalanine level above 8 mg/dl blood: diagnostic of PKU. Effective in newborn period; used also to monitor PKU diet; blood easily obtained by heel or finger puncture; inexpensive; used for wide-scale screening

APPENDIX

H Relationship of Drugs to Breast Milk and Effect on Infant

Drug	Excreted in Milk	Amount in Milk After Therapeutic Dose	Effect on Infant
ANALGESICS AND ANTIINFLAMMATORY DRUGS (NONNARCOTIC)			
Acetaminophen (Datril, Tylenol)	Yes		Detoxified in liver. Avoid in immediate postdelivery period, otherwise no problems with therapeutic dose.
Aspirin	Yes	1-3 mg/dl*	Long history of experience shows complications rare. Can cause interference with platelet aggregation and diminished factor XII (Hageman factor) at birth. When mother requires high, continuing level of medication for arthritis, aspirin is drug of choice. Observe infant for bruisability. Platelet aggregation can be evaluated. Salicylism only seen in maternal overdosing. Mother should increase vitamin C and vitamin K intake.
Indomethacin (Indocin)	Yes		Convulsions in breast-fed neonate (case report). Used to close patent ductus arteriosus. Insufficient data as to effect on other vessels. May be nephrotoxic.
Mefenamic acid (Ponstel)	Yes	Trace amounts†	No apparent effect on infant at therapeutic doses; infant able to excrete via urine.
Naproxen (Naproxyn, synaxyns, naprosine, naxen, proxen)	Yes	1% of maternal plasma; binds to plasma protein	Less toxic in adults than some other organic derivatives.
Propoxyphene (Darvon)	Yes	0.4% of maternal‡ dose	Only symptoms detectable would be failure to feed and drowsiness. On daily, around-the-clock dosage, infant could consume 1 mg/day.
ANTIBIOTICS			
Ampicillin (Polycillin, Amcill, Omnipen, Penbritin)	Yes	0.07 μg/ml	Sensitivity due to repeated exposure; diarrhea or secondary candidiasis.
Carbenicillin (Pyopen, Geopen)	Yes	0.265 μg/ml 1 hr after 1 g given	Levels not significant. Drug is given to neonate.
Cefazolin (Ancef, Kefzol)	Yes	1.5 μg/ml (0.075% of dose)	Probably not significant.
Cephalexin (Keflex)	No		

Modified from Lawrence RA: Breastfeeding: a guide for the medical profession, ed 2, St Louis, 1985, The CV Mosby Co pp. 509-529.
*Plasma level was 1-5 mg/dl.
†0.91 μg/ml mean maternal plasma level showed 0.21 μg/ml mean milk level. Mean infant plasma level was 0.08 μg/ml and mean urine level, 9.8 μg/ml.
‡Shown by animal experiments. Milk plasma ratio (M/P) = 1/2.

Drug	Excreted in Milk	Amount in Milk After Therapeutic Dose	Effect on Infant
Cephalothin (Keflin)	No		
Chloramphenicol (Chloromycetin)	Yes	Half blood level; 2.5 mg/dl	Gray syndrome. Infant does not excrete drug well, and small amounts may accumulate. Contraindicated. May be tolerated in older infant with mature glycuronide system.
Colistin (Colymycin)	Yes	0.05-0.09 mg/dl	Not absorbed orally.
Demeclocycline (Declomycin)	Yes	0.2-0.3 mg/dl	Not significant in therapeutic doses. Can be given to infants.
Erythromycin (Ilosone, E-Mycin, Erythrocin)	Yes	0.05-0.1 mg/dl; 3.6-6.2 μg/ml	Higher concentrations have been reported in milk than in plasma. Should not be given under 1 month of age because of risk of jaundice. Dose in milk higher when given IV to mother.
Gentamicin	Unknown		Not absorbed from gastrointestinal tract, may change gut flora. Drug is given to newborns directly.
Isoniazid (Nydrazid)	Yes	0.6-1.2 mg/dl*	Infant as risk for toxicity, but need for breast milk may outweigh risk.
Kanamycin (Kantrex)	Yes	18.4 μg/ml after 1 g given IM	Infant absorbs little from gastrointestinal tract. Infants can be given drug.
Lincomycin (Lincocin)	Yes	0.5-2.4 mg/dl	Not significant in therapeutic doses to affect child.
Mandelic acid	Yes	0.3 g/24 hr after dose of 12 g/day	Not significant in therapeutic doses to affect child.
Methacycline (Rondomycin)	Yes	½ plasma level; 50-260 μg/dl	Same precautions as with tetracycline.
Metronidazole (Flagyl)	Yes	Level comparable to serums†	Caution should be exercised because of its high milk concentrations. Contraindicated when infant under 6 months may cause neurologic disorders and blood dyscrasia.
Nitrofurantoin (Furadantin)	Yes	Trace to 0.5 μg/ml	Not significant in therapeutic doses to affect child except in G6PD deficiency.
Novobiocin (Albamycin, cathomycin)	Yes	0.36-0.54 mg/dl	Infant can be given drug directly.
Nystatin (Mycostatin)	No	Not absorbed orally	Can be given to infant directly
Oxacillin (Prostaphlin)	No		
Para-aminosalicylic acid	No		
Penicillin G, benzathine (Bicillin)	Yes	10-12 units/dl	Clinical need should supersede possible allergic responses.
Penicillin G, potassium	Yes	Up to 6 units/dl; 1.2-3.6 μg/dl	Infant can be given penicillin directly. Parents should be told to inform physician that infant has been exposed to penicillin because of potential sensitivity.
Streptomycin	Yes	Present for long periods in slight amounts when given as dihydrostreptomycin	Not to be given more than 2 weeks. Ototoxic and nephrotoxic with long use. Is given to infants directly.
Sulfisoxazole (Gantrisin)	Yes	Concentration similar to plasma level	To be avoided during first month after delivery; may cause kernicterus.
Tetracycline HC1 (Achromycin, Panmycin, Sumycin)	Yes	0.5-2.6 μg/ml after dose of 500 mg four times a day	Not enough to treat an infection in an infant. May cause discoloration of the teeth in the infant; the antibiotic, however, may be largely bound to the milk calcium. Do not give longer than 10 days or repeatedly.

*Same concentration in milk as in maternal serum.
†Gives serum levels in infants of 0.05 to 0.4 μg/ml.

Drug	Excreted in Milk	Amount in Milk After Therapeutic Dose	Effect on Infant
ANTICOAGULANTS			
Coumarin derivatives Dicumarol (bishydroxy-coumarin) Warfarin (Panwarfin)	Yes	Probably little but may be cumulative*	Monitor prothrombin time. Give vitamin K to infant. Discontinue if surgery or trauma occurs. Drug of choice if mother to continue nursing.
Heparin	No		Heparin ineffective orally.
ANTICONVULSANTS AND SEDATIVES†			
Barbital (Veronal)	Yes	8-10 mg/L after 500 mg dose	May produce sedation in infant, in general, barbiturates pass into milk but do not sedate infant. Watch for symptoms.
Phenytoin (Dilantin)	Yes	1.5 to 2.6 μg/ml after 300 mg/24 hr dose	One case of hemolytic reaction reported. Other infants appear to tolerate the small doses. Therapeutic plasma level 10-20 μg/ml.
Pentobarbital (Nembutal)	Yes		Depends on liver for detoxification so may accumulate in first week of life until infant is able to detoxify. No problem for older infant in usual doses.
Phenobarbital (Luminal)	Yes	0.1-0.5 mg when plasma level 0.6-1.8 mg	Sleepiness and decreased sucking possible. On usual analeptic doses infants alert and feed well. On hypnotic doses infants depressed and difficult to rouse.
Sodium bromide (Bromo-Seltzer and across-the-counter sleeping aids)	Yes	Up to 6.6 mg/dl	Drowsy, decreased crying, rash, decreased feeding.
ANTIHISTAMINICS Brompheniramine (Dimetane) Diphenhydramine (Benadryl)	Yes	No specific data available; all pass into milk	Drug is used in neonates. May cause sedation, decreased feeding, or may produce stimulation and tachycardia. Should avoid long-acting preparations, which may accumulate in infant. When combined with decongestants, may cause decrease in milk.
AUTONOMIC DRUGS			
Atropine sulfate‡	Yes	0.1 mg/dl	Hyperthermia, atropine toxicity, infants especially sensitive; also inhibits lactation. Infant dose 0.01 mg/kg.
Ergot (Cafergot)	Yes	Unknown	90% of infants had symptoms of ergotism: vomiting and diarrhea to weak pulse and unstable blood pressure. Short-term therapy for migraine should not exceed 6 mg. Cafergot also contains 100 mg caffeine.
Neostigmine	No		No known harm to infant.
Proprantheline bromide (Pro-Banthine)	No	Uncontrolled data indicate no measurable levels	Drug rapidly metabolized in maternal system to inactive metabolite. Mother should avoid long-acting preparations, however.
Scopolamine (Hyoscine)	Yes		Usually given as single dose and of no problem to neonate. No data on repeated doses.
CARDIOVASCULAR DRUGS			
Diazoxide (Hyperstat)			Arteriolar dilators and antihypertensive, only given IV, not active orally.

*Reports conflict.
†All barbitals appear in breast milk.
‡Ingredient in many prescription and nonprescription drugs.

Drug	Excreted in Milk	Amount in Milk After Therapeutic Dose	Effect on Infant
Digoxin	Yes	0.96-0.61 ng/m*	Dixogin 20% bound to protein; infant receives <1/100 of dose. If mother at toxic level of 5 ng/ml, milk would have a 4.4 ng/ml and infant would receive only 1/20 daily dose.
Hydralazine (Apresoline)	Yes		Jaundice, thrombocytopenia, electrolyte disturbances possible.
Methyldopa (Aldomet)†	Yes		Galactorrhea. No specific data except as affects mother's milk production.
Propranolol (Inderal)‡	Yes	40 ng/ml of maternal plasma§	Insignificant amount. Infants reported had no symptoms noted. Should watch for hypoglycemia and/or "β-blocking" effects.
Quinidine	Yes		Arrhythmia may occur.
Reserpine (Serpasil)‖	Yes		May produce galactorrhea, lethargy, diarrhea, or nasal stuffiness.
CATHARTICS			
Cascara	Yes	Low	Caused colic and diarrhea in infant.
Milk of magnesia	No	None	No effect.
Mineral oil	No	None	No effect.
Phenolphthalein	Unknown	Unknown¶	Reported to cause symptoms in some.
Rhubarb	Unknown	None	None in syrup form. Fresh rhubarb may give symptoms of colic and diarrhea.
Saline cathartics	No	None	No effect.
Senna	No	None	None.
Stool softeners and bulk-forming laxatives	No	None	No effect.
Suppositories (for constipation)	No	None	Not absorbed
Tuberculin test	No		Tuberculin-sensitive mothers can adoptively immunize their infants through breast milk, and that immunity may last several years.
X-ray films	No		No effect.
DIURETICS			
Acetazolamide (Diamox)	Probable	No specific data available but probably similar to sulfonamide	Acts as enzyme inhibitor on carbonic anhydrase non-bacteriostatic sulfonamide. Observe only for dehydration and electrolyte loss by monitoring urine and turgor.
Furosemide (sulfamoylanthranilic acid) (Lasix)	No		Drug is given to children under medical management.
Spironolactone (Aldactone)	Yes	Canrenone, a metabolite, appears	Acts as antagonist of aldosterone; causes sodium excretion and potassium retention. The metabolite apparently has some activity.
Thiazides (Diuril, Enduron, Esidrix, Hydrodiuril, Oretic, Thiuretic tables)	Yes	>0.1 mg/dl#	Risk of dehydration and electrolyte imbalance, especially sodium loss, which would require monitoring. Watching weight and wet diapers and taking an occasional specific gravity reading of the urine and serum sodium would indicate status of infant. Risk, however, is extremely low, May suppress lactation due to dehydration in mother.

*Peak level occurs 4-6 h after dose given. Maternal plasma level was higher, M/P = 0.9 and 0.8; infant's plasma level was 0.
†Adrenergic blocking agent.
‡β-blocking agent.
§Total daily dose to infant via milk is 15-20 μg.
‖Adrenergic blocking agent.
¶Reports differ.
#Linear relationship between plasma and milk. In 1 L of milk at 0.1 mg/dl there would be 1 mg/24 hr. Infant dose is 20 mg/kg /24 hr.

Drug	Excreted in Milk	Amount in Milk After Therapeutic Dose	Effect on Infant
ENVIRONMENTAL AGENTS			
Benzene hexachloride (BHC)	Yes	Varies by location	Not a reason to wean from breast. No need to test milk unless inordinate exposure.
Dichlorodiphenyltrichloroethane (DDT or DDE)	Yes	Varies by location	Not a reason to wean from breast. No need to test milk unless inordinate exposure.
Methyl mercury	Yes	500-1,000 ng/ml*	Infant blood level 600 ng ml in heavy exposure. Only in excessive exposure is testing and/or weaning necessary.
Polybrominated biphenyl (PBB)	Yes	Varies by location	If mother at high risk from the environment or the diet, milk sample should be measured. If level in milk is high, then breastfeeding should be discontinued. Those at risk are (1) workers who handle PBB/PCB and (2) individuals who eat game fish from contaminated waters. Crash diets mobilize fats and should be avoided especially if PBB or PCB present.
Polychlorinated biphenyl (PCB)	Yes	Varies by location	
^{90}Sr,^{89}Sr (strontium)	Yes	1/10 of that in maternal diet	Cow's milk has six times as much as human milk. Cow's milk-fed infant doubles amount in body in 1 month.
HEAVY METALS			
Arsenic	Yes	Can be measured for given woman	Can accumulate. Check infant's blood level if there is reason to suspect exposure.
Fluorine	Yes		Monitor for excessive dose.
Iron	Yes		
Lead	Unknown		Nursing contraindicated if maternal serum 40 μg; conflicting reports, breast milk not always cause of lead poisoning in breastfed infant.
Mercury	Yes		Hazardous to infant.
HORMONES AND CONTRACEPTIVES			
Chlorotrianisene (Tace)	Yes		Has estrogenic effect although does not change consistency of milk. May have feminizing effect on infant.
Contraceptives (oral) Ethinyl estradiol Mestranol 19-Nortestosterone Norethindrone (Norlutin) Norethynodrel (Enovid)	Yes		May diminish milk supply. May decrease vitamins, protein, and fat in milk. One author showed no difference when mothers took norethindrone. Most significant concern is long-range impact of hormone on young infant, which is not certain. Reports of feminization of infant.
Corticotropin	Yes		Destroyed in gastrointestinal tract of infant. No effect.
Cortisone	Yes		Animal studies show 50% lower weight than controls and retarded sexual development and exophthalmos.
Epinephrine (Adrenalin)	Yes		Destroyed in gastrointestinal tract of infant.
Estrogen	Yes	0.17 μg/dl after 1 g	Risks as with oral contraceptives.
Insulin	Unknown		Destroyed in intestinal tract.
Medroxyprogesterone acetate (Provera)	No		
Prednisone	Yes	0.07-0.23% dose/L after 5 mg dose†	Minimum amount not likely to cause effect on infant in short course.

*M/P = 8.6% in heavy exposure.
†0.16 μg/ml after 10 mg dose; 2.67 μg/ml after 2 hr.

Drug	Excreted in Milk	Amount in Milk After Therapeutic Dose	Effect on Infant
Pregnanediol	Yes		Unknown risk as with other female hormones over a long period of time.
Tolbutamide (Orinase)	Yes		Not recommended in the childbearing years.
NARCOTICS			
Codeine		0 to trace after 32 mg every 4 hr (6 doses)	No effect in therapeutic level and transient usage. Can accumulate. Individual variation. Watch for neonatal depression.
Heroin	Yes		13 of 22 infants had withdrawal. Historically breastfeeding had been used to wean addict's infant. This is no longer recommended.
Marijuana *(Cannabis)*	Yes		Shown in laboratory animals to produce structural changes in nursling's brain cells; impairs DNA and RNA formation. Infant at risk of inhaling smoke during feeding or when held by person who is smoking.
Meperidine (Demerol)	Yes	>0.1 mg/dl*	Trace amounts may accumulate if drug taken around the clock when infant is neonate. Watch for drowsiness and poor feeding
Methadone	Yes	0.03 μg/ml or 0.023-0.028 mg/24 hr†	When dosage not excessive, infant can be breast-fed if monitored for evidence of depression and failure to thrive.
Morphine	Yes	Trace	Single doses have minimum effect. Potential for accumulation. May be addicting to neonate. Breastfeeding no longer considered appropriate means of weaning infant of an addict.
Percodan (oxycodone [derived from opiate thebaine] aspirin, phenacetin, caffeine)	Yes		Consider for its component parts. In neonatal period sleepiness and failure to feed, which increase maternal engorgement and neonatal weight loss, have been observed, probably caused by oxycodone.
PSYCHOTROPIC AND MOOD-CHANGING DRUGS			
Alcohol	Yes	Similar to plasma level	Ordinarily no problem and can be therapeutic in moderation, infants are more susceptible to effects. Chronic drinking reported to cause obesity in infant. Ethanol in doses of 1-2 g/kg to mother causes depression of milk-ejection reflex (dose dependent). No acetaldehyde found in infants.
Amphetamine	Yes		Has caused stimulation in infants with jitteriness, irritability, sleeplessness. Long-acting preparations cumulative.
Benzodiazepines‡ Chlordiazepoxide HC1 (Librium)	Yes		Not sufficient to affect infant first week when glucuronyl system needed for detoxification. May accumulate. Older infant, no apparent problem.
Diazepam (Valium)	Yes	90 μg/L§	Detoxified in glucuronyl system. In first weeks of life may contribute to jaundice. Metabolite active. Effect on infant: hypoventilation, drowsiness, lethargy, and weight loss. Single doses over 10 mg contraindicated during nursing. Accumulation in infant possible.

*Plasma 0.07-0.1 mg/dl.
†Mother received 50 mg/24 hr; M/P = 0.83. Peak level 4 hr after oral dose. Results obscured if addict also taking the herbal root golden seal.
‡Alcohol enhances effect of this group.
§10 mg or less yields 45 mg of diazepam/ml and 85 ng of metabolite/ml. P/M ratio is variable. Mean P/M ratio of diazepam is 6.14; of metabolite is 3.64. Effect lasts about 4 days.

Drug	Excreted in Milk	Amount in Milk After Therapeutic Dose	Effect on Infant
Haloperidol (Haldol)	Yes	Unknown	A butyrophenone antidepressant: animal studies in nurslings show behavior abnormalities.
Lithium carbonate (Eskalith, Lithane, Lithonate)	Yes	⅓-½ maternal plasma level*	Measurable lithium in infant's serum. Infant kidney can clear lithium; however, lithium inhibits adenosine 3′:5:-cyclic monophosphate, significant for brain growth. Also affects amine metabolism. Real effects not measurable immediately. Report of cyanosis and poor muscle tone and ECG changes in nursing infant.
Monomine oxidate (MAO) inhibitors (Eutonyl, Nardil)			Inhibits lactation.
Meprobamate (Miltown, Equanil)	Yes	2-4 times maternal plasma level	If therapy continued, infant should be followed closely.
Phenothiazines			
Chlorpromazine (Thorazine)	Yes	⅓ plasma level†	Can be safely nursed; minimum in milk. Increase maternal prolactin. No symptoms in infants reported; 5-year follow-up showed infants normal.
Piperacetazine (Quide)	Yes	Minimum	Probably no effect
Thioridazine (Mellaril)	Yes	No information	Thioridazine is less potent in general than other phenothiazines. Probably quite safe.
Trifluoperazine (Stelazine)	Yes	Minimum	
Tricyclic antidepressants	Yes		Apparently no accumulation. No infants that have been observed showed symptoms. Watch for depression or failure to feed. Increase maternal prolactin secretion.
Amitriptyline HC1 (Elavil)	Yes	Minimum amounts	
Desipramine HC1 (Norpramin, Pertofrane)		Minimum amounts	
Imipramine HC1 (Tofranil)	Yes	0.1 mg/dl‡	
STIMULANTS			
Caffeine	Yes	1% of dose	Accumulates when intake moderate and continual. Causes jitteriness, wakefulness, and irritability. Caffeine present in many hot and cold drinks. Consider if infant very wakeful.
Theobromine	Yes	3.7-8.2 mg/L after 240 mg dose§	No adverse symptoms observed in the infants. Chocolate most common cause of exposure.
Theophylline	Yes	10% of maternal dose‖	Irritability, fretfulness.
THYROID AND ANTITHYROID MEDICATIONS			
Thiouracil	Yes	9-12 mg/dl¶	Same as for propylthiouracil
Thyroid and thyroxine	Yes		Does not produce adverse symptoms on long-range follow-up. Noted to improve milk supply of hypothyroid mothers. No contraindication.

*0.030 mmol/L in infant's serum, 0.57 mmole/L in infant's urine. Milk level was half of maternal serum level in one case report.
†If dose <200 mg, milk contains bare trace. Dose of 1200 mg showed trace.
‡Plasma level 0.2-1.3 mg/dl.
§113 g chocolate bar.
‖M/P = 0.7.
¶Maternal plasma level was 3.4 mg/dl after a 1 g dose; M/P = 3.

Drug	Excreted in Milk	Amount in Milk After Therapeutic Dose	Effect on Infant
MISCELLANEOUS			
DPT	Yes	Minimum	Does not interfere with immunization schedule.
Methotrexate	Yes	Minor route of excretion: M/P = 0.08/1.0	Antimetabolite. Infant would receive 0.26 μg/dl, which researchers consider nontoxic for infant.
Nicotine	Yes	Mean 91 ppb (20-512 ppb)*	Decreases milk production. No apparent effect on infant—perhaps a tolerance is developed in utero. Smoking may interfere with let-down reflex if smoking started before onset of a feeding.
Poliovirus vaccine	No		Live vaccine taken orally. Not necessary to withhold nursing 30 min before and after dose. Provide booster after infant no longer nursing.
Rh antibodies	Yes		Destroyed in gastrointestinal tract; not effective orally.
Rubella virus vaccine	Yes	Minimum	Will not confer passive immunity. Mother should not be given vaccine when at risk for pregnancy.

*At 1/2 -1 1/2 packs/day. Large variation from single donor.

I Resources

This Appendix includes community and national resources, national clearing-houses, journals and nursing organizations of interest to the maternity nurse.

COMMUNITY AND NATIONAL RESOURCES

AASK (Aid to the Adoption of Special Kids)
3530 Grand Avenue
Oakland, CA 94610
(415) 451-1748

AIDS Medical Foundation
10 East 13th Street, Suite LD
New York, NY 10003
(212) 206-0670

American Academy of Husband-Coached Childbirth
P.O. Box 5224
Sherman Oaks, CA 91413
(818) 788-6662
Teaches Robert A. Bradley's method of "Husband-Coached Childbirth," an offshoot of Grantly Dick-Read's method.

American Cancer Society
90 Park Avenue
New York, NY 10016
(212) 736-3030
Provides brochures on Papanicolaou (Pap) smears, smoking during pregnancy, and breast self-examination.

American Cleft Palate Association
331 Salk Hall
Pittsburgh, PA 15261
(412) 681-9620

American Fertility Foundation
2131 Magnolia Avenue
Suite 201
Birmingham, AL 35256
(205) 251-9764

American Foundation for Maternal and Child Health, Inc.
(research on the perinatal period)
30 Beekman Place
New York, NY 10022
(212) 759-5510

American Red Cross
17th and E Streets
Washington, DC 20006
(202) 737-8300

American Society for Psychoprophylaxis in Obstetrics (ASPO)
1840 Wilson Boulevard
Suite 204
Arlington, VA 22201
(703) 524-7802
Teaches Lamaze technique of prepared childbirth to interested couples; prepares qualified people for teaching this method. Offers brochures, publications, teaching materials, and audiovisual aids.

Association for the Aid of Crippled Children
345 East 46th Street
New York, NY 10017
Devoted to the prevention of crippling diseases and conditions and to improvement in the care of disabled children and youth and their adjustment in society.

Association of Birth Defects in Children
3201 E. Crystal Lake Avenue
Orlando, FL 32806

Association for Childbirth at Home, International
P.O. Box 39498
Los Angeles, CA 90039
(213) 667-0839
See also Childbirth

Association of Voluntary Sterilization, Inc. (AVS)
(provides information on sterilization and referral service)
122 E. 42nd Street
New York, NY 10168
(212) 351-2500

Black Male Youth Health Enhancement Project
Family Life Center
Shiloh Baptist Church
Washington, DC

Boston Women's Health Book Collective
47 Nichols Avenue
Watertown, MA 02172
(617) 921-0271

Centers for Disease Control
1600 Clifton Road, N.E.
Atlanta, GA 30333
(404) 329-1819 (404) 329-3286

Center for the Study of Multiple Birth
333 East Superior Street
Suite 463-5
Chicago, IL 60611
(312) 266-9093

Channing L. Bete Co., Inc.
Greenfield, MA 01301
Publishes material regarding childbearing in cartoon form.

Child Study Association of America
9 East 89th St.
New York, NY 10028
Provides parent education materials.

Compassionate Friends
(Following death of an infant)
P.O. Box 1347
Oak Brook, IL 60521
(312) 990-0010

COPE (Coping with the Overall Pregnancy/Parenting Experience)
37 Clarendon Street
Boston, MA 02116
(617) 357-5588

C/SEC, Inc. (Cesarean/Support Education and Concern)
22 Forest Road
Framingham, MA 01701
(617) 877-8266

Department DES
National Cancer Institute
Office of Cancer Communications
Bldg. 31, Room 10A19
Bethesda, MD 20892
(800) 4-CANCER

Ed-U-Press
760 Ostrum Ave.
Syracuse, NY 13210
Offers series of excellent cartoon books for adolescents and parenting classes.

Educational and Scientific Plastics, Ltd.
76 Holmethorpe Avenue
Holmethorpe, Red Hill Surrey, RH1, 2PF, England
Offers numerous plastic models.

Endometriosis Association
238 West Wisconsin Avenue
P.O. Box 92187
Milwaukee, WI 53202
(414) 962-8972

Environmental Protection Agency (EPA)
Public Information Center
Room PM 211-B
401 M Street, SW
Washington, DC 20460
(202) 382-7550

Equal Rights for Fathers
P.O. Box 90042
San Jose, CA 95109-3042
(415) 848-2323

Florence Crittenton Association of America
608 South Dearborn Street
Chicago, IL 60605
Unites in forming an effective and continuing organization; develops and maintains standards of service; in general, assists in bringing about a greater understanding of factors relating to unmarried mothers and adolescent girls with other problems in adjustment.

Home Oriented Maternity Experience (HOME)
511 New York Avenue
Takoma Park, MD 20012

Infant Stimulation/Mother Training Model (IS/MT)
University of Cincinnati College of Medicine
Cincinnati, Ohio

International Childbirth Education Association (ICEA)
P.O. Box 20048
Milwaukee, WI 55420
Assists individuals and childbirth groups who are interested in family-centered maternity: film and record directory, books and pamphlets and an annotated catalogue of resources.

LA LECHE LEAGUE
P.O. Box 1209
Franklin Park, IL 60131-8209
312-455-7730 (24-hour line)

Maternal Health Society
Box 46563, Station G
Vancouver, B.C. V6R 4G8

Maternity Center Association, Inc.
48 East 92nd Street
New York, NY 10028
(212) 269-7300
Publishes free brochure describing their many publications and pattern for knitted uterus.

National Abortion Rights Action League
1101 14th Street, NW
Washington, DC 20005
(202) 371-9779
Pro-choice political action group

National Coalition Against Domestic Violence
Suite 305
2401 Virginia Avenue, NW
Washington, DC 20037

National Coalition Against Sexual Assault
c/o Fern Ferguson, President
Volunteers of America of Illinois
8787 State Street, Suite 202
East St. Louis, IL 62203

Nurses Association of the American College of Obstetricians and Gynecologists
409 12th Street, SW
Washington, DC 20024-2191
(202) 638-0026

National Association of Childbirth Education, Inc. (NACE)
3940 Eleventh Street
Riverside, CA 92501

National Childbirth Trust
9 Queensborough Terrace
London, W2, England
Offers books, films, and other aids for use in classes or in labor.

National Conference of Catholic Charities
1346 Connecticut
Washington, DC 20036
Gives particular emphasis to service for children and youth; i.e., foster care, counseling (unmarried parents), adoption services (statewide), short-term counseling to families and youth, emergency material assistance.

National Foundation/March of Dimes
1275 Mamaroneck Avenue
White Plains, NY 10605
(914) 428-7100
Publishes a directory of genetic services. It is involved in professional education, as well as research on genetic defects. The Foundation also sponsors programs for purchase of teaching and disseminating information to the general public.

National Foundation for Jewish Genetic Diseases, Inc.
250 Park Avenue, Suite 1000
New York, NY 10177

National Institute of Child Health and Human Development (NICHD)
National Institutes of Health
9000 Rockville Pike
Bldg 31, Room 2A32
Bethesda, MD 20892
(301) 496-4000

National Organization of Mothers of Twins Clubs, Inc.
12404 Princess Jeanne, NE
Albuquerque, NM 87112
(505) 275-0955

National Right to Life Committee
419 7th Street, NW
Suite 402
Washington, DC 20004
(202) 626-8800
Pro-life political action group.

National Sudden Infant Death Syndrome Foundation
2320 Glenview Road
Glenview, IL 60025
(312) 657-8080

Parenthood After Thirty
451 Vermont
Berkeley, CA 94707
(415) 524-6635

Parents of Prematures
% Houston Organization for Parent Education, Inc.
2990 Richmond
Suite 204
Houston, TX 77098
(713) 524-3089

Parents Plus Parents-Too-Soon
Department of Public Health
Springfield, IL

Parents Without Partners
8807 Colesville Road
Silver Spring, MD 20910
(301) 588-9354

Patient Counseling Library
Budlong Press Co.
5428 N. Virginia Avenue
Chicago, IL, 60625
(212) 541-7800
Provides videotapes (e.g., "A doctor discusses. . .") suitable for clinics or waiting rooms covering topics such as pregnancy, infant care, sexuality, breastfeeding, and weight control.

Planned Parenthood Federation of America, Inc.
810 Seventh Avenue
New York, NY 10019
Provides leadership for universal acceptance of family planning as an essential element of responsible family life through education, service, and research.

Premenstrual Syndrome Action
P.O. 16292
Irving, CA 92713
(714) 854-4407

Reach to Recovery (breast cancer)
American Cancer Society

Resolve, Inc. (impaired fertility)
5 Water Street
Arlington, MA 02174
(617) 643-2424

Save the Children Federation, Inc.
345 East 46th Street
New York, NY 10017
Helps eliminate the causes of poverty among children in the United States and overseas while maintaining efforts to ameliorate the effects of poverty in those areas where the needs are greatest.

SHARE (Source of Help in Airing and Resolving Experiences) for parents who have suffered loss of newborn baby
% St. John's Hospital
800 E. Carpenter Street
Springfield, IL 62760
(217) 544-6464

SIECUS
Human Science Press
72 Fifth Avenue
New York, NY 10011
Provides publications (e.g., "Sexual relations in pregnancy and postpartum") and teaching aids.

Teen Obstetrical Perinatal Parenting Services Clinic (TOPPS)
University of Arkansas College of Medicine
Little Rock, Arkansas

Victims Anonymous
9514-9 Reseda Blvd. #607
Northridge, CA 91324
(818) 993-1139

VBAC (Vaginal Birth After Cesarean)
10 Great Plain Terrace
Needham, MA 01292

Women Against Rape
P.O. Box 02084
Columbus, OH 43202
(614) 291-9751

Women Against Violence Against Women (WAVAW)
543 North Fairfax Avenue
Los Angeles, CA 90036

Young Parents Young People (YPYP)
Chapel of the Cross-Lutheran Church
St. Louis, Missouri

❑ NATIONAL CLEARINGHOUSES

American Foundation for Maternal and Child Health
(research on the perinatal period)
300 Beekman Place
New York, NY 10022
(212) 759-5510

Food and Drug Administration (FDA)
Office of Consumer Affairs
Public Inquiries
5600 Fishers Lane (HFE-88)
Rockville, MD 20857
(301) 443-3170

National Maternal and Child Health Clearinghouse
3520 Prospect St., N.W., Ground Floor
Washington, DC 20057

Sudden Infant Death Syndrome Clearinghouse
8201 Greensboro Dr., Suite 600
McLean, VA 22102

❑ NURSING JOURNALS

Birth: Issues in Prenatal Care and Education (formerly **Birth and Family Journal**)
110 El Camino Real
Berkeley, CA 94705
(415) 658-5099
Quarterly publication, sponsored by International Childbirth Education Association (ICEA) and American Society of Psychoprophylaxis in Obstetrics (ASPO)

Bookmarks
ICEA Supplies Center
P.O. Box 20048
Minneapolis, MN 55420
Complimentary annotated catalogue of book reviews published several times per year.

Canadian Nurse
The Canadian Nurses' Association
50 The Driveway
Ottawa, Canada K2PIE2

The Female Patient
Division Excerpta Medica
301 Gibraltar Drive
P.O. Box 528
Morris Plains, NJ 07950

Journal of Nurse-Midwifery
Editor
82 Willow Ln.
Tenafly, NJ 07670

or

American Elsevier Publishing Co.
52 Vanderbilt Avenue
New York, NY 10017
Official publication of the American College of Nurse-Midwives

Journal of Obstetric, Gynecologic and Neonatal Nursing
Harper & Row, Publishers
Medical Department
2350 Virginia Avenue
Hagerstown, MD 21740
Journal of the Nurses' Association of the American College of Obstetricians and Gynecologists

Journal of Perinatal and Neonatal Nursing
Aspen Publishers, Inc.
7201 McKinney Circle
Frederick, MD 21701

Maternal/Newborn Advocate
The National Foundation/March of Dimes
P.O. Box 2000
White Plains, NY 10602
Complimentary quarterly publication of the National Foundation/March of Dimes

MCN The American Journal of Maternal Child Nursing
555 W. 57th Street
New York, NY 10019

Nurse Practitioner: A Journal of Primary Nursing Care
3845 42nd Ave., N.E.
Seattle, WA 98105

Nursing Research
555 W. 57th Street
New York, NY 10019

Perinatal Press
Perinatal Press Subscriptions
The Perinatal Center
Sutter Memorial Hospital
52nd and F Sts.
Sacramento, CA 95819

Women's Health Nursing Scan
J.B. Lippincott Co.
Downsville Pike, Rte 3, Box 20-B
Hagerstown, MD 21740

❑ NURSING ORGANIZATIONS

American College of Nurse Midwives
1522 K Street, NW
Suite 1120
Washington, DC 20005
(202) 347-5445

American Nurses Association
1101 14th Street, NW
Suite 200
Washington, DC 20005
(202) 789-1800

Canadian Nurses Association
50 The Driveway
Ottawa, Ont. K2P 1E2

Midwives Alliance of North America
United States and Canada
℅ Concord Midwifery Service
30 South Main Street
Concord, NH 03301
(603) 225-9586

National League for Nursing (NLN)
Ten Columbus Circle
New York, NY 10019
(212) 582-1022
See also Nurse-Widwifery

Nurses Association of the American College of Obstetricians and Gynecologists (NAACOG)
409 12th Street, S.W.
Washington, DC 20024-2191
(202) 638-0026
Toll free 1-800-533-8822

Index

Page numbers followed by *b* indicate boxed material. Page numbers followed by *f* indicate illustrations. Page numbers followed by *t* indicate tables.

E

M

Temperature Equivalents

Celsius	Fahrenheit	Celsius	Fahrenheit
34.0	93.2	38.6	101.4
34.2	93.6	38.8	101.8
34.4	93.9	39.0	102.2
34.6	94.3	39.2	102.5
34.8	94.6	39.4	102.9
35.0	95.0	39.6	103.2
35.2	95.4	30.8	103.6
35.4	95.7	40.0	104.0
35.6	96.1	40.2	104.3
35.8	96.4	40.4	104.7
36.0	96.8	40.6	105.1
36.2	97.1	40.8	105.4
36.4	97.5	41.0	105.8
36.6	97.8	41.2	106.1
36.8	98.2	41.4	106.5
37.0	98.6	41.6	106.8
37.2	98.9	41.8	107.2
37.4	99.3	42.0	107.6
37.6	99.6	42.2	108.0
37.8	100.0	42.4	108.3
38.0	100.4	42.6	108.7
38.2	100.7	42.8	109.0
38.4	101.1	43.0	109.4

To convert Fahrenheit to Celcius:
(Temperature minus 32) × 5/9
Example: To convert 98.6 degrees Fahrenheit to Celcius:
98.6 - 32 = 66.6 × 5/9
= 37 degrees

To convert Celcius to Fahrenheit:
9/5 × temperature + 32
Example: To convert 40 degrees Celsius to Fahrenheit:
9/5 × 40 = 72 + 32
= 104 degrees

Conversion of Pounds and Ounces To Grams for Newborn Weights*

Pounds \ Ounces	0	1	2	3	4	5	6	7	8	9	10	11	12	13	14	15	Pounds
0	—	28	57	85	113	142	170	198	227	255	283	312	430	369	397	425	0
1	454	482	510	539	567	595	624	652	680	709	737	765	794	822	850	879	1
2	907	936	964	992	1021	1049	1077	1106	1134	1162	1191	1219	1247	1276	1304	1332	2
3	1361	1389	1417	1446	1474	1503	1531	1559	1588	1616	1644	1673	1701	1729	1758	1786	3
4	1814	1843	1871	1899	1928	1956	1984	2013	2041	2070	2098	2126	2155	2183	2211	2240	4
5	2268	2296	2325	2353	2381	2410	2438	2466	2495	2523	2551	2580	2608	2637	2665	2693	5
6	2722	2750	2778	2807	2835	2863	2892	2920	2948	2977	3005	3033	3062	3090	3118	3147	6
7	3175	3203	3232	3260	3289	3317	3345	3374	3402	3430	3459	3487	3515	3544	3572	3600	7
8	3629	3657	3685	3714	3742	3770	3799	3827	3856	3884	3912	3941	3969	3997	4026	4054	8
9	4082	4111	4139	4167	4196	4224	4252	4281	4309	4337	4366	4394	4423	4451	4479	4508	9
10	4536	4564	4593	4621	4649	4678	4706	4734	4763	4791	4819	4848	4876	4904	4933	4961	10
11	4990	5018	5046	5075	5103	5131	5160	5188	5216	5245	5273	5301	5330	5358	5386	5415	11
12	5443	5471	5500	5528	5557	5585	5613	5642	5670	5698	5727	5755	5783	5812	5840	5868	12
13	5897	5925	5953	5982	6010	6038	6067	6095	6123	6152	6180	6209	6237	6265	6294	6322	13
14	6350	6379	6407	6435	6464	6492	6520	6549	6577	6605	6634	6662	6690	6719	6747	6776	14
15	6804	6832	6860	6889	6917	6945	6973	7002	7030	7059	7087	7115	7144	7172	7201	7228	15
	0	1	2	3	4	5	6	7	8	9	10	11	12	13	14	15	

Ounces

*To convert pounds and ounces to grams, multiply the pounds by 453.6 and the ounces by 28.35; add the totals.
To convert grams into pounds and decimals of a pound, multiply the grams by 0.0022
To convert grams into ounces, divide the grams by 28.35 (16 oz = 1 lb).